D0479485

*To my husband, Glenn M. Nelson, whose willingness to make a million
little sacrifices, read manuscripts, and continually offer encouragement
made my contribution to this book a possibility.*
Ramona Nelson

*To my father, Forest Thorpe, who supported education for women during
an age when it was deemed superfluous.*
Nancy Staggers

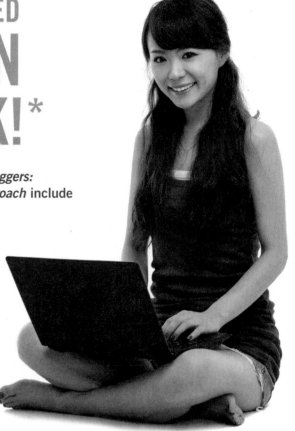
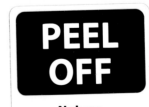
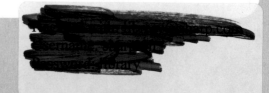

Health
Informatics

An Interprofessional Approach

Ramona Nelson, PhD, RN-BC, ANEF, FAAN
Professor Emerita
Slippery Rock University
Slippery Rock, Pennsylvania;
President, Ramona Nelson Consulting
Allison Park, Pennsylvania

Nancy Staggers, PhD, RN, FAAN
Professor, Informatics
University of Maryland School of Nursing
Baltimore, Maryland;
Adjunct Professor, College of Nursing and
  Department of Biomedical Informatics
University of Utah
Salt Lake City, Utah

ELSEVIER

ELSEVIER
MOSBY

3251 Riverport Lane
St. Louis, Missouri 63043

HEALTH INFORMATICS: AN INTERPROFESSIONAL APPROACH   ISBN: 978-0-323-10095-3

Library of Congress Cataloging-in-Publication Data

Health informatics (Saint Louis, Mo.)
  Health informatics : an interprofessional approach / [edited by] Ramona Nelson, Nancy Staggers.—1st edition.
    p. ; cm.
  Includes bibliographical references and index.
  ISBN 978-0-323-10095-3 (pbk.)
  I. Nelson, Ramona, editor of compilation.   II. Staggers, Nancy, editor of compilation.   III. Title.
  [DNLM: 1. Medical Informatics. W 26.5]
  R858.A1
  610.285—dc23
                                                                        2013011395

Vice President: Loren Wilson
Executive Content Strategist: Teri Hines Burnham
Content Development Specialist: Heather Rippetoe
Publishing Services Manager: Jeff Patterson
Project Manager: Megan Isenberg
Design Direction: Karen Pauls
Marketing Manager: Abby Hewitt

Printed in the United States of America

Last digit is the print number: 9   8   7   6   5   4   3   2   1

ABOUT THE AUTHORS

Ramona Nelson holds a baccalaureate degree in nursing from Duquesne University and a master's degree in both nursing and information science, as well as a PhD in education from the University of Pittsburgh. In addition, she completed a postdoctoral fellowship at the University of Utah. Prior to her current position as president of her own consulting company, Ramona was a Professor of Nursing and Chair of the Department of Nursing at Slippery Rock University. Her primary areas of interest include informatics education for health professionals, social media and empowered patients, and application of theoretical concepts in health informatics practice.

Her past publications include textbooks, monographs, book chapters, journal articles, World Wide Web publications, abstracts, and newsletters. Current books include *Social Media for Nurses* (2013) and *Introduction to Computers for Health Professionals* (2014), 6th ed. She was named a fellow in the American Academy of Nursing in 2004 and was inducted into the National League for Nursing Academy of Nursing Education Fellows in 2007. Because of her pioneering work in informatics she was invited to participate as a member of the task force charged with revising *Nursing Informatics: Scope and Standards of Practice*, published in 2008 by the American Nurses Association.

Nancy Staggers has been involved in health informatics for many years as an information technology executive and more recently as clinical informatics faculty. She received a PhD from the University of Maryland and subsequently led enterprise electronic health record installations in major organizations, including the Department of Defense. For her work on nursing informatics (NI) competencies and NI leadership, she was deemed a Nursing Informatics Pioneer by the American Medical Informatics Association Nursing Informatics Working Group in 2006. Nancy led the two most recent task forces in writing the American Nurses Association's *Nursing Informatics: Scope and Standards of Practice*. Nancy's research program centers on the usability of electronic health records and she publishes widely about the topic. Her recent research focuses on care transitions and hand-offs.

Antonia Arnaert, RN, MPH, MPA, PhD
Associate Professor
Ingram School of Nursing
McGill University
Montreal, Quebec

Nancy C. Brazelton, RN, MS
Director Application Services
Information Technology Services
University of Utah Health Care
Salt Lake City, Utah

Christine A. Caligtan, RN, MSN
Health Data and Patient Safety Clinical
    Specialist
Research & Development
PatientsLikeMe
Cambridge, Massachusetts

Diane Castelli, RN, MS, MSN
Telemedicine Product Development
    Manager
Medweb, LLC, PACs, and Telemedicine
    Software
San Francisco, California

**Helen B. Connors, PhD, RN, DrPS
    (Hon), FAAN**
Executive Director
University of Kansas Center for Health
    Informatics
Associate Dean/Integrated Technologies
    and Professor
University of Kansas, School of Nursing
Kansas City, Kansas

Vicky Elfrink Cordi, RN-BC, PhD
Clinical Associate Professor Emeritus
The Ohio State University
Columbus, Ohio;
Senior Associate
iTelehealth Inc.
Cocoa Beach, Florida

Mollie R. Cummins, PhD, RN
Associate Professor
College of Nursing
Adjunct Associate Professor
Department of Biomedical Informatics
University of Utah
Salt Lake City, Utah

Mical DeBrow, PhD, RN
Principal Consultant 2
Strategic Clinical Consulting
Siemens Medical Solutions
Malvern, Pennsylvania

Guilherme Del Fiol, MD, PhD
Assistant Professor
Department of Biomedical Informatics
University of Utah
Salt Lake City, Utah

Elizabeth S. Dickson, RN, BSN
Department of Veterans Affairs
Cheyenne, Wyoming;
Healthcare Informatics MS Student
College of Nursing
University of Colorado
Aurora, Colorado

**Patricia C. Dykes, DNSc, RN, FAAN,
    FACMI**
Senior Nurse Scientist
Program Director, Center for Patient Safety
    Research and Practice
Program Director, Center for Nursing
    Excellence
Brigham and Women's Hospital
Boston, Massachusetts

W. Scott Erdley, DNS, RN
Special Projects Simulation Education
    Specialist
Behling Simulation Center
University at Buffalo
Buffalo, New York;
Adjunct Professor, Department of Nursing
Niagara University
Niagara, New York

Lisa Gallagher, BSEE, CISM, CPHIMS
Vice President, Technology Solutions
Healthcare Information and Management
    Systems Society
Chicago, Illinois

Bryan Gibson, DPT, PhD
Research Assistant Professor
Division of Epidemiology
University of Utah
Salt Lake City, Utah

Luciana Schleder Gonçalves, BSN, MSc
Assistant Professor
Federal University of Parana, Brazil;
Fulbright/CAPES Scholar
Biomedical Informatics
University of Utah
Salt Lake City, Utah

Teresa Gore, DNP, FNP-BC, NP-C, CHSE
Vice President of Programs
International Nursing Association for
    Clinical Simulation and Learning
Associate Clinical Professor and Simulation
    Learning Coordinator
Auburn University School of Nursing
Auburn, Alabama

Paul Guillory, MS, BSN, RN-BC
Clinical Applications Coordinator
Clinical Informatics Service
Department of Veterans Affairs
Pacific Islands Health Care System
Honolulu, Hawaii

Andrea Haught, RN, MSN, PMP
Senior Associate
iTelehealth Inc.
Cocoa Beach, Florida

Susan D. Horn, PhD
Senior Scientist
Institute for Clinical Outcomes Research
International Severity Information Systems,
    Inc.
Adjunct Research Professor
College of Nursing
Adjunct Professor
Department of Biomedical Informatics
Department of Physical Medicine and
    Rehabilitation
Department of Family and Preventative
    Medicine
School of Medicine
University of Utah
Salt Lake City, Utah

Valerie Howard, EdD, MSN, RN
President, International Nursing
    Association for Clinical Simulation and
    Learning (INACSL)
Assistant Dean for External Affairs
Professor of Nursing
Director Regional Research and Innovation
    in Simulation Education (RISE) Center
School of Nursing and Health Sciences
Robert Morris University
Moon Township, Pennsylvania

David E. Jones
Doctoral Student
Department of Biomedical Informatics
University of Utah
Salt Lake City, Utah

Irene Joos, PhD, RN, MN, MSIS
Associate Professor
IST Department
Former Director of Online Learning
La Roche College
Pittsburgh, Pennsylvania

Kensaku Kawamoto, MD, PhD
Director
Knowledge Management and Mobilization
Assistant Professor
Department of Biomedical Informatics
University of Utah
Salt Lake City, Utah

Michael H. Kennedy, PhD, MHA, FACHE
Associate Professor and Director
Health Services Management Program
Department of Health Services and
    Information Management
East Carolina University
Greenville, North Carolina

Tae Youn Kim, PhD, RN
Associate Professor
Betty Irene Moore School of Nursing
University of California Davis
Sacramento, California

Gerald R. Ledlow, PhD, MHA, FACHE
Professor
Health Policy and Management
Jiann-Ping Hsu College of Public
    Health
Georgia Southern University
Statesboro, Georgia

Kim Leighton, PhD, RN
Associate Director
Simulation Center of Excellence
DeVry, Inc.
Downers Grove, Illinois

Leslie Lenert, MD, MS, FACP, FACMI
Ann G. and Jack Mark Presidential Chair
    in Internal Medicine
Associate Chair for Ambulatory
    Care
Department of Internal Medicine
Professor
Internal Medicine and Department of
    Biomedical Informatics
University of Utah School of Medicine
Salt Lake City, Utah

Ann Lyons, RN, MS
Clinical Analyst
University of Utah Hospitals and Clinics
Information Technology Services
Salt Lake City, Utah

Kathleen MacMahon, RN, MS, CNP
Telehealth Nurse Practitioner
American Telecare
Minneapolis, Minnesota

Michele Person Madison, JD
Partner
Morris, Manning and Martin, LLP
Atlanta, Georgia

E. LaVerne Manos, DNP, RN-BC
Director of Nursing Informatics
Director of Master of Science in Health
    Informatics Program
Director of Academic Electronic Health
    Record Program
University of Kansas Center for Health
    Informatics
Graduate Informatics Faculty, University of
    Kansas School of Nursing
Kansas City, Kansas

Karen S. Martin, RN, MSN, FAAN
Health Care Consultant
Martin Associates
Omaha, Nebraska

Cynthia M. Mascara, RN, MSN, MBA
Principal Consultant 2
Strategic Clinical Consulting
Siemens Medical Solutions
Malvern, Pennsylvania

Susan A. Matney, MSN, RN, FAAN
Medical Informaticist
HDD Team
3M Health Information Systems
Salt Lake City, Utah

Christine D. Meyer, PhD, RN-BC
Senior Consultant
McKesson Corporation
Alpharetta, Georgia

Sandra A. Mitchell, PhD, CRNP
Research Scientist
Outcomes Research Branch
Division of Cancer Control and Population
    Sciences
National Cancer Institute
Bethesda, Maryland

Judy Murphy, RN, FACMI, FHIMSS, FAAN
Deputy National Coordinator for
    Programs and Policy
Office of the National Coordinator for
    Health Information Technology
Department of Health & Human Services
Washington, DC

Daniel A. Nagel, RN, BScN, MSN
PhD Student
School of Nursing, Faculty of Health
    Sciences
University of Ottawa
Ottawa, Ontario

Scott P. Narus, PhD
Associate Professor
Department of Biomedical Informatics
University of Utah, School of Medicine
Medical Informatics Director
Information Systems – Medical Informatics
Intermountain Healthcare
Salt Lake City, Utah

Ramona Nelson, PhD, RN-BC, ANEF, FAAN
Professor Emerita
Slippery Rock University
Slippery Rock, Pennsylvania;
President
Ramona Nelson Consulting
Allison Park, Pennsylvania

Kumiko Ohashi, RN, Ph.D
Research Fellow
Division of General Internal Medicine &
    Primary Care
Brigham and Women's Hospital
Harvard Medical School
Boston, Massachusetts

Sally Okun, RN, MMHS
Vice President, Advocacy, Policy, and
    Patient Safety
PatientsLikeMe
Cambridge, Massachusetts

Hyeoun-Ae Park, PhD, RN, FAAN
Dean and Professor, Biostatistics and
    Health Informatics
College of Nursing, Seoul National
    University
Seoul, South Korea

Ginette A. Pepper, PhD, RN, FAAN
Director, Hartford Center of Geriatric
    Nursing Excellence
Professor and Helen Bamberger Colby
    Presidential Endowed Chair in
    Gerontologic Nursing
Associate Dean for Research and PhD
    Program
College of Nursing, University of Utah
Salt Lake City, Utah

Mitra Rocca, Dipl Med Inform
Senior Medical Informatician
Food and Drug Administration
Silver Spring, Maryland

Kay M. Sackett, EdD, RN
Associate Professor
Capstone College of Nursing
University of Alabama
Tuscaloosa, Alabama

Loretta Schlachta-Fairchild, RN, PhD, FACHE, LTC(ret), U.S. Army
President and CEO
iTelehealth Inc.
Cocoa Beach, Florida

Charlotte Seckman, PhD, RN-BC
Assistant Professor, Course Director
Organizational Systems and Adult Health
University of Maryland School of Nursing
Baltimore, Maryland

Joyce Sensmeier, MS, RN-BC, CPHIMS, FHIMSS, FAAN
Vice President, Informatics
Healthcare Information and Management
    Systems Society
Chicago, Illinois

Diane J. Skiba, PhD, FACMI, FAAN
Professor and Coordinator
Health Care Informatics Program
College of Nursing
University of Colorado
Aurora, Colorado

Catherine Janes Staes, BSN, MPH, PhD
Assistant Professor
Department of Biomedical Informatics
University of Utah School of Medicine
Salt Lake City, Utah

Nancy Staggers, PhD, RN, FAAN
Professor, Informatics
School of Nursing
University of Maryland
Baltimore, Maryland;
Adjunct Professor
College of Nursing
Department of Biomedical Informatics
University of Utah
Salt Lake City, Utah

Kathleen R. Stevens, RN, EdD, ANEF, FAAN
STTI Episteme Laureate
Professor and Director
Academic Center for Evidence-Based
    Practice and Improvement Science
    Research Network
School of Nursing
University of Texas Health Science Center
    San Antonio
San Antonio, Texas

Jim Turnbull, DHA
Chief Information Officer
University of Utah Health Care
Salt Lake City, Utah

Karen B. Utterback, MSN, RN
Vice President, Strategy and Marketing
McKesson Extended Care Solutions Group
Springfield, Missouri

Dianna Vice-Pasch, RN-BC, BSN, CCM, CTCP
MSN Student
Telemedicine Clinical Coordinator
University of Kentucky TeleCare
Lexington, Kentucky

Judith J. Warren, PhD, RN, BC, FAAN, FACMI
Christine A. Hartley Centennial Professor
Director of Nursing Informatics, KUMC
    Center for Healthcare Informatics
University of Kansas School of Nursing
Kansas City, Kansas

Charlene R. Weir, PhD, RN
Associate Professor
Department of Biomedical Informatics
University of Utah School of Medicine
Associate Director, Geriatric Research and
    Clinical Care
Salt Lake City Veterans Administration
    Medical Center
Salt Lake City, Utah

Marisa Wilson, DNSc, MHSc, RN-BC
Assistant Professor
Director, MS Programs
University of Maryland School of Nursing
Baltimore, Maryland

Kathy H. Wood, PhD, FHFMA
University Dean, Health
Colorado Technical University
Colorado Springs, Colorado

REVIEWERS AND ANCILLARY WRITERS

REVIEWERS

Donna Baker, APRN, BSN, MS, ACNS-BC, CNOR
Certified by the AANC and CCI for Perioperative Nursing
Adult Clinical Nurse Specialist
Clinical Process Consultant
Picis, Inc./OptumInsight

Carol Bickford, PhD, RN-BC, CPHIMS
Senior Policy Fellow
Department of Nursing Practice and Policy
American Nurses Association
Silver Spring, Maryland

Mary T. Boylston, RN, MSN, EdD, AHN-BC
Professor of Nursing
Eastern University
St. Davids, Pennsylvania

Jane M. Brokel, PhD, RN
Adjunct Faculty
College of Nursing
University of Iowa
Iowa City, Iowa;
Executive Committee & Advisory Council
Iowa Health Information Network
Iowa Department of Public Health
Des Moines, Iowa

Perry Gee, MSN, RN, PhD(c)
Betty Irene Moore School of Nursing
Faculty
Health Informatics Certificate Program
University of California, Davis
Davis, California

Dorothea E. McDowell, PhD, RN
Professor
Department of Nursing
Henson School of Science and Technology
Salisbury University
Salisbury, Maryland

Susan Pierce, EdD, MSN, RN, CNE
Professor
College of Nursing and Allied Health
Northwestern State University
Shreveport, Louisiana

Kathleen Smith, MScEd, RN-BC, FHIMSS
Managing Partner
ICCE, LLC
Olney, Maryland

ANCILLARY WRITERS

Linda M. Belsanti, RN, BSN, MS HI&M
UMASS Medical Center
Worcester, Massachusetts

Jane M. Brokel, PhD, RN
Adjunct Faculty
College of Nursing
University of Iowa
Iowa City, Iowa;
Executive Committee & Advisory Council
Iowa Health Information Network
Iowa Department of Public Health
Des Moines, Iowa

Gina Keckritz
Wordbench
Maryland Heights, Missouri

Ron Piscotty, MS, RN-BC
Instructor of Nursing
Oakland University
School of Nursing
Rochester, Michigan;
PhD in Nursing Candidate
University of Michigan
School of Nursing
Ann Arbor, Michigan

Over our many years spent working in the practice setting and teaching in the academic setting we have increasingly recognized the need for an informatics textbook that provides a solid overview of the field using an interprofessional perspective. When approached by Elsevier (Mosby) to create such a book, it was an opportunity that could not be missed. The book's title, *Health Informatics: An Interprofessional Approach*, was carefully selected to reflect the comprehensive nature of the book and the interprofessional focus of the content. Health informatics epitomizes a field where collaborations among disciplines are not just helpful but imperative for success. The contributors to this book are leaders in health informatics with expertise in a wide variety of health-related disciplines.

Health Informatics: An Interprofessional Approach provides the reader with a comprehensive understanding of how informatics relates to the healthcare industry. Each chapter opens with key terms, learning objectives, and an abstract giving the readers an overview of the topics covered within the chapter. The headings within each chapter provide a conceptual framework for understanding the focus of that chapter. Case studies with analytic questions demonstrate how informatics concepts apply in real-life situations. Each chapter ends with a conclusion and future directions, followed by references. At the end of every chapter, discussion questions encourage critical thinking and additional learning.

USES OF THE BOOK

This textbook is an excellent resource that can be used within and across various health disciplines. That is, it may be used for either intradisciplinary or interdisciplinary informatics courses. The text can span levels of education depending on program of study and the needs of faculty and students. Rather than being targeted at one level of education the content of this book is targeted to the interface of learning between undergraduate courses and core graduate-level courses. The book is designed for use with students enrolled in upper division or advanced undergraduate courses, RN to BSN/MSN programs, and graduate students in healthcare, especially DNP and PhD students. When used in graduate health informatics programs such as nursing informatics, this book is especially appropriate as a textbook for the initial core courses.

Vendors, Applications, Institutions, etc.

Throughout the book several specific vendors, applications, products, organizations, and institutions are discussed. They are included in this book for information purposes and are an important aspect of health informatics, however, at no time is the inclusion of this information an endorsement of a specific company, product or organization.

ORGANIZATION OF THE BOOK

The book is organized into nine units. The first unit, Background and Foundational Information, focuses on material that is fundamental to understanding the discipline as a whole. Content includes the history of health informatics, terms and definitions, theories models and conceptual frameworks underpinning health informatics, evidenced-based practice, practice-based evidence, and program evaluation.

The second unit, Information Systems in Healthcare Delivery, provides readers with an integrated approach to the major areas of healthcare practice, the related applications, and supporting technical infrastructure. Topics include electronic health records, ancillary application, telehealth, home health, clinical decision support, and public health informatics.

The third unit, Participatory Healthcare Informatics and Healthcare on the Internet, addresses the evolving empowered, engaged, and equipped epatient and related applications or technology such as social media and personal health records. Readers are introduced to the impact of these changes on the healthcare provider–patient relationship and the totality of healthcare delivery.

The fourth unit, Project Management: Tools and Procedures, provides the knowledge and skills needed to lead and guide informatics-related projects throughout the systems life cycle, including selecting systems, implementing and evaluating them as well as planning for downtimes. The unit concludes by exploring the policies and procedures needed to ensure the privacy and security of healthcare systems.

The fifth unit, Quality, Usability, and Standards in Informatics, explains the complex interrelationship between safety, usability, and standards. The unit focuses on creating a culture of safety that ensures that information systems are usable for patients, healthcare providers, and institutions.

The sixth unit, Governance and Organizational Structures for Informatics, deals with the local and national infrastructure required in health informatics. On the local level the unit addresses questions such as how to structure and lead an informatics or information technology (IT) department. On the national level it addresses questions about national policy issues and how leaders in health informatics can address these challenges.

The seventh unit, Education and Informatics, focuses on the role of education in informatics and the role of informatics in the education of healthcare providers. It includes chapters that discuss educational applications and issues, educational tools, simulation, distributive education, and informatics in the curriculum.

The eighth unit, International Informatics Efforts, contains a chapter on the international aspects of informatics. The last and ninth unit is titled The Present and Future. The chapter in this unit provides an overview of current trends and future directions, including nanotechnology.

The book is carefully edited to ensure an organized approach to the wide-ranging content. For example, content such as the Health Information Technology for Economic and Clinical Health (HITECH) Act that is affecting many different aspects of informatics is discussed in more than one chapter. However, each time it is discussed the content is focused on the topic of the individual chapter. At the same time, the sweeping impact of the HITECH Act is clarified throughout the book.

TEACHING AND LEARNING PACKAGE

Health informatics is a fast-changing field. Resources and emerging developments related to each chapter are available on the Evolve website. For example, new government reports and other important documents are posted or referenced for easy student access. These materials are targeted to all faculty, including those newer to the field as well as those with additional experience in the discipline of informatics.

For the Instructor

- **TEACH Lesson Plans** contain objectives and key terms from the text. Topics from the book are mapped to Quality and Safety Education for Nurses (QSEN) standards, American Association of Colleges of Nursing (AACN) Essentials Series, concept-based learning, and American Health Information Management Association (AHIMA) competencies. These lesson plans tie in all of the chapter resources for effective presentation of material and include additional highlights and learning activities tied to the content within the chapters.
- **PowerPoint Presentations** are available to accompany the TEACH Lesson Plans. Pulling content and figures from the text, the PowerPoint slides provide students with the highlights of the chapter and provide instructors with additional topics of conversation tied to the topic.
- A **test bank** containing more than 300 questions is compliant with the NCLEX standards and provides text page references and cognitive levels. The ExamView software allows instructors to create new tests; edit, add, and delete text questions; sort questions; and administer and grade online tests.
- The **Image Collection** contains all of the art from the text for use in lectures or to supplement the PowerPoint Presentations provided.
- **Online Activities** for each chapter provide additional assignments to deepen students' understanding of the content of the text.

For the Student

- **Student Review Questions** provide additional practice for students trying to master the content presented within the text.
- Most chapters have a **Bibliography and Additional Readings** to provide sources for additional research on the subject.
- **Web Resources** are available for most chapters. These links direct students to cutting-edge information and tools to encourage additional learning on the subject.

ACKNOWLEDGEMENTS

First, we would like to acknowledge Teri Hines Burnham, Executive Content Strategist, who spent hours convincing both Elsevier and us that this book could and should be written. Next, we would like to acknowledge Heather Rippetoe, Content Development Specialist, who provided support throughout the project. Heather was always available for support, ideas, and solutions when dealing with the problems, big and small, that are inherent in writing a book with nine units and 31 chapters. Next in the process were Megan Isenberg, Project Manager; Abby Hewitt, Marketing Manager; Jeff Patterson, Publishing Services Manager, and Karen Pauls, Designer. Their expertise was imperative for developing a polished and professional product.

Each chapter of this book is supported with Evolve resources. We also wish to acknowledge the support of Prathibha Mehta, Project Manager, and Thapasya Ramkumar, Multimedia Producer, for the Evolve resources, and ancillary writers Ron Piscotty, Gina Keckritz, Linda Belsanti, and Jane Brokel for their development of these resources.

Finally we would like to acknowledge the reviewers: Donna Baker, Carol Bickford, Mary Boylston, Jane Brokel, Perry Gee, Dorothea McDowell, Susan Pierce, and Kathleen Smith. Their many suggestions, tips, and comments were invaluable in creating this book.

CONTENTS

UNIT 6   GOVERNANCE AND ORGANIZATIONAL STRUCTURES FOR INFORMATICS

UNIT 8   INTERNATIONAL INFORMATICS EFFORTS

UNIT 9   THE PRESENT AND FUTURE

Background and Foundational Information

Introduction: The Evolution of Health Informatics

Ramona Nelson

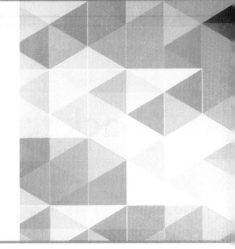

Over time the collaborative opportunities to create a more effective and efficient healthcare system will become more interesting and motivating than the historical struggles and hierarchical relations of the past.

OBJECTIVES

At the completion of this chapter the reader will be prepared to:
1. Analyze how historical events have influenced the definition and current scope of practice of health informatics in healthcare
2. Discuss the development of health informatics as a discipline, profession, and specialty
3. Analyze informatics-related professional organizations and their contributions to professional development and informatics

KEY TERMS

Biomedical informatics, 13
Clinical informatics, 11
Computer science, 3
Dental informatics, 6
Health informatics, 2

Informatics, 4
Information science, 3
Medical informatics, 5
Nursing informatics, 6

ABSTRACT

Health informatics has evolved as both a discipline or field of study and an area of specialization within the health professions. This chapter describes the historical process of that evolution as a basis for understanding the current status of health informatics as both a discipline and a specialty within healthcare. The historical roots within computer and information science are explored. The development of professional organizations, educational programs, and the knowledge base as documented in conference presentations, proceedings, journals, and books is described. The history of and process for naming the specialty and the discipline are then analyzed.

INTRODUCTION

Health informatics has evolved as a discipline and an area of specialization within the health professions. As both a practice specialty and a field of study, health informatics incorporates processes, procedures, theories, and concepts from computer and information sciences, the health sciences (e.g., nursing and medical science), and the social sciences (e.g., cognitive and organizational theory). Health informatics professionals use the tools of information technology to collect, store, process, and communicate health data, information, knowledge, and wisdom. The goals of health informatics are to support healthcare delivery and improve the health status of all. Information technology and related hardware, as well as software, are viewed as tools to be used by consumers, patients, and clients; healthcare providers; and administrators in achieving these goals. Health informatics incorporates processes, procedures, theories, and concepts from a number of different health professions and is therefore a unique interprofessional field of study as well as an area of specialization within the different health professions. This chapter explores the evolution of health informatics as both a discipline and a specialty practice within healthcare.

THE ROOTS OF INFORMATICS WITHIN THE COMPUTER AND INFORMATION SCIENCES

Health informatics emerged as a distinct specialty within healthcare over time as nurses, physicians, and other healthcare visionaries applied innovative developments in the computer and information sciences to complex problems in healthcare. Computer science brings to health informatics the technology and software coding required for this specialty while information science contributes the procedures and processes needed to develop and process data, information, and knowledge. The health professions provide the knowledge and wisdom to use computer and information science effectively in delivering healthcare and improving the health of all people. Understanding the scope and boundaries of health informatics begins with an appreciation of its roots within computer and information sciences.

Computer Science

Computer science is defined as the "systematic study of algorithmic methods for representing and transforming information, including their theory, design, implementation, application, and efficiency . . . The roots of computer science extend deeply into mathematics and engineering. Mathematics imparts analysis to the field; engineering imparts design."[1(para 1)] The word *computer* is derived from the Latin word *computare*, which means to count or sum up. The word first appeared in English in 1646, meaning a person who computes or processes mathematical data.

However, a key problem with these early human computers was that they made errors. In the early 1800s, Charles Babbage, a mathematician, became increasingly concerned with the high error rate in the calculation of mathematical tables. Impressed by existing work on calculating machines, he proposed the development of a "difference engine." As a result of his efforts to create a general-purpose, programmable computer employing punch cards, he is often identified as the first person to create a nonhuman computer or a programmable mechanical device aimed at solving problems.[2] While Babbage was not successful in building a functioning computer, the process of using punch cards to input data and obtain output did become an effective technology in other fields, such as rug making.

The Babbage approach to creating a computer included input and output but not storage. Herman Hollerith took this idea a step forward in the late 1800s when he used punch cards for input, processing, creating output, and storing data. Hollerith, like Babbage, was motivated by his concern with laborious, time-consuming, and error-prone human operations. In Hollerith's case, the problems were evident in the processes used for collecting and calculating the 1880 U.S. census and related data. His invention, which both sorted and tabulated data, "was the first wholly successful information processing system to replace pen and paper."[3(para 2)] In 1896, starting with this and related inventions, Hollerith founded the Tabulating Machine Company. In 1911 the Tabulating Machine Company merged with two other companies, creating the company that is now IBM. Hollerith's technology, developed for completing the U.S. census for 1890, was used well into the 1960s. By the 1960s automation was becoming part of healthcare and health informatics was beginning to emerge as a new discipline.

The move from a mechanical to an electronic digital computer is usually dated to the creation of ENIAC (Electronic Numerical Integrator and Computer) in the 1940s. This was a large machine requiring huge amounts of space, a specialized environment, and specially trained personnel. It initiated the concept of centralized computing and the information services department. Twenty years after ENIAC began functioning, the first Department of Computer Sciences in the United States was established in 1962 at Purdue University within the school's Division of Mathematical Sciences.[4] The foundational relationship between the science of mathematics and the development of computer science provides certain benefits for health informatics. The culture of mathematics brings to the study of informatics systematic, logical approaches, processes, and procedures for understanding natural phenomena and solving problems.

In the 1980s the personal computer (PC) emerged and forever changed the role of the user as well as the organizational infrastructure for supporting computerization within institutions. Computerization within healthcare institutions was no longer totally centralized and computer use was no longer limited to specially trained personnel. As healthcare providers became direct users of the computer, they began to discover a wide range of new uses for these tools. The increased interest in the value of computers and the increased level of computer literacy among a number of healthcare providers proved a major advantage to the creation of the informatics specialty. These same factors have also created a certain tension between centralized and decentralized infrastructures to support technology within healthcare settings.

Information Science

"Information science is a discipline that investigates the properties and behavior of information, the forces governing the flow of information, and the means of processing information for optimum accessibility and usability. It is concerned with that body of knowledge relating to the origination, collection, organization, storage, retrieval, interpretation, transmission, transformation, and utilization of information. This includes the investigation of information representations in both natural and artificial systems, the use of codes for efficient message transmission, and the study of information processing devices and techniques, such as computers and their programming systems."[5(p3)]

Establishing the beginning of information science is difficult since it emerged from the convergence of various disparate disciplines, including library, computer, communication, and behavioral sciences.[6] However, there are key dates and events that can be used to demonstrate the evolution of information science as a distinct specialty whose roots extend deeply into the profession of library science. These include the following:

- In 1937 the American Documentation Institute (ADI) was established. The initial organizational focus was the development of microfilm as an aid to information dissemination. Because of the expansion and diversification of its members, ADI changed its name to the American Society for Information Science in 1968 and then to the American Society for Information Science and Technology in 2000.[7]
- In 1948 the Royal Society of Great Britain held a conference bringing together "libraries, societies, and institutions responsible for publishing, abstracting, and information services to examine the possibility of improvement in existing methods of collection, indexing, and distribution of scientific literature, and for the extension of existing abstracting services."[8(p136)] The decision by this prestigious group to hold such a conference demonstrated the growing importance of managing information.
- In 1963 the first textbook that treated information science as a discrete discipline was published. The book was titled *Information Storage and Retrieval: Tools, Elements and Theories.*[6]
- In 1964 the National Library of Medicine (NLM) began using the computerized MEDLARS (Medical Literature Analysis and Retrieval System) as a mechanism to create *Index Medicus.*[9]
- In 1971 the NLM began offering national online access to MEDLINE.
- In 1972 the NLM began training physicians and other health scientists in the use of computer technology for medical education and the provision of healthcare. This was the beginning of its informatics training programs.[10] The NLM would go on to play a major role in the development of the health informatics specialty.

The relationship between library science and the development of information science provides certain benefits for health informatics. The culture of library science brings to the study of informatics policies and procedures for managing information, an awareness of the value of the information to the user of that information, and a culture of service. Evidence of this cultural value can be inferred from the guiding principles of the American Library Association outlined in Box 1-1.

Health Informatics

The development of health informatics is usually traced to the 1950s with the beginning uses of computers in healthcare.[11] This early period in the history of informatics extended into the 1960s and was characterized by experimenting with the use of this new technology in medicine and in nursing education.[12] For example, Robert Ledley, a dentist interested in biomedical research, published with Lee Lusted one of the first papers in this field. The paper, titled "Reasoning Foundations of Medical Diagnosis," discussed computer-based medical diagnosis.[13] Ledley went on to invent the computed tomography (CT) scanner in the 1970s. An example from nursing is the work of Connie Settlemeyer, a graduate student in the University of Pittsburgh School of Nursing in the late

BOX 1-1	AMERICAN LIBRARY ASSOCIATION: GUIDING PRINCIPLES

Advocacy for Libraries and the Profession
Diversity
Education and Lifelong Learning
Equitable Access to Information and Library Services
Intellectual Freedom
Literacy
Organizational Excellence
Transforming Libraries in a Dynamic and Increasingly Global Digital Information Environment

TABLE 1-1	CHARTING USING THE SOAPE FORMAT	
LETTER	**ITEM**	**DESCRIPTION**
S	Subjective data or observations	Data provided by the patient, family, or others that cannot be observed, such as pain
O	Objective data or observations	Data that can be observed, such as the condition of an incision (inflamed, open with purulent drainage)
A	Assessment	The conclusion, diagnosis, or interpretation of the data, such as wound infection
P	Plan	A list of goals and planned interventions
E	Evaluation	A description of the outcomes or responses to the interventions

1960s. Settlemeyer designed a mainframe-based computer-assisted instruction program for teaching students how to chart using the common problem-oriented format referred to as SOAPE or SOAP. See Table 1-1 for an overview of this format. This program was then used to teach undergraduate nursing students at the University of Pittsburgh throughout the 1970s.

During this same period the term *informatics* was established. Informatics is actually the English translation of terms used in other languages. Because of differences in language it is difficult to determine whether the initial use of the word *informatics* was referring to the discipline of informatics, information science, computer science, or a combination of these. A.I. Mikhailov at Moscow State University is credited with first using the Russian terms *informatik* and *informatikii*. In 1968, Mikhailov published the book *Oznovy Informatiki*, which was translated as *Foundations of Informatics*. In 1976, he published a second book, *Nauchnye Kummunikatsii i Informatika*, which was translated as *Scientific Communication and Informatics*. In this book he defined informatics as the science that "studies the structure and general properties of scientific information and the laws of all processes of scientific communication."[14(p39)]

In the 1960s the word *informatique* began to appear in the French literature. *Informatique* translates to English as informatics or computing, data processing, or the handling of information, especially by a computer. During these same years the German term *informatik* was used. *Informatik* translates as meaning computing, calculating, figuring, or reckoning. The term *medical informatics* began to appear in English publications in the early 1970s. While the term *medical informatics* was not explicitly defined in these initial publications, it was generally accepted to mean the use of a computer to process medical data and information.[14]

While the period previous to the 1970s was characterized by experimentation and the establishment of the term *informatics*, the next 10 to 15 years were characterized by the beginning use of computers in actual patient care and the development of health informatics as a discipline. Beginning in 1971, El Camino worked in partnership with Lockheed to install the world's first computer-aided medical information system, known as MIS.[15] A number of hospitals followed this example by installing information systems to manage business and inventory data.

At that time nurses, and unit secretaries under the direction of nurses, were responsible for completing the paper forms necessary to implement physicians' orders that had been handwritten on patients' charts. These paper forms were used to communicate the orders to other departments and to capture the hospital charges associated with these orders. As a result, the functions of "order entry" and "results reporting" were in some of the first hospital information systems with direct patient care implications. Nurses, along with employees in specialty departments such as labs and radiology, were some of the first healthcare providers directly affected by the use of this technology in healthcare. During this same decade computers were beginning to be used in specialty areas such as the cardiac lab as hemodynamic monitoring systems. In these environments computers were used to do calculations, returning accurate results within seconds. By the end of the 1970s both commercial and academic developments in computers, libraries, and healthcare had created a fertile environment for the growth and development of the new discipline of health informatics.

ESTABLISHING THE SPECIALTY OF HEALTH INFORMATICS

Over the next several decades, evidence that a new specialty was being established can be seen in the following:
1. Publications of health informatics books
2. Development of new journals
3. Establishment of professional organizations
4. Number of informatics conferences that are now recurring events
5. Creation of university-level educational programs
6. Development of certification programs

The history of each of these activities contributed to the development of the knowledge base that is unique to the discipline. Over time a result of these activities is an organized body of knowledge that is specific to the discipline. The newest information within the discipline is often presented at conferences. While a conference may have a theme and even subthemes, the focus is on presenting the newest information and not an organized body of knowledge. "The timeliest articles on computer applications in medicine [are] found in proceedings and transactions of meetings sponsored by professional and commercial organizations."[14(p46)] As journals develop, the information and knowledge specific to the discipline become more established and organized. As the knowledge increases, the organizational structure of that knowledge is recognized and accepted within the discipline. At this point in the development of any discipline, including health informatics, books play a key role in presenting the knowledge of the discipline in an organized format. For example, scan the table of contents of this book and notice the overall organization of the knowledge specific to this discipline. This general pattern of increasing organization within publications over time is demonstrated in Figure 1-1. As the discipline matures, these elements intersect with conferences and journal material coinciding and then feeding more formal material to books.

Books

Books related to computers and healthcare began appearing in the 1960s. Examples of these types of books are included in Box 1-2. However, the use of the word *informatics* in a

> **BOX 1-2   EARLY BOOKS ON COMPUTERS AND HEALTHCARE**
>
> *Computer Applications in the Behavioral Sciences* (1962) by Harold Borko
> *Computer Applications in Medicine* (1964) by Edward Eaton Mason and William G. Bulgren
> *Use of Computers in Biology and Medicine* (1965) by Robert Steven Ledley with the assistance of James Bruce Wilson
> *Computers in Biomedical Research* (1965) by Ralph W. Stacy and Bruce D. Waxman

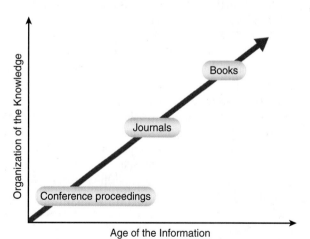

FIG 1-1 General trends in the development of knowledge within a discipline.

book title did not appear until 1971 when the International Federation for Documentation published *An Introductory Course on Informatics/Documentation* by A.I. Mikhailov and R.S. Giljarevskij. This was followed in 1977 by *Informatics and Medicine: An Advanced Course*, edited by P.L. Reichertz and G. Goos. In the 1980s books related to computers and nursing began to appear. The first of these books, *Nursing Information Systems* by Werley and Grier, established and explained the minimum data set in nursing practice.[16] This was quickly followed by one of the classic publications in informatics, *Computers in Nursing* by Rita Zielsorff.[17]

The 1980s were characterized by several publications dealing with computers and nursing. Well-recognized examples include the first edition of *Essentials of Computers* by Virginia Saba and Kathleen McCormick in 1987 and *Guidelines for Basic Computer Education in Nursing* by Diane Skiba and Judith Ronald. In 1988 the first book using the term nursing informatics in its title was published. This book, authored by Ball, Hannah, Newbold, and Douglas, was titled *Nursing Informatics: Where Caring and Technology Meet*.[18] In 1990 one of the first medical informatics textbooks, titled *Medical Informatics: Computer Applications in Health Care and Biomedicine*, was published by Shortliffe, Perreault, Wiederhold, and Fagan.[19] In this same year the first dental informatics book, *Dental Informatics: Strategic Issues for the Dental Profession*, part of the series Lecture Notes in Medical Informatics, was edited and published by John J. Salley, John L. Zimmerman, and Marion Ball. Today most if not all of the major publishers in the healthcare arena publish books related to health informatics. A search of offerings on Amazon or the Books in Print database can result in well over 1000 hits. However, because different editions, as well as hardback and paperback editions, are counted as separate books, it is impossible to get an accurate count of the total number of informatics books now in print. See Table 1-2 for a brief book list.

Journals

Following the same pattern as books, new journals began to be published in the 1960s and used the word *computer* as opposed to *informatics*. Homer Warner at the University of Utah edited the first peer-reviewed journal within the new discipline. This journal, titled *Computers in Biomedical Research*, began publishing in 1967.[14] Table 1-3 includes the names and beginning dates of other initial health informatics journals from this time period.

In 1982, the first edition of the journal *Computers in Nursing* was published as a newsletter. The newsletter became an official journal published by Lippincott in 1984. Today the journal is known as *CIN: Computers Informatics Nursing*. While these journals provided a publishing resource for the evolving discipline, articles were also being published in other professional journals. In 1960, a total of 38 articles were indexed under the subject "computers in medicine."[14] Since that date close to 15,000 articles have been indexed in MEDLINE and CINAHL using the key word "informatics."

TABLE 1-2	EXAMPLES OF INFORMATICS BOOKS	
TITLE	**AUTHORS OR EDITORS**	**EDITION AND DATE OF COPYRIGHT**
Biomedical Informatics: Computer Applications in Health Care and Biomedicine	Edward H. Shortliffe and James J. Cimino	3rd edition, 2006
Health Informatics: Practical Guide for Healthcare and Information Technology Professionals	Robert E. Hoyt, Nora Bailey, and Ann Yoshihashi	5th edition, 2012
Information Technology for the Health Professions	Lillian Burke and Barbara Weill	3rd edition, 2008
Essentials of Nursing Informatics	Virginia Saba and Kathleen McCormick	5th edition, 2012
Introduction to Computers for Healthcare Professionals	Irene Joos, Ramona Nelson, and Marjorie J. Smith	5th edition, 2010
Informatics and Nursing: Opportunities and Challenges	Jeanne Sewell and Linda Thede	4th edition, 2013

TABLE 1-3	EARLY JOURNALS IN HEALTH INFORMATICS	
NAME	**BEGINNING DATE**	**PUBLISHER**
Computers and Medicine	1972	American Medical Association
Journal of Clinical Computing	1972	Gallagher Printing
Journal of Medical Systems	1977	Plenum Press
MD Computing 1983	1983	Springer-Verlag

While the term *informatics* began appearing in the titles of articles in the early 1970s, it was not until 1986 that the first journal article using the term *nursing informatics* was indexed in MEDLINE as well as CINAHL. This article, titled "The NI Pyramid—A Model for Research in Nursing Informatics," presented a model for research in nursing informatics.[20] This model is described in Chapter 2 of this book. As with books, the number of journals has expanded significantly. As of

September 2012 the NLM catalog of journals included 119 informatics journals. Fifty-four of these journals are referenced in the National Center for Biotechnology Information (NCBI) database. Updated numbers can be seen by searching the database online at www.ncbi.nlm.nih.gov/nlmcatalog. Note that not all of the referenced journals are traditional print journals. The *Online Journal of Public Health Informatics* (http://firstmonday.org/htbin/cgiwrap/bin/ojs/index.php/ojphi/index), established in 2009, is and always has been an online journal. The journals in this growing database reflect the overall field of informatics as well as subspecialties within informatics. For example, one of the journals indexed in MEDLINE—*CIN: Computers Informatics Nursing*—is specific to nursing informatics. The proceedings from the International Medical Informatics Association (IMIA) Nursing Informatics Conferences were added to this list starting in late 2012.

Professional Organizations

Many of the early practitioners interested in the field of health informatics soon discovered there were no formal education programs or colleagues in their professional associations and local community who were also interested in the growing impact of computers. As a result, beginning in the late 1960s and early 1970s, professional organizations began to emerge, playing a significant role in the development of this specialty and providing a major source of education and networking for these early pioneers.[21] Initially informatics groups formed within other larger professional groups. For example, the American Medical Association (AMA) formed a committee on computers in medicine in 1969.[14] As these initial efforts expanded, professional organizations focused on health informatics began to split off from the larger organizations. At the same time that national and international groups were being established, a number of health informatics groups were established as smaller local groups.

The 1980s were a key decade for these activities. IMIA, which was established in 1967 as a technical committee of the International Federation for Information Processing (IFIP), became an independent organization in 1987. Prior to this, IMIA established Working Group 8 on Nursing Informatics in 1981 with representatives from 25 countries. The IMIA Nursing Informatics group continues to this day as a special interest group within IMIA. In the United States, the Symposium on Computer Applications in Medical Care (SCAMC) merged with the American Association for Medical Systems and Informatics (AAMSI) and the American College of Medical Informatics (ACMI) in 1989 to become the American Medical Informatics Association (AMIA). AMIA established a Special Interest Group: Computers in Nursing in the same year.

In 1986 the Hospital Management Systems Society (HMSS), an affiliate of the American Hospital Association (AHA), became the Healthcare Information and Management Systems Society (HIMSS), reflecting the growing influence of information systems and telecommunications

professionals within HIMSS as well as healthcare. In 1993 HIMSS became an independent, not-for-profit corporation.[22]

The American Nurses Association (ANA) established the Council on Computer Applications in Nursing in 1984, and the National League for Nursing (NLN) established the National Forum on Computers in Health Care and Nursing. Beginning in the 1980s and continuing over the next three decades, several local nursing informatics groups were formed. One of the largest and best known of these organizations is the Capital Area Roundtable on Informatics in Nursing (CARING) established in 1982. In 2010, the American Nurses Informatics Association (ANIA) from California and CARING from Washington, D.C. merged, creating ANIA-CARING, a national nursing informatics organization that includes five regions. With more than 3000 members in 34 countries and 50 states, ANIA is one of the largest nursing informatics organizations in existence.[23] Today a number of other local or regional nursing informatics groups continue to exist. In 2004, realizing the advantage of collaboration between these different nursing groups, 18 national and regional nursing informatics groups established the Alliance for Nursing Informatics (ANI) with the financial and leadership support of AMIA and HIMSS.[24] As of July 2012, there were 30 member groups. Box 1-3 lists examples of ANI's accomplishments.

An additional major informatics organization is the American Health Information Management Association. This Association has taken a slightly different path than the other significant informatics-related organizations. In 1928 the Association of Record Librarians of North America (ARLNA) was formed. One of the goals of this new organization was to improve the record of care provided to patients through the use of standards. Professionals within ARLNA were titled as registered record librarians (RRLs). In the mid-1940s the association changed its name to the American Association of Medical Record Librarians (AAMRL). However, this was not the last name change. As medical records

---

BOX 1-3   EXAMPLES OF THE ALLIANCE FOR NURSING INFORMATICS' ACCOMPLISHMENTS

Successfully asked Google to appoint a nurse to the Google Health Advisory Council.

Worked closely with Technology Informatics Guiding Educational Reform (TIGER) initiative to increase the knowledge and awareness of students and practicing nurses concerning informatics.

Provided expert testimony for the Institute of Medicine and the Robert Wood Johnson forum on the Future of Nursing.

Recommended numerous nursing experts for service on national committees and expert panels.

Submitted comments to the National Institute of Standards and Technology (NIST) on Usability Framework as well as a number of other such documents.

were increasingly computerized and as members assumed increasing responsibility within that process, the emphasis on information management became obvious. In 1991 the AAMRL changed its name to the American Health Information Management Association (AHIMA).[25] Today, AHIMA continues to play "a leadership role in the effective management of health data and medical records needed to deliver quality healthcare to the public."[26] Box 1-4 lists the major health informatics organizations and includes additional information on nursing informatics groups.

Given the number of health informatics–related professional organizations with similar names, it is not surprising that there is sometimes confusion, even among specialists in the field, concerning the missions and goals of the different groups. For example, because of the overlapping and complementary interests of AMIA and AHIMA, members of these organizations have at times expressed confusion about how the interests and activities of these organizations relate to one another. In response to this, AMIA and AHIMA jointly developed a document addressing potential questions

---

BOX 1-4   MAJOR HEALTH INFORMATICS AND NURSING INFORMATICS GROUPS

Health-Related Informatics Associations with Special Interest Groups

- American Medical Informatics Association (AMIA): www.amia.org
  - "AMIA leads the way in transforming health care through trusted science, education, and the practice of informatics, a scientific discipline."
  - Regular member dues are $300.
  - A significant number of members are involved in academic settings.
  - Publishes a monthly peer-reviewed journal: *Journal of the American Medical Informatics Association (JAMIA)*.
  - Is the official American representative to the International Medical Informatics Association (IMIA).
  - Includes a special interest group in nursing located at www.amia.org/programs/working-groups/nursing-informatics. This group is responsible for appointing the nursing representative to the IMIA—Nursing Informatics Special Interest Group.
- Healthcare Information and Management and Systems Society (HIMSS): www.himss.org/ASP/index.asp
  - "Advancing the best use of information and management systems for the betterment of health care."
  - Regular member dues are $160.
  - A significant number of members are involved in the practice setting or work for information technology (IT) vendors.
  - With more than 44,000 individual members, more than 570 corporate members, and more than 170 not-for-profit organizations, HIMSS offers a wide range of activities and services.
  - Includes a nursing informatics community located at www.himss.org/asp/nursingInformaticsCommunity.asp.

Health-Related Informatics Associations with Specific Areas of Interest

- American Telemedicine Association (ATA): www.americantelemed.org/
  - "Telemedicine will be fully integrated into healthcare systems to improve quality, access, equity and affordability of healthcare throughout the world."
  - Regular member dues are $220.
  - Members include individuals and organizations interested in telemedicine, including healthcare and academic institutions and corporations that provide products and services supporting remote healthcare.
  - Includes a telehealth nursing special interest group located at www.americantelemed.org/i4a/pages/index.cfm?pageid=3327.
- American Health Information Management Association (AHIMA): www.ahima.org
  - "Leading the advancement and ethical use of quality health information to promote health and wellness worldwide."
  - Regular dues are $160.
  - Members are employed mainly in medical records management.
- College of Healthcare Information Management Executives (CHIME): www.cio-chime.org/
  - "CHIME was created as a complement to HIMSS, intending to provide a specific focus for healthcare CIOs."
  - Regular dues are $405 for joint CHIME-HIMSS membership or $290 for CHIME-only membership.
  - Members are the highest-ranking IT executives within their organizations.

Nursing Informatics Associations

- Alliance for Nursing Informatics (ANI): www.allianceni.org/
  - "Transform health and health care through nursing informatics."
  - The organization is jointly sponsored by AMIA and HIMSS; there are no dues for members.
  - Regular membership is open to nursing informatics–related organizations. A list of the members with links to each organization is located at www.allianceni.org/members.asp. A comprehensive list of the local nursing informatics groups can be found in this list.
- American Nursing Informatics Association (ANIA): www.ania.org/
  - "To provide education, networking, and information resources that enrich and strengthen the roles in the field of nursing informatics."
  - Regular membership dues are $60.
  - Membership is open to individuals interested in nursing informatics and includes around 3000 members.

about the two professional associations and their relationship with one another. "AMIA is the professional home for informatics professionals who are concerned with basic research in the field or any of the biomedical or health application domains, either as researchers or practitioners. AHIMA is the professional home for health information management professionals, with a focus on those elements of informatics that fall under the health informatics area of applied research and practice."[27] The need for such a statement and the wide range of professional organizations focused on informatics reflect the interprofessional nature of informatics and the evolution of health informatics as a distinct area of specialization within the different health professions.

Educational Programs

During the 1950s selected medical schools at major universities began to fund medical computer centers to support the computing requirements of a variety of new biomedical research projects. During the 1960s and 1970s the federal government, mainly via the National Institutes of Health (NIH), played a major role in supporting these efforts. In 1962 NIH was authorized to spend an additional $2 million to fund regional biomedical instrumental centers. By 1968 there were 48 fully operational biomedical computer centers. By introducing medical students, interns, and residents to informatics, these centers were fertile ground for the future development of medical informatics as a specialty. Individual lectures, elective courses, and, in time, medical informatics programs began to develop. In 1968 James Sweeney at Tulane University became the first professor of computer medicine in the United States.[14] One of the earliest departments of medical informatics was established in 1964 at the University of Utah.[28]

Starting in the 1980s the NLM became more active in supporting medical informatics education through its extramural grants program. In 1984 the NLM began the Integrated Advanced Information Management Systems (IAIMS) grant program with the goal of helping health science institutions and medical centers integrate information systems to support patient healthcare, health professions education, and basic and clinical research. By 1986 the NLM was supporting five academic sites, training a total of 29 students.[29] Two decades later the NLM was supporting 18 sites around the nation, with 270 students.[29] While most of these informatics-related educational programs were located in medical schools and attracted mainly physicians, a number of programs offered master's and doctoral degrees that were interprofessional in their recruitment of students.

The early acceptance of other professions in these programs may have supported the position that medical informatics programs are interprofessional and that the term *medical* was meant to be inclusive of all health-related professions in the same way that the term *man* can refer to both men and women. However, a number, if not most, of the health professions did not and still do not consider the term *medical* as inclusive of all health-related specialties. This is especially true for nurses who continued to develop their own university-based educational programs and be recognized as a separate profession in their own right. By 2012 AMIA took a formal position that medical informatics and nursing informatics are both subspecialties; medical informatics is not an inclusive name for both.[30]

In 1977, the State University of New York at Buffalo offered the first computer-related course in a nursing program, a three-credit elective. Just one decade later, in 1988, the University of Maryland offered the first master's program in nursing informatics (NI). Within just a few years a doctoral degree with a focus in NI was offered. This was followed in 1990 by a master's program at the University of Utah and in 1995 by a graduate program at New York University.[31] Over the next several years a number of educational programs in NI were established. These programs reflected their unique setting as well as the strengths and interests of their individual faculty and varied from postbaccalaureate certificate programs to doctoral programs. Because of the wide variation in programs and the lack of any organization tracking them, it is impossible to determine how many nursing informatics programs have actually existed at any point in time.

In 2002 the AMIA Nursing Informatics Working Group (AMIA NI-WG) established a task force on NI curriculum that was charged with developing a working document on the status of graduate curricula in nursing informatics. The goal was to achieve a consensus on the requirements for a master's-level informatics program. The task force which identified 18 graduate programs that had been in existence for at least 2 years, issued their report in 2004, and concluded that:

> Despite several attempts, the task force did not reach consensus on a model that would represent the underlying themes and concepts, yet be flexible. The need for flexibility is important so that individual programs can determine the depth and breadth of the underlying themes and concepts, as well as the development of niche informatics areas, such as consumer informatics, telehealth, or educational applications. Such a model was deemed premature at this time. So a narrative organization of the concepts and themes and content was selected to represent the work of this task force.[32]

Today, as the number of nursing informatics educational programs and other informatics educational programs expand, a variety of degrees and certificates are offered. While nursing and medicine make up the largest groups within the healthcare specialties, a number of other healthcare disciplines have developed informatics programs specific to each discipline. For example, in 1996 Temple University established the nation's first department of dental informatics.[33]

The Health Information Technology for Economic and Clinical Health (HITECH) Act of 2009 included funding for a new educational program for health informatics specialists, a certificate (nondegree) program. Recognizing the shortage of informatics specialists, the designers of this 9-month program wanted to provide beginning formal education to health professionals to quickly increase the numbers of available informatics specialists. However, the creation of these programs means that additional avenues of informatics education are available, but it is unclear how these different levels of education should relate to each other and to the needs of healthcare. How employers will react to certificate program graduates will be a source of study in the future. Chapter 26 includes additional information on this program.

Certification

While attempts to create a consistent and systematic approach to educating health informatics professionals have not been successful, some level of success has been achieved in informatics specialty recognition, developing certification processes, and identifying competencies within a scope of practice.

Nursing was the first group to develop a certification process within health informatics. As a result, other groups have looked to nursing's process as a model. In 1992, the ANA designated NI a specialty within the practice of nursing. Subsequently, an ANA task force developed a monograph outlining the scope of practice and describing the specialty attributes of nursing informatics.[34] The scope of practice was followed a year later by a second monograph outlining the standards of practice and professional performance for nursing informatics.[35] These resources defining the scope and standards of practice provided the necessary groundwork for the development of a certification process. In 1995 a certification examination was created at the generalist practitioner level by the American Nurses Credentialing Center (ANCC). A baccalaureate degree in nursing (BSN) was and still is required to sit for the certification exam.

In 2001 a new task force was established to update and combine the scope and standards documents. That document was updated and revised again in 2008.[36] A key statement within the Scope and Standards of Nursing Informatics Practice is the goal of nursing informatics:

> The goal of Nursing Informatics (NI) is to improve the health of populations, communities, families, and individuals by optimizing information management and communication. These activities include the design and use of informatics solutions and technology to support all areas of nursing, including, but not limited to, the direct provision of care, establishing effective administrative systems, designing useful decision support systems managing and delivering educational experiences, supporting lifelong learning, and supporting nursing research.[36(p1)]

The NI certification examination is regularly revised to reflect evolving practice. Nurses who successfully complete the certification process include the letters RN-BC after their names to indicate they are registered nurses with board certification. The latest data available from March 8, 2010 list a total of 779 actively certified ANCC informatics nurses.[37]

While the ANCC offers only one level of certification for the informatics nurse, the 2008 ANA scope and standards of practice document makes a distinction between an informatics nurse and an informatics nurse specialist. An informatics nurse specialist requires graduate preparation while the informatics nurse does not require this level of preparation. However, with only one level of certification, this distinction is not always clear. For example, in 2002 Johnson & Johnson launched a campaign to deal with the predicted nursing shortage. The website DiscoverNursing.com is an online extension of that campaign. As of late 2012 the site included 104 specialties, including Informatics Nurse. The educational requirement listed on the site is a BSN. Results of a search of the Internet for available nursing informatics positions frequently show a requirement of a nurse with a BSN, or baccalaureate in a related field such as computer science, with a master's degree preferred.

The 2008 ANA task force that wrote the current scope and standards of practice recognized the wide variation in job titles, broad scope of responsibilities, and wide range of roles of informatics nurses. Rather than focus on roles and titles, the 2008 document identified nine functional areas within the nursing informatics scope of practice:

- Administration, leadership, and management
- Analysis
- Compliance and integrity management
- Consultation
- Coordination, facilitation, and integration
- Development
- Educational and professional development
- Policy development and advocacy
- Research and evaluation

NI specialists employed in research, administration, or education employ each of these functional areas to varying degrees, depending on the specific task at hand.[36] The task force's conclusion was further supported by a national informatics nurse role delineation and job analysis survey completed by ANCC in 2010 as a basis for updating the certification examination. This survey included 412 informatics-certified nurses from across the United States. Key findings of the survey are listed in Box 1-5. The majority of certified informatics nurse specialists are employed in healthcare settings providing leadership and support during the life cycle of a healthcare information system within healthcare institutions.[37] This is reflected in the content areas of the certification exam (Box 1-6). Students will want to keep in mind that certified NI specialists may not represent the specialty as a whole. Many NI specialists with graduate or doctoral degrees do not sit for the exam since it is targeted at a generic level and not typically used as an employment discriminator for individuals with these degrees.

The next group to develop a certification examination was HIMSS. In 2002, HIMSS launched CPHIMS, which stands for Certified Professional in Healthcare Information and Management Systems. The "examination is designed to test the knowledge, experience and judgment of IT professionals in healthcare informatics practice. Successful completion of the

BOX 1-5   KEY FINDINGS OF THE AMERICAN NURSES CREDENTIALING CENTER 2010 ROLE DELINEATION STUDY: INFORMATICS NURSE

Highest level of education: master's degree, 40 percent; baccalaureate, 35 percent

Average number of years working within the specialty of informatics: 5.81 years

Majority of respondents (62 percent) practiced within a hospital setting

Ten top work activities included:

- Modeling ethical behavior in use of systems and data
- Promoting adherence to confidentiality across the organization, health exchanges, or state and national registries
- Identifying issues related to privacy
- Serving on clinical committees
- Observing process flows
- Documenting process flows
- Analyzing existing system problems that affect nursing workflow
- Serving as a liaison between clinical, administrative, educational, and information technology groups within the organization
- Serving as a system or technical resource to client (definition of client: consumers, patients, nurses, other healthcare providers, vendors, and other organizations)
- Serving on a go-live implementation team

BOX 1-6   CONTENT AREAS IN THE AMERICAN NURSES CREDENTIALING CENTER CERTIFICATION EXAM FOR NURSING INFORMATICS

1. Information Management and Knowledge Generation (37.33%)
   A. Foundations of Nursing Informatics Knowledge
   B. Models and Theories
   C. Human–Computer Interactions
2. Professional Practice (27.67%)
   A. Nursing Informatics Practice
   B. Informatics and Health Care Industry Topics
   C. Regulatory Monitoring and Accreditation Requirements
   D. Education and Staff Development
3. System Life Cycle (22.00%)
   A. System
   B. System Analysis
   C. System Design, Development, and Customization
   D. System and Functional Testing
   E. System Implementation, Evaluation, Maintenance, and Support
4. Information Technology (14.00%)
   A. Hardware
   B. Software
   C. Communication Technologies
   D. Security, Privacy, and Confidentiality

examination verifies broad-based knowledge in healthcare information and management systems."[38(p2)] As with ANCC, the content tested on the CPHIMS examination was developed by conducting a role delineation study. However, with this exam, information technology (IT) professionals were surveyed to identify tasks that were performed routinely and considered important to competent practice. The content developed from the survey is divided into three major topics with subsections. Box 1-7 outlines the topic areas tested on this examination.

HIMSS's publications concerning the development of the certification examination do not describe how the IT professionals were selected. However, the qualifications to sit for the exam do indicate how the term *IT professional* is defined. These qualifications include (1) a baccalaureate degree, or global equivalent, plus 5 years of associated information and management systems experience, with 3 of those years in healthcare or (2) a graduate degree, or global equivalent, plus 3 years of associated information and management systems experience, with 2 of those years in healthcare. Associated information and management systems experience is defined as including experience in administration or management, clinical information systems, ehealth, information systems, or management engineering.

As with the ANCC exam, there is a heavy emphasis on systems life cycle. In addition, both certifications require recertification (including fees). ANCC has a 5-year period of certification and CPHIMS requires recertification in 3 years. As of 2011 there were 1651 individuals with CPHIMS certification. Of these individuals, 251 were healthcare providers, divided as follows:

- 68.5% Registered Nurse
- 18.3% Medical Doctor
- 8.8% Registered Pharmacist
- 4.4% Other[39]

AMIA is the third group to begin the process of formally recognizing an area of specialization related to informatics. A town hall discussion in 2005 at the AMIA annual meeting concluded that:

1. Informatics as a discipline is more than clinical informatics.
2. Clinical informatics is an interprofessional domain.
3. There is social value in formal clinical informatics training and certification.[40]

While the town hall discussion described clinical informatics as an interprofessional domain and AMIA adopted this as formal policy, the actual process for recognizing clinical informatics as a specialty since then has limited this recognition to clinical informatics as a medical specialty for physicians only. In 2007 AMIA was awarded a grant to develop two documents that are required by the American Board of Medical Specialties (ABMS) to establish a medical subspecialty. In 2009 the core content for the subspecialty of clinical informatics[41] and the program requirements for fellowship education in clinical informatics[42] were published. In July 2009 the American Board of Preventive Medicine (ABPM) agreed to sponsor the specialty application and in

---

BOX 1-7   CONTENT AREAS IN THE CERTIFIED PROFESSIONAL IN HEALTHCARE INFORMATION AND MANAGEMENT SYSTEMS CERTIFICATION EXAM FOR INFORMATION TECHNOLOGY PROFESSIONALS

1. General
   a. Healthcare Environment
   b. Technology Environment
2. Systems
   a. Analysis
   b. Design
   c. Selection, Implementation, Support, and Maintenance
   d. Testing and Evaluation
   e. Privacy and Security
3. Administration
   a. Leadership
   b. Management

March 2010 ABPM submitted the application to ABMS. After an extensive review, the proposal was approved by the ABMS Board in a vote on September 21, 2011. The certification exam is in development and the clinical informatics subspecialty board exam is expected to be administered for the first time in the fall of 2013.[43] The Accreditation Council for Graduate Medical Education will accredit the training programs in clinical informatics; however, this process is yet to be developed. During the first 5 years of the certification procedure, a grandfathering process will be used for physicians who have not completed a formal fellowship in clinical informatics.[44]

Finally, two other informatics-related certification examinations are in development as of late 2012. In 2010, the Office of the National Coordinator for Health Information Technology (ONC) awarded a $6 million grant to Northern Virginia Community College to support the development of a competency examination program for individuals who complete the community college–based certificate (nondegree) for training in Information Technology Professionals in Health Care.[45]

In addition, at its June 2011 meeting the AMIA Academic Forum created the Advanced Interprofessional Informatics Certification (AIIC) Task Force with the goal of exploring an alternate pathway for certification of other informatics professionals in parallel with the clinical informatics certification of physicians. The AIIC Task Force delivered a recommendation to the AMIA board of directors to pursue establishment of an Advanced Interprofessional Informatics Certification. Work is progressing on a white paper that will present a structure for describing and categorizing the varying roles, functions, and related certification needs among those working in the healthcare environment.[44]

As demonstrated by this review of events from published books to the development of credentialing processes, health informatics evolved as a fragmented interprofessional specialty from a variety of disciplines having their own histories, cultures, and established structures. Books are written with nursing informatics or medical informatics in the title, suggesting that these are texts for different health-related disciplines; however, core informatics domain knowledge spans these disciplines. Credentialing exams with overlapping content are developed by different informatics-related professional organizations and are targeted to select specialties within health informatics. The next section explores the implications of the history of health informatics.

RECOGNITION OF THE SPECIALTY

While health informatics has evolved as an interprofessional informatics specialty with a focus on healthcare, combining the words *interprofessional* and *specialty* may have created an oxymoron. First, the study of informatics is not limited to healthcare. Informatics as a field of study has been combined with a number of other professions. For example, Indiana University–Purdue University Indianapolis (http://informatics. iupui.edu/) has established a School of Informatics, which offers, along with a number of other programs, an undergraduate degree in informatics with the opportunity to specialize in biology, business, computer information technology, computer science, health science, human–computer interaction, or legal informatics among other options. Purdue also offers a graduate program in bioinformatics that will prepare the student to design and execute translational research linking data to medicine and drug discoveries, as well as a separate graduate program in health informatics that will prepare the student to analyze and protect patient data, increase healthcare efficiencies, and produce quality patient care.[46]

Second, while health informatics is considered an area of specialization with a focus on healthcare, the question of which discipline it falls within has never been established. In other words, is health informatics a specialty within (1) computer science, (2) information science, (3) each of the various healthcare disciplines, or (4) an interdisciplinary healthcare specialty with students from the different healthcare specialties combined, or (5) a new specialty distinct from its historical roots in the other disciplines? Currently, examples of educational programs representing each of these approaches can be found in colleges and universities across the United States. These programs vary from offering a certificate to an associate degree to offering a postdoctoral fellowship. As a result, the type and amount of previous education required for admission to these different health informatics programs can vary widely. In addition, there is limited consistency in the number of credits and types of courses required in programs of the same type. In recognition of these issues, key leaders within the professional organizations have attempted to establish the appropriate name of this specialty, describe the relationship of the specialty to other related fields of study, and develop a scope of practice with core competencies for the specialty.

NAMING THE SPECIALTY—NAMING THE DISCIPLINE

Earliest references in the late 1950s used the term *bioengineering*. However, as the computer emerged as integral to health informatics, a number of terms combining the disciplines of medicine and computing, including *medical computer science, medical computing,* and *computer medicine,* were used to reflect the new specialty.[14] As other healthcare disciplines continue to develop a focus on informatics, using the terms *medicine* or *medical* to include all specialties has become more controversial, as noted earlier in this chapter. Many disciplines solved this problem by combining the name of their field of practice with the word *informatics.* Box 1-8 provides several examples. This approach is consistent with the strong division of labor, often called scope of practice, and hierarchical structures in healthcare education and healthcare delivery. This approach is also based on the assumption that informatics is a subspecialty within a specific health-related profession. However, the approach of modifying the term *informatics* with a specific health-related discipline, area of interest, or specialization does not provide a name and definition for the discipline as a whole. As pointed out previously, over the years some have argued that *medicine* was an inclusive term covering all aspects, including all healthcare roles in preventing, diagnosing, and treating health problems, including disease. This is demonstrated by the current names of the international and national associations: the International Medical Informatics Association (IMIA) and the American Medical Informatics Association (AMIA). These are interdisciplinary informatics associations with members from various healthcare disciplines. The 3800 members of AMIA include both individual members such as physicians, nurses, dentists, biomedical engineers, medical librarians, those in information technology, and other health professionals and institutional or corporate members such as nonprofit organizations, universities, hospitals, libraries, and corporations with an interest in biomedical and health informatics.[47] Many educational programs changed their names to biomedical informatics to solve this issue and there have been suggestions to change the names of the IMIA and AMIA to use *biomedical* in place of the term *medical*;[30] however, not all members may consider the term *biomedical* as more inclusive than *medical informatics.*

Others have pointed out that the practice of medicine defines the scope of practice for a physician and therefore have suggested that *health* or *healthcare* is a more inclusive term since it includes all levels of wellness as well as disease and other health problems. For example, the Healthcare Information Management and Systems Society (HIMSS) can be described as an interprofessional informatics association but uses the term *healthcare.* The Scope and Standards of Nursing Informatics Practice, published by the ANA, states in the introduction:

Nursing Informatics (NI) is one example of a discipline-specific informatics practice within the broader category of health informatics.[36(p1)]

BOX 1-8	NAMING HEALTH INFORMATICS: RELATED DISCIPLINES

Biomedical Imaging Informatics
Biomedical Pattern Recognition
Clinical Informatics
Clinical Research Informatics
Consumer Health Informatics
Critical Care Informatics
Dental Informatics
Global Health Informatics
Health and Medical Informatics Education
Informatics in Genomic Medicine (IGM)
Intensive Care Informatics
Mental Health Informatics
Nursing Informatics
Open Source Health Informatics
Pediatric Health Informatics & Technology (PHIT)
Pharmacoinformatics or Pharmacy Informatics
Primary Care Informatics or Primary Healthcare Informatics
Public Health Informatics
Public Health/Population Informatics
Telemedicine and Mobile Computing Informatics
Translational Bioinformatics
Veterinary Informatics

Likewise the AMIA Nursing Informatics working group provides the following mission in describing its group:

To promote the advancement of nursing informatics within the larger interdisciplinary context of health informatics. The organization and its members pursue this goal in many arenas: professional practice, education, research, governmental and other service, professional organizations, and industry. The Working Group represents the interests of nursing informatics for its members and AMIA through member services and outreach functions, provides official representation to IMIA-NI and liaises to other national and international groups.[32]

The challenge has been and may still be to select a name that describes the discipline as a whole and yet acknowledges the different informatics disciplines and their relationship with the broader field of study. In 2002 Englebardt and Nelson used the term *health informatics* but presented two different "interdisciplinary" models in response to these issues. Figure 1-2 shows an umbrella model that recognizes the clear boundaries between the different health informatics disciplines at the same time as it demonstrates that it is the connections between the boundaries or the frame of the umbrella that create the discipline. Figure 1-3 uses a Venn diagram to describe health informatics as overlapping the different health informatics disciplines yet being distinct. However, neither model suggests a name that would be inclusive of the different health informatics specialties and their relationships.

In 2006 Shortliffe and Blois recommended the term *biomedical informatics* in Chapter 1 of a book that was retitled for the third edition, *Biomedical Informatics: Computer*

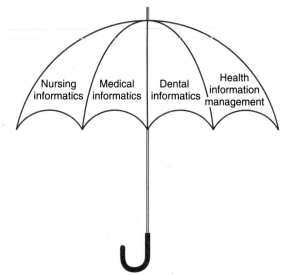

FIG 1-2 Umbrella Model of Health Informatics. (Copyright Ramona Nelson. Reprinted with permission.)

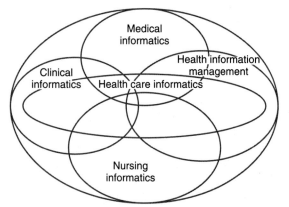

FIG 1-3 Venn Diagram Model. (Copyright Ramona Nelson. Reprinted with permission.)

Applications in Health Care and Biomedicine. "In an effort to be more inclusive and to embrace the biological applications with which many medical informatics groups had already been involved, the name medical informatics has gradually given way to biomedical informatics. Several academic groups have already changed their names, and a major medical informatics journal *Computers and Biomedical Research* was reborn as *The Journal of Biomedical Informatics.*"[19(p23)] In arriving at this position, Shortliffe and Blois explain within the chapter why they believe the terms *health* and *health informatics* are not inclusive but rather exclude key groups:

> Many observers have expressed concern that the adjective "medical" is too focused on physicians and fails to appreciate the relevance of this discipline to other health and life science professionals, although most people in the field do not intend that the word "medical" be viewed as being specifically physician-oriented or even illness-oriented. Thus, the term health informatics, or healthcare informatics, has gained some popularity, even though it has the disadvantage of tending to exclude applications to biology . . . and, as we will argue shortly, it tends to focus the field's name on an application domain (public health and prevention)

rather than the basic discipline and its broad range of applicability.[19(p23)]

The term *biomedical* and the rationale for selecting it resonated with a number of other leaders within AMIA. Six years later the *AMIA Board White Paper: Definition of Biomedical Informatics and Specifications of Core Competencies for Graduate Education in the Discipline* was formally approved by the AMIA Board on April 17, 2012 and published online in June 2012.[30] With the acceptance of this paper AMIA now defined biomedical informatics (BMI) as "the interdisciplinary field that studies and pursues the effective uses of biomedical data, information, and knowledge for scientific inquiry, problem solving and decision making, motivated by efforts to improve human health."[30(p3)] The areas of research and application within BMI range from molecules to populations and societies.

In selecting the term *biomedical informatics* the authors of the paper noted that they had adopted the newer position that the term *medical informatics* refers solely to the "component of research and practice in clinical informatics that focuses on disease and predominantly involves the role of physicians. Thus AMIA now uses *medical informatics* primarily as a parallel notion to other subfields of clinical informatics such as nursing informatics or dental informatics."[30(pp2–3)] The term *health informatics* is also seen as limited in scope. "BMI is the core scientific discipline that supports applied research and practice in several biomedical disciplines, including health informatics, which is composed of clinical informatics (including subfields such as medical, nursing, and dental informatics) and public health informatics."[30(p3)] Figure 1-4 demonstrates the relationships of these previously used terms now under the broad definition of BMI.

However, the authors of the AMIA paper may have realized that the term *biomedical informatics* may not have sounded inclusive to all health-related informatics disciplines in stating that "the phrase 'biomedical *and* health informatics' is often used to describe the full range of application and research topics for which BMI is the pertinent underlying scientific discipline" [emphasis added].[30(p1)]

Not all groups within healthcare identify biomedical as the inclusive term in that it contains the term *medical* as opposed to *health*. However, combining the terms *health and biomedical* informatics, as in the previous quote, may be more acceptable. For example, the Northwestern University Feinberg School of Medicine, Department of Preventive Medicine chose to name its program the Department of Health and Biomedical Informatics. This was after careful consideration of the evolution of the names for the discipline. A summary of this consideration is posted at www.preventivemedicine.northwestern.edu/divisions/hbmi/about.html and is illustrated in Figure 1-5. As can be seen in these two figures, a common consensus has not yet been achieved but there are more similarities than there are differences. In both diagrams informatics is the broader or parent discipline and nursing, medicine, dentistry, etc. are subspecialties within that broader field.

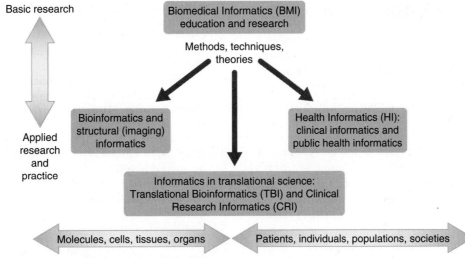

FIG 1-4 AMIA position: biomedical informatics and its areas of application and practice. (Redrawn from Kulikowski CA, Shortliffe EH, Currie LM, et al. AMIA Board white paper: definition of biomedical informatics and specification of core competencies for graduate education in the discipline. *J Am Med Inform Assoc.* 2012. With permission from BMJ Publishing Group Ltd.)

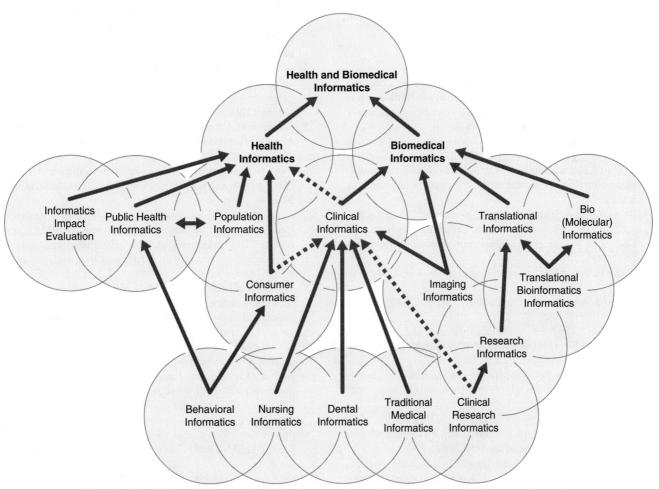

FIG 1-5 Hierarchy of Informatics. This diagram shows the relationships between various subdomains of Health and Biomedical Informatics. The domains are shown as blobs rather than as discrete boxes to emphasize the high degree of overlap among the domains. This hierarchy should be considered a snapshot in time rather than a definitive final solution. (Northwestern University Feinberg School of Medicine, Department of Preventive Medicine.)

CONCLUSION AND FUTURE DIRECTIONS

This chapter has traced the evolution of informatics as a specialty within healthcare and as a discipline. The history of health informatics has been strongly influenced by the history of the health professions and their current infrastructures, such as the educational systems, professional organizations, and professional cultures. As informatics-related education among the professions becomes more consistent and as computerization becomes more integrated into every aspect of healthcare, these historical struggles will become yesterday's story. The emphasis will move from defining the differences and establishing boundaries between the professions to creating an interprofessional approach to meet the health-related needs of individuals and societies. Within this environment, one can expect the healthcare-related specialties to move forward in reaching a working consensus on their individual roles as well as their ever-changing scope of practice within health and biomedical informatics. The focus will evolve to shared core competencies, knowledge, and skills versus emphasizing differences. Over time the collaborative opportunities to create a more effective and efficient healthcare system will become more interesting and motivating than the historical struggles and hierarchical relations of the past.

REFERENCES

1. UB School of Engineering and Applied Sciences. Computer science vs computer engineering. University at Buffalo School of Engineering and Applied Sciences. http://www.eng.buffalo.edu/undergrad/academics/degrees/cs-vs-cen.
2. Cesnik B, Kidd MR. History of health informatics: a global perspective. *Stud Health Technol Inform*. 2010;151:3-8.
3. da Cruz F, Herman Hollerith. Columbia University, Computing History. http://www.columbia.edu/cu/computinghistory/hollerith.html. 2011.
4. Rice J, Rosen S. History of the Department of Computer Sciences at Purdue University. Purdue University, Department of Computer Science. http://www.cs.purdue.edu/history/history.html. 1994.
5. Borko H. Information science: what is it? *Am Doc*. 1968;19(1):3-5.
6. Herner S. Brief history of information science. *J Am Soc Inform Sci*. 1984;35:157-163.
7. American Society for Information Science and Technology (ASIS&T). History of ASIS&T. ASIS&T. http://www.asist.org/history.html.
8. McNinch JH. The Royal Society Scientific Information Conference, London, June 21–July 2, 1948. *B Med Libr Assoc*. 1949;37(2):136-141.
9. U.S. National Library of Medicine. OLDMEDLINE data. U.S. National Library of Medicine. http://www.nlm.nih.gov/databases/databases_oldmedline.html. 2012.
10. U.S. National Library of Medicine. United States National Library of Medicine 1836–2011. U.S. National Library of Medicine. http://apps.nlm.nih.gov/175/milestones.cfm. 2011.
11. Dezelic G. A short review of medical informatics history. *Acta Inform Med*. 2007;March:43-48.
12. Masic L. A review of informatics and medical informatics history. *Acta Inform Med*. 2007;15(3):178-188.
13. Ledley R, Lusted LB. Reasoning foundations of medical diagnosis. *Science*. 1959;130(3366):9-21.
14. Collen MF. *A History of Medical Informatics in the United States*. Washington, DC: American Medical Informatics Association; 1995.
15. El Camino Hospital. About El Camino hospital: history & milestones. El Camino Hospital. http://www.elcaminohospital.org/About_El_Camino_Hospital/History_Milestones.
16. Werley H, Grier MR. *Nursing Information Systems*. New York, NY: Springer; 1980.
17. Zielstorff R. *Computers in Nursing*. Rockville, MD: Aspen Systems Corp; 1982.
18. Ball M, Hannah K, Newbold S, Douglas J. *Nursing Informatics: Where Caring and Technology Meet*. New York, NY: Springer-Verlag; 1988.
19. Shorttliffe E, Perreault LE, Wiederhold G, Fagan L. *Medical Informatics: Computer Applications in Health Care and Biomedicine*. Boston, MA: Addison-Wesley; 1990.
20. Schwirian PM. The NI pyramid: a model for research in nursing informatics. *Comput Nurs*. 1986;4(3):134-136.
21. Nelson R, Joos I. Resources for education in nursing informatics. In: Arnold JM, Pearson GA, eds. *Computer Applications in Nursing Education and Practice*. New York, NY: National League for Nursing; 1992:9-23.
22. HIMSS Legacy Workgroup: Chair Berry Ross. A history of the Healthcare Information and Management Systems Society. HIMSS. http://www.himss.org/content/files/HIMSS_HISTORY.pdf. 2007.
23. CIN: News Release. Leading nursing informatics organizations merge. *CIN–Comput Inform Nu*. 2010;28(2):126.
24. Greenwood K. The Alliance for Nursing History Informatics: a history. *CIN–Comput Inform Nu*. 2010;28(2):124-127.
25. Abdelhak M, Grostick S, Hanken M. *Health Information: Management of a Strategic Resource*. 4th ed. St. Louis, MO: Elsevier; 2012.
26. American Health Information Management Association (AHIMA). AHIMA facts. AHIMA. http://www.ahima.org/about/facts.aspx. 2012.
27. American Medical Informatics Association (AMIA), American Health Information Management Association (AHIMA). Joint AMIA/AHIMA summary of their relationship and links to the informatics field. AMIA. http://www.amia.org/joint-amia-ahima-summary. 2012.
28. University of Utah School of Medicine. Biomedical informatics: about us—an introduction. School of Medicine, Department of Biomedical Informatics. http://medicine.utah.edu/bmi/about/index.php. 2010.
29. U.S. National Library of Medicine (NLM). 1986–2006: two decades of progress: a brief report: major elements of NLM's work since its long range plan of 1986. NLM. http://www.nlm.nih.gov/pubs/plan/lrp06/report/decadesofprogress.html#18. 2007.
30. Kulikowski CA, Shortliffe EH, Currie LM, et al. AMIA Board white paper: definition of biomedical informatics and specification of core competencies for graduate education in the discipline. *J Am Med Inform Assoc*. 2012;19(6):931-938. Epub 2012 Jun 8.
31. Saba V, McCormick K. *Essentials of Nursing Informatics*. 5th ed. Columbus, OH: McGraw-Hill; 2012.
32. American Medical Informatics Association. Nursing Informatics Working Group. Educational Think Tank. Report of the Nursing Informatics Working Group Think Tank. AMIA. 2007.

33. University of Pittsburgh School of Dental Medicine, Center for Dental Informatics. University of Pittsburgh School of Dental Medicine establishes Center for Dental Informatics. University of Pittsburgh School of Dental Medicine. http://www.dental.pitt.edu/informatics/cdipr021402.html.

34. American Nurses Association. *Scope of Practice for Nursing Informatics.* Silver Spring, MD: Nursesbooks.org; 1994.

35. American Nurses Association. *Standards of Practice for Nursing Informatics.* Silver Spring, MD: Nursesbooks.org; 1995.

36. American Nurses Association. *Nursing Informatics: Scope & Standards of Practice.* Silver Spring, MD: Nursesbooks.org; 2008.

37. American Nurses Credentialing Center (ANCC). 2010 Role Delineation Study: informatics nurse: national survey results. ANCC. http://www.nursecredentialing.org/Documents/Certification/RDS/2010RDSSurveys/Informatics-RDS2012.aspx. 2011.

38. HIMSS, CPHIMS Technical Committee. Candidate handbook and application. HIMSS. http://www.himss.org/content/files/CPHIMS_Candidate_Handbook.pdf. 2011.

39. HIMSS, CPHIMS. CPHIMS statistics: January 27, 2002 thru December 15, 2011. HIMSS. http://www.himss.org/content/files/CPHIMS_Statistics.pdf. 2012.

40. Detmer D, Lumpkin JR, Williamson J. Defining the medical subspecialty of clinical informatics. *J Am Med Inform Assn.* 2009;16(2):167-168.

41. Gardner R, Overhage J, Steen E, et al. Core content for the subspecialty of clinical informatics. *J Am Med Inform Assn.* 2009; March/April:153-157.

42. Safran C, Shabot MM, Munger B, et al. Program requirements for fellowship education in the subspecialty of clinical informatics. *J Am Med Inform Assn.* 2009;16(2):158-166.

43. American Medical Informatics Association (AMIA): News Releases. Clinical informatics becomes a board-certified medical subspecialty following ABMS vote. AMIA. http://www.amia.org/news-and-publications/press-release/ci-is-subspecialty. 2011.

44. American Medical Informatics Association (AMIA): CI Medical Subspecialty. Frequently asked questions (FAQ): clinical informatics subspecialty. AMIA. http://www.amia.org/faq-clinical-informatics-medical-subspecialty.

45. Office of National Coordinator for Health Information Technology. Competency Examination Program: frequently asked questions. U.S. DHHS Office of the National Coordinator. http://healthit.hhs.gov/portal/server.pt?open=512&objID=1433&&PageID=16974&mode=2&in_hi_userid=11673&cached=true. 2010.

46. Purdue University Indianapolis School of Informatics. School of Informatics: degrees & courses. Indiana University Purdue University Indianapolis School of Informatics. http://informatics.iupui.edu/degrees/. 2012.

47. American Medical Informatics Association (AMIA). Homepage. AMIA. http://www.amia.org. 2012.

DISCUSSION QUESTIONS

1. Healthcare as a professional field of practice is often traced to the Middle Ages. Its historical roots are tied to the hierarchical structure of the church and the military. How does this history influence the current structure and relationships between the subspecialties within healthcare and biomedical informatics?

2. Which professional associations would be most appropriate for professionals interested in nursing informatics, pharmacy informatics, or public health informatics? Explain the combination selected and the rationale for each choice.

3. Is biomedical and health informatics a discipline or is this an area of subspecialization of interest to health professionals such as nurses, physicians, dentists, etc.?

4. Should there be one certification process and set of credentials for all biomedical and health informatics specialists, or should each of the health professions develop a certification process specific to that specialty?

5. What interprofessional name would you recommend and why?

CASE STUDY

In this case study you, as the reader, will need to fill in a number of the details. The case study begins at the point when you return to school for a graduate degree. Details related to your previous education, professional experience in healthcare, and goals in returning to school should be filled in from your own life story. The program of study for your graduate degree includes an Introduction to Informatics course. This is a required course for all students in the program. One of the first course requirements is that you join an informatics organization and complete a short paper explaining why and how you selected that specific organization. Be sure to explain how you analyzed the options and narrowed your choice to the one organization.

Discussion Questions

1. Talk to several faculty members or others with an interest in informatics to see what organizations they belong to and why. Ask how they became interested in informatics and see if you can match their history with informatics to what you learned about the history of informatics in this chapter.

2. Review the organization websites in Box 1-4 to determine which organization fits best with your interests. Explain how you matched your areas of interest to the information on the website of your chosen organization.

3. Discuss how you would use the information from questions 1 & 2 in selecting appropriate mentors.

Theoretical Foundations of Health Informatics

Ramona Nelson and Nancy Staggers

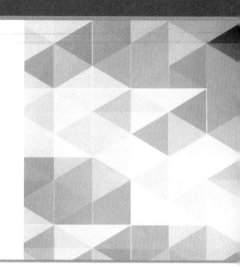

Health informatics specialists draw on a wide range of theories to guide their practice.

OBJECTIVES

At the completion of this chapter the reader will be prepared to:

1. Use major theories and models underpinning informatics to analyze health informatics–related phenomena

2. Use major theories and models underpinning informatics to predict health informatics–related phenomena

3. Use major theories and models underpinning informatics to manage health informatics–related phenomena

KEY TERMS

ABSTRACT

This chapter provides an overview of theories and models useful for health and nursing informatics. The chapter begins by defining and explaining components of grand, middle range, and micro theories. Specific theories relevant to informatics are outlined. Systems, chaos, and complexity theories provide the foundation for understanding each of the theories presented in the chapter. Recognizing the importance of teaching within the role of the informaticist, an overview of selected learning theories is included. Information models from Blum, Graves, and Nelson outline the data, information, knowledge, and wisdom continuum. Next, a selection of informatics models is summarized.

Change theories and the diffusion of innovation theory begin this section of the chapter. The final section discusses a commonly used model, the systems life cycle. A new model of the systems life cycle is described and its application is outlined.

INTRODUCTION

A theory explains the process by which certain phenomena occur.[1] Theories vary in scope depending on the extent and complexity of the phenomenon of interest. Grand theories are wide in scope and attempt to explain a complex phenomenon within the human experience. For example, a learning theory that attempted to explain all aspects of human learning would be considered a grand theory. Because of the complexity of the theory and the number of variables interacting in dependent, independent, and interdependent ways, these theories are difficult to test. However, grand theories can be foundational within a discipline or subdiscipline. For example, learning and teaching theories are foundational theories within the discipline of education.

Middle range theories are used to explain specific defined phenomena. They begin with an observation of the specific phenomena. For example, one might note how people react to change. But why and how does this phenomenon occur? A theory focused on the phenomenon of change would explain the process that occurs when people experience change and predict when and how they will respond in adjusting to the change.

Micro theories are limited in scope and specific to a situation. For example, one might describe the introduction of a new electronic health record (EHR) within a large ambulatory practice and even measure the variables within that situation that could be influencing the acceptance and use of the new system. In the past, micro theories with their limited scope have rarely been used to test theory. However, this may change with the development of Web 2.0 and the application of meta-analysis techniques to automatized natural language processing.

The development of a theory occurs in a recursive process moving on a continuum from the initial observation of the phenomenon to the development of a theory to explain that phenomenon. The continuum can be divided into several stages, including the following:

1. A specific phenomenon is observed and noted.
2. An idea is proposed to explain the development of the phenomenon.
3. Key concepts used to explain the phenomenon are identified and the processes by which the concepts interact are described.
4. A conceptual framework is developed to clarify the concepts and their relationships and interactions. Conceptual frameworks can be used to propose theories and generate research questions. The conceptual framework can also be used to develop a conceptual model. A conceptual model is a visual representation of the concepts and their relationships.
5. A theory and related hypothesis are proposed and tested.
6. Evidence accumulates and the theory gains general acceptance.

Theories can be combined with concepts and conceptual frameworks to create a theoretical framework. Theoretical frameworks are used to explain a combination of related phenomena. Many of the models used to guide the practice of health informatics and discussed in this chapter can be considered theoretical models or frameworks. Because theoretical frameworks explain a combination of related theories and concepts, they can be used to guide practice and generate additional research questions. With this definition, one can argue that the concept of a theoretical framework can be conceived as a bridge between a middle range theory and a grand theory. A theoretical model is a visual representation of a theoretical framework. Many of the models in healthcare and health informatics use a combination of theories in explaining phenomena of interest within these disciplines and fit the definition of a theoretical framework.

While the terms *theory* and *concept* are fairly consistently defined and used in the literature, the terms *conceptual* and *theoretical framework*, as well as the terms *conceptual* and *theoretical models*, are not. There is not a set of consistent criteria that can be applied to determine whether a model is conceptual or theoretical. As a result, researchers and informaticists will often publish models without clarifying that the proposed model is either conceptual or theoretical. In turn, it is possible for one reference to refer to a model as a conceptual framework while another uses the term *theory* when it refers to a model as a theoretical framework.

The building blocks of a theory are concepts. Concepts may be more abstract, such as fruit, or more concrete, such as apple. Concepts provide structure to a theory. For example, in Figure 2-1 the relationships between concepts are depicted. These concepts and the location of the concepts on the page demonstrate the structure of the theory. The interactions

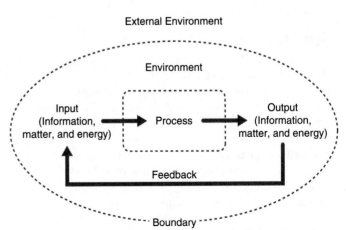

FIG 2-1 An open system interacting with the environment. (Copyright Ramona Nelson. Reprinted with permission.)

between the concepts in a theory explain the function or operations of that theory. For example, the electrical system of the heart is a concrete concept. Impulses travel through this system and produce a contraction of the atria and ventricles. The concept of the heart's electrical system and the description of how it functions provide a theory that can be used to explain how the heart beats.

Because a theory explains the "what" and "how" of a phenomenon, such as the conduction of a heartbeat, a theory can provide direction for planning interventions. Continuing the cardiac example, an impulse travels from the atrium across the atrioventricular (AV) node to the ventricles. If the atrium is beating too fast, as occurs with atrial fibrillation, there can be a fast ventricle response or tachycardia. Drugs that block or slow the rate of impulse transmission at the AV node can be used to treat tachycardia caused by atrial fibrillation with fast ventricle response. This is an example of using a theory to understand and manage a problem.

THEORIES AND MODELS UNDERLYING HEALTH INFORMATICS

As mentioned in Chapter 1, health informatics is an applied field of study incorporating theories from information science; computer science; the science for the specific discipline, such as medicine, nursing, or pharmacy; and the wide range of sciences used in healthcare delivery. As a result, health informatics specialists draw on a wide range of theories to guide their practice. This chapter focuses on selected theories that are of major importance to health informatics and those that are most directly applicable. These theories are vital to understanding and managing the challenges faced by health informatics specialists. In analyzing the selected theories the reader will discover that understanding these theories presents certain challenges. Some of the theories overlap, different theories are used to explain the same phenomena, and sometimes different theories have the same name. The theories of information are an example of each of these challenges.

The one theory that underlies all of the theories used in health informatics is systems theory. Therefore this is the first theory discussed in this chapter.

Systems Theory

A system is a set of related interacting parts enclosed in a boundary.[2] Examples of systems include computer systems, school systems, the healthcare system, and a person. Systems may be living or nonliving. For example, a person is a living system while a computer is a nonliving system.[3]

Systems may be either open or closed. Closed systems are enclosed within an impermeable boundary and do not interact with the environment. An example of a closed system is a chemical reaction enclosed in a glass structure with no interaction with the environment outside the glass. Open systems are enclosed within a semipermeable boundary and do interact with the environment. This chapter focuses on open systems, which can be used to understand technology

and the people who are interacting with the technology. Figure 2-1 demonstrates an open system interacting with the environment. Open systems take input (information, matter, and energy) from the environment, process the input, and then return output to the environment. The output then becomes feedback to the system. Open systems are sometimes referred to as closed. This reference does not mean that the system is truly a closed system but rather that the boundaries are less permeable and as a result input is limited. Concepts from systems theory can be applied in understanding the way people work with computers in a healthcare organization. These concepts can also be used to analyze individual elements such as software or the total picture of what happens when systems interact.

A common expression in computer science is "garbage in garbage out," or GIGO. GIGO refers to the input–output process. The counterconcept implied by this expression is that quality input is required to achieve quality output. While GIGO usually is used to refer to computer systems, it can apply to any open system. Some examples are the role of a poor diet in the development of health problems and the role of informed active participants when selecting a healthcare information system. In these examples garbage in can result in garbage out or quality data can support quality output. Not only is quality input required for quality output, but the system must also have effective procedures for processing those data. Systems theory provides a framework for looking at the inputs to a system, analyzing how the system processes those inputs, and measuring and evaluating the outputs from the system.

Characteristics of Systems

Open systems have three types of characteristics: purpose, structure, and functions. The purpose is the reason for the system's existence. The purpose of an institution or program is often outlined in the mission statement. For example, the purpose of a BSN educational program is to prepare professional nurses. Many times computer systems are referred to or classified by their purpose. The purpose of a radiology system is to support the radiology department; the purpose of a laboratory system is to support the laboratory department. A scheduling system is used to schedule either clients or staff.

It is quite possible for a system to have more than one purpose. For example, a hospital information system may have several different purposes. One of the purposes of a hospital information system is to provide interdepartmental communication. Another purpose is to maintain a census that can be used to bill for patient care.

One of the first steps in selecting a computer system for use in a healthcare organization is to identify the purposes of that system. Purpose answers the question: "Why select a system?" Many times there is a tendency to minimize this step with the assumption that everyone already agrees on the purposes of the system. When a system has several different purposes it is common for individuals to focus on the purposes most directly related to their area of responsibility.

Taking the time to specify and prioritize the purposes helps to ensure that the representatives from clinical, administration, and technology agree on the reasons for selecting a system and understand the full scope of the project.

Functions, on the other hand, focus on the question: "How will the system achieve its purpose?" Functions are sometimes mistaken for purpose. However, it is important to clarify why a system is needed and then identify what functions the system will carry out to achieve that purpose. For example, a hospital may achieve the interdepartmental communication purpose by maintaining an intranet as well as maintaining patient census data including admissions, discharges, and transfers for the institution through a computerized registration system. Each time a department accesses the patient's online record, the name and other identifying information are transmitted from a master file, ensuring consistency throughout the institution. Communication between departments is managed using these functions. For example, when a lab or radiology department has results to report, these results are uploaded for viewing by healthcare providers on the clinical units and also posted to the health information exchange for viewing by other involved healthcare providers. At the same time these results may also be posted to the personal health record for the patient's viewing. When selecting a computer system the functions for that system are carefully identified and defined in writing. These are listed as functional specifications. Functional specifications identify each function and describe how that function will be performed.

Systems are structured in order to perform their functions. Structure follows function and is influenced by the resources available to complete these functions. Note how healthcare teams are organized. The organizational structure varies with the purpose of the organization and the functions that are being performed. The organization of a nursing staff on a clinical unit demonstrates this concept. The staff may be organized using concepts such as primary nursing, case management, or functional nursing. A clinical unit in a nursing home setting staffed mainly by aides with a limited number of professional nurses is more likely to use a functional approach while an intensive care unit (ICU) in a major medical center staffed entirely with professional nurses is more likely to use a primary care approach. In each unit the primary purpose is to provide patient care. The staff is structured to ensure that the functions necessary for nursing care are completed. The same is true with information systems in healthcare. The structure that is effective in one institution may be completely inappropriate in a second institution.

Two different models operating concurrently can be used to conceptualize healthcare technical infrastructures. These are hierarchical and web. The hierarchical model is an older architectural model and the terms, such as *mainframe*, that are used to describe the model reflect that reality. The location and type of hardware used within a system often follow a hierarchical model; however, as computer systems are becoming more integrated, information flow increasingly follows a web model. The hierarchical model can be used to structure the distribution of the computer processing loads at the same time as the web model is used to structure communication of health-related data throughout the institution. The hierarchical model is demonstrated in Figure 2-2. Each individual computer is part of a local area network (LAN). The LANs join together to form a wide area network (WAN) that is connected to the mainframe computers. In Figure 2-2 the mainframe is the lead computer or lead part. This structure demonstrates a centralized approach to managing the computer structure.

When analyzing the hierarchical model the term *system* may refer to any level of the structure. In Figure 2-2 an individual computer may be referred to as a system or the whole diagram may be considered a system. Three terms are used to indicate the level of reference. These are subsystem, target system, and supersystem. A subsystem is any system within the target system. For example, if the target system is a LAN, each computer is a subsystem. The supersystem is the overall structure in which the target system exists. If the target system is a LAN, then Figure 2-2 represents a supersystem. The second model used to analyze the structure of a system is the web model. The interrelationships between the different LANs function like a web. Laboratory data may be shared with the pharmacy and the clinical units concurrently, just as the data collected by nursing, such as weight and height, may be shared with each department needing these data. The Internet is an example of a complex system that demonstrates both hierarchical and web structures interacting as a cohesive unit. As these examples demonstrate, a system includes structural elements from both the web model and the hierarchical model. Complex systems discussed later in this chapter can include a number of supersystems organized using both hierarchical and web structures. In addition, newer technology and concepts as demonstrated by the recent introduction of cloud computing will produce additional models and complex systems in the future.

Boundary, attributes, and environment are three concepts used to characterize structure. The boundary of a system forms the demarcation between the target system and the environment of the system. Input flows into the system by moving across the boundary and output flows into the environment across this boundary. Understanding boundary concepts assists in the development of healthcare information systems. For example, one of the techniques used in developing healthcare information systems is to divide the healthcare delivery system into modules or subsystems. This helps to establish the boundaries of a project and hopefully controls scope creep. Scope creep occurs when a project expands beyond its initial boundaries and the leader begins to lose control of the project.

Figure 2-2 can be used to demonstrate how these concepts can establish the boundaries of a project. Each computer in the diagram represents a target system for a specific project. For example, a healthcare institution could be planning for a new pharmacy information system. The new pharmacy

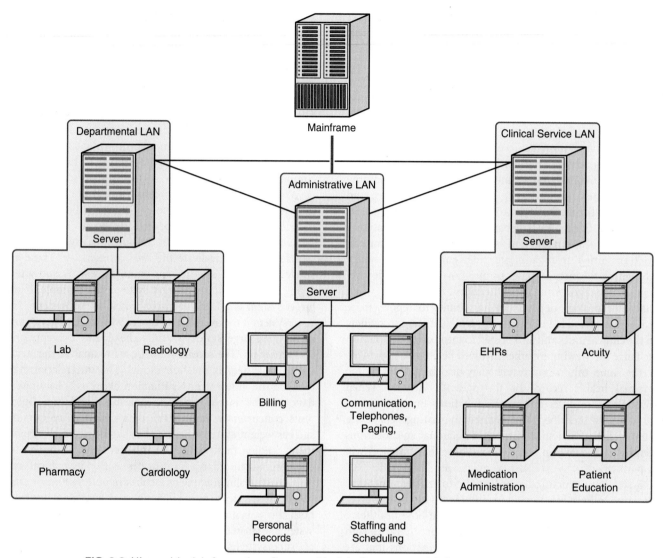

FIG 2-2 Hierarchical Information System Model. Departmental information systems; *LAN,* local area network. (Copyright Ramona Nelson. Reprinted with permission.)

system becomes the target system. However, as the model demonstrates, the pharmacy system interacts with other systems within the total system. The task group selecting the new pharmacy system will need to identify the functional specifications needed to automate the pharmacy and the functional specifications needed for the pharmacy system to interact with the other systems in the environment. Clearly, specifying the target system and the other systems in the environment that must interact or interface with the target will assist in defining the scope of the project. By defining the scope of the project it becomes possible to focus on the task at hand while planning for the integration of the pharmacy system with other systems in the institution. A key example is planning for the impact of the new pharmacy system in terms of the activities of nurses who are administering medications.

In planning for healthcare information systems, attributes of the system are identified. Attributes are the properties of the parts or components of the system. They define the specific data elements to be included in describing a system. For example, the attributes of a person include color of hair, weight, and IQ. When discussing computer hardware these attributes are usually referred to as specifications. A list of attributes or specifications can be seen in advertisements or the owner's manual for computer hardware and include such things as amount of random access memory (RAM), size of the hard drive, and even the size of the case covering the computer. Another example of a list of attributes can be seen on an intake or patient assessment form in a healthcare setting. The form lists the attributes of interest. A completed assessment form describes the individual patient's expression of these attributes.

Attributes and the expression of those attributes play a major role in the development of databases. Field names are a list of the attributes of interest for a specific system. The datum in each cell is the individual system's expression of that attribute. A record lists the attributes for each individual system. The record can also be seen as a subsystem of the total database system.

Systems and the Change Process

Both living and nonliving systems are constantly in a process of change. Six concepts are helpful in understanding the change process. These are dynamic homeostasis, equifinality, entropy, negentropy, specialization, and reverberation.

Dynamic homeostasis refers to the processes used by a system to maintain a steady state or balance. The normal fluctuations seen in body chemistry levels demonstrate dynamic homeostasis. Blood levels of the normal blood elements begin the drift down or up. Through a feedback loop the body begins to produce more of the decreasing elements and eliminate the excess elements. As the blood levels change, the feedback loop then kicks in to reverse the process. This same goal of maintaining a steady state can affect how clinical settings respond when changes are made or a new system is implemented.

Equifinality is the tendency of open systems to reach a characteristic final state from different initial conditions and in different ways. For example, two different clinics may be scheduled for the implementation of a new electronic health record. One unit may be using paper records and the other unit may have an outdated system. A year or two later both clinical units may be at the same point, comfortably using the new system. However, the process for reaching this point may have been very different.

Entropy is the tendency of all systems to break down into their simplest parts. As it breaks down the system becomes increasingly disorganized or random. In data transmission, entropy measures the loss of information when a signal is transmitted. Entropy is demonstrated in the tendency of all systems to wear out. Even with maintenance a healthcare information system will reach a point where it must be replaced. Healthcare information that is transferred across many different systems in many different formats can also demonstrate entropy, thereby causing confusion and conflict between different entities within the healthcare system.

Negentropy is the opposite of entropy. This is the tendency of living systems to grow and become more complex. This is demonstrated in the growth and development of an infant as well as in the increased size and complexity of today's healthcare system. With the increased growth and complexity of the healthcare system there has been an increase in the size and complexity of healthcare information systems. As systems grow and become more complex, they divide into subsystems and then subsubsystems. This is the process of differentiation and specialization. Note how the human body begins as a single cell and then differentiates into different body systems, each with specialized purposes, structures, and functions. This same process occurs with healthcare delivery systems as well as with healthcare information systems. As this process occurs, a lead part emerges. The lead part is at the top of the hierarchy and plays a primary role in organizing and maintaining vertical and horizontal data or information flow. Changes to the lead part can have a major impact across the total system. For example, if the chief information officer leaves an organization, the impact is much more significant than if a beginning-level systems analyst moves to another organization. If the mainframe in Figure 2-2 were to stop functioning, the impact would be much more significant than if an individual computer in one of the LANs were to stop functioning. Understanding the role of the lead part can be key in developing the backup, security, and disaster recovery plans for a healthcare information system.

Change within any part of the system will be reflected across the total system. This is referred to as reverberation. Reverberation is reflected in the intended and unintended consequences of system change. When planning for a new healthcare system, the team will attempt to identify the intended consequences or expected benefits to be achieved. While it is often impossible to identify a comprehensive list of unintended consequences, it is important for the team to consider the reality of unintended consequences. The potential for unintended consequences should be discussed during the planning stage; however, these will be more evident during the testing stage that precedes implementation or go-live. Many times unintended consequences are not considered until after go-live, when they become obvious. For example, email may be successfully introduced to improve communication in an organization. However, an unintended consequence can be the increased workload from irrelevant email messages. However, unintended consequences are not always negative. They can be either positive or negative. In the 1950s chaos theory was developed to explain the phenomena of unintended consequences.

Chaos Theory

While chaotic activity was noted by mathematicians and physicists starting in the 1880s, these observations were often considered to be the result of noise or imprecise measurement. The recognition of these observations as evidence of a new and developing theory is credited to Edward Lorenz, an American mathematician and meteorologist who made his initial discovery while using a computer simulation to predict weather patterns.[4] The computer program ran using decimals with six digits but the report writer used to print the output rounded the numbers to three digits. For example, the computer calculations might include a number such as 0.548394 or 0.548194. The printout would round both of these numbers to 0.548. Lorenz decided to take a shortcut and enter only three-digit numbers as well as start the program in the middle. He soon discovered that these minor changes created significantly different results over time. He reported these observations in the classic paper titled "Deterministic Nonperiodic Flow," published in the *Journal of the Atmospheric Sciences*. Interestingly, the word *chaos* is never used in the paper.

Chaos is defined as a physical "mathematical dynamic system which is: (a) deterministic (b) is recurrent and (c) has sensitive dependence on the initial state."[5(p164)] In turn, chaos theory can be defined as "the qualitative study of unstable aperiodic behavior in deterministic, nonlinear dynamical systems."[6(p2)] Chaotic systems embody several common characteristics.

First, chaotic systems are dynamic systems. In other words, while chaotic systems vary in their state of stability, they are in a constant state of change. The change is nonlinear. In a linear system the output is consistently proportional to the input. Increase the input and the output increases at the same rate. In a nonlinear system the output of the system is not proportional to the input. The reiterative feedback loop that exist within these systems have a major effect on how inputs will affect outputs. A minor change in input can create a major change in output. On the other hand, a major change in input can result in minor changes in output. This has been described as the butterfly effect. A butterfly flapping its wings in California over time can become a hurricane in New York. If the butterfly had been in a slightly different position or if any other input had been changed slightly, the hurricane may never have happened.

Second, while the output or behavior of a chaotic system will appear unstable, aperiodic, and even random, these systems are deterministic. Their output is determined by the initial input, reiterative feedback loops, and the dynamic changes that occur over time. "Although it looks disorganized like random behavior, it is deterministic like periodic behavior. However, the smallest difference in any system variable can make a very large difference to the future state of the system."[7(p15)] Over time fractal type patterns begin to emerge from these outputs. Fractals are repeating nonregular geometric shapes such as snowflakes, trees, or seashells. Thus out of chaos comes order.[8]

In itself chaos theory would have limited applicability to the issues of concern to health informatics; however, complexity theory, which is very applicable to these same issues, is based on chaos theory. Both chaos and complexity theory involve the study of dynamic nonlinear systems that change with time and demonstrate complex relationships between inputs and outputs due to reiterative feedback loops. "The quantitative study of these systems is chaos theory. Complexity theory is the qualitative aspect drawing upon insights and metaphors that are derived from chaos theory."[7(p14)]

Complexity Theory

As human beings we constantly work to understand and manage the world in which we live. The idea that a theory exists to describe, explain, and predict events and maybe even control outcomes in a complex organization such as a healthcare system is very seductive. But such a theory may not yet exist. Note the conflict evident in the following two conclusions. In 2005 Lela Holden published a concept analysis of complex adaptive systems. She concluded the abstract by stating: "Complexity science builds on the rich tradition in nursing that views patients and nursing care from a systems

BOX 2-1	QUESTIONING THE USE OF COMPLEXITY THEORY IN PUBLISHED LITERATURE

It is my contention that much of the work in complexity theory has indeed been pseudo-science, that is, many writers in this field have used the symbols and methods of complexity science (either erroneously or deliberately) to give the illusion of science even though they lack supporting evidence. . . . This proliferation of pseudo-science has, in turn, obscured the meaning and agenda of the science of complexity.

Phelan S. What is complexity science, really? *Emergence.* 2001;3(1):120.

There have been numerous references to complexity theory and complex systems in the recent healthcare literature, including nursing. However, exaggerated claims have (in my view) been made about how they can be applied to health service delivery, and there is a widespread tendency to misunderstand some of the concepts associated with complexity thinking (usually justified by describing the misconception as a metaphor). . . . In this paper I first outline some of the key ideas in the theory of complex adaptive systems, and then suggest that they have been distorted by a series of influential articles in the medical literature.

Paley J. Complex adaptive systems and nursing. *Nurs Inq.* 2007;14:233.

perspective."[9(p651)] In contrast Steven Phelan concluded his article with the following:

Complexity science is not:
- *General systems theory*
- *A postmodern science*
- *A set of metaphors or analogies based on resemblance thinking.*[10(p132)]

Additional evidence of this same issue is demonstrated in Box 2-1. The conflict between these experts demonstrates a lack of agreement within the professions concerning the abstract and operational definitions of concepts included in complexity theory. This suggests that complexity science is an area of study but not yet a theory. If the concepts within the theory cannot be defined consistently, a theory cannot be developed. However, some general ideas or principles from the study of complexity science are useful in understanding issues within informatics:
- Complex organizations adapt to their environment. They may or may not be successful but changes in the environment will produce changes in the organization. The larger and more diffuse the organization, the more likely it is to survive in some form. For example, individual hospitals, clinics, and third-party payers may go out of business but the healthcare system as a societal institution will continue to exist in ever-evolving ways.
- Complex systems are made up of self-organizing units. When a system adapts to change, the specific adaptations occur within the different parts or units of the overall system and are not dictated by a central source. A workaround is an example of this type of adaptive behavior.

- The adaptive response of a complex system to environmental change includes an element of unpredictability. The overall pattern of adaptation that emerges from the adaptive changes within each unit is unique to each organization and impossible to predict completely. For example, computerized provider order entry (CPOE) has changed the workflow for unit secretaries, nurses, physicians, hospital departments, etc. Each of these units within the system is creating adaptations at the same time as it is adjusting to changes occurring in the other units. A significant number of these changes (whether they were seen as positive or negative by individuals in the institution) are experienced as unintended consequences.

- The change process within complex systems is nonlinear. For example, a small inexpensive change on a computer screen may make that screen easier to understand and in turn prevent a number of very dangerous mistakes. On the other hand, a major implementation of a healthcare information system may be very expensive but not successful.

- The adaptive process within complex organizations demonstrates infinitely complex unique patterns. For example, the go-live process within or across complex organizations follows a similar but unique process each time a new system is installed, even when the same software is installed in a new site.

All systems, whether they are complex or simple, change and in the process interact with the environment. The basic framework of this interaction is shown in Figure 2-1. Input to the system consists of information, matter, and energy. These inputs are then processed and result in outputs. Understanding this process as it applies to informatics involves an understanding of information theory.

Information Theory

The term *information* has several different meanings. An example of this can be seen in Box 2-2, taken from *Merriam-Webster's Collegiate Dictionary*.[11] Just as the term *information* has more than one meaning, information theory refers to more than one theory.[12] In this chapter two theoretical models of information theory are examined: the Shannon-Weaver information-communication model and the Nelson data-information-knowledge-wisdom model that evolved from Blum's and Graves' initial work.

Shannon-Weaver Information-Communication Model

Information theory was formally established in 1948 with the publication of the landmark paper "The Mathematical Theory of Communication" by Claude Shannon.[13] The concepts in this model are presented in Figure 2-3. The sender is the originator of the message or the information source. The transmitter is the encoder that converts the content of the message to a code. The code can be letters, words, music, symbols, or a computer code. For example, the modem used with a computer acts as an encoder when it converts a file from a digital form to a form that can be sent over cable or phone lines. The telephone or cable line is the channel, or the medium used to carry the message. Examples of channels include sound waves, telephone lines, and paper. Each channel has its own physical limitations in terms of the size of the message that can be carried. Noise is anything that is not part of the message but that occupies space on the channel and is transmitted with the message. Examples of noise

---

BOX 2-2   DEFINITION OF INFORMATION

1: the communication or reception of knowledge or intelligence

2 a (1): knowledge obtained from investigation, study, or instruction (2): INTELLIGENCE, NEWS (3): FACTS, DATA

  b: the attribute inherent in and communicated by one of two or more alternative sequences or arrangements of something (as nucleotides in DNA or binary digits in a computer program) that produce specific effects

  c (1): a signal or character (as in a communication system or computer) representing data (2): something (as a message, experimental data, or a picture) which justifies change in a construct (as a plan or theory) that represents physical or mental experience or another construct

  d: a quantitative measure of the content of information; specifically: a numerical quantity that measures the uncertainty in the outcome of an experiment to be performed

3: the act of informing against a person

4: a formal accusation of a crime made by a prosecuting officer as distinguished from an indictment presented by a grand jury

Information. *Merriam-Webster's Collegiate Dictionary.* http://www.merriam-webster.com/dictionary/information. 2012.

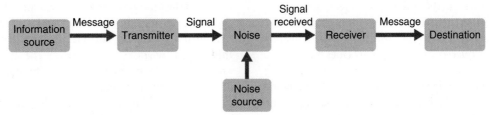

FIG 2-3 Schematic diagram of a general communication system. (Reprinted with corrections from Shannon C, Weaver W. The mathematical theory of communication. *Bell Syst Tech J.* 1948;27:379-423, 623-656. http://cm.bell-labs.com/cm/ms/what/shannonday/shannon1948.pdf. Reprinted with permission of Alcatel-Lucent USA Inc.)

include static on a telephone line and background sounds in a room. The decoder converts the message to a format that can be understood by the receiver. When listening to a phone call the telephone is a decoder. It converts the analog signal back into sound waves that are understood as words by the person listening. The person listening to the words is the destination.

Shannon, one of the authors of the Shannon-Weaver information-communication theory, was a telephone engineer. He was not concerned with the semantic meaning of the message but rather with the technical problems involved in signal transmission across a communication channel or telephone line. He used the concept of entropy to explain and measure the amount of information in a message. The amount of information in a message is measured by the extent to which the message decreases entropy. The unit of measurement is a bit. A bit is represented by a 0 (zero) or a 1 (one). The two sides of a coin can be used to explain this concept. If a coin is thrown into the air, it may land on either of two possible sides: heads up or tails up. This can be coded as 1 for heads up and 0 for tails up. Using this approach the message concerning which side is up can be transmitted with one bit. If there were four possible states, additional bits would be needed to transmit the message. For example, if the message is north, south, east, or west it could be coded as 00 for north, 11 for south, 01 for east, and 10 for west. Computer codes are built on this concept. For example, how many bits are needed to code the letters of the alphabet? What other symbols are used in communication and must be included when developing a code?

Warren Weaver, from the Sloan-Kettering Institute for Cancer Research, provided the interpretation for understanding the semantic meaning of a message.[13] He used Shannon's work to explain the interpersonal aspects of communication. For example, if the speaker is a physician who uses medical terms that are not known to the receiver (the patient), there is a communication problem caused by the method used to code the message. However, if the patient cannot hear well, he may not hear all of the words in the message. In this case the communication problem is caused by the patient's ear, which converts the sound waves into neurological impulses that the brain can decode.

The communication-information model provides an excellent framework for analyzing the effectiveness and efficiency of information transfer and communication. For example, a physician may use a computerized order entry system to enter orders. Is the order entry screen designed to capture and code all of the key elements for each order? Are all aspects of the message coded in a way that can be transmitted and decoded by the receiving computer? Does the message that is received by the receiving department include all of the key elements in the message sent? Does the screen designed at the receiver's end make it possible for the message to be decoded or understood by the receiver?

These questions demonstrate three levels of communication that can be used in analyzing communication problems.[14] The first level of communication is the technical level.

Do the system hardware and software function effectively and efficiently? The second level of communication is the semantic level. Does the message convey meaning? Does the receiver understand the message that was sent by the sender? The third level of communication is the effectiveness level. Does the message produce the intended result at the receiver's end? For example, did the provider order one medication but the patient received a different medication with a similar spelling? Some of these questions require a more in-depth look at how healthcare information is produced and used. Bruce Blum's definition of information provides a framework for this more in-depth analysis.

Blum Model

Bruce L. Blum developed his definition of information from an analysis of the accomplishments in medical computing.[15] In his analysis he identified three types of healthcare computing applications. Blum grouped applications according to the objects they processed. The three types of objects he identified are data, information, and knowledge. Blum defined data as uninterpreted elements such as a person's name, weight, or age. Information was defined as a collection of data that have been processed and then displayed as information such as weight over time. Knowledge results when data and information are identified and the relationships between the data and information are formalized. A knowledge base is more than the sum of the data and information pieces in that knowledge base. A knowledge base includes the interrelationships between the data and information within the knowledge base. A textbook can be seen as containing knowledge.[15] These concepts are well accepted across information science and are not limited to healthcare and health informatics.[16]

Graves Model

Judy Graves and Sheila Corcoran, in their classic article "The Study of Nursing Informatics," used the Blum concepts of data, information, and knowledge to explain the study of nursing informatics.[17] They incorporated Barbara A. Carper's four types of knowledge: empirical, ethical, personal, and aesthetic. Each of these represents a way of knowing and a structure for organizing knowledge. This article is considered the foundation for most definitions of nursing informatics.

Nelson Model

In 1989 Nelson extended the Blum and Graves and Corcoran data-to-knowledge continuum by including wisdom.[18] This initial publication provided only brief definitions of the concepts but later publications included a model.[19] Figure 2-4 demonstrates the most current version of this model. Within this model, wisdom is defined as the appropriate use of knowledge in managing or solving human problems. It is knowing when and how to use knowledge in managing patient needs or problems. Effectively using wisdom in managing a patient problem requires a combination of values, experience, and knowledge. The concepts of data, information, knowledge, and wisdom overlap and interrelate as demonstrated by the overlapping circles and arrows in the model.

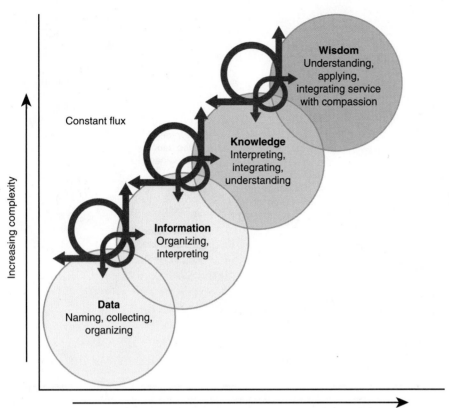

FIG 2-4 Revised Nelson data-to-wisdom continuum. (Copyright Ramona Nelson. Reprinted with permission.)

Of note, what is information in one context may be data in another. For example, a nursing student may view the liver function tests within the blood work results reported this morning and see only data or a group of numbers related to some strange-looking tests. However, the staff nurse looking at the same results will see the information and in turn see the implications for the patient's plan of care. The greater the knowledge base used to interpret data, the more information disclosed from that data and in turn the more data points that may be generated. Data processed to become information can create new data items. For example, if one collects the blood sugar levels for a diabetic patient over time, patterns begin to emerge. These patterns become new data items to be interpreted. One nurse may notice and describe the pattern but a nurse with more knowledge related to diabetes may identify a Somogyi-type pattern with important implications for the patient's treatment protocols. The concept of constant flux is illustrated by the curved arrows moving between the concepts. As one moves up the continuum there are increasing interactions and interrelationships within and between the circles, producing increased complexity of the elements within each circle. Therefore the concept of wisdom is much more complex than the concept of data.

The introduction of the concept of wisdom gained professional acceptance in 2008 when the American Nurses Association included this concept and the related model in *Nursing Informatics: Scope and Standards of Practice.*[20] In this document the model is used to frame the scope of practice for

nursing informatics. This change meant that the scope of practice for nursing informatics was no longer fully defined by the functionality of a computer and the types of applications processed by a computer. Rather the scope of practice is now defined by the goals of nursing and nurse–computer interactions in achieving these goals.

Using the concepts of data, information, knowledge, and wisdom makes it possible to classify the different levels of computing or automated systems. An information system such as a pharmacy information system takes in data and information, processes the data and information, and outputs information. A computerized decision support system uses knowledge and a set of rules for using that knowledge to interpret data and information and output suggested or actual recommendations. A healthcare application may recommend additional diagnostic tests based on a pattern of abnormal test results, such as increasing creatinine levels. With a decision support system the user decides whether the suggestion or recommendations will be implemented. A decision support system relies on the knowledge and wisdom of the user.

An electronic expert system goes one step further. An expert system implements the decision that has been programmed into the computer system without the intervention of the user. For example, an automated system that monitors a patient's overall status and then uses a set of predetermined parameters to trigger and implement the decision to call a code is an expert system. In this example, the data were

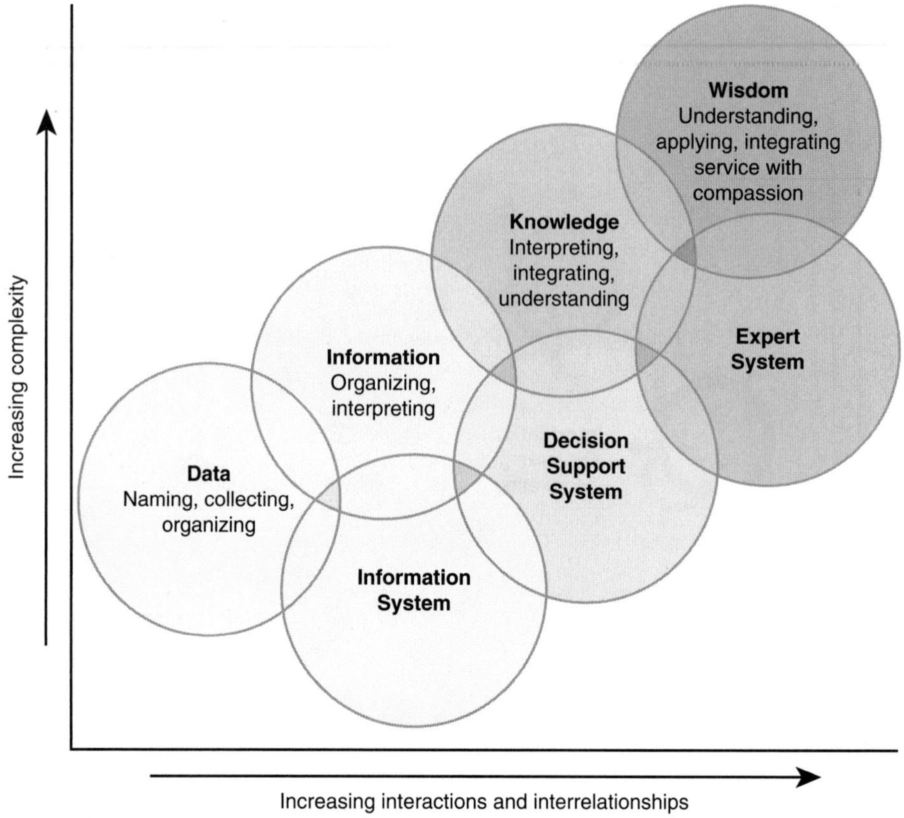

FIG 2-5 Moving from data to expert systems. (Modified from Englebardt S and Nelson R. *Health Care Informatics: An Interdisciplinary Approach.* St. Louis, MO: Mosby; 2002. Modified figure designed by Ramona Nelson and printed here with her permission.)

BOX 2-3   ATTRIBUTES OF DATA, INFORMATION, AND KNOWLEDGE

Data
   Descriptive—qualitative
   Measurable—quantitative

Information
Quality
   Accurate
   Coherent
   Comprehensive or complete
   Objective or free from bias
   Verifiable

Usable
   Appropriate or relevant
   Economical
   Clear or understandable

Format
   Quantifiable
   Precise
   Organized for specific use

Available
   Accessible
   Secure
   Timely or current

Knowledge
   Accurate
   Relevant
   Type

---

converted to information, a knowledge base was used to interpret that information, and the decision to implement an action based on this process has been automated. The relationships among the concepts of data, information, knowledge, and wisdom, as well as information, decision support, and expert computer systems, are demonstrated in Figure 2-5.

In the model the three types of electronic systems overlap, reflecting how such systems are used in actual practice. For example, an electronic system recommending that a medication order be changed to decrease costs might be consistently implemented with no further thought by the provider entering the orders. In this example, an application designed as a decision support system is being used as an expert system. Because there are limits to the amount of data and information the human mind can remember and process, each practitioner walks a tightrope between depending on the computer to assist in the management of a situation with a high cognitive load and delegating the decision to the computer application. This reality presents interesting and important practical and research questions concerning the effective and appropriate use of automated decision support systems in the provision of healthcare.

Effective computerized systems are dependent on the quality of data, information, and knowledge processed. Box 2-3 lists the attributes of data, information, and knowledge. These attributes provide a framework for developing evaluation forms that measure the quality of data, information, and knowledge. For example, healthcare data are presented as text, numbers, or a combination of text and numbers. Good-quality health data provide a complete description of the item being presented with accurate measurements.

Using these attributes, an evaluation form can be developed for judging the quality (including completeness) of a completed patient assessment form or for judging the quality of a healthcare website. The same process can be used with the attributes of knowledge. Think about the books or online references one might access in developing a treatment plan for a patient or consider a knowledge base that is built into a decision support system. What would result if the knowledge was incomplete or inaccurate or did not apply to the patient's specific problem, or if suggested approaches were out of date and no longer considered effective in treating the patient's problem? What if the knowledge was not presented in the appropriate format for use?

While this section has focused on computer systems, humans are also open systems that take in data, information, knowledge, and wisdom. Learning theory provides a framework for understanding how patients and healthcare providers as open learning systems take in, process, and output data, information, knowledge, and wisdom.

Learning Theory

Learning theory attempts to determine how people learn and to identify the factors that influence that process. Learning has been defined in a variety of ways, but for the purpose of this text learning is defined as an increase in knowledge, a change in attitude or values, or the development of new skills. Several different learning theories have been developed. Each theory reflects a different paradigm and approach to understanding and explaining the learning process. One example demonstrating the wide range of learning theories is the database of learning theories maintained by InstructionalDesign.org located at www.instructionaldesign.org/theories/index.html. This active site, initially developed by Greg Kearsley, includes summaries of more than 50 major theories of learning and instruction and continues to grow.[21]

Learning theories are not mutually exclusive. They often overlap and interrelate. However, this collection of learning theories cannot be used to create a comprehensive theory of the learning process. With these limitations in mind, this chapter focuses on four types of learning theories that demonstrate the major approaches to learning theory. These are cognitive or information processing theories, adult learning theories, constructionist theories, and learning styles.

Learning theories are important to the practice of health informatics for a variety of reasons. Health informatics specialists plan and implement educational programs to teach healthcare providers to use new and updated applications and systems. A well-designed and well-implemented educational program can result in competent healthcare providers when it is able to satisfy all learning styles. Understanding how people learn is especially helpful in designing computer screens and developing computer-related procedures that are safe and effective for healthcare providers. These theories are also helpful in understanding and building decision support systems that provide effective and appropriate support for healthcare providers who deal with a multitude of complex problems. Selected learning theories are presented in this chapter. Specific learning theories as they relate to specific topics are presented in other chapters.

Cognitive and Constructionist Learning Theories

Learning theories that are included under the heading of information processing theories divide learning into four steps, as follows:

1. How the learner takes input into the system
2. How that input is processed and constructed
3. What type of learned behaviors are exhibited as output
4. How feedback to the system is used to change or correct behavior

Data are taken into the system through the senses. First, if there is a sensory organ defect, data may be distorted or excluded. Second, data are moving across the semipermeable boundary of the system. There are limits to how much data can enter at one time. For example, if one is listening to a person who is talking too fast, some of the words will be missed. In addition, the learner will screen out data that are considered irrelevant or meaningless, such as background noise. Data limits are increased if the learner is under stress. Individuals who are anxious about learning to use a computer program will experience higher data limits and thereby less learning.

If new information is presented using several senses simultaneously, it is more likely to be taken in. For example, if a new concept is presented using slides that are explained by a speaker, the combination of both verbal and visual input makes it more likely that the learner will grasp the concept. As data enter the system the learner structures and interprets these data, producing meaningful information. Previous learning has a major effect on how the data are structured and interpreted. For example, if a healthcare provider is already comfortable using Windows and is now learning a new software program based on Windows, he or she will be able to structure and interpret the new information quickly using previously developed cognitive structures. This is one reason why consistency in screen development can be very important for patient safety. In contrast, if the new information cannot be related to previous learning, the learner will need to build interpreting structures as he or she takes in the new information. For example, if a person is reading new information, she may stop at the end of each sentence and think about the content in that sentence. She is building interpretive cognitive structures as they import the data. If this same learner is hearing the new information at the same time she is taking notes, she may have difficulty capturing the content she is trying to record. The more time that is needed to interpret and structure data, the slower the learner will be able to import data. Assessment of the learner's previous knowledge can help the instructor to identify these potential problems. Relating new information to previously learned information will help the learner to develop interpreting structures and in turn learn the information more effectively. Describing learning as a process of building interpretive cognitive structures while learning new content is consistent with constructionist theory explained below. By combining what is known with the new information the learner goes beyond the information that was provided in the learning experience. Using organizing structures such as outlines, providing examples, and explaining how new information relates to previously learned concepts encourages the learner to develop chunks and increases retention. An "aha moment" is the sudden understanding that occurs when the new information fits with previous learning and the student gains a new insight on the discussion.

Social constructivism focuses on how group interaction can be used to build new knowledge.[22] Group discussion in which learners share their perceptions and understanding through peer learning encourages new insight as well as retention of the newly constructed knowledge. There is limited research on how groups such as interprofessional health teams actually learn via the group construction process. Two studies at Massachusetts Institute of Technology (MIT) and Carnegie Mellon University (CMU) found converging evidence that groups participating in problem-solving activities demonstrate a general collective intelligence factor that explains a group's performance on a wide variety of tasks. "This 'c factor' is not strongly correlated with the average or maximum individual intelligence of group members but instead with the average social sensitivity of group members, the equality in distribution of conversational turn-taking and the proportion of females in the group."[23(p686)] Certain characteristics of the individuals within the group and the group's ability to work together as a whole can influence the effectiveness of the group. "A group's interactions drive its intelligence more than the brain power of individual members."[24] But practical approaches to assessing and measuring the learning within a group are for the most part an unexplored area. For example, few educators are prepared to give group tests and to measure learning based on these tests.

Information once taken into the system is retained in several different formats. The three most common formats are episodic order, hierarchical order, and linked. For example, life events are often retained in episodic order. A list of computer commands is also retained in episodic order. Psychomotor commands learned episodically can become automatic. An example of this can be seen in the simple behavior of typing or the more complex behavior of driving a car. Cognitive learning tends to be retained in hierarchical order. For example, penicillin is an antibiotic. An antibiotic is a drug. Finally, information is retained because it is linked or related to other information. For example, the concept "paper" is related to a printer. The process by which information is retained in long-term memory (LTM) can be reinforced by a variety of teaching techniques. Providing the student with an outline when presenting cognitive information helps to reinforce the learner retaining the information in hierarchical order. Telling stories or jokes can be used to reinforce links between concepts. Practice exercises that encourage repeated use of specific keystroke sequences or computer commands assist with long-term retention of psychomotor episodic learning.

While LTM can retain large amounts of information, two processes can interfere with the storage of information in

TABLE 2-1	PLANNING FOR LONG-TERM RETENTION OF NEW INFORMATION
PRINCIPLE	**EXAMPLE**
Distribute the learning over time	Online learning should be designed so that the content is divided into logical units, with learners encouraged to spread the learning over a period of time, and not all of the content is available from the beginning.
Plan to retain the information	Before teaching new content, explain to the learners why the information will be important to their performance and when they will need to recall the new information.
Review the materials	When presenting a list of new ideas, stop after each idea is explained and list each of the ideas that have already been explained. Include practice sessions or self-assessment tools that reinforce the learning.
Increase the time spent on the task	This does not mean increasing the time scheduled for class but increasing the amount of time the learner is actively working on the content to be learned with readings before class or exercises after class.

LTM. First, new information or learning may replace old information. For example, healthcare providers may become very proficient with an automated order-entry system. However, over time they may forget how to use the manual system to place orders. This can be a problem if the manual system is the backup plan for computer downtime. Second, previously learned information can interfere with the learning of new information. This can be seen when a new computer system is installed and new procedures are implemented. Experienced users of the old system must remember *not* to use the old procedures that were part of that system. This can be especially difficult if the previous learning has become automatic psychomotor commands. If the instructor for the new system includes clues to remind the experienced users of the change, the process of replacing old learning with new information can be reinforced.

When planning educational programs for healthcare users, the health informatics specialist must first plan for intake of the new information via short-term memory (STM) and then for transfer of the new information to LTM. Several factors assist in moving information from STM to LTM. A list of these factors and examples of each can be seen in Table 2-1. Information that is stored in LTM is used in critical thinking, problem solving, decision making, and a number of other mental processes.

Learned behaviors are exhibited as output. Three types of output or behaviors are usually considered: cognitive, affective, and psychomotor. Cognitive behaviors reflect intellectual skills. They include critical thinking, problem solving, decision making, and a number of other mental processes. These are the skills used when designing a protocol for a user of an automated healthcare information system or for troubleshooting a computer system that is not functioning correctly.

Affective skills relate to values and attitudes. Planning for the learning of appropriate values and attitudes is often overlooked and yet these can have a major impact on the implementation of an automated healthcare information system. Computerizing healthcare delivery requires change. This change can be stressful for healthcare providers. Training programs may focus exclusively on how to use the system without time to discuss how to integrate the new system into patient care. There may be limited discussion of the benefits of change and little support for the development of positive attitudes toward a new system. Development of positive values and attitudes can also be important to the ongoing maintenance of automated systems in healthcare.[19] A negative attitude toward a system encourages users to develop workarounds and shortcuts. Positive attitudes encourage users to suggest new and innovative uses for computer systems.

Psychomotor skills involve the integration of cognitive and motor skills. These types of skills require time and practice to develop. During the time period when these skills are being developed, productivity is often decreased and users can be frustrated. When new healthcare information systems are implemented, the institution is interested in measuring the impact of the new system. However, while new users are in the process of developing the psychomotor skills that are part of using the new system, it is ineffective to measure either the impact of a new system or user satisfaction. During this period the focus should be on supporting the users' adjustment, tracking, and troubleshooting problems. Any decision to make significant changes to a new system based on user feedback must be evaluated carefully.

Adult Learning Theories

In 1970 Knowles coined and defined the term *andragogy*.[25] Andragogy is the art and science of helping adults to learn. Knowles's model proposed that adults share a number of similar learning characteristics and that these characteristics can be used in planning adult educational programs. Table 2-2 lists a number of these characteristics and provides examples of how they can be used to plan for teaching adult users.[22,26-28]

Learning Styles

All learners are not alike. They learn in different ways. They vary in how they take in and process information. There are preferential differences in seeing and hearing new information. Some learners process information by reflecting while others process it by acting. Some learners approach reasoning logically while others are intuitive. Some learners learn by analyzing while others learn by visualizing. Learning theories concerning learning styles attempt to explain these differences. Experiential learning theory is one example.[29] The

TABLE 2-2	ADULT LEARNING CHARACTERISTICS AND RELATED APPLICATIONS
LEARNING CHARACTERISTICS	**APPLICATION**
Adults are self-directed.	If they do not see the relevance of new information, learners will not focus on remembering that information. Explain in practical terms when and how the new information will be used.
Adults have accumulated a number of life experiences and cognitive structures. These are used to interpret new learning.	When teaching a new system ask the learners to provide examples from their experience and use these examples to correct misconceptions as well as to reinforce how the new system will function.
Adults are practical and look for immediate application of learning.	Orientation to a new system should occur no more than 4 weeks before actual implementation.
Adults are more interested in learning how to solve problems than in retaining facts.	When teaching adults about computer applications use real-life examples and scripts that can be expected to occur on the clinical unit.
Adult learners expect to be treated with respect and have their previous learning acknowledged.	When explaining a new system ask the learners what they already know about the new system. Listen to their comments and concerns about the screen design and how it will or will not support safe practice.

first stage of Kolb's theory involves concrete experience. For example, the learner may view a demonstration of a new healthcare information system.

As the learner begins to understand how the system works, he begins to think about how the system would work in his healthcare setting. This is the second stage, or reflection. In this stage the learner reflects or thinks about the concrete experience. As the learner continues to think he begins to form abstract conceptualizations of how the system functions. This is the third stage. Finally, the learner is ready to try using the system. This is the fourth stage, when the learner uses his abstract conceptualization to guide action. In Kolb's model these four stages exist on two intersecting continuums. These are Concrete Experience ←→ Abstract Conceptualization (CE-AC) and Reflective Observation ←→ Active Experimentation (RO-AE). There are individual differences in how learners use each of these four stages in their individual learning approaches, but all learners ultimately learn by doing.

<table>
<tr><td>

BOX 2-4   **THEORY-BASED LEARNING PRINCIPLES**

- Each learner is an individual with his or her own approach to learning.
- Making new information meaningful to the individual learner supports retention.
- Only so much input or new information can be handled at one time.
- Scheduling learning over time and ensuring adequate time on task improves learning.
- Active engagement and participation in the learning task supports long-term retention.
- Conceptual learning is enhanced with concrete realistic examples.
- Learning is enhanced when the teaching method includes the cognitive, affective, and psychomotor domains in concert.
- Learning takes place intentionally and unintentionally.
- Learning is contagious. A core of knowledgeable users creates a learning environment.

</td></tr>
</table>

Using this model, Kolb developed a learning assessment tool to identify individual learning styles. The intersection of the two continuums forms four quadrants: Diverger, Assimilator, Converger, and Accommodator. In this model there are these four individual learning styles. The learner plots a score along the Concrete Experience/Abstract Conceptualization (CE-AC) scale and along the Reflective Observation/Active Experimentation (RO-AE) scale to identify which quadrant reflects his or her learning style.

A second, more widely used measure of individual learning styles is the Myers-Briggs Type Indicator.[30] This theory uses four continuums: Thinking ←→ Feeling, Sensing ←→ Intuition, Extroverted ←→ Introverted, and Judging ←→ Perceptive. A series of questions is used to determine where the learner falls on each of the four continuums. For example, a learner may be Thinking, Sensing, Extroverted, and Judging (TSEJ). The combination of where the learner falls on each of the four continuums is then used to form a composite picture of the learner's individual learning style.

A health informatics specialist plans and implements educational programs for a variety of groups within the healthcare delivery system. These may include physicians, nurses, unlicensed personnel, administrators, and others. These groups vary widely in learning ability, education, motivation, and experience. However, a great deal of variation exists among the learners within each group. Learning styles help to explain these differences and are helpful in planning instructional strategies that are effective for individual learners within a group. Each of the four types of learning theories discussed in this chapter provides insights into effective approaches to teaching. Box 2-4 lists examples of principles that can be derived from these theories.

Change Theory

Each of the theories presented in this chapter includes an element of change. Change theory is the study of change in individuals or social systems such as organizations. Understanding change theory provides a framework for effectively planning and implementing change in social systems and organizations. Healthcare information systems have a major impact on the structure and functions of healthcare delivery systems. They bring about significant change. The approach to managing the change process may result in a more effective and efficient healthcare delivery system or it may result in increased dissatisfaction and disruption. Health informatics specialists play a major role in planning for, guiding, and directing these changes.

The change process can be analyzed from two perspectives. The first perspective is demonstrated by Kurt Lewin's theory, which focuses on how a change agent can guide the change process. This is referred to as planned change. The second perspective focuses on the process by which people and social systems make changes. Research in this area has demonstrated that people in various cultures follow a similar pattern when incorporating innovation and change. Both of these perspectives provide a framework for understanding how people react to change and for guiding the change process.

Planned Change

Kurt Lewin is frequently recognized as the father of change theory.[31] His theory of planned change divides change into three stages: unfreezing, moving, and refreezing.[32] As demonstrated in the discussion of homeostasis, systems expend energy to stay in a steady state of stability. A system will remain stable when the restraining forces preventing change are stronger than the driving forces for change. Initiating change begins by increasing the driving forces and limiting the restraining forces, thereby increasing the instability of the system. This is the unfreezing stage. The first stage in the life cycle of an information system involves evaluating the current system and deciding what changes, if any, need to be made. The pros and cons for change reflect the driving and restraining forces for change. If changes are to be made, the restraining forces that maintain a stable system and resist change must be limited. At the same time the driving forces that encourage change must be increased. For example, pointing out to users the limitations and weaknesses with the current information management system increases the driving force for change. Asking for user input early in the process before decisions have been made decreases the restraining forces. Once a decision is made to initiate change the second stage, moving, begins.

The moving stage involves the implementation of the planned change. By definition this is an unstable period for the social system. Anxiety levels can be expected to increase. The social system attempts to minimize the impact or degree of change. This resistance to change may occur as missed meetings, failure to attend training classes, and failure to provide staff with information about the new system. If the resistance continues, it can cause the planned change to fail. Health informatics specialists as change agents must anticipate and minimize these resistive efforts. This can be as simple as providing food at meetings to a planned program of recognition for early adopters. For example, an article in the institution's newsletter describing and praising the pilot units for their leadership will encourage the driving forces for change.

Once the system is in place or the change has been implemented, additional energy is needed to maintain the change. This is the refreezing stage and it occurs during the maintenance phase of the information system life cycle. If managed effectively by the change agent, this phase is characterized by increased stability. In this stage the new system is in place and forces resistant to change are encouraged. Examples include training programs for new employees, a yearly review of all policies and procedures related to the new system, and continued recognition for those who become experts with the new system.

In today's healthcare environment it is not unusual to have several new information applications being implemented at the same time. Not all of these implementations will affect everyone to the same degree. Different individuals and clinical units can be at different stages of change with different implementations. Taken together, the overall scope of change will create a sense of anxiety or excitement throughout the organization. It is important for informatics specialists to monitor the amount of change and the resulting tension in placing and planning for ongoing implementations.

The informaticist may find helpful newer change models that have been built on Lewin's premises. For example, Conner's book *Managing at the Speed of Change* outlines key concepts to facilitate change in complex organizations:

- Create a burning platform for change (the burning need for change)
- Identify key stakeholders and clearly define their roles in the change
- Hold managers responsible and accountable for specific elements of change
- Assess organizational culture, capacity, resistance, and responsiveness to create an effective plan for change[33]

Diffusion of Innovation

The diffusion of innovation theory, developed by Everett Rogers, explains how individuals and communities respond to new ideas, practices, or objects.[34-36] Diffusion of innovation is the process by which an innovation is communicated through certain channels over time among members of a social system. Innovations may be either accepted or rejected. Healthcare automation, with new ideas and technology, involves ongoing diffusion of innovation. By understanding the diffusion of innovation process and the factors that influence this process, health informatics specialists can assist individuals and organizations in maximizing the benefits of automation.

Social systems consist of individuals within organizations. Both the individuals and the organization as a whole vary in how they respond to innovations. Based on their responses, individuals can be classified into five groups—innovators, early adopters, early majority, late majority, and laggards —with the number of individuals in each group following a

normal distribution. Innovators are the first 2.5% of individuals within a system to adapt to an innovation. These individuals tend to be more cosmopolitan. They are comfortable with uncertainty and above average in their understanding of complex technical concepts. These are the individuals who test out a new technology; however, they are too far ahead of the social group to be seen as leaders by other members of the social system. Some of their ideas become useful over time while others are just passing fads. As a result they are not usually able to sell others on trying new technology. This is the role of the early adopters.

Early adopters are the next 13.5 percent of individuals in the organization. They are perceived by others as discreet in their adoption of new ideas and therefore serve as role models for others. Because of their leadership role within the organization, the support of early adopters is key when introducing new approaches to automation. If the early adopters accept an innovation, the early majority are more likely to follow their example. The early majority are the next 34% of individuals in an organization. Members of the early majority are willing to adapt to innovation but not to lead. However, acceptance by the early majority means that the innovation is becoming well integrated in the organization. This is sometimes referred to as the tipping point.

The late majority is the next group to accept an innovation. The late majority makes up 34% of the individuals within the organization. Most of the uncertainty that is inherent in a new idea must be removed before this group will adapt to an innovation. They adopt the innovation not because of their interest in the innovation but rather as a result of peer pressure.

The late majority is followed by the last 16 percent of individuals in the organization. These are the laggards. Laggards focus on the local environment and on the past. They are resistant to change and will change only when there is no other alternative. They are suspicious of change and change agents. Change agents should not spend time encouraging laggards to change but rather should work at establishing policies and procedures that incorporate the innovation into the required operation of the organization.

Just as individuals vary in their response to innovation, organizations also vary. There are five internal organizational characteristics that can be used to understand how an organization will respond to an innovation.[37]

- *Centralization:* Organizations that are highly centralized with power concentrated in the hands of a few individuals tend to be less accepting of new ideas and therefore less innovative.
- *Complexity:* Organizations in which many of the individuals have a high level of knowledge and expertise tend to be more accepting of innovation. However, these types of organizations can have difficulty reaching a consensus on approaches to implementation.
- *Formalization:* Organizations that place a great deal of emphasis on rules and procedures tend to inhibit new ideas and innovation. However, once a decision has been made to move ahead this tendency toward rules

and procedures does make it easier to implement an innovation.

- *Interconnectedness:* Organizations in which there are strong interpersonal networks linking the individuals within the organization are better prepared to communicate and share innovation. This can be seen, for example, in organizations in which Web 2.0 tools are an integral part of organizational communication.
- *Organizational slack:* Organizations with uncommitted resources are better prepared to manage innovation. These resources may be people and/or money. With the current emphasis on cost control, healthcare institutions have less and less organizational slack.

While these characteristics help to explain how an organization as a whole will respond to innovation, they can be analyzed at both an individual and an organizational level. For example, adapting to new software involves a certain degree of complexity. Think about what is involved when an individual must select a new email application. Now think about what is involved if an organization decides to select a new clinical documentation application.

The perceived attributes of the innovation, the nature of organizational communication channels, the innovative decision process, and the efforts of change agents influence the possibility that an innovation will be adapted as well as the rate of adoption. There are five attributes that can be used to characterize an innovation.

- *Relative advantage:* Is the innovation seen as an improvement over the current approach? For example, has the need to standardize with one patient documentation system forced certain clinical units to give up certain functionality? Or is the new system seen as an upgrade with new functionality?
- *Compatibility:* Does the innovation fit with existing values, workflow, and individual expectations? For example, will the new application cause certain tasks to be shifted from one department to another?
- *Complexity:* Is the innovation easy to use and understand? If yes, the innovation can be seen as a minor change. If no, the innovation will be seen as a major change.
- *Trialability:* Can the innovation be tested or tried before individuals must make a commitment to it? While trialability can be an advantage in encouraging innovation, it can be difficult to trial a computer application in a large, complex organization such as a healthcare institution.
- *Observability:* Are the results of using the innovation visible to others?

If each of these five questions related to the five innovative attributes can be answered with a "yes," it is more likely that the innovation will be adopted and that the adoption will occur at a rapid rate. If, on the other hand, an innovation is not gaining acceptance, these characteristics can be used as a framework for evaluating the source of the problem. For example, it may take more time to document a patient assessment with the new system compared to the previous system. As a result nurses will prefer the previous system because of the relative advantage.

The decision of individuals and organizations to accept or reject an innovation is not an instantaneous event. The process involves five stages.[38] These stages can be demonstrated when a healthcare institution considers using blogs and wikis to support internal communication for all professional staff. The first stage of the innovation decision process is knowledge. In the knowledge stage the individual or organization becomes aware of the existence of the innovation. Managers become aware of other institutions that are using these tools and begin to learn about the possible advantages. Mass communication channels are usually most effective at this stage. For example, the institution's newsletter may carry a story about blogs and wikis and how staff might use these tools to support patient care and institutional goals. If the change agent does not have access to formal mass communication channels to reach all professional staff, the knowledge stage can be significantly delayed. While personal information moves quickly via informal communication channels, cognitive information does not move as quickly through these types of channels.

Once individuals become aware of an innovation they begin to develop an opinion or attitude about it. This is the persuasion stage. During the persuasion stage interpersonal channels of communication are more important and early adopters begin to play a key role. In the persuasion stage attitudes are not fixed but are in the process of being formed. The health informatics specialist should work closely with early adopters in developing and communicating positive attitudes to others in the organization.

Once these attitudes become more fixed, individuals make a decision to accept or reject the innovation. This is the decision stage. It is at this point that individuals will decide to try these tools for themselves. For each person this decision can occur at a different point. The early adopters will decide to try the system before the early majority. In testing out the system most people begin to discover new features or functions of the system. They also begin to discover potential problems. As they gain a better understanding of how to use the new functions they also discover challenges, modifications and adjustments that need to be made. The health informatics specialist needs to be sensitive to these modifications, as they will take on an added significance when formal and informal policies and procedures are developed. Once the decision has been made to accept the innovation, the implementation stage begins. The development of formal policies and procedures related to the innovation is a clear indication that the implementation stage is in place. The final stage is confirmation. At this point the innovation is no longer an innovation. It either has been rejected or has become the standard procedure. For example, certain key interinstitutional communication will depend on staff using these tools.

Using Change Theory

Effective change requires a champion or champions with a clear vision, a culture of trust, an organizational sense of pride, and the intense involvement of the people who must live with the change. The champion must have the institutional resources to support the change process. These resources include leadership skills; personnel, including change agents; money; and time. The change agent uses change theory to understand and manage reactions to change throughout the change process. Reactions to change may be negative, such as resistance, frustration, aggression, surface acceptance, indifference, ignoring, and organized resistance. Or the reaction to change can be positive, such as an increase in excitement and energy, a sense of pride, supporting and encouraging others, involvement in demonstrating how the innovation improves the organization, and overall acceptance. Change agents usually encounter both positive and negative reactions during the change process. It is usually more effective to support the positive reactions to change than it is to spend time and effort responding to the negative reactions.

THE SYSTEMS LIFE CYCLE MODEL

The most common change for informaticians is the introduction or modification of a health-related information system. A commonly used model of the stages within this change is the systems life cycle (SLC) or systems development life cycle model. This model is used in project management to describe stages or phases of an informatics project and it guides system implementation from initial feasibility through a more completed stage of maintenance and evaluation of the products. Most authors use the title "systems development life cycle" to describe the model. However, the term *development* is too limiting in health informatics because we often purchase systems or applications from vendors and customize them rather than developing them from scratch.

Various iterations of the systems life cycle have been published and no agreement exists about the numbers and types of stages in the life cycle. The number of stages ranges from three (preimplementation, implementation, and postimplementation) to at least seven. Project managers may even sort and combine phases to suit their needs according to the complexity and type of project being planned. In general, an SLC methodology follows the following steps:

1. *Feasibility and analysis.* The existing environment and systems are evaluated. A readiness assessment may be conducted. User needs and information system deficiencies are identified using informal or formal methods. New system requirements are defined. Deficiencies in the existing system are addressed with specific proposals for improvement.
2. *Planning.* The proposed system is planned and designed. Planning includes extensive work in myriad topics: physical construction, hardware, operating systems, programming, communications, implementation support, evaluation, and security issues. A workflow analysis and process reengineering may be completed as a basis for determining the scope of system functions and the flow of information and activities within care processes.
3. *Develop or purchase.* The new system is developed or purchased. New components and programs are obtained and installed. For vendor-supported solutions, extensive tailoring occurs. Users are trained in its use and all aspects are tested. Ideally, adjustments are made at this stage to correct gaps in the scope of system functions or work processes.
4. *Implementation.* The system is implemented via several possible techniques. The new system can be piloted, phased in according to application or location, or implemented all at once. The system is then used.
5. *Maintenance and evaluation.* Once the new system is up and running, it should be evaluated exhaustively. A maintenance phase begins to focus on maintaining system integrity, upgrades, and correcting issues that arise. Evaluation occurs at the end of the cycle.[39]

An entire life cycle can last many years. The average life cycle is about a decade, but some systems may be in place for longer periods; for example, the inpatient system in the military is nearly two decades old with few changes. Other systems may evolve continually for several decades with upgrades, module additions, and technology platform changes.

Staggers and Nelson Systems Life Cycle Model (SLCM)

The Staggers and Nelson SLCM depicted in Figure 2-6 incorporates the steps listed above, combines them with previous work from Thompson, Synder-Halpern, and Staggers, and expands the steps to include a new, important consideration: the depiction of the cycle as a spiral.[40] Once an organization completes the SLCM, it does not return in circular fashion to the assessment stage as most models indicate. Instead, reassessment occurs based on the organization's development into a new operating baseline (see Fig. 2-6). Two notions are used from work first published by Thompson and colleagues outlining an Expanded Systems Life Cycle.[40] The first is a step divided into purchase or development. The second is that evaluation occurs at every stage of the SLC versus relegating evaluation to the end of the cycle. The steps of the life cycle are outlined below.

1. *Analyze.* The existing environment and systems are evaluated. Major problems and deficiencies are identified using informal or formal methods. The feasibility of the system is determined and system requirements are defined. Informaticists may interview key system users or potential users and consult with information technology (IT) personnel. Formal research projects (e.g., observing users interacting with applications, determining workflow in specialty areas such as the operating room) or formal surveys or focus groups may be conducted to determine needs. Gaps are noted and current capabilities and limitations are outlined. Initial user and system requirements are formulated.
2. *Plan.* The proposed system is comprehensively planned. Planning includes strategic levels, such as whether the system will be developed internally, purchased and tailored, or designed and developed jointly with a vendor. The analysis and planning phases are the most time consuming of any project and are often estimated to require

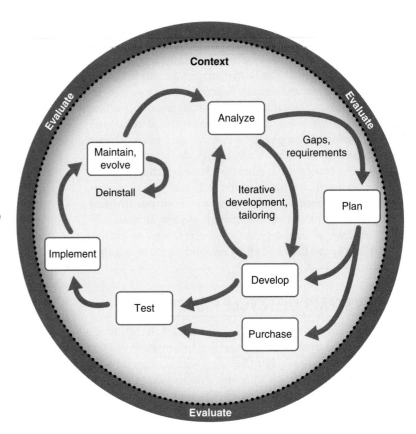

FIG 2-6 The Staggers and Nelson Systems Life Cycle Model.

70% of a project's time and resources from start to initial implementation.

Topics to consider in this step include planning for project governance, key stakeholders, hardware, operating systems, databases, interface engines, programming (if needed), tailoring methods, marketing and communications, support for go-live, support for extensive testing, project maintenance, evaluation and success factors, security and privacy, and systems integration and IT support such as integration into the call center, on-call support for clinicians, etc.

3. *Develop or purchase.* At this stage the system is purchased or the new system development begins. New components and programs are obtained and installed. For vendor-supported solutions, extensive tailoring occurs. This step may not be distinct from steps 1 and 2, depending on the type of development and tailoring the organization decides to employ. For instance, the organization may use user-centered techniques that include iterative design and evaluation with actual end-users. Training is designed but may be carried out as part of the implementation stage.

4. *Test.* In this step extensive testing occurs just before step 5 and go or no-go decisions are made about deadlines. Toward the end of this step marketing and communication efforts are accelerated to make users aware of the impending change.

5. *Implement or go-live.* The system is implemented using a selected method best suited to the organization and its tolerance for risk. User training is completed. The plan for conversion or go-live is implemented. For larger projects the go-live can include a command center to coordinate activities for the few days or weeks. Users begin to actually use the system for their activities such as patient care.

6. *Maintain and evolve.* Once the system has been formally acknowledged as passing user acceptance testing, typically at 90 or 120 days after go-live, it enters a maintenance stage. Here, the project is considered routine and is integrated into normal operations in IT, clinical, and business areas. However, the system is not static and evolves over time. For example, a project in the maintenance stage should have regular upgrades to maintain software currency and have system change requests completed.

7. *Evaluate.* Evaluation occurs at each step of the SLCM, as may be seen in Figure 2-6. The evaluation stage actually begins in the planning stage of the project. Evaluation techniques are discussed in Chapter 5.

8. *Return to analyze.* Unlike the methods depicted in most systems life cycle models, the organizational baseline has matured and does not return to the preimplementation baseline. Thus the SLCM is typically a spiral of ongoing analysis, refinement with installation of upgrades and enhancements, and new projects building on the initial work. Atypically, a project may have a formal end through deinstallation or replacement with a new system. If that occurs, it would be at this step in the SLCM.

TABLE 2-3	SELECTED MODELS OF NURSING INFORMATICS		
NAME	**AUTHOR**	**MAJOR CONCEPTS**	**REFERENCE**
The NI Pyramid Model	Patricia M. Schwirian, PhD, RN Professor Emerita School of Nursing The Ohio State University	The four primary concepts are raw nursing information, the technology, the users, and the goal or objective, arranged in a pyramid with a triangular base. Although the stated purpose was to describe concepts in NI, the model probably better describes human–computer interaction concepts.	Schwirian PM. The NI pyramid: A model for research in nursing informatics. *Comput Nurs.* 1986;4(3):134-136.
Turley's Nursing Informatics Model	James Turley, PhD, RN Associate Professor School of Health Information Sciences University of Texas Health Science Center at Houston	The five primary concepts are cognitive science, information science, computer science, informatics, and nursing science. The concepts of cognitive science, information science, and computer science are depicted as three overlapping circles with informatics at the junction of all three. Nursing science surrounds and provides a context for the overlapping circles.	Turley J. Toward a model for nursing informatics. *Image J Nurs Sch.* 1996;28(4):309-313.
Goosen's Framework for Nursing Informatics Research	William T.F. Goosen, RN, PhD Director Results 4 Care Netherlands	Goosen's model builds on and extends the Graves model. The concepts of data, information, knowledge, decision, action, and evaluation are depicted as six boxes with each of these concepts progressing to the next. Each of these six concepts interacts with the seventh concept in the model: Nursing Management and Processing to Patient Care.	Goosen W. Nursing informatics research. *Nurs Res.* 2000;8(2):42-54. Goosen W. Nursing information management and processing: a framework and definition for systems analysis, design and evaluation. *Int J Biomed Comput.* 1996;40(3):187-195.
The Informatics Research (IRO) Model	Judith Effken, PhD, RN, FACMI, FAAN Associate Professor, Nursing College of Nursing The University of Arizona	This model includes two component models. First is a five-phase systems development life cycle depicted as a circle in the center of the IRO model. This is surrounded by the process of evaluation, which occurs throughout the life cycle. The outer ring includes four constructs that interact with each other and the inner circle. These are (1) the client, (2) NI interventions, (3) outcomes, and (4) the cultural, economic, social, and physical context.	Effken J. An organizing framework for nursing informatics research. *CIN-Comput Inform Nu.* 2003;21(6):316-323.

NI, Nursing informatics.

ADDITIONAL INFORMATICS-RELATED MODELS

Although informatics is a fairly new discipline, various models have proven useful to leaders within this field. An overview of several key models and theories used within the discipline has been provided. Currently there is not one comprehensive, generally accepted theoretical or conceptual model of health or nursing informatics. A number of models have been introduced, some defining an overall model of informatics and some dealing with a specific aspect of informatics. For example, Graves and Corcoran, discussed earlier, defined an overall model while Garcia-Smith proposed an integrated model to predict a successful clinical information system (CIS) implementation.[41] Selected models are included in Table 2-3.

Informatics incorporates a number of other disciplines and, as a result, theories from those disciplines have been effectively used to guide research within the field of informatics. This chapter is an introduction to the use of theory in informatics and not a comprehensive analysis of theories that have or can be used to deal with questions of importance to informatics. Several theoretical and conceptual models used in health informatics are described elsewhere in this book and are not repeated in this section. For example, the model of biomedical informatics developed by the American Medical Informatics Association is included in Chapter 1. Staggers's model of human–computer interaction is included in Chapter 21. Both the Graves and Nelson models were discussed in this chapter. In the future one can expect to see additional models developed as the field of informatics continues to mature and as developments in healthcare as well as technology continue to evolve.

CONCLUSION AND FUTURE DIRECTIONS

Healthcare is an information-intensive service. Computerization and the use of technology provide an effective and efficient means to manage large volumes of data and information with knowledge and wisdom. However, the move to a fully electronic healthcare system is changing every aspect of healthcare. With this degree of change comes excitement, anxiety, resistance, and conflict. Health informatics specialists function at the very core of this change. They play a major role in implementing, managing, and leading healthcare organization as they move forward with automation. To play this role they work directly with the clinical, administrative, and technical people in the organization. For health informatics specialists to provide effective leadership, they must understand the institution's vision and values and the people and processes within these organizations. The theories presented in this chapter provide a foundation for supporting and managing the enormous degree of change experienced by the healthcare system and the people within any healthcare system.

REFERENCES

1. Hawking SW. *A Brief History of Time*. New York, NY: Bantam Books; 1988.
2. Von Bertalanffy L, Ruben BD, Kim JY, eds. *General Systems Theory and Human Communication*. Rochelle Park, NJ: Hayden Book Company; 1975.
3. Joos I, Nelson R, Lyness A. *Man, Health and Nursing*. Reston, VA: Reston Publishing Company; 1985.
4. Lorenz EN. Deterministic nonperiodic flow. *J Atmos Sci*. 1963; 20:130-141. doi:http://dx.doi.org/10.1175/1520-0469(1963)020 <0130:DNF>2.0.CO;2.
5. Smith L, Smith L. *Chaos: A Very Short Introduction*. New York, NY: Oxford University Press; 2007.
6. Kellert S. *In the Wake of Chaos: Unpredictable Order in Dynamical Systems*. Chicago, IL: University of Chicago Press; 1993.
7. Kernick D. *Complexity and Healthcare Organizations: A View from the Street*. Oxon, United Kingdom: Radcliffe-Medical Press Ltd; 2004.
8. Walker R. Quotations from Friedrich Nietzsche [1844–1900]. Working Minds. http://www.working-minds.com/FNquotes.htm. 2012.
9. Holden LM. Complex adaptive systems: concept analysis. *J Adv Nurs*. 2005;52(6):651-657.
10. Phelan S. What is complexity science, really? *Emergence*. 2001; (1):120-136. http://faculty.unlv.edu/phelan/Phelan_What%20is% 20complexity%20science.pdf.
11. Information. *Merriam-Webster's Collegiate Dictionary*. http:// www.merriam-webster.com/dictionary/information. 2012.
12. Robertson J. The fundamentals of information science: an online overview. http://www-ec.njit.edu/~robertso/infosci/index. html. 2004.
13. Shannon C, Weaver W. The mathematical theory of communication. *Bell Syst Tech J*. 1948;27:379-423, 623-656. http://cm.bell-labs.com/cm/ms/what/shannonday/shannon1948.pdf.
14. Hersh W. *Information Retrieval: A Health Care Perspective*. 3rd ed. New York, NY: Springer Science; 2009.
15. Blum B. *Clinical Information Systems*. New York, NY: Springer-Verlag; 1986.
16. Clarke R. Fundamentals of "information systems." Xamax Consultancy Pty Ltd. http://www.rogerclarke.com/SOS/ISFundas. html. 1999.
17. Graves J, Corcoran S. The study of nursing informatics. *Image*. 1989;21(4):227-230.
18. Nelson R, Joos I. On language in nursing: from data to wisdom. *PLN Visions*. 1989;Fall:6.
19. Nelson R. Major theories supporting health care informatics. In: Englebardt S, Nelson R, eds. *Health Care Informatics: An Interdisciplinary Approach*. St. Louis, MO: Mosby-Year Book; 2002: 3-27.
20. American Nurses Association. *Nursing Informatics: Scope and Standards of Practice*. Silver Spring, MD: Nursesbooks.org; 2008.
21. Kearsley G. *The theory into practice database*. Instructional Design. http://www.instructionaldesign.org/about.html. nd.
22. Harapnuik D. Inquisitivism or "the HHHMMM??? what does this button do?" approach to learning: the synthesis of cognitive theories into a novel approach to adult education. http://dte6. educ.ualberta.ca/tech_ed/publish/inquisitivism.htm. 1998.
23. Woolley A, Chabris C, Pentland A, Hashmi N, Malone T. Evidence for a collective intelligence factor in the performance of human groups. *Science*. 2010;330:686-689.
24. Marshall J. How to measure the wisdom of a crowd. Discovery News. http://news.discovery.com/human/group-intelligence-wisdom-crowd.html. 2010.
25. Knowles M. *The Modern Practice of Adult Education: Andragogy versus Pedagogy*. New York, NY: Association Press; 1970.
26. Harriman G. Adult learning. E-Learning Resources. http:// www.grayharriman.com/adult_learning.htm. 2004.
27. Conner M. Introduction to adult learning. http://marciaconner. com/resources/adult-learning. nd.
28. Conner ML. *Learning: The Critical Technology—A Whitepaper on Adult Education in the Information Age*. St. Louis, MO: Wave Technologies International; 1996.
29. Kolb D. *Experiential Learning: Experience as the Source of Learning and Development*. Englewood Cliffs, NJ: Prentice-Hall; 1984.
30. Myers IB, McCaulley MH. *Manual: A Guide to the Development and Use of the Myers Briggs Type Indicator*. Mountain View, CA: Consulting Psychologists Press; 1985.
31. Greathouse J. Kurt Lewin: 1890–1947. Muskingum College, Psychology Department. http://www.muskingum.edu/~psychology/psycweb/history/lewin.htm. 1997.
32. Schein E. Kurt Lewin's change theory in the field and in the classroom. Purdue University, College of Technology. http:// www2.tech.purdue.edu/Ols/courses/ols582/SWP-3821-32871445.pdf. 1999.
33. Conner D. *Managing at the Speed of Change*. New York, NY: Random House; 2006.
34. Rogers EM. *Diffusion of Innovation*. 4th ed. New York, NY: The Free Press; 1995.
35. Rogers EM, Scott KL. The diffusion of innovations model and outreach from the National Network of Libraries of Medicine to Native American communities. National Network of Libraries of Medicine. http://www.nnlm.nlm.nih.gov/pnr/eval/rogers. html. 1997.
36. Sapp S. Diffusion of innovation: part 1 and part 2. Iowa State University, Department of Sociology. http://www.soc.iastate. edu/sapp/soc415read.html. 2012.

37. Trujillo MF. Diffusion of ICT innovations for sustainable human development: problem definition. Tulane University Law School, Payson Center for International Development. http://payson.tulane.edu/research/E-DiffInnova/diff-prob.html. 2000.

38. Rogers EM. *Diffusion of Innovation*. 5th ed. New York, NY: The Free Press; 2003.

39. Rouse M. Systems development life cycle (SDLC). TechTarget. http://searchsoftwarequality.techtarget.com/definition/systems-development-life-cycle. 2009.

40. Thompson C, Synder-Halpern R, Staggers N. Analysis, processes, and techniques: case study. *Comput Nurs.* 1999;17(5): 203-206.

41. Garcia-Smith D. *Testing a Model to Predict Successful Clinical Information Systems* [doctoral dissertation]. The University of Arizona, College of Nursing. http://www.nursing.arizona.edu/Library/Garcia-Smith_Dianna.pdf. 2007.

DISCUSSION QUESTIONS

1. Using Shannon and Weaver's model of information as a framework, describe several ways in which miscommunication can occur between healthcare providers working together in a clinical setting. Use this same framework to suggest how technology could be used to decrease this miscommunication.

2. Use Blum's model of information to explain the nursing process and then identify the implication of this model for the development of decision support systems to support the nursing process.

3. Some have argued that the data-to-wisdom continuum cannot be used to define the scope of clinical practice because computers cannot process wisdom. Identify and describe whether this is a fallacy.

4. This chapter includes four types of learning theories. Use each of these types of learning theories to explain how to design and implement a staff education program to support a go-live implementation in a major medical center.

5. The responses of individuals to innovation have been classified into five groups. List and describe the five groups. Now describe how each group should be managed when planning for a major change within a healthcare institution.

6. List and explain the five internal organizational characteristics that can be used to predict how an organization will respond to a change in automation. Now use these same characteristics to predict how the American healthcare system will respond to the automation of healthcare over the next 5 years.

CASE STUDY

A good friend of yours is director of nursing at a 220-bed community hospital. Last year the hospital merged with a much larger medical center. One of the upsides, as well as one of the challenges, resulting from this change has been the rapid introduction of new computer systems. The goal is to bring the hospital "up to speed" within 3 years. At present CPOE is being implemented. The general medical and surgical units went live last month. The ICU and pediatrics and obstetrics units are scheduled to go-live next month. The plan is to work out any kinks or problems on the general units and then go-live in the specialty units.

Most of the physicians, nurse practitioners, and physician assistants initially complained but are now becoming more comfortable with the computers and are beginning to integrate the CPOE process into their daily routines. Several physicians are now requesting the ability to enter orders from their offices and others are looking into this option.

However, there are three physicians who have not commented during this process but are clearly resisting. For example, after performing rounds and returning to their offices they called the unit with verbal orders. After being counseled on this behavior they began to write the orders on scraps of paper and put these in the patient's charts or leave them at the nurses' station. When they were informed that these were not "legal orders" they began smuggling in order sheets from the nonactivated units. In addition, they have been coercing the staff nurses on the units to enter the orders for them. This has taken two forms. Sometimes they sign in and then ask the nurses to enter the orders. Other times they ask the nurses to put the orders in verbally and then they confirm the orders. The nurses feel caught between the hospital's goals and the need to maintain a good working relationship with these physicians.

Discussion Questions

1. How would you use the theories presented in this chapter to diagnosis the problems demonstrated in this case. List your diagnoses and explain your analysis.

2. What actions would you recommend to your friend and what reason (theories) would you use as a basis for your recommendations?

Evidence-Based Practice and Informatics

Kathleen R. Stevens and Sandra A. Mitchell

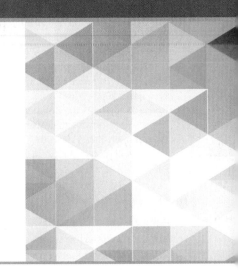

Informatics can greatly add to support of evidence-based practice (EBP), patient-centered care, and transitions of care across settings. Such technology can greatly assist in the exchange of health information for continuity and quality of care.

OBJECTIVES

At the completion of this chapter the reader will be prepared to:

1. Explore the trend in evidence-based quality improvement in terms of implications for all levels of healthcare organizations and across all professions
2. Review effective models in structuring evidence-based practice (EBP) initiatives
3. Identify informatics-based resources for increasing evidence-based quality improvement
4. Discuss the role of EBP in developing informatics-based solutions for managing patients' care needs

KEY TERMS

ABSTRACT

This chapter links evidence-based practice (EBP) and informatics by exploring the central, shared construct of *knowledge*. The discussion offers a foundation for understanding EBP and describes how it is supported through a variety of current informatics applications. The chapter concludes by exploring opportunities for applying informatics solutions to maximize EBP in healthcare. Specific information in the chapter includes (1) the rationale for EBP, (2) overview of EBP models, (3) a detailed example of how a model can be used to organize concepts related to EBP, (4) computerized databases supporting EBP, and (5) informatics-related opportunities for using EBP.

INTRODUCTION

Informatics solutions and tools hold great potential for enhancing evidence-based clinical decision making. The field of informatics and the concept of evidence-based practice (EBP) intersect at the crucial junction of knowledge for clinical decisions with the goal of transforming healthcare to be reliable, safe, and effective.

A foundational paradigm for informatics is the framework of data, information, knowledge, and wisdom discussed in Chapter 2. This framework holds that as data are organized into meaningful groupings, the information within those data can be seen and interpreted. The organization of information and the identification of the relationships between the facts within the information create knowledge. The effective use of knowledge, such as the process of providing personalized care to manage human healthcare needs, is wisdom. Computerization offers the opportunity to efficiently and effectively collect, organize, label, and deliver evidence-based information and knowledge at the point of decision making, so that clinicians can use concepts from EBP at the point of care.

Knowledge is at the heart of EBP. Within the EBP paradigm knowledge must be transformed through a number of

BOX 3-1 INSTITUTE OF MEDICINE FINDINGS ON 2001 LEVEL OF CURRENT CARE COMPARED WITH STANDARDS OF CARE

47% of myocardial infarction patients did not receive beta blockers

50% of children with asthma did not receive written instructions

48% of elderly did not receive annual influenza vaccine

63% of smokers were not advised to quit smoking

84% of Medicare patients with diabetes were not tested with the A1c blood test

Data from Institute of Medicine. Crossing the quality chasm: A new health system for the 21st Century [Committee on Health Care in America & Institute of Medicine]. Washington, DC: National Academies Press; 2001.

forms to increase its utility at the point of care.[1] The ultimate goal of EBP is improvement of systems and microsystems within healthcare, with these improvements based on science. Using computerized methods and resources to support the implementation of EBP holds great potential for improving healthcare. Delivering evidence to the point of patient care can align care processes with best practices that are supported by evidence.

The evolution of EBP underscores its potential impact on quality of care and health outcomes. In a well-known report, *To Err Is Human*, experts noted that almost 100,000 patients were being harmed annually by the healthcare system.[2] As an immediate response, national leaders identified the gap between what is known about best care and what is widely practiced in the report titled *Crossing the Quality Chasm*.[3] The 2001 report points to EBP as a critical solution to redesigning and improving healthcare.

Multiple reports point to the fact that healthcare is not as good or as safe as it could be. In the *Chasm* report, more than 100 surveys of quality of care were cited, showing that scores on the "report card" for healthcare performance was poor. Box 3-1 presents findings from these surveys comparing current care to what was deemed to be best care or standards of care. These results indicate that much improvement is needed if every patient is to receive high-quality care at all times.

Another report, the *National Healthcare Quality Report* (NHQR), produced online by the Agency for Healthcare Research and Quality (AHRQ), provides a snapshot of the quality of care across the country.[4] This national report has been published annually only since 2004. The survey demonstrates that while improvements have been detected, progress is occurring in only half of the quality indicators and the magnitude of improvement is agonizingly small—in the 2% to 4% range. Conclusions from the 2011 NHQR continue to point to persistent shortcomings in delivering care known to be most effective.[4]

Solutions to the healthcare quality gap are offered in the *Chasm* report.[3] The Institute of Medicine (IOM) expert panel issued recommendations for urgent action to redesign healthcare so that it is safe, timely, effective, efficient, equitable, and patient-centered, often referred to as the STEEEP principles.[3] Each of the STEEEP redesign principles is described further in Table 3-1.

The *Chasm* report continues to be a major influence, directing national efforts targeted at transforming healthcare. For example, the STEEEP recommendations are now reflected in health profession education programs. The American Association of Colleges of Nursing (AACN) educational competencies include requirements for programs to prepare nurses who contribute to quality improvement.[5] AACN *Essentials* specifies that professional nursing practice be grounded in translation of current evidence into practice and further point to the need for knowledge and skills in information management as being critical in the delivery of quality patient care.[5] Likewise, the Accreditation Council for Graduate Medical Education (ACGME) requires medical education in quality improvement.[6] The STEEEP principles are also reflected in clinical practice resources, such as the AHRQ Health Care Innovations Exchange, in which the elements of STEEEP are employed as selection criteria for inclusion in this unique clearinghouse.[7]

Quality of care and EBP are conceptually linked and form the hub of healthcare improvement. The descriptions and definitions of each reflect overlap of these concepts and offer reference points against which to expand the understanding

TABLE 3-1 DESCRIPTIONS OF THE STEEEP PRINCIPLES FOR REDESIGNING HEALTHCARE

PRINCIPLE	DESCRIPTION
Safe	Avoid injuries to patients from the care that is intended to help them.
Timely	Reduce waits and sometimes harmful delays for both those who receive and those who give care.
Effective	Provide services based on scientific knowledge to all who could benefit, and refrain from providing services to those not likely to benefit.
Efficient	Avoid waste, including waste of equipment, supplies, ideas, and energy.
Equitable	Provide care that does not vary in quality because of personal characteristics such as gender, ethnicity, geographic location, and socioeconomic status.
Patient-centered	Provide care that is respectful of and responsive to individual patient preferences, needs, and values, and ensure that patient values guide all clinical decisions.

Adapted from Institute of Medicine. Crossing the quality chasm: A new health system for the 21st Century [Committee on Health Care in America & Institute of Medicine]. Washington, DC: National Academies Press; 2001:39-40.

of these concepts. In particular, the focal point of both is the use of knowledge in practice.

The definition of quality of care includes two key connections to EBP and knowledge that in turn provide a strong linking point for informatics. First, quality healthcare services increase the likelihood that the goal of desired outcomes will be reached. This implies that processes of EBP must assist clinicians in *knowing* which options in health services are effective. The strongest cause-and-effect knowledge is discovered through research. Second, EBP is connected to quality insofar as healthcare is consistent with current knowledge. *Using knowledge* presumes accessibility to it at the point of care. The overlap of EBP and knowledge is further underscored by the definition of the STEEEP principle "effective." In the STEEEP framework, effectiveness is defined as evidence-based decision making, suggesting that "Patients should receive care based on the best available scientific knowledge."[3(p62)] *Knowledge* is the point of convergence across the areas of EBP, informatics, and improvement. Using informatics approaches can make evidence available and accessible at the point of care.

EBP is put into action during clinical decision making. The primary impetus for EBP in healthcare is that clinicians want to select the option that is most likely to be effective in improving the patient's health problem. This is the option that is supported by best available research evidence. Clients present a plethora of actual and potential health problems that need to be managed or resolved (e.g., living with asthma, succeeding in the face of learning disabilities, preventing obesity). Many clinical actions are not based on best available scientific knowledge and therefore offer the client care that is not as effective as it could be.[3] The essential role of the healthcare provider is to select and apply interventions that have the greatest potential to improve the client's situation and to implement the most effective strategies for changing the microsystem or system of care. Clinicians choose from and interpret a huge variety of clinical data and information while facing pressure to decrease uncertainty, risks to patients, and costs. Knowledge underlies these decisions and plays a primary role in the care provided.

Evidence-based clinical decision making can be described as a prescriptive approach to making choices in diagnostic and intervention care, based on the idea that research-based care improves outcomes most effectively. Research-based care provides evidence about which option is most likely to produce the desired outcome. EBP is seen as a key solution in closing the gap between what is known and what is practiced.

However, important questions lie between accepting this as true and the clinician's and system's ability to enact it: How do clinicians know which interventions will most likely diminish or resolve the health problem and help the client reach his or her health goal? What resources are available to apply EBP principles directly in clinical decision making? Answers to these questions begin by analyzing the different models of EBP.

EVIDENCE-BASED PRACTICE (EBP) MODELS

A number of EBP models are useful in understanding various aspects of EBP and elucidating connections between informatics and EBP. An overview of models in the field reflects several challenges for developing informatics approaches. A prime challenge is the complexity of issues surrounding standardized terminology in healthcare and the lack of a common framework across the field of EBP. Standardized terminology is requisite for naming, classifying, tagging, and locating evidence in order to use it in practice. A common framework could be used to consistently organize and implement EBP principles.

Prominent EBP models can be grouped into three categories of models for designing and implementing systematic approaches to strengthen evidence-based clinical decision making.[8] Table 3-2 describes the critical attributes and provides examples in three categories.

The first category includes models that focus on EBP, research use, and knowledge transformation principles. These models emphasize a systematic approach to synthesizing knowledge. These models specify a series of processes designed to:

1. Identify a question, topic, or problem in health care
2. Retrieve relevant evidence to address the identified issue
3. Critically appraise the level and strength of that evidence
4. Synthesize and apply the evidence to improve clinical outcomes

Some models emphasize the process by which research findings can be developed into a more useful form, such as a clinical practice guideline or standards of care, which can then be used to guide clinical decision making in the practice arena. Other models address outcomes evaluation to determine whether the EBP change has produced the expected clinical outcomes or to compare actual practice and ideal practice (thereby identifying unacceptable practice variation).

The second category includes models that offer an understanding of the mechanisms by which individual, small group, and organizational contexts affect the diffusion, uptake, and adoption of new knowledge and include innovation as essential to the design of EBP initiatives. These models propose that specific interventions serve to accelerate the adoption of practices that are based on best evidence. Examples of such interventions include the following:

- Facilitation
- Use of opinion leaders
- Real-time feedback about patient outcomes
- Audit feedback about clinicians' variation from established practice standards

Thus, within these models, feedback regarding both patient and practitioner outcomes is seen as a change strategy.

A third category of models and frameworks postulates that formalized, bidirectional, and ongoing interactions among practitioners, researchers, policy-makers, and consumers accelerate the application of new discoveries in clinical care. This ongoing interaction increases the likelihood that researchers will focus on problems of importance to

TABLE 3-2	MODELS FOR EVIDENCE-BASED PRACTICE (EBP)	
FOCUS	**DESCRIPTION**	**EXAMPLES OF MODELS**
EBP, research use, and knowledge transformation processes	Direct a systematic approach to synthesizing knowledge and transforming research findings to improve patient outcomes and the quality of care Address both individual practitioners and healthcare organizations Focus on increasing the meaningfulness and utility of research findings in clinical decision making	• ACE Star Model of Knowledge Transformation[1] • Advancing Research and Clinical Practice through Close Collaboration (ARCC) Model of Evidence-Based Practice in Nursing and Healthcare[9] • Johns Hopkins Nursing Evidence-Based Practice Model and Guidelines[10] • Iowa Model of Evidence-Based Practice[11] • Stetler Model of Research Utilization[12]
Strategic and organizational change theory to promote uptake and adoption of new knowledge	Trace mechanisms by which individual, small group, and organizational contexts affect diffusion, uptake, and adoption of new knowledge and innovation Premise is that interventions, outcomes evaluations, and feedback are important methods to promote practice change	• Promoting Action on Research Implementation in Health Services (PARiHS)[13-15] • Vratny and Shriver Model for Evidence-Based Practice[16] • Pettigrew and Whipp Model of Strategic Change[12] • Outcomes-Focused Knowledge Translation[17] • Determinants of Effective Implementation of Complex Innovations in Organizations[18] • Ottawa Model of Research Use[19,20]
Knowledge exchange and synthesis for application and inquiry	Structure ongoing interactions among practitioners, researchers, policy-makers, and consumers to facilitate the generation of clinically relevant knowledge and the application of knowledge in practice All parties are engaged in bidirectional collaboration across the translation continuum	• Collaborative Model for Knowledge Translation between Research and Practice Settings[21] • Framework for Translating Evidence into Action[22] • Knowledge Transfer and Exchange[23] • Canadian Institutes of Health Research Knowledge Translation within the Research Cycle Model or Knowledge Action Model[24-26] • Interactive Systems Framework for Dissemination and Implementation[27]

From Mitchell SA, Fisher CA, Hastings CE, et al. A thematic analysis of theoretical models for translational science in nursing: mapping the field. *Nursing Outlook*. 2010;58(6):287-300. Used with permission.

clinicians. Such models simultaneously address the generation of new knowledge (discovery) and the stimulation of uptake. This collaboration supports the exchange of expertise and knowledge to strengthen decision making and action for all involved parties.[8]

Each EBP model described previously brings forth perspectives that may prove valuable in designing and advancing informatics approaches to EBP. The following section examines the application of one of these models, the ACE Star Model of Knowledge Transformation, as a framework for exploring and expanding the informatics-EBP link.[1] In this chapter the ACE Star Model will be used to demonstrate how an EBP model can be used to:

1. Guide the transition from the discovery of new information and knowledge to the provision of care that is based on evidence
2. Identify how computerization and informatics principles can be used to make this transition realistically possible in a world in which information and knowledge is growing at an explosive rate

ACE STAR MODEL OF KNOWLEDGE TRANSFORMATION

The ACE Star Model of Knowledge Transformation provides a framework for converting research knowledge into a form

that has utility in the clinical decision making process. The ACE Star Model articulates a necessary process for reducing the volume and complexity of research knowledge, evolving one form of knowledge to the next, and incorporating a broad range of sources of knowledge throughout the EBP process.

The ACE Star Model addresses two major hurdles in employing EBP: (1) the volume of current professional knowledge and (2) the form of knowledge that healthcare professionals attempt to apply in practice. In both instances, informatics-based solutions have been created. The ACE Star Model explains the key concept of knowledge transformation. Knowledge transformation is defined as the conversion of research findings from discovery of primary research results, through a series of stages and forms, to increase the relevance, accessibility, and utility of evidence at the point of care to improve healthcare and health outcomes by way of evidence-based care.[1]

When considering the *volume* of knowledge, experts point out that "no unaided human being can read, recall, and act effectively on the volume of clinically relevant scientific literature."[3(p25)] It is estimated that, in medicine, more than 10,000 new research articles are published annually. Even the most enthusiastic clinician would find it challenging to stay abreast of this volume of literature. When considering the *form* of knowledge as a barrier, it is clear that most research

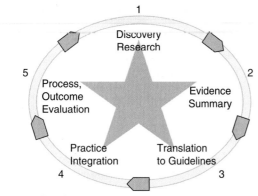

FIG 3-1 ACE Star Model of Knowledge Transformation. (Copyright Stevens KR. *ACE Star Model of EBP: Knowledge Transformation.* San Antonio, TX: Academic Center for Evidence-Based Practice, University of Texas Health Science Center at San Antonio; 2004. Used with expressed permission.)

reports are not directly clinically useful but must be converted to a form applicable at the point of care. Research results, often presented in the form of statistical results, exist in a larger body of knowledge. The complexity and congruence across all studies on a topic create a barrier when using this as a basis for clinical decision making. The ACE Star Model addresses the transformation that is necessary for converting research results from single study findings to guidelines that can be applied and measured for impact. Discussion of this model is expanded below, with specific electronic resources for each form of knowledge identified and described.

In the ACE Star Model, individual studies move through four cycles, ending in practice outcomes and patient outcomes. The knowledge transformation process occurs at five points, which can be conceptualized as a five-point star as shown in Figure 3-1.

These five points are discovery research, evidence summary, translation to guidelines, practice integration, and evaluation of process and outcome.[1] A description of each star point is provided below along with identification and descriptions of computerized resources and examples.

Point 1: Discovery Research

Primary research on point 1 represents the knowledge produced through primary discovery. In this stage knowledge is in the form of results from single research studies. Over the past 3 decades, health-related research has produced thousands of research studies on a wide variety of health-related issues. However, the clinical utility of this form of knowledge is low. The cluster of primary research studies on any given topic may include both strong and weak study designs, small and large samples, and conflicting or converging results, leaving the clinician to wonder which study is the best reflection of cause and effect in selecting effective interventions. Point 1 knowledge is less useful in clinical decision making

because there may be hundreds of research studies on a given topic, with the overall collection being unwieldy. Further, the group of studies does not necessarily converge on a consensus of the intervention most likely to produce the desired outcome. Instead, one study may show that the intervention was successful while another shows no difference between control and experimental conditions.

Initially health sciences researchers focused on applying results from primary research studies directly in patient care, detailing ways to move a single study into practice. However, since there may be multiple studies on a given topic, this strategy no longer is appropriate for many interventions. Table 3-3 illustrates part of the challenge in moving research into practice with this approach. In this example, the clinician seeks to locate current evidence about falls prevention in the elderly. A CINAHL literature search on the topic "falls prevention" returned more than 5600 articles to consider. Even when the search strategy was limited to "research," more than 2000 articles remained in the list. This volume of literature is far too great to have clinical utility.

Point 2: Evidence Summary

Table 3-3 illustrates the striking advantage of knowledge management through EBP stages, in particular, evidence summaries. Evidence summaries include evidence synthesis, systematic reviews (SRs), integrative reviews, and reviews of literature, with SRs being the most rigorous approach to evidence summary. Before evidence summaries were invented, the clinician was left to deal with the many articles located via a bibliographic database search—in this case, thousands of articles. However, if the research knowledge has been transformed through evidence synthesis, the resulting SR will contain the world's knowledge in a single article. The EBP solution to the complexity and volume of literature seen in point 1 is the point 2 evidence summary. In this second stage of knowledge transformation a team locates all primary

TABLE 3-3	LITERATURE SEARCH AND KNOWLEDGE FORMS ON "FALLS PREVENTION"		
STAR POINT FORM OF KNOWLEDGE		SEARCH	RESULTS
Point 1: Discovery Research		CINAHL search for "falls"	5639 citations
		Limit search to "research"	2092 citations
Point 2: Evidence Summary		Limit search to "systematic reviews"	168 citations
		Focus on "prevention in elderly"	1 systematic review

research on a given clinical topic and summarizes it into a single statement about the state of knowledge on the topic. This summary step is the main knowledge transformation that distinguishes EBP from simple research application and research use in clinical practice. The importance of this transformation cannot be understated: SRs have been described as the central link between research and clinical decision making.[28]

Returning to Table 3-3 and our example on falls above, once the literature search is narrowed to "systematic reviews," the volume of hits is decreased to 168 citations. Once a narrowed clinical topic is applied, the search yields a single SR on falls prevention in the elderly, thereby transforming almost 6000 pieces of knowledge into a single source.

To date there are many health-related topics on which a significant number of quality research studies do not yet exist to form the basis for SRs or for which the resources are not available to complete the work involved in an SR. Many informatics interventions and products are examples of this. In fact, Weir et al. contend that researchers rushed to perform experimental studies for computerized provider order entry (CPOE) before the phenomenon was understood.[29,30] Because of this, existing SRs confused available evidence due to inconsistent definitions and components of CPOE across studies. With newer areas such as informatics, qualitative and descriptive studies are needed first. Then, solid primary research and subsequent integrative reviews and SRs can be conducted to build the science of health informatics.

The ACE Star Model concentrates on evidence in the field with more available research than health informatics. The most widely used methods in rigorous evidence summaries produce an SR that reflects the methods established in the mid-1990s.[31] SRs transform research knowledge in a number of significant ways and their invention marked a major shift in the way that research evidence was brought to practice. Key advantages of SRs are summarized in Box 3-2.

An SR is a rigorous evidence summary that uses a scientific approach to combine results from a body of original research studies into a clinically meaningful whole, produces

new knowledge through synthesis, and typically uses the statistical procedure meta-analysis to combine findings across multiple studies. In this way evidence summaries remove the obstacle of voluminous and rapidly expanding bodies of research literature. Evidence summaries communicate the latest scientific findings in a palatable and accessible form that can be readily applied in making clinical decisions; that is, evidence summaries form the basis upon which to build EBP. When developing an evidence summary, one must keep in mind that nonsignificant findings can be as important to practice as positive results. However, nonsignificant findings tend not to be published and so are underrepresented in the literature.

Conducting sound evidence summaries requires scientific skill and extensive resources—often more than a year's worth of scientific work. SRs, not conducted to a high scientific standard, can lead to incorrect conclusions about the proven impact of a given intervention on targeted health outcomes. If done to rigorous standards, evidence summaries will review research across all relevant disciplines and across the globe, screen studies for relevance and quality of design, use multiple reviewers to abstract findings, and analyze the results to combine findings and examine the extent of bias in the set of research studies. For this reason evidence summaries are often conducted by scientific and clinical teams that are specifically prepared in the methodology. The dominant methodology for systematic reviews is published in the *Cochrane Handbook for Systematic Reviews of Interventions*.[31]

Resources and Examples

Major computerized resources for locating systematic reviews include the Cochrane Database of Systematic Reviews, the Agency for Healthcare Research and Quality, as well as the general professional literature. Systematic reviews in the Cochrane Library are produced by the Cochrane Collaboration. The International Cochrane Collaboration's mission is to ensure that current, accurate information about effectiveness of healthcare interventions is available worldwide.

A primary strategy for achieving this is through the production and dissemination of SRs of healthcare interventions. This group established the "systematic review" as a literature review, conducted using rigorous approaches that synthesize all high-quality research evidence to reflect current knowledge about a specific question. The scientific methods are specified by the Cochrane Collaboration and its design is considered the gold standard for evidence summaries.[32] After 4 decades of global collaborative work, the Cochrane Collaboration has posted more than 5000 SRs in the Cochrane Database of Systematic Reviews.[32]

Returning to the example of falls prevention, the single SR was located through a targeted search using the Cochrane and summarized in Box 3-3. The evidence summary offers powerful knowledge about what interventions are likely to be most successful. Note that in this example 62 trials (point 1 studies) were located, screened for relevance and quality, and meta-analyzed into a single set of conclusions. These conclusions indicate which interventions are most likely to be beneficial

---

BOX 3-2 ADVANTAGES OF SYSTEMATIC REVIEWS

A rigorous systematic review:
Reduces information into a manageable form
Establishes generalizability—participants, settings, treatment variations, study designs
Assesses consistencies across studies
Increases power in cause and effect
Reduces bias and improves true reflection of reality
Integrates information for decisions
Reduces time between research and implementation
Offers basis for continuous updates

From Mulrow CD. Rationale for systematic reviews. *BMJ.* 1994;309(6954):597-599. Reproduced with permission from BMJ Publishing Group Ltd.

in preventing falls in elderly people. However, the recommendations for practice from the SR are not yet action oriented. For this to happen, it is necessary to translate a conclusion into an actionable recommendation, moving the knowledge to point 3.

Point 3: Translation to Guidelines

In the third stage of EBP, translation, experts are called on to consider the evidence summary, fill in gaps with consensus expert opinion, and merge research knowledge with expertise to produce clinical practice guidelines (CPGs). This process translates the research evidence into clinical recommendations. The IOM defines clinical guidelines as "systematically developed statements to assist practitioner and patient decisions about appropriate health care for specific clinical circumstances."[33]

CPGs have evolved during the past 20 years from recommendations based largely on expert judgment to recommendations grounded primarily in evidence. Expert consensus is used in guideline development when research-based evidence is lacking.[34] CPGs are commonly produced and sponsored by a clinical specialty organization. Such guidelines are present throughout all organized healthcare in the form of clinical pathways, nursing care standards, and unit policies. An exemplar of the development of CPGs in nursing is Putting Evidence into Practice in Oncology.[35] This program engages scientists and expert clinicians in examining evidence, conducting evidence summaries, generating practice recommendations, and developing tools to implement the guidelines. These online guidelines are accessible to clinicians and are also published in nursing literature.[36]

Crucial criteria for well-developed CPGs are (1) the evidence is explicitly identified and (2) the evidence and recommendation are rated. To assist in rating evidence, several taxonomies have been developed. One such taxonomy was developed by the Center for Evidence Based Medicine in the United Kingdom. This rating system identifies SRs as the uppermost strength of evidence.[37]

Also included and counted as evidence is *consensus of expert opinion*, which is rated the weakest strength of all levels of evidence. However, if no other evidence exists, this may serve to support clinical decision making. Well-developed CPGs and care standards share several characteristics: A specified process is followed during guideline development; the guideline identifies the evidence upon which each recommendation is made, whether it is research or expert opinion; and the evidence is rated using a strength-of-evidence rating scale. Figure 3-2 illustrates a strength-of-evidence rating hierarchy.[38] The higher the evidence is placed on the pyramid, the more confident the clinician can be that the intervention will cause the targeted health effect.

A number of EBP approaches emphasize the usefulness of CPGs in bridging the gap between primary research findings and clinical decision making.[28] CPGs are systematically developed statements to assist practitioners and patients in decisions about appropriate healthcare for specific clinical circumstances.[33] CPGs are seen as tools to help move scientific evidence to the bedside. To increase the likelihood that the recommended action will have a positive impact on the clinical outcome, it is imperative that guidelines are based on best available evidence, systematically located, appraised, and synthesized (i.e., evidence based).

Resources and Examples

Locating CPGs can be challenging. Prior to the EBP movement, guidelines were developed and disseminated by clinical specialty organizations, particularly in medicine. These guidelines were not necessarily evidence based and often were based on consensus opinion of clinical experts. Today, the AHRQ provides the National Guideline Clearinghouse, a searchable database of more than 2500 CPGs entered by numerous sources. While this knowledge management database can be easily used to locate a wide variety of CPGs, the user must examine the information presented with the CPG to determine that the CPG is current, was developed systematically, and is based on best evidence.

Other guidelines can be located on the U.S. Preventive Services Task Force (USPSTF) segment of the AHRQ website.[39] These recommendations focus on screening tests, counseling, immunizations, and chemoprophylaxis and are based on evidence summary work performed by the AHRQ. The USPSTF was convened by the U.S. Public Health Service in 1984 to systematically review the evidence of effectiveness of a wide range of clinical preventive services.

Critical appraisal of the various forms of knowledge is important. However, for clinical decision making, appraisal of guidelines is crucial for effective clinical care. A number of standards for critical appraisal of CPGs have been established and can be used to examine CPGs as clinical agencies consider adoption into practice. Fundamental to the use of evidence-based CPGs is the clinician's critical appraisal of those under consideration for adoption. Systematic

**Strength of Evidence
Rating**

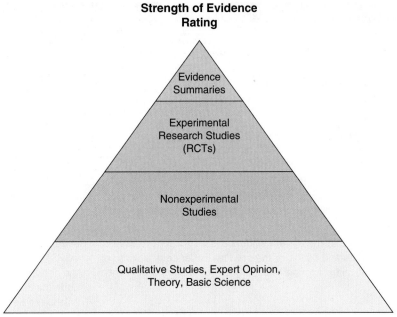

FIG 3-2 Strength of evidence hierarchy. *RCT*, Randomized controlled trial. (From Stevens KR, Clutter PC. Strength of evidence rating. Academic Center for Evidence-Based Practice. http://www.ACESTAR.uthscsa.edu. 2007. Accessed August 3, 2012. Used with permission.)

approaches have been developed, with a good example being the instrument used to assess practice guidelines developed by the AGREE (Appraisal of Guidelines for Research and Evaluation) enterprise.[40] The 23-item AGREE II instrument developed by this international collaboration is reliable and valid and outlines primary facets of the CPG to be appraised: scope and purpose, stakeholder involvement, rigor of development, clarity and presentation, application, and editorial independence. While the instrument is not easily used by the individual clinician, it is helpful to groups and organizations charged with adoption of specific CPGs. Box 3-4 identifies key elements to be examined when appraising a CPG.

Once located and critically appraised, a CPG can be considered for adoption into a specific clinical agency. Recommendations flowing from evidence are rated in terms of strength. The USPSTF uses a schema for rating its evidence-based recommendations.[39] It grades strength of recommendations according to one of five classifications (A, B, C, D, and I). The recommendation grade reflects the strength of evidence and magnitude of net benefit (benefits minus harms). Table 3-4 defines each grade and indicates the suggestion for practice.

Professional groups within the agency can move forward with confidence that all research evidence has been systematically gathered and amassed into a powerful conclusion of what will work. The evidence summary is vetted through clinical experts, and interpretations are made for direct clinical application. In instances where there is a gap in the evidence summary, the experts consider evidence of lower rating and finally add their own expertise into the fully developed CPG. Box 3-5 presents an example of point 3 in the form of a CPG for preventing falls in the elderly. Note that both the evidence and the recommendation are rated.

BOX 3-4 CRITICALLY APPRAISING A CLINICAL PRACTICE GUIDELINE

1. Why was this guideline developed?
2. What was the composition (expertise and disciplinary perspective) of the panel that developed the guideline?
3. What entity provided financial sponsorship?
4. What decision making processes were used in developing the guideline?
   a. What clinical question was the guideline developed to address?
   b. How was the evidence used in the guideline gathered and evaluated?
   c. Were gaps in the evidence explicitly identified?
   d. How explicitly is the available evidence linked to the recommendations in the guideline?
   e. If lower levels of evidence were incorporated (e.g., expert opinion) in the guideline, are these instances labeled explicitly and are the reasons for the inclusion of expert opinion, the line of reasoning, and the strength of extrapolation from other data clearly identified?
   f. How are patient preferences incorporated into the guideline?
   g. Is cost effectiveness considered?
   h. What is the mechanism and interval for updating the guideline?

A number of rating scales have been developed to convey the strength of the recommendation. Coupled with strength of evidence, the clinician can move forward with "Level 1" evidence and "Grade A" recommendation to support clinical decisions. The USPSTF adopted a system that links strength of evidence with strength of recommendation as follows:

TABLE 3-4 USPSTF GRADE, DEFINITION, AND SUGGESTION FOR PRACTICE

GRADE	DEFINITION	SUGGESTION FOR PRACTICE
A	The USPSTF recommends the service. There is high certainty that the net benefit is substantial.	Offer/provide this service.
B	The USPSTF recommends the service. There is high certainty that the net benefit is moderate or there is moderate certainty that the net benefit is moderate to substantial.	Offer/provide this service.
C	*Note: The following statement is undergoing revision.* Clinicians may provide this service to selected patients depending on individual circumstances. However, for most individuals without signs or symptoms there is likely to be only a small benefit from this service.	Offer/provide this service only if other considerations support the offering or providing of the service to an individual patient.
D	The USPSTF recommends against the service. There is moderate or high certainty that the service has no net benefit or that the harms outweigh the benefits.	Discourage the use of this service.
E	The USPSTF concludes that the current evidence is insufficient to assess the balance of benefits and harms of the service. Evidence is lacking, of poor quality, or conflicting, and the balance of benefits and harms cannot be determined.	Read the clinical considerations section of USPSTF Recommendation Statement. If the service is offered, patients should understand the uncertainty about the balance of benefits and harms.

From U.S. Preventive Services Task Force (USPSTF). U.S. Preventive Services Task Force ratings. USPSTF. http://www.uspreventiveservicestaskforce.org/uspstf07/ratingsv2.htm. 2007.
USPSTF, U.S. Preventive Services Task Force.

BOX 3-5 EXAMPLE OF STAR POINT 3: CLINICAL PRACTICE GUIDELINES FOR PREVENTING FALLS IN THE ELDERLY

Multifactorial Interventions

Strong—All older people with recurrent falls or assessed as being at increased risk of falling should be considered for an individualized multifactorial intervention. (Evidence level I)

Strong—In successful multifactorial intervention programs the following specific components are common (Evidence level I):

- Strength and balance training
- Home hazard assessment and intervention
- Vision assessment and referral
- Medication review with modification/withdrawal

From National Collaborating Centre for Nursing and Supportive Care. CPG for the Assessment and Prevention of Falls in Older People. London, United Kingdom: National Institute for Clinical Excellence; 2004. http://www.nice.org.uk/. Accessed June 27, 2012.

---

strength of the evidence as "A" (strongly recommends), "B" (recommends), "C" (no recommendation for or against), "D" (recommends against), or "I" (insufficient evidence to recommend for or against).[41] Box 3-6 presents three examples of USPSTF recommendations along with the grade of each recommendation.

As evidenced by the discussion, the translation of guidelines into practice is a labor-intensive process involving a significant cognitive load. In the busy world of healthcare, clinicians cannot routinely take the time to search out CPGs and translate their application to individual patients. However, using CPGs to design clinical decision support (CDS) systems can make it possible for busy clinicians to access evidence-based guidelines that have been individualized to the patient's needs and status at the point of care.

Point 4: Practice Integration

Once guidelines are produced, the recommended actions are clear. Next, the challenge is to integrate the clinical action into practice and thinking. This integration is accomplished through change at individual clinician, organizational, and policy levels. Integration inevitably involves change and integration of evidence into a myriad of health information technology (health IT) tools such as CDS, Infobuttons, order sets in electronic health records (EHRs), and evaluation of compliance using data warehouses or other big data sources. As advances and best practices emerge, it is essential that all members of the healthcare team be actively involved in making quality improvement and health IT changes. Healthcare providers, including nurses, are called on to be leaders and followers in contributing to such improvement at the individual level of care, as well as at the system level of care, together with other disciplines.[42]

Patient preference is taken into account at the point of integration, with patient and family circumstances guiding individualized EBP. Integration may not be straightforward because underlying evidence and science of healthcare is as yet incomplete. Also, computerized tools may not be available to assist in the process. As personal health records expand, health IT should be able to integrate patient preferences in a more electronic and systematic manner. In reviewing the USPSTF's highly developed, well-grounded recommendations presented in Box 3-6, it becomes clear that clinical judgment must be used and individualization to patient circumstances and preferences occurs in moving the

---

BOX 3-6	**EXAMPLES OF STAR POINT 3: USPSTF CLINICAL RECOMMENDATIONS AND GRADES**

Ocular Prophylaxis for Gonococcal Ophthalmia Neonatorum

Release Date: July 2011
  Summary of Recommendation
- The USPSTF recommends prophylactic ocular topical medication for all newborns for the prevention of gonococcal ophthalmia neonatorum.
Grade: *A Recommendation*

From U.S. Preventive Services Task Force (USPSTF). Ocular prophylaxis for gonococcal ophthalmia neonatorum. USPSTF. http://www.uspreventiveservicestaskforce.org/uspstf/uspsgononew.htm. 2011.

Prevention of Falls in Community-Dwelling Older Adults

Current Recommendations
  Release Date: May 2012
- The USPSTF recommends exercise or physical therapy and vitamin D supplementation to prevent falls in community-dwelling adults aged 65 years or older who are at increased risk for falls.
Grade: *B Recommendation*
- The USPSTF does not recommend automatically performing an in-depth multifactorial risk assessment in conjunction with comprehensive management of identified risks to prevent falls in community-dwelling adults aged 65 years or older because the likelihood of benefit is small. In determining whether this service is appropriate in individual cases, patients and clinicians should consider the balance of benefits and harms on the basis of the circumstances of prior falls, comorbid medical conditions, and patient values.
Grade: *C Recommendation*

From U.S. Preventive Services Task Force (USPSTF). Prevention of falls in community-dwelling older adults. USPSTF. http://www.uspreventiveservicestaskforce.org/uspstf/uspsfalls.htm. 2012.

Screening for Prostate Cancer

Current Recommendation
  Release Date: May 2012
- The USPSTF recommends against PSA-based screening for prostate cancer.
Grade: *D Recommendation*
  This recommendation applies to men in the general U.S. population, regardless of age. This recommendation does not include the use of the prostate-specific antigen (PSA) test for surveillance after diagnosis or treatment of prostate cancer; the use of the PSA test for this indication is outside the scope of the USPSTF.

From U.S. Preventive Services Task Force (USPSTF). Screening for prostate cancer. USPSTF. http://www.uspreventiveservicestaskforce.org/prostatecancerscreening.htm. 2012.

BOX 3-7	**EXAMPLE OF STAR POINT 4: AN INNOVATION**

Fall Prevention Toolkit Facilitates Customized Risk Assessment and Prevention Strategies, Reducing Inpatient Falls
What They Did
Periodic assessment, specific risk factors, customized interventions
Computerized program produces tailored prevention recommendations
Individualized care plan, educational handout, bedside alert poster

Did It Work?
Significantly reduced falls, particularly in >65

Evidence Rating
Strong: Cluster randomized study comparing fall rates

Adapted from Dykes P. Interprofessional nursing quality research initiative. AHRQ Health Care Innovations Exchange. http://www.innovations.ahrq.gov/content.aspx?id=3094. Accessed June 27, 2012.
AHRQ, Agency for Healthcare Research and Quality.

evidence-based recommendations into practice. It is at this point in the transformation of knowledge that the whole of the EBP definition becomes clear: EBP is the integration of best research knowledge, clinical expertise, and patient preference to produce best practice.

Resources and Examples

The AHRQ Health Care Innovations Exchange provides a venue for sharing "what works at our place" along with the evidence of how the innovation was tested.[7] The Health Care Innovations Exchange was created to speed the implementation of new and better ways of delivering healthcare. This online collection of more than 700 innovation profiles supports the AHRQ's mission to improve the quality of healthcare and reduce disparities. The Health Care Innovations Exchange offers front-line health professionals a variety of opportunities to share, learn about, and hasten adoption of tested innovations. It also contains more than 1500 quality tools suitable for a range of healthcare settings and populations. New innovation profiles and quality tools are continuously entered into the Exchange. Box 3-7 presents an example of an innovation profile.

Practice guidelines for individual agencies are commonly integrated throughout the organization in the form of policy and procedure manuals. Increasingly, agencies are raising the standard of excellence in local policies and procedures by moving toward EBP guidelines and away from non-EBP manuals. Health IT approaches to integrate EBP guidelines into care hold promise of placing such best practices into point-of-care decision making. For example, as clinical summaries and evidence-based order sets can be available in EHRs, credible practice guidelines can be linked and pushed forward in CDS applications.

Point 5: Evaluation

The fifth stage in knowledge transformation is evaluation. Practice changes are followed by evaluation of the impact on a wide variety of outcomes, including effectiveness of the care in producing desired patient outcomes, redesign of care, patient outcomes, population outcomes, efficiency and cost factors in the care (short term and long term), and satisfaction of both healthcare providers and patients. Evaluation of specific outcomes has risen to a high level of public interest.[3,4] As a result, quality indicators are being established for healthcare improvement and for public reporting. Additional information on how EHRs and computerization can be used to provide evaluation data (knowledge discovery and data mining) is provided in Chapter 4. Chapter 10 provides more detailed information about integrating EBP into CDS applications.

Resources and Examples

Among the significant entities establishing quality indicator sets is the AHRQ, through its *National Healthcare Quality Report* (NHQR).[4] This report tracks the healthcare system through quality measures, such as the percentage of heart attack patients who received recommended care when they reached the hospital or the percentage of children who received recommended vaccinations. The 2011 NHQR identifies trends in effectiveness of care, patient safety, timeliness of care, patient centeredness, efficiency of care, care coordination, and healthcare system infrastructure. The reports present, in chart form, the latest available findings on quality of and access to healthcare. Initiated in 2004, this annual report is designed as a chart book that contains data on more than 250 healthcare quality measures derived from more than 45 databases. Selection of tracked measures is guided by an advisory body representing many Health and Human Services agencies. Key selection criteria include measures that are the most important and scientifically supported. With these measures the NHQR provides an annual snapshot of how our healthcare system is performing and the extent to which healthcare quality and disparities have improved or worsened over time. Figure 3-3 is a graph of a quality measure from the NHQR.

Another influential entity establishing quality measures is the National Quality Forum (NQF), acting as a nonprofit organization that brings together a variety of healthcare stakeholders (e.g., consumer organizations, public and private purchasers, physicians, nurses, hospitals, accrediting and certifying bodies, supporting industries, and healthcare research and quality improvement organizations). The NQF's mission includes consensus building on priorities for performance improvement, endorsing national consensus standards for measuring and reporting on performance, and education and outreach.[43] An example of an NQF-endorsed measure for palliative care is presented in Box 3-8.

An important collection of quality measures is assembled in the National Quality Measures Clearinghouse (NQMC), an initiative of the AHRQ.[44] The NQMC is a database and website for information on evidence-based healthcare quality

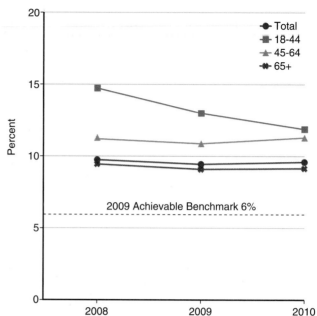

FIG 3-3 Example of star point 5. Hospice patients aged 18 and older who did *not* receive the correct amount of help for feelings of anxiety or sadness, by age, 2008-2010. (From Agency for Healthcare Research and Quality.)

BOX 3-8   EXAMPLE OF STAR POINT 5 FROM THE NATIONAL QUALITY FORUM

Palliative Care and End-of-Life Care Measures

1626: Patients admitted to the ICU who have care preferences documented.

Description: Percentage of vulnerable adults admitted to ICU who survive at least 48 hours who have their care preferences documented within 48 hours *or* documentation as to why this was not done.

Adapted from National Quality Forum (NQF). *NQF Measure Endorsement: 2012 Mid-Year Review.* Washington, DC: NQF; 2012. *ICU,* Intensive care unit.

---

measures and measure sets. Its purpose is to promote widespread access to quality measures by the healthcare community and other interested individuals. The key targets are practitioners, healthcare providers, health plans, integrated delivery systems, purchasers, and others. The aim is to provide an accessible mechanism for obtaining detailed information on quality measures and to further their dissemination, implementation, and use in order to inform healthcare decisions. Box 3-9 presents a measure from the NQMC. However, measuring the status of healthcare at any point in time does not complete the feedback circle where this information is used to improve practice. Computerized tools for analyzing the big data in these national databases and teasing out the factors influencing healthcare outcomes will provide a basis for evidence in the search for other levels of EBP.

> **BOX 3-9 EXAMPLE OF STAR POINT 5 FROM THE NATIONAL QUALITY MEASURES CLEARINGHOUSE**
>
> Fall Risk Management:
> % of Medicare members who discussed falls problems with their provider
> - 75 years of age or older; or
> - 56 to 74 years of age with balance or walking problems or a fall in past 12 months
> - Seen by provider in past year and
> - Discussed falls or balance problems
>
> Collected using Medicare Health Outcome Survey

From National Quality Measures Clearinghouse (NQMC). *Measure Summary: Fall Risk Management*. Rockville, MD: Agency for Healthcare Research and Quality; 2012.

CONCLUSION AND FUTURE DIRECTIONS

Informatics and IT hold great promise for achieving full integration of EBP into all care, for every patient, every time. The EBP frameworks provide a foundation upon which informatics solutions can be constructed to move evidence into practice. As seen in the examples addressing each point in the ACE Star Model, knowledge can be sorted and organized into its various forms. The national efforts that were cited have resulted in the availability of a number of significant web-based information resources to support each point on the ACE Star Model. However, translating information stored in these information resources to guide decision making at the point of care will require new and innovative knowledge management tools.

Informatics can greatly add to support of EBP, patient-centered care, and transitions of care across settings. Such technology can greatly assist in the exchange of health information for continuity and quality of care. Health informatics is also essential in improving healthcare decision making through the use of integrated datasets and knowledge management.

The success of improvement through best (evidence-based) practice could be boosted with greater understanding of the context in which such changes are being made. Once the knowledge is transformed into recommendations (best practices), integration of EBP into practice requires change at levels that include the patient and family, individual provider, microsystem, and macrosystem. The good intentions of an individual provider to use practice guidelines in decision making can be either supported or thwarted by the automated clinical information systems at the point of care.

Successful models of EBP are emerging. For example, the national team performance training, Team Strategies and Tools to Enhance Performance and Patient Safety (TeamSTEPPS), has been promoted across military healthcare since 1995, with a "civilian" rollout initiated in 2006.[45] The program is built on a solid evidential base from human factors engineering and solves urgent problems from defects arising from team-based care. The program has demonstrated improvements in communication and teamwork skills among healthcare professionals. However, it is clear from the history of adoption that context is having a large effect not only on uptake of TeamSTEPPS, but also on sustainment (H. King, personal communication, July 15, 2012). Decisions to adopt and sustain are thought to be heavily dependent on the organizational context and the information systems within that context. A culture of patient safety in an organization seems to determine the decision to adopt, as well as the sustainment processes and systems that support EBP. Other important organizational characteristics are the learning climate, culture, and high reliability of the available information management and communication tools.

Measurement and classification of information into databases for retrieval and analysis are only the first steps in building EBP decision support tools. In addition to identifying and measuring essential constructs, the foundational work of taxonomy development and classification schema is essential. Specialists in the field of informatics will continue to develop IT tools that are useful at the point of care by identifying, classifying, and guiding systems to capture context data previously lost in manual systems. When paired with data about individual patients, new evidence for performance improvement and organizational effectiveness can be detected.

In a recent report, the role of health IT in quality measurement was circumscribed.[46] Past quality processes were conducted via manual chart entry, manual chart abstraction, and analysis of administrative claims data. In locations with existing health IT, advances are seen. As information systems are created and expanded, the ability to pull meaningful data from the point of care is increasingly computerized. A major potential for health IT is to evolve existing measures into electronic measures and computerize data collection.[46]

The long-term goal for improving health IT–enabled quality measurement is to achieve a robust information infrastructure that supports national quality measurement and reporting strategies. Key goals include interoperability that ensures that EHRs can share information for care coordination, patient-centered care, and cost savings. Such interoperability relies on harmonizing standards. Information exchange, integrating interoperability standards into vendor products, and data linkage are critical for advancement.[46]

A number of challenges must be overcome to achieve the next generation of health IT–enabled quality measurement. First, consensus among quality stakeholders is required to move forward on topics such as the purpose of measurement; achieving patient-centricity in a fragmented health delivery system; alignment of incentives; ownership and funding; increased information exchange; and ensuring privacy, security, and confidentiality. Second, measurement challenges to be overcome include measures valuable to consumers, measures to assess value, measures for specialty uses, and accounting for variations in risk in measurement. Third, technology challenges to be overcome include expansion of emeasures; advancement in measure capture technologies; advancement in patient-focused technologies, health information exchange, interoperability, and standards; Internet connectivity; and aggregation and analysis. Importantly, the report concludes with a call for stakeholder input to inform pathways to achieving the next generation of quality improvement, an important opportunity in which healthcare providers can engage.[46]

Today's health informatics research agenda mirrors the agendas set in 1993 and 1998, includes an expansion to inter-disciplinary teams, and reflects farsighted goals related to research needed in evidence-based quality improvement.[47] The shifting emphasis on performance improvement and EBP results in the need for research that tests innovations in real-world settings. When the conditions for standardization and interoperability of EHRs are satisfied, patient-specific data can be connected across healthcare settings. Once this occurs, knowledge discovery about coordination and care processes can be expanded through the use of data generated routinely from care settings. By organizing the informatics approach of data, information, knowledge, and wisdom into the EBP knowledge transformation and application in real-world settings, the field of quality improvement and EBP translation into practice can be advanced.

REFERENCES

1. Stevens KR. *ACE Star Model of EBP: Knowledge Transformation.* San Antonio, TX: Academic Center for Evidence-Based Practice, University of Texas Health Science Center in San Antonio; 2004.
2. Institute of Medicine. *To Err Is Human: Building a Safer Health System.* Washington, DC: National Academies Press; 2000.
3. Institute of Medicine. *Crossing the Quality Chasm: A New Health System for the 21st Century.* Washington, DC: National Academies Press; 2001.
4. Agency for Healthcare Research and Quality (AHRQ). *National Healthcare Quality Report* AHRQ Publication No. 12-0005. Bethesda, MD: AHRQ; 2011.
5. American Association of Colleges of Nursing (AACN). *The Essentials of Baccalaureate Education for Professional Nursing Practice.* Washington, DC: AACN; 2008.
6. Accreditation Council for Graduate Medical Education (ACGME). *Common Program Requirements.* Chicago, IL: ACGME; 2007.
7. Agency for Healthcare Research and Quality (AHRQ). AHRQ Health Care Innovations Exchange. AHRQ. http://www.innovations.ahrq.gov/. 2012.
8. Mitchell SA, Fisher CA, Hastings CE, Silverman LB, Wallen GR. A thematic analysis of theoretical models for translational science in nursing: mapping the field. *Nurs Outlook.* 2010;58(6):287-300.
9. Melnyk BM, Fineout-Overholt E, Mays MZ. The evidence-based practice beliefs and implementation scales: psychometric properties of two new instruments. *Worldviews Evid Based Nurs.* 2008;5(4):208-216.
10. Newhouse RP, Dearholt SL, Poe SS, Pugh LC, White KM. *Johns Hopkins Nursing Evidence-Based Practice Model and Guidelines.* New York, NY: Sigma Theta Tau International Honor Society of Nursing; 2007.
11. Titler MG, Kleiber C, Steelman VJ, et al. The Iowa model of evidence-based practice to promote quality care. *Crit Care Nurs Clin North Am.* 2001;13(4):497-509.
12. Stetler CB, Ritchie J, Rycroft-Malone J, Schultz A, Charns M. Improving quality of care through routine, successful implementation of evidence-based practice at the bedside: an organizational case study protocol using the Pettigrew and Whipp model of strategic change. *Implement Sci.* 2007;2(1):3.
13. Kitson AL, Rycroft-Malone J, Harvey G, McCormack B, Seers K, Titchen A. Evaluating the successful implementation of evidence into practice using the PARiHS framework: theoretical and practical challenges. *Implement Sci.* 2008;3:1.
14. Rycroft-Malone J. The PARiHS framework: a framework for guiding the implementation of evidence-based practice. *J Nurs Care Qual.* 2004;19(4):297-304.
15. Rycroft-Malone J, Kitson A, Harvey G, et al. Ingredients for change: revisiting a conceptual framework. *Qual Saf Health Care.* 2002;11(2):174-180.
16. Vratny A, Shriver D. A conceptual model for growing evidence-based practice. *Nurs Adm Q.* 2007;31:162-170.
17. Doran DM, Sidani S. Outcomes-focused knowledge translation: a framework for knowledge translation and patient outcomes improvement. *Worldviews Evid Based Nurs.* 2007;4(1):3-13.
18. Weiner BJ, Lewis MA, Linnan LA. Using organization theory to understand the determinants of effective implementation of worksite health promotion programs. *Health Educ Res.* 2009;24(2):292-305.
19. Graham ID, Tetroe J. Some theoretical underpinnings of knowledge translation. *Acad Emerg Med.* 2007;14(11):936-941.
20. Logan J, Graham ID. Toward a comprehensive interdisciplinary model of health care research use. *Sci Commun.* 1998;20(2):227-246.
21. Baumbusch JL, Kirkham SR, Khan KB, et al. Pursuing common agendas: a collaborative model for knowledge translation between research and practice in clinical settings. *Res Nurs Health.* 2008;31(2):130-140.
22. Swinburn B, Gill T, Kumanyika S. Obesity prevention: a proposed framework for translating evidence into action. *Obes Rev.* 2005;6(1):23-33.
23. Mitton C, Adair CE, McKenzie E, Patten SB, Perry BW. Knowledge transfer and exchange: review and synthesis of the literature. *Milbank Q.* 2007;85(4):729-768.
24. Armstrong R, Waters E, Roberts H, et al. The role and theoretical evolution of knowledge translation and exchange in public health. *J Public Health.* 2006;28(4):384-389.
25. Brachaniec M, Tillier W, Dell F. The Institute of Musculoskeletal Health and Arthritis (IMHA) Knowledge Exchange Task Force: an innovative approach to knowledge translation. *J Can Chiropr Assoc.* 2006;50(1):8-13.
26. Graham ID, Logan J, Harrison MB, et al. Lost in knowledge translation: time for a map? *J Contin Educ Health Prof.* 2006;26:13-24.
27. Wandersman A, Duffy J, Flaspohler P, et al. Bridging the gap between prevention research and practice: the interactive systems framework for dissemination and implementation. *Am J Community Psychol.* 2008;41(3-4):171-181.
28. Institute of Medicine. *Knowing What Works in Health Care: A Roadmap for the Nation.* Washington, DC: National Academies Press; 2008.
29. Weir C, Staggers N, Laukert T. Reviewing the impact of computerized provider order entry on clinical outcomes: the quality of systematic reviews. *Int J Med Inform.* 2012;81:219-231.
30. Weir C, Staggers N, Phansalkar S. The state of the evidence for computerized provider order entry: a systematic review and

analysis of the quality of the literature. *Int J Med Inform.* 2009; 78(6):365-374.

31. Higgins JPT, Green S, eds. Cochrane handbook for systematic reviews of interventions. The Cochrane Collaboration. http://www.cochrane-handbook.org. 2011.

32. The Cochrane Collaboration. The Cochrane Database of Systematic Reviews. The Cochrane Collaboration. http://www.cochrane.org/policy-manual/223-cochrane-database-systematic-reviews. 2011.

33. Institute of Medicine (IOM). *Clinical Practice Guidelines We Can Trust.* Washington, DC: National Academies Press; 2011.

34. Clancy CM, Cronin K. Evidence-based decision making: global evidence, local decisions. *Health Aff.* 2005;24(1):151-162.

35. Oncology Nursing Society (ONS). Putting evidence into practice. ONS. http://www.ons.org/research/pep. 2012.

36. Mitchell SA, Beck SL, Hood LE, Moore K, Tanner ER. Putting evidence into practice: evidence-based interventions for fatigue during and following cancer and its treatment. *Clin J Oncol Nurs.* 2009;11(1):99-113.

37. Center for Evidence-Based Medicine (CEBM). Levels of evidence and grades of recommendations. CEBM. http://www.cebm.net/index.aspx?o=5653. Sept 2012.

38. Stevens KR, Clutter PC. Strength of evidence rating. Academic Center for Evidence-Based Practice. http://www.ACESTAR.uthscsa.edu. 2007. Accessed August 3, 2012.

39. U.S. Preventive Services Task Force (USPSTF). U.S. Preventive Services Task Force ratings. USPSTF. http://uspreventiveservicestaskforce.org/uspstf07/ratingsv2.htm. 2011. Accessed August 3, 2012.

40. Appraisal of Guidelines, Research, and Evaluation (AGREE). About the AGREE Enterprise. AGREE. http://www.agreetrust.org/. 2010.

41. Harris RP, Helfand M, Woolf SH, et al. Current methods of the U.S. Preventive Services Task Force: a review of the process. *Am J Prev Med.* 2001;20(3 suppl):21-35.

42. Institute of Medicine. *The Future of Nursing: Focus on Scope of Practice.* Washington, DC: National Academies Press; 2010.

43. National Quality Forum (NQF). http://www.qualityforum.org/Home.aspx. 2012.

44. Agency for Healthcare Research and Quality (AHRQ). *National Quality Measures Clearinghouse (NQMC).* Bethesda, MD: Agency for Healthcare Research and Quality; 2012.

45. Agency for Healthcare Research and Quality (AHRQ). *TeamSTEPPS™: National Implementation.* Rockville, MD: Agency for Healthcare Research and Quality (AHRQ). 2012. http://teamstepps.ahrq.gov/.

46. Anderson KM, Marsh CA, Flemming AC, Isenstein H, Reynolds J. *Quality Measurement Enabled by Health IT: Overview, Possibilities, and Challenges.* AHRQ Publication No. 12-0061-EF. Rockville, MD: Agency for Healthcare Research and Quality; 2012.

47. Bakken S, Stone PW, Larson EL. A nursing informatics research agenda for 2008-18: contextual influences and key components. *Nurs Outlook.* 2008;56:206-214.

DISCUSSION QUESTIONS

1. Review the three categories of EPB models and discuss how these models might be used to guide the development of EBP.

2. Discuss why automation is required if EBP is to become reality in busy clinical settings.

3. How can the design of a healthcare information system support or thwart the use of EPB guidelines at the point of care? Give examples from your own experience if possible.

4. Explore the AHRQ Health Care Innovations Exchange at www.innovations.ahrq.gov/index.aspx. Discuss how automation and informatics-based tools could be used to bring resources from this site to the point of care.

5. Analyze the following statement and determine whether you do or do not support it: "With the development of a fully integrated national health information system, big data reflecting patient outcomes will replace the role of research studies in developing EBP guidelines."

CASE STUDY

You are consulting with the education and practice development team in a large tertiary care hospital serving a region comprising mostly rural communities. The team is responsible for strengthening the implementation of evidence-based practice based on outcomes. Over the next 2 years, it must set performance objectives to (1) strengthen screening for pain, depression, and adverse health behaviors (smoking, excess alcohol intake, and body mass index [BMI] greater than 30) at intake for all adult admissions; (2) implement comprehensive geriatric assessment for all those over age 65 hospitalized for more than 7 days or readmitted within less than 3 days following discharge; and (3) promote care team performance.

The hospital has 200 adult admissions each week and has implemented a fully electronic health record. Guideline dissemination generally occurs through educational venues or via the electronic policy and procedure manual. The method of documentation for narrative notes is documentation by exception using SOAP (subjective, objective, assessment, and plan) and the hospital has also made extensive use of checklists to complement the documentation system.

Discussion Questions

1. Using clinical guidelines and standards of care, identify what data elements should be included in the EHR assessment and evaluation screens if these goals are to be achieved.

2. Identify how information system defaults and alerts could be used to achieve these goals.

3. Once screening has been improved, what are the next steps in improving patient outcomes?

4. How could the EHR be designed to support these outcome-related goals?

Knowledge Discovery, Data Mining, and Practice-Based Evidence

Mollie R. Cummins, Ginette A. Pepper, and Susan D. Horn

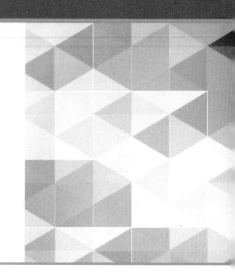

The next step to comparative effectiveness research is to conduct more prospective large-scale observational cohort studies with the rigor described here for knowledge discovery and data mining (KDDM) and practice-based evidence (PBE) studies.

OBJECTIVES

At the completion of this chapter the reader will be prepared to:

1. Define the goals and processes employed in knowledge discovery and data mining (KDDM) and practice-based evidence (PBE) designs

2. Analyze the strengths and weaknesses of observational designs in general and of KDDM and PBE specifically

3. Identify the roles and activities of the informatics specialist in KDDM and PBE in healthcare environments

KEY TERMS

Comparative effectiveness research, 69
Confusion matrix, 62
Data mining, 61
Knowledge discovery and data mining (KDDM), 56

Machine learning, 56
Natural language processing (NLP), 58
Practice-based evidence (PBE), 56
Preprocessing, 56

ABSTRACT

The advent of the electronic health record (EHR) and other large electronic datasets has revolutionized efficient access to comprehensive data across large numbers of patients and the concomitant capacity to detect subtle patterns in these data even with missing or less than optimal data quality. This chapter introduces two approaches to knowledge building from clinical data: (1) knowledge discovery and data mining (KDDM) and (2) practice-based evidence (PBE). The use of machine learning methods in retrospective analysis of routinely collected clinical data characterizes KDDM. KDDM enables us to efficiently and effectively analyze large amounts of data and develop clinical knowledge models for decision support. PBE integrates health information technology (health IT) products with cohort identification, prospective data collection, and extensive front-line clinician and patient input for comparative effectiveness research. PBE can uncover best practices and combinations of treatments for specific types of patients while achieving many of the presumed advantages of randomized controlled trials (RCTs).

INTRODUCTION

Leaders need to foster a shared learning culture for improving healthcare. This extends beyond the local department or institution to a value for creating generalizable knowledge to improve care worldwide. Sound, rigorous methods are needed by researchers and health professionals to create this knowledge and address practical questions about risks, benefits, and costs of interventions as they occur in actual clinical practice. Typical questions are as follows:

- Are treatments used in daily practice associated with intended outcomes?
- Can we predict adverse events in time to prevent or ameliorate them?
- What treatments work best for which patients?

- With limited financial resources, what are the best interventions to use for specific types of patients?
- What types of individuals are at risk for certain conditions?

Answers to these questions can help clinicians, patients, researchers, healthcare administrators, and policy-makers to learn from and improve real-world, everyday clinical practice. Two important emerging approaches to knowledge building from clinical data are KDDM and PBE, both of which are described in this chapter.

Research Designs for Knowledge Discovery

The gold standard research design for answering questions about the efficacy of treatments is an experimental design, often referred to as a randomized controlled trial (RCT). An RCT requires random assignment of patients to treatment condition as well as other design features, such as tightly controlled inclusion criteria, to assure as much as posible that the only difference between the experimental and control groups is the treatment (or placebo) that each group receives. The strength of the RCT is the degree of confidence in causal inferences, in other words, that the therapeutic intervention caused the clinical effects (or lack of effects). Drawbacks of the RCT include the time and expense required to conduct a comparison of a small number of treatment options and the limited generalizability of the results to patients, settings, intervention procedures, and measures that differ from the specific conditions in the study condition. Further, RCTs have little value in generating unique hypotheses and possibilities.

Observational research designs can also yield valuable information to characterize disease risk and generate hypotheses about potentially effective treatments. In addition, observational research is essential to determine the effectiveness of treatments or how well treatments work in actual practice. In observational studies the investigator merely records what occurs under naturalistic conditions, such as which individual gets what therapy and what outcomes result or which variables are associated with what outcomes. Of course, with observational studies the patients who receive different treatments generally differ on many other variables (selection bias) since treatments were determined by clinician judgment rather than random assignment and selection. For example, one therapy may be prescribed for sicker patients under natural conditions or may not be accessible to uninsured patients. Since diagnostic approaches vary in clinical practice, patients with the same diagnosis may have considerable differences in the actual condition.

Observational studies can be either prospective (data are generated after the study commences) or retrospective (data were generated before the study). Chart review has traditonally been the most common approach to retrospective observational research. However, chart review previously required tedious and time-consuming data extraction and the requisite data may be missing, inconsistent, or of poor quality. Prospective studies have the advantage that the measurements can be standardized, but recording both research data and clinical data constitutes a documentation burden for clinicians that cannot be accommodated in typical clinical settings unless the research and clinical data elements are combined to become the standard for documentation.

EHRs and Knowledge Discovery

The advent of the EHR and other large electronic datasets has revolutionized observational studies by increasing the potential for efficient access to comprehensive data, reflecting large numbers of patients and the capacity to detect subtle patterns in the data, even with missing or less than optimal data quality. With very large samples available from EHRs at relatively low cost, it is often possible to compensate with statistical controls for the lack of randomization in the practice setting. With electronic data, standardized data collection is facilitated and data validity can be enhanced, minimizing the documentation burden by using clinical data for research purposes.

Increased adoption of EHRs and other health information systems has resulted in vast amounts of structured and textual data. Stored on servers in a data warehouse (a large data repository integrating data across clinical, administrative, and other systems), the data may be a partial or complete copy of all data collected in the course of care provision. The data can include billing information, physician and nursing notes, laboratory results, radiology images, and numerous other diverse types of data. In some settings data describing individual patients and their characteristics, health issues, treatments, and outcomes has accumulated for years, forming longitudinal records. The clinical record can also be linked to repositories of genetic or familial data.[1-3] These data constitute an incredible resource that is underused for scientific research in biomedicine and nursing.

The potential of using these data stores for the advancement of scientific knowledge and patient care is widely acknowledged. However, the lack of availability of tools and technology to adequately manage the data deluge has proven to be an Achilles' heel. Very large data resources, typically on the terabyte scale or larger, require highly specialized approaches to storage, management, extraction, and analysis. Moreover, the data may not be useful. Data quality can be poor and require substantial additional processing prior to use.

Clinical concepts are typically represented in the EHR in a way that supports healthcare delivery but not necessarily research. For example, pain might be qualitatively described in a patient's note and EHR as "mild" or "better." This may meet the immediate need for documentation and care but it does not allow the researcher to measure differences in pain over time and across patients, as would measurement using a pain scale. Clinical concepts may not be adequately measured or represented in a way that enables scientific

TABLE 4-1	CHARACTERISTICS OF KNOWLEDGE DISCOVERY AND DATA MINING (KDDM) AND PRACTICE-BASED EVIDENCE (PBE)	
CHARACTERISTIC	**KDDM**	**PBE**
Description	Application of machine learning and statistical methods for pattern discovery	Participatory research approach requiring documentation of predefined process and outcome data and analysis
Goal	Develop models to predict future events or infer missing information	Determine the effectiveness of multiple interventions on multiple outcomes in actual practice environment
Design classification	Observational (descriptive)	Observational (descriptive)
Temporal aspects	Retrospective	Prospective
Typical sample size	1000-1,000,000 or more, depending on project and available data	800-2000+

analysis. Data quality affects the feasibility of secondary analysis.

Knowledge Building Using Health IT

Two observational approaches to knowledge building from health IT can be employed for research and clinical performance improvement. One approach is based on machine learning applied to retrospective analysis of routinely collected clinical data and a second approach is based on increasing integration of health IT with cohort identification, front-line knowledge, and prospective data collection for research and clinical care.

Knowledge discovery and data mining (KDDM), the first approach, uses pattern discovery in large amounts of clinical and biomedical data and entails the use of software tools that facilitate the extraction, sampling, and large-scale cleaning and preprocessing of data. KDDM also makes use of specialized analytic methods, characteristically machine learning methods, to identify patterns in a semiautomated fashion. This level of analysis far exceeds the types of descriptive summaries typically presented by dashboard applications, such as a clinical summary for a patient. Instead, KDDM is used to build tools that support clinical decision making, generate hypotheses for scientific evaluation, and identify links between genotype and phenotype. KDDM can also be used to "patch" weaknesses in clinical data that pose a barrier to research. For example, if poor data quality is a barrier to automatic identification of patients with type II diabetes from diagnostic codes, a machine learning approach could be used to more completely and accurately identify the patients on the basis of text documents and laboratory and medication data.

Practice-based evidence (PBE) is an example of the second approach. PBE studies are observational cohort studies that attempt to mitigate the weaknesses traditionally associated with observational designs. This is accomplished by exhaustive attention to determining patient characteristics that may confound conclusions about the effectiveness of an intervention.

For example, observational studies might indicate that aerobic exercise is superior to nonaerobic exercise in preventing falls. But if the prescribers tend to order nonaerobic exercise for those who are more debilitated, severity of illness is a confounder and should be controlled in the analysis. PBE studies use large samples and diverse sources of patients to improve sample representativeness, power, and external validity. Generally there are 800 or more subjects, which is considerably more than in a typical RCT but far less than in a KDDM study. PBE uses approaches similar to community-based participatory research by including front-line clinicians and patients in the design, execution, and analysis of studies, as well as their data elements, to improve relevance to real-world practice. Finally, PBE uses detailed standardized structured documentation of interventions, which is ideally incorporated into the standard electronic documentation.

This method requires training and quality control checks for reliability of the measures of the actual process of care. Statistical analysis involves determining bivariate and multivariate correlations among patient characteristics, intervention process steps, and outcomes. PBE can uncover best practices and combinations of treatments for specific types of patients while achieving many of the presumed advantages of RCTs, especially the presumed advantage that RCTs control for patient differences through randomization. Front-line clinicians treating the study patients lead the study design and analyses of the data prospectively based on clinical expertise, rather than relying on machines to detect patterns as in KDDM. The characteristics of KDDM and PBE are summarized in Table 4-1. Both techniques are detailed in the following sections.

KNOWLEDGE DISCOVERY AND DATA MINING

KDDM is a process in which machine learning and statistical methods are applied to analyze large amounts of data. Frequently, the goal of analysis is to develop models that predict future events or infer missing information based on available data. Methods of KDDM are preferred for this type of endeavor because they are effective for analyzing very large repositories of clinical data and for analyzing complex, non-linear relationships. Models developed on the basis of routinely collected clinical data are advantageous for several reasons:

1. KDDM models access and leverage the valuable information contained in large repositories of clinical data
2. Models can be developed from very large sample sizes or entire populations
3. Models based on routinely collected data can be implemented in computerized systems to support decision making for individual patients
4. Models induced directly from data using machine learning methods often perform better than models manually developed by human experts

For example, Walton and colleagues developed a model that forecasts an impending respiratory syncytial virus (RSV) outbreak.[4] RSV is a virus that causes bronchiolitis in children, and severe cases warrant hospitalization. RSV outbreaks cause dramatic increases in census at pediatric hospitals, so advance warning of an impending RSV outbreak would allow pediatric hospitals to plan staffing and supplies. Some evidence indicates that weather is related to outbreaks of RSV and RSV outbreaks are known to follow a biennial pattern, information that may be useful for predicting outbreaks in advance. Given these circumstances the authors built a model using historical data that predicts RSV outbreaks up to 3 weeks in advance. These types of models can be especially effective in designing clinical decision support (CDS) systems. CDS systems are computer applications that assist healthcare providers in making clinical decisions about patients and are explained in detail in Chapter 10. The design of individual CDS systems varies and can be as simple as an alert that warns about potential drug–drug interaction.[5] Every CDS system is based on some underlying algorithm or rules and on existing or entered patient data. These rules must be specified in machine-readable code that is compatible with patient data stored in an EHR or other applications. Historically, clinical practice guidelines have not been expressed as a set of adequately explicit rules and could not be executed by a machine. See, for example, Lyng and Pederson and Isern and Moreno for a detailed discussion of this issue.[6,7] While a human being can reason on the basis of conditions such as "moderate improvement" or "diminished level of consciousness," a machine cannot. CDS models must consist of rules, conditions, and dependencies described in terms of machine-interpretable relationships and specific data values. Moreover, the algorithms and rules must be executable over the data as they are coded in the information system.

For example, gender may be included in a set of rules. If the rule is based on a gender variable coded with the values male, female, or unknown, it will not work in a system where gender is coded as 0, 1, 2, 3, or null, where 0 = male, 1 = female, 2 = transgender, 3 = unknown, and null = missing. While relatively simple changes could adapt the rule set for use in a system with different coding of gender, other variables pose a greater challenge. Some necessary variables may not exist as coded data in an information system or may be represented in a variety of ways that cannot be resolved as easily as gender can be.

In recent years there has been a substantial effort to develop computer-interpretable guidelines—guidelines that are expressed as an adequately explicit set of rules—with some success.[8] KDDM is also advantageous in this situation because it develops *only* machine-executable algorithms or rules, based on native data. Every model could potentially be used in a CDS system. Moreover, in situations where there is insufficient evidence to fully specify rules, the rules can be induced from a large sample of real-life examples using KDDM.

Retrieving a Dataset for Analysis

The process of KDDM, depicted in Figure 4-1, encompasses multiple steps and actions. Data must first be extracted from the clinical data warehouse. To review, data warehouses are a complex, vast collection of databases and it is usually necessary to join a number of tables to construct a usable dataset for KDDM purposes. To accomplish this investigators must collaborate closely with informatics specialists to develop effective queries, queries that select the clinical data relevant to the specific KDDM project with a sufficient but not overwhelming sample size.

To request the appropriate data, investigators and clinicians first need to understand how the concepts of interest are represented (coded) in the health IT product. In many health IT products, for example, laboratory tests are coded according to the standard Logical Observation Identifier Names and Codes (LOINC) terminology.[9] To ensure that the extracted dataset contains urinalysis data, for example, it will be necessary to first determine how and where a urinalysis is coded. For example, in the case of Veterans Health Administration (VHA) data, this may entail identification of the LOINC codes used to represent urinalysis results. For less precise concepts, such as mental health diagnoses, multiple codes may be relevant. Some data may not be structured and may be captured only in text documents such as discharge summaries. Information extraction from these documents can be accomplished and represents an active area of research and development.[10]

Queries written in a specialized programming language (Structured Query Language or SQL) are used to retrieve data from the data warehouse according to a researcher's specifications. Currently, investigators and healthcare organization IT personnel collaborate to develop effective queries. The code used to execute the query is saved as a file and can be reused in the future or repeatedly reused on a scheduled basis. In some cases healthcare organizations opt to support ongoing investigator data needs by creating separate repositories of aggregated, processed clinical data that relate to a particular clinical domain. In the VHA, investigators in infectious disease have developed procedures to aggregate a specialized set of nationwide patient data related to methicillin-resistant *Staphylococcus aureus* (MRSA).[11] These

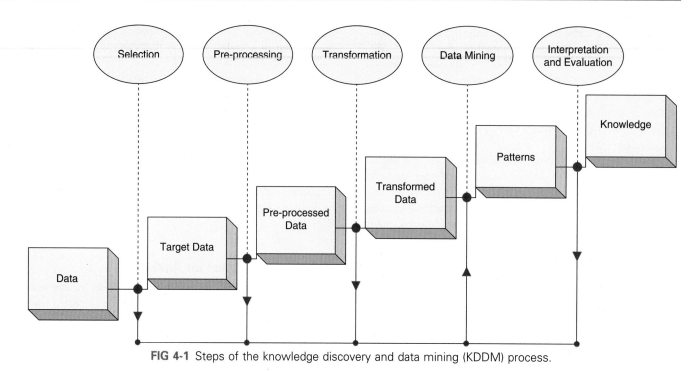

FIG 4-1 Steps of the knowledge discovery and data mining (KDDM) process.

specialized repositories of data can be more readily analyzed on an ongoing basis to support quality improvement, health services research, and clinical research.

The amount of data retrieved from clinical data warehouses can be enormous, especially when data originate from multiple sites. Investigators will want to define a sampling plan that limits the number of selected records, according to the needs of the study or project. For KDDM, it may not be possible to import the data fully into analytic software as a single flat file. Fortunately, many statistical and machine learning software packages can be used to analyze data contained within an SQL database. For example, SAS Enterprise Miner can be used to analyze data within an SQL database using Open Database Connectivity (ODBC).[12] Clinicians or investigators who are new to KDDM should plan to collaborate with statistical and informatics personnel to plan an optimal approach.

Preprocessing Clinical Data

EHRs include both coded (structured) data and text data that must be cleaned and processed prior to analysis. EHRs collect and store data according to a coding system consisting of one or more terminologies (Box 4-1). While standard terminologies exist, many systems make use of a local terminology, a distinct set of variables, and a distinct coding system for those variables that are not necessarily shared across systems. Different sites, clinics, or hospitals within a healthcare organization could use different terminologies, coding data in different ways. Within a single site, changes in information systems and terminologies over time can also result in variations in data coding. When data are aggregated across time and across sites, the variations in terminology result in a dataset that

represents similar concepts in multiple ways. For example, one large healthcare organization recognized that within its clinical data the relatively simple concepts of "yes" and "no" were represented using 30 unique coding schemes.[13] Unlike data collected using a prospective approach, clinical data often require extensive cleaning and preprocessing. Thus preprocessing constitutes the majority of effort in the clinical KDDM process shown in Figure 4-1.

Preprocessing Text Data

In clinical records, the richest and most descriptive data are often unstructured, captured only in the text notes entered by clinicians. Text data can be analyzed in a large number of clinical records using a specialized approach known as natural language processing (NLP) or, more specifically, information extraction.[14] Methods of information extraction identify pieces of meaningful information in sequences of text, pieces of information that represent concepts and can be coded as such for further analysis. Machine interpretation of text written in the form of natural language is not straightforward because natural language is rife with spelling errors, acronyms, and abbreviations, among other issues.[14] Consequently, information extraction is usually a computationally expensive, multistep process in which text data are passed through a pipeline of sequential NLP procedures. These procedures deal with common NLP challenges such as word disambiguation and negation and may involve the use of machine learning methods. However, each pipeline may differ according to the NLP task at hand.[15] Unstructured Information Management Architecture (UIMA) (http://uima.apache.org) is one example of an NLP pipeline framework. Information extraction for clinical text is an active area of research and development. However, information extraction tools are not commonly used outside of informatics research settings and text data are included infrequently in KDDM projects. This technique is another example of an area where researchers or clinicians need to partner with informaticists.

Preprocessing Coded (Structured) Data

In a set of consistently coded clinical data, the data should be analyzed using descriptive statistics and visualization with respect to the following:

- *Distribution:* Normally distributed data are most amenable to modeling. If the data distribution is skewed, the data can be transformed using a function of the original data or using nonparametric statistical methods.
- *Frequency:* The frequency of specific values for categorical variables may reveal a need for additional preprocessing. It is not uncommon for identical concepts to be represented using multiple values. Also, some values are so rare that their exclusion from analysis should be considered.
- *Missingness:* Missingness can be meaningful. For example, a missing hemoglobin A1c (HgA1c) laboratory test may indicate that a patient does not have diabetes. In that case, a binary variable indicating whether or not HgA1c values are missing can be added to the dataset. In other circumstances, the values are simply missing at random. If values are missing at random, they can be replaced using a number of statistical imputation approaches.
- *Sparsity:* Sparse data are data for which binary values are mostly zero. Categorical variables with a large number of possible values contribute to sparsity. For example, a field called "primary diagnosis" has a set of possible values equal to the number of diagnoses found in the ICD-9 coding system. Upon 1 of n encoding, the number of possible values becomes the number of new columns added to the dataset. Some diagnoses will be more common than others. For uncommon diagnoses the value of "primary diagnosis" will almost always equal zero. The value of "1" will be found in only a small percentage of records.
- *Outliers:* Outliers, data points that fall far outside the distribution of data, should be considered for elimination or further analysis prior to modeling.
- *Identifiers:* Codes or other values that uniquely identify patients should be excluded from the modeling process.

- *Erroneous data:* Absurd, impossible data values are routinely found in clinical data. These can be treated as randomly missing values and replaced.

Descriptive analysis is facilitated by many software packages. For example, Figure 4-2 depicts a screenshot from Weka, a freely available data mining software package.[16] In this software, when a variable from the dataset is selected, basic descriptive statistics and a graph of the frequency distribution are displayed. A variety of filters can then be applied to address issues with the data.

The considerations in preprocessing the data at this stage are numerous and readers are referred to an excellent text by Dorian Pyle, *Data Preparation for Data Mining.*[17] Preprocessing is always best accomplished through a joint effort by the analyst and one or more domain experts, such as clinicians who are familiar with the concepts the data represent. The domain experts can lend valuable insight to the analyst, who must develop an optimal representation of each variable. Review of the data at this point may reveal conceptual gaps, the absence of data, or the lack of quality data that represent important concepts. For example, age and functional status (e.g., activities of daily living) might be important data to include in a project related to the prediction of patient falls in the hospital. By mapping concepts to variables, or vice versa, teams can communicate about gaps and weaknesses in the data.

Sampling and Partitioning

Once the data have been fully cleaned and preprocessed they must be sampled and partitioned. Sampling is the step in which a smaller subset of the data is chosen for analysis. Sampling is important because excessive amounts of data slow computer processing time during analysis. Sampling for classification tasks is typically random or stratified on class membership.

Partitioning refers to the assignment of individual records or rows in a dataset for a specific purpose: model development (training, incremental testing of models during development) or model validation (data held out from the development process for the purpose of unbiased performance estimation). There are multiple approaches to sampling and partitioning, and the suitability of the approach depends on the nature of the project and the quantity of available data. If very large amounts of data are available, large sets can be sampled for model development and validation. If more limited amounts of data are available, it will be necessary to optimize the use of that data through resampling approaches such as bootstrapping or cross-validation.[18]

Within the model development dataset, cross-validation can be used to maximize the amount of data used for both training and testing. In cross-validation the data are partitioned into n folds. Then, in a series of n experiments, $n - 1$ folds are used to train models, and the remaining fold, which is unique in each experiment, is used for testing. In that way, each record is available for both training and testing but there is no duplication of records in the testing dataset. Cross-validation is commonly performed with either 10 or

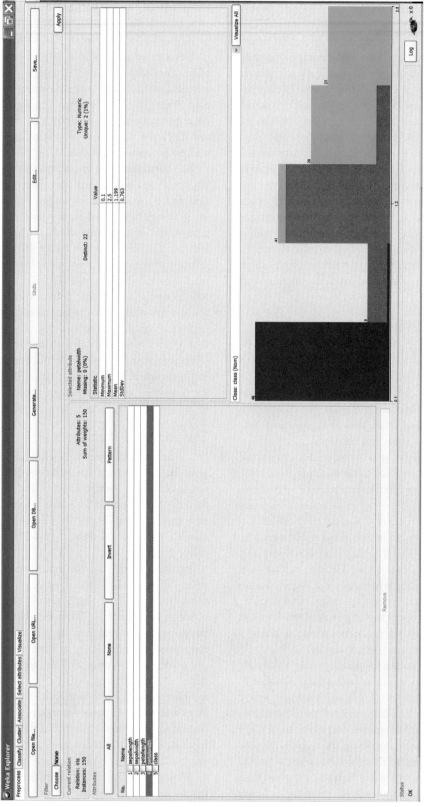

FIG 4-2 Weka GUI Explorer. (From Hall M, Frank E, Holmes G, Pfahringer B, Reutemann P, Witten I. The WEKA data mining software: an update. *SIGKDD Explorations.* 2009;11(1):10-18.)

100 folds. In very small datasets, leave-one-out cross-validation can be implemented, wherein the number of folds equals the number of records. This maximizes the amount of data available for training within each of the n experiments.

Data Mining

Data mining is the step in the knowledge discovery process where patterns are enumerated over a set of data.[19] The methods used to accomplish this enumeration are varied and include both machine learning and statistical approaches.

Statistical Approaches

Statistical approaches fit a model to the data. Bayesian networks, a class of models based on Bayes theorem, constitute one popular approach. Bayesian models are robust, tolerate missing data, and can be computed quickly over a set of data. The simplest implementation, Naive Bayes, has been shown to perform well despite its assumption of independence between input variables. Another important approach is logistic or linear regression.

Machine Learning

Machine learning methods are computer algorithms that learn to perform a task on the basis of examples. In data mining the task is typically prediction or regression (predict a real number) or classification (predict class membership). Machine learning algorithms vary in the way they learn to perform tasks. Many algorithms begin with an initial working theory of how a set of input data predict an output (a.k.a. target), a future event, or an unknown value. The algorithm then makes incremental adjustments to the working theory, based on examples of both the input and the target. The examples are contained in a set of training data. A complete discussion of machine learning and specific machine learning algorithms is beyond the scope of this chapter. However, key methods and characteristics are summarized in Table 4-2. All of the methods listed in Table 4-2 are commonly implemented in general-purpose data mining software.

Multiple variant algorithms can be used to implement each approach, and specialized method-specific software is available to support more flexible configurations. Machine learning algorithms also can be implemented in a variety of programming languages. Data mining software allows users to implement versions of these algorithms via point-and-click graphic user interfaces. However, these algorithms can also be written and executed using packages such as R, MATLAB, and Octave. It is important that users understand how to apply each unique method properly in order to produce optimal models and avoid spurious results.

Evaluating Data Mining Models

The most critical step in evaluation, the partitioning of data, occurs early in KDDM (Fig. 4-3). Performance estimates are calculated by comparing a model's predictions to actual

TABLE 4-2	EXAMPLES OF DATA MINING METHODS
METHOD	**DESCRIPTION**
Decision trees	Recursive partitioning of data based on an information criterion (entropy, information gain, etc.) Common algorithms: C4.5, CART (classification and regression trees) Easily intepreted Require pruning based on coverage to avoid overfit More difficult to calibrate to new populations and settings
Decision rules	Classification rules in the form of if-then-else rule sets Easily interpreted Require pruning based on coverage to avoid overfit Closely related to decision trees; decision trees can be easily converted to decision rules
Artificial neural networks	Networks of processing units Output a probability of class membership Computationally expensive Effective for modeling complex, nonlinear solutions Not easily interpreted
Support vector machines	Linear functions implemented in a transformed feature space Computationally efficient Effective for modeling complex, nonlinear solutions Not easily interpreted
Random forests	"Ensemble" method that combines the output of multiple decision trees Scalable (computationally feasible even with very large amounts of data) Not easily interpreted
Bayesian networks	Probabilistic models based on Bayes theorem Models are easily calibrated for use with new settings and populations Models may assume conditional independence among variables Not as scalable as other methods; may not work well with very large amounts of data due to the way in which Bayesian networks are computed

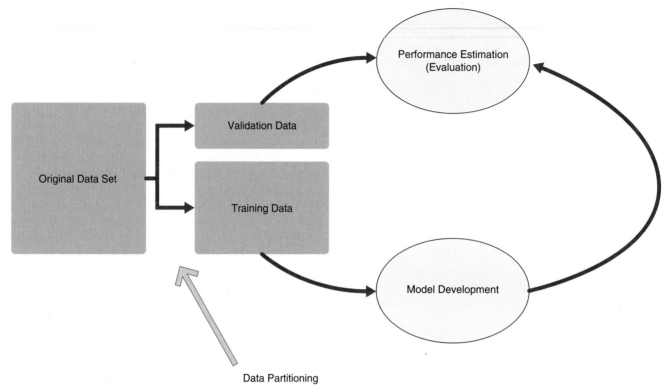

FIG 4-3 The relationship of data partitioning to both model development and evaluation.

values on a set of data for which the actual values are known. If this comparison is made using the training data—that is, the same data used to parameterize the model—the performance estimates will be optimistically biased. It is critical that a sizable sample of the original data is set aside and not used in any way to train or calibrate models. This held-out sample of data is often termed the validation set or testing set. Used solely for performance estimation, the held-out data will yield unbiased estimates.

Performance measures are based on a comparison of the predicted and actual values in a set of held-out testing data. In classification, this comparison yields a confusion matrix that can be used to derive performance measures, similar to the performance measures used in evaluating clinical diagnostic tests: true-positive rate, false-positive rate, true-negative rate, false-negative rate, sensitivity, specificity, likelihood ratios, etc. (Fig. 4-4). The specific performance measures should be selected with respect to the goals of the KDDM project. For example, if a model is developed as a screening tool, sensitivity may be of particular interest. If a model is developed for a CDS tool, alert fatigue is an important consideration and so the false-positive rate may be of particular interest.

To evaluate and compare overall model performance, the receiver operating characteristic (ROC) curve and the area under the ROC curve are important measures of performance. The ROC curve, depicted in Figure 4-5, is obtained by plotting the false-positive fraction and true-positive fraction, based on cumulative comparison of predicted and actual values at increasing values of probability. The resulting curve shows the trade-off between sensitivity and specificity

exhibited by a classifier at any given threshold. The area under the ROC curve is the probability that a randomly chosen positive case will be selected as more likely to be positive than a randomly selected negative case.[20] As such, it serves as an overall measure of model performance. An area under the ROC curve ($Az = 0.5$) is equivalent to random chance. Better performance is indicated by higher values of Az. Interpretation of the area under the ROC curve, especially in relation to other models or classifiers, requires the calculation of confidence intervals.

For models that predict a real number (e.g., glucose level), performance measures are simply based on the difference between the predicted value and the true value in a set of held-out testing data for which the true values are known. From these differences various measurements of error can be calculated: mean squared error, root mean squared error, etc. Measurement of correlation is also important (e.g., r^2), as is visualization of predicted and actual values.

PRACTICE-BASED EVIDENCE

PBE Features and Challenges

The term *practice-based evidence (PBE) design* should not be confused with evidence-based practice (EBP). EBP refers to a process for identifying the evidence supporting specific approaches to clinical practice and conducting practice according to the best evidence. Once identified, best clinical practices may be standardized in practice guidelines. In EBP the highest level of evidence is often considered to be the RCT, as mentioned earlier. By contrast, PBE is an innovative prospective research design that uses data gathered from

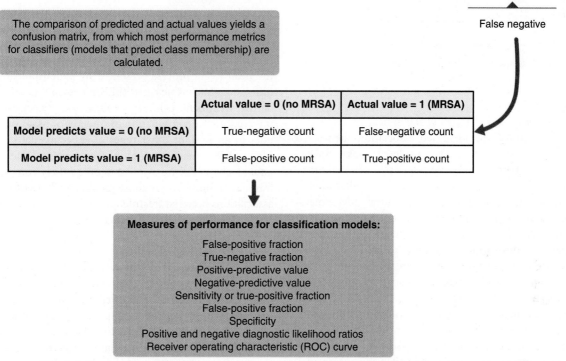

A model has been developed to predict whether or not a patient is colonized with MRSA upon admission to a tertiary health care facility. The model outputs a probability of MRSA colonization, from which a prediction of MRSA status can be generated . . . The model's predictions are compared to actual patient MRSA status in order to estimate the model's performance.

Case ID	Known MRSA Status	Probability of MRSA	Predicted MRSA Status
5478	0	0.23	0
2222	1	0.85	1
6123	1	0.85	1
0805	1	0.46	0

False negative

The comparison of predicted and actual values yields a confusion matrix, from which most performance metrics for classifiers (models that predict class membership) are calculated.

	Actual value = 0 (no MRSA)	Actual value = 1 (MRSA)
Model predicts value = 0 (no MRSA)	True-negative count	False-negative count
Model predicts value = 1 (MRSA)	False-positive count	True-positive count

Measures of performance for classification models:

False-positive fraction
True-negative fraction
Positive-predictive value
Negative-predictive value
Sensitivity or true-positive fraction
False-positive fraction
Specificity
Positive and negative diagnostic likelihood ratios
Receiver operating characteristic (ROC) curve

FIG 4-4 The process of calculating performance estimates from a comparison of predicted and actual values for a classification model of methicillin-resistant *Staphylococcus aureus* (MRSA) status on admission.

current practice to identify what care processes work in the real world. *EBP is about using evidence to guide practice. PBE is about obtaining evidence from practice.*

PBE studies are observational cohort studies that attempt to mitigate the weaknesses usually associated with traditional observational designs in four main ways:

1. Exhaustive attention to patient characteristics to address confounds or alternative explanations of treatment effectiveness
2. Use of large samples and diverse sources of patients to improve sample representativeness, power, and external validity
3. Use of detailed standardized structured documentation of interventions with training and quality control checks for reliability of the measures of the actual process of care

4. Inclusion of front-line clinicians and patients in the design, execution, and analysis of studies and their data elements to improve ecological validity

PBE studies require comprehensive data acquisition. By using bivariate and multivariate associations among patient characteristics, process steps, and outcomes, PBE studies can uncover best practices and combinations of treatments for specific types of patients while achieving many of the presumed advantages of RCTs, especially advantages derived from controlling for patient differences through randomization.

PBE study designs are structured to minimize the potential for false associations between treatments and outcomes. These studies focus on minimizing biasing effects of possible alternative factors or explanations when estimating the complex associations between treatments and outcomes within

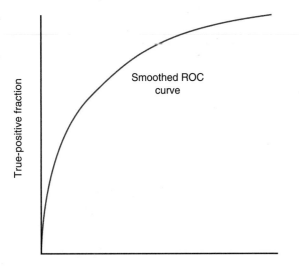

FIG 4-5 Smoothed receiver operating characteristic (ROC) curve.

a specific context of care.[21] Heeding the aphorism "correlation is not causation," the identified associations between treatment and outcome are not considered causal links. However, to the extent that the research design can measure and statistically control for these confounders or alternative explanations, the associations still inform causal judgments.

In other words, the PBE approach does not infer causality directly like RCTs, but the strength of the evidence that a causal link exists comes from several sources. First, alternative hypotheses regarding possible causes are tested using the large number of available variables to identify additional potential variables that may be influencing outcomes. Results can be used to drill down to discover potential alternative causes and to generate additional specific hypotheses. Analyses continue until the project team is satisfied that they cannot think of any other variables to explain the outcomes. Second, one can test the predictive validity of significant PBE findings by introducing findings into clinical practice and assessing whether outcomes change when treatments change, as predicted by PBE models. Third, studies can be repeated in different health care settings and assessed to determine if the findings remain the same.

Underlying the common criticism of observational studies (that they demonstrate association but not causation) is an unchallenged assumption that the evidence for causation is dichotomous; that is, something either is or is not the cause. Instead, the evidence for causation should be viewed as a continuum that extends from mere association to undeniable causation. While observational studies cannot prove causation in some absolute sense, by chipping away at potential confounders and by testing for predictive validity in follow-up studies we move upward on the continuum from mere association to causation. PBE studies offer a methodology for moving up this continuum.

Research design involves a balance of internal validity (the validity of the causal inference that the treatment is the "true"

cause of the outcome) and external validity (the validity that the causal inference can be generalized to other subjects, forms of the treatment, measures of the outcome, practitioners, and settings). Essentially, PBE designs trade away the internal validity of RCTs for external validity.[22] PBE designs have high external validity because they include virtually all patients with or at risk for the condition under study, as well as potential confounders that could alter treatment responses. PBE designs attempt to minimize threats to internal validity by trying to collect information on all patient variables—demographic, medical, nursing, functional, and socioeconomic—that might account for differences in outcome. By doing so, PBE designs minimize the need for compensating statistical techniques such as instrumental variables and propensity scoring to mitigate selection bias effects, unknown sources of variance, and threats to internal validity.

PBE study designs attempt to capture the complexity of the health care process presented by patient and treatment differences in routine care; PBE studies do not alter or standardize treatment regimes to evaluate the efficacy of a specific intervention or combination of interventions, as one usually does in an RCT or other types of experimental designs.[23,24] PBE studies measure multiple concurrent interventions, patient characteristics, and outcomes. This comprehensive framework provides for consequential analyses of significant associations between treatment combinations and outcomes, controlling for patient differences.

Steps in a PBE Study

Table 4-3 outlines the steps involved in conducting a PBE study and gives a brief description of what each step involves. Once a clinical issue is identified, PBE methods begin with the formation of a multidisciplinary team, often with representatives of multiple sites. Participation of informaticists on the team is critical to ensure that the electronic documentation facilitates data capture for the research and clinical practice without undue documentation burden. Details follow about several of the steps in a PBE study.

Create a Multisite, Multidisciplinary Project Clinical Team (PCT)

One factor that distinguishes PBE studies from most other observational studies is the extensive involvement of front-line clinicians and patients. Front-line clinicians and patients are engaged in *all* aspects of PBE projects; they identify all data elements to be included in the PBE project based on initial study hypotheses, extensive literature review, and clinical experience and training, as well as patient experience. Many relevant details about patients, treatments, and outcomes may be recorded in existing EHRs; however, the project clinical team (PCT) often identifies additional critical variables that must be collected in supplemental standardized documentation developed specifically for the PBE study. Clinicians and patients also participate in data analyses leading to publication. Front-to-back clinician and patient participation fosters high levels of clinician and patient buy-in that

TABLE 4-3	STEPS IN A PRACTICE-BASED EVIDENCE (PBE) STUDY
STEP	**DESCRIPTION**
1. Create a multisite, multidisciplinary project clinical team (PCT)	PCT (a) identifies outcomes of interest, (b) identifies individual components of the care process, (c) creates a common intervention vocabulary and dictionary, (d) identifies key patient characteristics and risk factors, (e) proposes hypotheses for testing, and (f) participates in data collection, analyses, and dissemination of findings. The PCT builds on theoretical understanding, research evidence to date, existing guidelines, and clinical expertise and experience about factors that may influence outcomes.
2. Control for differences in patient severity, including comorbidities, treatment processes, and outcomes	Comprehensive severity measure should be an age- and disease-specific measure of physiologic and psychosocial complexity. It is used to control for selection bias and confounding by indication. An example is the Comprehensive Severity Index (CSI) that is disease- and age-specific and composed of more than 2200 clinical indicators.
3. Implement intensive data collection and check reliability	Capture data on patient characteristics, care processes, and outcomes drawn from medical records and study-specific data collection instruments. Data collectors are tested for interrater reliability.
4. Create a study database	Study database consists of merged, cleaned data and is suitable for statistical analyses.
5. Test hypotheses successively	Hypotheses are based on questions that motivated the study originally, previous studies, existing guidelines, and, above all, hypotheses proposed by the PCT. Bivariate and multivariate analysis approaches include multiple regression, analysis of variance, logistic and Cox proportional hazard regression, hierarchical mixed models, and other methods consistent with measurement properties of key variables.
6. Validate and implement study findings	Implement findings in practice to test predictive validity. In this step findings from the first five steps are implemented and evaluated to determine whether the new or modified interventions replicate results identified in earlier phases and outcomes improve as predicted. After the validation of specific PBE findings, the findings are ready to be incorporated into routine care and clinical guidelines.

contribute to data completeness and clinical ownership of study findings, even when findings challenge conventional wisdom and practice. Such ownership is essential to knowledge translation and best practice.

Control for Differences in Patient Severity of Illness

Controls for Patient Factors. PBE designs require recording the treatment that each subject receives as determined by clinicians in practice rather than randomizing subjects to neutralize the effect of patient differences. PBE studies address patient differences by *measuring* a wide variety of patient characteristics that go beyond race, gender, age, payer, and other variables that can be exported from administrative, registry, or EHR databases and then accounting for patient differences through statistical control.

The goal is to measure essentially all variables that contribute to outcomes to have the information needed to control for patient differences. This is the major reason for including front-line clinicians and patients in PBE study design and implementation; by including clinicians and patients from multiple sites, spread geographically across the country and world, a comprehensive set of patient factors is suggested for PBE studies. There always remains the possibility that some patient characteristic may be overlooked, but unlike most observational cohort studies, such as those based on preexisting administrative data, PBE's exhaustive patient characterization minimizes significantly the chances of not being able

to resolve unknown sources of variance due to patient differences.

One critical component of the PBE study design is the use of the Comprehensive Severity Index (CSI).[21,25-34] In PBE studies the CSI is used to measure how ill a patient is at the time of presentation for care as well as over time within a setting. Degree of illness is defined as extent of deviation from "normal values." CSI is "physiologically-based, age- and disease-specific, independent of treatments, and provides an objective, consistent method to define patient severity of illness levels based on over 2,200 signs, symptoms, and physical findings related to a patient's disease(s), not just diagnostic information, such as ICD-9-CM coding alone."[35(p S132)] However, patient diagnosis codes and data management rules are used to calculate severity scores for each patient overall and separately for each of a patient's diseases (principal and each secondary diagnosis).

CSI and other measures of patient key characteristics, such as level and completeness of spinal cord injury, severity of stroke disability, or severity of traumatic brain injury, etc., to control for patient differences; using these patient differences can help to account for treatment selection bias or confounding by indication in analyses. The validity of CSI has been studied for over 30 years in various clinical settings and conditions such as inpatient adult and pediatric conditions, ambulatory care, rehabilitation care, hospice care, and long-term care settings.[26-33]

Controls for Treatment and Process Factors. Treatment in clinical settings is often determined by facility standards, regional differences, and clinician training. Therefore, like patient differences, treatment differences must be recorded during a PBE study. The goal is to find measurable factors that describe each treatment to be compared. Examples include the medications dispensed and their dosage; rehabilitation therapies performed and duration on each day of treatment; content, mode, and amount of patient education; and nutritional consumption.

PBE identifies better practices by examining how different approaches to care are associated with outcomes of care, while controlling for patient variables. PBE does not require providers to follow treatment protocols or exclude certain treatment practices. However, characteristics of treatment, including timing and dose, require detailed documentation. These characteristics must be defined by the PBE team and measured in a structured, standard manner for all participating sites and their clinicians. Consistency is critical for minimizing variation in data collection and documentation.[35]

PBE studies require that clinicians accurately describe the actual interventions they use during real-world patient care. However, the level of detail found in routine documentation of interventions may be insufficient. Each PBE team must assess the level of detail afforded by routine documentation and determine whether supplemental documentation is necessary.[35] Further, point-of-care documentation or EHR data are pilot tested to ensure complete representation of variables. PBE studies require engagement from all members of the multi-disciplinary patient care team to ensure that data collection is sufficiently comprehensive.

Pilot testing ensures that point-of-care documentation or EHR data collection captures all elements that clinicians suggest may affect the outcomes of their patients. *If a variable is not measured, it cannot be used in subsequent analyses.* PBE studies require effort from all types of clinicians and healthcare providers involved with a patient's care to ensure that data acquisition is as comprehensive as necessary.

Controls for Outcome Factors. Multiple outcomes can be addressed in a single PBE project; projects are not limited to one primary outcome, as is the case in other study designs. In particular, PBE studies incorporate widely accepted, standard measures. For example, the Braden Scale for risk of pressure ulcer development is commonly collected in PBE studies, and has been used as both a control and an outcome variable.[33-35] PBE projects incorporate as many standard measures as possible, but also include outcome measures specific to the study topic. These measures can be found in administrative databases, the EHR, or collected prospectively. Additional patient outcomes commonly assessed in PBE studies are condition-specific complications, condition-specific long-term medical outcomes (based on clinician assessment or patient self-report), condition-specific patient-centered measures of activities and participation in society, patient satisfaction, quality of life, and cost.[36]

While PBE project teams endeavor to include as many standard outcome measures as possible, they also include other measures specific to the study topic. Some outcomes (e.g., discharge destination [home, community, institution], length of stay, or death) are commonly available in administrative databases. Some outcome variables (e.g., repeat stroke, deep vein thrombosis, pain, electrolyte imbalance, anemia) are found in traditional paper charts or EHR documentation but typically are available only up to discharge from the care setting.

Implement Intensive Data Collection and Check Reliability

Using the data elements identified in step 2, historical data are collected by the research team from the EHR. Direct care providers document the specific elements of treatment at point of care. For example, if the treatment includes physical therapy, the type, intensity, and duration are precisely recorded during each therapy session. If the nurse provides patient counseling or education, the teaching methods, instructional materials, topical content, and duration of each teaching session are recorded. The informatics specialist is a critical partner in designing the data capture to prevent the need for parallel documentation for the research record and clinical record. If the documentation is too burdensome, clinicians will not comply with documentation requirements and the data will be incomplete. So the design of the data collection is critical to the success of this research approach. The fact that these data collection formats are defined by the front-line clinicians helps to ensure that the data collection formats are specifically designed so that data can be documented easily and quickly.

Create a Study Database

The elements of data collected are compiled into a study-specific database with the assistance of informatics personnel. PBE studies usually do not require the informed consent of patients unless a follow-up interview or other activity is planned that is not part of the "standard of care" in that setting. Since the usual care is not altered but only recorded, patients are not usually aware of the study. In fact, consent may not be required because care is not changed. However, to ensure the correct protocol is followed, researchers are always best served by contacting their local institutional review boards for study approval and compliance with the latest guidance. Data sources include existing or new clinician documentation of care delivered. Patients drop out of a PBE study if they leave the care setting before completion of treatment or drop out during follow-up.[36] Patients who withdraw from a treatment do not distort results of PBE study findings because PBE studies follow patients throughout the care process, taking date and time measurements on all therapies. Hence if a patient withdraws from care of the study, investigators can use the existing data in the analyses, controlling for time in the study. Patients who withdraw exist in both RCTs and PBE studies, but PBE studies have a huge advantage due to their large sample size and number of information points so that much better and more complete comparison of subjects who complete therapy and subjects who withdraw is possible.

Successively Test Hypotheses

PBE studies use multivariable analyses to identify variables most strongly associated with outcomes. Detailed characterization of patients and treatments allows researchers to specify direct effects, indirect effects, and interactions that might not otherwise become apparent with less detailed data. CSI (overall or its individual components or individual severity indicators) is used in data analysis to represent the role of comorbid and co-occurring conditions along with the principal diagnosis. If a positive outcome is found to be associated with a specific treatment or combination of treatments, the subsequent methodological approach is to include confounding patient variables or combinations of variables in the analysis in an attempt to "disconfirm" the association. The association may remain robust or variables may be identified that explain the outcome more adequately.

In PBE studies, ordinary least squares multiple regression is used to examine associations between variables describing patient demographic and health characteristics and process variables with each patient's outcome measure at discharge or at follow-up intervals. Data include many clinical and therapeutic variables and a selection procedure is applied to decide on significant variables to retain in regressions. Only variables suggested by the PCT based on the literature and team members' education and clinical experience and with frequencies equal to or greater than 10 to 20 patients in the sample are usually allowed to be included in regression models. The most parsimonious model for each outcome is created by allowing only significant variables to remain in the model. Independent variables entering regression models are checked for multicolinearity; no correlations greater than 0.70 are allowed.

To account for possible clustering (correlation) of patients within facilities or healthcare providers or patients themselves over time, hierarchical linear mixed-model analyses with repeated measures are used. Mixed models permit data to exhibit correlation and nonconstant variability across patients with specified treatment facility or healthcare provider as a random-effects parameter. Hierarchical linear mixed models are tested for differences from the regression models using likelihood ratio tests. To avoid the possibility of overspecification of the regression models, a ratio of number of observations per maximum number of significant variables of 10:1 is maintained.

Analyses conducted using PBE databases are iterative. Counterintuitive findings are investigated thoroughly. In fact, counterintuitive and unexpected findings often lead to new discoveries of important associations of treatments with outcomes.

Large numbers of patients (usually greater than 1000 and often greater than 2000) and considerable computing power are required to perform PBE analyses. When multiple outcomes are of interest and there is little information on effect size of each predictor variable, sample size is based on the project team's desire to find small, medium, or large effects of patient and process variables.

Validate and Implement Findings

See the exemplar in Box 4-2 that shows how a PBE study of stroke rehabilitation culminated in validation studies and

---

BOX 4-2 PRACTICE-BASED EVIDENCE EXEMPLAR: STROKE REHABILITATION

An integrated healthcare system determined that outcomes for patients following a stroke were highly variable. Rehabilitation professionals in the geographic region were polled to determine the local standards of care and concluded that the interventions were quite diverse. A regional task force was convened representing eight hospitals from two care delivery systems as well as an independent hospital. The task force was led by a rehabilitation nurse and a physical therapist and initiated a PBE study to determine what combinations of medical devices, therapies (e.g., physical therapy, occupational therapy, speech therapy), medications, feeding, and nutritional approaches worked best for various subtypes of stroke patients in real-world practices. A multidisciplinary project clinical team of physicians, nurses, social workers, psychologists, physical therapists, occupational therapists, recreational therapists, and speech-language therapists was convened. Poststroke patients and caregivers were also invited to participate.

The first decisions of the group addressed the outcome variables, including the Functional Independence Measure (FIM) scale score, length of stay in rehabilitation, discharge disposition, mortality, and morbidity (contracture, deep vein thrombosis, major bleeding, pulmonary embolism, pressure ulcer, pneumonia). Each profession identified possible interventions and developed documentation for the components of the intervention and the intensity (e.g., number of repetitions for each exercise maneuver and time required). Documentation was incorporated into the standard electronic documentation. Over a 2-year period 1461 patients ranging from 18.4 to 95.6 years of age were studied. Patient-related data collected included age, gender, race, payer, stroke risk factors, and FIM scores. Detailed process and outcome data were collected. Severity of illness was determined using the CSI scale. There were significant differences in the average severity of illness at the eight sites. There was also heterogeneity in the intensity of therapies, use of tube feedings, and use of psychotropic and opioid medication. Following control for severity of illness, univariate and multivariate analysis of the data determined that factors were positively and negatively associated with the FIM scores at discharge.

Continued

BOX 4-2	PRACTICE-BASED EVIDENCE EXEMPLAR: STROKE REHABILITATION—cont'd

CATEGORIES OF FACTORS	POSITIVE ASSOCIATION WITH FIM SCORE (↑ INDEPENDENCE)	NEGATIVE ASSOCIATION WITH FIM SCORE (↓ INDEPENDENCE)
Patient factors	Bed motility in first 3 hours	Age
	Advanced gait activity in first 3 hours	Severe motor and cognitive impairment at admission
	Home management by OT	
Therapy factors	Bed motility in first 3 hours	Days until rehabilitation onset
	Advanced gait activity in first 3 hours	
Nutrition	Enteral feeding	
Medications	Atypical antipsychotics	Tricyclic antidepressants
	Neurotropic pain treated with medications	Older SSRIs

OT, Occupational therapist; *SSRI,* selective serotonin reuptake inhibitors.

After additional studies to replicate findings, the participating hospitals initiated the following policy changes in the treatment of stroke patients. Several of these are novel interventions that would not have been identified without the PBE study method. Continuous quality improvement monitoring was implemented to document adherence and outcomes.

- *Early rehabilitation admission:* patients are admitted to rehabilitation as soon as possible and therapies begin in the intensive care unit if possible
- *Early gait training by physical therapy:* patients are put in harness on treadmill for safety but gait training is initiated as soon as possible even in the most affected patients
- *Early feeding:* if patients are not able to eat full diet, early enteral feedings (nutritional supplements, tube feeding) are initiated
- *Opioids for pain:* opioids are ordered at admission for any time the patient misses therapy due to pain

Source: Horn SD, DeJong G, Smout RJ, Gassaway J, James R, Conroy B. Stroke rehabilitation patients, practice, and outcomes: is earlier and more aggressive therapy better? *Arch Phys Med Rehab.* 2005;86(12 suppl 2):S101-S114.

changes in the standard of care in a healthcare system. Because PBE studies are observational research designs, the conclusions require prospective validation before they can be incorporated into clinical guidelines and standards of care, despite rigorous attempts to challenge the causal nature of relationships during the hypothesis testing step (step 5). Validation of PBE findings can use a continuous quality improvement approach consisting of systematic implementation of the interventions found to be better in conjunction with monitoring of their outcomes. If the findings from the outcome assessment replicate the findings of the initial retrospective stage in multiple settings and populations, the intervention would be a candidate for incorporation into clinical guidelines as a care process that has established efficacy and effectiveness. This is in contrast to interventions that only have RCT evidence, which generally indicates only efficacy.

Limitations and Strengths of PBE Studies

PBE methods work best in situations where one wishes to study existing clinical practice. Unless a treatment is used frequently enough, it may not appear statistically significant unless its effect size is large. However, there are no limitations related to conditions or settings for use of PBE study methods. Of course, the technique can be time consuming in terms of conducting the initial PBE steps as well as data extraction. Although the relevant variables may change, PBE study designs have been found to work in various practice settings, including acute and ambulatory care, inpatient and outpatient rehabilitation, hospice, and long-term care, and for adult and pediatric patients.

CONCLUSION AND FUTURE DIRECTIONS

Knowledge discovery and data mining is a process that can be used to glean important insights and develop useful, data-driven models from collected healthcare data. With each patient and each healthcare event, data describing numerous aspects of care accumulate. Large warehouses of clinical data are now commonplace, and as time passes the data will become increasingly longitudinal in nature. This future direction presents an enormous opportunity, as large repositories of clinical data can be used to gain insight into the relationship between the characteristics of patient, diagnoses, interventions, and outcomes. They can be used to identify prospective patient cohorts for scientific research. They can be used to assist healthcare providers with clinical decisions and avoid medical error. However, the sheer size and complexity of the data necessitate specialized approaches to data management and analysis. The methods of knowledge discovery and data mining enable us to analyze the data efficiently and effectively and develop clinical knowledge models for decision support.

As more healthcare systems move toward EHRs, data acquisition will become easier and less costly; data elements needed for PBE studies can be hard-coded in EHRs in structured, exportable formats while also being used for clinical documentation of care. This concept has been implemented already in health systems in Israel and in various PBE studies in the U.S.[37] However, transitioning to EHRs, as many health systems are doing, presents its own challenges, especially for data-intensive PBE studies. While EHRs can facilitate data acquisition, they are not always research-friendly because many desired data elements are in text such as clinical notes that cannot be exported easily. If EHR data cannot be exported directly, they must be abstracted manually, a task that can be more labor intensive than abstracting paper charts. In addition, EHR modifications for optimization of point-of-care data documentation and abstraction are costly and time consuming, potentially slowing down planning and implementation of PBE studies based on routine electronic data capture. Over time, new EHR exporting and reporting software will emerge that will make EHR data abstraction less labor intensive.

PBE methods collect and analyze a comprehensive set of patient, treatment, facility, and outcome variables, enabling study of comparative effectiveness among treatments. Moreover, the PBE approach leverages the knowledge of front-line practicing clinicians and patients. This multidisciplinary team approach to comparative effectiveness research ensures inclusion of a wide spectrum of variables so that differences in patient characteristics and treatments are measured and can be controlled for statistically.[35] PBE requires interprofessional collaboration to identify the data elements for the study. The information specialist helps to identify sources of the data in the record and integrate new elements into the EHR. However, even with optimal integration, data collection for PBE studies may alter the documentation process by incorporating unprecedented detail on care processes. Hence, leaders must foster a shared learning culture in all departments toward improvement in healthcare. This extends beyond the local department or institution to a value for creating generalizable knowledge to improve care worldwide.

The number and quality of studies is often insufficient to support clinical practice in complex environments with diverse populations, and recent developments in nonrandomized research methodologies have strengthened their value. The next step for comparative effectiveness research is to conduct more rigorous, prospective large-scale observational cohort studies. From a PBE perspective, rigor entails controlled measurement of outcomes related to multiple intervention combinations and a variety of patient characteristics in diverse clinical settings.[35] The research question and the type of knowledge that is needed are what determine the most appropriate design for a specific study. KDDM and PBE are methodological alternatives to RCT or other methods. KDDM and PBE provide additional sources of systematic outcomes information to improve upon the anecdotal and informal knowledge base that underlies much of clinical

practice. Providers are looking for ways to evaluate current practice and improve clinical decision making that do not disrupt their delivery of care to patients. PBE studies address questions in the real world where multiple variables and factors can affect the outcomes; they can fit seamlessly into everyday clinical documentation, and therefore have the potential to influence and improve real-world clinical care for the benefit of patients.

The nature of the research question and type of knowledge needed determine the design of a study. KDDM and PBE do not replace the RCT or other methods but rather provide additional sources of systematic outcomes information that improve on the anecdotal and informal knowledge base underlying clinical practice. PBE studies undertaken by clinical teams have enormous power to enable providers to evaluate current practice and improve clinical decision making. These studies answer questions in the real world where multiple variables and factors can affect the outcomes and therefore have the potential to influence and improve real-world clinical care for the benefit of patients.

REFERENCES

1. Duvall SL, Fraser AM, Rowe K, Thomas A, Mineau GP. Evaluation of record linkage between a large healthcare provider and the Utah Population Database. *J Am Med Inform Assoc.* 2012;19(e1):e54-e59.
2. Slattery ML, Kerber RA. A comprehensive evaluation of family history and breast cancer risk: the Utah Population Database. *JAMA.* 1993;270(13):1563-1568.
3. Hu H, Correll M, Kvecher L, et al. DW4TR: a data warehouse for translational research. *J Biomed Inform.* 2011;44(6):1004-1019.
4. Walton NA, Poynton MR, Gesteland PH, Maloney C, Staes C, Facelli JC. Predicting the start week of respiratory syncytial virus outbreaks using real time weather variables. *BMC Med Inform Decis Mak.* 2010;10:68.
5. Smithburger PL, Buckley MS, Bejian S, Burenheide K, Kane-Gill SL. A critical evaluation of clinical decision support for the detection of drug-drug interactions. *Expert Opin Drug Saf.* 2011;10(6):871-882.
6. Lyng KM, Pedersen BS. Participatory design for computerization of clinical practice guidelines. *J Biomed Inform.* 2011;44(5):909-918.
7. Isern D, Moreno A. Computer-based execution of clinical guidelines: a review. *Int J Med Inform.* 2008;77(12):787-808.
8. Sonnenberg FA, Hagerty CG. Computer-interpretable clinical practice guidelines: where are we and where are we going? *Yearb Med Inform.* 2006:145-158.
9. McDonald CJ, Huff SM, Suico JG, et al. LOINC, a universal standard for identifying laboratory observations: a 5-year update. *Clin Chem.* 2003;49(4):624-633.
10. Meystre S, Haug PJ. Natural language processing to extract medical problems from electronic clinical documents: performance evaluation. *J Biomed Inform.* 2006;39(6):589-599.
11. Jones MM, DuVall SL, Spuhl J, Samore MH, Nielson C, Rubin M. Identification of methicillin-resistant *Staphylococcus aureus* within the nation's Veterans Affairs Medical Centers using natural language processing. *BMC Med Inform Decis Mak.* 2012;12(1):34.

12. SAS Institute. SAS/ACCESS Interface to Teradata (white paper). 2002; 1-42.

13. Lincoln MJ. VA Enterprise Terminology Project (presentation). Salt Lake City, UT: University of Utah Department of Biomedical Informatics Seminar Series; 2006.

14. Meystre SM, Savova GK, Kipper-Schuler KC, Hurdle JF. Extracting information from textual documents in the electronic health record: a review of recent research. *Yearb Med Inform*. 2008: 128-144.

15. Nadkarni PM, Ohno-Machado L, Chapman WW. Natural language processing: an introduction. *J Am Med Inform Assoc*. 2011;18(5):544-551.

16. Hall M, Frank E, Holmes G, Pfahringer B, Reutemann P, Witten I. The WEKA data mining software: an update. *SIGKDD Explorations*. 2009;11(1):10-18.

17. Pyle D. *Data Preparation for Data Mining*. San Francisco, CA: Morgan Kaufmann Publishers; 1999.

18. Sahiner B, Chan HP, Hadjiiski L. Classifier performance estimation under the constraint of a finite sample size: resampling schemes applied to neural network classifiers. *Neural Netw*. 2008;21(2-3):476-483.

19. Fayyad UMP-SG, Smyth P. From data mining to knowledge discovery: an overview. In: Fayyad UMP-SG, Smyth P, Uthurasamy R, eds. *Advances in Knowledge Discovery and Data Mining*. Menlo Park, CA: AAAI Press/The MIT Press; 1996: 1-34.

20. Hanley JA, McNeil BJ. The meaning and use of the area under a receiver operating characteristic (ROC) curve. *Radiology*. 1982;143(1):29-36.

21. Horn SD, DeJong G, Ryser DK, Veazie PJ, Teraoka J. Another look at observational studies in rehabilitation research: going beyond the holy grail of the randomized controlled trial. *Arch Phys Med Rehabil*. 2005;86(12 suppl 2):S8-S15.

22. Mitchell M, Jolley J. *Research Design Explained*. 4th ed. New York, NY: Harcourt; 2001.

23. Horn S, Gassaway J. Practice-based evidence study design for comparative effectiveness research. *Med Care*. 2007;45(suppl 2):S50-S57.

24. Horn SD, Gassaway J. Practice-based evidence: incorporating clinical heterogeneity and patient-reported outcomes for comparative effectiveness research. *Med Care*. 2010;48(6 suppl 1):S17-S22.

25. Horn SD, Sharkey PD, Kelly HW, Uden DL. Newness of drugs and use of HMO services by asthma patients. *Ann Pharmacother*. 2001;35:990-996.

26. Averill RF, McGuire TE, Manning BE, et al. A study of the relationship between severity of illness and hospital cost in New Jersey hospitals. *Health Serv Res*. 1992;27:587-606; discussion 607-612.

27. Clemmer TP, Spuhler VJ, Oniki TA, Horn SD. Results of a collaborative quality improvement program on outcomes and costs in a tertiary critical care unit. *Crit Care Med*. 1999;27: 1768-1774.

28. Horn SD, Torres Jr A, Willson D, Dean JM, Gassaway J, Smout R. Development of a pediatric age- and disease-specific severity measure. *J Pediatrics*. 2002;141:496-503.

29. Willson DF, Horn SD, Smout R, Gassaway J, Torres A. Severity assessment in children hospitalized with bronchiolitis using the pediatric component of the Comprehensive Severity Index. *Pediatr Crit Care Med*. 2000;1:127-132.

30. Ryser DK, Egger MJ, Horn SD, Handrahan D, Gandhi P, Bigler ED. Measuring medical complexity during inpatient rehabilitation after traumatic brain injury. *Arch Phys Med Rehabil*. 2005;86:1108-1117.

31. Horn SD, Sharkey PD, Buckle JM, Backofen JE, Averill RF, Horn RA. The relationship between severity of illness and hospital length of stay and mortality. *Med Care*. 1991;29:305-317.

32. Gassaway JV, Horn SD, DeJong G, Smout RJ, Clark C. Applying the clinical practice improvement approach to stroke rehabilitation: methods used and baseline results. *Arch Phys Med Rehabil*. 2005;86(12 suppl 2):S16-S33.

33. Carter MJ, Fife CE, Walker D, Thomson B. Estimating the applicability of wound care randomized controlled trials to general wound-care populations by estimating the percentage of individuals excluded from a typical wound-care population in such trials. *Adv Skin Wound Care*. 2009;22(7):316-324.

34. Rosenbaum PR. *Observational Studies*. New York, NY: Springer; 2002.

35. Horn SD, DeJong G, et al. Practice-based evidence research in rehabilitation: an alternative to randomized controlled trials and traditional observational studies. *Arch Phys Med Rehabil*. 2012;93(8 Suppl):S127-S137.

36. Deutscher D, Horn SD, Dickstein R, et al. Associations between treatment processes, patient characteristics, and outcomes in outpatient physical therapy practice. *Arch Phys Med Rehabil*. 2009;90(8):1349-1363.

37. Deutscher D, Hart DL, Dickstein R, Horn SD, Gutvirtz M. Implementing an integrated electronic outcomes and electronic health record process to create a foundation for clinical practice improvement. *Phys Ther*. 2008;88(2):270-285.

■ DISCUSSION QUESTIONS

1. How does the KDDM process relate to clinical decision support?

2. Why is it necessary to process coded and text data before using data mining methods?

3. How does evaluation of data mining models differ for prediction of class membership versus real numbers?

4. What is the meaning of the following adage: "Garbage in, garbage out"?

5. How does preprocessing differ for coded versus text data?

6. What are the limitations of observational studies and how does PBE address these?

7. Why is the informaticist a critical member of the PBE team? What essential skills should this team member have?

8. You are a member of a PBE team that will study the prevention and management of ventilator-associated pneumonia. Describe how you would apply the steps of PBE to this problem.

9. In what ways is PBE superior and inferior to RCTs?

10. Compare and contrast KDDM and PBE for secondary use of electronic health data.

CASE STUDY

Pressure Ulcer Case Study*

A PBE study involving 95 long-term care facilities in the United States determined that nursing and clinical nursing assistant (CNA) interventions for pressure ulcer (PrU) prevention and management were highly variable among facilities and that nearly 30% of patients at risk for developing a PrU developed an ulcer during the 12-week study. Characteristics and interventions associated with higher and lower likelihood of PrU development are summarized in the table below.

Research findings were used to develop PrU prevention protocols that included standardized CNA documentation of important data elements and CDS tools. Four long-term care facilities that participated in the study and shared a common electronic medical record system (all members of the same provider network) took the first step in changing practice by sharing study findings with clinical staff including CNAs, who spend the most one-on-one treatment time with nursing home residents and thus are often the first members of the care team to observe changes in residents' nutritional intake, urinary incontinence, mood state, etc. Concurrently, local study leaders worked with their software vendor to incorporate standard documentation for nurses and CNAs and the CDS tools for staff.

Negative Association with Likelihood of Developing a PrU (less likely)

Patient factors

Patient new to long-term care

Treatment factors

Use of disposable briefs for urinary incontinence for >14 days

Nutrition

Use of oral medical nutritional supplements for >21 days

Tube feeding for >21 days

IV fluid supplementation

Medications

Antidepressant medication

Facility staffing patterns

RN hours ≥0.5 hours/resident/day

CNA hours ≥2.25 hours/resident/day

LPN turnover rate <25%

Positive Association with Likelihood of Developing a PrU (more likely)

Patient factors

Higher admission severity of illness

History of PrU in previous 90 days

Significant weight loss

Oral eating problems

Treatment factors

Use of urinary catheter

Use of positioning devices

Discussion Questions

1. What are the steps of the PBE process related to this case study?
2. As the informatics specialist working with the clinical team in the four long-term care facilities, identify the following:
   a. Elements to incorporate into the documentation by CNAs and managers that address factors identified in the original study
   b. CDS tools that could be incorporated into computer systems
3. How can the cost effectiveness of the new documentation requirements and standards of care be efficiently evaluated?

IV, Intravenous; *LPN*, licensed practical nurse; *RN*, registered nurse.
*This case study is fictional; factors are consistent with findings reported in Sharkey S, Hudak S, Horn SD, Spector W. Leveraging certified nursing assistant documentation and knowledge to improve clinical decision making: the on-time quality improvement program to prevent pressure ulcers. *Adv Skin Wound Care.* 2011;24(4):182-188.

Program Evaluation and Research Techniques

Charlene R. Weir

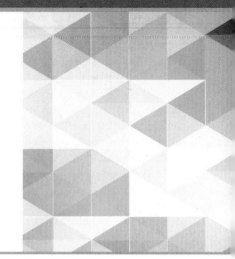

Evaluation of health information technology (health IT) programs and projects can range from simple user satisfaction for a new menu or full-scale analysis of usage, cost, compliance, patient outcomes, and observation of usage to data about patient's rate of improvement.

OBJECTIVES

At the completion of this chapter the reader will be prepared to:

1. Identify the main components of program evaluation
2. Discuss the differences between formative and summative evaluation
3. Apply the three levels of theory relevant to program evaluation
4. Discriminate program evaluation from program planning and research
5. Synthesize the core components of program evaluation with the unique characteristics of informatics interventions

KEY TERMS

ABSTRACT

Evaluation is an essential component in the life cycle of all health IT applications and the key to successful translation of these applications into clinical settings. In planning an evaluation the central questions regarding purpose, scope, and focus of the system must be asked. This chapter focuses on the larger principles of program evaluation with the goal of informing health IT evaluations in clinical settings. The reader is expected to gain sufficient background in health IT evaluation to lead or participate in program evaluation for applications or systems.

Formative evaluation and summative evaluation are discussed. Three levels of theory are presented, including scientific theory, implementation models, and program theory (logic models). Specific scientific theories include social cognitive theories, diffusion of innovation, cognitive engineering theories, and information theory. Four implementation models are reviewed: PRECEDE-PROCEED, PARiHS, RE-AIM, and quality improvement. Program theory models are discussed, with an emphasis on logic models.

A review of methods and tools is presented. Relevant research designs are presented for health IT evaluations, including time series, multiple baseline, and regression discontinuity. Methods of data collection specific to health IT evaluations, including ethnographic observation, interviews, and surveys, are then reviewed.

INTRODUCTION

The outcome of evaluation is information that is both useful at the program level and generalizable enough to contribute to the building of science. In the applied sciences, such as informatics, evaluation is critical to the growth of both the specialty and the science. In this chapter program evaluation is defined as the "systematic collection of information about the activities, characteristics, and results of programs to make judgments about the program, improve or further develop program effectiveness, inform decisions about future programming, and/or increase understanding."[1] Health IT interventions are nearly always embedded in the larger processes of care delivery and are unique for three reasons. First, stakeholders' knowledge about the capabilities of health IT systems may be limited at the beginning of a project. Second, the health IT product often changes substantially during the implementation process. Third, true implementation often takes 6 months or longer, with users maturing in knowledge and skills and external influences, such as new regulations or organizational initiatives, occurring over that period. Identification of the unique contribution of the health IT application therefore is often difficult and evaluation goals frequently go beyond the health IT component alone. In this chapter the health IT component of evaluation is integrated with overall program evaluation; unique issues are highlighted for evaluating health IT itself. The chapter is organized into three sections: (1) purposes of evaluation, (2) theories and frameworks, and (3) methods, tools, and techniques.

PURPOSES OF EVALUATION

The purpose of evaluation determines the methods, approaches, tools, and dissemination practices for the entire project being evaluated. Therefore identifying the purpose is a crucial first step. Mark, Henry, and Julnes have provided four main evaluation purposes, which are listed in Box 5-1.

Usually an evaluation project is not restricted to just one of these purposes. Teasing out which purposes are more important is a process for the evaluator and the involved stakeholders. The following sections represent a series of questions that can clarify the process.

Formative versus Summative Evaluation

Will the results of the evaluation be used to improve the program or to focus on determining whether the goals of the program have been met? This question refers to a common classification of evaluation activities that fall into two types: (1) formative evaluation and (2) summative evaluation. The difference is in how the information is used. The results of the formative evaluation are used as feedback to the program for continuous improvement.[2,3] The results of the summative evaluation are used to evaluate the merit of the program. Formative evaluation is a term coined by Scriven in 1967 and expanded on by a number of other authors to mean an assessment of how well the program is being implemented and to describe the experience of participants.[4] Topics for formative evaluation include the fidelity of the intervention, the quality of implementation, the

| BOX 5-1 | MAIN PURPOSES OF PROGRAM EVALUATION |

- Program and organizational improvement
- Assessment of merit or worth
- Knowledge development
- Oversight and compliance

Adapted from Mark M, Henry G, Julnes G. Evaluation: An Integrative Framework for Understanding, Guiding and Improving Policies and Programs. San Francisco, CA: Jossey-Bass; 2000.

characteristics of the organizational context, and the types of personnel. Needs assessments and feasibility analyses are included in this general category. Box 5-2 outlines several questions that fall into the category of formative evaluation for health IT.

In contrast, summative evaluation refers to an assessment of the outcomes and impact of the program. Cost-effectiveness and adverse events analyses are included in this category. Some questions that fall into the summative evaluation category are listed in Box 5-3.

Dividing the evaluation process into the formative and summative components is somewhat arbitrary, as they can be and often are conducted concurrently. They do not necessarily differ in terms of methods or even in terms of the content of the information collected. Formative evaluation is especially important for health IT products where the overall goal is improvement. Because health IT products are "disruptive technologies," they both transform the working environment and are themselves transformed during the process of implementation.[5] Many writers in the informatics field have noted the paucity of information on implementation processes in published studies. In a meta-analysis of health IT by researchers at RAND, the authors noted:

> In summary, we identified no study or collection of studies, outside of those from a handful of health IT leaders that would allow a reader to make a determination about the generalizable knowledge of the system's reported benefit. This limitation in generalizable knowledge is not simply a matter of study design and internal validity. Even if further randomized, controlled trials are performed, the generalizability of the evidence would remain low unless additional systematic, comprehensive, and relevant descriptions and measurements are made regarding how the technology is

| BOX 5-2 | QUESTIONS TO POSE DURING FORMATIVE EVALUATION |

- What is the nature and scope of the problem that is being addressed by health IT?
- What is the extent and seriousness of the need?
- How well is the technology working and what is the best way to deliver it?
- How are participants (and users) experiencing the program?
- How did the intervention change after implementation?

utilized, the individuals using it, and the environment it is used in.[6(p4)]

Although written in 2006, this statement is still relevant today.

Generalizability and Scope

Will the results of the evaluation be used to inform stakeholders of whether a particular program is "working" and is in compliance with regulations and mandates? This question refers to issues of the generalizability and scope of the project. It is also a question of whether the evaluation is more of a program evaluation or a research study. An evaluation of a locally developed project usually would be considered a program evaluation. In contrast, if the program was designed to test a hypothesis or research question and described, measured, or manipulated variables that could be generalized to a larger population, then the results of the evaluation study are more like research. However, both approaches use systematic tools and methods. For example, if the program to be evaluated is a local implementation of alerts and decision support for providers at the point of care to evaluate skin breakdown, then the stakeholders are the administrators, nurses, and patients who are affected by use of the decision support program. The evaluation questions would address the use of the program, the impact on resources, satisfaction, and perhaps clinical outcomes. The evaluation would likely use a before and after format and a more informal approach to assess whether the decision support worked. However, if the evaluation question is whether or not computerized guidelines affect behavior in general and under what conditions, then the specific stakeholders matter less and the ability to generalize beyond the contextual situation matters more. A more formal, research-based approach is then used. This question is really about what is to be learned. Vygotsky called these two approaches "patterning" versus "puzzling."[7] In the patterning approach to evaluation the comparison is between what went before at the local level, whereas in the puzzling approach the task is to do an in-depth comparison between different options and puzzle through the differences.

Another way to address this issue is to imagine that evaluation activities fall along a continuum from "program evaluation" to "evaluation research." Program evaluation tends to have a wide scope, using multiple methods with a diverse range of outcomes. Evaluation research tends to be more targeted, using more selected methods and fewer outcomes. On the program evaluation end of the continuum, evaluation can encompass a range of activities including but not limited to program model development, needs assessment, tracking and performance monitoring, and continuous quality improvement. On the research end of the continuum, activities include theory testing, statistical evaluation of models, and hypothesis testing. At both ends of the continuum and in between, however, evaluators can use a variety of research designs, rigorous measurement methods, and statistical analyses.

Program Continuance versus Growth

Will the results of the evaluation be used to make a decision about continuing the program as is or about expanding it to a larger or different setting if it has generalizable knowledge? Answering the question of whether a program will be continued requires a focus on the concerns and goals of stakeholders as well as special attention to the contextual issues of cost, burden, user satisfaction, adoption, and effectiveness. Answering this question also requires an assessment about the manner in which the program was implemented and its feasibility in terms of resources and efforts. Does the program require ongoing and intense training of staff and technicians? Does it require unique hardware requirements that are a one-time or ongoing cost? Does the program have "legs" (i.e., can it exist on its own once implemented)? Are the benefits accrued available immediately or is it a long-term process?

One specific example to determine whether the program should be continued is to assess whether or not it contributes to the institution being a "learning organization."[8,9] This approach focuses on performance improvement and the following four areas of concern (modified for health IT):

1. What are the mental models and implicit theories held by the different stakeholders about the health IT product?
2. How does the health IT product promote mastery or personal control over the work environment?
3. What is the system-level impact of the health IT product? How does the intervention support a system thinking approach?
4. How does the health IT product create a unified vision of the information environment? Addressing this question requires understanding how individuals view the future computerized environment and whether or not they have come to a shared vision.

THEORIES AND FRAMEWORKS

The use of theory in evaluation studies is controversial among evaluators as well as in the informatics community. On the one hand, some authors note that evaluation studies are local, limited in scope, and not intended to be generalizable. On the other hand, other authors argue that theory is necessary to frame the issues adequately, promote generalizable knowledge, and clarify measurement. This author would argue that theory should be used for the latter reason. Theoretical perspectives clarify the constructs and methods of measuring constructs as well as bring forward an understanding of mechanisms of action.

For the purposes of this chapter, theoretical perspectives will be divided into three levels of complexity. At the most complex level are the *social science*, *cognitive engineering*, and *information science theories*. These theories are well established, have a strong evidence base, and use validated measures and well-understood mechanisms of action. This chapter discusses some well-known social science theories as well as two health IT–specific adaptations of these theories that have significant validation. At the next level are the *program implementation models*, which are less complex and basically consist of a conceptual model. The models are often used to describe processes but few studies attempt to validate the models or test models against each other. Finally, at the most basic level are the *program theory models*, which are program specific and intended to represent the goals and content of a specific project. *All* evaluations for health IT products should develop a program theory model to guide the evaluation process itself. The descriptions below are brief and are intended to provide an overview of the possibilities at each level.

Social Science Theories

There are myriad theories relevant to both the design of interventions and products and the structure of the evaluation. A more detailed description of such theories as they apply to informatics is found in Chapter 2. A short description is provided here for the purpose of context. These social science theories include social cognitive theories, diffusion of innovation theory, cognitive engineering theories, and information theories.

Social Cognitive Theories

The social cognitive theories include the theory of planned behavior,[10] its close relative the theory of reasoned action,[11] and Bandura's social cognitive theory.[12] These theories predict intentions and behavior as a function of beliefs about the value of an outcome, the likelihood that the outcome will occur given the behavior, and the expectations of others and self-efficacy beliefs about the personal ability to engage in the activity. The empirical validation of these theories is substantial and they have been used to predict intentions and behavior across a wide variety of settings.

Diffusion of Innovations Theory

Another very commonly used model in informatics is diffusion of innovations theory by Rogers.[13,14] In this model characteristics of the innovation, the type of communication

channels, the duration, and the social system are predictors of the rate of diffusion. The central premise is that diffusion is the process by which an innovation is communicated through certain channels over time among the members of a social system organization. Individuals pass through five stages: knowledge, persuasion, decision, implementation, and confirmation. Social norms, roles, and the type of communication channels all affect the rate of adoption of an innovation. Characteristics of an innovation that affect the rate of adoption include relative advantage as compared to other options; trialability, or the ease with which it can be tested; compatibility with other work areas; complexity of the innovation; and observability, or the ease with which the innovation is visible.

Cognitive Engineering Theories

The cognitive engineering theories have also been widely used in informatics, particularly naturalistic decision making (NDM),[15-17] control theory,[18] and situation awareness (SA).[19] These theories focus more on the interaction between the context and the individual and are more likely to predict decision making, perception, and other cognitive variables. NDM is a broad and inclusive paradigm. SA is narrower and is particularly useful in supporting design.

SA combines the cognitive processes of orientation, attention, categorization or sense-making, and planning into three levels of performance. These activities are thought to be critical to human performance in complex environments. Endsley refers to a three-level system of awareness: (1) perception, (2) comprehension, and (3) projection. She defines shared SA as the group understanding of the situation.[19] For example, in one recent study of health IT, higher SA was significantly associated with more integrated displays for intensive care unit (ICU) nursing staff.[20,21] Table 5-1 presents the core components of SA and associated definitions.

TABLE 5-1	LEVELS OF SITUATIONAL AWARENESS	
LEVEL	**DESCRIPTION**
Perception of the elements in the environment	What is present, active, salient, and important in the environment? Attention will be driven by task needs.
Comprehension of the current situation	Classification of the event is a function of activation of long-term memory. Meaning is driven by the cognitive process of classification and task identification.
Projection of future status	Expectations of outcomes in the future. Driven by implicit theories and knowledge about the causal mechanisms underlying events.

Information Theories

One of the most influential theories is *information theory* published in 1948 by Claude Shannon.[22] Shannon focused on the mathematical aspects of the theory. Weaver, an oncologist, focused on the semantic meaning of the theory.[23] Information theory identifies the degree of uncertainty in messages as a function of the capacity of the system to transmit those messages given a certain amount of noise and entropy. The transmission of information is broken down into *source, sender, channel, receiver,* and *destination*. Because information theory is essentially a theory of communication, information is defined relative to three levels of analysis:

1. At the *technical* or statistical level, information is defined as a measure of entropy or uncertainty in the situation. The question at this level is: How accurately are the symbols used in the communication being transmitted?

2. At the *semantic* level, information is defined as a reduction of uncertainty at the level of human meaning. The question here is: How well do the symbols that were transmitted convey the correct meaning?

3. At the *effectiveness* level, information is defined as a change in the goal state of the system. The question here is: How well does the perceived meaning effect the desired outcome?[24]

This simple framework can provide an effective evaluation model for any system that evaluates the flow of information. For example, Weir and McCarthy used information theory to develop implementation indicators for a computerized provider order entry (CPOE) project.[25]

Information foraging theory is a relatively new theory of information searching that has proven very useful for analyzing web searching.[26] Information foraging theory is built on foraging theory, which studies how animals search for food. Pirolli and Card noticed similar patterns in the processes used by animals to search for food and the processes used by humans to search for information on the Internet. The basic assumption is that all information searches are goal directed and constitute a calibration between the energy cost of searching and the estimated value of information retrieved. The four concepts listed in Box 5-4 are important to measure. Empirical work on foraging theory has validated its core concepts.[27]

Information Technology Theories

Two well-developed information technology theories are specifically used in the IT domain. As is true of many IT theories, they are compiled from several existing theories from the basic sciences to improve their fit in an applied setting.

Information System Success

An IT model that integrates several formal theories is DeLone and McLean's multifactorial model of IT success developed with the goal of improving scientific generalization.[28] Their theory was originally developed in 1992 and revised in 2003 based on significant empirical support. The model is based on Shannon and Weaver's communication theory[23] and Mason's information "influence" theory.[29] DeLone and McLean used Shannon and Weaver's three levels of information: (1) technical (accuracy and efficiency of the communication system), (2) semantic (communicating meaning), and (3) effectiveness (impact on receiver). These three levels correspond to DeLone and McLean's constructs of (1) "systems quality," (2) "information quality," and (3) impact (use, user satisfaction, and outcomes). DeLone and McLean revised the model in 2003 to include recent literature and added a fourth level—"service quality"—referring to the degree to which users are supported by IT staff. Figure 5-1 depicts an adaptation of the updated 2003 model that adds user satisfaction, user characteristics, and task effectiveness to the original model.

Unified Theory of Acceptance and Use of Technology (UTAUT)

An adaptation of the social cognitive theories within the field of informatics is the unified theory of acceptance and use of technology (UTAUT).[30] UTAUT, depicted in Figure 5-2, explains users' intentions to use an information system as a function of performance expectancy or self-efficacy beliefs, effort expectancies, social influence, and facilitating conditions. Significant moderators of these variables of intentions

---

BOX 5-4	**FOUR CONCEPTS OF FORAGING THEORY**

1. Information and its perceived value
2. Information patches or the temporal and spatial location of information clusters
3. Information scent or the presence of cues value and location of information
4. Information diet or the decision to pursue one source over another

---

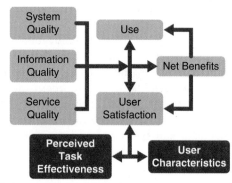

FIG 5-1 A model of information system success (Adapted from *Journal of Management Information Systems*, vol. 19, no. 4 [Spring 1993]: 9-30. Copyright © 1993 by M.E. Sharpe, Inc. Reprinted with permission. All Rights Reserved. Not for Reproduction.)

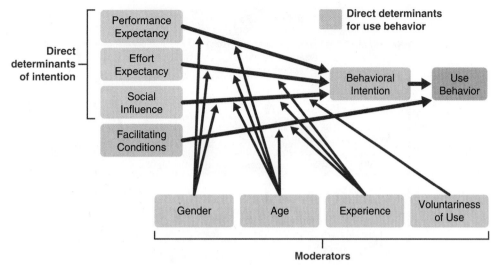

FIG 5-2 An example of unified theory of acceptance and use of technology. (From Venkatesh V, Morris M, Davis G, Davis F. User acceptance of information technology: toward a unified view. *MIS Quart.* 2003;27[3]:425-478.)

are gender, age, and the degree to which usage is mandated. This model integrates social cognitive theory,[12] theory of reasoned action,[11] and diffusion of innovations theory.[13]

Venkatesh and Davis conducted a systematic measurement meta-analysis that tested eight major models of adoption to clarify and integrate the adoption literature.[31] All of the evaluated models were based to some degree on the social cognitive models described above but adapted to the question of IT adoption and use. Empirical studies showed that UTAUT explained around 70% of the variance in intention to use, significantly greater than any of the initial models alone. Two key findings of this work are important. First, Venkatesh et al. found that the variables associated with initial intentions to use are different than the variables associated with later intentions.[30,32,33] Specifically, the perceived work effectiveness constructs (perceived usefulness, extrinsic motivation, job fit, relative advantage, and outcome expectations) were found to be highly predictive of intentions over time. In contrast, variables such as attitudes, perceived behavioral control, ease of use, self-efficacy, and anxiety were predictors only of early intentions to use.

Second, the authors found that the variables predictive of intentions to use are not the same as the variables predictive of usage behavior itself.[30] They found that the "effort factor scale" (resources, knowledge, compatible systems, and support) was the only construct other than intention to significantly predict usage behavior. Finally, these authors found that the model differed significantly depending on whether usage was mandated or by choice. In settings where usage was mandated, social norms had a stronger relationship to intentions to use than the other variables.

Program Implementation Models

Program implementation models refer to generalized, large-scale implementation theories that are focused on performance improvement and institution-wide change. Four models are reviewed here: PRECEDE-PROCEED, PARiHS, RE-AIM, and quality improvement.

PRECEDE-PROCEED Model

The letters in the PRECEDE-PROCEED model represent the following terms: PRECEDE—Predisposing, Reinforcing, and Enabling Constructs in Educational Diagnosis and Evaluation; PROCEED—Policy, Regulatory, and Organizational Constructs in Educational and Environmental Development. This model was originally developed to guide the design of system-level educational interventions as well as evaluating program outcomes. It is a model that addresses change at several levels, ranging from the individual to the organization level. According to the model the interaction between the three types of variables produces change: *predisposing factors* that lay the foundation for success (e.g., electronic health records or strong leadership), *reinforcing factors* that follow and strengthen behavior (e.g., incentives and feedback), and *enabling factors* that activate and support the change process (e.g., support, training, computerized reminders, and templates or exciting content). The model has been applied in a variety of settings, ranging from public health interventions, education, and geriatric quality improvement and alerting studies.[34] Figure 5-3 illustrates the model applied to a health IT product.

Promoting Action on Research Implementation in Health Services (PARiHS)

The PARiHS framework outlines three general areas associated with implementation (Fig. 5-4):

1. *Evidence*: Establishing the efficiency and effectiveness of the intervention through expert contribution, literature reviews, surveys, usability testing, and cognitive task analyses

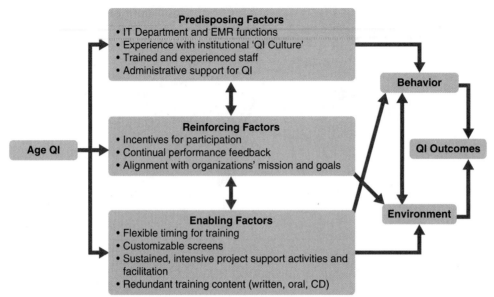

FIG 5-3 An adaptation of the PRECEDE-PROCEED model for a health IT product. (From Green LW, Kreuter MW. *Health Program Planning: An Educational and Ecological Approach.* 4th ed. Mountain View, CA: McGraw-Hill; 2005. Republished with permission of McGraw-Hill Companies Inc.)

Promoting Action on Research Implementation in Health Services (PARiHS)

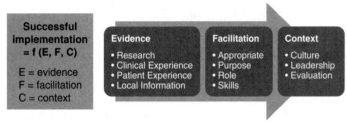

FIG 5-4 The PARiHS model. (From Kitson AL, Rycroft-Malone J, Harvey G, McCormack B, Seers K, Titchen A. Evaluating the successful implementation of evidence into practice using the PARiHS framework: theoretical and practical challenges. *Implement Sci.* 2008;3:1.)

2. *Context:* Enhancing leadership support and integrating with the culture through focus groups and interviews
3. *Facilitation of the implementation process:* Skill level and role of facilitator in promoting action as well as frequency of supportive interactions[35]

These three elements are defined across several subelements, with higher ratings suggestive of more successful implementation. For instance, a high level of evidence may include the presence of randomized controlled trials (i.e., the gold standard in research), high levels of consensus among clinicians, and collaborative relationships between patients and providers. Context is evaluated in terms of readiness for implementation, including consideration of the context's culture, leadership style, and measurement practices. High ratings of context may indicate an environment focused on continuing education, effective teamwork, and consistent

evaluation and feedback. Finally, the most successful facilitation is characterized by high levels of respect for the implementation setting, a clearly defined agenda and facilitator role, and supportive flexibility.[36] Successful implementation (*SI*) is thus conceptualized as a function (*f*) of evidence (*E*), context (*C*), and facilitation (*F*), or SI = f(E, C, F).[37] The PARiHS framework suggests a continuous multidirectional approach to evaluation of implementation. Importantly, evaluation is a cyclic and interactive process instead of a linear approach.

Reach Effectiveness Adoption Implementation Maintenance (RE-AIM)

RE-AIM was designed to address the significant barriers associated with implementation of any new intervention and is particularly useful for informatics. Most interventions meet with significant resistance and any useful evaluation should measure the barriers associated with the constructs (Reach, Effectiveness, Adoption, Implementation, and Maintenance). These constructs serve as a good format for evaluation.[38,39] First, did the intervention actually *reach* the intended target population? In other words, how many providers had the opportunity to use the system? Or, how many patients had access to a new website? Second, for *effectiveness*, did the intervention actually do what it was intended to do? Did the wound care decision support actually work as intended every time? Did it identify the patients it was supposed to identify? Or, did the algorithms miss some key variables in real life? Third, for *adoption*, what proportion of the targeted staff, settings, or institutions actually used the program? What was the breadth and depth of usage? Did they use it for all relevant patients or only for some? Fourth, for *implementation*, was the intervention the same across settings and time? With most health IT products there is constant change to the software, the skill level of users, and the settings in which they are used. These should be documented and addressed in the evaluation. Finally, for *maintenance*, some period of time should be identified a priori to assess maintenance and whether usage continues and by whom and in what form. For health IT interventions it is especially useful to look for unintended consequences as well as workarounds during implementation and maintenance in particular.

Quality Improvement

Evaluation activities using a quality improvement framework are often based on Donabedian's classic structure-process-outcome (SPO) model for assessing healthcare quality.[40,41] Donabedian defines structural measures of quality as the professional and organizational resources associated with the provision of care, such as IT staff credentials, CPOE systems, or staffing ratios. Process measures include the tasks and decisions imbedded in care, such as the time to provision of antibiotics or the proportion of patients on deep vein thrombosis (DVT) prevention protocols. Finally, outcomes are defined as the final or semifinal measurable outcomes of care, such as the number of amputations due to diabetes, the number of patients with DVT, or the number of patients with drug-resistant pneumonia. These three categories of variables are thought to be mutually interdependent and reinforcing. A model for patient safety and quality research design (PSQRD) expands on this well-known, original SPO model.[42] For more details on this model, see Chapter 20.

Program Theory Models

Program theory models are the most basic and practical of the evaluation models. They are the implicit theories of stakeholders and participants of the proposed program. A detailed program theory identifies variables, the timing of measures and observations, and the key expectations that reflect their understandings. Most importantly, a program theory model serves as a shared vision between the evaluator team and the participants, creating a unified conceptual model that guides all evaluation activities.

Six Steps

Program theory evaluation is recommended practice for all program evaluation and an important approach regardless of whether the program is the implementation of a new documentation system or an institution-wide information system. Invariably, various participants will have different ideas about what the program is and why it works.[43] Creation of a program theory model serves to align the various stakeholders into a single view. The Centers for Disease Control and Prevention's six-step program evaluation framework is one of the best examples in current use.[44] It recommends the following six steps:

1. *Engage stakeholders* to ensure that *all* partners have contributed to the goals of the program and the metrics to measure its success.

2. *Describe the program systematically* to identify goals, objectives, activities, resources, and context. This description process involves all stakeholders.
3. *Focus the evaluation design* to assess usefulness, feasibility, ethics, and accuracy.
4. *Gather credible evidence* by collecting data, conducting interviews, and measuring outcomes using a good research design.
5. *Justify conclusions* using comparisons against standards, statistical evidence, or expert review.
6. *Ensure use and share lessons learned* by planning and implementing dissemination activities.

Logic Models

A logic model is a representation of components and mechanisms of the program as noted by the authors of the W.K. Kellogg Foundation's guide to logic models:

> Basically, a logic model is a systematic and visual way to present and share your understanding of the relationship among the resources you have to operate your program, the activities you plan, and the changes or results you hope to achieve. The most basic logic model is a picture of how you believe your program will work. It uses words and/or pictures to describe the sequence of activities thought to bring about change and how these activities are linked to the results the program is expected to achieve.[45(p1)]

The basic structure of a logic model is illustrated in Figure 5-5. The logic model starts with a category of "inputs," which include staff, resources, prior success, and stakeholders. In health IT the inputs are the programs, software, the IT staff, hardware, networks, and training. "Outputs" include the activities that are going to be conducted, such as training, implementation, software design, and other computer activities. Participation refers to the individual involved. Outcomes are divided into short, medium, and long outcomes or short-term versus long-term outcomes. The goal is to make sure that the components of the program are easy to see and the mechanisms are made explicit.

The specific methods used to apply a model are not prescribed (although creating a logic model is recommended). Use of a wide range of methods and tools is encouraged. Engaging the stakeholders is the first step and that process could involve needs assessment, functionality requirements analyses, cognitive task analyses, contextual inquiry, and ethnographic observation, to name a few approaches. In all cases, the result is the ability to provide a deep description of the program, the expected mechanisms, and the desired outcomes. Once there is agreement on the characteristics of the program at both the superficial level and the deeper structure, designing the evaluation is straightforward. Agreement among stakeholders is needed not only to identify concepts to measure, but also to determine how to meaningfully measure them.

In a health IT product implementation, agreement, especially about goals and metrics, should be made early in the program implementation process. Because health IT products are unique, creating a shared vision and a common

Program Action – Logic Model

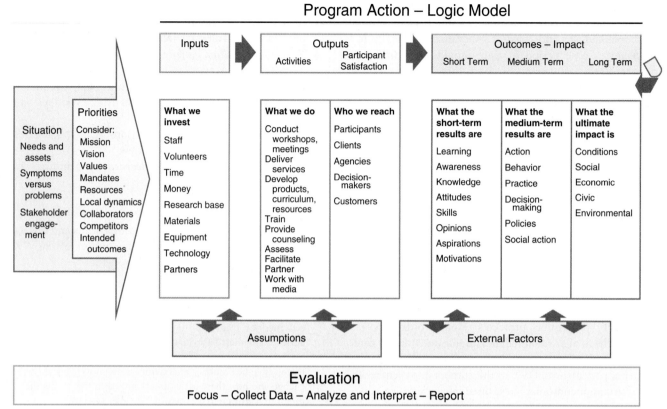

FIG 5-5 Example of a logic model structure. (From University of Wisconsin–Extension, Cooperative Extension, Program Development and Evaluation website. Logic model. http://www.uwex.edu/ces/pdande/evaluation/evallogicmodel.html. 2010.)

understanding of the meaning of the evaluation can be challenging. Using an iterative process for implementation can mitigate this problem where design and implementation go hand in hand and the stakeholder's vision is addressed repeatedly throughout the process.

METHODS, TOOLS, AND TECHNIQUES

The need for variety in methods is driven by the diversity in population, types of projects, and purposes that are characteristic of research in informatics. Many evaluation projects are classified as either qualitative or quantitative. This division may be somewhat artificial and limited but using the terms *qualitative* and *quantitative* to organize methods helps to make them relatively easy to understand. A central thesis of this section is that the choice of method should fit the question and multiple methods are commonly used in evaluations.

Quantitative versus Qualitative Questions

Because evaluation is often a continuous process throughout the life of a project, the systems life cycle is used to organize this discussion. Evaluation activities commonly occur during the planning, implementation, and maintenance stages of a project (see Chapter 2 for more details about these stages and others in the systems life cycle). At each stage both quantitative and qualitative questions might be asked. At the beginning of a project the goal is to identify resources,

feasibility, values, extent of the problem to be solved, and types of needs. The methods used to answer these questions are essentially local and project specific. During the project, evaluation questions focus on the intensity, quality, and depth of the implementation as well as the evolution of the project team and community. Finally, in the maintenance phase of the project the questions focus on outcomes, cost–benefit value, or overall consequences.

Table 5-2 presents a matrix that outlines the different stages of a project and the types of questions that might be asked during each stage. The questions are illustrations of possible evaluation questions and loosely categorized as either qualitative or quantitative.

Qualitative Methods

Many individuals believe that qualitative methods refer to research procedures that collect subjective human-generated data. However, subjective data can be quantitative, such as the subjective responses to carefully constructed usability questionnaires used as outcome end points. Diagnostic codes are another example of quantitative forms of subjective data. Qualitative methods, rather, refer to procedures and methods that produce narrative or observational descriptive data that are not intended for transformation into numbers. Narrative data refer to information in the form of stories, themes, meanings, and metaphors. Collecting this information requires the use of systematic procedures where the purpose is to understand and explore while minimizing bias. There

TABLE 5-2	EVALUATION RESEARCH QUESTIONS BY STAGE OF PROJECT AND TYPE OF QUESTION	
	TYPES OF QUESTIONS	
STAGE OF PROJECT	**QUALITATIVE**	**QUANTITATIVE**
Planning	What are the values of the different stakeholders? What are the expectations and goals of participants?	What is the prevalence of the problem being addressed by the health IT product? What are the resources available? What is the relationship between experiencing a factor and having a negative outcome? What are the intensity and depth of use of health IT tools?
Implementation	How are participants experiencing the change? How does the health IT product change the way individuals relate to or communicate with each other?	How many individuals are participating? What changes in performance have been visible? What is the compliance rate? How many resources are being used during implementation (when and where)?
Maintenance	How has the culture of the situation changed? What themes underscore the participants' experience? What metaphors describe the change? What are the participants' personal stories?	Is there a significant change in outcomes for patients? Did compliance rates increase (for addressing the initial problem)? What is the rate of adverse events? Is there a significant change in efficiency? Is there a correlation between usage and outcomes?

IT, Information technology.

are several very good guides to conducting qualitative research for health IT evaluation studies.[46]

Structured and Semistructured Interviews

In-person interviews can be some of the best sources of information about an individual's unique perspectives, issues, and values. Interviews vary from a very structured set of questions conducted under controlled conditions to a very informal set of questions asked in an open-ended manner. Typically, evaluators audio-record the interviews and conduct thematic or content coding on the results. For example, user interviews that focus on how health IT affects workflow are especially useful. Some interviews have a specific focus, such as in the critical incident method.[47] In this method an individual recalls a critical incident and describes it in detail for the interviewer. In other cases the interview may focus on the individual's personal perceptions and motivations, such as in motivational interviewing.[48] Finally, cognitive task analysis (CTA) is a group of specialized interviews and observations where the goal is to deconstruct a task or work situation into component parts and functions.[49-51] A CTA usually consists of targeting a task or work process and having the participant walk through or simulate the actions, identifying the goals, strategies, and information needs. These latter methods are useful for user experience studies outlined in Chapter 21.

Observation and Protocol Analysis

An interview may not provide enough information and therefore observing users in action at work is necessary to fully understand the interactions of context, users, and health IT. Observation can take many forms, from using a video camera to a combination of observation and interview where individuals "think aloud" while they work. The think-aloud procedures need to be analyzed both qualitatively for themes and quantitatively for content, timing, and frequency.[52]

Interviews, CTAs, and observation are essential in almost every health IT evaluation of users. Technology interventions are not uniform and cannot simply be inserted into the workflow in a "plug and play" manner. In addition, the current state of the literature in the field lacks clarity about the mechanisms of action or even delineating the key components of health IT. Thus understanding the user's response to the system is essential. For more information about the user experience, see Chapter 21.

Ethnography and Participant Observation

Ethnography and participant observation are derived from the field of anthropology, where the goal is to understand the larger cultural system through observer immersion. The degree of immersion can vary, as can some of the data collection methods, but the overall strategy includes interacting with all aspects of the context. Usually ethnography requires considerable time, multiple observations, interviews, and living and working in the situation if possible. It also includes reading historical documents, exploring artifacts in current use (e.g., memos, minutes), and generally striving to understand a community. These methods are particularly useful in a clinical setting, where understanding the culture is essential.[46,53]

Less intensive ethnographic methods are also possible and reasonable for health IT evaluations. Focused ethnography is a method of observing actions in a particular context. For example, nurses were observed during patient care hand-offs and their interactions with electronic health records were recorded. From these observations design implications for hand-off forms were derived.[54,55]

Quantitative Methods
Research Designs

Quantitative designs range from epidemiologic, descriptive studies to randomized controlled trials. Three study designs presented may be particularly useful for health IT and clinical settings. Each of these designs takes advantage of the conditions that are commonly found in health IT projects, including automatically collected data, the ubiquitous use of pre-post design, and outcome-based targets for interventions.

Time Series Analysis

This design is an extension of the simple pre-post format but requires multiple measures in time prior to and after an intervention such as health IT. Evidence of the impact is found in the differences in mathematical slopes between measures during the pre-test and post-test periods. This design has significantly more validity than a simple pre-post one-time measure design and can be very feasible in clinical settings where data collection is automatic and can be done for long periods with little increase in costs. For example, top-level administrators might institute a decision support computerized program to improve patient care for pain management. A straightforward design is to measure the rate of compliance to pain management recommendations during several periods about 12 months prior and several periods up to 12 months after implementation, controlling for hospital occupancy, patient acuity, and staffing ratios. This design is highly recommended for health IT implementations where data can be captured electronically and reliably over long periods.[56,57]

Regression Discontinuity Design

A regression discontinuity design is similar to a time series analysis but is a formal statistical analysis of the pattern of change over time for two groups. This design is particularly suited to community engagement interventions, such as for low vaccination rates in children or seat belt reminders. Participants are divided into two nonoverlapping groups based on their prescores on the outcome of interest. The example used above of compliance with pain management guidelines in an inpatient surgical unit may also be applicable. Providers with greater than 50% compliance to pain guidelines are put in one group and those with less than 50% compliance with pain guidelines are in the other group. Those with the lowest compliance receive a decision support intervention such as a computerized alert and a decision support system to assess and treat pain while the rest do not. Post measures are taken some time after the intervention and the difference between the predicted scores of the low compliance group and their actual scores as compared to the nonintervention group are noted. The validity of this design is nearly as high as a randomized controlled trial, but this design is much easier to implement because those who need the intervention

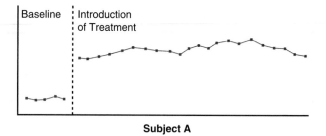

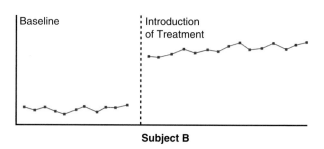

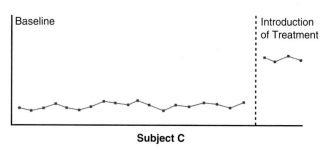

FIG 5-6 Example of a multiple baseline study.

receive it. However, this design requires large numbers, which may not be available except in a system-wide or multisite implementation.[58]

Multiple Baseline with Single Subject Design

This design adds significant value to the standard pre-post comparison by staggering implementation systematically (e.g., at 3-month intervals) over many settings but the measurement for *all* settings starts at the same time. In other words, measurement begins at the same time across five clinics but implementation is staggered every 3 months. Figure 5-6 illustrates the pattern of responses that might be observed. The strength of the evidence is high if outcomes improved after implementation in each setting and they followed the same pattern.[59]

Instruments

Data are commonly gathered through the use of instruments. User satisfaction, social network analyses, and cost-effectiveness tools are discussed briefly below.

User Satisfaction Instruments

User satisfaction is commonly measured as part of health IT evaluations but is a complex concept. On the one hand it is thought to be a proxy for adoption and on the other hand it is used as a proxy for system effectiveness. In the first conception, the constructs of interest would be usability and ease of use and whether others use it (usability and social norms). In the second conception, the constructs of interest would refer to how well the system helped to accomplish task goals (usefulness). One of the most common instruments for evaluating user satisfaction is the UTAUT.[31] This well-validated instrument assesses perceived usefulness, social norms and expectations, perceived effort, self-efficacy, ease of use, and intentions to use. Reliability for these six scales ranges from 0.92 to 0.95.

A second measure of user satisfaction focuses on service quality (SERVQUAL) and assesses the degree and quality of IT service. Five scales have been validated: reliability, assurance, tangibles, empathy, and responsiveness. These five scales have been found to have reliability of 0.81 to 0.94.[60]

A third measure is the system usability scale (SUS), which is widely used outside health IT.[61] It is a 10-item questionnaire applicable to any health IT product. Bangor and colleagues endorsed the SUS above other available instruments because it is technology agnostic (applicable to a variety of products) and easy to administer and the resulting score is easily interpreted.[62] The authors provide a case study of product iterations and corresponding SUS ratings that demonstrate the sensitivity of the SUS to improvements in usability.

Social Network Analysis

Methods that assess the linkages between people, activities, and locations are likely to be very useful for understanding a community and its structure. Social network analysis (SNA) is a general set of tools that calculates the connections between people based on ratings of similarity, frequency of interaction, or some other metric. The resultant pattern of connection is displayed as a visual network of interacting individuals. Each node is an individual and the lines between nodes reflect the interactions. Although SNA uses numbers to calculate the form of the networked display, it is essentially a qualitative technique because the researcher must interpret the patterns of connections and describe them in narrative form. Conducting an SNA is useful if the goal is to understand how an information system affected communication between individuals. It is also useful to visualize nonpeople connections, such as the relationship between search terms or geographical distances.[63] For example, Benham-Hutchins used SNA to examine patient care hand-offs from the emergency department to inpatient areas, finding that each hand-off entailed 11 to 20 healthcare providers.[64]

Cost-Effectiveness Analysis

Cost-effectiveness analysis (CEA) attempts to quantify the relative costs of two or more options. Simply measuring additional resources, start-up costs, and labor would be a rudimentary cost analysis. A CEA is different than a cost–benefit analysis, which gives specific monetary analysis. A simple CEA shows a ratio of the cost divided by the change in health outcomes or behavior. For example, a CEA might compare

the cost of paying a librarian to answer clinicians' questions as compared to installing Infobuttons per the number of known questions. Most CEA program evaluations will assess resource use, training, increased staff hiring, and other cost-related information. This would not necessarily be a full economic analysis that would require a consultation with an economist. The specific resources used could be delineated in the logic model, unless it was part of hypothesis testing in a more formal survey. The reader is directed to a textbook if further information is needed.[37]

CONCLUSION AND FUTURE DIRECTIONS

Evaluation of health IT programs and projects can range from simple user satisfaction for a new menu to full-scale analysis of usage, cost, compliance, patient outcomes, observation of usage, and data about patients' rate of improvement. Starting with a general theoretical perspective and distilling it to a specific program model is the first step in evaluation. Once overall goals and general constructs have been identified, then decisions about measurement and design can be made. In this chapter evaluation approaches were framed, focusing on health IT program evaluation to orient the reader to the resources and opportunities in the evaluation domain. Health IT evaluations are typically multidimensional, longitudinal, and complex. Health IT interventions and programs present a unique challenge, as they are rarely independent of other factors. Rather, they are usually embedded in a larger program. The challenge is to integrate the goals of the entire program while clarifying the impact and importance of the health IT component. In the future, health IT evaluations should become more theory driven and the complex nature of evaluations will be acknowledged more readily.

As health IT becomes integrated at all levels of the information context of an institution, evaluation strategies will necessarily broaden in scope. Outcomes will not only include those related to health IT but span the whole process. The result will be richer analyses and a deeper understanding of the mechanisms by which health IT has its impact. The incorporation of theory into evaluation will also result in more generalizable knowledge and the development of health IT evaluation science. Health practitioners and informaticists will be at the heart of these program evaluations due to their central place in healthcare, IT, and informatics departments.

REFERENCES

1. Patton MQ. *Utilization-Focused Evaluation*. 4th ed. London: Sage; 2008.
2. Ainsworth L, Viegut D. *Common Formative Assessments*. Thousand Oaks, CA: Corwin Press; 2006.
3. Fetterman D. *Foundations of Empowerment Evaluation*. Thousand Oaks, CA: Sage Publications; 2001.
4. Scriven M. The methodology of evaluation. In: Stake R, ed. *Curriculum Evaluation, American Educational Research Association, Monograph Series on Evaluation, No 1*. Chicago: Rand McNally; 1967.

5. Christensen C. *The Innovator's Dilemma*. New York, NY: HarperBusiness; 2003.

6. Shekelle P. *Costs and Benefits of Health Information Technology*. Santa Monica, CA: Southern California Evidence-Based Practice Center; 2006.

7. Vygotsky L. *Mind and Society*. Cambridge, MA: Harvard University Press; 1978.

8. Preskill H, Torres R. Building capacity for organizational learning through evaluative inquiry. *Evaluation*. 1999;5(1):42-60.

9. Senge P. *The Fifth Discipline: The Art and Practice of the Learning Organization*. New York, NY: Doubleday; 1990.

10. Ajzen I. The theory of planned behavior. *Organ Behav Hum Decis Process*. 1991;50:179-211.

11. Fishbein M, Ajzen I. *Belief, Attitude, Intention, and Behavior: An Introduction to Theory and Research*. Reading, MA: Addison-Wesley; 1975.

12. Bandura A. Human agency in social cognitive theory. *Am Psychol*. 1989;44:1175-1184.

13. Rogers EM. *Diffusion of Innovations*. New York, NY: Free Press; 1983.

14. Cooper, RB, Zmud, RW. Information Technology Implementation Research: A Technological Diffusion Approach. *Management Science*. 1990:36:123-139.

15. Klein G. An overview of natural decision making applications. In: Zsambok CE, Klein G, eds. *Naturalist Decision Making*. Mahwah, NJ: Lawrence Erlbaum Associates; 1997.

16. Kushniruk AW, Patel VL. Cognitive and usability engineering methods for the evaluation of clinical information systems. *J Biomed Inform*. 2004;37(1):56-76.

17. Zsambok C, Klein G. *Naturalistic Decision Making*. Mahwah, NJ: Lawrence Erlbaum; 1997.

18. Åström K, Murray R. *Feedback Systems: An Introduction for Scientists and Engineers*. Princeton, NJ: Princeton University Press; 2008.

19. Endsley M, Garland D. *Situation Awareness Analysis and Measurement*. Mahway, NJ: Lawrence Erlbaum; 2000.

20. Koch S, Weir C, Haar M, et al. ICU nurses' information needs and recommendations for integrated displays to improve nurses' situational awareness. *J Am Med Inform Assn*. 2012;March 21 [e-pub].

21. Koch SH, Weir C, Westenskow D, et al. Evaluation of the effect of information integration in displays for ICU nurses on situation awareness and task completion time: a prospective randomized controlled study. *J Am Med Inform Assn*. In press.

22. Shannon C. A mathematical theory of communication. *Bell Syst Tech J*. 1948;27:379-423, 623-656.

23. Shannon C, Weaver W. *The Mathematical Theory of Communication*. Urbana, IL: University of Illinois Press; 1949.

24. Krippendorf K. *Information Theory: Structural Models for Qualitative Data*. Thousand Oaks, CA: Sage Publications; 1986.

25. Weir CR, McCarthy CA. Using implementation safety indicators for CPOE implementation. *Jt Comm J Qual Patient Saf*. 2009;35(1):21-28.

26. Pirolli P, Card S. Information foraging. *Psychol Rev*. 1999;106(4):643-675.

27. Pirolli P. *Information Foraging Theory: Adaptive Interaction with Information*. Oxford, United Kingdom: Oxford University Press; 2007.

28. DeLone W, McLean E. The DeLone and McLean model of information systems success: a ten-year update. *J Man Inf Syst*. 2003;19(4):9-30.

29. Mason R. Measuring information output: a communication systems approach. *Information & Management*. 1978;1(5):219-234.

30. Venkatesh V, Morris M, Davis G, Davis F. User acceptance of information technology: toward a unified view. *MIS Quart*. 2003;27(3):425-478.

31. Venkatesh V, Davis F. A theoretical extension of the technology acceptance model: four longitudinal field studies. *Manage Sci*. 2000;46(2):186-204.

32. Agarwal R, Prasad J. A conceptual and operational definition of personal innovativeness in the domain of information technology. *Inform Syst Res*. 1998;9(2):204-215.

33. Karahanna E, Straub D, Chervany N. Information technology adoption across time: a cross-sectional comparison of pre-adoption and post-adoption beliefs. *MIS Quart*. 1999;23(2):183-213.

34. Green L, Kreuter M. *Health Program Planning: An Educational and Ecological Approach*. 4th ed. Mountain View, CA: Mayfield Publishers; 2005.

35. Stetler CB, Damschroder LJ, Helfrich CD, Hagedorn HJ. A guide for applying a revised version of the PARiHS framework for implementation. *Implement Sci*. 2011;6:99. doi:1748-5908-6-99 [pii].

36. Kitson A, Harvey G, McCormack B. Enabling the implementation of evidence based practice: a conceptual framework. *Qual Health Care*. 1998;7(3):149-158.

37. Kitson AL, Rycroft-Malone J, Harvey G, McCormack B, Seers K, Titchen A. Evaluating the successful implementation of evidence into practice using the PARiHS framework: theoretical and practical challenges. *Implement Sci*. 2008;3:1.

38. Gaglio B, Glasgow R. Evaluation approaches for dissemination and implementation research. In: Brownson R, Colditz G, Proctor E, eds. *Dissemination and Implementation Research in Health: Translating Science to Practice*. New York, NY: Oxford University Press; 2012:327-356.

39. Glasgow R, Vogt T, Boles S. Evaluating the public health impact of health promotion interventions: the RE-AIM framework. *Am J Public Health*. 1999;89(9):1922-1927.

40. Donabedian A. *Explorations in Quality Assessment and Monitoring: The Definition of Quality and Approaches to Its Assessment. Vol. 1*. Ann Arbor, MI: Health Administration Press; 1980.

41. Donabedian A. The quality of care: how can it be assessed? *JAMA*. 1988;260:1743-1748.

42. Brown C, Hofer T, Johal A, et al. An epistemology of patient safety research: a framework for study design and interpretation. Part 1: conceptualising and developing interventions. *Qual Saf Health Care*. 2008;17(3):158-162.

43. Friedman C. Information technology leadership in academic medical centers: a tale of four cultures. *Acad Med*. 1999;74(7):795-799.

44. Centers for Disease Control and Prevention. framework for program evaluation in public health. *MMWR*. 1999;48(RR11):1-40.

45. W.K. Kellogg Foundation. *Using Logic Models to Bring Together Planning, Evaluation, and Action: Logic Model Development Guide*. Battle Creek, MI: W.K. Kellogg Foundation; 2004.

46. Patton, M. *Qualitative Research and Evaluation Methods*. 3rd ed. Newberry Park, CA: Sage Publications; 2001.

47. Flanagan JC. The critical incident technique. *Psychol Bull*. 1954;51(4):327-358.

48. Miller WR, Rollnick S. *Motivational Interviewing: Preparing People to Change*. 2nd ed. New York, NY: Guilford Press; 2002.

49. Crandall B, Klein G, Hoffman R. *Working Minds: A Practitioner's Guide to Cognitive Task Analysis*. Cambridge, MA: MIT Press; 2006.

50. Hoffman RR, Militello LG. *Perspectives on Cognitive Task Analysis*. New York, NY: Psychology Press Taylor and Francis Group; 2009.

51. Schraagen J, Chipman S, Shalin V. *Cognitive Task Analysis*. Mahway, NJ: Lawrence Erlbaum Associates; 2000.

52. Ericsson K, Simon H. *Protocol Analysis: Verbal Reports as Data*. Rev. ed. Cambridge, MA: MIT Press; 1993.

53. Kaplan B, Maxwell J. Qualitative research methods for evaluating computer information systems. In: Anderson JG, Aydin CE, Jay SJ, eds. *Evaluating Health Care Information Systems: Approaches and Applications*. Thousand Oaks, CA: Sage; 1994: 45-68.

54. Staggers N, Clark L, Blaz J, Kapsandoy S. Nurses' information management and use of electronic tools during acute care handoffs. *Western J Nurs Res*. 2012;34(2):151-171.

55. Staggers N, Clark L, Blaz J, Kapsandoy S. Why patient summaries in electronic health records do not provide the cognitive support necessary for nurses' handoffs on medical and surgical units: insights from interviews and observations. *Health Informatics J*. 2011;17(3):209-223.

56. Harris A, McGregor J, Perencevich E, et al. The use and interpretation of quasi-experimental studies in medical informatics. *J Am Med Inform Assoc*. 2006;13:16-23.

57. Ramsay C, Matowe L, Grill R, Grimshaw J, Thomas R. Interrupted time series designs in health technology assessment: lessons from two systematic reviews of behavior change strategies. *Int J Technol Assess*. 2003;19(4):613-623.

58. Lee H, Monk T. Using regression discontinuity design for program evaluation. *American Statistical Association–Proceedings of the Survey Research Methods Section*. ASA; 2008. Retrieved from http://www.amstat.org/sections/srms/Proceedings/.

59. Shadish WR, Cook TD, Campbell DT. *Experimental and Quasi-Experimental Designs for Generalized Causal Inference*. Boston, MA: Houghton Mifflin; 2002.

60. Pitt L, Watso NR, Kavan C. Service quality: a measure of information systems effectiveness. *MIS Quart*. 1995;19(2):173-188.

61. Sauro J. Measuring usability with the system usability scale (SUS). Measuring Usability LLC. http://www.measuringusability.com/sus.php. February 2, 2011. Accessed September 27, 2012.

62. Bangor A, Kortum P, Miller JT. An empirical evaluation of the system usability scale. *Int J Hum-Comput Int*. 2008;24(6):574-594.

63. Durland M, Fredericks K, eds. *New Directions in Evaluation: Social Network Analysis*. Hoboken, NJ: Jossey-Bass/AEA; 2005.

64. Benham-Hutchins MM, Effken JA. Multi-professional patterns and methods of communication during patient handoffs. *Int J Med Inform*. 2010;79(4):252-267.

DISCUSSION QUESTIONS

1. Of the levels of theory discussed in this chapter, what level would be most appropriate for evaluation of electronic health records? Would the level of theory be different if the intervention was for an application targeting a new scheduling system in a clinic? Why?

2. What is the difference between program evaluation and program evaluation research?

3. Assume that you are conducting an evaluation of a new decision support system for preventative alerts. What kind of designs would you use in a program evaluation study?

4. Using the life cycle as a framework, explain when and why you would use a formative or summative evaluation approach.

5. What are the basic differences between a research study and a program evaluation?

6. Review the following article: Harris A, McGregor J, Perencevich E, et al. The use and interpretation of quasi-experimental studies in medical informatics. *J Am Med Inform Assoc*. 2006;13:16-23. Explain how you might apply these research designs in structuring a program evaluation.

CASE STUDY

A 410-bed hospital has been using a homegrown provider order entry system for 5 years. It has recently decided to put in bar code administration software to scan medications at the time of delivery in order to decrease medical error. The administration is concerned about medication errors, top-level administration is concerned about meeting The Joint Commission accreditation standards, and the IT department is worried that the scanners may not be reliable and may break, increasing their costs. The plan is to have a scanner in each patient's room; nurses will scan the medication when they get to the room and also scan their own badges and the patient's arm band. The application makes it possible to print out a list of the patients with their scan patterns and the nurses sometimes carry this printout because patient's arm bands can be difficult to locate or nurses do not want to disturb patients while they are sleeping. The bar code software was purchased from a vendor and the facility has spent about a year refining it. The IT department is responsible for implementation and has decided that it will implement each of the four inpatient settings one at a time at 6-month intervals.

The hospital administration wants to conduct an evaluation study. You are assigned to be the lead on the evaluation.

Discussion Questions

1. What is the key evaluation question for this project?
2. Who are the stakeholders?
3. What level of theory is most appropriate?
4. What are specific elements to measure by stakeholder group?

UNIT 2

Information Systems in Healthcare Delivery

Electronic Health Records and Applications for Managing Patient Care

Charlotte Seckman

In the future the electronic health record (EHR) will play a pivotal role in personalized medicine as a medium for data, information, and knowledge exchange and for exploration.

OBJECTIVES

At the completion of this chapter the reader will be prepared to:

1. Discuss terms and definitions associated with the electronic health record (EHR)
2. Describe the essential components and attributes of an EHR
3. Define Meaningful Use in the context of EHR adoption and the impact on health practitioners
4. Examine EHR applications used in the clinical setting
5. Analyze the benefits of an EHR related to cost, access, quality, safety, and effectiveness
6. Evaluate stakeholder perspectives and key issues that affect EHR adoption
7. Explore future directions for EHR adoption and integration

KEY TERMS

Ancillary system, 95
Bar Code Medication Administration (BCMA), 93
Clinical documentation, 94
Computerized provider order entry (CPOE), 92
Data integrity, 99
Disruptive technology, 100
Electronic health record (EHR), 88

Electronic medical record (EMR), 88
Electronic Medication Administration Record (eMAR), 93
Health Information Technology for Economic and Clinical Health (HITECH) Act, 90
Niche applications, 95
Radio frequency identification (RFID), 94
Stakeholders, 97

ABSTRACT

Over the past decades the electronic health record (EHR) is one of the most significant innovations introduced in healthcare. Today almost all healthcare providers are using automation in the sharing of patient data and information across facilities locally, nationally, and perhaps internationally. Although there is concern about how to establish a nationwide interoperable system and many issues still need to be resolved related to EHR implementation and adoption, the long-term benefits to organizations, healthcare providers, and patients and consumers cannot be ignored. This chapter explores the evolving nature of the EHR along with essential components and functions, how these components are used in the clinical setting, and benefits related to cost, access, quality, safety, and efficiency of care. A discussion of key issues that influence the implementation and adoption of these systems and future directions concludes this chapter.

INTRODUCTION

The complex nature of the current U.S. healthcare system has created a challenging environment for managing patient data and information. Traditional paper systems can be easier to use for documenting a single episode of care but access to these records is limited, reporting is extremely cumbersome, and trending of data across patient visits or types is nearly impossible. Provider specialty practices create treatment silos that often hinder continuity of care. Healthcare providers and hospitals endeavor to keep current with billing regulations to receive optimal reimbursement. This requires vigilant monitoring of private insurance contracts and changes in governmental mandates. Some clinicians find it difficult to maintain competencies and gain access to information about the latest medical techniques and research. Add to this the introduction of personal computers, mobile devices, and the Internet, which have boosted consumer demands and a variety of healthcare delivery concerns.

The robust nature of the EHR has the potential to address many of these issues and transform the way we collect, store, access, process, manage, and report patient data. Government initiatives and financial incentives are being offered to expedite the implementation and expansion of EHR systems. However, despite all of the attention on this technology, there are still different views on what an EHR is, what it does or should do, and how it should be used.

Early Terms and Definitions

Multiple labels and definitions have been used throughout the years to refer to electronic systems used in healthcare. Early terms focused on using the words *computer* and *record* to merge the idea of a paper chart with technology, but computers provided much more functionality than traditional methods. These early terms were not sufficient to describe this emerging phenomenon. Specific early terms and acronyms such as computer patient records (CPRs), computer-based patient records (CBPRs), and computer health records (CHRs) were used to identify systems that contained select automated components of the patient's medical record. The acronym CPR was not popular in the health community since it also represents the term *cardiopulmonary resuscitation*. Generic names like hospital information system (HIS) or medical information system (MIS) were adopted to represent the management of a larger body of data and information throughout a specific hospital or healthcare system.

Later definitions for electronic systems in healthcare often focused on the system's distinctive purpose, content, ownership, and functional differences. This is especially true for technology used in specialty areas such as nursing, pharmacy, laboratory, radiology, and other support departments. For example, a laboratory information system (LIS) would be used to collect, store, process, and manage laboratory data and would be controlled by the laboratory department personnel whereas a pharmacy system would provide medication inventory, control, and dispensing for pharmacy personnel. Specific clinical departmental systems will be discussed in more detail later in the chapter. Terms such as CBPR or CPR referred to a larger collection of information about the patient, such as orders, medications, treatments, laboratory and diagnostic test results, and other information related

to overall patient care. Although the terms imply a patient-owned record, access and input to the record were typically controlled by the healthcare provider. As computer technology continued to progress and more functionality became available, a need surfaced for clarity and refinement in terms and definitions relating to EHR systems.

Electronic Medical Record (EMR) versus Electronic Health Record (EHR)

More recently, terms such as electronic medical record (EMR) and electronic health record (EHR) have emerged. These are often used interchangeably but it is important to understand the differences between them. Sewell and Thede defined the EMR as "an electronic version of the traditional record used by the healthcare provider."[1(p320)] Hebda and Czar described an EMR as an electronic information resource used in healthcare to capture patient data.[2] In essence, an EMR can be viewed as the electronic version of a patient's paper chart. The EMR is what most clinicians think of as the automated medical record system used in the clinical setting and it represents an episodic view of patient encounters. This type of system, seen in hospitals, hospital corporations, and clinician practices, is predominately controlled by the healthcare provider. The EMR is not just one system but may include interfaces with multiple other systems and applications used by the facility such as registration, patient scheduling, order entry, clinical documentation, radiology, laboratory, and other departmental systems. The patient usually does not interact with or provide input to the EMR, although some software vendors are working to incorporate portals that provide patient access to test results, scheduling features, email interaction with clinicians, and the ability to add and update health information.

How is this different from an EHR? In 2008 the National Alliance for Health Information Technology, as a division of the U.S. Department of Health & Human Services (HHS), convened to clarify and define key health information technology (health IT) terms. The EHR was defined as "An electronic record of health-related information on an individual that conforms to nationally recognized interoperability standards and that can be created, managed, and consulted by authorized clinicians and staff across more than one health care organization."[3] This suggests the availability and use of communication standards, such as nomenclatures, vocabularies, and coding structures, in order to share patient data across multiple organizations.[4] It also implies data sharing across multiple facilities. In comparison, the EMR is limited to information exchange within a single organization or practice whereas the EHR has the ability to exchange information outside the healthcare delivery system.[5]

The Healthcare Information and Management Systems Society (HIMSS) provides a similar definition of the EHR as a longitudinal electronic record of patient health information produced by encounters in one or more care settings.[6] The implication is that every person will have a birth to death (and even prenatal and postmortem) record of health-related information in electronic form from multiple sources, such as physician office visits, inpatient and outpatient hospital encounters, medications, allergies, and other medical services to support care. This means that components of the EMR would ultimately be part of the EHR. Other definitions stress the importance of the EHR as a way to automate and streamline workflow for healthcare providers, support patient care activities, and provide decision support, quality management, and outcomes reporting.[7-11] Despite the clarification provided by these definitions, many are still using the terms EMR and EHR interchangeably. Also, these definitions are often directed toward the needs of the healthcare provider and lack reference to patient and consumer interaction or integration of personal health records.

At this point it is important to mention the personal health record (PHR) as a component of the EHR. This type of record is primarily patient or consumer controlled and is discussed in more detail in Chapter 15. The ultimate goal is that PHR development conform to nationally recognized standards and be integrated into larger systems allowing the individual to view, manage, and share personal health information with providers. As part of the EHR, this could provide a more comprehensive record of a person's medical history and overall health.

In summary, EHR has become the preferred term for the lifetime patient record that would include data from a variety of healthcare specialties and provide interactive access and input by the patient. The term EHR is distinct in meaning from the term EMR. As with other expressions in the past, the term EMR may eventually fade away. Although some disagreement exists on exactly what the terms EHR and EMR mean or how an interoperable lifetime patient record will work, the EHR is clearly a complex tool that will continue to grow and evolve.[12]

EHR COMPONENTS, FUNCTIONS, AND ATTRIBUTES

Present-day electronic systems in most organizations typically include patient demographics, financial data, order information, laboratory and diagnostic test results, medications and allergies, problem lists, and clinical documentation. Beyond these basic features, an EHR should also incorporate clinical events monitors, preventive care recommendations, and decision support tools that enhance the efficiency and effectiveness of patient care.

In 2003 the HHS formed a group called the EHR Collaborative to support rapid adoption and to develop standards for EHR design in preparation for this initiative.[13] This group included sponsors from the following organizations:

- American Health Information Management Association (AHIMA)
- American Medical Association (AMA)
- American Nurses Association (ANA)
- American Medical Informatics Association (AMIA)
- College of Healthcare Information Management Executives (CHIME)
- eHealth Initiative (eHI)

- Healthcare Information and Management Systems Society (HIMSS)
- National Alliance for Health Information Technology (NAHIT)

The EHR Collaborative held forums and gathered input from stakeholder communities such as healthcare providers, insurance companies, IT vendors, researchers, pharmacists, public health organizations, and consumers. EHR Collaborative organizations, along with the IOM and Health Level Seven (HL7), were tasked to design a standard for EHRs. As a result the IOM released a report on July 31, 2003, called *Key Capabilities of an Electronic Health Record System.*[14] This report identified eight essential care delivery components for an EHR, with an emphasis on functions that promote patient safety, quality, and efficiency. More recently the U.S. Department of Defense added dentistry and optometry records as EHR components needed to provide a more comprehensive picture of overall health status.[15] See Table 6-1 for a list of essential EHR components and their descriptions. Each component of an EHR incorporates unique functions and attributes that contribute to the integration of a comprehensive patient record.

In addition to the various components and functions, there are 12 key attributes prescribed by the IOM[14] as the gold standard components of an EHR. These attributes serve as guidelines to organizations and vendors involved in the design and implementation of EHRs and include the information shown in Box 6-1.

SOCIOTECHNICAL PERSPECTIVES

Since the late 1990s, the design, implementation, and adoption of EHR systems has received a great deal of attention as a method to reduce medical errors, increase patient safety, and improve the quality of care.[16-18] The underlying assumption is that an EHR will save time, provide real-time access to patient information at the point of care, facilitate the work of the clinician, provide decision support capabilities, support clinical care and research, and improve quality and safety of care.[9,19-22] This section explores factors that influence EHR adoption, Meaningful Use, and the health practitioner's role in EHR adoption.

EHR Adoption

As discussed in Chapter 24, a presidential executive order in 2004 called for widespread adoption of interoperable EHRs. More recent regulation also guides EHRs in the United States. Numerous strategies and incentives are being used to expedite implementation, adoption, and meaningful use of EHR systems.

Meaningful Use

National mandates and guidelines from collaborative working groups were not enough to accelerate the development and adoption of health IT. In 2009 the American Recovery and Reinvestment Act (ARRA) was passed and included a critical

TABLE 6-1	SUMMARY OF THE EHR ESSENTIAL COMPONENTS AND FUNCTIONS FOR CARE DELIVERY	
COMPONENT	**ESSENTIAL FUNCTIONS**	**APPLICATION EXAMPLES**
Administrative processes	Ability to conduct all financial and administrative functions associated with institutional operations and patient management.	Admissions/registration Scheduling Claims processing Administrative reporting
Communication and connectivity	Provides a medium for electronic communication between healthcare providers and patients.	Email Text/web messaging Integrated health records Telemedicine
Decision support	Provides reminders, alerts, and resource links to improve the diagnosis and care of the patient.	Medication dosing, allergies Risk screening/prevention Clinical guidelines Resource links
Dentistry and optometry	Ability to incorporate dental records and vision prescriptions.	Dental records Vision records
Health information and data	Ability to enter and access key information needed to make clinical decisions.	Patient demographics Problem lists Medical/nursing diagnoses Medications/allergies Results reporting
Order entry management	Ability to enter all types of orders via the computer system.	Laboratory Pharmacy Radiology Other orders
Patient support	Provides patient education and self-monitoring tools.	Discharge instructions Computer-based learning Telemonitoring
Results management	Provides the ability to manage current and historical information related to all types of diagnostic reports.	Laboratory tests Radiology reports Other procedures
Population health management	Provides data collection tools to support public and private reporting requirements.	Public health system Disease surveillance Bioterrorism

Adapted from Institute of Medicine, Committee on Data Standards for Patient Safety: Board of Health Care Services. *Key Capabilities of an Electronic Health Record System: Letter Report*. Washington, DC: The National Academies Press; 2003.
EHR, Electronic health record.

component addressing healthcare technology called the Health Information Technology for Economic and Clinical Health (HITECH) Act. The HITECH Act authorized programs designed to improve healthcare quality, safety, and efficiency using health IT.[23] More details about the HITECH Act and Meaningful Use criteria can be found in Chapters 24 and 25. Of importance to this chapter, the provision was targeted to stimulate the adoption of EHRs and the development of secure health information exchange (HIE) networks. It includes incentives for healthcare providers (primarily physicians) through Meaningful Use of certified EHRs. The purpose of Meaningful Use is more than just to implement an EHR but also to leverage the technology to improve quality, safety, and efficiency in patient care. Meaningful Use objectives are being implemented in several stages. The first stage focuses on electronic data capture and tracking,

coordination of care, and sharing of health information.[24,25] Box 6-2 summarizes core and optional Meaningful Use objectives for Stage 1.

Requirements for Stage 2 Meaningful Use were released by the Federal Register in August 2012, with reporting to begin as early as fiscal year 2014. The focus of this stage is to encourage patient engagement and the robust use of health IT through continuous quality improvement efforts, HIE networks, and structured data capture. Similar to Stage 1, healthcare providers and hospitals will need to address a set of 17 core and 3 of 6 optional Meaningful Use objectives. In a broader sense, the expectation for Stage 2 involves expanded EHR functionality to support quality improvement, patient safety, structured information exchange, population health, and research.[26] Stage 3 criteria will expand on the objectives for the first two stages to further support quality initiatives;

BOX 6-1   THE INSTITUTE OF MEDICINE'S KEY ATTRIBUTES OF AN ELECTRONIC HEALTH RECORD (EHR)

1. Provides active and inactive problem lists for each encounter that link to orders and results; meets documentation and coding standards
2. Incorporates accepted measures to support health status and functional levels
3. Ability to document clinical decision information; automates, tracks and shares clinical decision process/rationale with other caregivers
4. Provides longitudinal and timely linkages with other pertinent records
5. Guarantees confidentiality, privacy and audit trails
6. Provides continuous authorized user access
7. Supports simultaneous user views
8. Access to local and remote information
9. Facilitates clinical problem solving
10. Supports direct entry by physicians
11. Cost measuring/quality assurance
12. Supports existing/evolving clinical specialty needs

Adapted from Institute of Medicine, Committee on Data Standards for Patient Safety: Board of Health Care Services. *Key Capabilities of an Electronic Health Record System: Letter Report.* Washington, DC: The National Academies Press; 2003.

improve safety, efficiency, and patient outcomes; address population health requirements; provide enhanced decision support; and promote patient-centered HIE.

EMR Adoption Model

In 2005 the HIMSS Analytics group developed an EMR Adoption Model to track the progress of health IT adoption rates in hospitals and, more recently, ambulatory facilities.[27] The systems and functions required for each stage for U.S. hospitals are shown in Table 6-2. Although originally developed for the United States, the EMR Adoption Model is also being used in Europe and Canada.[28,29] This model provides realistic and achievable measures in seven stages that coincide with Meaningful Use requirements. The model assists organizations by providing a sequenced implementation structure for IT adoption to align with business strategies, benchmarking data to compare progress with other facilities, and an approach that maps to Meaningful Use objectives. EMR Adoption Models for physician practice and ambulatory facilities are similar, with modifications specific to those settings.

Health Practitioner Role in EHR Adoption and Meaningful Use

Although early incentives are directed toward hospitals, clinics, and physician practice, all health practitioners will be

BOX 6-2   STAGE 1: MEANINGFUL USE OBJECTIVES

CORE SET OF MEANINGFUL USE OBJECTIVES

1. Use of computerized provider order entry (CPOE) for medication orders by licensed prescriber
2. Implement drug–drug, drug–allergy checks
3. Transmit prescriptions electronically
4. Record patient demographic information
5. Maintain current problem and diagnoses list
6. Maintain active medication and medication allergy list
7. Record and chart changes in vital signs
8. Record smoking status (13 years or older)
9. Implement one clinical decision support rule related to specialty
10. Report clinical quality measures to CMS or State (where appropriate)
11. Provide electronic summary of care when patient transitions to another setting or care provider
12. Provide patients with an electronic copy of health information upon request
13. Provide patients with electronic copy of discharge instructions or summaries of office visits
14. Protect electronic health information using appropriate technical capabilities.

OPTIONAL OBJECTIVES (5 OF 10 REQUIRED)

1. Incorporate clinical lab test results as structured data
2. Implement drug formulary checks
3. Support medication reconciliation
4. Record advance directives (65 years or older)
5. Provide patient-specific education resources
6. Generate summary of care records for transition of care or referral to another provider
7. Submit electronic data to immunization registries
8. Submit syndromic surveillance data to public health agencies
9. Provide patients electronic access to health information
10. Generate lists with patient conditions for quality improvement, reduction of disparities, research or outreach

From U.S. Department of Health and Human Services, Centers for Medicare & Medicaid Services Medicare and Medicaid Programs. Electronic Health Record Incentive Program final rule. *Federal Register.* 2010;75(144):44313-44588. http://edocket.acess.gpo.gov/2010/pdf/2010-17207.pdf.
CMS, Centers for Medicare & Medicaid Services.

TABLE 6-2	HIMSS ANALYTICS UNITED STATES EMR ADOPTION MODEL 2005-2012
STAGE	**CUMULATIVE CAPABILITIES**
Stage 7	Complete electronic medical record (EMR); CCD transactions to share data; data warehousing in use; data continuity with Emergency Department, Ambulatory, Outpatient
Stage 6	Physician documentation (structured templates); full CDS system (variance & compliance); full radiology-picture archiving and communication system (R-PACS)
Stage 5	Closed-loop medication administration
Stage 4	Computerized provider order entry (CPOE); CDS system (clinical protocols)
Stage 3	Clinical documentation (flow sheets); CDS system (error checking); picture archiving and communication system (PACS) available outside Radiology
Stage 2	Clinical Data Repository (CDR); controlled medical vocabulary CDS system; may have document imaging; health information exchange
Stage 1	Ancillaries—Lab, Radiology, Pharmacy—all installed
Stage 0	All three ancillaries not installed

Adapted from Healthcare Information and Management Systems Society (HIMSS). EHR: Electronic health record. HIMSS. http://www.himssanalytics.org/stagesGraph.asp.
CCD, Continuity of Care Document; *CDS*, clinical decision support; *HIMSS*, Healthcare Information and Management Systems Society.

integral to the collection of Meaningful Use data through the use of EHR technology.[30] For example, nursing care is a primary reason for hospitalization so nurses' roles in addressing the Meaningful Use objectives should not be underestimated. Nurses are the single largest group of employees in the hospital setting, where labor costs are often bundled with room and supply fees.[31] With the threat of a nursing shortage, executives are pressured to find ways to increase productivity while they struggle to recruit and retain qualified healthcare personnel. The adoption of an EHR system can enhance access to patient information, provide more accurate and complete documentation, improve data availability, and provide decision support capabilities often leading to increased staff productivity and satisfaction.[2,21,32] Many health practitioners are involved in providing care coordination and patient education, key objectives of the Meaningful Use requirements. Health practitioners assist in designing clinical decision support (CDS) systems that can be used to enhance patient adherence to disease management. Other activities include developing data set standards to improve outcomes, increase patient safety, and evaluate quality of care. Many are engaged in local, regional, and national strategic

initiatives to improve care coordination using EHRs and an HIE.[25,33,34] How the HITECH Act will affect the role of each group of health professionals in the future is yet to be determined. What is clear is that patient care should be a collaborative effort guided by interdisciplinary teams that work together with the patient to provide the best possible outcomes. A typical EHR is designed to allow access and input by a variety of healthcare providers as a way to manage this care. In the same way, fulfillment of the Meaningful Use objectives requires active involvement and contributions from multiple disciplines in order to produce high-quality patient outcomes.

EHR APPLICATIONS USED IN THE CLINICAL SETTING

An EHR is composed of multiple applications and in different settings may differ in terms of integration between the components, data presentation, usability, and clinical workflow. This section discusses the various applications currently used in the clinical setting, including computerized provider order entry (CPOE), Electronic Medication Administration Record (eMAR), Bar Code Medication Administration (BCMA), clinical documentation, specialty applications, and clinical decision support (CDS).

Computerized Provider Order Entry (CPOE)

Computerized provider order entry (CPOE) is a component of the larger EHR system. The "P" in CPOE originally stood for "physician" but since advanced practice registered nurses, physician assistants, and other healthcare providers also write orders, this "P" has changed to "prescriber," "practitioner," or "provider." CPOE is software designed to allow clinicians to enter a variety of orders, such as medications, dietary services, consults, admission and discharge orders, nursing orders, lab requisitions, and other diagnostic tests, via a computer.

For many years handwritten orders were interpreted and entered into the computer system by unit secretaries, nurses, and pharmacists. Transcription errors such as a misplaced decimal point and illegible handwriting were major causes of error. Incomplete orders were a problem that caused additional steps in the nursing workflow. The idea behind CPOE was for prescribers, such as physicians, dentists, osteopathic doctors, anesthesiologists, nurse practitioners, and physician assistants, to enter orders directly into the computer. During the ordering process, alerts, such as drug allergy warnings, and other decision support rules should be available to assist the healthcare provider. Once an order is entered, the CPOE system interfaces or integrates with other EHR components, such as a laboratory or pharmacy system, to process the order. In fact, the term *order entry* can be misleading, as CPOE is truly an orders management system that allows orders to be entered, processed, tracked, updated, and completed.

The 1999 IOM report *To Err Is Human: Building a Safer Health System*[18] and demands from special interest groups put pressure on physicians and other prescribers to enter their orders directly into EHRs. Financial incentives offered through the HITECH Act and Stages 1 and 2 Meaningful Use objectives were designed to enforce the use of some aspects of CPOE and systematic adoption of EHR functionality. The mandate for EHR adoption, and specifically CPOE, as a means of reducing medical errors continues to receive a lot of attention.[17,18,35] Studies have consistently demonstrated the benefits of CPOE on reducing medication errors. Early landmark studies found that the implementation of CPOE decreased the length of hospital stay, lowered costs, improved quality of care, improved the appropriateness of drug dosing, and decreased the number of allergic reactions.[35-38] Mekhjian et al.[39] conducted a pre- and post-CPOE implementation comparison study at a large university medical center and found significant reductions in transcription errors, faster medication turnaround times, and timely reporting of results. Bates et al.[40] went further by evaluating the impact of CPOE with decision support tools on different types of medication errors and reported a significant reduction in overall errors. Other studies that focused on CPOE implementation suggest that medical and medication errors can be reduced along with improving data integrity, accuracy, workflow, and patient outcomes.[41-44] In essence, CPOE combined with clinical decision support capabilities such as checking for drug interactions, drug–allergy interactions, and dosing ranges can significantly reduce many serious medication errors.[45]

Physician resistance, financial constraints, and other issues make CPOE compliance challenging. In a landmark study, Ash, Berg, and Coiera[17] identified unintended consequences of CPOE that lead to medical errors related to (1) the process of entering and retrieving information and (2) methods of communication and coordination. Koppel et al.[46] also researched CPOE-related factors that may increase the risk of medication errors and found that new errors were reported because of fragmented data and processes, lack of integration among systems, and human–computer interaction issues.

Using CPOE can be time consuming during order entry, and design efficiencies are needed to entice clinicians to enter their own orders. For example, prior to CPOE many providers used standard handwritten order sheets for their patient population. Order sets were developed to include all or most of the information required to process multiple orders at one time. In a study comparing the use of traditional order entry methods and standardized order sets, researchers reported the potential to reduce errors, decrease order entry time, and eliminate variations in order presentation.[47]

The lack of decision support or overuse of alerts was another issue. Payne et al.[48] found that in 42,641 orders generated there was an 88% override rate for critical drug interaction alerts and a 69% override rate for drug–allergy interaction alerts among ordering practitioners. This prompted concern that too many alerts could cause the ordering healthcare provider to become immune to the warnings and ignore them. Recommendations to address unintended consequences, user resistance, and discussion support issues focused on providing education to healthcare providers and consumers, designing systems that support communication

and clinical workflow, early user participation in the implementation process, continuous safety monitoring, and the use of qualitative multidisciplinary research methods to provide deeper insight into the benefits and issues surrounding CPOE and EHRs generally.[49,50]

Electronic Medication Administration Record (eMAR)

The Electronic Medication Administration Record (eMAR) provides a medium to view and document medication use for individual patients. This system takes the place of using medication cards or a Kardex. When medication orders are entered into the CPOE system, this information is sent to the pharmacy system for verification and dispensing by the pharmacist. New orders appear on the patient's medication list in the eMAR and include information about the drug name, administration time, dose, and route. Usually the eMAR contains all types of medication and intravenous fluid orders, with the ability to sort the list in a variety of ways. For example, users can display scheduled, as needed (prn), pending, past due, or completed medications and can query the list for specific entries. Some systems will color-code medication order types for quick sorting and identification. Efforts to decrease medication administration errors use an eMAR in combination with bar-coding devices. An example of an eMAR screen is shown in Figure 6-1.

Bar Code Medication Administration (BCMA)

Bar Code Medication Administration (BCMA) is a method used to address patient safety and reduce errors that occur during the actual administration of medicines. This system is most effective when combined with CPOE, a pharmacy dispensing system, and the eMAR. Although CPOE has been successful in reducing transcription-related medication errors, it was not designed to prevent errors that may occur during the actual dispensing of a drug to the patient. In 2004 the U.S. Food and Drug Administration (FDA) indicated that the use of BCMA had the potential to reduce medication errors and recommended that bar-coding become standard on patient identification bands and medication labels.[51] Bar codes can then be read by optical scanners or bar code readers. The research findings in the area of BCMA support its advantages. Poon et al.[52] conducted a before and after, quasi-experimental study to evaluate the effectiveness of BCMA and eMARs. They reported a significant reduction in medication error rates as well as avoidance of numerous potential adverse drug events. Other studies report similar results and found that BCMA was easy to use, saved time, and improved medication documentation.[53-56]

The medication administration process with BCMA in the clinical setting starts with the nurse scanning his or her badge, the patient's wristband bar code, and the medication bar code. The scanner verifies the five "rights" of medication administration—right patient, right drug, right dose, right time, and right route—and documents the actual administration in the eMAR. Radio frequency identification (RFID) is also being used for medication administration. This

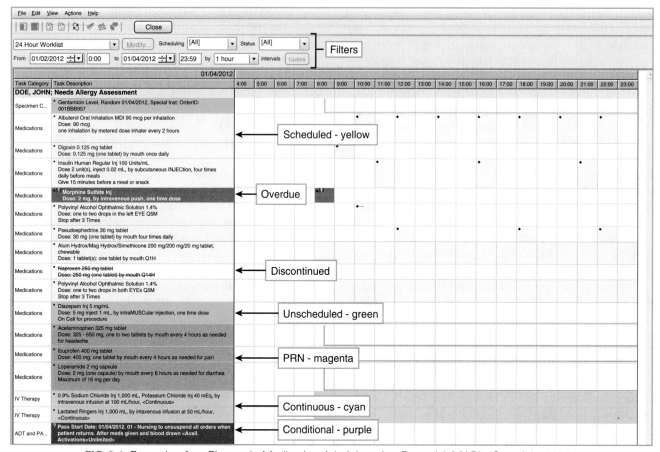

FIG 6-1 Example of an Electronic Medication Administration Record (eMAR). (Copyright 2012 Allscripts. Used with permission.)

technology uses electronic tags embedded in an identification badge or band to track and monitor activities. Passive RFID works in a similar way to regular bar-coding with the use of a scanner. Active RFID does not require a scanner; rather, it automatically transmits signals to a computer or wireless device without disturbing the patient. This technology is becoming more common in hospitals to track patient care activities, including medication dispensing and administration.[57]

Clinical Documentation

Clinical documentation software provides a medium for recording, managing, and reporting patient care activities by a variety of disciplines. The format for documenting may differ by application and organizational preference. Although many clinicians still embrace the richness of narrative notes, advantages exist to using standardized vocabularies and taxonomies for documenting patient care, as discussed in detail in Chapter 22. Structured notes using standardized language may come in the form of pull-down menus, decision trees, or key words embedded in a sentence. Some systems contain functionality to store and retrieve predefined notes of normal findings. Some organizations may use "charting by exception" wherein normal values and entries are predefined and selected

according to established guidelines so clinicians need to document only abnormal findings.

Clinical documentation systems should have functionality to support workflow processes and the creation of plans of care. Often electronic flow sheets or grids are used to record vital signs and other procedures quickly. An effective documentation system includes decision support rules that alert the clinician about abnormal values, missing content, or additional assessments that are needed. Rules can also be written to remind healthcare providers to verify essential information (e.g., new orders or allergies). Many systems provide the ability to graph numeric data, such as vital signs and lab values. Problem lists, allergies, medications, and other critical information about a patient can be extracted and displayed on a single summary screen to assist the busy clinician. Depending on the type of data collected, various clinical, administrative, and research reports can be generated.

Overall, clinical documentation systems should support better communication between healthcare providers, promote professional accountability, and streamline workflow. Access to literature sources, policies and procedures, clinical guidelines, and standards of care can be functionally incorporated to support evidence-based practice (EBP) through the use of applications such as Infobuttons or the EBP InfoBot (discussed under Clinical Decision Support below). Additional information about EBP is included in Chapter 3. Electronic documentation makes it easier to search, query, and extract data for reports. This information can be used for quality improvement initiatives, critical incident reviews, resource management, long-term planning, and research and to address the requirements of the accreditation process.

Specialty Applications

Many of the basic EHR components such as CPOE, eMAR, and clinical documentation are available to all healthcare providers, but sometimes there is a need for unique functionality beyond what is provided in these applications. Specialty or niche applications are software programs created to address the requirements of specific departments and groups of users. Although many niche applications can function as stand-alone systems, integration with or interface to the hospital-wide EHR is preferred in order to decrease redundancy, enhance communication, and provide a more comprehensive patient record. Some examples of specialty department systems include perioperative or surgical services, maternity care, neonatal intensive care, and the emergency department (ED).

A surgical information system (SIS) incorporates functionality to improve clinical, operational, and financial outcomes throughout the entire perioperative experience. Functionality may include operating room scheduling; management of equipment, supplies, and inventory; documentation for nurses and anesthesiologists; patient and specimen tracking; and administrative reporting capabilities.

A maternity care information system (MCIS) is another type of niche system used to address the needs of obstetrics staff. An MCIS is used to support clinical protocols for maternity care, track mother and baby progress, capture fetal-uterine monitoring data, and record results of Doppler blood flow and other diagnostic tests. Key features of this system include electronic forms for documenting and reporting all aspects of antenatal, intrapartum, and postnatal care as well as normal, healthy, or adverse pregnancy outcomes. Likewise, a neonatal information system (NIS) that interfaces with the EHR would contain much of the same information found in the primary system. Unique to an NIS would be growth charts, nutritional calculations, monitor parameters, and coding structures specific to the needs of critically ill newborns. Clinical staff in these specialty units can benefit from user-defined logbooks, resource utilization, quality improvement, and statistical reports designed for their specific needs.

The ED has unique computer needs related to clinical workflow, documentation of triage and patient encounters, tracking of patient location and treatment progress, charge capture and reimbursement management, clinical rules for risk mitigation, and patient education and referral. Once again, not unlike other niche systems, the emergency department information system (EDIS) is designed to improve clinical, operational, and financial outcomes throughout the entire ED experience. However, EDISs are often integrated into a facility's EHR since EDs are the portal into acute care; these integrated data are then readily available to acute care providers and areas.

Clinical Decision Support (CDS)

Clinical decision support (CDS) systems are tools and applications that assist the healthcare provider with some aspect of decision making. These applications are discussed in detail in Chapter 10. Of importance here, CDS systems are crucial components of EHRs, linked to at least CPOE in the form of warnings related to duplicate orders, allergies, and medication dosing errors. A CDS system could also provide alerts related to changes in a patient's condition and reminders about important tasks such as follow-up visits, preventive care, immunizations, and updates to critical patient information.[58]

Some EHRs may contain external web links to resources to assist with clinical decision making (see, for example, the discussion of Infobuttons in Chapter 10). Many healthcare systems also have internal intranets that provide links to policies and procedures, clinical guidelines, and evidence-based protocols. In 2006 the National Institutes of Health (NIH) in collaboration with the National Library of Medicine (NLM) developed a decision support application called the Evidence-Based Practice (EBP) InfoBot.[59] This system was designed to augment a patient's EHR automatically by searching various literature sources and providing information that could be used to develop plans of care and assist with decision making. Operating behind the scenes are rule sets programmed to extract key data from the patient's medical record, map free text data to standardized terminology, and create a series of EBP-type queries from extracted data. These questions are used to search multiple NLM databases, internal standards of care and guidelines, and other external clinical resources, and then provide a summary of the information based on clinical user group preference directly into the EHR. The application functions in real time and provides flexibility to adapt to the requirements of the decision maker. Overall, the EBP InfoBot decreased provider search time, reduced information overload, and provided current and timely resources to support decision making at the bedside. An example of the EBP InfoBot summary screen is shown in Figure 6-2. Ideally, at a minimum, the CDS in EHRs should be accurate, be available to the clinician at the point of care, provide timely and up-to-date information, and easily be incorporated into daily care processes and workflow.

Ancillary Systems

An ancillary system usually refers to software applications used by patient care support departments such as laboratory, radiology, and pharmacy. Other departments such as cardiology, respiratory, physical therapy, and material management may have their own software applications as well. Laboratory information systems (LISs) and radiology

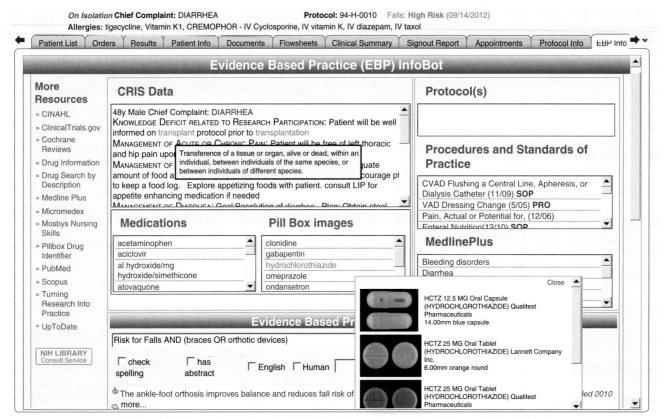

FIG 6-2 Evidence-Based Practice InfoBot. (From the National Library of Medicine.)

information systems (RISs) were available long before the concept of EHR systems was introduced. Both LISs and RISs are designed to address the specific needs of the department related to collecting, processing, and reporting test results along with managing resources and costs. The LIS consists of several components related to the laboratory subdepartments, including hematology, chemistry, microbiology, blood bank, and pathology. The LIS may also interface with other devices, such as blood analyzers, for direct input of blood test results.

Coding structures are used to track and identify resources and provide cost data for billing. Logical Observation Identifier Names and Codes (LOINC) is a universal coding system used to identify laboratory and other clinical observations, while the Systematized Nomenclature of Medicine (SNOMED) coding structure is commonly used in pathology. These standard languages are discussed in more detail in Chapter 22.

The RIS is similar to the LIS in that it incorporates data from multiple services that include x-rays, fluoroscopy, mammography, ultrasound, magnetic resonance imaging (MRI) scans, computed tomography (CT) scans, and other special procedures. It also uses coding structures such as Current Procedural Terminology (CPT) or International Classification of Diseases (ICD) to identify procedures, resources, and billing. However, the global standard for the transmission, storage, and display of medical imaging information is Digital Imaging and Communications in Medicine (DICOM). The

RIS may integrate data from a picture archiving and communication system (PACS), which stores digital versions of diagnostic images for display in the EHR.

The pharmacy department typically has a system to assist with inventory, prescription management, billing, and dispensing of medications. The FDA requires that all drugs be registered and reported using a National Drug Code (NDC). The NDC and SNOMED C axis are examples of coding structures that would be used in a pharmacy system. RxNorm is another standard mandated by the Office of the National Coordinator for Health related to Meaningful Use reporting and data exchange. Clinical screening can be done by monitoring medication usage throughout the hospital and identifying potential adverse drug events. Prescriptions can be tracked along with printing of labels and medication instructions for patients or staff. The pharmacy system can provide patient drug profiles that include current and past medications, allergies, and contraindications. These features are designed to enhance patient safety. A closed-loop medication management system connects the pharmacy system to the CPOE, eMAR, and bar-coding systems.

EHR BENEFITS

Most health policy initiatives are designed to address a triad of concerns that focus on cost, access, and quality. For example, concerns regarding the increasing cost of prescription drugs became the focus of Medicare reform legislation in 2003. Recent policy directed toward the adoption of EHR systems also highlights these concerns. The HITECH Act (2009) and the Patient Protection and Affordable Care Act (2010) addressed the need for EHR adoption to improve the quality, safety, and efficiency of care. With this in mind, the benefits of an EHR will be presented in terms of cost; access; and quality, safety, and efficiency of care delivery.

Cost

Cost savings is always a big motivator, especially if a healthcare provider or institution wants to stay in business. Numerous studies focusing on direct cost savings related to EHR use reported a positive financial return on investment for the healthcare organization.[60-64] Other cost benefits include increased productivity, efficiency in billing, improved reimbursement rates, improved verification of coverage, faster turnaround for accounts, lower medical record costs, support for pay-for-performance bonuses, and enhanced regulatory requirement compliance.[61,65,66] Benefits to patient care were also seen related to lower costs associated with disease management and decreased length of stay.[65,67]

Access

There is no doubt that an EHR provides better and faster access to patient care information. Looking for paper charts that mysteriously disappear from the nurses' station or waiting for medical records to retrieve an old record are events of the past. An EHR allows simultaneous access to patient records and restricts users' access to only the information that they are permitted to view. Many systems contain functionality such as graphs and charts that trend on demand and tools that facilitate comparison of current and past data. Another benefit is that clinicians have access to drug information, decision support tools, and literature searches to supplement patient care. Alerts and triggers that warn users of drug interactions and allergies can prevent medication errors. Clinical research often involves reviewing chart data and can be a cumbersome process if done manually. The EHR provides a more effective and efficient method to access and aggregate data for research. As EHR adoption continues to expand this will improve data access across multiple facilities and provide better continuity of care.

Quality, Safety, and Efficiency of Care Delivery

One of the main reasons to adopt an EHR is the potential to improve the quality, safety, and efficiency of care delivery. Quality is an ambiguous term that has a variety of meanings. Quality as it relates to EHR technology is fostered through better management of health information and improved data integrity. This may take the form of providing data that are readable, organized, accurate, and complete. Quality could also refer to increased staff and patient satisfaction, improved care coordination, and support for benchmarking. Safety and efficiency are much easier to quantify. Reducing medication errors has been a major focus of CPOE implementation. Systems that support clinical decision making and provide early warnings of changes in patient status can be used to avert medical errors. Diagnosis and treatment options can be explored through the use of decision support technology. Clinical and operational efficiencies in communication, workflow, documentation, and administrative functions are reported benefits of EHR adoption.

STAKEHOLDER PERSPECTIVES

In most organizations the implementation of an EHR will affect multiple groups or stakeholders that share a vested interest in the outcome of this endeavor. Stakeholders may have similar concerns about the technology but different needs and approaches for resolution. It is important to consider many perspectives; essential stakeholders may include consumers, nurses and other healthcare providers, healthcare administration and organizations, insurance payers, and state and national governments.

Consumers

The general attitude of consumers toward health IT is positive but consumers are embracing this innovation with some skepticism. According to a large survey conducted by the Louisville Health Information Exchange (LouHIE), consumers were most interested in "time-savings, streamlined registration, tracking their own records, safer emergency care, improved care quality, and reduced duplicate services."[68(p46)] Although the EHR has the potential to address these items, security and privacy of personal information is a major concern. In a national survey conducted by the California HealthCare Foundation in 2008, consumers indicated a desire to be more engaged in healthcare decisions and have access to online medical information.[69] Consumers also reported that health IT has the potential to improve quality and efficiency of care throughout the healthcare system and that concerns about privacy should not hinder organizations from moving ahead with EHR adoption. From a consumer perspective an EHR system should provide the ability to customize care through appointment reminders, health risk assessments, and timely access to personal health information. The availability of online educational resources can also improve consumers' understanding of their health status and treatment choices.

Nurses

Nurses constitute one of the largest groups of users of the EHR and their perspective is critical to the successful integration of current and future technology. There are mixed reviews on user satisfaction related to individual systems but nurses are encouraged to embrace the EHR as a way to enhance consistency and quality of care.[70-72] Seckman and Mills[73] reported that nurses' perception of an EHR was positive over a 5-year period and that overall the system increased productivity, improved performance, enhanced effectiveness, was easy to use, and supported clinical care and research.

Other reported benefits involve improvements related to centralized access to patient information, clinical documentation, monitoring patient status, and resources for patient education.

Nurses are responsible for distributing medications to patients under their care. Because the EMR and EHR usually interfaces with a pharmacy system, eMAR, and bar-coding technology, the potential exists to decrease administration-related medication errors. Knowledge-based systems may include functionality that integrates clinical guidelines or protocols to assist nurses in the development of critical pathways and plans of care.

Nurse leaders struggle to measure quality outcomes required by The Joint Commission (TJC), the Centers for Medicare & Medicaid Services (CMS), and other regulatory agencies. The EHR provides the ability to access data and compare across institutions for benchmarking. Stefan[74] suggested several quality metrics that nurse leaders should evaluate when implementing an EHR, including timely access and documentation of patient information, EBP alerts, impact on length of stay, discharge follow-up with patients, and accuracy of documentation for reimbursement and regulatory agencies.

Healthcare Providers

In a recent study of EHR use in primary care practices, physicians and staff reported increased efficiencies related to billing and care coordination, access to current and past medical records, storing of patient information, and overall office operations.[75] Doyle et al.[76] concurred with these findings and concluded that EHRs used in the healthcare provider's examination room facilitate a partnership between physician and patient through collaboration of treatment plan options and increase patient teaching by sharing of online medical information. In other studies physicians also reported improvements in prescribing and medication safety when eprescribing and decision support tools were available.[77,78] EHRs that provide tools for comprehensive documentation, warnings for changes in patient status, medication alerts, and follow-up and preventive care reminders improve decision making, which can reduce liability for the physician.[79] In addition, automated reporting capabilities enhance compliance to quality and regulatory requirements.[80]

Overall, healthcare providers reported favorable opinions about the EHR, citing many potential benefits related to clinical, organizational, and consumer outcomes.[65] Clinical benefits are often seen through the reduction of medical and medication errors, better health and disease management, and enhanced quality of care. Financial needs of the physician practice are streamlined and more efficient with electronic access to payer information and reporting to facilitate compliance with regulatory requirements. Workflow, communication, and coordination of care activities improve when there is easier access to records and other resources. Consumers also benefit from EHR technology when there is collaborative interaction between patients and physicians,

more timely access to personal health information, and online access to educational materials.

Healthcare Organizations

A current question for healthcare organizations is how to stay financially viable in a healthcare environment determined to control escalating healthcare costs. Added to this burden is the mandate to implement comprehensive EHR systems to meet Meaningful Use criteria and reap the benefits of available incentives. Depending on the size and complexity of each organization, costs for implementing EHR technology are a significant investment. Beyond the initial expense for the hardware and software are fees associated with consultants and programmers to assist with implementation, licensing, maintenance, and providing staff time away from regular duties to participate in the process. For the healthcare executive, implementing EHR systems has the potential to improve operational efficiency, strengthen communication throughout the organization, increase patient safety, support compliance with regulatory requirements, improve medical record security and storage, improve care coordination, enhance the quality of care, and provide faster turnaround for procedure authorization, billing, and claims submission.

Healthcare executives and leaders must look at leveraging this technology not only to control costs, but also to improve the quality of care. The successful implementation of information systems requires an understanding of the technical, cultural, and organization factors that influence change. Additional information related to successful implementation of health-related information systems can be found in Chapter 17. Healthcare executives must also reflect beyond single-facility implementation to the possible benefits of system integration that will foster collaboration at local, national, and international levels.

Insurance Payers

The EHR provides several benefits for insurance companies through better disease management and reporting of services. Pay for performance requirements are supported and can be submitted in a timely manner. Claims that are incorrectly coded or that lack coding standards can confuse payers when they attempt to reimburse organizations for services. Systems that integrate patient data with coding and billing structures can provide data to control costs and manage expensive procedures.

State and National Governments

Over the past 20 years the cost of healthcare in the U.S. has risen to nearly $2.6 trillion and is expected to grow faster than the national income.[81] One proposed measure for cost containment focuses on improving coordination and quality of care. The implementation of a nationwide interoperable EHR is recommended as a solution that would significantly reduce medical errors, improve care quality, and save the U.S. healthcare system major expense.[18,82] The U.S. is behind other developed nations in deploying technology of this magnitude. A major challenge is how to support the sharing of patient data across multiple organizations, requiring a nationwide technology infrastructure and communication standards, such as standardized nomenclatures, vocabularies, and coding structures.[4] Although the initial expenditures for such a system would be high, the anticipated benefits to our nation would be the ability to identify and address safety issues in a timely fashion, notify patients and populations at risk for disease or environmental exposure, detect epidemics, and prepare for bioterrorism attacks.[83] A clinical dataset of essential information would be available, allowing researchers to explore preventive and curative solutions that address the nation's health and healthcare issues. Ultimately, the adoption of a nationwide EHR system would assist government agencies to improve overall healthcare for all U.S. citizens.

KEY ISSUES

The actual and potential benefits of an EHR are promising but challenges also exist. This section focuses on several issues associated with EHR adoption related to cost, ownership, data integrity, privacy and confidentiality, standards, organizational culture, and human factors.

Cost

The cost to implement and maintain an EHR is a major barrier. Physicians in private practice can expect to spend between $54,000 and $100,000 or more to purchase and implement a certified EHR.[24] This does not include the per-year maintenance costs or hiring of technical staff to keep the system running on a daily basis. If a practice is using paper records, additional staff may be needed to enter previous patient data into the new system. Providers with a noncertified EHR will need to replace or update the system to meet standards and data conversion may be necessary to move from the old system to the new system.

Hospitals and other healthcare organizations have the same issues. EHR technology expenses can range from $1 million to $100 million or more depending on the size of the facility, software vendor selection, and functionality purchased. Annual maintenance is an added expense that can be approximately 20% of the purchase price and easily cost more than $1 million annually. In both scenarios, financial planning for initial and ongoing training, technical support, and software upgrades must be considered. The bottom line is that implementing and maintaining an IT system is very expensive. Currently each healthcare organization purchases its own EHR; connections to other facilities are less common, although this trend is changing with the use of HIE. It is unclear who will be responsible for the electronic links that will form the infrastructure for local, regional, or national EHRs of the future.

Ownership

Ownership of the patient record is another issue. Traditional health records have always been the property of the service institution. Patient access to this record could be permitted but sometimes at a cost. A comprehensive,

interoperable EHR would cross institutional boundaries and include patient interaction, making ownership more complex. Since healthcare providers use a lot of the same data, many questions are currently unanswered, such as: What data would be shared? How would users access these data? Who would be responsible for updating and ensuring data accuracy? Who would store the shared data? Would patients and consumers have access to the data or a subset of the data? What role would the government play in monitoring the access, quality, security, privacy, and confidentiality of patient records? Consumer consent and access are critical elements of the EHR adoption initiative, which has implications for healthcare organizations and the issue of ownership. Healthcare providers may be uncomfortable with the prospect of patients reading their notes and alter what and how they document to accommodate consumer access. Consumer consent is required for health professionals to retrieve or share patient records to ensure that personal information is not accessed inappropriately. This rule could affect quality of care if the consumer is concerned about confidentiality and denies permission. Ultimately, ownership may be driven by who has control and access to the data.

Data Integrity

Data integrity refers to the accuracy and consistency of stored and transmitted data that can be compromised when information is entered incorrectly or deliberately altered or when the system protections are not working correctly or suddenly fail. As EHR adoption expands to include data from multiple healthcare entities, more opportunities for human error exist. Poor screen designs that are confusing and cumbersome and lack of system training often lead to data entry errors. How this will be monitored and who is responsible for correcting inaccurate information will be an issue. Critical patient information, such as allergies and medications, should always be validated and updated at each episode of care. Education on how to use the EHR should be provided to all staff prior to implementing a new system, when changes are made to an existing system, and during orientation for new employees. Stringent security measures that include audit trails, penalties for fraudulent activities, and detailed policies and procedures are other measures that protect data integrity.

Data integrity can also be affected if a system is not working correctly or suddenly fails. Unfortunately, users do not always recognize when a feature is not functioning, such as a broken alert or incorrect calculations, and this leads to inaccuracies in data. When an interface from one application to another is not working, this also may not be readily noticeable. For example, a physician is able to enter orders using CPOE but the interface to the pharmacy department system fails and medication orders are not received or dispensed, which ultimately affects patient care. A nurse may discover this problem only when it is time to administer medications and he or she learns that they are missing from the unit. When the interface resumes functioning the orders will cross over, but depending on the time the order was placed, some data may be lost or corrupted. Appropriate downtime procedures (discussed in Chapter 18) and support mechanisms, such as a customer help desk to track and resolve issues, along with rigorous system testing is extremely important to ensuring data integrity.

Privacy and Confidentiality

Despite advances in technology and robust software that limits access to computerized health information, privacy and confidentiality continue to be major concerns for both the healthcare professional and consumer. With the expansion of the EHR and HIE as a driving force to automate and share health information, clinicians may find government and regulatory requirements for controlled access to patient information too restrictive or an invasion of privacy. In this respect, providers may be less inclined to use the EHR or more cautious when documenting patient care in order to avoid litigation. Like facilities, consumers can also be bombarded with PHR computer attacks, such as viruses, spyware, and hackers. Some consumers do not trust that health IT will be any different than traditional healthcare and fear a large-scale EHR system could allow access to personal data without adequate protection against unauthorized use of information. Some consumers prefer that sensitive health information (such as psychiatric care) never be shared, which creates problems because this can represent critical information missing from a medical record. Before a nationwide interoperable EHR can be implemented, issues related to privacy and confidentiality need to be resolved. This topic is discussed in more detail in Chapter 19.

Standards

In a famous commentary on hospitals in 1863, Florence Nightingale wrote: "In attempting to arrive at the truth, I have applied everywhere for information, but in scarcely an instance have I been able to obtain hospital records fit for any purposes of comparison. If they could be obtained they would enable us to decide many other questions besides the ones alluded to. They would show subscribers how their money was being spent, what amount of good was really being done with it, or whether the money was not doing mischief rather than good."[84(p176)] Almost 150 years later these same issues with extracting data for comparisons still exist. Healthcare professionals have been discussing the need for standardized vocabularies and terminologies for many decades. Implementation has been hindered by numerous factors related to disagreement on which terminologies to use, lack of standards to harmonize multiple coding structures, cultural and language barriers, interpretation of meaning, threats to autonomy, and user resistance. The benefits of standardization allow for a mutual understanding of terms and improved communication among healthcare professionals along with a common way to collect and aggregate data. A universal language would allow us to consistently capture, represent, access, and communicate clinical data, information, and knowledge across all settings. While progress is underway, standards continue to be an issue for EHR adoption.

Organizational Culture

The healthcare environment is filled with many cultures, subcultures, and traditions and the implementation of an EHR can be disruptive to the socio-cultural system. A disruptive technology is an innovation that replaces long-held traditional ideas and ways of doing things. This type of technology can improve or replace a product in ways that are unexpected and often opens up new market demand, which leads to lower-priced products or products designed for a different set of consumers. Cellphones, email, Twitter, and Facebook have significantly changed our interpersonal, professional, and business communications. In this respect, a disruptive technology such as the EHR may challenge and alter social and cultural norms. How these cultures respond to change will vary based on belief systems, values, roles within the healthcare team, and computer knowledge.

Healthcare organizations are challenged with issues surrounding the evolving nature of EHR technology, one of the most important of which is user acceptance. Whether in a hospital setting or private practice, nurses, physicians, and other caregivers are required to use an EHR as part of their daily routine but some find it difficult to comply. Reasons for this vary from lack of computer skills, complexity of application, lack of available hardware, or difficulty adjusting to change. Caregivers often indicate that documenting in the computer interferes with routine workflow or takes away from valuable time with patients. When CPOE was enforced by some institutions, physicians complained that entering orders in the computer was a task beneath them since this was traditionally secretarial work. This also had an impact on the role of nurses since they no longer had to interpret and validate handwritten orders. Physicians entered these orders in isolation and the computer forced them to be more specific during the entry process. Nurses' workflow changed since they no longer had a paper form to alert them when new orders became available. Checking the computer more often was disruptive to care and procedures were needed to avoid mistakes and delays. These types of reasons for resistance must be addressed for an EHR adoption to be successful. Acceptance of this technology is dependent on effective leadership, user involvement, the ability of the system to integrate with workflow, and timely education and technical support.

Human Factors

A significant amount of time is spent by all healthcare providers in processing and documenting patient-related data but using an EHR system for these activities can be perceived as a frustrating experience.[85] Research on human–computer interaction has identified several issues related to the usability of EHRs. Despont-Gros, Mueller, and Lovis,[86] in their review of human–computer interaction models, reported user acceptance to be a reliable concept to reflect evaluation of clinical information systems. Problems with usability related to complex human–computer interfaces, poorly designed decision support tools, and lack of training are recognized as obstacles that lead to significant medical errors and resistance to accept the technology.[17,85,87,88]

The complexities of EHR technology add concerns that new types of errors are beginning to emerge. Many clinicians complain that information systems increase their workload, which decreases productivity and efficiency. Ash, Berg, and Coiera[17] reported that EMR systems can have a negative impact on communication and teamwork due to the linear processing of computer systems, which conflicts with the more fluid iterative and interruptive nature of providing care. They also concluded that cognitive workload increased with unnecessary clerical tasks, overly structured data entry requirements, and fragmented patient data retrieval formats. In a study of physician groups who used an EMR, the investigators reported that adequate technical support and training were critical for the successful integration and acceptance of new technology.[88] Addressing issues related to human factors is complex and requires early user involvement and attention to system design and testing. Human factors concepts are discussed in detail in Chapter 21.

CONCLUSION AND FUTURE DIRECTIONS

EHR has become the preferred term for the lifetime patient record that would include healthcare data from the consumer and a variety of provider sources. The IOM identified eight essential care delivery components for all EHRs: (1) administrative processes, (2) communication and connectivity, (3) decision support, (4) health information and data, (5) order entry management, (6) patient support, (7) results management, and (8) population health management.[14] Dentistry and optometry records were added to this list by the Department of Defense.[15]

Common EHR applications used in the clinical setting include CPOE, eMAR, BCMA, clinical documentation, specialty applications, and CDS. The HITECH Act (2009) established programs to accelerate EHR adoption, one of which offers financial incentives for hospitals and healthcare providers who adopt certified EHR technology and comply with Meaningful Use objectives. How the HITECH Act will address the needs of health practitioners is unclear but many are actively involved in local, regional, and national initiatives to improve the quality, safety, and efficiency of care using technology. Current research findings indicate that EHR benefits related to cost, access, quality, safety, and efficiency of care delivery support healthcare policy initiatives driving adoption. Despite the many advances in technology, there are still numerous issues to resolve associated with implementation costs, ownership, data integrity, privacy and confidentiality, organizational culture, human factors, and development of an infrastructure to support a nationwide EHR. Future directions are promising for the EHR for personalizing care, supporting research efforts, and mobilizing care coordination across national and international boundaries.

In the future the EHR will play a pivotal role in personalized medicine as a medium for data, information, and knowledge exchange and for exploration. Advanced computing and systems integration will provide powerful evaluation tools to facilitate healthcare providers and consumers in the decision making process. The Human Genome Project, in which findings were accelerated through the use of computer technology, will contribute knowledge that could lead to genetic profiling and the creation of individualized care. Genetic testing, along with access to an interoperable EHR, can be used to diagnose, prevent, and treat preexisting and potential health issues based on our unique biological responses. In the future an individual's genome sequence may be part of a comprehensive medical record, not unlike recording medications and allergies.[89]

Customized medications will likely eliminate prescribing drugs or doses that do not work, minimize side effects, and decrease costs. Other treatments, such as diet and exercise, can be personalized to avoid a lot of guesswork and trial and error. For example, if a patient's genetic code reveals a risk for colon cancer, preventive measures can start earlier. More frequent exams, colonoscopies, and diets that promote colon health can be the focus of care. In addition to personalizing care, the EHR will contain a wealth of information related to disease, interventions, and treatment responses that can be used for research. Data mining of these huge databases can reveal patterns and predictions on how to reverse or prevent disease.

The EHR continues to be an evolving concept with global and national implications. As of early 2012 EHR adoption in U.S. hospitals was progressing, with approximately 43.9% at Stage 3 and another 30% at Stage 4 or above.[27] The rate of adoption by physician practices and clinics was much lower, with only 10.9% at Stage 3. Although hospitals may be in a better position to fulfill Meaningful Use objectives, additional support and guidance may be needed to achieve nationwide implementation goals projected for 2015. Many other countries, such as Canada, Australia, England, and Finland, have focused their efforts toward building an infrastructure and developing systems that support health information at a national level.[90] The European Commission has launched several initiatives to improve the safety and quality of care through information sharing at an international level, such as the eHealth Action Plan that supports standardization of EHR content and structure and the Smart Open Services (SOS) project that recommends allowing healthcare provider access to critical medical information for consumers traveling abroad.[91,92] EHR adoption has the potential to reach beyond the borders of this nation to meet the needs of a mobile society.

REFERENCES

1. Sewell J, Thede L. *Informatics and Nursing: Opportunities and Challenges.* 3rd ed. Philadelphia, PA: Lippincott, Williams, & Wilkins; 2013.
2. Hebda T, Czar P. *Handbook of Informatics for Nurses and Healthcare Professionals.* 5th ed. Boston, MA: Pearson; 2012.
3. National Library of Medicine (NLM). Medline/PubMed search and electronic health record information resources. NLM.

http://www.nlm.nih.gov/services/queries/ehr.html. Updated 2011. Accessed April 30, 2012.

4. Seckman C, Romano C. Electronic health record. In: Feldman H, ed. *Nursing Leadership: A Concise Encyclopedia*. 2nd ed. New York, NY: Springer; 2012:126-128.

5. National Alliance for Health Information Technology. Defining key health information technology terms. April 28, 2008. http://www.himss.org/content/files/HITTermsFinalReport.pdf.

6. Healthcare Information and Management Systems Society (HIMSS). EHR: electronic health record. HIMSS. http://www.himss.org/asp/topics_ehr.asp. Updated 2012. Accessed February 18, 2012.

7. Barey E. The electronic health record and clinical informatics. In: McGonigle D, Mastrian K, eds. *Nursing Informatics and the Foundation of Knowledge*. 2nd ed. Burlington, MA: Jones & Bartlett; 2012:285-301.

8. Hunter K. Electronic health record. In: Englebardt S, Nelson R, eds. *Health Care Informatics: An Interdisciplinary Approach*. Philadelphia, PA: Elsevier; 2001:209-230.

9. Keyhani S, Hebert P, Ross J, Federman A, Zhu C, Siu A. Electronic health record components and the quality of care. *Med Care*. 2008;46(12):1267-1272.

10. Dowding D, Turley M, Garrido T. The impact of an electronic health record on nurse sensitive patient outcomes: an interrupted time series analysis. *J Am Med Inform Assoc*. 2012; 19(4):615-620.

11. Kelley T, Brandon D, Docherty S. Electronic nursing documentation as a strategy to improve quality of patient care. *J Nurs Scholarship*. 2011;43(2):154-162.

12. Whetton S. *Health Informatics: A Socio-Technical Perspective*. Oxford, United Kingdom: Oxford University Press; 2005.

13. eHealth Initiative. EHR collaborative. http://www.ehrcollaborative.org/overview.htm. Updated 2004. Accessed June 20, 2012.

14. Institute of Medicine. Key capabilities of an electronic health record system: letter report from the Committee on Data Standards for Patient Safety: Board of Health Care Services. 2003. http://www.nap.edu/catalog.php?record_id=10781.

15. Anderson H. EHR pioneers try to stay out front. *Health Data Manag*. 2007;15(5):26-34.

16. Bates W, Teich J, Lee J, et al. The impact of computerized physician order entry on medication error prevention. *J Am Med Inform Assoc*. 1999;6(4):313-321.

17. Ash JS, Berg M, Coiera E. Patient care information systems-related errors. *J Am Med Inform Assoc*. 2004;11(2):104-112.

18. Kohn LT, Corrigan JM, Donaldson MS. *To Err Is Human: Building a Safer Health System*. Washington, DC: Institute of Medicine; 2000.

19. Ammenwerth E, Kutscha U, Kutscha A, Mahler C, Eichstadter R, Haux R. Nursing process documentation systems in clinical routine prerequisites and experiences. *Int J Med Inform*. 2001; 64:187-200.

20. Ammenwerth E, Mansmann U, Iller C, Eichstadter R. Factors affecting and affected by user acceptance of computer-based nursing documentation: results of a two-year study. *J Am Med Inform Assoc*. 2003;10:69-84.

21. Case J, Mowry M, Welebob E. The nursing shortage: can technology help? June 2002. http://www.wflboces.org/uploads/sdm/nursingshortagetechnologyfull.pdf.

22. Parsons A, McCullough C, Wang J, Shih S. Validity of electronic health record–derived quality measurement for performance monitoring. *J Am Med Inform Assoc*. 2012. doi:10.1136/amiajnl-2011-000557.

23. U.S. Department of Health and Human Services (HHS). The office of the national coordinator for health information technology: electronic health records and meaningful use. HHS. http://healthit.hhs.gov/portal/server.pt?open=512&objID=2996&mode=2. Updated 2011. Accessed June 12, 2012.

24. Harris C. An overview of the Meaningful Use final rule. Healthcare Information and Management Systems Society. http://www.himss.org/content/files/MU_Final_Rule_overview_PPT.pdf. Updated 2010. Accessed June 15, 2012.

25. Murphy J. HITECH programs supporting the journey to meaningful use of EHRS. *Comput Inform Nurs*. 2011;29(2):130-131. doi:10.1097/NCN.0b013e318210f0fc.

26. Centers for Medicare & Medicaid Services. Medicare and Medicaid program: electronic health record incentive program—Stage 2 final rule. 2012;42 CFR Parts 412, 413, 422, and 495. CMS-0044-F RIN 0938-AQ84.

27. HIMSS Analytics. HIMSS analytics introduces framework for ambulatory health IT adoption. HIMSS Analytics. http://www.himssanalytics.org/about/NewsDetail.aspx?nid=80352. Updated 2012. Accessed June 27, 2012.

28. HIMSS Analytics. News & Exclusives: BCS and HIMSS Analytics Europe to collaborate on EMR Adoption Model project. http://www.himssanalytics.org/about/NewsDetail.aspx?nid=80024. Accessed May 5, 2012.

29. Hoyt J. State of the industry: informatics perspectives on the EMR adoption model. Healthcare Information and Management Systems Society. http://www.himss.org/ASP/ContentRedirector.asp?ContentId=75059&type=HIMSSNewsItem&src=cii20101108. Updated 2010. Accessed July 1, 2012.

30. Greenwood K, Murphy J, Sensmeier J, Westra B. Nursing profession reengineered for leadership in landmark report: special report for the Alliance for Nursing Informatics member organizations. *Comput Inform Nurs*. 2011;29(2):66-67.

31. Farrell A, Taylor S. Electronic health record vendor applications. In: Saba V, McCormick K, eds. *Essentials of Nursing Informatics*. 5th ed. New York, NY: McGraw-Hill; 2011:317-339.

32. Cipriano P. The future of nursing and health IT: the quality elixir. *Nurs Econ*. 2011;29(5):286-289.

33. Harrison RL, Lyerla F. Using nursing clinical decision support systems to achieve Meaningful Use. *Comput Inform Nurs*. 2012;30(7):380-385. doi:10.1097/NCN.0b013e31823eb813.

34. Westra BL, Subramanian A, Hart CM, et al. Achieving "meaningful use" of electronic health records through the integration of the nursing management minimum data set. *J Nurs Adm*. 2010;40(7-8):336-343. doi:10.1097/NNA.0b013e3181e93994.

35. Bates DW, Teich JM, Lee J, et al. The impact of computerized physician order entry on medication error prevention. *J Am Med Inform Assoc*. 1999;6(4):313-321.

36. Bates DW, Leape LL, Cullen DJ, et al. Effect of computerized physician order entry and a team intervention on prevention of serious medication errors. *JAMA*. 1998;280(15):1311-1316.

37. Evans RS, Pestotnik SL, Classen DC, et al. A computer-assisted management program for antibiotics and other antiinfective agents. *N Engl J Med*. 1998;338(4):232-238. doi:10.1056/NEJM199801223380406.

38. Gandhi TK, Weingart SN, Seger AC, et al. Outpatient prescribing errors and the impact of computerized prescribing. *J Gen Intern Med*. 2005;20(9):837-841. doi:10.1111/j.1525-1497.2005.0194.x.

39. Mekhjian HS, Kumar RR, Kuehn L, et al. Immediate benefits realized following implementation of physician order entry at an academic medical center. *J Am Med Inform Assoc*. 2002;9(5):529-539.

40. Bates DW, Cohne M, Leape LL, Overhage M, Shabot MM, Sheridan T. Reducing the frequency of errors in medicine using information technology. *J Am Med Inform Assoc*. 2001;8(4): 299-308.

41. Spalding SC, Mayer PH, Ginde AA, Lowenstein SR, Yaron M. Impact of computerized physician order entry on ED patient length of stay. *Am J Emerg Med*. 2011;29(2):207-211. doi:10.1016/j.ajem.2009.10.007.

42. Altuwaijri MM, Bahanshal A, Almehaid M. Implementation of computerized physician order entry in National Guard hospitals: assessment of critical success factors. *J Family Community Med*. 2011;18(3):143-151. doi:10.4103/2230-8229.90014.

43. Chapman AK, Lehmann CU, Donohue PK, Aucott SW. Implementation of computerized provider order entry in a neonatal intensive care unit: impact on admission workflow. *Int J Med Inform*. 2012;81(5):291-295. doi:10.1016/j.ijmedinf.2011.12.006.

44. Adam TJ, Waitman R, Jones I, Aronsky D. The effect of computerized provider order entry (CPOE) on ordering patterns for chest pain patients in the emergency department. *AMIA Annu Symp Proc*. 2011;2011:38-47.

45. Hughes RG, ed. *Patient Safety and Quality: An Evidence-Based Handbook for Nurses*. Rockville, MD: Agency for Healthcare Research and Quality; 2006.

46. Koppel R, Metlay J, Cohen A, et al. Role of computerized physician order entry systems in facilitating medication errors. *J Am Med Inform Assoc*. 2005;293(10):1197-1203.

47. Seckman C, Romano C, Defensor R, Benham-Hutchins M. Design efficiencies and satisfaction of computerized physician order entry: a comparison of two order entry methods. Presented at the 16th Annual Summer Institute in Nursing Informatics held July 19-22, 2006 at the University of Maryland School of Nursing.

48. Payne TH, Nichol WP, Hoey P, Savarino J. Characteristics and override rates of order checks in a practitioner order entry system. *Proc AMIA Symp*. 2002:602-606.

49. Ash JS, Bates DW. Factors and forces affecting EHR system adoption: report of a 2044 ACMI discussion. *J Am Med Inform Assoc*. 2005;12(1):8-12.

50. Ash J, Sittig D, Dykstra R, Campbell E, Guappone K. The unintended consequences of computerized provider order entry: findings from a mixed methods exploration. *Int J Med Inform*. 2009;78S:S69-S76.

51. U.S. Food and Drug Administration (FDA). HHS announces new requirements for bar codes on drugs and blood to reduce risks of medication errors. FDA. http://www.fda.gov/NewsEvents/Newsroom/PressAnnouncements/2004/ucm108250.htm. Updated 2009. Accessed July 2, 2012.

52. Poon EG, Keohane CA, Yoon CS, et al. Effect of bar-code technology on the safety of medication administration. *N Engl J Med*. 2010;362(18):1698-1707. doi:10.1056/NEJMsa0907115.

53. Chou S, Yan H, Huang H, Tseng K, Kuo S. Establishing and evaluating bar-code technology in blood sampling system: a model based on human centered design method. Proceedings from the NI2012: 11th International Congress on Nursing Informatics, Montreal, Canada; 2012:79-82.

54. Tseng K, Feng R, Chou S, Lin S, Yan H, Huang H. Implementation and evaluation of the effectiveness of the bar-coded medication administration system in a medical center. Proceedings from the NI2012: 11th International Congress on Nursing Informatics, Montreal, Canada; 2012:416.

55. Helmons PJ, Wargel LN, Daniels CE. Effect of bar-code-assisted medication administration on medication administration errors and accuracy in multiple patient care areas. *Am J Health Syst Pharm*. 2009;66(13):1202-1210. doi:10.2146/ajhp080357.

56. Dwibedi N, Sansgiry SS, Frost CP, et al. Effect of bar-code-assisted medication administration on nurses' activities in an intensive care unit: a time-motion study. *Am J Health Syst Pharm*. 2011;68(11):1026-1031. doi:10.2146/ajhp100382; 10.2146/ajhp100382.

57. Versel N. Emergency room patients tracked with RFID tags. *Information Week*. http://www.informationweek.com/healthcare/electronic-medical-records/emergency-room-patients-tracked-with-rfi/231901224?queryText=emergency room patients tracked with RFID tags. Updated 2011. Accessed July 2, 2012.

58. Coiera E, Lau Y, Tsafnat G, Sintchenko V, Magrabi F. The changing nature of clinical decision support systems: a focus on consumers, genomics, public health and decision safety. *IMIA Yearbook of Medical Informatics 2009*. 2009:84-95.

59. Demner-Fushman D, Seckman C, Fisher C, Hauser S, Clayton J, Thoma G. A prototype system to support evidence-based practice. *AMIA Annual Symposium Proceedings*. 2008:151-155.

60. Wang SJ, Middleton B, Prosser LA, et al. A cost–benefit analysis of electronic medical records in primary care. *Am J Med*. 2003; 114(5):397-403.

61. Li K, Naganawa S, Wang K, et al. Study of the cost–benefit analysis of electronic medical record systems in general hospital in China. *J Med Syst*. 2012;36(5):3283-3291. doi:10.1007/s10916-011-9819-6.

62. Maviglia SM, Yoo JY, Franz C, et al. Cost–benefit analysis of a hospital pharmacy bar code solution. *Arch Intern Med*. 2007;167(8):788-794. doi:10.1001/archinte.167.8.788.

63. Shekelle PG, Morton SC, Keeler EB. Costs and benefits of health information technology. *Evid Rep Technol Assess (Full Rep)*. 2006;(132):1-71.

64. Grieger DL, Cohen SH, Krusch DA. A pilot study to document the return on investment for implementing an ambulatory electronic health record at an academic medical center. *J Am Coll Surg*. 2007;205(1):89-96. doi:10.1016/j.jamcollsurg.2007.02.074.

65. Menachemi N, Collum TH. Benefits and drawbacks of electronic health record systems. *Risk Manag Healthc Policy*. 2011; 4:47-55.

66. Uslu A, Stausberg J. Value of the electronic patient record: an analysis of the literature. *J Biomed Inform*. 2008;41:675-682.

67. Miskulin DC, Weiner DE, Tighiouart H, et al. Computerized decision support for EPO dosing in hemodialysis patients. *Am J Kidney Dis*. 2009;54(6):1081-1088. doi:10.1053/j.ajkd.2009.07.010.

68. Cox B, Thornewill J. The consumer's view of the electronic health record: engaging patients in EHR adoption. *J Healthc Inf Manag*. 2008;22(2):43-47.

69. Undern T. Consumers and health information technology: a national survey. California Healthcare Foundation, Oakland, CA April 2010. http://www.chcf.org/~/media/MEDIA%20LIBRARY%20Files/PDF/C/PDF%20ConsumersHealthInfo-TechnologyNationalSurvey.pdf.

70. Orlovsky C. The endless nursing benefits of electronic medical records. NurseZone.com. http://www.nursezone.com/nursing-news-events/devices-and-technology/The-Endless-Nursing-Benefits-of-Electronic-Medical-Records_24676.aspx. Updated 2005. Accessed July 5, 2012.

71. Cherry BJ, Ford EW, Peterson LT. Experiences with electronic health records: early adopters in long-term care facilities. *Health Care Manage Rev*. 2011;36(3):265-274. doi:10.1097/HMR.0b013e31820e110f; 10.1097/HMR.0b013e31820e110f.

72. Chisolm DJ, Purnell TS, Cohen DM, McAlearney AS. Clinician perceptions of an electronic medical record during the first year of implementation in emergency services. *Pediatr Emerg Care.* 2010;26(2):107-110. doi:10.1097/PEC.0b013e3181ce2f99.

73. Seckman C, Mills M. *Clinicians' Perceptions of Usability of an Electronic Medical Record over Time* [dissertation]. College Park, MD: University of Maryland; 2008.

74. Stefan S. Using clinical EHR metrics to demonstrate quality outcomes. *Nurs Manage.* 2011;42(3):17-19. doi:10.1097/01.NUMA.0000394062.30819.61.

75. Goetz Goldberg D, Kuzel AJ, Feng LB, DeShazo JP, Love LE. EHRs in primary care practices: benefits, challenges, and successful strategies. *Am J Manag Care.* 2012;18(2):e48-e54.

76. Doyle RJ, Wang N, Anthony D, Borkan J, Shield RR, Goldman RE. Computers in the examination room and the electronic health record: physicians' perceived impact on clinical encounters before and after full installation and implementation. *Fam Pract.* 2012. doi:10.1093/fampra/cms015.

77. Abramson EL, Barron Y, Quaresimo J, Kaushal R. Electronic prescribing within an electronic health record reduces ambulatory prescribing errors. *Jt Comm J Qual Patient Saf.* 2011;37(10):470-478.

78. Kaushal R, Kern LM, Barron Y, Quaresimo J, Abramson EL. Electronic prescribing improves medication safety in community-based office practices. *J Gen Intern Med.* 2010;25(6):530-536. doi:10.1007/s11606-009-1238-8.

79. Mitchell RN. Physician adoption of EHR in an all-digital hospital. Advance for Health Information Professionals. http://health-information.advanceweb.com/Article/Physician-Adoption-of-EHR-in-an-All-digital-Hospital.aspx. Published March 28, 2007. Accessed July 8, 2012.

80. Bell B, Thornton K. From promise to reality: achieving the value of an EHR. *Healthc Financ Manage.* 2011;65(2):50-56.

81. Kaiser Family Foundation. U.S. health care costs. KaiserEDU.org. http://www.kaiseredu.org/issue-modules/us-health-care-costs/background-brief.aspx. Updated 2012. Accessed June 2, 2012.

82. Kumar S, Aldrich K. Overcoming barriers to electronic medical record (EMR) implementation in the U.S. healthcare system: a comparative study. *Health Informatics J.* 2010;16(4):306-318. doi:10.1177/1460458210380523.

83. Office of the National Coordinator. EHR benefits for our country's health. HealthIT.gov. http://www.healthit.gov/patients-families/ehr-benefits-our-countrys-health. Updated 2012. Accessed June 15, 2012.

84. Nightingale F. Notes on Hospitals. London, United Kingdom: Longman, Green, Longman, Roberts, and Green; 1863. http://archive.org/stream/notesonhospital01nighgoog#page/n218/mode/2up.

85. Gillespie G. EHR game changer focuses on taking invisible path to change. *Health Data Manag.* 2012;20(6):48-49.

86. Despont-Gros C, Mueller H, Lovis C. Evaluating user interactions with clinical information systems: a model based on human-computer interaction models. *J Biomed Inform.* 2004;38:244-255.

87. Gardner E. EHR success all in the details. *Health Data Manag.* 2012;20(5):30-32.

88. Miller RH, Sim I. Physicians' use of electronic medical records: barriers and solutions. *Health Affair.* 2004;21(2):116-126.

89. Frist B. Personalized medicine. The Hill's Congress Blog. http://thehill.com/blogs/congress-blog/healthcare/237155-personalized-medicine. Published July 10, 2012.

90. Hayrinen K, Saranto K, Nykanen P. Definition, structure, content, use and impacts of electronic health records: a review of the research literature. *Int J Med Inform.* 2008;77:291-304.

91. European Commission. eHealth initiatives to support medical assistance while traveling and living abroad. Europa. http://europa.eu/rapid/pressReleasesAction.do?reference=IP/08/1075&format=HTML&aged=0&language=EN&guiLanguage=en. Updated 2008. Accessed February, 12, 2012.

92. Europe's Information Society. The right prescription for Europe's eHealth. Europe's Information Society. http://ec.europa.eu/information_society/activities/health/policy/index_en.htm. Updated 2012. Accessed February 16, 2012.

■ DISCUSSION QUESTIONS

1. In September 2012 the American Health Information Management Association (AHIMA) released a new guide to help consumers understand medical records. A press release can be viewed at www.ahima.org/downloads/pdfs/pr/press-releases/consumer%20onc%20presentation.pdf and the guide can be viewed at http://myphr.com/HealthLiteracy/understanding.aspx. Discuss the significance of using the term *medical record* as opposed to *health record*.

2. Historically, patient records maintained by healthcare institutions did not contain financial data such as charges or incident reports. Should this segregation of patient data be maintained with the implementation of EHRs?

3. Increasingly patients expect full access to their EMRs and EHRs. What limitations, if any, would be in the best interest of patients? For example, should healthcare providers have access to new test results for 3 full business days before these are posted for patient viewing?

4. How does the introduction of a computerized provider order entry (CPOE) system affect communication between healthcare providers (e.g., between pharmacists and physicians or nurses, between nurses and physicians)? What modifications, if any, should be made in the workflow of the different healthcare providers to adjust for this change in communication patterns?

5. Discuss the advantages and disadvantages associated with implementing and using a regional and national EHR.

CASE STUDY

A large healthcare enterprise in the Mid-Atlantic region that was created by a merger owns two acute care hospitals, a rehabilitation center, an outpatient surgical center, and three long-term care facilities. Each of these institutions uses a different EMR system. Admitting privileges extend to 550 physicians who have office systems that interface with at least one of the acute care EMR systems. The vision is to create an environment to support communication, care coordination, and data sharing across the organization in preparation for a regional EHR system. The organization also wants to move quickly in order to take advantage of the incentives offered by the government and meet mandatory requirements. Executives have decided to focus on the acute care facilities first and use lessons learned there to integrate the other centers at a later time. Hospital A uses certified EHR applications and has implemented ancillary systems, CPOE, and clinical documentation whereas Hospital B has a highly customized, beloved old mainframe computer that is outdated and no longer supported by the vendor. Instead of selecting a new system for both hospitals, the software programs used in Hospital A will be implemented in Hospital B.

Discussion Questions

1. You are the Vice-President of Patient Services for both acute care hospitals. Who would you identify as stakeholders in the implementation and why? What steps would you take to minimize user resistance?

2. According to the U.S. EMR Adoption Model, at what stage of implementation would you classify Hospital A? After both hospitals are using the same system, what would you recommend implementing next?

3. The healthcare enterprise needs to do more than implement certified systems in order to receive government incentives and address regulatory requirements. Identify at least five core objectives related to Meaningful Use that the hospitals need to execute.

Applications for Managing Institutions Delivering Healthcare

Michael H. Kennedy, Kathy H. Wood, and Gerald R. Ledlow

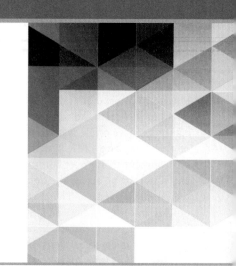

If a healthcare system cannot effectively track the total cost of all materials used to treat an individual patient and aggregate data to determine the cost of treating groups of patients, managing the cost of healthcare is not possible.

OBJECTIVES

At the completion of this chapter the reader will be prepared to:

1. Outline the evolution of financial information systems (FISs) in healthcare organizations
2. Discuss the basic FISs and their application in healthcare organizations
3. Compare and contrast practice management systems (PMSs) and integrated healthcare systems
4. Describe and explain the attributes of an efficient materials management (supply chain) system in a healthcare organization
5. Appraise how a quality supply chain system supports the operation and management of clinical systems
6. Describe the human resources management actions associated with the subsystems typically deployed with a human resources information system
7. Define business intelligence
8. Distinguish between enterprise-level and application-level business intelligence

KEY TERMS

ABSTRACT

This chapter addresses the administrative applications within health information systems that are designed to facilitate the delivery of healthcare, such as financial, practice management, supply chain and materials management, human resources, and business intelligence systems.

INTRODUCTION

Health information systems are "complexes or systems of processing data, information and knowledge in health care environments."[1(p270)] These environments comprise a variety of settings, including hospitals, ambulatory settings, long-term care facilities, and managed care organizations.

Typically, the applications within health information systems are categorized as clinical or administrative. This chapter focuses on the administrative applications within health information systems designed to facilitate the management of healthcare delivery. The chapter considers in turn financial, practice management, materials management, human resources, and business intelligence systems.

Vendor Resource Guides

The applications required to process information in healthcare settings are primarily provided by vendors. The vendor market for hospital information systems alone in 2011 had total revenues of $12 billion, with the top five vendors in terms of revenue being McKesson ($3.2 billion), Cerner ($2.2 billion), Siemens ($1.7 billion), Allscripts ($1.4 billion), and Epic Systems Corporation (nearly $1 billion). These revenue statistics exclude vendors that do not sell a comprehensive suite of applications designed to automate both the administrative and the clinical departments in a hospital.[2]

Vendors that deploy a comprehensive suite of applications are referred to as enterprise vendors. The Healthcare Information and Management Systems Society (HIMSS) (www.himss.org) publishes annually a white paper titled "Essentials of the U.S. Hospital IT Market," which lists the top enterprise healthcare information technology (IT) vendors for the U.S. hospital market. Top niche vendors promoting specialized applications are listed separately. When specialty vendors and vendors targeting nonhospital markets are included, the health information system marketplace becomes a confusing morass of products whose capabilities are difficult to assess.

Fortunately, professional organizations like the HIMSS, hard copy and online content publishers like Health Data Management (www.healthdatamanagement.com), and trade and technology research companies like Gartner (www.gartner.com) and KLAS (www.klasresearch.com) help stakeholders to make more informed decisions.

HIMSS provides an online conference exhibitors guide (http://onlinebuyersguide.himss.org) in the form of a searchable database with an exhaustive list of healthcare IT companies, products, and services. Clicking on a product category results in the retrieval of vendor names, contact information, and brief descriptions of the products and services offered. HIMSS Analytics (www.himssanalytics.org) is a wholly owned not-for-profit subsidiary of HIMSS that offers services to providers and healthcare IT companies. Hospitals and other providers that participate in an annual study gain access to the HIMSS Analytics Database and a number of benefits free of charge, including an Electronic Medical Record Adoption Model Score, an American Recovery and Reinvestment Act Hospital Scorecard, benchmarking reports, up to four market overview reports, and the *Annual Report of the U.S. Hospital IT Market*. The HIMSS Analytics Database is available by subscription to healthcare IT companies, which may also purchase ad hoc data reports.

In addition to publishing a monthly magazine of the same name and maintaining an extensive website, Health Data Management maintains a resource guide (http://marketplace.healthdatamanagement.com) by subject category. Similar to the HIMSS online conference exhibitors guide, clicking on a subject category returns vendor names, contact information, and brief descriptions of the products and services offered.

Gartner and KLAS provide fee-based ratings services. Gartner states, "We deliver the technology-related insight necessary for our clients to make the right decisions, every day."[3] KLAS declares that its mission is "to improve healthcare technology delivery by honestly, accurately, and impartially measuring vendor performance for our provider partners."[4] This is done by monitoring vendor performance based on feedback from healthcare providers and by conducting independent analyses of products and services. KLAS publishes a *Best in KLAS Awards* report annually for software, professional services, and medical equipment. KLAS's reports should be used with some caution, as the vendors cited by KLAS represent the rankings of just one ratings service, but they do serve as a resource. Additional information about these services is included in Chapter 16.

MAJOR TYPES OF APPLICATIONS

Financial Systems

A financial information system (FIS) is a system that stores and records fiscal (financial) operations within an organization that are then used for reporting and decision making. There are various "financial" types of functions that healthcare organizations, like any other business, must perform to remain viable. These involve the following components:

- A customer (patient) purchasing the product (receiving the service)
- Salespeople (healthcare personnel) providing the service or product
- A facility to receive the service or product (healthcare facility)
- Supplies needed for a procedure (materials management)
- Payment received by the healthcare organization for the product (service) received (receivables)
- Monies received to be deposited in accounts (accounting)
- Payment made to healthcare personnel and support staff for services performed (payroll)
- Expenses paid (payables) to external constituents that made it possible to perform a procedure (mortgage, utilities, etc.)

The architecture of a typical FIS is illustrated in Figure 7-1. As Rogoski noted, FISs can no longer be regarded as "back-office" systems.[5] Although it is true that financial functions are usually not a matter of life or death for the patient, an ill-fitted FIS can be life or death for the fiscal viability of the organization. Therefore one must choose wisely and update the FIS often to keep up with the ever-changing regulations and variations that affect the revenue and profitability of the organization.

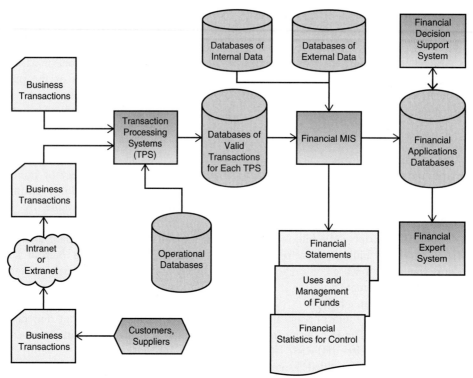

FIG 7-1 Financial information system architecture. (Healthcare Financial Management Association Certification Professional Practicum PowerPoint.)

Evolution of Healthcare FISs

Automated FISs were the first type of systems to be used in many healthcare facilities. The main purpose of these initial FISs was basic bookkeeping and payroll. Basic accounting systems were then put into place to help with the billing function. As Latham quotes: "Cash is king, so cash flow is the lifeblood of the kingdom."[6(p1)] To get cash flow, charges must be captured and collected from the patient or the patient's third-party payment system. Entering charges and creating claims to send to insurance companies and patients were some of the first, and easiest, functions for an FIS. Payroll was also a very simple function for an FIS to perform. There was no need for analytics or importing to spreadsheets and reporting functions were limited.[6] Healthcare organizations embraced the basic financial functions to remain financially viable. Figure 7-1 shows how financial transactions fit within the FISs.

Some of the basic financial systems required by healthcare organizations and other businesses are general ledger, payroll, patient accounting, claims processing, claims denial management, contracts management, and fixed asset management.

General Ledger. The general ledger consists of *all* financial transactions made by the healthcare organization. This is similar to a personal checking ledger where any checks written or deposits made are recorded in the account. Numerous financial areas need to be tracked and as a result a healthcare organization will also maintain various subsidiary ledgers. Each of these ledgers tracks customer and vendor names,

dates of transactions, types of transactions, and balances remaining. The FIS managing the general ledger must be able to track and report information in a variety of ways to meet the needs of the decision makers. Types of financial data that need to be tracked include the following:

- *Assets:* Assets are property items that can be converted easily into cash. Assets are classified as tangible and intangible. Tangible assets include current and fixed assets such as inventory or buildings and equipment. Intangible assets include nonphysical resources such as copyrights or computer systems.
- *Accounts payable:* Accounts payable are the monies that are owed to vendors and suppliers for items purchased on credit (very similar to using a personal credit card and then paying back the amount on a monthly basis). These usually occur in the form of invoices or statements. This would fall under the category of disbursements in many systems. Since many vendors offer discounts when paid by a certain date, the FIS needs to be able to track the dates that payments need to be made in order to receive the discount or avoid the penalties that may be applied for late payments.
- *Accounts receivable:* The opposite of accounts payable, accounts receivable are monies that are owed to the institution. The vast majority of the dollars owed to the healthcare organization come in the form of patient-generated revenues. Once claims have been submitted to insurance companies (if the patient is covered by insurance), the

remaining balance is sent to the patient for payment. The FIS has to be able to track the amount owed by the insurance, minus any negotiated rate such as managed care contracting, and the remaining balance owed by the patient. Ideally, the system estimates the amounts owed up front so the collection process can begin at the time of the visit.

Payroll Application. The application that handles compensation payments to employees is the payroll system. This is also referred to as a disbursement system. The FIS application must be able to deduct taxes, benefits, possibly savings amounts, and other deductions. At the onset of FISs for payroll, the minimal functions could be performed. In today's more advanced systems, automatic payroll deposits and much more can be performed. In addition, overtime pay, pay rates, and payroll histories must be tracked and reported. At the end of the calendar year the system must be able to generate W2 forms for the employee to use in income tax preparation.

Patient Accounting Application. A patient accounting application tracks the accounting transactions related to patient services. All charges that are incurred as a result of the patient visit need to be tracked and added to the patient's financial record. This can include inpatient fees if the patient is hospitalized; healthcare provider (physicians, nurse practitioners, etc.) and medication fees associated with the treatment; and procedure costs, including surgeries, radiology, and whatever else is necessary for the care of the patient. The procedural and diagnostic codes also become part of the patient billing record in order to complete the information necessary for the insurance payer to submit payment for the claim. Without critical information such as charges and coding, the claim process is delayed, resulting in reduced cash flow for the healthcare organization.

The collection process can begin at the time of the visit. This statement implies that the patient can receive services without paying anything up front. This is the reality in emergency situations. Because of the Emergency Medical Treatment and Active Labor Act (EMTALA), patients must be treated in the case of emergency regardless of their ability to pay. This can lead to hundreds of thousands of dollars outstanding that the healthcare facility will try to collect after the service has been performed. Therefore the collection process in healthcare is much different than the process in a traditional business that requires payment before the product or service is provided. Hence the FIS also needs to be able to track outstanding balances and assist in tracking these for the patient accounts personnel who will be attempting to collect the balances. The older the balances are, the more difficult they are to collect. The FIS needs to be able to differentiate the balances based on several factors, including, but not limited to, amount, payer, age of the account, and so forth. The features needed in today's FISs are much more complex than in the past. For example, today managers may need to track the revenue generated by staff as a measure of productivity.

Claims Processing and Management System. As patients present for registration and admission, a single healthcare facility must be prepared to bill numerous insurance companies (third-party payers) representing hundreds of coverage and payment plans across government and private insurance. Some patients have primary coverage and supplemental coverage (e.g., Medicare as primary insurer and another insurer for supplemental coverage). Other patients receiving charity care or those with no insurance are categorized as private pay patients.

Claims processing and management is the submission of the insurance claim or bill to the third-party payer, either manually or electronically, and the follow-up on the payment from the payer. The application must be able to keep each of the payer types separate and know the requirements of how to bill the claims, who to bill for the balances, or if the balances need to be written off and not billed to anyone. Collections can be very challenging for the healthcare facility. Many new standards have been adopted for claims processing but there are still numerous different standards and requirements that must be followed for the various insurance companies and plans.

Sending "clean" claims is the key to getting payment quickly. Clean claims are those claims that contain all critical information such as patient demographics, charges and procedures performed, procedural and diagnostic coding, and other information required by the insurance company in order to remit prompt payment. Timely claims processing and collection are key to the fiscal health of institutions so they can meet the financial obligations in their disbursements and accounts payable functions. The claims processing application must review the claim before it is submitted to ensure that all necessary data fields are complete and accurate. If the claim is not clean, it will be denied, creating a delay and generating increased labor costs to correct errors before payment can be received for the service provided.

Claims Denial Management Application. Denials from insurance companies are tracked and require follow-up. The claims denial management application can prevent denials imposed by the insurance carrier in a variety of ways. For example, the application can issue an alert on a request by clinical personnel for a patient to stay an additional day in his or her current patient status (i.e., observation, inpatient) if that request is likely to be denied by the insurer. The submitted insurance claim for a patient's stay may also be denied for improper coding or missing information. When the denial occurs, the application needs to be able to track the update and the progress on having the denial reversed. Because a claim or request was denied initially does not mean that the decision cannot be reversed. Persistence and proper documentation can be the deciding factors leading to reversal. Documentation must be detailed and included with the denial reversal request in order to be effective.[7] In addition, the communications that took place between each area of patient care must be documented, collected, and stored in an orderly manner for the proof to be shown. This is just one example of why the FIS must be carefully integrated with the clinical systems.

Contract Management Application. Healthcare organizations have a variety of contracts they must track, including those for supply chain management (SCM) and managed care. These types of contracts affect the bottom line of the organization, so the contracts must be tracked and managed in order for the organization to obtain maximum financial gain. SCM contracts include group purchasing, where healthcare systems negotiate a price for using a standard vendor. Vendor price comparisons and usage need to be tracked and the system must ensure that employees are adhering to the purchasing policies. Additional SCM functions can include providing incentives for healthcare providers to reduce the cost of their preferred supplies. For example, some surgeons may have particular instruments or supplies they prefer for surgical procedures. These supplies may be much more expensive than an alternative brand. The FIS could help the organization track the supply costs and the costs for procedures and provide reports for physicians to accompany requests for their assistance in reducing those costs.

Managed care contracting can be very challenging and complex. The contracts can be numerous and each contract can have different terms. The FIS needs to be able to track these contracts and manage the terms and results of each contract individually. For example, when a patient is covered by a nongovernmental insurance plan, the insurance company may have negotiated an agreed-upon amount for reimbursement per service or per patient. The insurance and patients need to be billed according to that contract's terms and any negotiated discount should not be billed.

Fixed Asset Management Application. Fixed asset management applications manage the fixed assets in a healthcare facility that cannot be converted to cash easily, sold, or used for the care of a patient, such as land, buildings, equipment, fixtures and fittings, motor vehicles, office equipment, computers, software, and so forth. Each fixed asset needs to be tracked by location, person, age, and other factors. In a healthcare organization, the assets can be issued to a person, a procedure room, a department, and others. The FIS therefore needs to be able to handle the vast number of assets and the various areas in which the assets can be located. This system tracks depreciation, maintenance agreements, warranties related to the assets, and when the asset needs to be replaced.

Even though healthcare FISs during the first decade of the twenty-first century supported a number of improvements in the business processes, including patient scheduling, laboratory and ancillary reporting, medical record keeping and reporting, and billing and accounting, many opportunities still remain to improve efficiency, productivity, and quality, such as fiscal decision support.[8]

Financial Reporting

One of the primary functions of an FIS is providing the reports that demonstrate the financial condition of the organization. The most common reports for healthcare

TABLE 7-1 FINANCIAL STATEMENTS

FOR PROFIT	NOT FOR PROFIT
Balance Sheet	Statement of Financial Position
Income Statement	Statement of Operations
Statement of Cash Flows	Statement of Cash Flows

TABLE 7-2 INCOME STATEMENT

Revenue	$1,195,450.25	100.00%
Cost of Goods Sold	870,175.83	72.79%
Gross Margin	$ 325,274.42	27.21%
Overhead	29,879.65	2.50%
Net Ordinary Income (Loss)	$ 295,394.77	24.71%
Interest Expense	1,269.08	0.11%
Interest Income	5,387.08	0.45%
Net Income (Loss)	$ 299,512.77	25.05%

From Healthcare Financial Management Association Certification Professional Practicum PowerPoint.

organizations are summarized in Table 7-1. Note that the titles may vary depending on whether the organization is for profit or not for profit.

The income statement or statement of operations is a good representation of the bottom line, or money left over (net income or loss), of the organization (Table 7-2). This report lists all revenues (monies coming in) and expenses (monies going out) and these are often compared to prior years and to the budget plan.

The balance sheet or statement of financial position shows a glimpse of the organization's financial condition at any given point in time (Table 7-3). The FIS needs to pull the financial data from assets, liabilities, and equity to present the report so the organization can determine whether the numbers in the categories are balanced. Balance sheet data are based on a fundamental accounting equation (Assets = Liabilities + Owner's equity), so each side must "balance" to show the financial condition of the organization.

The cash flow statements show whether the organization will be successful in paying its bills (have more money than it owes). Table 7-4 provides an example of a cash flow statement. Figure 7-2 illustrates how the cash flow statement reconciles with the income statement.

A healthcare organization keeps track of certain financial ratios to help it evaluate its financial condition; these can be important when borrowing for future capital investments. The FIS must be able to calculate and report ratios on demand so that at any given time the organization can assess its financial condition. Ratios are classified into several categories, such as solvency, debt, management or turnover, profitability, and market value. Several ratios are unique to the healthcare

TABLE 7-3 BALANCE SHEET

ASSETS		CLAIMS ON ASSETS	
Current Assets		**Current Liabilities**	
Cash	$ 123,000	Accounts Payable	$ 100,000
Marketable Securities	$ 200,000	Notes Payable	$ 150,000
Accounts Receivable	$ 345,000		
Inventories	$ 100,000	*Total Current Liabilities*	$ 250,000
		Long-Term Note	$ 300,000
Total Current Assets	$ 768,000		
		Total Liabilities	$ 550,000
Long-Term Assets		Owner's Equity	$ 843,000
Building (Gross)	$ 350,000		
Accumulated Depreciation	$ (50,000)	**Total Claims**	$1,393,000
Net Building	$ 300,000		
Land	$ 325,000		
Total Long-Term Assets	$ 625,000		
Total Assets	$1,393,000		

From Healthcare Financial Management Association Certification Professional Practicum PowerPoint.

TABLE 7-4 STATEMENT OF CASH FLOWS

Cash Flow from Operations	**$1,800.00**
Net Income	**$259.00**
Adjustments	**$1,541.00**
Depreciation Expense	$(100.00)
Accounts Payable	$130.00
Credit Card Account	$50.00
Patient Credits	$0.00
Sales Tax Payable	$1.23
Accounts Receivable	$986.77
Inventory Asset	$473.00
Cash Flow from Investing	$(1,000.00)
Equipment	$(1,000.00)
Cash Flow from Financing	$1,500.00
Opening Balance Equity	$2,000.00
Owner's Equity	$(500.00)
Draw	$(500.00)
Investment	$0.00
Net Change in Cash	**$2,300.00**

From Healthcare Financial Management Association Certification Professional Practicum PowerPoint.

industry (Table 7-5), such as length of stay and bed occupancy. Average length of stay in the U.S. for most procedures is 4.8 days. Decision makers can analyze the length of stay for their hospitals to determine whether they are on track for most procedures. Keep in mind, however, that a shorter length of stay does not necessarily mean lower costs. Bed occupancy provides a quick glance at how many inpatient beds are being used. The occupancy is typically higher during flu season and other epidemics. The other ratios reported in Table 7-5 are typical of financial ratios for any organization. Accounts receivable days in a healthcare organization are generally higher than in other organizations since the services are provided before payment is made by the patient or insurance company.

Challenges with FISs

One of the challenges that large healthcare organizations face with the implementation of FISs is ensuring that the various systems in place at numerous locations are integrated. Larger healthcare organizations can include 20 or more facilities. Within each of these facilities can be numerous subfacilities. The different financial systems, applications, and SCM systems can become very complicated when they are merged and the information systems do not interface well.[5]

The purpose of healthcare organizations is to provide quality patient care. While generating maximum revenue is not its defining purpose, an organization must generate income to stay in business and advance new programs and services. What this means is that patient care systems can be seen by some as a higher priority than FISs. Decision makers may have a more challenging time realizing the return on investment or understanding the importance of the investment in FISs since IT software applications such as patient accounting or revenue are considered an intangible asset. The key is to ensure the integration of the various applications.[9] If an information system meets the requirements needed for patient care and it includes integrated applications such as patient accounting, the organization will have the best of both worlds. True integration supports the effective transfer of captured data across all applications. This leads to improved efficiency and enhanced cash flow, and the total cost of ownership is lower.[9]

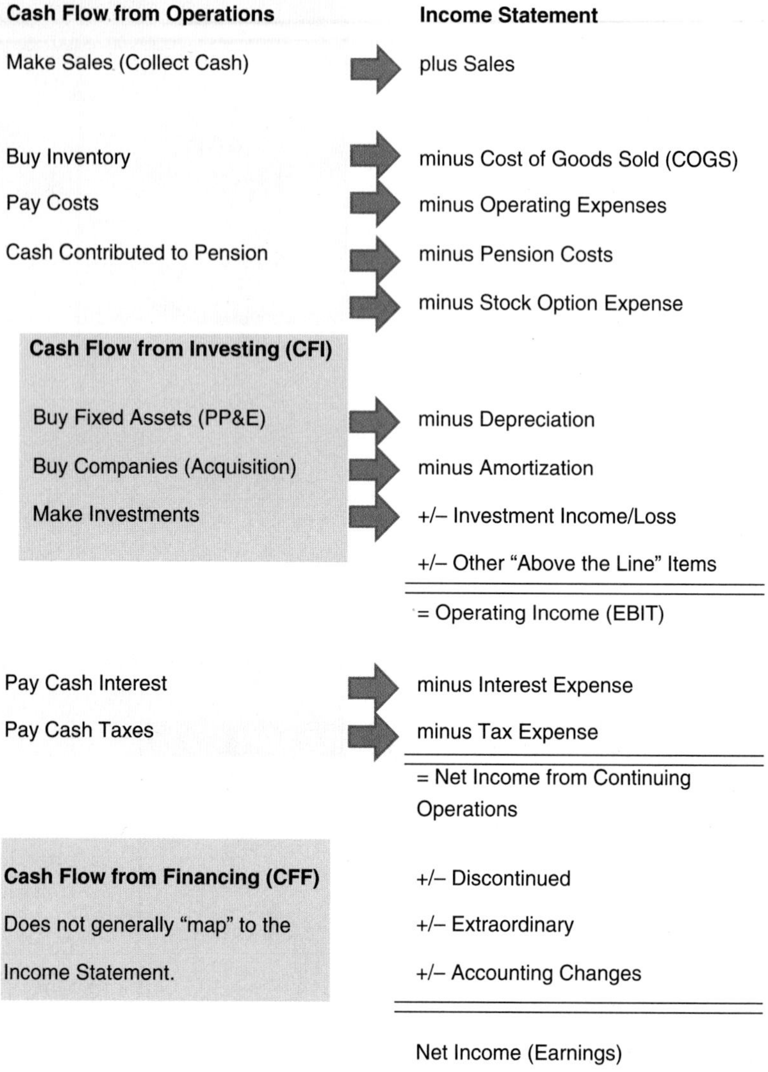

Cash Flow from Operations

Make Sales (Collect Cash) ➡ plus Sales

Buy Inventory ➡ minus Cost of Goods Sold (COGS)

Pay Costs ➡ minus Operating Expenses

Cash Contributed to Pension ➡ minus Pension Costs

➡ minus Stock Option Expense

Income Statement

Cash Flow from Investing (CFI)

Buy Fixed Assets (PP&E) ➡ minus Depreciation

Buy Companies (Acquisition) ➡ minus Amortization

Make Investments ➡ +/– Investment Income/Loss

+/– Other "Above the Line" Items

= Operating Income (EBIT)

Pay Cash Interest ➡ minus Interest Expense

Pay Cash Taxes ➡ minus Tax Expense

= Net Income from Continuing Operations

Cash Flow from Financing (CFF)

Does not generally "map" to the Income Statement.

+/– Discontinued

+/– Extraordinary

+/– Accounting Changes

Net Income (Earnings)

FIG 7-2 Statement of cash flows and reconciliation with income statement. (Healthcare Financial Management Association Certification Professional Practicum PowerPoint.)

TABLE 7-5 SAMPLE OF FINANCIAL RATIOS				
RATIO MEASURE	HOSPITAL #1	HOSPITAL #2	HOSPITAL #3	HOSPITAL #4
Sample size (n)	248	577	450-480	561
Average length of stay (days)	N/A	4.15	4.41	N/A
Maintained bed occupancy (%)	N/A	59.13	57.73	N/A
Operating margin (%)	2.6	2.64	2.93	2.4
Excess margin (%)	3.9	5.11	3.71	4.0
Debt services coverage (x)	3.5	3.05	N/A	3.7
Current ratio (x)	N/A	2.30	2.3	N/A
Cash on hand (days)	180.5	150.70	N/A	164.6
Cushion ratio (x)	13.6	6.06	N/A	14.2
Accounts receivable (days)	43.8	46.38	50.1	44.5
Average payment period (days)	63.4	49.88	N/A	56.8
Average age of plant (years)	10.2	9.51	N/A	10.0
Debt-to-capitalization (%)	42.1	34.17	50.74	38.1
Capital expense (%)	N/A	6.85	3.25	N/A

Healthcare Financial Management Association Certification Professional Practicum PowerPoint.
x, Denotes ratios whose result commonly is greater than 1.

FIS Integration

Financial systems matured much faster than clinical systems.[10] Integration within the FIS and across clinical systems eliminates duplication of effort, which also reduces the number of potential errors. Williams points out the following benefits from integration:

- A transition is provided between front-end and back-end operations.
- Information required for billing such as demographics and insurance can be gathered and verified at the point of service or admission and the information is immediately available for patient care and financial personnel.
- Eligibility checking for insurance can be done online; automated charging is supported, eliminating the need for charge entry.
- Availability of clinical records with detailed charges that has been secured through proper access allows staff to respond to questions from patients, payers, or others without having to pull paper charts.[10]

All of these features of integration result in an improvement to the bottom line, which is what healthcare finance is about. In addition to the basic accounting systems such as general ledger, accounts payable, and accounts receivable, FISs handle more complex functions such as activity or project management. Advanced revenue cycle IT, or new generation, is often referred to as integrated "bolt-ons."[9] TechTarget describes a bolt-on as a product or system similar to an add-on but one that can be attached *securely* to an existing system (http://whatis.techtarget.com). Besides integrated bolt-ons, there are workflow rules engines, advanced executive scorecards, and single database clinical and revenue cycle systems.[9] Workflow rules engines help to manage workflow. For example, documents can be stored in a document management system and email or event reminders can be automatically sent to the people involved with the tasks. Advanced executive scorecards are strategic management tools that aggregate data from electronic health records

(EHRs) in concert with an FIS, thereby providing a snapshot of how the company is performing in certain areas. These "scores" can be compared to other companies in the same line of work.

A single database clinical and revenue cycle system is a system used to ensure accuracy, availability, and data integrity for patient care and billing for the healthcare organization. When changes are made to information contained within the database, those changes are managed throughout the system. In other words, the user does not need to make the change in multiple locations; the database management system will do that for the user to ensure that all necessary changes have been made. This is particularly important when dealing with procedures, documentation for those procedures, and the charges that accompany those procedures. In line with the original accounting systems, these advanced systems are designed to improve billing by reducing billing errors, improve the timeliness of billing to cash collected and the cost to collect, provide real-time eligibility, and provide improvements to current operational efficiencies via other functions.[9]

Improvement in cash flow has remained a constant goal since the onset of FIS. Adaptability and flexibility in healthcare are the key to successful patient care and quality and the same applies to FIS choices. An example of the revenue cycle is provided in Figure 7-3.

One of the more recent IT tools used to positively affect the revenue cycle is a communication management system. The variety of communications (e.g., patient care, insurance coverage, patient admission), the method of communication (e.g., face to face, phone, fax, Internet), and the number of people engaged in communications make organizing and tracking communications a complex process. As Cruze points out, communications surrounding care of the patient and payment can be very difficult to track and retrieve.[7] A centralized management tracking system could assist in this area. An audit trail needs to be very detailed and include all

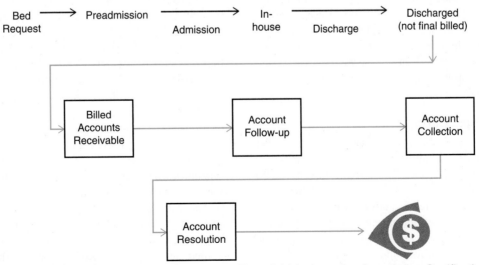

FIG 7-3 Revenue cycle function. (Healthcare Financial Management Association Certification Professional Practicum PowerPoint.)

communications that capture and travel with the patient as well as the authorizations associated with each step. In other words, these communications need to be captured, indexed, and archived for future retrieval.[7]

Efficiency Tools

Decision makers need tools to capture productivity for various activities within the financial services area of the organization. For example, collecting balances from the patient may fall within the responsibilities of a handful of employees. At the front end, patients who have been preregistered can be asked for payment on the estimated amount owed. At the back end, patients who have a remaining balance after insurance has paid will need to pay that balance. How does an organization know which employees are having success at collecting payments? The reporting tools need to provide a snapshot of the data so the decision makers can immediately analyze financial events within a particular area.

In addition to reporting tools, the application needs to be able to assist end-users with the questions that need to be asked, and when. For example, if a patient has an outstanding balance from a previous visit, the patient access personnel may need to know whether they should request payment. Information needed should be readily available and easy to access. When adaptable and flexible designs between clinical and financial systems are combined, powerful analytics are deployed via the web to every desktop; many activities are self-service, freeing up valuable time and resources for the healthcare organization.[9]

Operations have become more complex. For example, charge capture has increased in complexity just as medical care has.[9] As a result, there needs to be a more seamless flow of charges as a natural by-product of the care process to help reduce lost, late, or duplicate charges. These new functions require an investment in a new system to handle revenue cycle management.[11] A dashboard provides a visual analysis of specific data points so an organization can gauge how it is performing in certain areas (it is called a dashboard since it resembles the visual data points provided on an automobile dashboard). In addition, Moore points out features needed in an FIS to increase efficiency, including integrated compliance (i.e., coding edits), flexibility to override default values when the decision maker deems it necessary, ease of use (which increases employee efficiency), and executive dashboard capabilities.[11]

Practice Management Systems

Practice management systems (PMSs) are very similar to the information systems supporting integrated healthcare systems, only on a smaller scale. These applications focus on the services provided in a healthcare provider's office compared to the services provided in a large healthcare system or hospital. Similar to the hospital revenue cycle management system, the PMS is designed to collect patient demographic information, insurance information, appointment scheduling, the reason for the visit, patient care procedures performed for the patient, charging information for the billing

process, and collection and follow-up. As with inpatient or acute care systems, PMSs require integration. The primary differences between PMSs and information systems supporting hospitals are specific provider scheduling templates and types of visits, transaction or line-item provider billing compared to account-driven hospital billing, and provider-based medical record content (orders, referrals, provider documentation, problem lists) that differs from the typical comprehensive hospital medical record.[12] The charges from a medical practice office are connected to codes used for practice management billing and include Healthcare Common Procedure Coding System (HCPCS) and Current Procedural Terminology (CPT). Therefore the information system must be able to generate claims using this type of coding, usually through an electronic submission. Electronic medical records (EMRs) have become much more common modules within a PMS as the U.S. government has implemented incentives supporting EHRs (discussed in Chapter 6). An explanation of the difference between an EMR and an EHR can be found at www.healthit.gov/buzz-blog/electronic-health-and-medical-records/emr-vs-ehr-difference/. Information on the episodes of care maintained in the EMR can be passed along to the hospital or health center should the patient need to be admitted. Sharing this information helps to ensure that the information in the EMR becomes part of the EHR. However, this is often not a "plug and play" environment. Creating a successful interface to share data between the EMR of a practice and a hospital or health center information system is a complex process. Chapter 12 includes additional information on health information exchanges (HIEs) and health information organizations (HIOs) and the issues involved with these.

In outpatient settings healthcare providers can spend much of their time documenting the details of the patient visit. There are a variety of ways to accomplish this, including documenting and recording what is being said and done while the patient is in the examination room, dictating and transcribing based on written notes, or using voice recognition software during or after the visit. Traditionally, visit notes were often transcribed by a third party, leaving room for error through misreading of handwriting or mishearing of dictation. There is also a time delay until the documentation becomes part of the patient record because of the multiple processes required. As well, the healthcare provider is required to review and sign off on the final documentation but time constraints can encourage the provider to rush and perhaps overlook some details.

A method using more enhanced technology and providing quicker turnaround is voice recognition. These software capabilities have greatly improved over the last few years. Voice recognition eliminates the need for a third party and allows healthcare providers to input information themselves, saving steps, time, and money. The application allows text to be viewed in real time and providers can edit and approve it immediately. The time savings can result in much more timely billing and improved cash flow versus waiting for dictated notes to be approved after being transcribed.

BOX 7-1 **BENEFITS OF IMPLEMENTING AN ONLINE PAYMENT TOOL**

For Patients and Provider Offices
- Self-management of their open accounts
- Ability to pay outstanding balances
- Secure communication on a 24/7 basis with the business office (the practice will determine the turnaround time of communications to the patient)
- Ability to update address or demographic changes
- Ability to update changes to insurance coverage (which often occur annually)
- Preregister for services or appointments
- Enhanced customer service capabilities
- Ability for staff to accept payments in person or over the phone
- Ability for staff to view the patient statement exactly as submitted to the patient, which helps to improve communications and efficiencies for payment collection

Data from Conley C. Improve patient satisfaction and collections with efficient payment processes. Healthcare Financial Management Association. http://www.hfma.org/Publications/E-Bulletins/Patient-Friendly-Billing/Archives/2009/January/Improve-Patient-Satisfaction-and-Collections-with-Efficient-Payment-Processes/. January 1, 2009. Accessed December 18, 2011.

Patient Outreach System

Some practices specialize in providing preventive care to manage patients with chronic illnesses. In these practices an electronic registry of the clinic's entire patient population can be used in a patient outreach system. The registry includes the demographic and medical record information needed to notify patients and an automated reminder capability.[13] Patient outreach systems should incorporate evidence-based, specialty-specific protocols—or recommended care guidelines—for chronic and preventive care. Then, once the outreach system identifies patients due for preventive screenings and follow-up care for chronic diseases, the patients are contacted via an automated phone messaging system or another computerized method.

Online Billing and Payment Tool

Collections in a practice can be just as challenging as collections in a hospital except that few emergency cases occur in a provider practice setting, allowing office staff to determine the acceptability of denying services to a patient until a payment plan has been established. In addition to routine collection practices, implementing an online billing and payment tool (e.g., using a credit card to pay online) can help to improve the management and collection of fees owed by patients.[14] Conley states that the healthcare facility can realize increased patient satisfaction and improved staff efficiencies by implementing an online payment tool.[14] Benefits for the patient and the provider's office are outlined in Box 7-1.

Hospital–Healthcare Provider Connection

PMSs integrated with the hospital information system can be more efficient for healthcare providers in a clinic or private practice. According to Cash, physicians, nurse practitioners, physician assistants, and others with staff privileges who participate in the hospital network have certain expectations about the IT, including that it should:

- Provide a single sign-on to an integrated information system from all key system entry points
- Automate the provider's day as much as possible using mobile access (automation means that access is available wherever the clinician is and that the information is in a useful format)
- Have 24/7 support for any device, anywhere
- Provide a dashboard to view critical clinical and financial information with the ability to act on it immediately[15]

Healthcare provider dissatisfaction can occur if the information system:

- Slows him or her down in the task at hand
- Reduces the ability to bill insurance or the patient
- Adds more administrative duties to already maxed-out schedules (remember that providers want to practice medicine and leave administrative tasks to office personnel)

A Matter of Perspective

All healthcare providers have patient care as a top priority. While the provider's focus may be on care of the patient, office personnel must focus on receiving maximum payment for the care of that patient. The records stored at the practitioner level must be accessible and transferable to the hospital in the case of an admission or referral. Health information exchanges are making this possible for referrals, consultations, admissions, discharges, and transfers. IT solutions such as EMRs, digital storage of patient data, voice recognition software, and emailing of correspondence can offer efficiency, cost savings, and improved patient care, which should be the priorities of practice management.[16]

Materials Management

Materials management in healthcare is the storage, inventory control, quality control, and operational management of supplies, pharmaceuticals, equipment, and other items used in the delivery of patient care or the management of the patient care system. It is a subset of the larger function of SCM; the supply chain also includes the acquisition of materials of care and the logistics or movement of those materials to caregiving facilities and organizations. Routinely, health systems deploy information system solutions to support SCM.

Healthcare Supply Chain and Informatics

The acquisition, logistics, and management of materials in healthcare are complex and require a sophisticated information system to provide effective, efficient, and efficacious materials as needed. Typically materials management, also known as central supply in the hospital, bears the burden of having the right item at the right place at the right time. The healthcare supply chain is complex, with requirements that go across, for example, the equipment for operating suites, pharmaceuticals, and medical and surgical supplies for all settings. In any health system with hospitals, clinics, and

	B	C	F	G	H	I
1	Description	Vendor	Qty On Hand	Qty On Order	Min-Max	Packaging
2	INDICATOR CHEM PARACETIC ACID LIQ CSC	3M MED PROD DIV-ALL	51.00 PO	8.00 PO	56.00PO / 21.00CS	CS 4.00 PO 50.00 EA
3	BLADE CLIPPER DISP CSC	3M MED PROD DIV-ALL	21.00 CS	14.00 CS	23.00CS / 35.00CS	CS 50.00 EA
4	CARD MONITORING COMPLY RECORD SYSTEM CSC	3M MED PROD DIV-ALL	12.00 BX	0.00 BX	8.00BX / 3.00CS	CS 4.00 BX 250.00 EA
5	TAPE CLOTH ADH 1INX10YD CSC	3M MED PROD DIV-ALL	13.00 BX	0.00 BX	4.00BX / 1.00CS	CS 10.00 BX 12.00 RL
6	TAPE INDIC STEAM W/DISPENSER 1IN CSC	3M MED PROD DIV-ALL	18.00 RL	38.00 RL	40.00RL / 3.00CS	CS 18.00 RL
7	TAPE INDIC GAS .75X60YD CSC	3M MED PROD DIV-ALL	75.00 RL	0.00 RL	2.00RL / 1.00CS	CS 24.00 RL
8	TAPE PLAS TRANSPORE .50INX10YD CSC	3M MED PROD DIV-ALL	28.00 BX	0.00 BX	21.00BX / 3.00CS	CS 10.00 BX 24.00 EA
9	TAPE PLAS TRANSPORE 1INX10YD CSC	3M MED PROD DIV-ALL	413.00 BX	41.00 BX	573.00BX / 86.00CS	CS 10.00 BX 12.00 EA
10	TAPE SILK DURAPORE 2INX10YD CSC	3M MED PROD DIV-ALL	353.00 BX	671.00 BX	803.00BX / 121.00CS	CS 10.00 BX 6.00 RL
11	TAPE SILK DURAPORE 1INX10YD CSC	3M MED PROD DIV-ALL	611.00 BX	0.00 BX	619.00BX / 93.00CS	CS 10.00 BX 12.00 RL
12	TAPE PAPER MICROPOR DISPNSR 1X10YD CSC	3M MED PROD DIV-ALL	21.00 BX	0.00 BX	19.00BX / 3.00CS	CS 10.00 BX 12.00 RL
13	WRAP COBAN NS 1INX5YD CSC	3M MED PROD DIV-ALL	37.00 CS	0.00 CS	32.00CS / 49.00CS	CS 6.00 PK 5.00 RL
14	DRESSING STRIP STER 1/8X3IN CSC	3M MED PROD DIV-ALL	6.00 BX	0.00 BX	5.00BX / 2.00CS	CS 4.00 BX 50.00 EA
15	DRESSING STRIP STER .25 X 4IN CSC	3M MED PROD DIV-ALL	29.00 BX	0.00 BX	20.00BX / 8.00CS	CS 4.00 BX 50.00 EA
16	SPLINT CONFORMABLE 5INX30IN CSC	3M MED PROD DIV-ALL	9.00 CS	0.00 CS	6.00CS / 9.00CS	CS 10.00 EA
17	DRESSING STRIP STER .5X4IN CSC	3M MED PROD DIV-ALL	64.00 BX	15.00 BX	84.00BX / 32.00CS	CS 4.00 BX 50.00 EA
18	SPLINT CONFORMABLE 2INX10IN CSC	3M MED PROD DIV-ALL	1.00 CS	1.00 CS	2.00CS / 3.00CS	CS 10.00 EA
19	DRESSING TEGADERM 2.375X2.75IN CSC	3M MED PROD DIV-ALL	235.00 BX	0.00 BX	233.00BX / 87.00CS	CS 4.00 BX 100.00 EA
20	DRESSING TEGADERM 4X4.75IN CSC	3M MED PROD DIV-ALL	113.00 BX	0.00 BX	122.00BX / 46.00CS	CS 4.00 BX 50.00 EA
21	DRESSING TEGADERM 4X10IN CSC	3M MED PROD DIV-ALL	11.00 BX	3.00 BX	17.00BX / 6.00CS	CS 4.00 BX 20.00 EA
22	DRESSING TEGADERM 6X8IN CSC	3M MED PROD DIV-ALL	0.00 BX	3.00 BX	11.00BX / 2.00CS	CS 8.00 BX 10.00 EA
23	INDIC BIOLOG FLASH 1HR 270 DEG. CSC	3M MED PROD DIV-ALL	30.00 BX	0.00 BX	28.00BX / 10.00CS	CS 4.00 BX 50.00 EA
24	INDIC BIOLOG STEAM CSC	3M MED PROD DIV-ALL	11.00 BX	0.00 BX	7.00BX / 3.00CS	CS 4.00 BX 100.00 EA
25	WRAP COBAN NS 2INX5YD CSC	3M MED PROD DIV-ALL	775.00 RL	0.00 RL	688.00RL / 29.00CS	CS 36.00 RL
26	FILM NO STING BARRIER SWAB CSC	3M MED PROD DIV-ALL	6.00 BX	0.00 BX	4.00BX / 2.00CS	CS 4.00 BX 25.00 EA

Sample Item Master / Vendors / Volumetric Table

Ready   100%

FIG 7-4 Extract sample of a supply item master file. (Dr. Jerry Ledlow, personal files.)

employees ordering from the supply chain, thousands of transactions occur daily across hundreds of vendors.

The sophistication in automating this process has increased tremendously in the past 2 decades. Applications now include electronic catalogs; information systems such as enterprise resource planning (ERP) systems from vendors such as Lawson (www.lawson.com) or McKesson (www.mckesson.com); warehousing and inventory control systems from vendors such as TECSYS (www.tecsys.com) and Manhattan (www.manh.com); exchanges from vendors such as Global Health Exchange (GHX) (www.ghx.com); and integration with other systems from vendors such as clinical, revenue management, and finance. An innovative technology in this area is radio frequency identification (RFID); more information can be found at www.advantech-inc.com/index.html.

These systems have improved supply chain performance and management in healthcare, with more innovations expected in the future. The healthcare supply chain is an untapped resource of financial savings and revenue enhancement opportunities.[17] Recognizing these opportunities, HIMSS advocated for more improvements in a white paper titled *Healthcare ERP and SCM Information Systems: Strategies and Solutions.* HIMSS indicated that ERP systems will be tools for quality and safety because they integrate capabilities such as procure-to-pay, order-to-cash, and financial reporting cycles. These functions should help institutions match needed materials with care in a more timely and cost-effective manner.

Integrated Applications in Supply Chain Management

The importance of these ERP and SCM systems should be apparent, including the technology associated with them, such as bar code scanners and electronic medication cabinets (e.g., Omnicell, www.omnicell.com; Pyxis, www.carefusion.com/medical-products/medication-management/medication-technologies/pyxis-medstation-system.aspx). The basic components of an integrated healthcare supply chain system include the following:

- **Supply item master file:** A list (hard copy or electronic) of all items used in the delivery of care for a healthcare organization that can be requested by healthcare service providers and managers. This file typically contains between 30,000 and 100,000 items. Figure 7-4 shows a supply item master file.
- **Charge description master file:** A list of all prices for services (e.g., Diagnosis-Related Groups [DRGs], HCPCS, and CPT) or goods provided to patients that serves as the basis for billing.
- **Vendor master file:** A list of all manufacturers or distributors (vendors) that provide the materials needed for the healthcare organization along with the associated contract terms and prices for specific items. This file typically contains 200 to 500 different vendors or suppliers.
- **Transaction history file:** A running log of all material transactions of the healthcare organization. In a computerized system, it is a running list of all supplies and materials being used to deliver care or manage the operations of the institution.

These four files must be integrated to support the operations and management of the supply chain. The integration necessary in the modern healthcare organization is illustrated in Figure 7-5 as a diagram of interfaces across supply chain, clinical, and financial systems.[18]

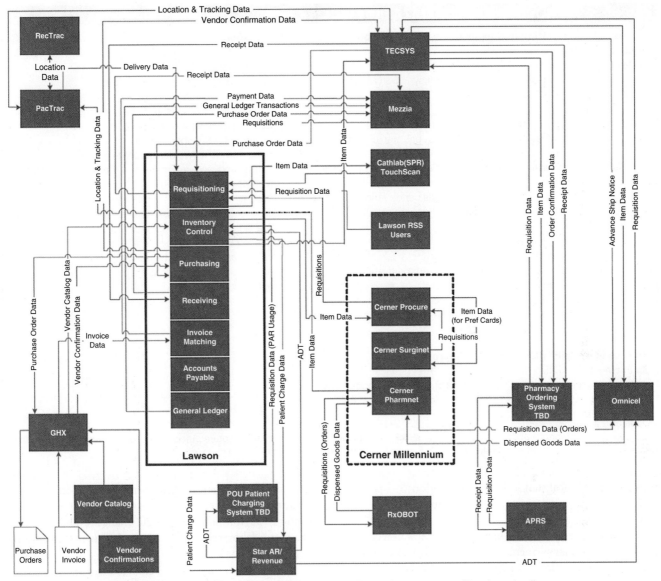

FIG 7-5 Wire diagram of healthcare supply chain information systems. (Dr. Jerry Ledlow, personal files.)

Supply Cost Capture

"In all industries, not just healthcare, three out of four chief executive officers consider their supply chains to be essential to gaining competitive advantage within their markets."[19(p2),20] According to Moore, if the trend in the cost of the healthcare supply chain continues to grow at the current rate, supply chain could equal labor cost in annual operating expenses for hospitals and health systems between 2020 and 2025.[21] Clearly, maximizing efficiency of the healthcare supply chain is an increasing concern.

Consider supply charge capture events in which patient-specific supplies are ordered for the care of that patient and the items are then billed separately to the patient. "Every year, hospitals lose millions of dollars when items used in the course of a patient's care somehow slip through the system without ever being charged or reimbursed."[22(p1)] Point-of-use technology, or capturing charges when supplies or materials

are used, allows healthcare institutions to increase productivity, increase accountability, and reduce downtime through improvements in their internal supply chain. Automated dispensing machines for medications or supplies can be used to decentralize store operations, capture charges, and bring supplies and materials to employees without compromising security and accountability.[23] These systems, if integrated with a solid business process, can enhance efficiency and effectiveness of the healthcare supply chain.

Strategic factors associated with supply success and enhancement are important as well. These include the following:

- Information system usefulness, electronic purchasing, and integration
- Leadership supply chain expertise
- Supply chain expenditures
- Provider level of collaboration

BOX 7-2 PROCESS STANDARDIZATION

Process Standardization in Conjunction with Utilization of an Information System

- Develop standard (or *more standardized*) processes for:
  - Item Master and CDM maintenance and synchronization
  - Supply stock selection, reduction, compression and management
  - Supply charge item capture (accurate and timely)
  - Accountability measures for Central Supply and clinical units
  - Standardize clinical/floor stocked supplies replenishment processes
  - Daily reconciliation of pharmaceuticals and medical/surgical supply items, especially supply charge capture items
    - Taking into consideration:
      - Clinical unit needs
      - Physical layout variations may require modification to an accepted standard
      - The business process must be efficient before a technological solution can be integrated into the process
      - "One size" solution will not fit all

Process Standardization in Process Improvement: Balancing Trade-Offs

- Competing goals exist between various stakeholder groups; trade-offs will be required to find the proper balance that best meets all needs.

- Clinician Goals
  - Does not impede caregivers or patient care delivery
  - Minimize rework
  - Right supplies, right place, right time
- Supply Chain Managers/Central Supply Goals
  - Improve accuracy for supplies consumed
  - Improve timeliness for supply consumption
  - Efficient use of labor
- Revenue and Cost Avoidance Goals
  - Procure and acquire material wisely with contracted compliance goals
  - Efficient management of materials considering utilization rates, preferences, expiration dates and Food and Drug Administration requirements
  - Reduce number of supply charge capture items
  - Improve accuracy for charge capture
  - Improve timeliness for charge capture
  - Improve charge capture rate

From Ledlow JR, Stephens JH, Fowler HH. Sticker shock: an exploration of supply charge capture outcomes. *Hospital Topics.* 2011;89(1):9. Reprinted by permission of the publisher (Taylor & Francis Ltd, http://www.tandf.co.uk/journals). *CDM*, Charge description master.

- Nurse and clinical staff level of collaboration
- Leadership team's political and social capital
- Capital funds availability[19]

This section has provided a high-level overview of technology in materials management. Box 7-2 details specific considerations for automating SCM and materials management.[24]

Human Resources Information Systems

Human resources information systems (HRISs) leverage the power of IT to manage human resources. They integrate "software, hardware, support functions and system policies and procedures into an automated process designed to support the strategic and operational activities of the human resources department and managers throughout the organization."[25(p58)] The authors distinguish between operational, tactical, and strategic HRISs. Operational HRISs collect and report data about employees and the personnel infrastructure to support routine and repetitive decision making while meeting the requirements of government regulations. Tactical HRISs support the design of the personnel infrastructure and decisions about the recruitment, training, and compensation of persons filling jobs in the organization. Strategic HRISs support activities with a longer horizon such as workforce planning and labor negotiations. In contrast, Targowski and Deshpande state that generic HRISs typically include the following subsystems defined by function: recruitment and selection; personnel administration; time, labor, and knowledge management; training and development; pension administration; compensation and benefits administration; payroll interface; performance evaluation; outplacement; labor relations; organization management; and health and safety.[26]

Human Resources Information Systems as a Competitive Advantage

Khatri argues that the management of human resources in healthcare organizations is a central function because the healthcare and administrative services delivered are based on the knowledge of staff delivering these services.[27] Human resources management should focus on employee training as well as developing and refining the work systems to improve the work climate and the quality of service to customers. Although healthcare organizations should include the effective management of human resources as part of strategic planning, most fail to do so. Khatri offers three reasons why many healthcare organizations do not employ optimal human resource practices. First, he argues that human resource activities are institutionalized and undervalued in many healthcare organizations. Second, the clinical culture of healthcare focuses on the clinical delivery of care with less attention paid to the effective management of resources. Finally, low skills in the human resource function have limited the ability of human resource managers to engage effectively in strategic and operational planning. Khatri's premise is that improving

BOX 7-3	SAMPLE VENDORS OFFERING COMPREHENSIVE HUMAN RESOURCES INFORMATION SYSTEMS

- Lawson Healthcare Solutions Suite (www.lawson.com/solutions/software/human-capital-management/human-capital-management)
- McKesson Enterprise Resource Planning Solution (http://www.mckesson.com/en_us/McKesson.com/For%2BHealthcare%2BProviders/Hospitals/Enterprise%2BResource%2BPlanning/Enterprise%2BResource%2BPlanning.html)
- Oracle PeopleSoft Enterprise (www.oracle.com/us/products/applications/peoplesoft-enterprise/overview/index.html)

human resource capabilities should help human resource managers engage more effectively in managing human resources.

Khatri further proposed five dimensions of human resources capability. The first four are a competent human resources executive in the C-suite, a skilled human resources staff, an organizational culture that elevates human resources to a central function, and commitment to continuous learning. An integrated, computerized HRIS is the final capability.

Human Resources Information Systems Vendors

KLAS analyzed whether HRISs deployed in healthcare institutions have similar capabilities and whether HRISs have developed additional capabilities in the intervening years. The reports should be used with some caution, as the vendors cited by KLAS represent the rankings of just one ratings service; however, this strategy does pare down a much more extensive list of HRIS vendors to just a handful to assess the capabilities representative of these systems. Three examples with comprehensive solutions are listed alphabetically in Box 7-3.

Two vendors offer component solutions that provide some but not all of the components of a complete human resources information system. Although not cited as current *Best in KLAS Award* winners, the component solutions these vendors offer compete with those of the enterprise human resources suites for the component services that they offer.

- API Healthcare Human Resources and Payroll (http://www.apihealthcare.com/health-systems/)
- Kronos Workforce HR/Payroll (http://www.kronos.com/)

Human Resources Subsystems

The human resources subsystems described below reflect a modification of the subsystems described by Targowski and Deshpande and represent a taxonomy of functions typically described by the vendor websites for HRISs.[26]

Personnel Administration. The centralized and integrated management of employee data is a key feature of HRISs. Personnel records are maintained and updated with information such as employee identification and demographics, dates of service, position and job code, location code, and employment status (permanent or temporary, full time or part time). Systems also maintain records of licensure, credentials, certifications, and skill proficiency levels. Increasingly, self-service capabilities allow employees to maintain a personal profile with the ability to access and modify personal information such as name, address, contact information, marital status, and information about dependent family members.

Managing Human Resources Strategically and Operationally. HRISs can be used to address in whole or in part the challenge of managing human resources from a strategic and operational perspective. First, strategic management of human resources can be accomplished by accurately reflecting the organizational structure of the healthcare institution. This can be completed by using a wiring diagram to illustrate the hierarchy of positions in the organization, the job descriptions associated with each position, and whether the positions are filled or vacant. This analysis is then used to support the recruiting process for vacant positions. Functions that support this process include posting job announcements and application forms; providing status reports for submitted applications; maintaining interview schedules; and providing selection tools such as dynamic interview guides, multistage testing, computer adaptive testing, and minisimulations. Once a decision is made, the formal job offer letter and new employee benefits can be viewed online. Vendors who offer these types of functionality include Oracle's PeopleSoft (www.oracle.com/us/products/applications/peoplesoft-enterprise/human-capital-management/053291.html) and Kronos (www.kronos.com/Hiring-Software/Workforce-Talent-acquisition/Overview.aspx).

HRISs should also have the capability to assist employees in transitioning out of the organization when discharged, displaced by reductions in the workforce, or retiring.[26]

Staffing and Scheduling. Staffing and scheduling replaces the subsystem "time, labor, and knowledge management" as a more accurate representation of the activities supported by this HRIS subsystem. Staffing and scheduling are two different activities. Staffing involves the assignment of personnel to job positions while ensuring that they are qualified by virtue of degree, licensure, certification, training, and experience. Scheduling involves the assignment of qualified personnel to a scheduling template within a work area in the organization to fulfill the mission of that organization. Scheduling of personnel such as nursing staff is extremely challenging, so much so that nurse scheduling can be considered a definitive representative of the archetypal multishift scheduling problem found in operations research and management sciences literature.

Each of the vendors discussed in Box 7-3 offers both staffing and scheduling modules. Other modules manage scheduling for nurse education and facilitate self-scheduling in conjunction with temporary staff management to fill openings in the schedule. Another vendor, Unibased USA RMS, has been the Best in KLAS award winner for enterprise scheduling for the past eight years (http://www.unibased.com/enterprisescheduling.html).

Key requirements for staffing and scheduling include cost-effective staffing while meeting constraints imposed by required qualifications, scheduling visibility, and matching the level and number of caregivers to patient classification and acuity levels as mandated by law or regulation. An example of an enterprise staffing and scheduling product focused on nurse scheduling is McKesson's ANSOS One-Staff. Functions provided by these systems include the following:

- Staff schedules derived from patient acuity and workload data collected by the software
- Hospital schedules automatically generated to meet core coverage goals while enforcing scheduling rules customized to meet schedule constraints and accommodate individual scheduling preferences
- Synchronous staffing data provided to managers to ensure that nurse-to-patient staff ratios are met
- Web-based self-scheduling
- Productivity and labor cost reporting[28]

Once scheduled, employees' time and attendance are tracked. Key elements include accurate time collection, implementation of user-defined pay rules, compliance with a variety of labor laws, and expeditious identification of productivity or overtime issues.

Just as schedules must be explicitly developed, time-off policies must be proactively managed because of their effect on the schedule. These time-off policies are designed to meet the requirements of federal labor laws such as the Family and Medical Leave Act (FMLA) and state and local laws. In addition to meeting legal and regulatory constraints, time-off policies must enforce organizational policy for vacation, maternity leave, and sick leave. The software used to do this is referred to as "leave management" or "absence management" and is typically a rules-based application designed to manage absence requests while interfacing with workload scheduling.

Because of the difficulty of scheduling in healthcare, innovative scheduling solutions are becoming increasingly common. API Healthcare provides software incorporating three solutions:

- Open shift management: This is a web-based self-scheduling solution in which the nurse manager broadcasts openings in the schedule to qualified staff via a number of instant communication tools. Staff members respond by tendering schedule and shift requests for consideration and approval.
- Incentive management: This involves the use of monetary and point-based rewards for staff who volunteer to fill openings in the schedule.
- Predictive scheduling: Predictive modeling is used to forecast bed demand while accounting for variables such as bed turnover, changes in patient acuity, workload distribution, and variability caused by shift, day of the week, month, and seasonality.[29]

Another vendor, CareWare (www.caresystemsinc.com/), is a relatively new entry into the health care staffing and scheduling arena, with a suite of products that manage time and attendance, assess patient acuity and estimated nurse workload, and employ intelligent scheduling algorithms to create optimal nursing schedules.

Training and Development. The three comprehensive vendors featured in Box 7-3 also addressed staff training and development. IT solutions should be able to be used as the infrastructure to plan and manage employee training, to serve as the delivery mechanism synchronously and online, and to link training with the developmental plan for each employee by identifying shortfalls in skills and competencies and then recording when those shortfalls have been remediated.[26]

Compensation, Benefits, and Pension Administration–Payroll Interface. "Compensation and benefit plans vary from company to company. They include various plans like flexible and non-flexible healthcare plans, short and long-term disability plans, saving plans, retirement plans, pension plans and Flexible Spending Accounts."[26(p46)] When coupled with personnel administration and staffing and scheduling systems and supported by timekeeping and absence management software, management of compensation, benefits, and pension administration becomes more accurate and less time consuming.

One example of a vendor offering integrated compensation, benefits, and payroll applications is Oracle's PeopleSoft (www.oracle.com/us/products/applications/peoplesoft-enterprise/human-capital-management/053949.html). This type of system permits managers to view and update employees records online, receive alerts and decision support when changes in salary and benefits are being considered, receive reports on individuals as well as groups of employees, and permit employees to view and maintain their own records as appropriate. For example, employees may record the renewal of a license or changes in addresses.

Performance Evaluation. "Talent management" and "performance management" are terms used by several vendors. From the healthcare provider's perspective the focus is on recruiting and training employees and developing competencies required to fulfill institutional goals and objectives. The individual career goals of employees are also considered. Information capabilities in this area include the following:

- Profiling employee competencies and any gaps
- Identifying when employee and organizational goals are met
- Identifying top performers
- Manager capabilities such as a dashboard to display unit performance

Lawson's Performance Management is an example of this kind of software.[30]

Underrepresented Subsystems. Labor relations and health and safety have received less attention from vendors developing information for managing human resources. On the other hand, web-based expense and travel applications have become more prevalent in healthcare organizations. These areas may represent future directions for ERP systems.

Business Intelligence Systems

For the past 2 decades healthcare institutions have been building data warehouses and integrating data. Along with the technical aspects, data warehousing includes improving data quality, developing protocols for governance, and determining how to select and employ the appropriate analytic measures. This is difficult because of practice variation and changes to the standards of practice over time. Dick Gibson, the CIO of Legacy Health, notes, "We generate and use data like any other industry, but health care does not lend itself to the use of discrete data because the outcomes are necessarily fuzzy and ongoing. Airlines have seats, schedules and know if you landed on time. In health care, we know if you are alive but the big money goes to broad sets of descriptive terms around patient care that are very qualitative."[31(p29)] These descriptive terms can be captured more succinctly by the use of diagnostic and procedural codes but data quality and integration is a problem because of the number of procedures and number of providers engaged in the delivery of care.[31]

Many organizations are turning to business intelligence (BI) software to provide tools to effectively manage and leverage their massive amounts of data. BI software is purported to lead to an improvement in financial (particularly revenue cycle) and operational performance, as well as patient care.[32] Implementing BI in healthcare that successfully integrates financial and clinical data is regarded as one of the four pillars of the Value Project undertaken by the Healthcare Financial Management Association.[33] Business intelligence is defined as the "acquisition, correlation, and transformation of data into insightful and actionable information through analytics, enabling an organization and its business partners to make better, timelier decisions."[34(p142)] However, Glaser and Stone warn that for the BI to be most effective, the following must happen.[32] For the analysis to be understood, the BI tools must be placed in the hands of the people who actually do the work; training must be done initially and throughout the project so that users will have time to use the basic functions and expand their knowledge; questions that arise throughout the analysis must be reviewed and answered; and the BI should be used for long-term planning. Glaser and Stone describe the BI platform as "a stack—one technology on top of another."[32(p69)] Their description was used to construct Figure 7-6. Effective management of this stackable technology involves making the business case for BI; establishing implementation targets; enlisting BI champions; governing effectively; and establishing BI roles to include data stewards, data owners, business users, and data managers.[32]

As with the other information systems discussed in this chapter, BI systems may be part of an enterprise system, provided as component software, or employed at application level. Most of the major healthcare information system vendors have BI software imbedded in their products. For example, McKesson has Enterprise Intelligence, Cerner has Knowledge Solutions, Seimens has Decision Support Solutions, and Allscripts has Integrated Performance Management.

KLAS lists the following vendors in this category of software but they are not part of an enterprise healthcare

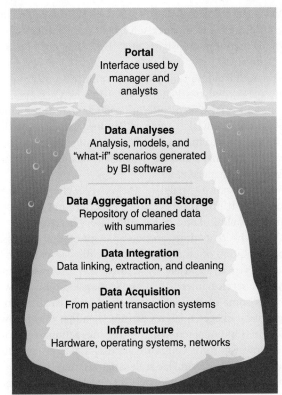

FIG 7-6 Business intelligence (BI) platform. (Data from Glaser J, Stone J. Effective use of business intelligence. *Healthc Financ Manage.* 2008;62[2]:68-72.)

information system. Instead, they provide BI solutions intended to support analytics in conjunction with enterprise software or they provide analytics for a segment of the healthcare marketplace.

- Dimensional Insight's The Diver Solution (www.dimins. com) provides BI and performance management solutions whose applications specific to healthcare include productivity reporting, provider network management, outcomes measurement, disease management, usage review, and Meaningful Use. Other applications that could have utility in healthcare include customer service, finance, human resources, sales and marketing, and supply chain analytics. Capabilities include data discovery and integration without the need to build a data warehouse, interactive dashboards and scoreboards available through a web-based portal, a consolidated view of enterprise data, a variety of data visualization options, and access through a variety of mobile devices.
- IBM Cognos Business Intelligence (www-01.ibm.com/ software/analytics/cognos/) offers a tailored line of BI software products, with Cognos Enterprise providing large-scale BI and performance management with capabilities similar to those described for Dimensional Insight, Cognos Express targeting midsize companies and work groups, and Cognos Insight providing desktop analytics for the individual user. IBM also owns the SPPS suite of statistical products.

- Information Builders WebFOCUS (www.informationbuilders. com/products/webfocus) advertises capabilities similar to Dimensional Insight and IBM Cognos Business Intelligence.
- Omnicell Pandora Clinicals (www.omnicell.com/Products/ Business_Analytics/Pandora_Analytics.aspx) is part of Pandora Analytics, a suite of products that also includes Pandora Financials. Omnicell Pandora Clinicals provides the analytics to manage medication compliance and clinical operations. Pandora Financials facilitates cost and inventory management.
- Vitera Practice Analytics (http://www.viterahealthcare. com/solutions/intergy/Pages/PracticeAnalytics.aspx) provides clinical and BI for ambulatory practices.

Given the cost, time, and complexity of the large-scale implementation of enterprise BI, application-level BI should be employed strategically to address "key processes, functions, or service lines."[35(p95)] Application-level BI software provides some of the data integration and visualization of enterprise packages, analyzes existing data that may be overlooked in traditional reporting, and creates actionable knowledge. However, some caution is necessary. Glaser and Stone note that ad hoc, smaller-scale analysis may lead to the creation of data silos, inefficient or repetitive management of data, and unnecessary duplication.[32] These are appropriate cautions but application-level BI can complement the development of enterprise BI by producing results in the interim as the enterprise capabilities are developed.[35]

CONCLUSION AND FUTURE DIRECTIONS

Given the magnitude of the investment in health information systems and the fact that administrative applications are more mature than clinical applications, a salient question is whether these administrative applications have made healthcare delivery more productive. In "Unraveling the IT Productivity Paradox—Lessons for Healthcare," Jones, Heaton, Rudin, and Schneider explore the paradoxical relationship between "the rapid increase in IT use and the simultaneous slowdown in productivity."[36(p2243)] Several lessons emerge from the authors' analysis:

- Mismeasurement partially contributed to the paradox. The authors suggest that "assessment of the value of healthcare outputs could be improved through the more sophisticated use of clinical data to understand access, convenience, and health outcomes."[36(p2244)]
- New information technology often requires redesign of the processes that were previously tailored to the technology or manual system just replaced.
- New information technology that fails to be user-centered compromises productivity.
- Finally, healthcare organizations can no longer afford to have an abundance of untapped data that fails to improve decision making. Improvements in healthcare information systems, BI, and analytics must continue to improve the quality of decision making.

Administrative systems in this chapter were listed as separate applications because they evolved independently of clinical systems. Many of the future benefits will accrue from integrating data from all systems. For example, if a healthcare system cannot effectively track the total cost of all materials used to treat an individual patient and aggregate data to determine the cost of treating groups of patients, managing the cost of healthcare is not possible. As new information becomes available for decision making, healthcare professionals on both the administrative and the clinical sides of the organization will need to learn new interprofessional approaches to using these data in making decisions.

REFERENCES

1. Haux R. Health information systems—past, present, and future. *Int J Med Inform*. 2006;75:268-281.
2. Ciotti V, Mathis B, Ames E. Top HIS vendors by 2011 revenue. *Health Data Manag*. 2012;20(5):16, 18.
3. Gartner, Inc. Why Gartner? Gartner. http://www.gartner.com/technology/why_gartner.jsp. Accessed October 1, 2012.
4. KLAS. About KLAS. KLAS. http://www.klasresearch.com/about/company.aspx. Accessed October 16, 2012.
5. Rogoski RR. Counting on efficiency: healthcare organizations in growth mode need financial information systems that can accommodate expansion. *Health Manag Technol*. 2006;27(3):10-12, 14.
6. Latham H. The healthcare CFO: squeezing more from IT. *Health Manag Technol*. 2009;30(1):10-11.
7. Cruze G. Saying it isn't so: how documentation can decrease denials. *Healthc Financ Manage*. 2008;62(2):84-89.
8. Thompson S, Dean MD. Advancing information technology in health care. *Communications of the ACM*. 2009;52(6):118-121.
9. Hammer D, Franklin D. Beyond bolt-ons: breakthroughs in revenue cycle information systems. *Healthc Financ Manage*. 2008;62(2):52-60.
10. Williams B. Gaining with integration: three healthcare organizations use integrated financial-clinical systems to achieve ROI, process improvement and patient care objectives. *Health Manag Technol*. 2002;23(6):10, 12-13, 15.
11. Moore R. Rural healthcare system drops AR days and cleans up claims. *Health Manag Technol*. 2010;31(7):16-17.
12. Sorrentino PA, Sanderson BB. Managing the physician revenue cycle. *Healthc Financ Manage*. 2001;65(12):88-90, 92, 94.
13. Curtis E, Schelhammer S. Patient outreach system helps clinic boost care visits, revenues. Healthcare Financial Management Association. http://www.hfma.org/Publications/Leadership-Publication/Archives/E-Bulletins/2011/August/Patient-Outreach-System-Helps-Clinic-Boost-Care-Visits-Revenues/. 2011. Accessed December 18, 2011.
14. Conley C. Improve patient satisfaction and collections with efficient payment processes. Healthcare Financial Management Association.http://www.hfma.org/Publications/E-Bulletins/Patient-Friendly-Billing/Archives/2009/January/Improve-Patient-Satisfaction-and-Collections-with-Efficient-Payment-Processes/. 2009. Accessed December 18, 2011.
15. Cash J. Technology can make or break the hospital-physician relationship. *Healthc Financ Manage*. 2008;62(12):104-109.
16. Gates P, Urquhart J. The electronic, "paperless" medical office: has it arrived? *Intern Med J*. 2007;37:108-111.

17. Roark DC. Managing the healthcare supply chain. *Nurs Manage.* 2005;36(2):36-40.
18. Corry AP, Ledlow GR, Shockley S. Designing the standard for a healthy supply chain. September 12, 2005. Available at: http://mthink.com/article/designing-standard-for-healthy-supply-chain/. Accessed November 30, 2011.
19. Ledlow G, Corry A, Cwiek M. Optimize Your Healthcare Supply Chain Performance: A Strategic Approach. Chicago, IL: Health Administration Press; 2007.
20. Poirer C, Quinn F. A survey of supply chain progress. *Supply Chain Management Review.* 2004;8(8):24-31.
21. Moore V. Clinical supply chain. Paper presented at: American College of Healthcare Executives National Congress; 2008; Chicago, IL.
22. Bacon S, Pexton C. Improving patient charge capture at Yale-New Haven. iSixSigma. http://www.isixsigma.com/index.php?option=com_k2&view=item&id=997:&Itemid=49. 2010. Accessed April 29, 2010.
23. Evahan Technology. Point of use technology in the supply chain. Ferret. http://www.ferret.com.au/c/Evahan/Point-of-use-technology-in-the-supply-chain-n698823. 2005. Accessed April 30, 2010.
24. Ledlow JR, Stephens JH, Fowler HH. Sticker shock: an exploration of supply charge capture outcomes. *Hosp Top.* 2011;89(1):9.
25. Chauhan A, Sharma S, Tyagi T. Role of HRIS in improving modern HR operations. *Review of Management.* 2011;1(2):58-70.
26. Targowski AS, Deshpande SP. The utility and selection of an HRIS. *Adv Competitiveness Res.* 2001;9(1):42-56.
27. Khatri N. Building HR capability in health care organizations. *Health Care Manage R.* 2006;31(1):45-54.
28. McKesson. ANSOS One-Staff. McKesson. http://www.mckesson.com/en_us/McKesson.com/For%2BHealthcare%2BProviders/Hospitals/Workforce%2BManagement%2BSolutions/ANSOS%2BOne-Staff/ANSOS%2BOne-Staff.html. Accessed October 15, 2012.
29. API Healthcare. Staffing and scheduling. API Healthcare. http://www.apihealthcare.com/health-systems/staffing-scheduling. Accessed October 15, 2012.
30. Lawson. Performance management. Lawson Corporation. http://www.lawson.com/Solutions/Software/Human-Capital-Management/Talent-Management/Performance-Management/Performance-Management. Accessed October 15, 2012.
31. Erickson J. BI's march to health care. *Inform Manage.* 2009;19(7):29-34.
32. Glaser J, Stone J. Effective use of business intelligence. *Healthc Financ Manage.* 2008;62(2):68-72.
33. Clarke R. Rethinking business intelligence. *Healthc Financ Manage.* 2012;66(2):120.
34. Giniat EJ. Using business intelligence for competitive advantage. *Healthc Financ Manage.* 2011;65(9):142-146.
35. Hennen J. Targeted business intelligence pays off. *Healthc Financ Manage.* 2009;63(3):92-98.
36. Jones SS, Heaton PS, Rudin RS, Schneider EC. Unraveling the IT productivity paradox—lessons for healthcare. *New Engl J Med.* 2012;366(24):2243-2245.

DISCUSSION QUESTIONS

1. Explain why healthcare facilities would require the use of an FIS and provide examples of this type of system.
2. Describe how a decision maker would use the FIS reporting function to make decisions and provide a summary of what the various reports tell the decision maker.
3. Explain the importance of physicians using a PMS and provide examples of tools that can be used at the point of care.
4. Describe and defend three principles of a quality SCM system with regard to patient care and support of clinicians providing care.
5. Discuss how self-service applications are typically deployed in HRISs.
6. Discuss the advantages and disadvantages of using BI at application level as opposed to enterprise level.

CASE STUDY

Michael H. Kennedy, Kim Crickmore,* and Lynne Miles*

Managing the flow of patients and bed capacity is challenging for any hospital, especially for unscheduled admissions. For Zed Medical Center, a large regional referral center in the South and a member of the University HealthSystem Consortium, the challenge is even greater. As the flagship hospital for a multihospital system with more than 750 licensed beds and a Level 1 trauma center with 50-plus trauma beds, approximately 70% of annual admissions are unscheduled.

The Assistant Vice-President for Operations has a PhD in Nursing, is a Fellow of the Advisory Board Company, and has more than 20 years' tenure at Zed Medical Center. Three of the ten departments under her purview (Patient Care Coordinator, Bed Control, and Patient Transfers) are directly engaged in managing patient flow and bed capacity. The division is also responsible for systemwide care coordination for patients discharged to skilled nursing facilities, to home health, and to home without planned service delivery. Current operational goals include (1) decreasing the current length of stay by 0.3 days from 5.7 to 5.4 days and (2) "ED to 3"—a slogan incorporating the intention to place patients from the emergency department into a bed within 3 hours of the decision to admit. With the Centers for Medicare & Medicaid Services in the process of clarifying penalties for readmissions within 30 days, Zed Medical Center has begun to prepare by determining its baseline percentage of readmissions within 30 days.

*Kim Crickmore and Lynne Miles are Advisory Board members for the East Carolina University Health Services Management Program.

The eight staff members assigned to Patient Transfers coordinate with hospitals within the region wanting to transfer patients to Zed Medical Center. They take calls, connect outside transfers with accepting physicians, and arrange transport. The accepting physician determines the patient's needed level of care, special care needs (e.g., diabetic), and the time frame for transfer. The Patient Transfer Department uses the software package CentralLogic (www.centrallogic.com/), specifically the ForeFront module (www.centrallogic.com/products/forefront), to manage the transfer and admission of patients. After a patient has been accepted for admission by the admitting physician, Bed Control makes the bed assignment. The staff members of Bed Control assign incoming patients to specific beds once the Patient Placement Facilitators from the Patient Care Coordinator Department identify the nursing unit to which patients should be assigned. This determination is made based on the level of care required, physician preferences in choice of nursing unit, and the scope of care supported by the nursing units. The Bed Control Department uses the Capacity Management Suite (www.teletracking.com/solutions/products/index.html) of TeleTracking software (www.teletracking.com/). The PreAdmitTracking module keeps track of bed status through the use of an "electric bedboard," which provides a graphical user interface through which planned admissions, transfers, and discharges can be annotated. The status of a bed freed by patient discharge for which a cleaning request has been made is also noted (dirty, in progress, cleaned). The Bed Tracking module uses the medical center's paging network to notify the environmental services staff of a cleaning request and the head nurse of the unit that a patient is incoming. The TransportTracking module automatically dispatches patient transport requests via phone or pager.

Discussion Questions

1. How are patients prioritized for bed assignment?
2. Describe some of the advantages and disadvantages of this new software. Include the stated organizational goals in your answer.
3. Discuss how this software might share data with other institutional applications to provide a dashboard view of census-type activity.

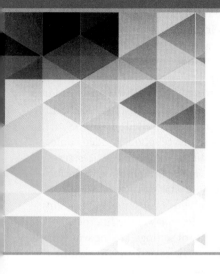

Telehealth and Applications for Delivering Care at a Distance

Loretta Schlachta-Fairchild, Mitra Rocca, Vicky Elfrink Cordi,
Andrea Haught, Diane Castelli, Kathleen MacMahon,
Dianna Vice-Pasch, Daniel A. Nagel, and Antonia Arnaert

Growth in telehealth could result in a future where access to healthcare is not limited
by geographic region, time, or availability of skilled healthcare professionals.

OBJECTIVES

At the completion of this chapter the reader will be prepared to:
1. Discuss the historical milestones and leading organizations in the development of telehealth
2. Explain the two overarching types of telehealth technology interactions and provide examples of telehealth technologies for each type
3. Describe the clinical practice considerations for telehealth-delivered care for health professionals
4. Analyze operational and organizational success factors and barriers for telehealth within healthcare organizations

5. Discuss practice and policy considerations for health professionals, including competency, licensure and interstate practice, malpractice, and reimbursement for telehealth
6. Describe the use of telehealth to enable self-care in consumer informatics
7. Discuss future trends in telehealth

KEY TERMS

ABSTRACT

Rapid advances in technology development and telehealth adoption are opening new opportunities for healthcare providers to leverage these technologies in achieving improved patient outcomes. Telehealth provides access to care and the ability to export clinical expertise to those patients who require care, regardless of the patients' geographic location. This chapter presents telehealth technologies and programs as well as telehealth practice considerations such as licensure and malpractice challenges. As telehealth advances, healthcare providers will require competencies and knowledge to incorporate safe and effective clinical practice using telehealth technologies into their daily workflow.

INTRODUCTION

Rapid advances in technology development and telehealth adoption are opening new opportunities for healthcare providers to leverage these technologies in achieving improved patient outcomes. Before we discuss these technologies and outcomes, it is important to explore the definitions of telehealth-related terminology.

Telehealth encompasses a broad definition of telecommunications and information technology–enabled healthcare services and technologies. Often used interchangeably with the terms *telemedicine, ehealth,* or *mhealth* (mobile health), telehealth is "the use of electronic information and telecommunications technologies to support long-distance clinical health care, patient and professional health-related education, public health, and health administration."[1] Telehealth is being used in this text to encompass all of these other terms. Telemedicine is the use of medical information exchanged from one site to another via electronic communications for the health and education of the patient or healthcare provider and for the purpose of improving patient care, treatment, and services.[2] Telenursing is the use of telehealth technology to deliver nursing care and conduct nursing practice.[3,4]

Telehealth enables the delivery of clinical care to those who are in need regardless of the geographic location of the patient or the healthcare provider. Well-established telehealth programs and evidence-based research supports the effective use of telehealth across most disciplines and specialties within healthcare (i.e., teleradiology, teledermatology, telepathology, telenursing, etc.).[5-10] Telehealth services provide access to health assessment, diagnosis, intervention, consultation, supervision, and information across distance.[11] As a result telehealth is now being integrated into routine care delivery of patients around the globe. Figure 8-1 depicts how telehealth can change healthcare delivery. Telehealth services can be classified as clinical or nonclinical. Clinical telehealth services include but are not limited to diagnosis, patient communication and education, disease management, triage and advice, remote monitoring, caregiver support, and provider-to-provider teleconsultations. Nonclinical telehealth services include but are not limited to distance education for healthcare consumers or clinicians, video conferencing or conference call meetings, research, healthcare administration, and healthcare management.

Providing care to underserved populations can be a challenge, especially in rural areas or where there is a shortage of healthcare professionals. Patients may face physical, financial, geographic, and other barriers to accessing care. However, telehealth can overcome many of these barriers. Telehealth proponents seek to improve quality, access, equity, and affordability of healthcare in the United States and throughout the world by using telehealth.[11] Healthcare professionals who use telehealth can export their clinical expertise to patients regardless of geographic location.

Telehealth technologies include configurations as simple as a telephone conversation between a healthcare provider and a patient or as sophisticated as a doctor performing robotic surgery on a patient across continents. Telehealth technologies include but are not limited to telephones; facsimile machines; email systems; cellphones; video conferencing; web-based, remote patient monitoring devices; transmission of still images; and Internet applications (ehealth) including patient portals, remote vital signs monitoring, continuing medical education, and direct consumer applications such as online physician consultations via the Internet.

Telehealth is used in a variety of settings, among which are rural hospitals, home health agencies and patients at home, prisons, dialysis centers, and nursing homes; telehealth is also used to provide care to astronauts in space.[11,12] The benefits of remote monitoring, diagnosis, and intervention have been proven in numerous scientific studies and include increased access to care, decreased costs of healthcare and increased healthcare provider productivity, and a high level of patient satisfaction.[3,13] Furthermore, the advantages of telehealth to patients are numerous and include the following:

- Decreased travel time or distance and removal of travel barriers
- Immediate access to care
- Early detection of disease processes or health issues
- Ownership of healthcare and feelings of empowerment
- Long-term health and independence
- Caregiver reassurance
- Patient satisfaction with healthcare

Examples of Successful Telehealth Programs

The following three examples of telehealth programs demonstrate the wide range of such programs currently providing services to patients at a distance.

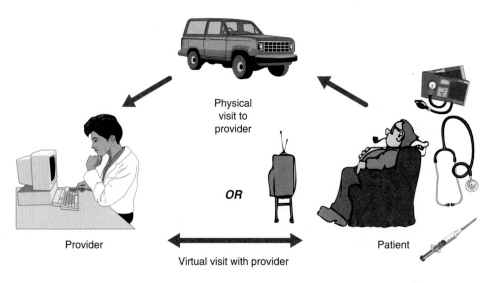

Physical visit to provider

OR

Provider

Virtual visit with provider

Patient

Telehealth enables the export of clinical expertise virtually to patients who need it

FIG 8-1 How telehealth changes healthcare delivery. (Copyright 2010 iTelehealth Inc. All Rights Reserved.)

- Rochester General Health System, Rochester, New York, developed a clinic-based telehealth program in 2008. Its healthcare providers use a video conferencing system for live patient consults with remote physician specialists. They have the capability to send video images and 12-lead digital electrocardiograms. The Director of Telehealth coordinates and schedules 34 physicians and 5 midlevel healthcare providers who see patients remotely. Rochester General's telehealth program developed a rigorous 1-day training session for all end-users.

- Sea Coast Mission Telehealth Program, Bar Harbor, Maine, provides seagoing health services to islanders living on four islands with no healthcare providers available.[14] Daily use of live video conferencing from a 72-foot boat called the *Sunbeam V* occurs with the support of a boat crew that includes a nurse. The telehealth program coordinator, an early adopter of telehealth, described herself as "technically challenged" during the site's implementation. Since then she has developed excellent clinical and technical skills to work proficiently in an austere environment. In this setting attention to a patient's health condition can at times be urgent, requiring immediate diagnosis and treatment. The goal is to diagnose sick patients in a timely manner so that they can be transferred off the island for access to a higher level of medical care on the mainland. Maine Sea Coast Mission's most recent project has been to implement health centers with video conferencing systems on four islands (Frenchboro, Matinicus, Swan's Island, and Isle au Haut), thereby providing access to remote health and education services year-round (Sharon Daley, RN, personal communication, March 2010).

- University of Miami, Miller School of Medicine, Miami, Florida, provides both live video conferencing and store-and-forward capability as part of its telehealth program. Its program reached out in 2010 to provide medical support after the earthquake in Haiti. One unique program is the Teledermatology Program for private cruise ships. The program uses expert dermatologists to evaluate an array of skin problems such as lesions, burns, infections, and rashes seen by emergency physicians on board cruise ships. The Clinical Telehealth Coordinator provides online training to cruise ship staff for using a digital camera and image capturing and transmission via a dermatology software application. Images are then reviewed by the dermatologist and patient reports with diagnosis and recommendations are sent back electronically to the emergency physician within a specific time frame.[15]

Telehealth Historic Milestones

In contrast to the common perception that telehealth is new and futuristic, it actually has a long history. The first documented report of healthcare delivery at a distance dates back to 1897 in *The Lancet*, when a case of croup was diagnosed over the telephone. In the United States modern telehealth programs began in 1964, with a closed-circuit television link between the Nebraska Psychiatric Institute and the Norfolk State Hospital for teleconsultations. Shortly thereafter, in 1965, a cardiac surgeon in the U.S. transmitted a live video feed of a surgical case to spectators in Geneva, Switzerland, via satellite. The surgeon discussed his case and answered live questions from the spectators in Geneva.[16]

The National Aeronautics and Space Administration (NASA) led telehealth initiatives in the 1960s with the transmission of physiologic signals from astronauts in space to command centers on Earth. NASA also funded several telehealth research programs in the late 1960s and early 1970s that contributed to the profession as a whole.[17] A landmark study completed by Kaiser Permanente in 1997 concluded that "technology in healthcare can be an asset for patients and providers and has the potential to save costs; therefore, this technology must be a part of continuous planning for quality improvement."[18(p45)] The researchers were emphatic about the benefits of telehealth, inspiring many of today's telehealth programs.

From July 2003 to December 2007 the U.S. Department of Veterans Affairs (VA) conducted a home telecare program analysis to coordinate care of chronically ill veterans and reduce long-term care admissions. The program evaluation was highly successful, realizing a reduction in long-term care bed days and inpatient hospital admissions among participants. Further, the veteran participants reported a high level of satisfaction. Costs to provide the program were and are substantially less than other VA programs or nursing home care. The program is now known as Care Coordination/Home Telehealth (CCHT) and is a routinely offered VA service to support aging veterans with chronic conditions.[19]

In the United Kingdom the Whole System Demonstrator (WSD) program was launched by the National Health Service in 2008 in order to determine the effectiveness of telehealth. As of its start date, the study was the largest randomized controlled trial of telehealth in the world, involving more than 6000 participants. The study confirmed that telehealth promotes well-being and should be a part of any complete healthcare system.[20]

Leading Telehealth Organizations

Starting in the 1990s, a number of professional, industry, and government organizations have provided the leadership needed to initiate effective telehealth programs. These leaders include the American Nurses Association (ANA), United States federal government agencies, the American Telemedicine Association (ATA), and the International Council of Nurses (ICN).

American Nurses Association (ANA)

With the advent of technology and rapidly emerging telehealth practice in the twentieth century, healthcare professionals sought guidance on incorporating telehealth into their care offerings. Multidisciplinary standards were needed to create a cohesive unity for telehealth across professions. To address the expansion and to create unified definitions and policies and a standard of care, the ANA brought together the Interdisciplinary Telehealth Standards Working Group. This group was composed of 41 representatives from different healthcare organizations and professional associations. The report of the interdisciplinary team, *Core Principles on Telehealth*, represents a "sense of the profession" as a whole.[21] The purpose of the core principles is to create a baseline standard of care in order to provide quality care as well as protect patients from harm.

United States Federal Government Agencies

NASA, the VA, the U.S. Department of Defense (DOD), and other government agencies have continued to lead the U.S. in telehealth research and programs. As an early adopter of telehealth, the VA operates the nation's largest telehealth program. The widespread adoption and positive research findings led the U.S. government to establish the Office for the Advancement of Telehealth (OAT), a division of the Office of Rural Health Policy within Health Resources and Services Administration (HRSA) at the U.S. Department of Health & Human Services (HHS). OAT promotes the use of telehealth technologies for healthcare delivery, education, and health information services and increases the use and quality of telehealth delivery through the following activities:

- Fostering partnerships within HRSA and with other federal agencies, states, and private sector groups to create telehealth projects
- Administering telehealth grant programs
- Providing technical assistance
- Evaluating the use of telehealth technologies and programs
- Developing telehealth policy initiatives to improve access to quality health services
- Promoting knowledge exchange about "best telehealth practices"[1]

American Telemedicine Association (ATA)

The American Telemedicine Association (ATA) is a nonprofit organization founded in 1993 and headquartered in Washington, D.C. The mission of ATA is to "promote professional, ethical and equitable improvement in healthcare delivery through telecommunications and information technology" through education, research, and communication.[22] ATA is a mission-driven, nonprofit organization that seeks to incorporate telehealth seamlessly into healthcare so that it is not necessarily a separate program but integrated into healthcare delivery as a whole.

International Council of Nurses (ICN)

Representing more than 200 national nursing organizations, including the ANA, Canadian Nurses Association, and associations of more than 198 other countries, the ICN initiated the Telenursing Network in 2008. As telenursing advances, this virtual collaboration is serving to share competencies and other jointly developed telenursing resources.

TELEHEALTH TECHNOLOGIES

Telehealth technologies enable the exchange of all types of data (i.e., voice, video, pictures of wounds, pathology or radiology images, device readings, etc.) between patients and healthcare providers or between healthcare providers on behalf of patients. Early telehealth technologies were "stand-alone" systems in which a telehealth encounter occurred and data were stored in a telehealth system database. With the increasing adoption of electronic health records (EHRs), telehealth technologies are being increasingly integrated with the EHR. Telehealth services can be delivered using two overarching types of technologies: synchronous (or real-time) technologies or asynchronous (or store-and-forward) technology.

Synchronous or "Real-Time" Technologies

Synchronous, real-time telehealth uses live, interactive telecommunications technology and/or patient monitoring technologies to connect a healthcare provider to a patient for direct care, to other healthcare providers for consultation and collaboration, or to a combination of the two.[23] The most commonly used synchronous telehealth employs video conferencing or telephone-based interaction.

Video Conferencing

Video conferencing integrates audio, video, computing, and communications technologies to allow people in different locations to electronically collaborate face to face, in real time, and share all types of information, including data, documents, sound, and picture. Use of interactive video conferencing in telehealth allows for patient–healthcare provider consultations, healthcare provider–specialist discussions, and health education. The technology requires live presence of the healthcare provider and patient or healthcare provider and medical specialist in an interactive environment.

A real-time live environment can include the following:

- Video conferencing units with a codec (*co*mpressor–*dec*ompressor) capable of encoding and decoding the video conferencing stream.
- Peripheral cameras such as high-definition cameras that have remote control pan, tilt, and zoom (PTZ) features.
- Video display devices such as computer monitors, television sets such as HD Plasma or LCD displays, and LCD projectors. These display devices are used to show the images received from the video conferencing codec.
- Audio components (microphones and speakers), a network connection, and the user interface. Prior to the availability of high-bandwidth Internet connections, signals were carried over point-to-point connections established via Integrated Services Digital Network (ISDN) lines and plain old telephone service (POTS). The Internet has now simplified some of the connectivity issues and the high-bandwidth requirement of video conferencing.

Patient Monitoring Technologies

Patient monitoring technologies, including home telehealth (also known as telehomecare), use devices to remotely collect and send biometric data to a home health agency or a remote diagnostic testing facility (RDTF) for interpretation by a healthcare provider. Such applications might include a specific vital sign device, such as blood glucose monitor, digital scale, thermometer, heart electrocardiogram (ECG), blood pressure monitor, pulse oximeter, or peak flow meters, or a variety of monitoring devices for homebound patients. Such services can be used to supplement the use of visiting nurses.[3] Use of monitoring devices will also allow patients to become more involved in and in many cases to oversee the monitoring process.[24]

Patient monitoring technologies for home telehealth consist of two major components: hardware and software. The hardware includes a base station where the patient interacts by entering data and answering questions and applies various medical devices that are used to gather patient data. The software enables healthcare providers and technicians to configure the hardware, receive data, and monitor the patient.

The telecommunications used can be *wired,* such as POTS or direct service line (DSL), or *wireless,* such as cellular (sometimes seen as code division multiple access, or CDMA), broadband, satellite, Bluetooth, infrared (IrDA), WiFi (or IEEE Standard 802.11), mobile broadband wireless access (MBWA or IEEE Standard 802.20), or Worldwide Interoperability for Microwave Access (WiMAX or IEEE Standard 802.16). mhealth and mobile health are umbrella terms that incorporate mobile or wireless telecommunications for transmitting telehealth-related data and services. Both the telecommunication and the hardware can be incorporated in the medical device.

Figure 8-2 provides a diagram of the components of a telehealth system.

1. Personal health devices monitor basic vital signs such as blood pressure, weight, pulse, oxygen level, and blood sugar values and transmit data via a wired or wireless connection via devices or sensors.
2. The aggregation and computation manager is a critical component of the connected health system, enabling individual monitoring devices to log data in an EHR for personal and clinician review. The aggregation manager collects and transmits data from an individual's personal health devices to a server using wired or wireless connections. The aggregation manager itself can be a cellphone, a personal computer, a dedicated device, or a personal health record (PHR).
3. The health service center is a physical location where a patient's digital information is collected, stored, analyzed, and distributed. It can be the doctor's office, the home of a family member, or another type of healthcare-related facility.

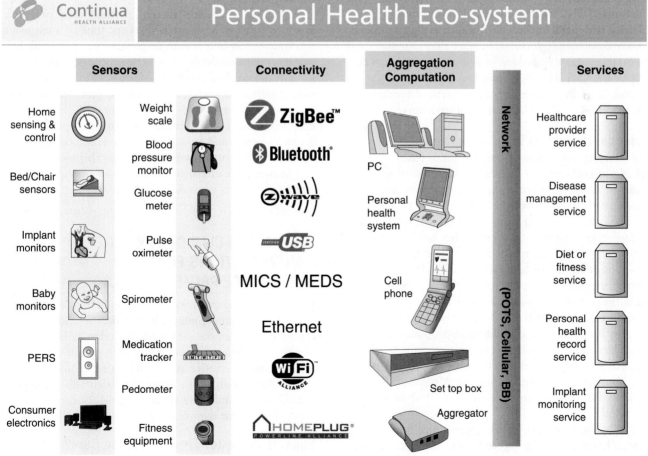

FIG 8-2 Personal health ecosystem. *BB,* Broadband; *PERS,* Personal Emergency Response System; *POTS,* plain old telephone service. (Copyright 2010 Continua Health Alliance. All Rights Reserved.)

Asynchronous or "Store-and-Forward" Technology

"Store-and-forward" technology allows for electronic transmission of telehealth-related information, video, images, and audio files. It can be used when healthcare providers and patients are not available at the same time. The sending healthcare provider or patient prepares an electronic consult package, which includes the patient's history, related diagnoses, and digital images such as x-rays, video, and photos. This package is either emailed or placed on a web server for the receiving healthcare provider to access when his or her schedule allows. The receiving healthcare provider then reviews the package, follows up with clarification questions, and provides a diagnosis, recommendations, and a treatment plan. The receiving healthcare provider's response is transmitted electronically back to the sending healthcare provider or patient. Store and forward technologies can be used in dermatology, radiology, pathology, dentistry, cardiology, wound care, home monitoring, pediatrics, and ophthalmology as well as other areas.

A store-and-forward technical environment can include the following:
- A personal desktop, laptop computer, tablet, or smartphone for the sender
- A personal desktop, laptop computer, tablet, or smartphone for the receiver
- Telecommunication technologies such as local area network (LAN), wireless communications, etc.
- Digital peripheral medical devices such as digital cameras, x-ray equipment, glucometers, vital sign monitors, and wearable sensors embedded in T-shirts or wristwatches
- Software such as a web-based application, encrypted email, specially designed store-and-forward software, an EHR, a PHR, and an electronic data repository

Technical Standards in Telehealth

Until recently the demand for telehealth-based medical devices was not sufficient to create unified, global technical standards. However, technical standards that were developed for associated markets have benefited telehealth. For example, use of American National Standards Institute (ANSI) H.32x standards has enabled wide-scale video conferencing interoperability, which led to further growth in nonhealthcare businesses. Not only has telehealth benefited from the video conferencing standards, but it is also benefiting from a reduction in the cost of equipment as well as the improved ability to conduct interactions between parties independent of the particular hardware used. In addition, development of Health Level Seven (HL7), which provides global interoperability standards for health information technology (health IT), and Digital Imaging and Communications in Medicine (DICOM) standards for imaging has also been of great benefit for telehealth.[3]

In 2006 the Continua Health Alliance was formed by a group of healthcare technology industry companies to establish interoperable personal telehealth solutions and to develop technical design guidelines. The goal is to agree on a set of common technical guidelines that will enable vendors to build interoperable sensors, home networks, telehealth platforms, and health and wellness services. The Continua Health Alliance also has developed a technical certification program based on these guidelines. Technologies that are certified by Continua Health Alliance have been technically tested and validated to work together and be interoperable.[25]

An example of such a standard is ZigBee/IEEE 802.15. This standard is targeted at applications that require a low data rate, long battery life, and secure networking. ZigBee/IEEE 802.15 has become a useful wireless connectivity standard for home or facility-based telehealth. ZigBee is a low-powered network capability that allows telehealth devices and sensors to operate longer and with smaller power sources, enabling miniature sensors to transmit health data. ZigBee is also a very low cost and easily installed network capability, providing usability and requiring minimal technical support. The ZigBee Alliance offers two specifications (ZigBee and ZigBee RF4CE) that serve as the base networking system to facilitate its interoperable market standards.[26]

Telehealth and Health Information Technology

A need exists to integrate all relevant medical device images and data from the telehealth technology with the patient's EHR. The interoperability of these systems could dramatically streamline a healthcare provider's workflow and improve the healthcare.

A key to telehealth success is healthcare providers' access to patients' health records at the time of a telehealth encounter—just as it is with in-person care. Telehealth networks serve to establish a link between provider EHRs, and securely moving health-related information that is exchanged among patients, hospitals, and healthcare providers as needed for care and treatment. Telehealth in HIE initiatives is expected to lead to the next generation of interoperability for health IT across and among healthcare enterprises. Existing telehealth infrastructure will also serve as a highway for EHRs and information exchange between and among rural and remote areas.[27]

TELEHEALTH CLINICAL PRACTICE CONSIDERATIONS FOR HEALTHCARE PROFESSIONALS

Healthcare providers have used the telephone as a communication tool for patient interaction for decades. Adding to the complexity of remote care delivery today, it is becoming increasingly common to use computers, remote monitoring devices, and interactive audio and video conferencing for patient interaction. With expanding telehealth technology capability, new and more efficient models of care are facilitated, allowing for removal of time and distance barriers.

Equal to or Better Than In-Person Care?

Telehealth is considered to be so effective that in 1997 the World Health Organization (WHO) announced that it has become part of the WHO's "health for all" strategy and should be made available to all people.[28] Physician–patient encounters via telehealth have been supported by research to be as effective as standard face-to-face visits held in a physician's office or clinic. In 2008 Dr. Gregory Jicha, assistant professor of neurology at the University of Kentucky's Sanders-Brown Center on Aging, led a study called Telemedicine Assessment of Cognition in Rural Kentucky. "The goal of the project was to adapt and validate the UDS [National Institute on Aging's Uniform Data Set, a standard set of questions asked of every patient being screened for Alzheimer disease] and other measures for diagnosing mild cognitive impairment (MCI) and early dementia in the telemedicine setting. An important aspect of the goal was to determine whether the telemedicine consultations were as effective as face-to-face meetings with a doctor."[29(p32)] Jicha stated that "developing and validating this telemedicine approach for diagnosing and treating MCI and early dementia will become a model for clinician-researchers at other centers serving rural populations."[29(p32)] Per Jicha's perception of using telemedicine to expand healthcare resources, "the bottom line is, our goal is to ensure that though telemedicine is not *better* than an in-person evaluation, it's *as good as* an in-person evaluation."[29(p34)]

Beginning in 2008, two studies (one in the United Kingdom and the other in Quebec, Canada) concluded that "telemedicine is increasingly seen as an efficient and cost-effective means for improving clinical outcomes and increasing patient involvement in their own care."[30(p59)] Both studies demonstrated two important factors that influence healthcare professionals' acceptance of telemedicine: training and support.

Telehealth Clinical Competency

As healthcare providers' use of ever wider and broader technological tools increases, so does the need to ensure telehealth competency to provide safe and optimal patient care. As healthcare further embraces telehealth to gain efficiencies, improve access to care, and reduce costs, there must be a focus on educating and preparing healthcare providers in telehealth technology, techniques, skills, coordination, and "on camera" communications. A telehealth clinical encounter involves multiple new components and competencies, including coordinating healthcare provider and patient scheduling, knowledgeable telepresenting skills (i.e., steps needed to facilitate a telemedicine encounter between a patient and remote healthcare provider), the exchange of prior medical record and new telehealth information, and an understanding of video and audio technology.

From initial academic preparation through ongoing continuing education requirements, healthcare providers practice in a dynamic field with ongoing changes in care delivery. All healthcare providers are required and expected to maintain and update clinical competency in the care they render to patients. Telehealth also requires competency for optimal healthcare delivery. A number of professional associations have stepped forward to identify the specific competencies required. As described earlier in this chapter, the ANA and 41 major healthcare provider organizations developed and

endorsed core principles for telehealth delivery in 1998.[21] A year later the ANA created and published *Competencies for Telehealth Technologies in Nursing*.[31] In 2001, with further expansion in telehealth, the ANA endorsed the development of telehealth protocols.[32] These protocols were developed to encompass the needs and concerns of both clients and practitioners. On an international level the ICN published the research-based, validated *International Competencies for Telenursing* based on an international survey of practicing telenurses in 36 countries around the globe.[4]

The *National Initiative for Telehealth Framework of Guidelines* (NIFTE Guidelines) was a critical milestone in development of telehealth not just for those who authored the guidelines in Canada, but globally.[33] This highly important and superbly designed framework was developed in Canada by a multistakeholder interdisciplinary group. The NIFTE Guidelines are designed to assist individuals and organizations to develop telehealth policies, standards, and procedures. NIFTE examines and offers principles and suggested guidelines for five overarching content areas related to telehealth:

- Clinical standards and outcomes
- Human resources
- Organizational readiness
- Organizational leadership
- Technology and equipment

In addition, Canadian nurses have provided more than a decade of telenursing leadership and developed extensive practice guidelines for nurses who are becoming or presently in the role of telenurse.[34]

In November 2011 the ATA developed an expert opinion consensus document on interactive video conferencing. The Expert Consensus Recommendations for Videoconferencing-Based Telepresenting defines the requirements for serving as a telepresenter in a live, synchronous telehealth encounter. As with all patient interactions, processes for patient registration, consent, clinical information, reimbursement information, and privacy are applicable to telehealth encounters.[35] The ATA has also developed Telemedicine Standards and Guidelines for Diabetes, Telemental Health, Teledermatology, Home Telehealth, and Telepathology.

Confidentiality, Privacy, and Informed Patients

Patient confidentiality and privacy are paramount when using technology for the transmission of health data and live video presentation of the patient to geographic environments at a distance from the patient's location. The requirements for ensuring confidentiality, privacy, and informing patients receiving care via telehealth are the same as for in-person care. This is particularly true when the possibility exists of others being present in a room but off-camera. Attending to the presence of others at either the sending or receiving locations is an additional, important privacy task for healthcare providers using telehealth. Another important concern is ensuring that patients are being adequately informed and educated regarding telehealth consultation and assessment and evaluation via video conferencing technology.[4,32]

Scope of Clinical Practice

For healthcare professionals the use of technology does not alter or change the practitioner's inherent standards of practice, ethics, scope of practice, or legalities of practice.[32,34] Healthcare professionals may use telehealth for patient consultations or for consultation with other healthcare providers. When telehealth is used for patient consultations, the healthcare professional's credentialing and clinical privileges at the site where the patient is located must be completed. The practitioner will need education, training, and technical support for the necessary technologies before, during, and after telehealth consultations.

The decision to refer a patient to a healthcare professional for consultation via telemedicine or telehealth is determined by multiple factors. Referrals for a telehealth consult need to consider the following factors:

1. Does the service requested provide telemedicine or telehealth access as an option?
2. What is the level of the practitioner's expertise and comfort with telemedicine or telehealth?
3. Is the patient's diagnosis appropriate for telemedicine or telehealth consultation?
4. Going forward, who will manage the patient's plan of care and how will this be managed?

As with any in-person patient encounter, documentation is of major importance. Appropriate documentation for telemedicine consults at both the sending and the receiving sites is essential for providing accurate and optimal continuity of care for the patient. Both sites need current patient demographic information, billing information, and consultant notes. Referring practitioners need consultant notes in a timely manner to carry out the patient's plan of care. After a telehealth consult, evaluation of telehealth processes and patient satisfaction is essential. The quality assurance and evaluation processes identify how to improve telehealth procedures, safety, effectiveness, and quality of care.[32]

Types of Clinical Telehealth Applications

In the past 15 years, telehealth specialty areas, such as telecardiology, teledentistry, teledermatology, home telehealth and remote monitoring, teleICU, telemental health, teleopthalmology, telepediatrics, teleradiology, telestroke, telewoundcare, and teletrauma, have been successfully developed and implemented in a variety of healthcare settings. Other telehealth programs outside the hospital setting include emergency preparedness, disaster response, correctional telemedicine, forensic telemedicine, telerehabilitation, and school telehealth.

A complete remote physical examination can be achieved by viewing images and hearing sounds. Healthcare providers can assess and treat a variety of health care problems such as cardiac or respiratory illnesses by listening to digital heart, lung, or bowel sounds live; by sending the data over a video conferencing system; or by using a computer with Internet connection to the computer of another clinician, who can then assess the information. The healthcare provider can use video scopes to conduct ear, nose, throat, oral cavity, eye, pelvic, or rectal exams; cameras or microscopes for skin examinations; radiology images to diagnose orthopedic injuries; and computed tomography (CT) scans of the head to rule out bleeding, brain injuries, or skull fractures. Teleradiology is one of the most commonly used and accepted telehealth applications, where digital images are captured and transmitted to the radiologist, who makes a diagnosis, sends a report, and stores the image. Healthcare providers can send complete readings for a 12-lead digital electrocardiogram to a cardiologist to diagnose heart problems or send a digital spirometry reading to a pulmonologist to diagnose respiratory lung capacity.

TELEHEALTH OPERATIONAL AND ORGANIZATIONAL SUCCESS FACTORS AND BARRIERS

Despite the advancements in telehealth technologies, significant barriers and gaps exist in the successful implementation of robust, integrated healthcare technology delivery systems.

B.E.L.T. Framework

In planning for implementation of telehealth technology, four main components must be considered: bandwidth, education, leadership, and technology (B.E.L.T.). The B.E.L.T. framework (Fig. 8-3) is a metaphoric representation of these four interrelated components and may be used to guide planning at macro, meso, or micro levels of implementation.

Bandwidth includes elements of telecommunication technology, including information transmission and connectivity to move and store digital data. Infrastructure and telecommunication architecture in some geographic areas may limit use of telehealth applications and have direct implications for access to and delivery of healthcare. This is particularly problematic for rural, isolated, and underserved regions.[36]

Education encompasses the preparation of both the existing workforce and future healthcare providers in developing

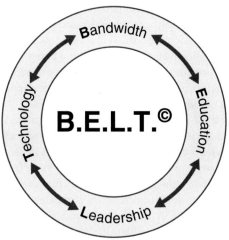

FIG 8-3 The B.E.L.T. framework. (Copyright McGill University School of Nursing. Montreal, Quebec.)

competencies in the adoption and use of telehealth technologies. Although research has been done in some areas of competency development, particularly in healthcare informatics and telenursing, scant research has been done in the broader use of telehealth technology to inform curriculum development and education of healthcare providers.[4,37] Patient safety in telehealth technology use is one aspect of healthcare delivery that is essential to professional practice and relates to competencies in clinical decision making.

Leadership reflects a broad range of management, change theory, and policy aspects that affect operationalizing telehealth technologies. Barriers to successful telehealth adoption frequently relate to factors such as resistance to technology, information security, stakeholder support, reimbursement, and financial commitment.[36,37]

Technology spans a large number of considerations such as the types of telehealth software, hardware, and devices available for care delivery and the choice of appropriate telehealth technology. To date, telehealth platforms have limited capacity to address the range of health conditions experienced across the population lifespan, resulting in a narrow focus on overall individual health, fragmentation of care, and duplication of effort for data retrieval and documentation. Since many current telehealth technologies are not interoperable and cannot be integrated into a single environment to support holistic care, data silos are created where information on the same individual may be contained in different systems and cannot be accessed in an efficient, seamless manner. This further fragments care, leads to duplication of services (e.g., repeat of blood work, diagnostics, or information retrieval), and creates unnecessary cost to the patient and to the healthcare system. Another limitation is that most current telehealth technologies focus on direct delivery of clinical services to individuals and do not readily support the broader goals of primary healthcare, such as enhancing health promotion, prevention opportunities, or generating necessary epidemiologic data needed to evaluate and inform healthcare delivery.

Operationalizing Telehealth

Several important steps exist for the success of telehealth programs and services. The first is planning, which includes a needs assessment and analysis to define patient populations and healthcare problems in which telehealth services can have a positive impact. A workplace environment with staff prepared to implement telehealth using specific standards and guidelines is the second important factor for success. Technology preparedness is a third factor for successful telehealth services. For successful telemedicine implementation, appropriate "user-friendly" technology that allows for creative use and quality as well as responsive and accessible technical support are crucial factors.[38] The final, critical step is learning how to implement, manage, and support a telehealth project or program. This becomes more complicated when more clinical specialties are involved. New telehealth programs should begin with one focused specialty application, such as teledermatology, and not add other specialties until the initial

program has been implemented successfully. Specific procedures are listed in Table 8-1, and project steps are outlined below.

Telehealth Acceptance and Training

Technology education trends have moved toward online courses or certificate education programs in telehealth to reach out to more healthcare providers throughout the United States and globally. Online and on-site telehealth training courses are available through several Telehealth Resource Centers (TRCs), federally funded by OAT. Additional information about these resource centers can be found at www.telehealthresourcecenter.org. The ATA located at www.americantelemed.org provides annual meetings with scientific research presentations, special interest group meetings, educational webinars, educational products, training program accreditations, and white papers and policies.

According to Duclos et al. "the acceptance of a telehealth program by providers who use it is crucial to its success."[39] Healthcare providers who use telehealth in their practice should know how telehealth technologies work and should understand their capabilities in providing patients with better access to healthcare services.

Opportunities abound for clinicians to become adept at using telehealth technologies beginning with a basic proficiency in using room-based video conferencing systems on personal computers (PCs) and mobile video conferencing systems on iPads and smartphones. It is advantageous for healthcare providers to learn to use medical devices with video scopes attached for patient assessments and video or digital cameras for exams. Healthcare providers need to be comfortable using a variety of audio, video, and medical device tools, video conferencing systems, and computer hardware and software applications. New technical challenges often emerge for clinicians, such as using a video ophthalmoscope to view retinal images inside the eye and on a display monitor. Hearing new heart sounds from a digital stethoscope with different high- and low-pitched sounds due to magnification can be another challenge. Clinicians may encounter workflow changes with telehealth software applications in paperless environments, such as digital ECG and spirometry readings that identify patients' heart rhythm and lung measurements. Technology literacy training may also be required for clinicians. Technology literacy includes knowledge of basic computer skills and communication technologies, basic skills to navigate the Internet for up-to-date health information, and the ability to access web-based telehealth software applications. For example, healthcare providers who are fluent in using digital cameras to take dermatology images and who are Internet savvy can access online resources to identify a skin lesion or obtain the latest treatment for the lesion online.

In the 2005 International Telenursing Survey, telenurses were found to have various job skills and to work in more than 30 clinical telehealth settings ranging from nurse call centers to urban and rural hospitals, public and private health clinics, schools, prisons, community health centers, military

TABLE 8-1   TELEHEALTH PROCEDURES

1. PREPARATION	2. PROVIDER AND PATIENT "REAL-TIME" TELEHEALTH ENCOUNTER	3. FOLLOW-UP, QUALITY, AND SAFETY
Provider credentialing completed at patient site and remote site	Provider is knowledgeable and competent in healthcare needs being addressed during patient-to-provider telemedicine visit	Review plan of care conveyed by provider or consultant and instructions provided regarding treatment plans, with time for patient and family questions and answers
Referral reviewed as appropriate for specialty service and accepted by telespecialist	Introduce patient to all individuals that will be in the patient room and to any individuals at the evaluating physician's location	Complete any necessary forms (e.g., patient consent to treat form; HIPAA forms) and share reimbursement information with both patient and physician sites
Knowledgeable regarding scheduling procedures and policies of facility and scheduling resources	Identify camera and microphone locations to patient and explain any potential for audio or video delay	Provide patient and family with consulting physician contact information, as needed for follow-up
Obtain and review preconsult clinical information and testing	Presenting site provider is knowledgeable of exam requirements, including patient preparation, patient positioning, and use of peripheral devices (i.e., electronic stethoscopes, Doppler, digital cameras, etc.)	Schedule follow-up appointments, treatments, etc. as ordered by physician
Obtain reimbursement information, such as copies of insurance cards, Medicare cards, etc.	Provide support to patient and family and be alert to nonverbal body language	Provide the referring primary care provider with the telemedicine encounter documentation
Provide patient with the appropriate forms for "consent to treat" and HIPAA compliance information	Provide time within the clinical visit for patient and family questions and answers	Evaluate outcomes of the telemedicine encounter, quality of encounter, and patient satisfaction and assess for improvements for future telemedicine encounters; clinical effectiveness is one of the factors associated with success in telemedicine
Contact patient to explain a telemedicine encounter and provide directions to the telemedicine site	Educate patient and family of their right and ability to terminate the telemedicine clinical visit at any time	
Ensure that equipment and technology has been tested and is in safe working order, provider and patient have clear audio and video of each other, extraneous noises are reduced, and any necessary peripheral devices and supplies are accessible at time of encounter		
Assess and prepare for cultural, language, or disability issues		
Establish a backup plan and be prepared to enact it in the event of technical problems		

facilities, native tribe reservations, and private physician and nurse practitioner practices.[40] Specific telehealth knowledge regarding equipment, workflow, clinical processes, and technology training is different for each clinical setting.

Scheduling dedicated time for healthcare providers' telehealth training is an obstacle and is one of the major barriers to a successful telehealth program. Actual hands-on training is beneficial, using telehealth case scenarios similar to those the healthcare provider would typically encounter. As mentioned earlier, clinical workflow is modified when telehealth technologies are implemented. Healthcare providers can adjust by continuing to use the same patient exam rooms for the telehealth patient, using similar medical devices for in-person and telehealth exams, training with telehealth technologies, and interacting with the same physicians and specialists for telehealth consultations as for in-person referrals.

Telehealth Implementation

There are three phases for successful telehealth program implementation: preimplementation, implementation, and postimplementation.

Preimplementation Phase

Implementing telehealth technologies in any clinical setting is no different than implementing other twenty-first century technologies. As with any informatics project, a team effort is critical to its success. Clinicians will first need to decide what types of telehealth programs provide access to remote healthcare specialists for their patients. Important preimplementation steps are listed in Box 8-1. Forming an administrative or executive team is advisable to oversee the project goals, budget, progress, and growth. The facility may already have a formal committee in place to oversee all IT projects and, if so, can tailor the governance to incorporate telehealth. The executive team should include the following:

- Hospital or facility administrator
- Clinical director (often a physician)
- Chief information officer
- Director of information technology and/or director of education
- Telehealth and telecommunications administrator
- Vendor account managers (may be only at the operational level below)

A second level of management for the telehealth program is a more operational interdisciplinary team including the following:

- Project manager
- Clinical champion (often a physician)
- Telehealth director or program manager
- Information technology engineer or support technician
- System administrator (if software is involved)

Super users and vendor trainers will also initiate, train, and support new staff for the telehealth project. The interdisciplinary teams are the change agents that assist in developing policies, procedures, project evaluation criteria, and permission forms prior to beginning the telehealth program.

Implementation Phase

Once the equipment is configured or tailored, the implementation phase involves equipment and software testing with mock telehealth patients and remote specialists and then piloting the project by identifying a patient needing a teleconsult. Equipment testing with mock patients should encompass all staff testing all of the telehealth equipment available. Equipment testing should also be conducted periodically after the initial implementation. After identifying differences between standard and telehealth patient encounters, daily use of telehealth equipment for routine patient exams is recommended so that providers become knowledgeable and comfortable using the various telehealth examination tools (electronic stethoscope, video otoscope or ophthalmoscope, digital ECG or spirometry software, video exam camera, telehealth software applications, and audio or video conferencing systems). The goal is for a clinician to present a patient, capture and send patient data, retrieve patient information from stored telehealth software applications, and respond to cases and add patient encounters if needed.

Postimplementation Phase

As with any other informatics project, evaluation criteria address adequacy of training; implementation, equipment, technology, or training issues; and program outcomes. A program of quality assurance and process improvement should be part of the evaluation process so that iterative progress toward implementation phase telehealth program success can be achieved.

Telehealth programs of any size experience similarities in success and failure. Table 8-2 lists common success factors and barriers to successful telehealth program implementation.

TELEHEALTH CHALLENGES: LICENSURE AND REGULATORY ISSUES FOR HEALTHCARE PROFESSIONALS

Telehealth enables physicians, advanced practice registered nurses (APRNs), nurses, pharmacists, and other allied health professionals to offer their clinical services remotely. State lines and geographic boundaries have no effect on the potential of the technology to deliver telehealth services. For example, radiologists can read x-ray reports from other countries, mental health professionals can provide care telephonically or with real-time video, and chronically ill patients can be monitored from a distance with telehealth. Despite technological advances, legal and regulatory challenges exist. Provider licensure and the credentialing and privileging processes in facilities remain the biggest hurdles to telehealth adoption in the United States.

BOX 8-1   TELEHEALTH PREIMPLEMENTATION STEPS

- Identify remote physician specialists and other clinical consultants who are willing to provide remote assessment and advice for treatment
- Meet standards and requirements for safe use of telemedicine equipment: installation in designated telehealth rooms; biomedical and electrical engineering help may be required
- Select appropriate telehealth equipment to use for telehealth examinations, including disposable accessories such as nonlatex gloves, gel, measurement tapes, alcohol wipes, gowns and cover sheets, and extra camera batteries
- Identify electrical and cable sources for power outlets and secure Internet access
- Designate telehealth exam rooms or areas
- Identify 24/7 technical support for clinicians at both sending and receiving sites
- Develop policies and procedures
- Train interdisciplinary team and staff end-users on telehealth equipment
- Set up and test telehealth scenarios prior to beginning telehealth consultation

TABLE 8-2 SUCCESS FACTORS AND BARRIERS TO TELEHEALTH IMPLEMENTATION

KEY SUCCESS FACTORS FOR TELEHEALTH	BARRIERS TO SUCCESSFUL TELEHEALTH IMPLEMENTATION
High-level organizational members (board of directors, administrator, medical director, champion physician, nurse administrator, nurse educator, program director) who have identified a need for telehealth and are able to provide support and finances throughout all phases of implementation, training, and maintenance of the telehealth program	No designated or dedicated project manager; not enough time or resources dedicated to manage project
Designated and dedicated telehealth project manager or coordinator	Interdisciplinary team not designated or prepared properly
Designated interdisciplinary telehealth team	Funding limited
Adequate facility network infrastructure to support the telehealth system or method selected and prepare setup for the telehealth program prior to installation	Lack of communication between administrative management, interdisciplinary team, and participants
Project management to include and allow time for professional telehealth education and refresher training classes, including participation for professional telehealth conferences, telehealth webinars, telehealth video training, and provision of telehealth resource information	Failure to identify remote clinical partners to whom to refer patients or to provide telehealth services; may be due to reimbursement issues, lack of understanding as to how telehealth works, practice and licensing issues in that state
Initiate telehealth program at local facility and then introduce to affiliated remote facilities	Poor telehealth equipment selection for specialty; poor quality and usability of telehealth equipment purchased
Provide staff with educational tools such as workflow diagrams, charts, digital photos, manuals, and descriptive pathways for how to initiate an urgent or nonurgent telehealth consult	Missing parts of equipment and supplies during installation or patient encounter
Provide education, training, and program development for teleconsultants	No designated telehealth area due to limited room availability
Schedule appointments for follow-up teleconsults with dates and times for physician and patient	Ergonomically poor placement of equipment, limited connectivity or lighting in telehealth area, poor cable management, limited counter size, small room, no storage cart for equipment, equipment not secure
Patient privacy and confidential information forms should be completed prior to teleconsult	No pretraining on telehealth system prior to telehealth installation
Provide on-site dedicated technical support throughout all phases of implementation and provide online support for main site, remote site, and teleconsultants	Healthcare providers not familiar with computer literacy (i.e., basic use of keyboard, personal computer, mouse, navigating software, data, or handling images captured) Training not formalized, no schedule confirmed to allow for all participants to be trained, not enough time provided for hands-on training or practice of case scenarios Staff resistant to training, no incentives, and no understanding of telehealth or technology advantages Off-hour shifts not trained or invited to participate in training sessions

Licensure

Both the 1997 and 2001 Telemedicine Reports to Congress by OAT identified licensure as a major barrier to the development of telemedicine and telehealth.[41] The cost and procedural complexity of current professional licensing policies precludes widespread adoption of telehealth. Currently, many health professionals must attain separate licenses in each state where services are rendered. Licensure authority defines who has the legal responsibility to grant a health professional the permission to practice his or her profession.[42] Under Article X of the U.S. Constitution, states have the authority to

regulate activities that affect the health, safety, and welfare of their citizens.[42,43] Regulating the delivery of healthcare services is one such activity. Exceptions to state licensure requirements include physician-to-physician consultations, educational and medical training programs, border state recognition programs, government employees practicing in military or federally funded facilities such as VA hospitals and clinics, and natural disaster and emergency situations.[42,43]

Legislation such as the 2011 Servicemembers' Telemedicine and E-Health Portability Act (STEP Act) facilitates the provision of telemedicine and telehealth services. The STEP Act removes the individual state licensing requirements to allow a licensed medical professional in one state to treat a patient in another.[41] As of this writing, the STEP Act rules apply only to military and federal personnel, although it is a beginning in terms of advancing telehealth services into the mainstream. Fortunately, major advancements are occurring to streamline licensure requirements. These regulatory alternatives include licensure by endorsement, state compacts and mutual recognition, reciprocity, registration, and limited licensure (Table 8-3).

Nursing has been the most successful healthcare provider group to adopt the mutual recognition model, referred to as the multistate Nurse Licensure Compact.[42] The Nurse Licensure Compact law became effective on January 1, 2000, with three states initially participating. As of February 2013, 24 compact states existed. Compact status applies only to registered nurse (RN) licensure. If an RN holds a license in one of the 24 compact states, he or she may practice in *any* of the 24 compact states, greatly facilitating telehealth interactions across state boundaries. International nurses on a visa who apply for licensure in a compact state may declare either the country of origin or the compact state as the primary place of residency. If the foreign country is declared as the primary place of residency, a single-state license will be issued by the compact state.[44] A mutual recognition model is being

discussed for APRNs at the time of this writing. The target date to complete that work is 2015. However, currently, APRNs who practice using telehealth across state boundaries must first apply for RN licensure (or endorsement) in the distant state and then apply for advanced practice status, which involves extensive credentialing and privileging processes.[45]

Credentialing and Privileging

Credentialing is the process of establishing the qualifications of licensed professionals and assessing their background and legitimacy. For example, if a physician does a telehealth consult from a hospital in State X but the patient resides in a skilled nursing facility in State Y, that physician must be credentialed by both facilities (i.e., the hospital and skilled nursing facility), as well as be licensed in both States X and Y. Each facility could have very different processes and rules for becoming credentialed. Similar to the need for licensing in multiple states, the need for credentialing in multiple, separate healthcare facilities is an obstacle to telehealth services. In May 2011 the Centers for Medicare & Medicaid Services (CMS) modified the existing credentialing and privileging regulations effective July 5, 2011. The new rule under part 42 CFR 410.78 of the CMS regulations allows hospitals

TABLE 8-3	TELEHEALTH PROFESSIONAL LICENSURE OPTIONS
LICENSURE OPTION	**DESCRIPTION**
Endorsement	Allows a state to grant licenses to health professionals licensed in other states that have equivalent standards. States may require additional documentation or qualifications before endorsing a license issued by another state.[43]
Mutual recognition	The distant state's licensing board accepts the licensing policies of the health professional's home state.[45] Federal healthcare agencies operate under this type of system. An analogous licensing system would be the mutual recognition of driver's licenses between states.
Reciprocity	A process in which two states voluntarily enter into a reciprocal agreement to allow the health professional to practice in each state without having to become licensed in both states. It does not involve additional review of the health professional's credentials, as endorsement does, and it does not require the participating states to agree to a standardized set of rules or procedures, as mutual recognition does. The negative aspect of this model is that it leaves the healthcare provider subject to different regulations in each state and therefore subject to different sets of laws. This can lead to legal issues of liability and wider exposure to potential malpractice opportunity.[46]
Registration	The health professional licensed in one state informs the authorities of other states that he or she wishes to practice in those states part-time. The provider is licensed in the home (originating) state but still is accountable to uphold the legal stipulations and regulations of the guest (distant) states. Similar to reciprocity, the provider would still be subject to the guest state's malpractice rules as well as the home state's rules and regulations.
Limited licensure	The health professional obtains his or her medical licensure in the home state and then obtains a second "limited" licensure in the guest state. The limited license allows for specific scope of services to be delivered under particular circumstances.[46]
National licensure	Individual states would voluntarily incorporate the same set of national standards into their laws. Given that most medical professionals pass the same national exam within their particular discipline, it stands to reason that standards of care and practice guidelines should not differ from state to state. Regulatory processes could be retained at the state or national level. For example, the American Medical Association could take full responsibility for the licensing of all physicians at a national level and similarly nurses could be licensed to practice nationally by their national organization, and likewise with other health professions (pharmacists, dentists, physical therapists, etc.). However, disciplinary actions or other procedural activities could be administered at the state level.

or Critical Access Hospitals (CAHs) to use information from a distant-site hospital or other accredited telemedicine entity when making credentialing or privileging decisions for the distant-site physicians and practitioners.[42] Regarding the legal risks and liabilities associated with these changes, the governing body of each hospital and CAH must weigh the risks and benefits of opting for this more streamlined process of credentialing and privileging telemedicine providers.[42] Modifications still need to be made to allow Medicare and Medicaid beneficiaries who reside in urban or metropolitan areas to be eligible to receive the same services.

Reimbursement

Telemedicine is often viewed as a cost-effective alternative to the more traditional face-to-face method of providing medical care.[42] As such, states in the U.S. have the option to determine whether or not to cover telemedicine- and telehealth-delivered care, what types of telehealth to cover, where in the state it can be covered, how it is provided and covered, what types of telehealth practitioners and providers may be covered and reimbursed (as long as such practitioners and providers are "recognized" and qualified according to Medicare and Medicaid statute and regulation), and how much to reimburse for telemedicine services (as long as such payments do not exceed the Federal Upper Limits).[46]

Reimbursement by insurance companies for medical services is based on Medicare's Current Procedural Terminology (CPT) codes billing system. As of 2012, Medicare telehealth services can be furnished only to an eligible telehealth beneficiary from an eligible originating site. In general, originating sites must be located in a rural Health Professional Shortage Area (HPSA) or in a county outside of a Metropolitan Statistical Area (MSA). The originating sites authorized by the statute include hospitals, skilled nursing facilities, offices of physicians or licensed healthcare practitioners, rural health clinics, community mental health centers, CAHs, CAH-based dialysis centers, and federally qualified health centers.[47] Medicaid reimbursement for telehealth varies by state, with some states electing not to reimburse for telehealth services. Internationally, in countries that provide government-based universal health care, telehealth adoption is flourishing and reimbursement has become a national budgetary decision. Providing more access to more citizens while at the same time reducing costs and more efficiently distributing clinical expertise using technology is a desired goal for any country's health service. Thus countries such as Canada, those in the European Union, Japan, China, and India are all expanding their telehealth capabilities and services.

Malpractice and Liability

Legal issues of liability and malpractice are burdensome for the telemedicine practitioner, as they "face additional vulnerability and uncertainty related to malpractice exposure in multiple states and would likely face additional expenses for malpractice insurance and for other costs should a suit be filed in a distant state."[48] Legal issues involve traditional jurisdictional issues, including the following:

- The place of treatment dilemma
- Lack of an established, bona fide doctor–patient relationship similar to the situation with cybermedicine (medical care via the Internet)
- Violating a particular state's specific regulations related to standards of care
- Failing to secure appropriate informed consent from a patient
- Negligence that may arise from technical glitches such as distorted images or poor sound quality of a particular device resulting in injury or misdiagnosis[42]

The traditional concepts of negligence, duty of care, and practicing within one's scope of legal license still apply to telehealth as they do in traditional face-to-face encounters. Initial case law in telemedicine and telehealth to date has been limited, primarily involving telephone triage and teleradiology. In telephone triage, if advice was given and a poor patient outcome occurred, the triage service and professionals are at risk for malpractice. In teleradiology (as is the case with in-person and in-house radiology readings), if a diagnosis of a lump or a mass is missed on an image, the radiology service and professional would be at risk for malpractice. As telehealth usage increases, further legal cases will illuminate and clarify these issues.

TELEHEALTH AND DIRECT PATIENT HEALTH SERVICES

While telehealth applications typically involve provider-to-provider teleconsults, patients and other healthcare consumers can use telehealth directly to support their healthcare decision making. Specifically, applications facilitate direct, online patient telemedicine care; provide remote patient telehealth visits and monitoring; and link consumers with online healthcare information.[49] As the technology used to deliver telehealth services becomes easier to use and more affordable, the technology is increasingly being used by patients in interaction with their healthcare providers and at times in directing their own care.

Patient-to-Provider Telehealth-Delivered Care

Increasingly, individuals find it difficult to obtain timely care for urgent health concerns from their healthcare provider. A survey of California hospitals found that 50% of the patients who visited an emergency department thought that their medical concerns could have been dealt with by their regular physicians; however, they were unable to obtain timely access to care.[50] Online telehealth direct care is a solution to this growing problem and the use of video conferencing for telehealth visits is increasing. Manhattan Research's Taking the Pulse U.S. v11.0 study indicated that nearly 7% of physicians use online video conferencing to communicate with their patients.[49] Physicians consider telehealth a method for consulting with patients about nonurgent issues or connecting with geographically dispersed patient populations that may not have nearby access to specialists. The study also found that certain specialty healthcare providers, such as psychiatrists and oncologists, are more likely to use video conferencing with their patients.

Adapt TeleHealth is an example of this approach. Once a community or clinic has identified that it has a need for psychiatric services, it contracts with Adapt TeleHealth to meet its mental health needs. It purchases a consistent number of hours per week, which are fulfilled by an Adapt TeleHealth mental health provider. Other direct patient care technologies focus more on providing a platform for a healthcare provider's office to provide telemedicine care. Companies such as Secure Telehealth (www.securetelehealth.com/telehealth-uses.html), TelaDoc (www.teladoc.com), and Online Care Anywhere (www.onlinecareanywheremn.com) are examples of platforms for direct online medical care.

Asynchronous applications using store-and-forward technologies or online diagnostic surveys are gaining in popularity. Virtuwell (www.virtuwell.com) from HealthPartners in Minnesota is available 24/7 and uses an online survey asking consumers to identify their chief concern. Responses are sent to a nurse practitioner who reviews the information and responds within 30 minutes. Responses are provided via text or email and include a diagnosis, potential remedies, and tips for preventing the condition in the future. If a prescription is needed, the nurse practitioner can send it to a local pharmacy. Forty common conditions, including bladder infections, lice, and yeast infections, are treated by Virtuwell's nurse practitioners.

Another asynchronous telemedicine company is RelayHealth, an online solution to connect consumers with their healthcare providers. Providers license RelayHealth web-based software, with capability for patient visits and consultations, prescription renewal, appointment scheduling, personal health record management, delivery of lab results, referral requests, and access to medically reviewed information.

Remote Telehealth Home Visits and Biosensors

Telehealth systems previously used interactive video conferencing between healthcare providers and patients; however, the ability to self-manage care is a driving fiscal concern.[51,52] Machlin and Woodwell noted that nearly two thirds of publicly insured adults in the U.S. under the age of 65 have one or more chronic conditions and that nearly 75% of all healthcare dollars were spent on managing these chronic conditions.[53] Use of telehealth technologies for remote home care and biosensor monitoring instruments are gaining momentum to address chronic illnesses and to promote safety for seniors living alone.

Remote Telehealth Home Visits and Monitoring

As mentioned earlier, the most widespread telehealth program in the United States is the VA national telehealth program, CCHT. Built around Wagner's Chronic Care Model, CCHT is characterized by "the use of health informatics, disease management and home telehealth technologies . . . with the specific intent of providing the right care in the right place at the right time."[19(p1120)] The range of technologies for CCHT includes videophones, messaging devices, biometric devices, digital cameras, and telemonitoring devices.[52] The videophones and video telemonitors facilitate synchronous face-to-face encounters with a healthcare provider through regular telephone lines or through computer links and the Internet. Biometric devices and digital images are also part of the comprehensive CCHT system and are used to gather timely healthcare data employing asynchronous store-and-forward technologies.

Two specific examples of technologies used with the VA and the general public are HealthBuddy (www.bosch-telehealth.com/en/us/products/health_buddy/health_buddy.html) and miLife (www.americantelecare.com). MiLife, adopted for use by the VA in 2011, offers live, interactive video combined with remote monitoring. In between video visits, veterans measure and transmit vital signs and other physiologic measurements with devices in their homes, answer self-assessment questions, and receive disease-specific educational information.

HealthBuddy does not include a video visit component but otherwise works in a similar way. Patients access the system and update their health status by answering a series of questions about their health and well-being using the HealthBuddy application. The data are sent over a telephone line or Ethernet Internet connection to a secure data center; the data are then available for review by a healthcare provider via the HealthBuddy desktop system. Peripheral monitoring devices such as blood glucose meters, blood pressure monitor, peak flow meters, pulse oximeters, and weight scales are also supported.

Both miLife and HealthBuddy allow nurses, social workers, and other healthcare provider coordinators to prioritize their patient caseload and develop treatment plans based on the patient's risk. Emerging research findings show that telehealth home visits and home monitoring are care and cost effective.[19,54]

Biometric Sensors

A number of healthcare applications use information and communication core components to help patients stay safe in their homes and communicate vital healthcare data to providers.[52] Box 8-2 provides an overview of biometric sensors. Peripheral health monitoring tools such as blood glucose monitors, pulse oximeters, blood pressure and ECG monitors, and electronic scales, already described as components of a telehomecare visit, fit this definition. They are the backbone of a viable remote disease management program.

More recently, a group of assistive technology devices dubbed "sensor technologies" have emerged and add a layer of connectedness between patients and their healthcare providers by monitoring patients' activity levels and physiologic parameters. Sensor technology has the potential to not only manage disease but also promote a safe and healthy environment for seniors.[52] A Frame Digital (www.aframedigital.com) has engineered a low-stigma, intuitive, wristwatch-based sensor system with an intelligent learning and predictive modeling platform that acquires physiologic data from

BOX 8-2 BIOMETRIC SENSOR OVERVIEW

Purposes
- Detect changes in patterns that signal improvement or early failings
- Signal need for urgent or emergency help
- Integrate with websites or mobile units to promote communication
- Have ubiquitous monitoring for peace of mind for older adult and family
- Keep an inventory of supply levels for medications and other resources
- Coach and monitor exercise effectiveness and participation in games

Information Potentials
- Physical: motion, location, activity
- Physiologic/medical: pulse, temperature, sweat, blood chemistry
- Social: telephone or web interaction counts or identification
- Memory support: monitoring cooking stoves, adherence to regimens
- Communication safety issues: stove use, fire, unsecured doors

Communication
- Devices and protocols networked to connect to computers
- Statistical and computational paradigms for analysis
- Applications for interaction with emergency rescues, healthcare providers, and social network

Monitoring Target Examples
- Restlessness as indicator of disturbed sleep
- Gait changes as indicator of drug side effect or physical debility
- Extended bedrest as indicator of depression or physical debility
- Pill counts as indicator of adherence or side effect issues

the wearer every 30 seconds. After collecting sufficient data points, the system learns the physiologic normal for the individual. If deviations from normal occur, an alert is sent to a neighbor, relative, friend, or emergency responder. Personalized, tailored remote monitoring and intelligent alerting is the hallmark of this innovative system.

One example of sensor technology that may be used in the future to promote a safe and healthy environment is the smart home. The "smart home or intelligent house"[52(p237)] is expected to use radio frequency identification (RFID) technology.[55] RFID technology uses a microchip to uniquely identify and track objects, record and update information, and make all of this accessible through a global network.[56] Depending on their use, RFIDs can be active or passive and are capable of being ingested, implanted, or attached externally. While concerns about potential privacy and security breaches exist, RFID benefits include unlimited sight connection and rapid information processing, predicting better utility than other

technologies such as bar-coding. Treatment-based applications such as monitoring handwashing practices, transmitting neuromuscular stimulation data, and authenticating medications have the potential to transition from the hospital to the smart home.

Sensor technology also supports next-generation healthcare by virtue of its mobility. Two forms of mobile sensors are wearable embedded technologies and wearable attached technologies.[52] Clothing with "smart fabrics" and embedded sensors is currently in use for measuring body temperature and heart activity or signaling a risk for falls. Recently, companies have designed sensors to integrate with smartphones. One example of an integrated sensor comes from WIN Human Recorder Co. Ltd. in Japan.[57] Consumers wear a small, portable sensor attached to the body and readings are accessed easily via a cellphone or a networked computer. The WIN Human Recorder is capable of monitoring electrocardiography signals, heart rate, brain waves, accelerated velocity, body temperature, respiration, and pulse waves. Biosensor fabrics will have the capacity to analyze blood chemistry levels from collected perspiration or immunosensors integrated in dressings will be able to detect healing.

Telehealth Technology and Healthcare Consumers

The proportion of American adults seeking information about a health concern from a source other than their physician dropped to 50 percent in 2010, down from 56 percent in 2007.[58] At first glance, readers may assume that consumers are not seeking information about their healthcare needs; however, the drop is actually attributed to an 18% decline in their use of print sources: books, magazines, and newspapers. Adults, especially the elderly and those with chronic disease conditions, have increased their Internet use for seeking health information, contributing to their engagement in self-care.[58] Online healthcare resources have the potential to aid consumers by supporting shared decision making with healthcare providers, providing personalized self-management tools and resources, building social support health networks, delivering tailored accurate health information, and increasing health literacy.[59]

Health information websites have been available to consumers since the mid-1990s.[60] Websites such as WebMD, a publicly traded company, and the National Institutes of Health's MedlinePlus, a federal government site, have provided healthcare information to a broad population of consumers, including the general public, employers, employees, health plans, and healthcare providers. More recently, however, some health websites have moved beyond one-way communication and developed innovative features and interactive tools that enable consumers to greatly increase their self-knowledge and promote greater safety and independence. Tools such as drug interaction checkers, symptom checkers, various health-related calculators, pill identifiers, patient forums, fitness trackers, and PHRs are becoming more prevalent and helping consumers to gain more control over their health.[60]

Everyday Health (www.everydayhealth.com) is an example of an interactive, consumer-based website. Everyday Health has partnered with experts from Harvard University, Cleveland Clinic, and the American Association of Family Practitioners to provide consumers with healthcare information and has also developed interactive consumer-oriented tools. Consumers can use assessment and tracking tools and online calculators, speak live with a pharmacist, find drugs and treatments, and create a personal plan for health. Additional information concerning interactive consumer-oriented recourses is included in Chapters 13 and 14.

eHealth Literacy: Critical Element for Telehealth Adoption

The proliferation of online healthcare resources has caused the development of a national and international quality standards agenda to help health professionals and consumers alike access and evaluate high-quality online health information that is accurate, current, valid, appropriate, intelligible, and free of bias.[61-63]

Health consumer advocates espouse the need for ehealth literacy as a way of evaluating the information and services delivered using IT tools.[64] Consumers must have basic reading skills in their search for online healthcare resources and use of telehealth tools. They also must have the following skills:

- Visual literacy: ability to understand graphs and read a label or other visual information
- Computer literacy: ability to operate a computer
- Information literacy: ability to obtain and apply relevant information
- Digital literacy: competency with digital devices of all types; technical skills to operate these devices and conceptual knowledge to understand their functionality; ability to creatively and critically use these devices to access, manipulate, evaluate, and apply data, information, knowledge, and wisdom in activities of daily living; ability to apply basic emotional intelligence in collaborating and communicating with others; ethical values and sense of community responsibility to use digital devices for the enjoyment and benefit of society[65]

eHealth literacy skills are critical for future telehealth adoption for both consumers and healthcare providers alike.

CONCLUSION AND FUTURE DIRECTIONS

Telehealth, considered futuristic by some, is actually not a new concept, dating back to 1897. Currently, telehealth services are being provided in diverse settings from islands off the coast of Maine to across the U.S. for remote care of military veterans. Two major types of telehealth exist: asynchronous and synchronous. Applications include teleradiology, teleconsulting, telepathology, telesensors, and remote home visits. Telehealth has the potential to decrease care costs and speed treatments but the field also has challenges, including issues regarding licensure, standards, reimbursement, credentialing and privileging, and lack of integration with other health IT, especially EHRs.

Growth in telehealth could result in a future where access to healthcare is not limited by geographic region, time, or availability of skilled health professionals. The potential to realize comprehensive, integrated, and seamless delivery of healthcare services through virtual environments, capable of spanning a broad range of prevention and health promotion interventions, already has been made possible through advances in telehealth technology. Conditions exist for expanding telehealth to other sectors for sustainable telehealth: rising healthcare costs, increasing prevalence of chronic diseases, an aging population, demands for improved access to healthcare, and global shortages of health professionals.[36,37,66-69] Creation of telehealth ecosystems and novel healthcare models requires interdisciplinary and intersectoral approaches spanning technology, education, and health management (Fig. 8-4).

The CuRE framework in Figure 8-4 depicts the Canada-India Centre of Excellence for uHealth Research and Education (CuRE). It provides a uhealth (ubiquitous health) view for operationalizing future global collaboration in advancing telehealth.

Policy decisions to adopt and implement telehealth technology in healthcare delivery are influenced by many drivers, such as global socioeconomic contexts, political motivations, capacity of technology to address healthcare needs, and fundamental understandings of telehealth capabilities.[66,70] Inconsistencies in telehealth research methods and data reporting have had an impact on empirical data available to evaluate telehealth technology in the areas of cost–benefit, effectiveness, and patient engagement.[67,68] Issues of authentication, data security, and practical aspects of telecommunication infrastructure remain critical challenges for the adoption and broader use of telehealth technologies.[71,72]

A consistent and coordinated approach in tracking healthcare technology use is lacking; therefore the effectiveness of

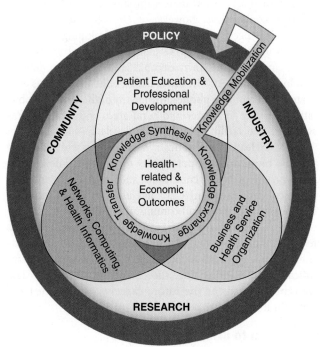

FIG 8-4 Components of telehealth. (Copyright 2012 Daniel Nagel and Antonia Arnaert. All Rights Reserved.)

telehealth is difficult to determine. Much available information on use and trends has been generated through industry and market analysis rather than through independent research. Significant challenges exist in tracking telehealth technology use and trends in healthcare, including the following:

1. How telehealth is defined; terms such as *telehealth, telemedicine*, and *informatics* are frequently and inconsistently used interchangeably in the literature
2. The variety in modalities of telehealth technologies being used and the capacity to which they are used
3. The vastly different contexts in which telehealth may be employed, such as varying models and settings for healthcare delivery, geographic regions, and cultural settings[66,70,72]

Telehealth Industry Growth

One market research firm valued the market for remote patient monitoring, one form of telehealth care, in the United States at about $7.1 billion in 2010 and anticipated this market will grow to $22.2 billion by 2015.[73] Healthcare technology usage in Canada during 2010 includes delivery of 260,000 telehealth encounters and 2500 patients enrolled in telehomecare services, reflecting a 35% annual growth during the previous 5 years.[74] In Europe, outpatient telehealth services are provided by either public or private hospitals. A report provided to the European Commission in 2011 indicated that 8% of hospitals provided telemonitoring to patients.[74] Continued global growth in telehealth is anticipated as technology evolves and the need for cost-effective healthcare delivery increases in both developed and developing countries.[36,37,66,75]

Rapid advances in technology, such as electronic platforms for healthcare services and technologies used in transmitting data, continue to expand the reach of healthcare delivery and the potential services available. Initially telehealth relied on Internet connections; however, a shift to more mhealth formats has occurred, particularly in developing countries. Growth in the mobile phone industry in countries such as China and India has increased 321% compared to 46% in developed countries.[76] In India, use of cellular phones is estimated at 742 million phones, with many of these new "mobile citizens" living in poorer and rural areas with scarce infrastructure and facilities, low literacy levels, and low Internet access.[77] mHealth capabilities now provide a wide range of wireless monitoring opportunities to transmit information for a variety of health conditions, such as diabetes and cardiovascular diseases. mHealth has also increased access to healthcare for persons and communities in rural and isolated regions.[66] A recent endorsement of 4G standards in wireless telecommunications by the International Telecommunications Union, a branch of the United Nations, will have significant implications for speed and quantity of data transmission and for the future capacity of mhealth technologies in healthcare delivery.

Telehealth to uHealth

At present a lack of integrated, secure technology "spaces" exists to facilitate migration of data between the various telehealth platforms, ehealth technologies, and mhealth devices for effective and efficient support of healthcare delivery. This gap in interoperability largely reflects industry strategies to protect proprietary rights; however, the lack of interoperability between technologies limits sharing of health information and the ability to implement a cohesive model of healthcare delivery in a virtual environment.[36]

Advancements in "cloud computing" technology, a more integrated wireless telecommunication architecture that supports accessible and seamless transmission and storage of digital data, may make it possible to facilitate a connection between healthcare information systems and to expand the capacity of healthcare delivery.[71,72]

More recent research and development has focused on *ubiquitous* (*u*health) technologies that integrate core components of computers, wireless networks, sensors, and other modalities (such as mhealth devices) to create an environment to monitor, respond to, and assist in meeting the healthcare needs of individuals.[78,79] An example of the utility of uhealth is the development of smart home systems that provide persons who have health concerns with a safer environment in which to live more independently.[78] As the number of people living longer with complex health conditions grows and the elderly population increases, uhealth innovations can be used to detect changes in health status, communicate pertinent patient information, and alert healthcare providers to facilitate efficient interventions.[79]

Improve Healthcare Provider Shortages and Access to Care

As telehealth expands, further integration with informatics will continue. Telehealth encounters will be integrated within PHRs and EHRs. Self-care data will also be integrated into data repositories for individuals and populations. As the global population increases, the supply and distribution of healthcare providers can be optimized using telehealth to provide services regardless of the geographic location of those in need. Shortages in primary care providers and nurses, for example, can benefit from redistribution of portions of clinical expertise using telehealth as the export mechanism.[4,40]

Future migration of telehealth to uhealth will require practicing healthcare provider licensure models that are not only interstate, but also international, enabling healthcare providers to practice in countries that have healthcare needs that can be met using telehealth technologies. This will require cooperation on the part of politicians, governments, and policy-makers on behalf of fully operationalized telehealth.[70,80]

REFERENCES

1. Health Resources and Services Administration (HRSA). Telehealth. HRSA. http://www.hrsa.gov/ruralhealth/about/telehealth/. 2012. Accessed January 21, 2012.
2. American Telemedicine Association (ATA). Telemedicine defined. ATA. http://www.americantelemed.org/i4a/pages/index.cfm?pageid=3333. 2012. Accessed February 10, 2012.

3. American Telemedicine Association (ATA). What is telemedicine? ATA. http://www.americantelemed.org/files/public/abouttelemedicine/What_Is_Telemedicine.pdf. 2012. Accessed January 22, 2012.

4. Schlachta-Fairchild L. *International Competencies for Telenursing*. Geneva, Switzerland: International Council of Nurses; 2008.

5. Krupinski E, Nypaver M, Poropatich R, Ellis D, Safwat R, Sapci H. Clinical applications in telemedicine/telehealth. *Telemedicine Journal and e-Health*. 2002:8(1):13-34.

6. University of Calgary, Health Telematics Unit. *State of the Science Report: Socioeconomic Impact of Telehealth Evidence Now for Health Care in the Future*. American Telemedicine Association. http://www.americantelemed.org/files/public/membergroups/hometelehealth/Canadian%20Telehealth%20Lit%20Search.pdf. 2003. Accessed July 25, 2012.

7. Schlachta-Fairchild L, Elfrink V, Deickman A. Patient safety, telenursing, and telehealth. In: Hughes R, ed. *Patient Safety and Quality: An Evidence-Based Handbook for Nurses*. Rockville, MD: Agency for Health Care Research and Quality; 2008: 1277-1316.

8. European Commission (EC). Telemedicine for the benefit of patients, health care systems and society. EC. http://ec.europa.eu/information_society/activities/health/docs/policy/telemedicine/telemedecine-swp_sec-2009-943.pdf. 2009. Accessed July 25, 2012.

9. American Heart Association/American Stroke Association. AHA/ASA scientific statement: a review of the evidence for the use of telemedicine within stroke systems of care. *Stroke*. 2009;40:2616-2634.

10. European Coordination Committee of the Radiological, Electromedical and Healthcare IT Industry (COCIR). COCIR telemedicine toolkit supporting effective deployment of telehealth and mobile health. COCIR. http://www.cocir.org/uploads/documents/Telemedicine%20Toolkit%20LINK2.pdf. 2011. Accessed July 25, 2012.

11. Medicaid CHIP Programs. Telemedicine and telehealth overview. Medicaid.gov. http://www.medicaid.gov/Medicaid-CHIP-Program-Information/By-Topics/Delivery-Systems/Telemedicine.html. 2012. Accessed February 1, 2012.

12. Telehealth Leadership Initiative (TLI). What is telehealth? TLI. http://www.telehealthleadership.org/telehealth101.html. 2008. Accessed January 26, 2012.

13. American Telecare. Telehealth: frequently asked questions. American Telecare. http://www.americantelecare.com/support_Main.html. 2012. Accessed January 26, 2012.

14. Helseth C. Telemedicine reaches beyond clinic walls: networks help extend access. *The Rural Monitor*. 2011. http://www.raconline.org/newsletter/summer11/feature.php#story2.

15. University of Miami Telehealth. Teledermatology. University of Miami, Miller School of Medicine. http://telehealth.med.miami.edu/featured/teledermatology/. 2012. Accessed July 25, 2012.

16. Darkins A, Cary M. *Telemedicine and Telehealth: Principles, Policies, Performance, and Pitfalls*. New York, NY: Springer Publishing Company; 2000.

17. House AM, Roberts JM. Telemedicine in Canada. *Can Med Assoc J*. 1977;117(4):386-388.

18. Johnston B, Wheeler L, Deuser J, Sousa K. Outcomes of the Kaiser Permanente tele-home research project. *Arch Fam Med*. 2000;9(1):40-45.

19. Darkins A, Ryan P, Kobb R, et al. Care coordination/home telehealth, and disease management to support the care of veteran patients with chronic conditions. *Telemed J e-Health*. 2008;14 (10):1118-1126.

20. Department of Health (United Kingdom). Whole system demonstrator programme: headline findings. Department of Health. http://www.dh.gov.uk/en/Publicationsandstatistics/Publications/PublicationsPolicyAndGuidance/DH_131684. 2011. Accessed January 27, 2012.

21. American Nurses Association. *Core Principles on Telehealth*. Washington, DC: American Nurses Publishing; 1998.

22. American Telemedicine Association (ATA). About ATA. ATA. http://www.americantelemed.org/i4a/pages/index.cfm?pageID=3281. 2012. Accessed February 12, 2012.

23. American Electronics Association. eHealth 201: designing the virtual hospital. TechAmerica. http://www.techamerica.org/content/wp-content/uploads/2009/07/aea_cs_ehealth_telemedicine.pdf . 2007. Accessed January 4, 2012.

24. Demiris G. Patient-centered applications: use of information technology to promote disease management and wellness. *J Am Med Inform Assn*. 2008;15:8-13.

25. Continua Health Alliance. Mission and purpose. Continua Health Alliance. http://www.continuaalliance.org/about-the-alliance/mission-and-objectives.html. 2012. Accessed February 10, 2012.

26. ZigBee Alliance. Specifications. ZigBee Alliance. http://www.zigbee.org/Specifications.aspx. 2012. Accessed February 11, 2012.

27. Thielst C. The crossroads of telehealth, electronic health records & health information exchange. The Northwest Regional Telehealth Resource Center. http://thielst.typepad.com/files/crossroads-of-telehealth-white-paper.pdf. 2010. Accessed February 10, 2012.

28. World Health Organization (WHO). Telehealth and telemedicine will henceforth be part of the strategy for health for all [press release]. Geneva, Switzerland: WHO; 1997.

29. Worley J. Long distance and up close: UK telemedicine in the vanguard of patient care. University of Kentucky, Odyssey. http://www.research.uky.edu/odyssey/spring10/jicha.html. 2010. Accessed February 2, 2012.

30. Gagnon MP, Orruno E, Asua J, Abdeljelil AB, Emparanza J. Using a modified technology acceptance model to evaluate health care professionals' adoption of a new telemonitoring system. *Telemed J e-Health*. 2012;18(1):54-59.

31. American Nurses Association. *Competencies for Telehealth Technologies in Nursing*. Washington, DC: American Nurses Publishing; 1999.

32. American Nurses Association. *Developing Telehealth Protocols: A Blueprint for Success*. Washington, DC: American Nurses Publishing; 2001.

33. Canadian Society for Telehealth. Canadian National Initiative for Telehealth releases Framework of Guidelines for Telehealth. Virtual Medical Worlds. http://www.hoise.com/vmw/03/articles/vmw/LV-VM-11-03-9.html. 2003. Accessed March 13, 2012.

34. College of Registered Nurses of Nova Scotia (CRNNS). Telenursing practice guidelines. CRNNS. http://www.crnns.ca/documents/TelenursingPractice2008.pdf. 2008. Accessed March 18, 2012.

35. American Telemedicine Association (ATA). Expert consensus recommendations for videoconferencing-based telepresenting. ATA. http://www.americantelemed.org. 2011. Accessed January 25, 2012.

36. Hein MA. Telemedicine: An Important Force in the Transformation of Health Care. Washington, DC: International Trade Administration, US Department of Commerce; 2009.

37. Care WD, Gregory DM, Chermonas WM. Nursing, technology, and informatics: understanding the past and embracing the future. In: McIntyre M, McDonald C, eds. Realities of Canadian Nursing: Professional, Practice, and Power Issues. Philadelphia, PA: Wolters Kluwer, Lippincott Williams & Wilkins; 2010.

38. Jennett P, Yeo M, Pauls M, Graham J. Organizational readiness for telemedicine: implications for success and failure. *Journal of Telemedicine and Telecare.* 2003;9:27-30.

39. Duclos C, Hook J, Rodriquez M. Telehealth in community clinics: three case studies in implementation. California Health-Care Foundation. http://www.chcf.org/~?media%library%files/PDF%20TelehealthClinicCaseStudies.pdf. 2010. Accessed February 12, 2012.

40. Schlachta-Fairchild L, Elfrink V. *International Telenursing Survey Report.* Frederick, MD: iTelehealth Inc; 2009.

41. Robbings D. Removing barriers for the advancement of telemedicine. Ebookbrowse. http://ebookbrowse.com/telemedicine-barriers-and-opportunities-doc-d109174564. 2001. Accessed February 2, 2012.

42. Pong RW, Hogenbirk JC. Licensing physicians for telehealth practice: issues and policy options. *Health Law Review.* 2002;8(1):3-14.

43. American Medical Association (AMA). Physician licensure: an update of trends. AMA. http://www.ama-assn.org/ama/pub/about-ama/our-people/member-groups-sections/young-physicians-section/advocacy-resources/physician-licensure-an-update-trends.page. 2012. Accessed January 12, 2012.

44. Telehealth Resource Center (TRC). Licensure and scope of practice. TRC. http://www.telehealthresourcecenter.org. 2011. Accessed January 28, 2012.

45. Philipsen N, Haynes D. The multi-state nursing licensure compact: making nurses mobile. *The Journal for Nurse Practitioners.* 2007;3(1):36-40.

46. U.S. Government Printing Office (GPO). Medicare and Medicaid programs: changes affecting hospital and critical access hospital conditions of participation: telemedicine and privileging. GPO. http://www.gpo.gov/fdsys/pkg/FR-2011-05-05/html/2011-10875.htm. 2011. Accessed February 10, 2012.

47. Medicaid.gov. Telemedicine. Medicaid.gov. http://www.medicaid.gov/Medicaid-CHIP-Program-Information/By-Topics/Delivery-Systems/Telemedicine.html. 2012. Accessed February 4, 2012.

48. Chee J. Tele-medical malpractice: negligence in the practice of telemedicine and related issues. The Center for Telehealth and E-Health Law. http://www.ctel.org/research/TeleMedical%20Malpractice%20Negligence%20in%20the%20Practice%20of%20Telemedicine%20and%20Related%20Issues.pdf. 2010. Accessed December 22, 2011.

49. Manhattan Research Group. Seven percent of U.S. physicians use video chat to communicate with patients. FierceHealthcare. http://www.fiercehealthcare.com/press-releases/seven-percent-us-physicians-use-video-chat-communicate-patients-1#ixzz1lGE7d5Ls. 2012. Accessed February 2, 2012.

50. Puskin D, Johnson B, Speedie S. Telemedicine, telehealth, and health information technology: an ATA issue paper. American Telemedicine Association. http://www.americantelemed.org/files/public/policy/HIT_Paper.pdf. 2006. Accessed February 2, 2012.

51. Lau C, Churchill S, Kim J, Matsen F, Yongmin K. Asynchronous web-based patient centered home telemedicine system. *IEEE T Bio-med Eng.* 2002;49(12):1452-1462.

52. Jordan-Marsh M. *Health Technology Literacy: A Transdisciplinary Framework for Consumer-Oriented Practice.* Sudbury, MA: Jones & Bartlett; 2011.

53. Machlin S, Woodwell D. *Health Care Expenses for Chronic Conditions among Non-Elderly Adults: Variations by Insurance Coverage, 2005-06 (Average Estimates): Statistical Brief #243.* Rockville,

MD: Agency for Healthcare Research and Quality; 2009. http://meps.ahrq.gov/mepsweb/data_files/publications/st243/stat243.pdf. Accessed February 6, 2012.

54. Newman M, McMahon T. Fiscal impact of AB 415: potential cost savings from expansion of telehealth prepared for Center for Connected Health Policy. American Well. http://www.americanwell.com/pdf/FiscalImpactofAB415PotentialCostSavingsfromExpansionofTelehealth.pdf. 2011. Accessed February 6, 2012.

55. Pang Soojung-Kim A. Smart homes and sociable devices: RFID takes off. In: Davis M, Hemberger K, eds. *Technology Horizon Program, Institute for the Future.* http://www.iftf.org/uploads/media/SR-926D_RFID_SmartHomes_SociableDevices.pdf. 2005. Accessed February 7, 2012.

56. The Learning Space. An overview of RFID in ICTS: device to device communication. The Open University, Scotland. http://openlearn.open.ac.uk/mod/oucontent/view.php?id=397529&section=7.2. 2012. Accessed February 7, 2012.

57. Kato S. Wearable health monitoring sensor debuts in Japanese market. Tech-On: Tech & Industry Analysis from Asia. http://techon.nikkeibp.co.jp/english/NEWS_EN/20100119/179393. 2010. Accessed September 25, 2012.

58. Center for Studying Health System Change. Surprising decline in consumers seeking health information. Center for Studying Health System Change. http://www.hschange.com/CONTENT/1261/. 2011. Accessed February 8, 2012.

59. Healthy People 2020. Health communication and health information technology. HealthyPeople.gov. http://healthypeople.gov/2020/topicsobjectives2020/overview.aspx?topicId=18. 2010. Accessed February 8, 2012.

60. Toner R. Consumer health websites accelerate consumer-driven health care value based purchasing. Thomas Jefferson University, Jefferson Digital Commons. http://jdc.jefferson.edu/cgi/viewcontent.cgi?article=1041&context=vbp&sei-redir=1&referer=http%3A%2F%2Fwww.google.com%2Furl%3Fsa%3Dt%26rct%3Dj%26q%3Dhistory%2520of%2520health%2520consumer%2520websites%26source%3Dweb%26cd%3D3%26sqi%3D2%26ved%3D0CEMQFjAC%26url%3Dhttp%253A%252F%252Fjdc.jefferson.edu%252Fcgi%252Fviewcontent.cgi%253Farticle%253D1041%2526context%253Dvbp%26ei%3DefYyT7iEOYLx0gGZ5o3kBw%26usg%3DAFQjCNGf0dlOmsTSJkvO6zj0cU8b6QY4Cg#search=%22history%20health%20consumer%20websites%22. 2009. Accessed February 9, 2012.

61. Health on the Net. HONCode in brief. Health on the Net Foundation. http://www.hon.ch/HONcode/Patients/Visitor/visitor.html. 2008. Accessed February 8, 2012.

62. Lorence D, Abraham J. A study of undue pain and surfing: using hierarchical criteria to assess web site quality. *Health Informatics J.* 2008;14(3):155-173.

63. Toms EG, Latter C. How consumers search for health information. *Health Informatics J.* 2007;13(3):223-235.

64. Glassman P. Health literacy. National Library of Medicine. http://nnlm.gov/outreach/consumer/hlthlit.html. 2011. Accessed February 9, 2012.

65. Nelson R, Joos IM, Wolf D. Social Media for Nurses. New York, NY: Springer Publishing; 2013.

66. Mechael PN. The case for mhealth in developing countries. *Innovations.* 2009;4(1):103-118.

67. Pare G, Jaana M, Sicotte C. Systematic review of home telemonitoring for chronic diseases: the evidence base. *J Am Med Inform Assn.* 2007;14(3):269-277.

68. Polisena J, Coyle D, Coyle K, McGill S. Home telehealth for chronic disease management: a systematic review and analysis of economic evaluations. *Int J Technol Assess*. 2009;25(3):339-349.

69. Vinson MH, McCallum R, Thornlow DK, Champagne MT. Design, implementation, and evaluation of population-specific telehealth nursing services. *Nurs Econ*. 2011;29(5):265-277.

70. Miller EA. Solving the disjuncture between research and practice: telehealth trends in the 21st century. *Health Policy*. 2007;82(2):133-141.

71. Nkosi MT, Mekuria SM. Cloud computing for enhanced mobile applications. *Cloud Computing Technology and Science*. 2010;31: 629-633. doi:10.1109/CloudCom.2010.31:629-633.

72. Thuemmlar C, Fan L, Buchanan W, Lo O, Ekonomou E, Khedim S. E-health: chances and challenges of distributed, service oriented architectures. *Journal of Cyber Security and Mobility*. 2012;37-52.

73. Kalorama Information. Remote patient monitoring systems may help overstressed ICUs. Kalorama Information. http://www.kaloramainformation.com/about/release.asp?id=2339:. 2011. Accessed January 16, 2012.

74. European Commission (EC). eHealth benchmarking III: SMART 2009/002: 2011. EC. http://ec.europa.eu/information_society/eeurope/i2010/docs/benchmarking/ehealth_benchmarking_3_final_report.pdf. 2011. Accessed February 5, 2012.

75. Canada Health Infoway. Telehealth benefits and adoption: connecting people and providers across Canada. Canada Health Infoway. https://www2.infoway-inforoute.ca/Documents/telehealth_report_2010_en.pdf. 2010. Accessed November 24, 2011.

76. Vital Wave Consulting. 10 Facts about mobile markets in developing countries. Vital Wave Consulting. http://www.vitalwaveconsulting.com/pdf/10FactsMobile.pdf. 2008. Accessed February 8, 2012.

77. Schwartz M. Mobiles will revolutionize seven sectors in rural India—Nokia, CKS. Centre for Knowledge Societies. http://www.cks.in/html/cks_pdfs/Mobiles%20will%20revolutionise%20seven%20sectors%20in%20rural%20India.pdf. 2007. Accessed February 8, 2012.

78. Agoulmine N, Deen MJ, Lee JS, Meyyappan M. U-Health smart home: innovative solutions for the management of the elderly and chronic diseases. *IEEE Nanotechnology Magazine*. 2011;5(3):6-11.

79. Otto C, Milenkovic A, Sanders C, Jovanov E. System architecture of a wireless body area sensor network for ubiquitous health monitoring. *Journal of Mobile Multimedia*. 2006;1(4):307-326.

80. Schlachta-Fairchild L, Castelli D, Pyke R. International telenursing: a strategic tool for nursing shortage and access to nursing care. In: Jordanova M, Lievens F, eds. *Proceedings of Medetel, the International Society of Telemedicine and eHealth Annual Conference*. Luxembourg: Luxexpo; 2008:399-405.

DISCUSSION QUESTIONS

1. What licensure model would be most useful to support telehealth clinical practice across international boundaries, for example, Canadian doctors or nurses (virtually) seeing and treating U.S. patients or U.S. pharmacists and occupational therapists (virtually) seeing and treating Australian patients?

2. How do the different models for delivering healthcare, including covering the cost of that healthcare, affect the telehealth programs in different countries?

3. What actions can individual healthcare providers take in the next 3 years to advance the benefits of telehealth for their profession?

4. Why has telehealth adoption taken so long in the healthcare industry when Skype, cellphones, and other video conferencing applications have been used in personal and business interactions for decades?

5. How much does usability affect you and your friends when deciding to accept or not use a new technology? Does this also apply in your role as healthcare provider?

6. What actions can individual healthcare providers take to improve their patients' ehealth literacy?

7. What needs to occur on an international basis in order for uhealth to be operationalized?

8. What are the first five steps you would take to start a telehealth program or application in the healthcare facility where you work?

9. What key success criteria for telehealth programs are "must have" and what criteria are "nice to have" when considering a new telehealth initiative?

10. What factor or factors will be most important in driving the exponential growth of telehealth in the future?

CASE STUDY

Mrs. Smith is 82 years old and is diagnosed with hypertension, diabetes, and congestive heart failure. Her two children live in California, while she lives in North Carolina in a small family home on 10 acres of land in the Blue Ridge Mountains. Mrs. Smith has been in the hospital four times in the last year due to congestive heart failure. As her eyesight and mobility get worse with age, she found it a challenge to stay on her medical plan and to do her shopping for the right foods she knows she should be eating. Mrs. Smith's health plan, Purple Cross of North Carolina, assigned a nurse case manager to address her situation. Purple Cross provided a digital scale and a remote monitoring device that recorded Mrs. Smith's condition every day by uploading her weight and transmitting the answers to a series of questions on a touch screen kiosk. The case manager also coordinated delivery of Meals on Wheels, providing low-sodium, diabetic-compliant dinners to Mrs. Smith on an ongoing basis. The case manager calls Mrs. Smith twice a week, taking the time to educate her about her medications, her activities, and the disease-specific elements that will keep her healthy and out of the hospital. When the case manager identifies that Mrs. Smith can no longer organize her daily medications, a digital medication dispenser will be provided that will keep her on her medication regimen. The medication dispenser will be preloaded with Mrs. Smith's medications and will issue a subtle doorbell tone when it is time to take her medicines. With the combination of remote and real-time (telephonic) support persons and technologies, Mrs. Smith is able to remain in her home and avoid further inpatient admissions.

Discussion Questions

1. Which components are critical to Mrs. Smith staying safely in her home?
2. Describe whether Mrs. Smith's regimen might be augmented using mhealth applications.

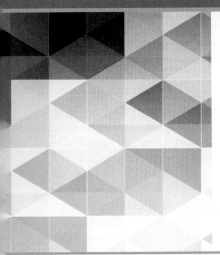

Home Health and Related Community-Based Systems

Karen S. Martin and Karen B. Utterback

No matter how dreary and gray our homes are, we people of flesh and blood would rather live there than in any other country, be it ever so beautiful. There is no place like home.

Baum LF. The Wonderful Wizard of Oz. *Chicago, IL: George M. Hill Co.; 1900.*

OBJECTIVES

At the completion of this chapter the reader will be prepared to:
1. Describe home health, palliative care and hospice, public health, nurse-managed health centers, and other practice models

2. Summarize the supporting electronic health records (EHRs) and information systems used at practice sites
3. Specify the value of the clinical data and information that can be generated by information systems used at practice sites

KEY TERMS

ABSTRACT

Home care and related community-based systems located in the United States are changing rapidly. Information technology is accelerating those changes. This chapter will address: (1) home health, palliative care and hospice, public health, nurse-managed health centers, and other practice models; (2) the electronic health records (EHRs) and information systems used at practice sites; and (3) the value of the clinical data and information that can be generated by these information systems. Core values of community-based clinicians include patient-centered care and services that are of high quality, efficient, and cost effective. Information systems began with billing systems and evolved to point-of-care solutions in the 1990s. Outcome and Assessment Information Set (OASIS) and patient experience surveys are examples of home health standardized datasets. Using standardized terminologies is another strategy that complements community-based core values. The Omaha System, one of the standardized terminologies recognized by the American Nurses Association, is described and a clinical example illustrates how practice, documentation, and information management can enhance the quality of care.

INTRODUCTION

Home care and related community-based systems located in the United States are changing rapidly and becoming increasingly visible to the healthcare community. Information technology (IT) and related technological advances are accelerating these changes. Numerous references describe home health research, economics, and patient personal preference, suggesting that the home is the optimal location for diverse health and nursing services.[1-6] Patient residences include houses, apartments, dormitories, trailers, boarding and care homes, hospice houses, assisted living facilities, shelters, and cars. Although residences are the primary location where care is provided, many home care and related community-based organizations offer services at workplaces, schools, churches, community buildings, and other sites.

This chapter addresses home health, palliative care and hospice, public health, nurse-managed health centers, and other practice models; the supporting electronic health records (EHRs) and information systems used at the practice sites; and the value of the clinical data and information that can be generated by these information systems. The assessment, planning, intervention, and evaluation services that are part of these models range from promoting wellness and preventing disease to care of the sick and dying. Ideally these services are captured in EHRs so that they can be quantified, analyzed, and used to measure the outcomes of care. Formal caregivers include nurses, social workers, physical and occupational therapists, speech-language pathologists, registered dietitians, home health aides, chaplains, physicians, and others. A team approach and interprofessional collaboration are required to address the intensity of the patient's and family's needs.

EVOLUTION AND MILESTONES

Home health and community-based systems have a long and distinguished history in this country. In the early years care for those who were ill or dying was typically informal and provided by the women who lived in the household or neighborhood. Home health provided by formal caregivers originated in the 1800s and was based on the district nursing model developed by William Rathbone in England. In many communities the initial programs evolved into visiting nurse associations. The movement expanded rapidly in the United States, resulting in the formation of 71 agencies prior to 1900 and 600 by 1909.[7-9]

In 1893 Lillian Wald and Mary Brewster established the Henry Street Settlement House in New York City and developed a comprehensive program that was staffed by nurses and social workers. One of Wald's more impressive innovations was to convince the Metropolitan Life Insurance Company to include home visits as a benefit and to examine the cost effectiveness of care, a partnership that continued until 1952.[7,9,10]

Public health departments were established and expanded during the early years of the twentieth century. Health department staff members were primarily nurses who focused on immigrants, milk banks for mothers and babies, communicable disease, and environmental issues. They were concerned about consistent practice standards, the patient record, and the collection of statistics.[10,11]

Home health services were included as a major benefit when Medicare legislation was enacted in 1965 and resulted in significant changes nationally. The benefit was designed to provide intermittent, shorter visits with temporary lengths of stay to persons age 65 and older; health promotion and long-term care services were not reimbursed. Although nurses continued to represent the largest group of agency staff members, involvement of other professions was required. When a patient was admitted to service, the home health agency was required to develop a plan of care, obtain the signature of a physician, and follow additional regulations.[12]

Hospice care was introduced in the 1970s. Florence Wald is acknowledged as the founder of the hospice movement; she established the Connecticut Hospice with interprofessional staff. The concept of hospice grew from a commitment to provide compassionate and dignified care to people who were at the end stage of life; the program offered care in the comfort of home with an emphasis on quality of life. Medicaid reimbursement for hospice care began in 1980 and Medicare reimbursement began in 1983; reimbursement determines many aspects of the hospice programs.[11,13]

Nurses employed in home health and community-based settings were concerned about documentation, standardization, and accountability in addition to practice. Their concerns were similar to those of other healthcare professionals. Physicians advanced systems for nomenclature and classification beginning with the International Classification of Diseases (ICD) in 1893. In 1966 Avedis Donabedian, a physician, described the well-known structure, process, and outcome framework for evaluating the quality of medical care.[14] Another physician, Lawrence Weed, developed a problem-oriented medical record in 1968 that was adaptable to computerization.[15] In 1986 Mary Elizabeth Tinetti developed and published a tool to measure mobility problems in elderly patients.[16] In 1990 Pamela Duncan developed a balance measure referred to as functional reach that is especially useful for her physical therapist colleagues who work in community settings. Functional reach can serve as a measure of frailty in elders to predict fall risk and help identify appropriate interventions.[17]

PRACTICE MODELS

Home Health

Home health is the delivery of intermittent health-related services in patients' places of residence with the goal of promoting self-care and independence rather than institutionalization. The intensity of services has increased dramatically as hospital stays have become shorter and patients are discharged with serious illnesses or soon after surgery and with complex treatment needs. The care delivered often focuses on supporting a safe transition back to the home following an episode of illness or exacerbation that required an inpatient or extended care facility stay.

Home health interventions include medication reconciliation; teaching and coaching to improve the ability of patients, families, and caregivers to manage independently; coordination of care with other healthcare providers and community resources; and early detection of decline or exacerbation. Common treatments and procedures now include ventilators, renal hemodialysis, and intravenous therapy for antibiotics, chemotherapy, and analgesia as well as delivery of total parenteral nutrition and blood products.

According to the Centers for Medicare & Medicaid Services (CMS) and the National Association for Home Care & Hospice, an estimated 11,633 Medicare-certified home health agencies operated across the country in 2011.[3,18] As the largest payer, Medicare accounted for 41% of total home health reimbursement. Medicaid, state and local governments, private pay, and private insurance are the other sources. Home health agencies provided services to approximately 12 million patients who ranged in age from infants to elders. Persons 65 years and older accounted for more than 86% of all home health patients. Recipients of home health services had diverse needs but circulatory disease was the most common diagnosis, followed by endocrine and nutritional diseases (diabetes) and diseases of the musculoskeletal system.

Palliative Care and Hospice

Palliative care and hospice involve the delivery of services by teams of interprofessional clinicians for those who have exhausted curative treatment measures or have life expectancies of 6 months or less. Both involve holistic care, an emphasis on dignity, and being surrounded by the comfort of home and family. However, the programs have differences. Typically, palliative care services focus on comfort, quality of life, and end-of-life or advanced care planning. Hospice involves symptom management with the goal of providing as much comfort and dignity as possible at the end of life. Hospice programs include bereavement follow-up for families after a patient's death. In this country a stigma may be associated with end-of-life care. It is associated with giving up and the refusal to accept death as a natural process, although this is changing as evidenced by the growth in hospice programs.

According to the Hospice Association of America[2] and the National Association for Home Care & Hospice,[3] there were approximately 3533 Medicare-certified hospices in 2011. Slightly more than 1 million patients received Medicare-certified hospice services in 2008, with an average stay of 83 days. The average length of stay is increasing as hospice becomes more widely accepted. As the largest payer, Medicare accounted for 84% of hospice expenditures in 2008, with Medicaid and private insurance paying the rest.

Public Health

The basis of public health practice is the individual, family, and community. Public health nurses and other clinicians provide services that address and include health education and wellness campaigns, immunization clinics, screening events, parent–child health and safety, communicable disease, family planning, environmental health, substance use, and sexually transmitted disease. Approximately 2800 city, county, metropolitan, district, and tribal health departments exist in the U.S. Since 2008, local health departments have lost 34,000 of 155,000 positions due to layoffs and attrition. Many public health nursing positions have been lost due to budget cuts.[19] In this chapter the emphasis is on computerization to support these types of public health services that are provided to individuals and families in the community.

Public health services can also be directed toward the community with a focus on the whole population and primary prevention. Principles of public health and epidemiology or causality, as well as community assessment and public policy, are usually components of these types of public health programs. Chapter 11 focuses on public health informatics with an emphasis on population health of communities and countries and global health.

Nurse-Managed Health Centers

Community health nurses as well as advanced practice registered nurses, including clinical nurse specialists, nurse practitioners, and certified nurse midwives, provide care at urban and rural centers called nurse-managed health centers. These centers may have collaborative agreements with physicians and other interprofessional colleagues. Many centers are part of or associated with educational institutions and provide clinical experiences for students and are located in underserved areas. Target populations include pregnant teens, fragile elders, low-income mothers and children, and others who may be underinsured or uninsured. Nurse-managed health centers offer primary care services, preventive care, chronic illness care, and care for specific conditions such as obesity. More than 250 centers exist in the U.S.; Philadelphia has more than any other city.[20]

Other Practice Sites

School, faith community, and occupational health nurses as well as other clinicians provide healthcare in noninstitutional settings. School nurses typically participate in classroom instruction, screen the school setting for safety hazards, provide medications in collaboration with parents and healthcare providers, monitor immunization status, and provide and follow up on screening procedures. Faith community nurses may function as case managers when they help their parishioners to obtain needed healthcare services, food, shelter, and supplies. Some provide educational and surveillance interventions for those who have chronic illnesses such as diabetes and cardiovascular disease. Occupational health nurses are often employed by businesses with a high risk of injury or with an emphasis on health promotion and wellness such as smoking cessation, weight loss, and regular exercise.

Similarities among Practice Models

Because community-based clinicians have the opportunity to work with patients and their families over time, they embrace core values that influence their practice. Interprofessional collaboration and a seamless healthcare environment are essential. Practice is based on the consumer movement: people have rights and responsibilities, must be knowledgeable about their own healthcare, and must participate as partners in healthcare decisions. These values are linked to themes of access, cost, quality, and IT.

The power of the patient and family is an important core value. When a nurse or other healthcare professional enters a patient's home, the patient and family are in charge, not the clinician. Clinicians immediately observe indicators and collect data about patients' lifestyles, resources, and motivation. While providing care clinicians identify patients' strengths and incorporate those strengths in the care process. The goal of community-based practice settings is to provide patient-centered care and include patients, their families, and their caregivers in care planning and delivery. In the hospital or long-term care facility, the nurse gives medications, changes dressings, and controls many aspects of care. In the home, nurses assist patients to provide their own care or assist family members or informal caregivers to provide that care.[11,21,22]

Clinicians who work in community settings need skills that demonstrate dedication, flexibility, and independence. Although they develop plans for their day and for each visit or encounter, those plans often need to be adapted and modified. It may not be possible to accomplish Plan A, so Plan B, C, or D may be substituted at a moment's notice. Colleagues, equipment, and references are not readily available to the extent that they are in hospitals and long-term care facilities. Selected help and supplies may be available in the trunk of a car or via cellphone, EHR, Internet, or pager request. Clinicians always need to consider their safety. Environments may be difficult, dysfunctional, or even dangerous. Many patients and families welcome clinicians, although that does not always happen. Clinicians need to develop and rely on their basic education, ongoing education, life experiences, and common sense to function self-sufficiently and to enjoy their work responsibilities.

The Triple Aim model for healthcare was published in 2008 (Box 9-1). However, the primary concepts of the model have been the foundation and core values of home health and related community-based services from their inception: services that are patient centered, of high quality, efficient, and cost effective. Although the size, staffing, organization, board structure, and financial arrangements of the practice models summarized in this chapter vary markedly, all deal with limited financial resources. In contrast to clinicians who work in hospitals or long-term care facilities, clinicians who work in community settings must be very knowledgeable about costs and funding. Frequently they help patients and families understand and manage health-related financial issues. In many situations Medicare and Medicaid funding regulations are the primary determinant of the type and length of home health and hospice services. Private insurance companies determine their own guidelines but typically follow Medicare's policies. Ever-changing regulations and reimbursement patterns, interest in private pay services, and the aging population contribute to altered services. Agencies that provide Medicare- and Medicaid-certified services must meet strict national regulations. Most states have additional licensing rules.[12]

STANDARDIZED DATASETS

Standardized datasets are used frequently in home health settings and are becoming more common in hospice and other community-based settings. The concept of a standardized dataset in the community began more than 20 years ago with the Resident Assessment Instrument (RAI). The adoption of this approach began in response to a public outcry about the poor quality of care occurring in long-term or extended nursing facilities and to the government's effort to bring visibility and transparency to care provided in these institutions. Over time the use of standardized datasets has expanded from long-term care to home health, renal dialysis units, and other care settings. This approach provides a means to collect patient characteristics and measurements in a standardized manner that allows data aggregation for analysis. The aggregated data offer the opportunity for data-driven decision making related to care delivery and correlating payment systems to a predicted level of care needed by the patient.[23]

Standardized datasets have evolved largely in the absence of adoption of standardized point-of-care and reference terminologies in practice settings. While standardized terminologies have existed for more than 40 years, adoption in practice has been limited and even more limited among the information systems commonly purchased by home health, hospice, and other community-based care settings. While standardized datasets have served an important and valuable purpose over the last 30-plus years, they will not position healthcare providers to achieve the care communication and coordination necessary to transform healthcare and achieve the Triple Aim for healthcare (see Box 9-1). These local datasets will continue to exist but they will not provide a successful strategy to help the health system evolve into one that is designed to deliver optimal best practices and evidence-based care by an interprofessional care team.[24]

| BOX 9-1 | THE TRIPLE AIM FOR HEALTHCARE |

- Better care for individuals, described by the six dimensions of healthcare performance: safety, effectiveness, patient-centeredness, timeliness, efficiency, and equity.
- Better health for populations, through attacking "the upstream causes of so much of our ill health," such as poor nutrition, physical inactivity, and substance abuse.
- Reducing per-capita costs.

Adapted from Berwick DM, Nolan TW, Whittington J. The Triple Aim: care, health, and cost. *Health Affair.* 2008;27(3):759-769.

Outcome and Assessment Information Set (OASIS)

The Outcome and Assessment Information Set (OASIS) is the standardized dataset that home health agency clinicians complete with their patients.[25] It is designed to determine payment and measure the quality and outcomes of practice. OASIS consists of 80-plus questions and response sets; collection requirements vary according to specific times during the process of care (i.e., admission, transfer, resumption of care, follow-up, or discharge). An example of a question is M1240: Has the patient had a formal Pain Assessment using a standardized pain assessment tool? A second example is M1242: Frequency of Pain interfering with patient's activities or movement.

Public reporting, another benefit of the data and outcomes collected using the OASIS dataset, began in 2003. It allows the general public to compare the outcomes of home health agencies in a local community to the state and national outcome averages.[26]

The OASIS dataset has undergone three major revisions and is currently known as OASIS-C.[25] Each major revision has involved modifications to the data collected, including exclusions, modifications, and additions. The latest iteration of the expanded dataset included reporting on key process measures. These measures represent measures that are harmonized across care settings for purposes of data collection and analysis. The next revision of OASIS is expected to include changes to support implementation of the ICD-10-CM planned for October 1, 2014.

Continuity Assessment Record and Evaluation (CARE) Tool

The Continuity Assessment Record and Evaluation (CARE) Tool evolved as part of the Post Acute Care Payment Reform Demonstration to establish a standardized dataset that can predict the appropriate level of care or care setting that supports optimal patient outcomes at the lowest possible cost.[27] The patient information section of the CARE Tool includes four domains: medical, functional, cognitive impairments, and social and environmental factors. The tool contains two types of core items (asked for every patient) and supplemental items (asked for patients with specific conditions). A sample is available at www.pacdemo.rti.org/UserFiles/File/Home_Health_Admission_CARE_Tool_Sample_12-10-09.pdf. In addition, the CARE Tool is designed to collect the costs of providing care to the Medicare and medically complex patient populations by including the Cost and Resource Utilization (CRU) data collection instrument that correlates patient characteristics with the costs of care in various settings.

The CARE project resulted from the Deficit Reduction Act of 2005, which directed the CMS to develop a Payment Reform Demonstration using standardized patient information to examine the consistency of payment to Medicare populations in various settings. It was expanded to include Medicaid and State Children's Health Insurance Program (SCHIP) in 2007. The final report of the CARE project was completed in 2012. It supports using a standardized approach to collecting and measuring patient characteristics across care settings. This approach has the potential to change payment methodologies between and among care settings to better align the care delivered and paid for with the desired value-based purchasing initiatives.[27]

Hospice Quality Measures

The Affordable Care Act of 2010 required that the Secretary of Health and Human Services publish, no later than October 1, 2012, the selected quality measures that must be reported by hospice programs. However, the approach to develop a standardized dataset for hospice agencies has been industry driven rather than mandated by the CMS. The Conditions of Participation for Hospice, effective in 2008, describe the expectation that the hospice industry determine the appropriate measures to collect and report nationally.[28] This approach reflects the fact that hospices had been collecting and reporting key quality measures through their associations and other data analysis partners for almost 20 years.[29] The CMS has mandated that hospices begin their reporting processes with two measures: one that is patient related and one that is structural. It is expected that the number of measures will increase as the industry continues to identify, propose, and refine a dataset. That dataset will probably incorporate frequently used tools such as the National Data Set for Hospice, Family Evaluations of Care, Survey of Team Attitudes and Relationships, and End Result Outcome Measures. The dataset may also reflect the results of the Prepare, Embrace, Attend, Communicate, Empower (PEACE) demonstration projects in the Carolinas and New York as well as the Palliative Care Quality Measures Project and the Assessment, Intervention, Measurement (AIM) Project.[30] Currently, a date has not been set for public reporting of hospice quality measures but penalties for failing to submit agreed-upon data are scheduled to begin in 2014.

Patient Experience Surveys

Home health agencies, skilled nursing facilities, and dialysis centers are required to submit patient experience surveys. These surveys, referred to as Consumer Assessment of Healthcare Providers and Systems (CAHPS), are designed to measure the interpersonal value of healthcare experienced by patients and contribute to their ability to make informed decisions about health plans and care providers.[31] Surveys provide an additional source of standardized data for aggregation and offer visibility and transparency about the care provided. It is expected that they will become increasingly important in the future because patient experience represents one of the key tenets of the Triple Aim for healthcare (see Box 9-1).

SUPPORTING HOME HEALTH WITH ELECTRONIC HEALTH RECORDS AND HEALTH INFORMATION TECHNOLOGY

Challenges related to distance, communication, productivity, and interprofessional practice are inherent in home health and related community-based services. Because of these challenges, agency providers are embracing technology that facilitates communication and collaboration, such as cellular telephones, telehealth, remote patient monitoring, fall detection device technology, sophisticated information systems, and point-of-care devices. The point-of-care devices are designed to make patient records available in the home when care is being provided and capture clinicians' documentation in real time, thereby supporting that care. These are national and global trends.[22,25,32-35]

The core values and practice models of community-based services have direct implications for technology and information systems. Systems must be designed to support the data, information, knowledge, and wisdom continuum as described in Chapter 2 and have interprofessional practice with the patient, family, and community as the central focus.[36-39]

Information systems used in community practice settings are evolving into next-generation systems. Software vendors are exploring the relationship of the design and function of their systems to improve their capabilities to support interprofessional practice, communication and collaboration, clinical decision support, and the ability to share information across care settings. Vendors and their healthcare provider customers not only are starting to share information with other providers, but also are encouraging patients to use personal health records to store their data in a longitudinal care record and plan.[37,40] In addition, information systems are viewed as a critical factor to achieving the Triple Aim for healthcare (see Box 9-1). Next-generation systems are expected to support the simplicity and connectivity that are essential to connecting caregivers across diverse locations and care settings. Interoperability and data exchange are required if all members of the healthcare team engage in a ubiquitous approach to care planning, collaboration, transparency, and efficiency in health care.[41]

Information systems were adopted by home health agencies in the early 1980s. The development and use of these systems in home health, hospice, and other community-based settings have generally evolved in the following historical sequence to (1) support billing, (2) collect data at the point of patient care to support the financial needs of the business, (3) manage and support collection of standard clinical datasets, and (4) provide clinical decision support. This evolution is analogous to the progression described in the data, information, knowledge, and wisdom continuum.

Billing Solutions

Initially, data within systems moved in one direction from the home health, hospice, or community-based agency to the third-party payer as an electronic claim. The payer, upon receiving the claim, reviewed and paid the claim. As financial systems and electronic capabilities advanced, bidirectional exchange of claims information management became commonplace. This allowed the payer to receive the electronic claim and return an acknowledgement of payment to the healthcare provider electronically.

Point-of-Care Solutions

The next milestone for information systems used by home health agencies and, to a lesser degree, hospices occurred as agencies recognized the value of capturing the clinicians' documentation that supported the interaction with the patient at the point of care. The principal value of these systems was to enable electronic capture of the service date and time for billing and payroll purposes.

In 1998 the value of point-of-care systems changed for home health agencies as a result of Medicare's transition from a cost-based reimbursement system to a prospective payment system. The prospective payment system was predicated on the use of a standardized assessment dataset designed to predict the patient's resource needs; the results of the dataset were associated with a payment rate. The standardized dataset became known as the Outcome and Assessment Information Set (OASIS) and was discussed earlier in this chapter.

Agencies that were computerized expected their software vendors to incorporate the OASIS dataset into their point-of-care systems to enable their clinicians to capture the information once, prepare, and then submit to their respective states for aggregation by the CMS. Home health agencies that had not adopted point-of-care solutions experienced a significant data entry burden to remain in compliance with regulations. As a result, agencies accelerated their adoption of point-of-care information systems and EHRs as a strategy to reduce the regulatory burden and streamline their operations.

In addition to supporting the change in payment methodology, the collection of the OASIS dataset created an opportunity to introduce an outcomes-based quality improvement (OBQI) process to home health. OBQI is a risk-adjusted and outcome reporting tool used across time and is viewed as a means to further move the risk from the payer to the healthcare provider by assigning a value-based purchasing facet to the model. OBQI represents the next step in evolving the payment system from fee for service to capitation or payment for care of a population. Figure 9-1 depicts a continuum that illustrates the onset of CMS reimbursement through the transition of payment risk from the payer to the healthcare provider.

As adoption of OBQI grew, provider agency managers and administrators recognized the value of mining OASIS data and converting it to information in order to support business and operational decision making in their organizations. The information was transformed into knowledge involving the care their staff delivered, potential opportunities for improvement, and marketing their successes.[36,39]

Currently, hospice agencies do not have a mandated standardized dataset and reporting requirements. However, hospices have worked closely with the CMS, their associations, and benchmarking companies to establish and develop a set of standard data points for collection. They are poised to move along the data, information, knowledge, and wisdom continuum and embrace information systems that can support their evolution. A natural result of having

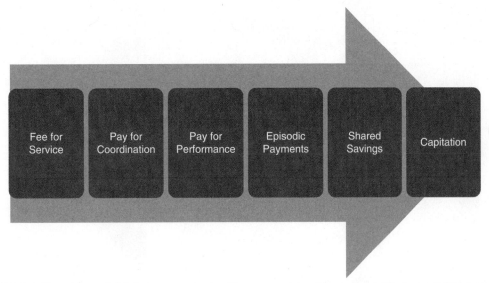

| Fee for Service | Pay for Coordination | Pay for Performance | Episodic Payments | Shared Savings | Capitation |

FIG 9-1 Transition of risk from payer to healthcare provider. (Centers for Medicare & Medicaid Services [CMS]. Oasis-C educational resources. CMS. http://www.cms.gov/Medicare/Quality-Initiatives-Patient-Assessment-Instruments/HomeHealthQualityInits/EducationalResources.html. 2010.)

information represented by OASIS and OBQI is the desire to understand the following three questions:

- What is causing the outcomes?
- How can the outcomes be improved?
- How much improvement can realistically be expected?

Efforts to answer these questions have identified the need to know more about the processes being used to deliver care, specifically what care processes contributed to positive clinical outcomes. The knowledge of the outcomes has resulted in a need for increased predictability, visibility, and transparency in the use of best practices and evidence-based practice protocols.

In 2010 the OASIS dataset was revised to improve the quality of responses to outcome questions. Specifically, 16 process measures were added to the dataset. The data collected about these process measures are intended to clarify how best practices and evidence-based practice affect outcomes.[42-43] As illustrated in Figure 9-2, the CMS and other payers are using this knowledge to transition to payment methodologies that support value-based purchasing, bundled payments, and accountable care, each of which are contributing to the increasing need for payer and agency provider collaboration to ensure the best possible patient outcomes at the lowest possible costs.[44-45] This transition has already had an impact on practice and is predicted to have an even greater impact in the future.

Clinical Decision Support (CDS) Systems

Clinical decision support (CDS) systems may be the next frontier for home health and other related community-based practice settings. Rouse described these systems as applications that analyze data and help healthcare providers make clinical decisions.[46] CDS systems generally use one of two approaches: (1) presenting best practices and evidence-based practice options to the clinician by finding and displaying what is known about the patient to a knowledge base using rule sets and an interface engine, or (2) using a process of machine learning that presents or displays best practices and evidence-based practice options to the clinician after analyzing the data entered and comparing them to similar patterns or scenarios that exist in the system. These systems have been challenging to implement because they are dependent on understanding the clinicians' workflow. Clinicians' workflow usually varies among clients and lacks structured clinical concepts, characteristics that are required to develop a knowledge base or machine learning.[46] In addition, standardized terminologies are required to develop effective CDS systems. The next goal for CDS systems is to achieve rapid learning systems that can support quick and widespread adoption of evidence-based practice. When these learning systems are used, the time needed to implement best practices and evidence-based practice will be significantly reduced. Reaching this goal will require health information networks that are capable of collecting and supporting analysis of large amounts of data in simple, clear terms and returning the findings to clinicians though CDS systems at the point of care.[40] See Chapter 10 for a more detailed discussion of CDS systems.

STANDARDIZED TERMINOLOGIES

The American Nurses Association (ANA) recognizes 12 reference and point-of-care or interface terminologies. These terminologies are described in detail in Chapter 22 and the references that accompany that chapter. As noted by the Alliance for Nursing Informatics, the use of standardized nursing

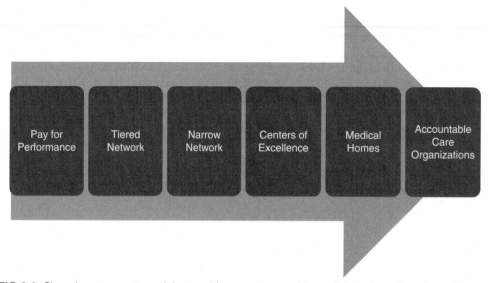

FIG 9-2 Changing payment models to achieve payer–provider collaboration. (Data from Nugent M. Achieving payer-provider collaboration in payment reform. Navigant. http://www.navigant. com/Insights/Library/Industry_News/Achieving_Payer_Provider_Collaboration_091911. September 19, 2011.)

and other health terminologies "is necessary and a prerequisite for decision support, discovery of disparities, outcomes reporting, improving performance, maintaining accurate lists of problems and medications, and the general use of and reuse of information needed for quality, safety, and efficiency."[47(p66)] It is critical that point-of-care terminologies are mapped to reference terminologies to enable current and future interoperability and data sharing described in this chapter. The point-of-care terminologies recognized by the ANA have been or are being mapped.

Ideally students are introduced to the 12 terminologies in their entry programs and clinical sites during their basic education and become somewhat familiar with them. In addition, students should understand the difference between reference terminologies, including Systematized Nomenclature of Medicine—Clinical Terms (SNOMED CT) and Logical Observation Identifier Names and Codes (LOINC), and point-of-care terminologies as discussed in Chapter 22.

Similarities and differences are evident when the terminologies are compared and contrasted.[48-50] Those that are especially pertinent to this chapter are summarized. Many authors note that while point-of-care terminologies were initially intended for use in specific settings (i.e., community, acute, or long-term care), healthcare delivery has changed dramatically and boundaries have blurred. It is possible to implement most of the terminologies across the continuum of care. Developing a structure that is computer compatible was not an initial goal in the development of all point-of-care terminologies. With the IT explosion and proliferation of software vendors, relationships are evolving between the terminologies and software developers of clinical information systems. When discussing point-of-care terminologies it is important to remember the distinction between the terminologies and the individual software applications that may incorporate a terminology. One terminology may become the foundation of systems for multiple developers and vendors.

OMAHA SYSTEM

The Omaha System is an example of a point-of-care terminology recognized by the ANA that is mapped to SNOMED CT and LOINC. Omaha was initially developed for home health use and is used in this chapter to demonstrate the use of a point-of-care terminology in the practice models discussed in this chapter. It was also initially developed to operationalize the nursing problem-solving process and to provide a practical, easily understood, computer-compatible guide for daily use in community settings. From the initial home health, hospice, public health, and school health focus, adoption began to expand in the 1990s with both automated applications and paper-and-pen forms. Current use represents the continuum of care and has extended far beyond the early community-based settings. More than 9000 interprofessional clinicians, educators, and researchers use the Omaha System in the U.S. and a number of other countries and more than 2000 clinicians use paper-and-pen forms. Details about the application, users, clinical examples (case studies), inclusion in reference terminologies, research, best practices and evidence-based practice, and listserv are described in publications and on the website (www.omahasystem.org).[22,52]

Description

The Omaha System consists of the Problem Classification Scheme, the Intervention Scheme, and the Problem Rating Scale for Outcomes. Reliability, validity, and usability were established when the fourth federally funded research project was completed in 1993 (Box 9-2). The three components, designed to be used together, are comprehensive, relatively

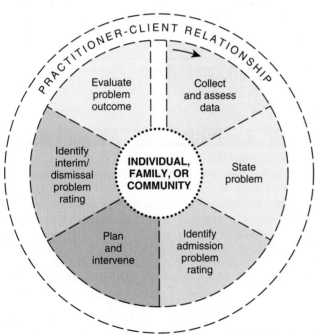

FIG 9-3 Omaha System model of the problem-solving process. (From Martin KS. The Omaha System: *A key to practice, documentation, and information management.* Reprinted 2nd ed. Omaha, NE: Health Connections Press; 2005.)

simple, hierarchical, multidimensional, and computer compatible. Since the first developmental research project in 1975, the Omaha System has existed in the public domain; thus the terms, definitions, and codes are not held under copyright. They are available for use without permission from the publisher or developers and without a licensing fee. However, the terms and structure must be used as published.[22,52]

The conceptual model is based on the dynamic, interactive nature of the problem-solving process, the clinician–client relationship, and concepts of diagnostic reasoning, clinical judgment, and quality improvement (Figure 9-3). The patient as an individual, a family, or a community appears at the center of the model, reflecting a patient-centered approach. The central location suggests the many ways in which the system can be used, the importance of the patient, and the essential partnership between patients and clinicians.

The system was intended for use by nurses and all members of healthcare delivery teams. The goals of the research were to (1) develop a structured and comprehensive system that could be both understood and used by members of various disciplines and (2) foster collaborative practice. Therefore the system was designed to guide practice decisions, sort and document pertinent patient data uniformly, and provide a framework for an agency-wide, interprofessional clinical information management system capable of meeting the daily needs of clinicians, managers, and administrators.[22,52-54]

Problem Classification Scheme

The Problem Classification Scheme is a comprehensive, orderly, nonexhaustive, mutually exclusive taxonomy designed to identify diverse patients' health-related concerns. Its simple and concrete terms are used to organize a comprehensive assessment, an important standard of interprofessional practice. The Problem Classification Scheme consists of four levels. Four domains appear at the first level and represent priority areas. Forty-two terms, referred to as client problems or areas of patient needs and strengths, appear at the second level. The third level consists of two sets of problem modifiers: health promotion, potential and actual, as well as individual, family, and community. Clusters of signs and symptoms describe actual problems at the fourth level. The content and relationship of the domain and problem levels are outlined in Box 9-3 and are further illustrated by the clinical example in Box 9-4. Understanding the meaning of and relationships among the terms is a prerequisite to using the scheme accurately and consistently to collect, sort, document, analyze, quantify, and communicate patient needs and strengths.

Intervention Scheme

The Intervention Scheme is a comprehensive, orderly, nonexhaustive, mutually exclusive taxonomy designed for use with specific problems. It consists of three levels of actions or activities that are the basis for care planning and intervention, providing the structure and terms to organize care plans and actual care. An important standard of interprofessional practice is providing interventions and leaving a data trail about the care that was provided. Four broad categories of interventions appear at the first level of the Intervention Scheme. An alphabetical list of 75 targets or objects of action and 1 "other" appear at the second level. Client-specific information

---

BOX 9-3　DOMAINS AND PROBLEMS OF THE OMAHA SYSTEM PROBLEM CLASSIFICATION SCHEME

Environmental Domain

Material resources and physical surroundings both inside and outside the living area, neighborhood, and broader community:

- Income
- Sanitation
- Residence
- Neighborhood/workplace safety

Psychosocial Domain

Patterns of behavior, emotion, communication, relationships, and development:

- Communication with community resources
- Social contact
- Role change
- Interpersonal relationship
- Spirituality
- Grief
- Mental health
- Sexuality
- Caretaking/parenting
- Neglect
- Abuse
- Growth and development

Physiological Domain

Functions and processes that maintain life:

- Hearing
- Vision
- Speech and language
- Oral health
- Cognition
- Pain
- Consciousness
- Skin
- Neuro-musculo-skeletal function
- Respiration
- Circulation
- Digestion-hydration
- Bowel function
- Urinary function
- Reproductive function
- Pregnancy
- Postpartum
- Communicable/infectious condition

Health-Related Behaviors Domain

Patterns of activity that maintain or promote wellness, promote recovery, and decrease the risk of disease:

- Nutrition
- Sleep and rest patterns
- Physical activity
- Personal care
- Substance use
- Family planning
- Health care supervision
- Medication regimen

From Martin KS. *The Omaha System: A Key to Practice, Documentation, and Information Management.* Reprinted 2nd ed. Omaha, NE: Health Connections Press; 2005.

BOX 9-4　JOHN T. LITTLE: MAN WHO RECEIVED HOME HEALTH SERVICES

Kelly S. Nelson, PT, DPT, PCS
Assistant Professor, Department of Physical Therapy and Assistant Director, Creighton Pediatric Therapy
School of Pharmacy and Health Professions, Creighton University
Omaha, Nebraska

Information Obtained during the First Visit/Encounter

John T. Little, aged 79 years, had a fracture of his left femur that was surgically repaired with a pin two weeks ago. John spent five days in the acute care hospital followed by nine days at the subacute rehabilitation facility. He was discharged to his home yesterday.

During the home health nurse's first visit, John's wife seemed relatively well informed. In John's presence she stated, "I am going to need help caring for him. It's a difficult time for us." The nurse summarized the agency's services including interprofessional providers, and the goals of care for both Mr. and Mrs. Little. The couple agreed when the nurse suggested that a home health aide visit to provide personal care.

John was resting in a hospital bed with an overhead trapeze and removable side rails. The equipment was set up before he came home. He moved in the bed with difficulty and needed assistance to roll or sit up. Mrs. Little could not find the mobility technique instructions that they were given yesterday. John, his wife, and the nurse discussed plans and goals for the physical therapist's visit later today and the occupational therapist's visit tomorrow.

The nurse indicated that the surgical site and John's skin were in excellent condition, and offered evidence-based suggestions about bed mobility and prevention of skin shearing and breakdown. Mrs. Little reported that she could manage John's diet, fluid intake, and elimination. She said she would appreciate the use of a raised toilet seat and a shower chair.

Although John was reluctant to admit that he had pain, he rated it as a 4 on a 0 to 10 pain scale. Mrs. Little administered pain medication at least three times a day and as needed, indicating that she "would not wait for John to look miserable." She described how she evaluated John's pain and would use the pain scale as the nurse instructed. The nurse showed Mrs. Little a web site describing evidence-based pain management, and gave her some printed instructional materials. Mrs. Little agreed to keep the nurse informed as John's need for pain medications changed and if other symptoms such as constipation occurred. The nurse mentioned several methods for achieving non-pharmacological pain relief and asked the couple to discuss their preferences before the nurse's next visit. They said they would do so.

BOX 9-4 **JOHN T. LITTLE: MAN WHO RECEIVED HOME HEALTH SERVICES—cont'd**

Application of the Omaha System:
Domain: Physiological
Problem: Pain (High Priority Problem)
Problem Classification Scheme
Modifiers: Individual and Actual
- Signs/Symptoms of Actual: expresses discomfort/pain
- compensated movement/guarding

Intervention Scheme
Category: Teaching, Guidance, and Counseling
Targets and client-specific information:
- anatomy/physiology (diagnosis and surgery in relation to pain, joint, and pain management)
- relaxation/breathing techniques (consider options and decide)
Category: Surveillance
Targets and client-specific information:
- signs/symptoms—mental/emotional (attitude, emotions)
- signs/symptoms—physical (ability/willingness to move)

Problem Rating Scale for Outcomes
Knowledge: 3—basic knowledge (knows pain causes, need for medication, but not other options)
Behavior: 3—inconsistent knowledge (not tried additional options for pain relief, but willing)
Status: 3—moderate signs/symptoms (caused by injury and surgery)

Problem: Neuro-Musculo-Skeletal Function
(High Priority Problem)
Problem Classification Scheme
Modifiers: Individual and Actual
Signs/Symptoms of Actual:
- limited range of motion
- gait/ambulation disturbance
- difficulty transferring
- fractures

Intervention Scheme
Category: Teaching, Guidance, and Counseling
Targets and client-specific information:
- occupational therapy care (plan of care)
- physical therapy care (plan of care)
Category: Surveillance
- durable medical equipment (bed set-up adequate, needs raised toilet seat and shower chair)
- mobility/transfers (bed mobility)
- signs/symptoms—physical (surgical site, skin condition)

Problem Rating Scale for Outcomes
Knowledge: 3—basic knowledge (recalls some instructions, can't find handout)

Behavior: 2—rarely appropriate behavior (limited mobility/activity)
Status: 2—severe signs/symptoms (minimal activity)

Domain: Health-Related Behaviors
Problem: Personal CARE (High Priority Problem)
Problem Classification Scheme
Modifiers: Individual and Actual
Signs/Symptoms of Actual:
- difficulty with bathing
- difficulty with toileting activities
- difficulty dressing lower body
- difficulty dressing upper body
- difficulty shampooing/combing hair

Intervention Scheme
Category: Case Management
Targets and client-specific information:
- paraprofessional/aide care (schedule 3 times/week)

Problem Rating Scale for Outcomes
Knowledge: 4—adequate knowledge (knows help needed)
Behavior: 4—usually appropriate behavior (requested assistance)
Status: 2—severe signs/symptoms (care is difficult because of John's physical condition)

Problem: Medication Regimen
Problem Classification Scheme
Modifiers: Individual and Actual
Signs/Symptoms of Actual:
- unable to take medications without help

Intervention Scheme
Category: Teaching, Guidance, and Counseling
Targets and client-specific information:
- medication action/side effects (reports of pain, movement, non-verbal cues)
- medication administration (scheduling doses appropriately)
Category: Surveillance
Targets and client-specific information:
- signs/symptoms—physical (discussed effectiveness, constipation, other symptoms; will use pain scale)

Problem Rating Scale for Outcomes
Knowledge: 4—adequate knowledge (informed about pain medication, watch for changing needs)
Behavior: 4—usually appropriate behavior (good administration schedule)
Status: 3—moderate signs/symptoms (pain scale = 4)

---

generated by practitioners is at the third level. The contents of the category and target levels are outlined in Boxes 9-5 and 9-6, respectively, and are further illustrated by the clinical example in Box 9-4. The Intervention Scheme enables practitioners to describe, quantify, and communicate their practice, including improving or restoring health, describing deterioration, or preventing illness.

Problem Rating Scale for Outcomes

The Problem Rating Scale for Outcomes consists of three five-point, Likert-type scales used to measure the entire range of severity for the concepts of Knowledge, Behavior, and Status. Each of the subscales is a continuum that provides a framework for measuring and comparing problem-specific patient outcomes at regular or predictable times. Evaluation

---

BOX 9-5   **CATEGORIES OF THE OMAHA SYSTEM INTERVENTION SCHEME**

Teaching, Guidance, and Counseling

Activities designed to provide information and materials, encourage action and responsibility for self-care and coping, and assist the individual, family, or community to make decisions and solve problems.

Treatments and Procedures

Technical activities such as wound care, specimen collection, resistive exercises, and medication prescriptions that are designed to prevent, decrease, or alleviate signs and symptoms for the individual, family, or community.

Case Management

Activities such as coordination, advocacy, and referral that facilitate service delivery; promote assertiveness; guide the individual, family, or community toward use of appropriate community resources; and improve communication among health and human service providers.

Surveillance

Activities such as detection, measurement, critical analysis, and monitoring intended to identify the individual, family, or community's status in relation to a given condition or phenomenon.

From Martin KS. *The Omaha System: A Key to Practice, Documentation, and Information Management.* Reprinted 2nd ed. Omaha, NE: Health Connections Press; 2005.

TABLE 9-1   **OMAHA SYSTEM PROBLEM RATING SCALE FOR OUTCOMES**

CONCEPT	1	2	3	4	5
Knowledge: Ability of client to remember and interpret information	No knowledge	Minimal knowledge	Basic knowledge	Adequate knowledge	Superior knowledge
Behavior: Observable responses, actions, or activities of client fitting occasion or purpose	Not appropriate behavior	Rarely appropriate behavior	Inconsistently appropriate behavior	Usually appropriate behavior	Consistently appropriate behavior
Status: Condition of client in relation to objective and subjective defining characteristics	Extreme signs/ symptoms	Severe signs/ symptoms	Moderate signs/ symptoms	Minimal signs/ symptoms	No signs/ symptoms

From Martin KS. *The Omaha System: A Key to Practice, Documentation, and Information Management.* Reprinted 2nd ed. Omaha, NE: Health Connections Press; 2005.

---

is an important interprofessional standard of practice. Suggested times include admission, specific interim points, and discharge. The ratings are a guide for the clinician as patient care is planned and provided. The ratings offer a method to monitor and quantify patient progress throughout the period of service. The content and relationships of the scale are outlined in Table 9-1 and are further illustrated by the clinical example in Box 9-4. Using the Problem Rating Scale for Outcomes with the other two schemes creates a comprehensive problem-solving model for practice, education, and research.

Clinical Example from Practice

The John T. Little clinical example (Box 9-4) depicts the use of the Omaha System with a patient and his home health nurse. It describes evidence-based and community-based practice, introduces the system as a standardized terminology, summarizes interprofessional practice, and offers details about EHRs, standards, and other concepts. Many additional references describe the application and value of using point-of-care documentation.[22,32-35,51,52]

Interpretation of the Clinical Example

The clinical example illustrates the following:

1. *Patient-centered care and the power of the patient and the family:* These are core values of home health and other

community-based services. The nurse asks for John and Mrs. Little to provide information about his status and asks them to share their preferences about pain relief during the next visit.

2. *Evidence-based practice:* The nurse follows the agency's evidence-based standards of practice in relation to skin care and medication management.

3. *Interprofessional practice:* The nurse, John, and Mrs. Little discuss plans for the home health aide, physical therapist, and occupational therapist.

4. *Practice and documentation using a standardized terminology:* The nurse uses the Omaha System to guide the assessment (Problem Classification Scheme), care plan (Intervention Scheme), and care delivery (Intervention Scheme). In addition, the nurse selects baseline Knowledge, Behavior, and Status ratings (Problem Rating Scale for Outcomes) that will guide evaluation during future visits. Other members of the care team will also use the system. Although not described in the clinical example, the nurse would have completed the OASIS dataset and entered billing, supplies, and other data.

5. *Practice, documentation, and information management linkages:*

   a. All members of the care team use one integrated EHR for documentation and can follow the data trail about

BOX 9-6   TARGETS OF THE OMAHA SYSTEM INTERVENTION SCHEME

- anatomy/physiology
- anger management
- behavior modification
- bladder care
- bonding/attachment
- bowel care
- cardiac care
- caretaking/parenting skills
- cast care
- communication
- community outreach worker services
- continuity of care
- coping skills
- day care/respite
- dietary management
- discipline
- dressing change/wound care
- durable medical equipment
- education
- employment
- end-of-life care
- environment
- exercises
- family planning care
- feeding procedures
- finances
- gait training
- genetics
- growth/development care
- home
- homemaking/housekeeping
- infection precautions
- interaction
- interpreter/translator services
- laboratory findings
- legal system
- medical/dental care
- medication action/side effects

- medication administration
- medication coordination/ordering
- medication prescription
- medication set-up
- mobility/transfers
- nursing care
- nutritionist care
- occupational therapy care
- ostomy care
- other community resources
- paraprofessional/aide care
- personal hygiene
- physical therapy care
- positioning
- recreational therapy care
- relaxation/breathing techniques
- respiratory care
- respiratory therapy care
- rest/sleep
- safety
- screening procedures
- sickness/injury care
- signs/symptoms—mental/emotional
- signs/symptoms—physical
- skin care
- social work/counseling care
- specimen collection
- speech and language pathology care
- spiritual care
- stimulation/nurturance
- stress management
- substance use cessation
- supplies
- support group
- support system
- transportation
- wellness
- other

From Martin KS. *The Omaha System: A Key to Practice, Documentation, and Information Management.* Reprinted 2nd ed. Omaha, NE: Health Connections Press; 2005.

John's progress. They can revise the care plan and interventions as needed to improve the quality of care they provide.

b. John's data will be analyzed and added to aggregate data. Outcome reports will be available to members of the care team as well as to agency managers and administrators. As data are transformed to information and knowledge, quality of care can be monitored and improved as part of the agency's quality improvement program.

c. Requests for orders and regular reports will be sent to John's referring medical staff, who are external members of the care team.

6. *External monitoring and quality control:*

a. Aggregate data about John and the home health agency's other patients will be submitted to CMS and other external third-party payers for reimbursement. In turn,

they may select John's EHR for review and a site visitor may accompany a team member on a home visit to observe John's care.

b. John's EHR may be selected for review by accreditation site visitors. They may also make a home visit to observe care. Many home health agencies are accredited by The Joint Commission, Community Health Accreditation Program (CHAP), or the Accreditation Commission for Health Care. The number of health departments that are accredited is increasing.

Examples of EHR Screen Images

Three screen images are presented in Figure 9-4 to illustrate a limited portion of John T. Little's EHR. Specifically, they depict pain assessment, problem identification, and care planning. The images are examples that enable the reader to visualize the application of concepts presented in this chapter. Note that the focus of the images varies but does not depict John's entire clinical record or other software modules that the home health agency would use. The images are part of McKesson Corporation's information system. McKesson Corporation and nine additional vendors are listed in Box 9-7 as examples of companies that sell information system solutions to diverse home health, hospice, and other community-based organizations in the U.S. Note that these 10 companies are examples only; many additional companies sell information systems and niche software to similar organizations.

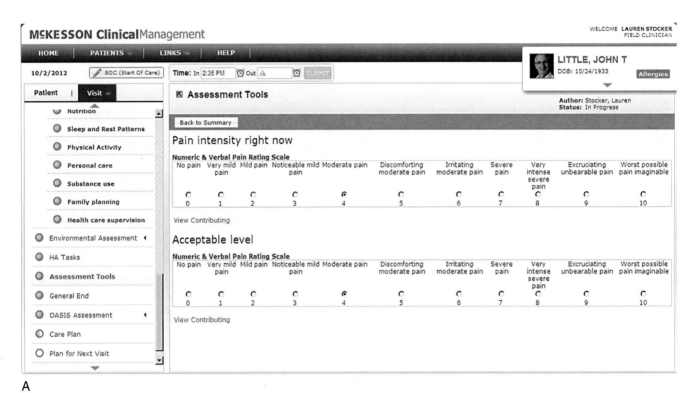

A

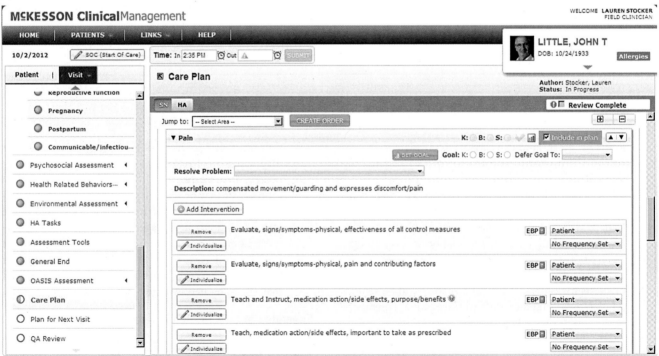

B

FIG 9-4 A, Pain assessment. **B,** Problem identification.

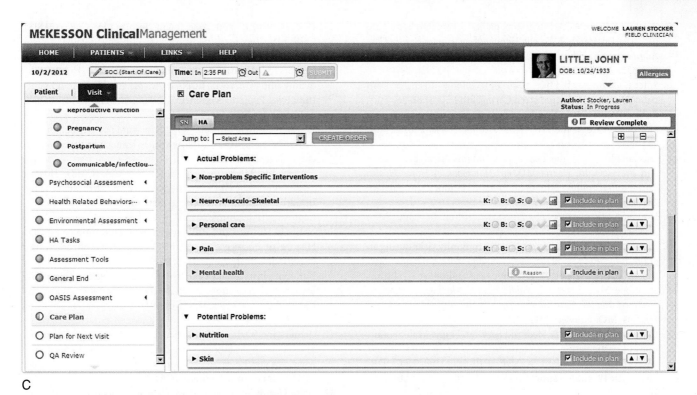

FIG 9-4, cont'd C, Care planning. (Copyright McKesson Corporation.)

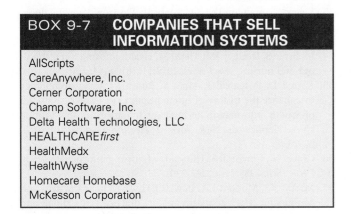

CONCLUSION AND FUTURE DIRECTIONS

The healthcare delivery system in the United States is under enormous pressure to change and create a more transparent, collaborative, efficient, and patient-centered system.[55] Adoption of EHRs and enabling the exchange of clinical information between members of the care team and across disparate systems are critical to achieving the goals of the U.S. Department of Health & Human Services, the Office of the National Coordinator for Health Information Technology, and the Triple Aim for healthcare.[40]

Home health, hospice, and other community-based care providers are actively engaged in envisioning and testing models of care. The evolving communication and collaboration models are designed to support safe transitions between care settings, effectively manage patient populations, and participate in accountable care organizations to achieve better clinical outcomes, better patient experiences, and lower costs. Data generated by information system solutions and capable of being transformed into information, knowledge, and wisdom are key to each of these initiatives. The information system solutions should support patients across the care continuum and into their homes to ultimately enable them to successfully self-manage their care needs. It is critical to seamlessly share and update a common plan of care, including medications, allergies, problems, planned interventions, and goals and results.[24]

When considering the longer term, there is an opportunity to aggregate information about common patient populations, create knowledge of effective care teams and treatment approaches, and share the knowledge in real time or near real time with the care team. Rapid learning systems and delivering wisdom to the healthcare community represent the opportunity ahead.

REFERENCES

1. Buhler-Wilkerson K. Care of the chronically ill at home: an unresolved dilemma in health policy for the United States. *Milbank Q.* 2007;85(4):611-639.
2. Hospice Association of America (HAA). Hospice facts and statistics. Washington, DC: HAA; 2010. http://nahc.org/facts/HospiceStats10.pdf.
3. National Association for Home Care & Hospice (NAHC). Basic statistics about home care. Washington, DC: NAHC; 2010. http://nahc.org/facts/10HC_Stats.pdf.
4. Naylor MD, Van Cleave J. The transitional care model for older adults. In: Meleis AI, ed. *Transitions Theory: Middle Range and Situational Specific Theories in Research and Practice.* New York, NY: Springer Publishing; 2010:459-464.

5. Perry KM, Parente CA. Integrating palliative care into home care practice. In: Harris MD, ed. *Handbook of Home Health Care Administration*. 5th ed. Sudbury, MA: Jones and Bartlett; 2010: 863-875.

6. Suter P, Hennessey B. Effective use of technology to engage both patients and provider partners. *Caring*. 2011;30(8):81-86.

7. Buhler-Wilkerson K. No place like home: a history of nursing and home care in the U.S. *Home Healthc Nurse*. 2002;20(10): 641-647.

8. Dieckmann JL. Home health care: an historical perspective and overview. In: Harris MD, ed. *Handbook of Home Health Care Administration*. 5th ed. Sudbury, MA: Jones and Bartlett; 2010:3-19.

9. Donahue MP. *Nursing: The Finest Art*. 3rd ed. St. Louis, MO: Elsevier; 2011.

10. Bhavnagri NP, Krolikowski S. Home-community visits during an era of reform (1870-1920). *Early Childhood Research and Practice*. 2000;2(1):1-29. http://ecrp.uiuc.edu/v2nl/bhavnagri.html.

11. Stanhope M, Lancaster J. *Public Health Nursing: Population-Centered Health Care in the Community*. 8th ed. Maryland Heights, MO: Elsevier; 2012.

12. Centers for Medicare & Medicaid Services. Home health conditions of participation. U.S. Government Printing Office. http://www.gpo.gov/fdsys/pkg/USCODE-2010-title42/pdf/USCODE-2010-title42-chap7-subchapXVIII-partE-sec1395bbb.pdf. 2012.

13. Zerwekh JV. *Nursing Care at the End of Life: Palliative Care for Patients and Families*. Philadelphia, PA: F.A. Davis; 2006.

14. Donabedian A. Evaluating the quality of medical care. *Milbank Q*. 1966;44(2):166-206.

15. Weed L. Special article: medical records that guide and teach. *New Engl J Med*. 1968;278(12):593-600, 652-657.

16. Tinetti ME. Performance-oriented assessment of mobility problems in elderly patients. *J Am Geriatr Soc*. 1986;34(2):119-126.

17. Duncan PW. Functional reach: a new clinical measure of balance. *J Gerontol*. 1990;45(6):M192-M197.

18. Centers for Medicare & Medicaid Services (CMS). National health expenditures 2010 highlights. CMS. http://www.cms.gov/Research-Statistics-Data-and-Systems/Statistics-Trends-and-Reports/NationalHealthExpendData/downloads/highlights.pdf. 2011.

19. National Association of County & City Health Officials (NACCHO). More than half of local health departments cut services in the first half of 2011. NACCHO. http://www.naccho.org/press/releases/100411.cfm. 2011.

20. National Nursing Centers Consortium (NNCC). http://www.nncc.us/site/index.php/about-nncc/who-we-are. 2012.

21. Humphrey CJ, Milone-Nuzzo P. Transitioning nurses to home care. In: Harris MD, ed. *Handbook of Home Health Care Administration*. 5th ed. Sudbury, MA: Jones and Bartlett; 2010: 515-527.

22. Martin KS. *The Omaha System: A Key to Practice, Documentation, and Information Management*. Reprinted 2nd ed. Omaha, NE: Health Connections Press; 2005.

23. Anderson R, Leonard MA, Mansell J, et al. Brief history of resident assessment instrument/minimum data set. American Health Information Management Association, Long-Term Care Insights. https://newsletters.ahima.org/newsletters/LTC_Insights/2010/Summer/transition.html#history. 2010.

24. Office of the National Coordinator for Health Information Technology. Long Term Post Acute Care Workgroup—Roadmap. Standards & Interoperability Framework. http://wiki.siframework.org/LTPAC+WG+Roadmap. 2012.

25. CGS. Outcome and Assessment Information Set (OASIS). CGS. http://www.cgsmedicare.com/hhh/coverage/oasis.html. 2012.

26. Centers for Medicare & Medicaid Services (CMS). Home health quality initiative. CMS. http://www.cms.gov/Medicare/Quality-Initiatives-Patient-Assessment-Instruments/HomeHealthQualityInits/index.html. 2012.

27. Research Triangle Institute (RTI). Post acute care payment reform demonstration. RTI. http://www.pacdemo.rti.org/meetinginfo.cfm?cid=caretool. 2012.

28. Centers for Medicare & Medicaid Services (CMS). Hospice quality reporting. CMS. http://www.cms.gov/Medicare/Quality-Initiatives-Patient-Assessment-Instruments/Hospice-Quality-Reporting/Index.html. 2012.

29. National Hospice and Palliative Care Organization (NHPCO). History of hospice care. NHPCO. http://www.nhpco.org/i4a/pages/index.cfm?pageid=3285. 2012.

30. National Hospice and Palliative Care Organization (NHPCO). Performance measure overview. NHPCO. http://www.nhpco.org/files/public/Statistics_Research/NHPCO_research_flier.pdf. 2012.

31. Centers for Medicare & Medicaid Services (CMS). Consumer assessment of healthcare providers and systems. CMS. http://www.cms.gov/Research-Statistics-Data-and-Systems/Research/CAHPS/Index.html?redirect=/CAHPS/. 2012.

32. Delta Health Technologies. Excellence in therapy report. Delta Health Technologies. http://deltahealthtech.com/assets/docs/DeltaExcellenceinTherapy.pdf. 2011.

33. Kelley TF, Brandon DH, Docherty SL. Electronic nursing documentation as a strategy to improve quality of patient care. *J Nurs Scholarship*. 2011;43(2):154-162.

34. McBride S, Delaney JM, Tietze M. Health information technology and nursing. *Am J Nurs*. 2012;112(8):36-44.

35. Russell D, Rosenfeld P, Ames S, Rosati RJ. Using technology to enhance the quality of home health care: three case studies of health information technology initiatives at the Visiting Nurse Service of New York. *J Healthc Qual*. 2010;32(5): 22-29.

36. Graves JR, Corcoran S. The study of nursing informatics. *Image J Nurs Sch*. 1989;21(4):227-230.

37. Martin KS, Monsen KA, Bowles KH. The Omaha System and Meaningful Use: applications for practice, education, and research. *Comput Inform Nurs*. 2011;29(1):52-58.

38. Monsen KA, Foster DJ, Gomez T, et al. Evidence-based standardized care plans for use internationally to improve home care practice and population health. *Applied Clinical Informatics*. 2011;2(3):373-383.

39. Nelson R, Joos I. On language in nursing: from data to wisdom. *Pennsylvania League for Nursing Visions*. 1989;1(5):6.

40. Office of the National Coordinator Health Information Technology. Federal health information technology strategic plan. U.S. Department of Health & Human Services. http://healthit.hhs.gov/portal/server.pt/community/federal_health_it_stratigic_plan_overview/1211. 2011.

41. Mandl KD. Escaping the EHR trap: the future of health IT. *New Engl J Med*. 2012;366(24):2240-2240.

42. Centers for Medicare & Medicaid Services (CMS). OASIS-C educational resources. CMS. http://www.cms.gov/Medicare/Quality-Initiatives-Patient-Assessment-Instruments/HomeHealthQualityInits/EducationalResources.html. 2010.

43. Laff L. OASIS-C: Managing the bumps in the road. Laff Associates. http://www.laffassociates.com/home.cfm/page/articles_Presentations.html. 2010.

44. Laff L. OASIS-C process measures . . . what is CMS thinking? Laff Associates. http://www.laffassociates.com/assets/pdfs/OASIS-C%20ACHC.pdf. 2009.

45. Nugent M. Achieving payer-provider collaboration in payment reform. Navigant. http://www.navigant.com/Insights/library/Industry_news/achieving_payer_provider_collaboration_091911. 2011.

46. Rouse M. Clinical decision support—definition. SearchHealthIT. http://searchhealthit.techtarget.com/definition/clinical-decision-support-system-CDSS#. 2010.

47. Sensmeier J. Clinical transformation: blending people, process, and technology. *Nursing Management (IT Solutions)*. 2011;42(10): 2-4.

48. American Nurses Association (ANA). ANA recognized terminologies that support nursing practice. *Nursing World*. http://www.nursingworld.org/Terminologies. 2012.

49. Lundberg CB, Brokel JM, Bulechek GM, et al. Selecting a standardized language to increase collaboration between research and practice. *Online Journal of Nursing Informatics*. 2008;12(2):1-18. http://ojni.org/12_2/lundberg.pdf.

50. Schwirian PM, Thede LQ. Informatics: the standardized nursing terminologies: a national survey of nurses' experiences and attitudes—survey II: participants, familiarity, and information sources. *Online Journal of Issues in Nursing*. 2012;17(2). http://www.nursingworld.org/MainMenuCategories/ANAMarketplace/ANAPeriodicals/OJNI/TableofContents/Vol-17-2012/No2-May-2012/Standardized-Nursing-Terminologies-SURVEY-II.html.

51. Thede LQ, Sewell JP. Informatics and nursing: competencies and applications. 3rd ed. Philadelphia, PA: Lippincott, Williams, & Wilkins. 2010.

52. Omaha System. http://www.omahasystem.org. 2012.

53. Gavin JH, Martin KS, Stassen DL, Bowles KH. The Omaha System: coded data that describe patient care. *J AHIMA*. 2008; 79(3):44-49.

54. Westra BL, Dey S, Fang G, et al. Interpretable predictive models for knowledge discovery from home-care electronic health records. *Journal of Healthcare Engineering*. 2011;2(1):55-74.

55. Federal Register. Patient Protection and Affordability Care Act. 2011;76(136). http://www.gpo.gov/fdsys/pkg/FR-2011-07-15/pdf/2011-17610.pdf.

DISCUSSION QUESTIONS

1. The focus of this chapter is home health and related community-based systems. What are your experiences with such settings? Do you expect to have more contact with them in the future?

2. Patient-centered care is an important theme in this chapter. Think about your experiences in practice settings. Describe whether you consider your experiences to be patient centered.

3. Describe your interest in and experience with standardized terminologies. List at least three positive and three negative experiences with standardized terminologies. What can be done to transform the negative experiences to positive ones?

4. Describe your interest in and experience with point-of-care documentation. List at least three positive and three negative experiences with point-of-care documentation. What can be done to transform the negative experiences to positive ones?

CASE STUDY

The ABC Home Health Agency is a nonprofit, Medicare-certified organization established in the mid-1950s in a small Midwestern city. It is accredited by the Accreditation Commission for Health Care, Inc. The agency offers a continuum of preventive and therapeutic services that have an individual, family, and community focus. Clinicians provide services to patients ranging in age from infants to elders. The agency employs supervisory, administrative, IT, and support staff as well as 45 clinicians: 25 nurses, 10 home care aides, 5 homemakers, 3 physical therapists, 1 occupational therapist, and 1 social worker. Staff members are on call 24 hours a day.

ABC Home Health Agency services include (1) skilled home health and hospice; (2) home care aide and homemaker; (3) private duty, including nursing, personal care, and respite care; (4) wellness, flu, and immunization clinics; (5) school health; (6) jail health; and (7) durable medical equipment.

There are two hospitals with about 100 beds and 15 physicians within the service area. The Agency has a good working relationship with both hospitals and the physicians. Many patients followed by the Agency have been referred from

these services. Last year the Agency provided 20,345 home visits.

The Agency has used an automated billing, statistical, and financial management information system for 15 years. However, all patient records are maintained in paper-and-pen format. Clinicians use a semistructured format consisting of subjective, objective, assessment, and plan (SOAP) sections. The previous director, who has just retired, did not believe that the cost of implementing an electronic health record (EHR) was justified. You have just been hired as the new director. The board of directors asks you to investigate purchasing an EHR and submit your recommendations to them.

Discussion Questions

1. Why would it be important to introduce the clinicians to standardized terminologies and involve them in discussions about EHRs before contacting potential software vendors, or should you use the reverse approach?

2. What steps would you need to complete before reporting to the board of directors?

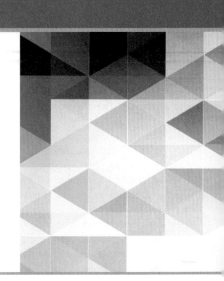

Clinical Decision Support Systems in Healthcare

Kensaku Kawamoto and Guilherme Del Fiol

Since shortly after computers were first introduced into clinical settings in the 1960s and 1970s, clinical decision support (CDS) has been shown to be a powerful tool for positively affecting care delivery and patient outcomes.

OBJECTIVES

At the completion of this chapter the reader will be prepared to:
1. Describe why clinical decision support is needed and its impact
2. Explain the major types of clinical decision support
3. Analyze best practices for clinical decision support
4. Synthesize the current adoption status and the barriers to the wide adoption of clinical decision support
5. Outline recent progress toward disseminating clinical decision support on a national level

KEY TERMS

ABSTRACT

Clinical decision support (CDS) is a key component of a variety of health information systems and a core component of electronic health records (EHRs). By providing the right information to the right person at the right time and at the right location, CDS systems can support effective clinical decision making and improve clinical care. CDS, encompassing various types of intervention modalities, has been shown to be effective for many decades. Important considerations in implementing CDSs include the application of best practices and the incorporation of knowledge management capabilities. Despite its benefits, significant challenges limit the widespread adoption and impact of CDS. These challenges include a healthcare payment model that has traditionally rewarded volume over quality and the difficulty of scaling CDS capabilities across healthcare systems and their information systems. In recent years several prominent efforts ensued to develop standards-based approaches to disseminating CDS on a national level. Moving forward, a need exists to capitalize on these ongoing initiatives to make advanced CDS available on a national scale.

INTRODUCTION

Since the early days of information technology in healthcare, the ultimate goals have been to help clinicians in their decision making process to prevent errors, to maximize efficiency, to enable evidence-based care, and ultimately to improve health and healthcare. Over time, tools that support the clinical decision making process have been generally designated as clinical decision support (CDS) systems.

According to the Institute of Medicine (IOM) report *To Err Is Human*, as many as 98,000 people die in hospitals in the United States every year due to preventable healthcare errors.[1] Many have considered this a conservative number since actual numbers are hard to obtain. Ten years after the IOM report was issued, little has changed. *Consumer Reports*, addressing the same question, reported that "based on our review of the scant evidence, we believe that preventable medical harm still accounts for more than 100,000 deaths each year—a million lives over the past decade."[2(p2)] Furthermore, a study by McGlynn et al. showed that, on average, patients in the United States receive only 54.9% of recommended processes of medical care.[3] To a great extent errors in healthcare are caused by process errors, information overload, and knowledge gaps.[1,4] Several factors further aggravate this problem, including rapidly evolving domain knowledge, an aging population having multiple comorbidities, and an increasingly complex healthcare delivery system. Ultimately this leads to a clinical information overload that significantly exceeds the human cognitive capacity.[5,6]

Many healthcare errors can be prevented, particularly through process improvement measures enabled by computerized information systems coupled with CDS tools. In addition, a large number of studies have shown that CDS tools help clinicians and patients to adopt evidence-based care whenever applicable.[7] As a result, several relevant reports and regulations have called for the use of health information technology (health IT) to support healthcare decision making, such as the IOM's *Crossing the Quality Chasm*,[8] the National Quality Forum's (NQF's) *Driving Quality and Performance Measurement—A Foundation for Clinical Decision Support*,[9] the United States EHR Meaningful Use incentive program,[10] and the IOM's *The Future of Nursing: Leading Change, Advancing Health*.[11]

Definition of CDS

Multiple definitions of CDS have been proposed, but in general these definitions have evolved from a narrow scope, typically focused on alerts and reminders, to a broader scope that encompasses a much wider set of tools that provides patient-specific information to support clinical decision making. According to Osheroff, CDS comprises a variety of tools and interventions that "provide clinicians, staff, patients, or other individuals with knowledge and person-specific information, intelligently filtered or presented at appropriate times, to enhance health and health care."[12(p141)] Similarly, the NQF defined CDS as "any tool or technique that enhances decision-making by clinicians, patients, or their surrogates in the delivery or management of health care."[9(p1)] In light of these definitions CDS can be applied to support several aspects of patient care decision making, such as the following:

- Reminding about a specific care need (e.g., patient due for an immunization)
- Alerting about a specific care action that may impose risk to the patient (e.g., a drug interaction)
- Providing intelligent views of a patient's record that help to cultivate a better understanding of the patient's status (e.g., intensive care reports, chronic disease management dashboards)
- Providing tools that assist in carrying out and documenting decisions more efficiently and accurately (e.g., documentation tools, order sets, medication reconciliation tools)
- Providing clinicians and patients with seamless access to patient-specific reference information available in online knowledge resources

History

Since the early 1970s, when the first studies demonstrating the impact of CDS were published by groups at the Regenstrief Institute in Indiana and the Latter-Day Saints (LDS) Hospital in Salt Lake City, CDS has become one of the holy grails of health informatics. Although designed more than 3 to 4 decades ago, these examples of CDS are still relevant and some of them are still in use.

De Dombal's Computer-Aided Diagnosis of Acute Abdominal Pain

According to a systematic review by Johnston et al.,[13] the first study to compare CDS with clinician performance was published in 1972 by de Dombal et al. on the diagnosis of acute abdominal pain.[14] The system comprised a Bayesian knowledge base and provided diagnostic probabilities as output.[15] An evaluation was conducted over an 11-month period at a general hospital in the United Kingdom, during which patient admissions due to acute abdominal pain were assessed independently by a physician and by the computer-aided diagnostic system.[14] The system's overall diagnostic accuracy was significantly higher than that of the most senior member of the clinical team (91.8% versus 79.6%). The results of this seminal study demonstrated the strong potential of using computers to assist patient care decision making.

Computer Reminders at Regenstrief Institute

One of the seminal randomized trials assessing the impact of a broad CDS intervention was published in 1976 by McDonald.[16] In this study physicians at the Regenstrief Institute received patient-specific reminders about 390 patient management protocols on a myriad of clinical conditions. These reminders were automatically generated by the computer based on the patients' EHRs and logic encoded in computable form. When a patient had a clinic visit, applicable reminders were printed and attached to the patient's chart. The study showed that physicians reacted to 51% of the events when exposed to reminders versus 21% when not exposed to reminders.

CDS Examples from the HELP System

A comprehensive set of CDS examples is provided by the HELP System, a clinical information system developed in the late 1960s and still in use at the LDS Hospital in Salt Lake City, Utah.[17] The HELP System includes a broad range of CDS tools that can be classified into the following four categories:

1. *Alerts* as a response to the presence of certain clinical data, such as life-threatening laboratory test results
2. Tools that *critique* clinicians' decisions, such as the presence of drug interactions in medication orders
3. Tools that provide on-demand diagnostic or therapeutic *suggestions*, such as computer protocols for ventilator management and antiinfective selection assistance
4. *Retrospective* quality assurance tools.

Several of these CDS tools have demonstrated a significant impact on clinicians' decisions and patient outcomes, such as appropriate use of perioperative antibiotics, reducing postoperative wound infections, reduced hospital stay when clinicians received alerts for life-threatening conditions, and increased survival rate in acute respiratory distress syndrome (ARDS) patients on the computer protocols for ventilator management. A compendium of the HELP CDS tools and a summary of the effect of these tools on clinicians' decisions and patient outcomes are available in an article by Haug et al.[17]

CDS TYPES AND EXAMPLES

Several taxonomies have been developed to classify CDS systems. A recent taxonomy was developed by the NQF as an extension of a functional taxonomy developed by researchers at Partners HealthCare.[18] The taxonomy is composed of four functional categories: triggers, input data, interventions, and action steps. *Triggers* are the events that initiate a CDS rule (e.g., a drug prescription). According to the NQF taxonomy, CDS can be triggered by an explicit request from a user, updates to a patient's data, user interactions with an EHR system, and a specific time. *Input data* are the additional data used in the background to constrain or modify the CDS, such as patient conditions, medications, diagnostic tests, and the care plan. *Interventions* are the possible actions that result from the CDS system, such as sending a message to a clinician, displaying relevant clinical knowledge or patient information, and logging that a particular event took place. *Action steps* are actionable alternatives offered to the CDS user, such as collecting or documenting information (e.g., reason to override an alert, completion of care recommended by CDS), requesting an order, and acknowledging a CDS recommendation. The complete NQF taxonomy is available

in the NQF consensus report *Driving Quality and Performance Measurement—A Foundation for Clinical Decision Support.*[9]

One of the most current and comprehensive taxonomies was developed by Wright et al. through a Delphi method with 11 CDS experts.[19] The taxonomy classifies CDS types from the user ("front end") perspective into six overarching categories: medication dosing support, order facilitators, point-of-care alerts and reminders, relevant information display, expert systems, and workflow support. Each of these categories is broken down into subtypes, leading to a total of 53 CDS types. The following sections describe each of the six overarching categories and provide real-life examples.

Medication Dosing Support

This category includes tools that assist clinicians in finding and monitoring the most appropriate doses for medication orders. Tools vary from simple "pick lists" with allowed dose options to more complex dose calculation algorithms based on parameters such as patient weight, height, renal function, and hepatic function (Fig. 10-1). Researchers at the Brigham and Women's Hospital have designed several medication dosing support tools for a broad range of medications within their computerized provider order entry (CPOE) system.[20]

Order Facilitators

Broader than medication dosing support tools, order facilitators are tools that assist clinicians in the order entry process in general. Order sets are perhaps the most common example in this category.[21] They assist clinicians by providing a set

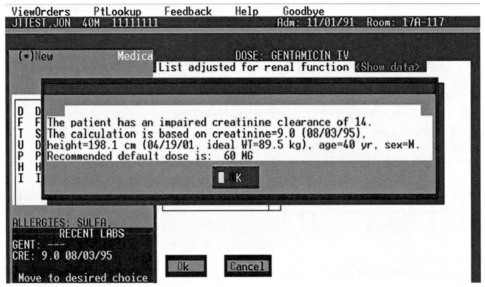

FIG 10-1 Dose adjustment recommendation for a gentamicin order in a patient with impaired renal function. The adjusted dose takes the patient's creatinine clearance and weight into account. (From the computerized provider order entry system at Brigham and Women's Hospital, Boston.)

of commonly used orders for a specific condition (e.g., community-acquired pneumonia) or service (e.g., hospital admission orders, postoperative orders). In addition to expediting the order entry process, order sets may help to reduce errors and promote consistent care, reducing unnecessary variability, enabling more complete orders, and reducing the need for verbal orders. Most currently available CPOE systems provide order set capabilities.[18] Figure 10-2 depicts a community-acquired pneumonia order set within the HELP2 system at Intermountain Healthcare.[21]

Point-of-Care Alerts and Reminders

Point-of-care alerts and reminders raise the clinician's or the patient's attention to important conditions or recommendations based on the patient's clinical data. One of the most common types of CDS, available in most CPOE and drug prescription systems, is an alert that notifies clinicians when a drug being prescribed interacts with other drugs the patient is already receiving. Similar examples include alerts of duplicate therapy, drug allergies, and a patient's condition that contraindicates the use of a particular drug. Similar to alerts, reminders are messages that aim to raise the clinician's attention to a particular patient's need to receive certain care, such as immunizations, cancer screening, fall prevention, and pain assessment. Figure 10-3 shows a set of patient care reminders

generated by the VistA EHR system at the Veterans Health Administration (VHA).

When designed appropriately, alerts have shown significant reduction in errors.[20] However, overuse of the alert mechanism may lead to a problem known as alert fatigue.[22] Figure 10-4 illustrates one way in which drug–drug interaction alerts may be presented without interrupting clinicians' workflow and therefore minimize alert fatigue. Other approaches to reducing alert fatigue include prioritizing alert display and improving the precision of the alert logic through contextual information about the patient, healthcare provider, and care setting to prevent false-positive alerts.[23]

Relevant Information Display

A different category of CDS is motivated by clinicians' information overload in the process of care, in terms of both patient information and domain knowledge. This broad category includes CDS tools that provide seamless access to relevant patient information or summarize prominent aspects of a patient's record to help clinicians understand the patient's condition and status. Intensive care daily reports that assist clinicians in patient rounds are one example of such tools. Another example is disease management dashboards that summarize relevant data for managing a specific condition. Figure 10-5 shows a disease management dashboard

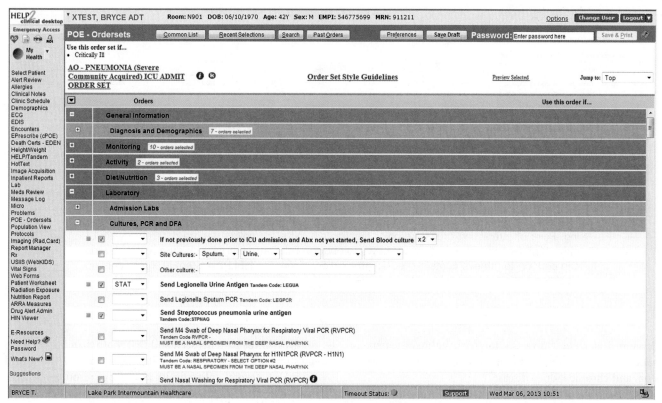

FIG 10-2 Computerized provider order entry system with a community-acquired pneumonia order set. (From the HELP2 system at Intermountain Healthcare, Salt Lake City.)

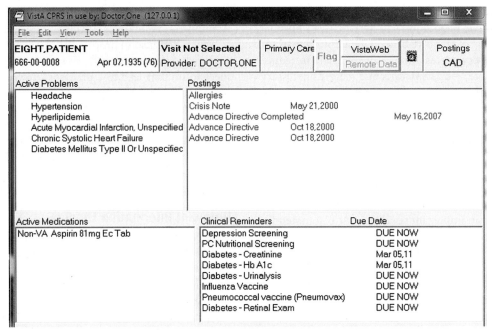

FIG 10-3 A set of care reminders (bottom right of screen) presented within the Veterans Health Administration's VistA Computerized Patient Record System. (Copyright Veterans Health Administration. All Rights Reserved.)

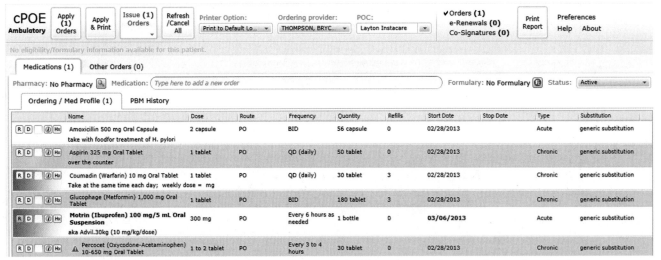

FIG 10-4 A medication prescription system coupled with noninterruptive drug interaction checking. Pairs of interacting drugs are color highlighted. Different colors denote different levels of interaction severity. The figure also shows Infobutton links adjacent to each drug that clinicians can click on to retrieve context-specific information. (From the HELP2 system at Intermountain Healthcare, Salt Lake City.)

developed at Duke University to assist the management of patients with chronic conditions such as diabetes, hypertension, and chronic kidney disease.[24]

In addition to the need for seamless access to relevant patient information, clinicians frequently raise domain knowledge questions when making patient care decisions. Research has shown that clinicians raise about two questions for every three patients seen and that more than half of these questions go unanswered.[25] With the advent of the World Wide Web, several online health knowledge resources became accessible through desktop and mobile devices. Although these resources have been shown to provide answers to most of the clinicians' questions, significant barriers limit their use at the point of care.[26] In essence, the amount of time

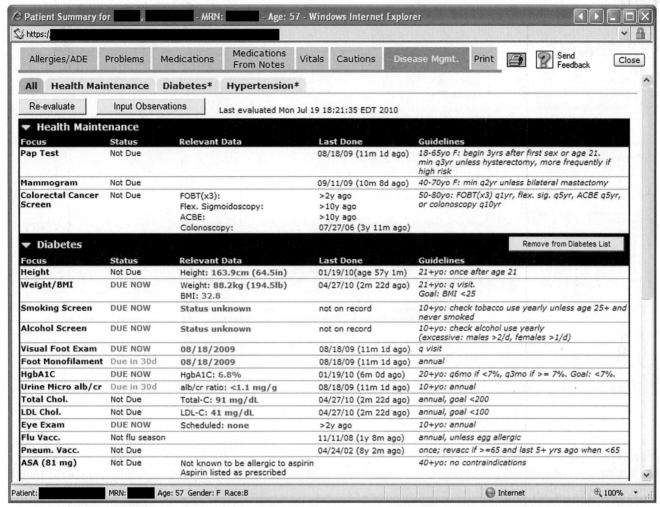

FIG 10-5 Chronic disease management module in use at the Duke University Health System. The system presents relevant data associated with evidence-based care recommendations. (Copyright Duke University Health System. All Rights Reserved.)

it typically takes for clinicians to find their answers is not compatible with the busy clinical workflow.[27] To facilitate access to these resources and reduce barriers to their use in patient care, researchers have been enabling access to these resources within EHR systems through an increasingly popular approach to CDS known as "Infobuttons."[28] Leveraging contextual attributes about the patient, clinician, care setting, and clinical task at hand within an EHR, Infobuttons anticipate clinicians' information needs and provide automated links to relevant online knowledge resources. For example, a physician prescribing a medication for a patient who has chronic kidney disease might want to know whether this medication is contraindicated or whether its dose needs to be adjusted based on the patient's condition. An Infobutton positioned beside the drug name within the EHR would provide access to this kind of information from an external drug knowledge resource. Figure 10-6 shows an example of Infobuttons within the HELP2 drug prescription module used at Intermountain Healthcare.[29]

Expert Systems

Expert systems provide diagnostic or therapeutic advice based on patient parameters. They typically contain more sophisticated computer logic than other forms of CDS and are less frequently found in commercial EHR systems.[19] Within informatics, the term *expert system* is also used to classify automated systems that go beyond decision support and actually automate the decision-making process. This use of the term is described in Chapter 2.

The antibiotic assistant and ventilator management protocols described in the section titled CDS Examples from the HELP System are examples of this category of CDS. Another example is diagnostic decision support systems such as Iliad,[30] Quick Medical Reference (QMR),[31] and DXplain.[32] These systems propose a list of candidate diagnoses based on a patient's signs and symptoms. Although diagnostic CDS tools have achieved a quite reasonable level of diagnostic accuracy, especially for differential diagnoses,[33] their use has been limited primarily to educational purposes.[34,35]

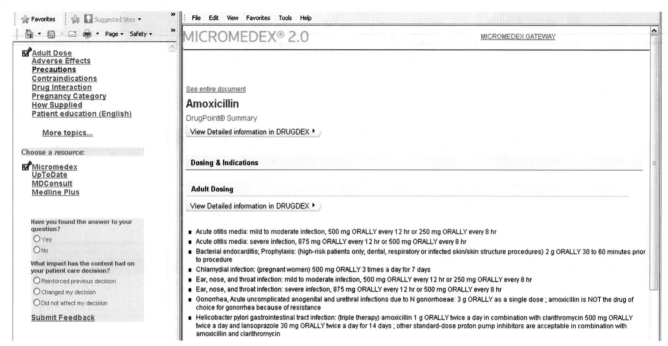

FIG 10-6 User interface presented to a physician who clicks on an Infobutton beside the drug amoxicillin, when prescribed to an adult patient. The left side has a navigation panel with automated context-specific links to relevant resources. The right side contains the content itself, which was retrieved from external online resources. (Copyright 2012 Truven Health Analytics Inc. and Intermountain Healthcare. All Rights Reserved.)

Workflow Support

The last category of CDS tools comprises tools that aid in important steps of the patient care workflow, such as care transitions, patient documentation, and orders. These workflow steps are susceptible to various types of errors and inefficiency that can be tackled with CDS. For example, medication errors in care transitions can be prevented with medication reconciliation tools;[36] structured documentation templates may provide consistent and efficient documentation;[37] and automatic steps in the ordering workflow, such as order approval, routing, and termination, may improve the overall efficiency and safety of the ordering process.[38,39]

CDS IMPACT

Evidence of Effectiveness

Numerous research studies have evaluated the impact of CDS. In 2011 Jaspers and colleagues synthesized the findings from 17 high-quality systematic reviews of the impact of CDS on healthcare practitioner performance and patient outcomes.[7] Within these systematic reviews 57% of 91 unique studies reported improved practitioner performance and 30% of 82 unique studies reported improved patient outcomes.[7] Improved practitioner performance was not always associated with a statistically significant improvement in patient outcomes, at least in part because studies of CDS interventions often lack large sample sizes and the associated statistical power required to reliably identify improvements in patient outcome metrics.

Examples of CDS Impact Studies

As one classic example of a CDS intervention resulting in positive outcomes, a study at Brigham and Women's Hospital in Boston, found that a CPOE system with various CDS capabilities reduced nonintercepted serious medication errors by 86%, with increasing benefits seen with the introduction of additional CDS capabilities.[20] In another classic example, also described in the section titled CDS Examples from the HELP System, the use of a rule-based CDS system for the mechanical ventilation of patients with ARDS resulted in a 60% survival rate compared to an expected survival rate of approximately 35%.[40] In another example, the impact of the antibiotic assistant developed by Evans and colleagues was assessed in a pre-post study. Compared to the preintervention period, use of the antibiotic assistant led to significant improvements in a variety of clinical measures, including antibiotic-susceptibility mismatches and adverse events caused by antiinfective agents.[41] Moreover, patients who received antiinfective therapy according to the regimens recommended by the CDS system had significantly reduced length of stay (10.0 days versus 16.7 days, $p <0.001$) and significantly lower total hospital costs ($26,315 versus $44,865, $p <0.001$) compared to patients who were not always managed according to the CDS system's recommendations.[41]

Not all CDS interventions result in the desired outcomes, however. For example, in a randomized controlled trial involving 29 health centers, an external CDS system for diabetes management accessible through the EHR system did not result in any clinically significant changes in practitioner performance or patient outcomes.[42] In another example, a stand-alone CDS system designed to guide referrals for patients at increased risk for hereditary breast cancer was found to have limited impact in a randomized controlled trial involving 86 primary care practices, due largely to the limited use of the tool by clinicians.[43] Last, a randomized controlled trial involving 60 primary care practices found no significant impact when a CDS system for asthma and angina management was made available to intervention clinicians as a separate path within their practices' EHR systems.[44]

Financial Impact of CDS

As with any investment, a healthcare institution should consider the expected financial impact when making decisions related to CDS investment. To the extent that CDS can facilitate desired changes in clinical practice patterns and patient outcomes, CDS can lead to positive returns on investment, for example, by reducing medical errors and lengths of stay. The VHA estimated that its health IT investments have resulted in more than $3 billion in net benefits, with CDS serving as an important catalyst for the return on investment.[45] In this analysis, mechanisms by which CDS provided a financial return on investment to the VHA included reduced costs for preventable adverse drug events, reduced inpatient costs for avoided admissions, and reduced laboratory and radiology costs for redundant and unnecessary tests.[46]

In assessing the financial impact of CDS, an important issue to consider is that the financial benefits of CDS may accrue to stakeholders other than those investing in CDS. For instance, if a healthcare delivery organization invests in CDS to support influenza and pneumococcal vaccinations and the rate of hospitalizations for these conditions decreases, the organization may lose money because of the decrease in revenue-generating hospitalizations, whereas society, patients, and health insurers would likely benefit from the investment. In another example, if a healthcare delivery organization invests in CDS systems to ensure that low back pain results in expensive diagnostic imaging and surgical procedures only when clearly warranted, it may lose money because of the decrease in revenue-generating radiologic exams and surgeries; again, society, patients, and health insurers would likely benefit from the investment. Thus when assessing the financial impact of CDS, it is important to assess the impact in terms of the different stakeholders involved, particularly patients, healthcare delivery organizations, and health insurers.

In the case of organizations such as the VHA that serve as both a healthcare delivery organization and a health insurer, the financial incentives of the major stakeholder groups may align well. Other health organizations' incentives do not align as well but, as discussed later, healthcare payment models are beginning to change toward models in which the financial incentives of the key stakeholders are better aligned. Currently, however, because of the healthcare payment models in the United States, the issue of misaligned financial incentives will likely continue to be an important issue in relation to the financial case for CDS.

CDS Adoption

Despite four decades of substantial evidence demonstrating the ability of well-implemented CDS to improve practitioner performance and patient outcomes, most commercial EHR systems and healthcare delivery organizations in the United States have implemented only basic CDS capabilities, such as alerts for drug–drug interactions and drug–allergy contraindications.[12] According to a systematic review, 24% of all studies on the impact of health IT on patient care were conducted at four healthcare organizations in the United States: the Regenstrief Institute, Brigham and Women's Hospital/Partners HealthCare, the U.S. Department of Veterans Affairs, and LDS Hospital/Intermountain Health Care.[46] Characteristics common to these four organizations are use of homegrown EHR systems that have been developed and implemented gradually; a strong informatics culture; and strong clinician engagement in the system design, development, and implementation process. Unfortunately, the approach taken at these organizations with internally developed systems is unlikely to be feasible for disseminating CDS to most healthcare settings. Hence the broad dissemination of CDS remains one of the most significant challenges and prominent areas of research in healthcare informatics.

Challenges and Barriers to CDS Adoption

The dissemination of CDS is limited by a significant set of barriers, which collectively make CDS interventions not easily replicable. The most prominent barriers are include:

- *Lack of incentives:* As discussed earlier, a key reason for the limited adoption of CDS is a healthcare payment model that has often failed to reward the provision of higher quality care and therefore investments in quality-enhancing technologies such as CDS. Within healthcare systems, CDS interventions often do not provide financial benefit to the individuals and organizations investing resources to implement CDS. Financial models with multiple vested interests are one of the most significant barriers to wide adoption of CDS.

- *Implementation challenges:* Successful CDS requires a well-designed implementation plan supported by a strong organizational culture and strategy. In fact, a recent meta-analysis identified local user involvement in the CDS development process as one of the key factors associated with successful CDS.[47] Unlike typical information system implementations, CDS implementations are an ongoing cycle requiring constant monitoring and updating of the underlying clinical logic to reflect changes in domain knowledge, local practices, workflow, and regulations. Ideally CDS should be seen as an integral component of a healthcare organization's quality and value improvement strategy, operationalized as an organization-wide clinical knowledge management effort.[48,49]

- *Low EHR adoption:* Because CDS generally requires that a core information system such as an EHR or CPOE system be in place first, a barrier to CDS adoption has historically been the limited adoption of EHR and CPOE systems. Although this is changing rather rapidly due to national

Medicare and Medicaid incentives, in 2011 less than 40% of outpatient physicians were estimated to be using EHRs in the United States.[50]

- *Multiple data sources with little information exchange:* Most CDS logic requires data that are typically fragmented across multiple data sources, such as laboratory; pharmacy; radiology; billing; admission, discharge, and transfer (ADT); and EHR systems. Moreover, a patient may have relevant data for CDS stored with many different healthcare organizations. These data sources are typically not shared with the EHR providing the CDS or not shared in a format that can be readily used by the CDS. As a result, many implementations of CDS require additional data entry by users. In turn, little or no need for data entry has often been suggested as a facilitator of successful CDS interventions.[47,51] Therefore a fundamental requirement for CDS adoption is the ability to exchange information with multiple data sources, ideally through a standards-based approach.
- *Lack of adequate CDS tools and capabilities in most EHR systems:* As mentioned earlier, most EHR systems offer only basic CDS capabilities and do not necessarily replicate successful CDS interventions developed and evaluated with "homegrown" or internally developed EHR systems. This limitation compromises the impact of CDS in most healthcare organizations that rely on commercial EHR systems.
- *"Cookbook medicine":* There is a belief among many physicians that the use of CDS reduces medicine from an art to a "cookbook" approach to patient care.[52] However, with the increased emphasis on evidence-based practice, standards of care, and best practices, this attitude is changing.
- *Lack of a framework for sharing CDS logic and capabilities:* As discussed later in this chapter, another important barrier to widespread CDS adoption has been the limited ability to scale most existing CDS logic and capabilities across healthcare organizations and health information systems.[12] This includes the lack of a business model for sharing CDS logic and capabilities, lack of a legal framework covering potential liability implications associated with CDS recommendations, lack of a widely adopted formalism for representing and sharing CDS knowledge, and lack of widely available, standards-based CDS tools and infrastructure.

CDS BEST PRACTICES

While CDS interventions can have profound impacts on clinical care, in a significant minority of cases they fail to result in meaningful improvements. Given the significant effort and cost that can be associated with implementing a CDS intervention, there has been major interest in identifying best practices for CDS to help maximize the likelihood that a CDS initiative will lead to the desired outcomes. In other words, substantial work has been done to make CDS more of a science than an art. These best practices also aim at contributing to the replicability and wide dissemination of CDS interventions.

As an important source of CDS best practices, seasoned experts have compiled guides for CDS best practices, two of which will be discussed here. First, in 2003 Dr. David Bates and colleagues published "Ten Commandments for Effective Clinical Decision Support: Making the Practice of Evidence-Based Medicine a Reality."[53] These 10 commandments are as follows:

1. Speed is everything
2. Anticipate needs and deliver in real time
3. Fit into the user's workflow
4. Little things can make a big difference
5. Recognize that physicians will strongly resist stopping
6. Changing direction is easier than stopping
7. Simple interventions work best
8. Ask for additional information only when you really need it
9. Monitor impact, get feedback, and respond
10. Manage and maintain your knowledge-based systems.[53]

A second notable source of CDS best practices is *Improving Outcomes with CDS: An Implementer's Guide*, which was authored by experts in the field and published in 2011 by the Healthcare Information and Management Systems Society (HIMSS).[54] This book synthesizes best practices into worksheets to guide the reader through the CDS implementation and evaluation process. It also provides a practical framework for designing and implementing CDS interventions that follows what is known as the "CDS Five Rights," which refers to providing the right information to the right person using the right CDS intervention format, delivered through the right channel and at the right point in the workflow.

As a complement to these best practices guides, some researchers have attempted to quantitatively analyze the features of CDS interventions strongly associated with, and which therefore potentially explain, the success or failure of those interventions. In particular, a systematic review led by Kawamoto analyzed 70 randomized controlled trials of clinician-directed CDS interventions to assess the degree to which the trial outcomes correlated with the presence or absence of CDS intervention features suggested as important by domain experts.[51] Through a multiple logistic regression analysis, this study found that a single feature was by far the most critical: the automatic provision of CDS as a part of clinician workflow (adjusted odds ratio 112.1, $p < 0.00001$). While there were CDS interventions that included this feature and yet had no impact, all CDS interventions not having this feature failed to result in a significant improvement in clinical practice. What this finding suggests is that unless a CDS intervention is provided automatically to end-users as a part of their routine workflow, there is a high likelihood that the CDS intervention will remain unused and therefore will not have an opportunity to affect patient care positively. In addition, this study found that the provision of CDS at the time and location of decision making as well as the provision of a recommendation, rather than just an assessment, was an additional independent predictor of a positive outcome.

RECENT PROGRESS TOWARD DISSEMINATING CDS ON A NATIONAL LEVEL

As noted throughout the chapter, CDS has the potential to significantly enhance the efficiency and effectiveness of healthcare delivery. Indeed, while CDS is not a silver bullet, it is a critical and largely underused resource for improving care and reducing costs, especially when implemented according to known best practices. Thus a critical challenge is disseminating comprehensive CDS on a national level. A number of initiatives are being developed to tackle the challenges and barriers to CDS adoption. In the following sections a series of relevant initiatives and progress that should contribute toward overall CDS adoption are reviewed.

Value-Based Payment Models

The recent trend with perhaps the most significant potential to spur nationwide adoption of advanced CDS is the current shift of healthcare payment from a fee-for-service model to approaches rewarding the delivery of better quality and better outcomes at lower cost. Driven by the fundamental problem that the historical fee-for-service payment model leads to unsustainable and relentless increases in healthcare costs, health insurers are increasingly moving toward models of payment in which healthcare delivery organizations are reimbursed less for care volume and more for care value (outcomes relative to costs). For example, a RAND technical report from 2011 catalogs nearly 100 implemented and proposed payment reform programs and predicts accelerated payment reform moving forward.[55] Thus while it is difficult to predict how quickly and how deeply these changes will ultimately come into place, this shift will likely have a profound impact on the degree to which healthcare delivery organizations are motivated to implement CDS-supported process changes in order to improve care quality and reduce care costs.

Meaningful Use Incentives for EHR and CDS Adoption

In 2009 the U.S. federal government established a law providing approximately $30 billion in incentives for clinicians and hospitals to make "Meaningful Use" of EHR systems.[10] As of 2012, the regulations related to this law have been relatively limited with respect to CDS, requiring only that compliant EHR systems implement a handful of CDS interventions and support a standard approach for integrating context-relevant information resources, typically referred to as Infobuttons.[56] Perhaps most important is that Meaningful Use is providing powerful incentives for healthcare delivery organizations to adopt EHR systems. As EHR systems are critical enablers of robust and widely distributable CDS, this federal program significantly increases the prospect of a national base of EHR systems through which advanced CDS capabilities can be shared and widely used.

Statewide Health Information Exchanges

As noted in Chapter 12, health information exchanges (HIEs) enable the secure exchange of health information across healthcare providers in a defined region, often through secure web portals to enable authorized clinical access. Beyond EHR systems, HIEs can provide a platform for CDS to be delivered to clinicians on a widespread scale. The U.S. federal government has invested more than $500 million in recent years in support of statewide HIEs.[57] As such, this increase in the potential capabilities and reach of HIEs presents an additional opportunity for enabling CDS on a national scale.

CDS Standards

In general, there are two complementary approaches to sharing CDS across a large number of healthcare delivery organizations: (1) sharing structured CDS knowledge resources (e.g., order sets, alert definitions) and (2) sharing a CDS capability over a secure Internet connection (e.g., sending anonymous patient data to a secure web server, which returns evidence-based care recommendations).[58] In both approaches a critical element is that common standards be used by the various interacting health information systems so that the approach can scale widely and be implemented at relatively low cost. In recognizing this need, a number of CDS standards required for a national approach to CDS have recently been developed and adopted by international standards development organizations such as Health Level Seven (HL7). Interested readers can obtain further details regarding the current state of CDS standards in a recent review article.[59]

National CDS and Knowledge Management Initiatives

To underscore the degree to which the national dissemination of advanced CDS has become an explicit priority for many relevant stakeholder groups, a number of efforts were initiated in recent years in which the nationwide dissemination of CDS is the explicit goal. The CDS Consortium, for example, is a public-private collaborative effort sponsored by the Agency for Healthcare Research and Quality to assess, define, demonstrate, and evaluate best practices for knowledge management and CDS that can scale across multiple healthcare settings and EHR technology platforms.[60] This effort includes demonstrations of how CDS interventions developed at one institution can be accessed over a secure Internet connection and integrated with the different EHR systems of different healthcare delivery organizations. The CDS Consortium research contract began on March 5, 2008, with a 5-year grant ending July 2013 (www.partners.org/cird/cdsc/default.asp).[61]

Furthermore, the NQF, responsible for the development of the various quality measures required for EHR Meaningful Use compliance, has also placed significant focus on how CDS could improve healthcare providers' performance with regard to the national quality measures developed by the group.[9] Also, the U.S. Office of the National Coordinator for Health Information Technology recently sponsored an effort known as Advancing CDS; one of the primary deliverables was to develop a proposed national framework for CDS content sharing and to pilot an initial implementation of that framework.[62] Finally, a multistakeholder effort known as Health eDecisions is actively working to identify, define, and harmonize standards that facilitate the emergence of systems and services whereby shareable CDS interventions can be implemented at scale.[63] Of note, an important goal of this effort is to develop and validate a standards-based approach to CDS scaling that can be incorporated into future Meaningful Use regulations.

Open Source, Freely Available Resources

As a practical matter, the implementation of a common standards-based approach to CDS can be facilitated by resources that are freely available in the public domain. In recognition of this potential enabling role of open source, freely available CDS resources, several CDS stakeholders have launched efforts to collaboratively develop such resources. One of these initiatives is known as OpenInfobutton (www.openinfobutton.org), sponsored by the VHA to develop an open source solution for supporting context-sensitive information retrieval in a standards-compliant manner.[64] An additional initiative in this area is OpenCDS (www.opencds.org), which is a multistakeholder collaborative effort to develop standards-based, open source resources to enable CDS at scale.[64]

RESEARCH CHALLENGES

Despite 4 decades of research, we are still in the infancy of CDS and notable challenges still need to be addressed to fully realize its benefits. To help focus effort toward achieving this goal, Sittig et al. compiled a list of top 10 grand challenges in CDS through a consensus-building process (Box 10-1).[65]

One particular area of interest receiving significant attention is the desire to leverage large and heterogeneous data sources, also known as "big data," through advanced analytic and visualization methods.[66] To develop research on big data, the U.S. federal government has allocated a significant amount of research funding to the National Science Foundation (NSF) and the National Institutes of Health (NIH).

Another area of growing interest is CDS interventions to promote patient-centered care (PCC), defined by the IOM as "care that is respectful of and responsive to individual patient preferences, needs and values, ensuring that patient values guide all clinical decisions."[8] Intelligent tools are needed to help patients understand their conditions and care alternatives, prioritize and carry out their care goals, and engage in shared decision making with their providers. A systematic review reported by the Agency for Healthcare Research and Quality (AHRQ) found an overall positive effect of health IT interventions for PCC on healthcare processes, clinical outcomes, responsiveness to the needs and preferences of individual patients, promoting

---

BOX 10-1   TOP 10 GRAND CHALLENGES IN CLINICAL DECISION SUPPORT

Improve the Effectiveness of CDS Interventions

1. The need for improvements in human–computer interfaces for delivering CDS
2. Tools that automatically summarize the patient's clinical data, helping clinicians to understand the patient's condition and status
3. Prioritize and personalize CDS recommendations to the user
4. Account for patient's comorbidities
5. Leverage the large amount of narrative text typically available in EHR systems

Create New CDS Interventions

1. Helping organizations to prioritize CDS content development and implementation
2. Leverage large clinical databases to create CDS

The third category addresses some of the barriers to the wide adoption of CDS.

Disseminate Existing CDS Knowledge and Interventions

1. Disseminating CDS best practices
2. Creating a framework for sharing CDS knowledge and capabilities
3. Creating online CDS repositories

Adapted from Sittig DF, Wright A, Osheroff JA, et al. Grand challenges in clinical decision support. *J Biomed Inform.* 2008;41(2):387-392.

---

shared decision making, and improving patient–clinician communication.[67] Yet studies reported a number of barriers for using these applications to enable PCC, such as lack of usability, low computer literacy in patient and clinicians, lack of standardization, workflow issues, and problems with reimbursement.

CONCLUSION AND FUTURE DIRECTIONS

Since shortly after computers were introduced into clinical settings in the 1960s and 1970s, CDS has been shown to be a powerful tool for positively affecting care delivery and patient outcomes. What has been lacking, however, has been a business environment conducive to widespread CDS, as well as technical approaches that enable CDS knowledge sharing on a widespread scale. Today there are a number of changes taking place that address both of these critical challenges. Therefore there is a real opportunity for relevant healthcare stakeholders to come together and realize the vision of advanced CDS that is available ubiquitously and at low cost to support improved healthcare across the nation.

Acknowledgments: Kensaku Kawamoto was recently a consultant to the RAND Corporation, Partners HealthCare, and Inflexxion on grant-funded research initiatives related to clinical decision support. Guillherme Del Fiol was supported by grant number K01HS018352 from the Agency for Healthcare Research and Quality (AHRQ).

REFERENCES

1. Institute of Medicine (IOM). *To Err Is Human: Building a Safer Health System.* Washington, DC: IOM; 1999.

2. Jewell K, McGiffert L. Consumer Reports. To err is human—to delay is deadly. 2009. http://safepatientproject.org/safepatientproject.org/pdf/safepatientproject.org-ToDelayIsDeadly.pdf. Accessed November 13, 2012.

3. McGlynn EA, Asch SM, Adams J, et al. The quality of health care delivered to adults in the United States. *N Engl J Med.* 2003;348 (26):2635-2645.

4. Leape LL, Bates DW, Cullen DJ, et al. Systems analysis of adverse drug events: ADE Prevention Study Group. *JAMA.* 1995;274(1): 35-43.

5. Stead WW, Searle JR, Fessler HE, Smith JW, Shortliffe EH. Biomedical informatics: changing what physicians need to know and how they learn. *Acad Med.* 2011;86(4):429-434.

6. Smith R. Strategies for coping with information overload. *BMJ.* 2010;341:c7126.

7. Jaspers MW, Smeulers M, Vermeulen H, Peute LW. Effects of clinical decision-support systems on practitioner performance and patient outcomes: a synthesis of high-quality systematic review findings. *J Am Med Inform Assoc.* 2011;18(3):327-334.

8. Institute of Medicine (IOM). *Crossing the Quality Chasm: A New Health System for the 21st Century.* Washington, DC: IOM; 2001.

9. National Quality Forum (NQF). *Driving Quality and Performance Measurement—A Foundation for Clinical Decision Support: A Consensus Report.* Washington, DC: NQF; 2010. http://www.qualityforum.org/WorkArea/linkit.aspx?Link Identifier=id&ItemID=52608. Accessed May 2012.

10. Jha AK. Meaningful use of electronic health records: the road ahead. *JAMA.* 2010;304(15):1709-1710.

11. Institute of Medicine (IOM). *The Future of Nursing: Leading Change, Advancing Health.* Washington, DC: IOM; 2010.

12. Osheroff JA, Teich JM, Middleton B, Steen EB, Wright A, Detmer DE. A roadmap for national action on clinical decision support. *J Am Med Inform Assoc.* 2007;14(2):141-145.

13. Johnston ME, Langton KB, Haynes RB, Mathieu A. Effects of computer-based clinical decision support systems on clinician performance and patient outcome: a critical appraisal of research. *Ann Intern Med.* 1994;120(2):135-142.

14. de Dombal FT, Leaper DJ, Staniland JR, et al. Computer-aided diagnosis of acute abdominal pain. *Br Med J.* 1972;2(5804): 9-13.

15. Horrocks JC, McCann AP, Staniland JR, Leaper DJ, de Dombal FT. Computer-aided diagnosis: description of an adaptable system, and operational experience with 2,034 cases. *Br Med J.* 1972;2(5804):5-9.

16. McDonald CJ. Protocol-based computer reminders, the quality of care and the non-perfectability of man. *N Engl J Med.* 1976; 295(24):1351-1355.

17. Haug PJ, Gardner RM, Tate KE, et al. Decision support in medicine: examples from the HELP system. *Comput Biomed Res.* 1994;27(5):396-418.

18. Wright A, Goldberg H, Hongsermeier T, Middleton B. A description and functional taxonomy of rule-based decision support content at a large integrated delivery network. *J Am Med Inform Assoc.* 2007;14(4):489-496.

19. Wright A, Sittig DF, Ash JS, et al. Development and evaluation of a comprehensive clinical decision support taxonomy: comparison of front-end tools in commercial and internally developed electronic health record systems. *J Am Med Inform Assoc.* 2011;18(3):232-242.

20. Bates DW, Teich JM, Lee J, et al. The impact of computerized physician order entry on medication error prevention. *J Am Med Inform Assoc.* 1999;6(4):313-321.

21. Del Fiol G, Rocha RA, Bradshaw RL, Hulse NC, Roemer LK. An XML model that enables the development of complex order sets by clinical experts. *IEEE Trans Inf Technol Biomed.* 2005;9(2): 216-228.

22. Ash JS, Sittig DF, Campbell EM, Guappone KP, Dykstra RH. Some unintended consequences of clinical decision support systems. *AMIA Annu Symp Proc.* 2007:26-30.

23. Duke JD, Bolchini D. A successful model and visual design for creating context-aware drug-drug interaction alerts. *AMIA Annu Symp Proc.* 2011:339-348.

24. Lobach DF, Kawamoto K, Anstrom KJ, Russell ML, Woods P, Smith D. Development, deployment and usability of a point-of-care decision support system for chronic disease management using the recently-approved HL7 decision support service standard. *Stud Health Technol Inform.* 2007;129(Pt 2):861-865.

25. Covell DG, Uman GC, Manning PR. Information needs in office practice: are they being met? *Ann Intern Med.* 1985;103(4): 596-599.

26. Ely JW, Osheroff JA, Chambliss ML, Ebell MH, Rosenbaum ME. Answering physicians' clinical questions: obstacles and potential solutions. *J Am Med Inform Assoc.* 2005;12(2):217-224.

27. Hersh WR, Hickam DH. How well do physicians use electronic information retrieval systems? A framework for investigation and systematic review. *JAMA.* 1998;280(15):1347-1352.

28. Cimino JJ, Elhanan G, Zeng Q. Supporting infobuttons with terminological knowledge. *Proc AMIA Annu Fall Symp.* 1997:528-532.

29. Del Fiol G, Haug PJ, Cimino JJ, Narus SP, Norlin C, Mitchell JA. Effectiveness of topic-specific infobuttons: a randomized controlled trial. *J Am Med Inform Assoc.* 2008;15(6):752-759.

30. Warner Jr HR, Bouhaddou O. Innovation review: Iliad—a medical diagnostic support program. *Top Health Inf Manage.* 1994;14(4):51-58.

31. Bankowitz RA, McNeil MA, Challinor SM, Parker RC, Kapoor WN, Miller RA. A computer-assisted medical diagnostic consultation service: implementation and prospective evaluation of a prototype. *Ann Intern Med.* 1989;110(10):824-832.

32. Barnett GO, Cimino JJ, Hupp JA, Hoffer EP. DXplain: an evolving diagnostic decision-support system. *JAMA.* 1987;258(1):67-74.

33. Berner ES, Webster GD, Shugerman AA, et al. Performance of four computer-based diagnostic systems. *N Engl J Med.* 1994; 330(25):1792-1796.

34. Lange LL, Haak SW, Lincoln MJ, et al. Use of Iliad to improve diagnostic performance of nurse practitioner students. *J Nurs Educ.* 1997;36(1):36-45.

35. Miller RA, Masarie Jr FE. Use of the Quick Medical Reference (QMR) program as a tool for medical education. *Methods Inf Med.* 1989;28(4):340-345.

36. Bassi J, Lau F, Bardal S. Use of information technology in medication reconciliation: a scoping review. *Ann Pharmacother.* 2010;44(5):885-897.

37. Rosenbloom ST, Denny JC, Xu H, Lorenzi N, Stead WW, Johnson KB. Data from clinical notes: a perspective on the tension between structure and flexible documentation. *J Am Med Inform Assoc.* 2011;18(2):181-186.

38. Buising KL, Thursky KA, Robertson MB, et al. Electronic antibiotic stewardship—reduced consumption of broad-spectrum antibiotics using a computerized antimicrobial approval system in a hospital setting. *J Antimicrob Chemother.* 2008;62(3):608-616.

39. Topal J, Conklin S, Camp K, Morris V, Balcezak T, Herbert P. Prevention of nosocomial catheter-associated urinary tract infections through computerized feedback to physicians and a nurse-directed protocol. *Am J Med Qual.* 2005;20(3):121-126.

40. Thomsen GE, Pope D, East TD, et al. Clinical performance of a rule-based decision support system for mechanical ventilation of ARDS patients. *Proc Annu Symp Comput Appl Med Care.* 1993:339-343.

41. Evans RS, Pestotnik SL, Classen DC, et al. A computer-assisted management program for antibiotics and other antiinfective agents. *N Engl J Med.* 1998;338(4):232-238.

42. Hetlevik I, Holmen J, Krüger O, Kristensen P, Iverson H, Furuseth K. Implementing clinical guidelines in the treatment of diabetes mellitus in general practice: evaluation of effort, process, and patient outcome related to implementation of a computer-based decision support system. *Int J Technol Assess Health Care.* 2000;16(1):210-227.

43. Wilson BJ, Torrance N, Mollison J, et al. Cluster randomized trial of a multifaceted primary care decision-support intervention for inherited breast cancer risk. *Fam Pract.* 2006;23(5):537-544.

44. Eccles M, McColl E, Steen N, et al. Effect of computerised evidence based guidelines on management of asthma and angina in adults in primary care: cluster randomised controlled trial. *BMJ.* 2002;325(7370):941.

45. Byrne CM, Mercincavage LM, Pan EC, Vincent AG, Johnston DS, Middleton B. The value from investments in health information technology at the U.S. Department of Veterans Affairs. *Health Aff.* 2010;29(4):629-638.

46. Chaudhry B, Wang J, Wu S, et al. Systematic review: impact of health information technology on quality, efficiency, and costs of medical care. *Ann Intern Med.* 2006;144(10):742-752.

47. Bright TJ, Wong A, Dhurjati R, et al. Effect of clinical decision-support systems: a systematic review. *Ann Intern Med.* 2012;157(1):29-43.

48. Rocha RA, Bradshaw RL, Hulse NC, Rocha BHSC. The clinical knowledge management infrastructure of Intermountain Healthcare. In: Greenes RA, ed. Clinical Decision Support: The Road Ahead. Burlington, VT: Academic Press; 2007:469-502.

49. Hongsermeier T, Kashyap V, Sordo M. Knowledge management infrastructure: evolution at partners healthcare system. In: Greenes RA, ed. *Clinical Decision Support: The Road Ahead.* Burlington, VT: Academic Press; 2007:447-467.

50. Decker SL, Jamoom EW, Sisk JE. Physicians in nonprimary care and small practices and those age 55 and older lag in adopting electronic health record systems. *Health Aff.* 2012;31(5):1108-1114.

51. Kawamoto K, Houlihan CA, Balas EA, Lobach DF. Improving clinical practice using clinical decision support systems: a systematic review of trials to identify features critical to success. *BMJ.* 2005;330(7494):765-768.

52. Cabana MD, Rand CS, Powe NR, et al. Why don't physicians follow clinical practice guidelines? A framework for improvement. *JAMA.* 1999;282(15):1458-1465.

53. Bates DW, Kuperman GJ, Wang S, et al. Ten commandments for effective clinical decision support: making the practice of evidence-based medicine a reality. *J Am Med Inform Assoc.* 2003;10(6):523-530.

54. Osheroff JA, Teich JM, Levick D, et al. *Improving Outcomes with Clinical Decision Support: An Implementer's Guide.* 2nd ed. Chicago, IL: Health Information Management and Systems Society; 2011.

55. Schneider EC, Hussey PS, Schnyer C. *Payment Reform: Analysis of Models and Performance Measurement Implications.* Arlington, VA: RAND Corporation; 2011.

56. Health Level Seven (HL7). HL7 context-aware information retrieval (Infobutton) standard. HL7. http://www.hl7.org/v3ballot2010may/html/domains/uvds/uvds_Context-aware KnowledgeRetrieval(Infobutton).htm. 2010. Accessed July 1, 2012.

57. U.S. Office of the National Coordinator for Health Information Technology. State health information exchange cooperative agreement program. HealthIT.gov. http://healthit.hhs.gov/portal/server.pt?open=512&objID=1488&mode=2. Accessed July 1, 2012.

58. Kawamoto K. Integration of knowledge resources into applications to enable clinical decision support: architectural considerations. In: Greenes RA, ed. *Clinical Decision Support: The Road Ahead.* Boston, MA: Elsevier; 2007:503-538.

59. Kawamoto K, Del Fiol G, Lobach DF, Jenders RA. Standards for scalable clinical decision support: need, current and emerging standards, gaps, and proposal for progress. *Open Med Inform J.* 2010;4:235-244.

60. Middleton B. The clinical decision support consortium. *Studi Health Technol Inform.* 2009;150:26-30.

61. Safe Patient Project. www.SafePatientProject.org. Accessed November 13, 2012.

62. U.S. Office of the National Coordinator for Health Information Technology. CDS sharing. HealthIT.gov. http://healthit.hhs.gov/portal/server.pt/community/healthit_hhs_gov__cds_sharing/3789. Accessed July 1, 2012.

63. Standards and Interoperability Framework. Health eDecisions homepage. S&I Framework. http://wiki.siframework.org/Health+eDecisions+Homepage. Accessed July 1, 2012.

64. Del Fiol G, Kawamoto K, Cimino JJ. Open-source, standards-based software to enable decision support. *AMIA Ann Fall Symp.* 2011;2127.

65. Sittig DF, Wright A, Osheroff JA, et al. Grand challenges in clinical decision support. *J Biomed Inform.* 2008;41(2):387-392.

66. Ohno-Machado L. Big science, big data, and a big role for biomedical informatics. *J Am Med Inform Assoc.* 2012;19(e1).

67. Agency for Healthcare Research and Quality. Enabling patient-centered care through health information technology. 2012. http://www.ahrq.gov/clinic/tp/pcchittp.htm. Accessed November 13, 2012.

DISCUSSION QUESTIONS

1. Describe examples of CDS that are available within your organization.
2. Describe the most important barriers to CDS adoption at your organization.
3. How will healthcare reimbursement reform affect healthcare organizations' use of CDS moving forward?
4. What recommendations do you have for the use of CDS to improve care value at your organization?
5. What opportunities do you see for CDS to facilitate the work of healthcare professionals?
6. When implementing a CDS system what should the appropriate relationship be between local values and standards and national standards?

CASE STUDY

Imagine that you have been appointed as Director of Clinical Decision Support at a healthcare delivery system. This healthcare system consists of several large hospitals and multiple outpatient clinics and uses the same EHR system across the enterprise. There has been limited CDS activity at the institution prior to your arrival. Now, with Meaningful Use and the increasing need to provide increased care value, the appropriate use of CDS is an institutional priority. The current CDS available at your institution consists primarily of off-the-shelf drug–drug interaction and drug–allergy alerting, which is the source of significant clinician complaints due to the rate of false-positive alerts. There is a strong sense within the institution's administration that IT in general and CDS specifically should be leveraged to improve care value and to enable the institution to influence its clinical practice patterns more systematically and more rapidly. You have a reasonable budget and adequate staff to make meaningful changes and you do have support from key institutional stakeholders, including healthcare system executives, the nursing informatics officer, and the chief medical informatics officer. You have been asked to devise a strategic plan for CDS at your institution within 3 months of your arrival and to have concrete "wins" within 12 to 18 months.

Discussion Questions

1. Describe the approaches you would use to ensure that all aspects of patient care were considered when developing a CDS system. How would you prioritize the efforts of your CDS team? Potential areas on which to focus include areas in which payment rates are tied to national quality measures, CDS interventions that meet Meaningful Use requirements, readmissions for congestive heart failure and other care events for which payers increasingly are not reimbursing, and areas that have been identified as institutional priorities for clinical improvement.
2. How would you balance the need to deliver desired CDS capabilities quickly against the benefits of establishing robust infrastructure to enable future deliverables to be implemented more quickly?
3. Identify one area for quality and value improvement. Define the CDS interventions that you would implement to address this area of need. Describe how your approach aligns with the best practices discussed in this chapter, such as the CDS Five Rights, the CDS 10 commandments, and the desire to use standards-based, scalable approaches. How would you systematically measure the impact of these CDS interventions?

Public Health Informatics

Catherine Janes Staes, Marisa Wilson, and Leslie Lenert

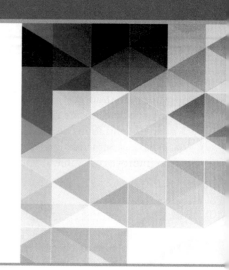

"*Public health is what we, as a society, do collectively to assure the conditions in which people can be healthy.*"

Institute of Medicine, Future of Public Health for the 21st Century, *p. 1*

OBJECTIVES

At the completion of this chapter the reader will be prepared to:

1. Summarize critical public health functions and common workflows that may be supported by information technology
2. Analyze the sociopolitical context for public health and other factors that may influence the implementation of informatics solutions
3. Critique key public health applications for infectious and chronic diseases
4. Describe current efforts to improve the exchange of information between public health and clinical systems
5. Explain why cloud computing is critical to the future of public health informatics

KEY TERMS

ABSTRACT

The chapter includes a description of the importance and unique features of public health practice and explores the differences between clinical and public health practice. It includes social and political challenges that affect public health informatics. A list of several major public health data systems is provided to help the reader understand the scope of information generated and used by public health, but these data systems alone are not informatics applications that transform data to knowledge. To illustrate public health informatics applications, the chapter includes a description of surveillance systems, immunization information systems, and the role of public health in a health information exchange. The chapter includes a description of the workflows associated with these systems and the value of information technology (IT), decision support, and standards. The next section describes the opportunities to leverage the electronic health record (EHR) to meet and promote public health goals. EHRs can be used to manage a population of patients in a single clinical practice or in a more complex medical home model. EHR data are used to generate and track quality performance measures important for preventing disease, reducing healthcare costs, and improving outcomes such as the Healthcare Effectiveness Data and Information Set (HEDIS) measures that concern antibiotic use, influenza vaccination, cancer screening, body mass index assessment, and other quality metrics. In addition, EHRs can be used to deliver patient-specific alerts for preventive or screening interventions. Finally, there is a discussion about the future of public health informatics and the need to leverage new technologies and paradigms to meet new challenges and resource constraints in the twenty-first century.

INTRODUCTION

Public health informatics is the specialty whereby informatics methods and tools are used to solve public health problems or support population and public health goals. This definition transcends the walls of a public health department and recognizes that population and public health practice occurs in the community, in clinical sites, and in a variety of other settings outside the domain of a health department. Rapidly evolving technologies, standards, and partnerships have created new opportunities for monitoring and improving population health and preventing injury and disease. This chapter explains how informatics concepts can be applied to populations, with the goals of limiting contagion and promoting health.

PUBLIC HEALTH: A POPULATION PERSPECTIVE

Public health is the science, art, and practice of protecting and improving the health of populations. It has contributed substantially to improvements in health status throughout the world. For example, during the twentieth century life expectancy at birth among U.S. residents increased 62%, from 47.3 years in 1900 to 76.8 years in 2000. Unprecedented improvements in population health status were observed at every stage of life across a variety of different metrics.[1] While the average lifespan of persons in the U.S. lengthened by 30 years, 25 years of this gain are attributable to advances in public health.[2] Advances in medical diagnostic modalities, antibiotics, and other treatments and therapies are important, but the following great public health achievements of the twentieth century illustrate the breadth of other strategies that have had an impact on health in the United States:

- Vaccinations
- Motor vehicle safety
- Safer workplaces
- Control of infectious diseases
- Decline in deaths from coronary heart disease and stroke
- Safer and healthier foods and healthier mothers and babies
- Family planning
- Fluoridation of drinking water
- Recognition of tobacco use as a health hazard[3]

As an example, the recognition of tobacco use as a health hazard and the subsequent public health antismoking campaigns resulted in changes in social norms to prevent initiation of tobacco use, promote cessation of tobacco use, and reduce exposure to environmental tobacco smoke.[3] Since the 1964 Surgeon General's report on the health risks of smoking, the prevalence of smoking among adults has decreased, and during the years 1964 to 1992 an estimated 1.6 million deaths caused by smoking were prevented.[4]

Despite the unprecedented improvements in sanitation and control of infectious diseases, the achievements of the twentieth century, and the fact that the U.S. spends more money on healthcare than any other nation in the world, the U.S. population still ranks near the bottom on most standard measures of health status when compared with other developed nations.[5] In a call to do better, Schroeder states that the pathways to better health do not generally depend on better healthcare and that even in those instances in which healthcare is important, too many Americans do not receive it, receive it too late, or receive poor-quality care.[5] In particular, though, Schroeder calls for improved efforts to address the behavioral patterns that affect health in the twenty-first century. Given that smoking and the constellation of poor diet and physical inactivity were the "actual cause" for about one third of all deaths in the United States in 2000,[6] public health efforts in the twenty-first century need to tackle these and other modifiable behavioral risk factors to substantively affect population health. Going forward, public health priorities and activities will continue to evolve as the following occur:

- New problems arise, such as the anthrax or violent bioterrorism events seen on and after September 11, 2001, West Nile virus, severe acute respiratory syndrome (SARS), and the influenza H1N1 pandemic
- New priorities are recognized, such as the need to address the rising rates of obesity and behavioral risk factors and the need to improve preparedness for natural and human-made disasters
- There is a continued need to prevent and control infectious and chronic diseases, injuries, and behaviors such as smoking that cause high rates of morbidity and mortality

To address these challenges, public health involves a diverse set of professionals and agencies that all have one common goal: to improve people's health and protect them from health risks. The professionals specialize in public health nursing, behavioral science and health education, epidemiology, environmental health, injury control, biostatistics, emergency medical services, health services, international health, maternal and child health, nutrition, public health laboratory practice, public health policy, and public health clinical practice. The agencies involved include local (city and county), state, and tribal health departments and federal agencies such as the Centers for Disease Control and Prevention (CDC), the Food and Drug Administration (FDA), the Environmental Protection Agency (EPA), the Census Bureau, and so forth. The CDC includes the National Center for Health Statistics, the National Institute for Occupational Safety and Health, and other centers that focus on domains such as injuries, infectious disease, genomics, global health, and so forth. These governmental public health agencies partner with healthcare delivery systems and others to assure the conditions for population health (Fig. 11-1).

When asked to define public health people often mention service functions, such as "where you go to get your child immunized or to get a birth or death record," or job duties, such as "employing disease detectives that respond to outbreaks and inspectors that check restaurants." While correct, these responses are incomplete. Public health agencies provide direct clinical services similar to any healthcare organization but also provide services, such as outbreak management and

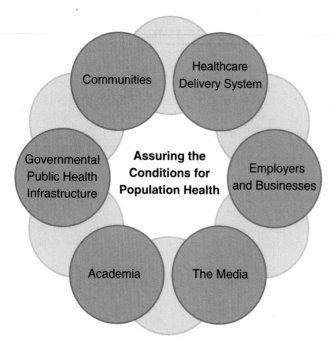

FIG 11-1 The public health system: government and some of its potential partners. (From Committee on Assuring the Health of the Public in the 21st Century. *The Future of the Public's Health in the 21st Century.* Washington, DC: The National Academies Press; Copyright 2002, National Academy of Sciences.

surveillance, that are not otherwise performed in a community.[7] A broad spectrum of public health practice is largely invisible to the general public because much of the goal of *public health* is to stop hazardous situations from arising.[8] When public health strategies function well, hazardous events do not occur, which creates a paradox: You often do not get grateful patients or communities when problems are prevented.[8] Some less visible examples of public health activities include monitoring of air and water, prevention and control of injuries, building of safe roadways, protection of the food supply, proper disposal of solid and liquid waste and medications, rat control and mosquito abatement, surveillance of

infectious and chronic diseases, and prevention and preparedness research (Fig. 11-2). This diverse set of activities can be summarized in the core functions and essential services for effective public health systems that were defined by the Institute of Medicine (IOM) Committee for the Study of the Future of Public Health. There are many opportunities to use informatics strategies with these services.

The IOM framework developed in 1988 holds true today.[8] Public health systems should perform three core functions: (1) assessment: "every health department should regularly and systematically collect, assemble, analyze, and make available information on the health of the community, including statistics on health status, community health needs, and epidemiologic and other studies of health problems"[8(p7)]; (2) policy development: "every health department should exercise its responsibility to serve the public interest in the development of comprehensive public health policies by promoting use of the scientific knowledge base in decision-making"[8(p8)]; and (3) assurance: "public health agencies should assure their constituents that the services necessary to achieve agreed upon goals are provided, either by encouraging actions by other entities (private or public sector), by requiring such action through regulation, or by providing services directly."[8(p8)] Each agency should involve key policymakers and the general public in determining a set of high-priority personal and communitywide health services that governments will guarantee to every member of the community. This guarantee should include subsidization or direct provision of high-priority personal health services for those unable to afford them."[(p8)] The essential services related to these functions are described in Box 11-1.

Public health practice differs from clinical practice in important ways that will help to illustrate core public health principles. Most notably, public health is focused on prevention and the health of populations *before* they are ill rather than treating individuals *after* they become injured or ill. The primary goal of clinical care is to obtain the best possible outcome for the individual receiving care. This paradigm leads to saving "one life at a time." In contrast, the primary goal of public health practice is to affect population health

FIG 11-2 The visible and invisible work of public health. (Copyright 2010 Catherine Staes. Reprinted with permission.)

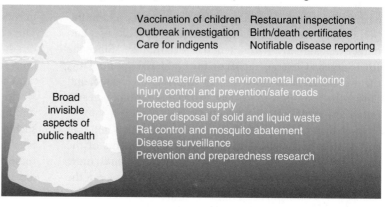

BOX 11-1 CORE FUNCTIONS AND THE 10 ESSENTIAL SERVICES FOR EFFECTIVE PUBLIC HEALTH SYSTEMS

Core Function: Assessment
Essential Services
- Monitor health status to identify community health problems.
- Diagnose and investigate health problems and health hazards in the community.

Core Function: Policy Development
Essential Services
- Inform, educate, and empower people about health issues.
- Mobilize community partnerships to identify and solve health problems.
- Develop policies and plans that support individual and community health efforts.

Core Function: Assurance
Essential Services
- Enforce laws and regulations that protect health and ensure safety.
- Link people to needed personal health services and assure the provision of healthcare when otherwise unavailable.
- Assure a competent public health and personal healthcare workforce.
- Evaluate effectiveness, accessibility, and quality of personal and population-based health services.
- Research for new insights and innovative solutions to health problems.

From Committee for the Study of the Future of Public Health. *The Future of Public Health*. Washington, DC: The National Academies Press; 1988.

---

and ensure a healthy community. This is performed by encouraging healthy behaviors, focusing on prevention, and balancing individual autonomy with limitations on individuals that protect the individuals or others. For example, this balance is seen in smoking and helmet laws designed to limit exposures to known risks for injury and disease. The policies and strategies are designed to save "millions of lives at a time."

The diagnostic tools used in the two domains differ. Clinical providers measure the health of an individual using tools ranging from a stethoscope to sophisticated imaging or laboratory modalities. In contrast, epidemiologists and public health officers measure the vital status of a community using birth and death records, surveys, and surveillance data to understand the distribution and determinants of disease *and health* in their community. A list of the major surveys performed by the National Center for Health Statistics is available on its website.[9] Other important systems will be described later in the chapter.

The breadth of entities involved in medical and public health practice differs. A clinical provider primarily interacts with people and data associated with hospitals, laboratories, and other clinical care settings. In contrast, public health practitioners may perform work in a clinical setting but the assessment, policy development, and assurance functions often involve schools, the legislature, the workplace, correctional facilities, food establishments, water systems, the community at large, and many other settings.

Public health interventions focus on events earlier in the causal pathway of disease (Fig. 11-3). While medical care addresses the diagnosis and treatment of disease, public health interventions focus on creating a safe environment to avoid or reduce exposure to hazards, promote healthy behaviors, and reduce the prevalence of risky behaviors and other risk factors. For example, public health practitioners focus on safely removing leaded paint in a child's home to avoid lead poisoning and they advocate or require the use of helmets to prevent head injuries.

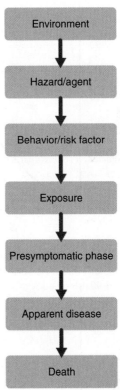

FIG 11-3 Causal pathway of disease. (Reproduced from Public health 101 for informaticians, Koo D, O'Carroll P, LaVenture M, 8, 585-97, 2001 with permission from BMJ Publishing Group Ltd.)

Public health practice differs from clinical practice in one additional significant manner. The risk reduction strategies employed by public health are based on a population perspective to determine priorities and evaluate success. Three models for risk reduction are discussed extensively in *The Future of the Public's Health in the 21st Century*[10] and illustrated in Figure 11-4. These models are based on three central realities in the development of effective population-based prevention

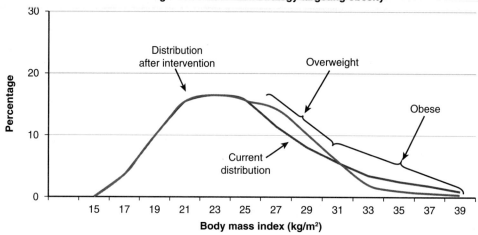

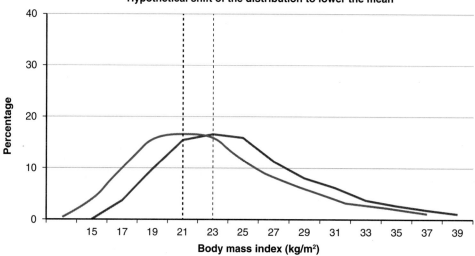

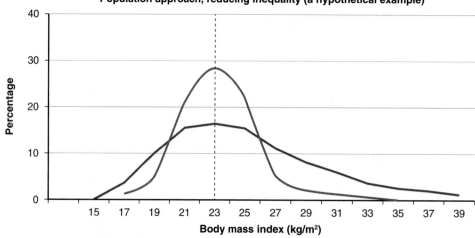

FIG 11-4 Models for risk reduction. (Printed with permission from Committee on Assuring the Health of the Public in the 21st Century. *The Future of the Public's Health in the 21st Century.* The National Academies Press; Copyright 2002, National Academy of Sciences.)

strategies. First, disease risk is a continuum rather than a dichotomy. There is no clear division between risk for disease and no risk for disease regarding levels of blood pressure, cholesterol, alcohol consumption, tobacco consumption, physical activity, diet and weight, lead exposure, and other risk factors. Second, most often only a small percentage of any population is at the extremes of high or low risk. The majority of people fall in the middle of the distribution of risk. Exposure of a large number of people to a small risk can yield a more absolute number of cases of a condition than exposure of a small number of people to a high risk. Third, an individual's risk of illness cannot be considered in isolation from the disease risk for the population to which he or she belongs.

Figure 11-4 illustrates the hypothetical impact on the distribution of risk in a population when efforts are focused on only those at highest risk (see Fig. 11-4, A), when strategies are employed to shift the mean level of risk for the entire population (see Fig. 11-4, B), or when strategies attempt to limit variation in risk and tighten the distribution around the population mean (see Fig. 11-4, C). American society experienced the second approach to disease prevention and health promotion when measures were taken to promote sanitation and food and water safety in the early twentieth century and more recently when implementing policies about seat belt use, unleaded gasoline, and vaccination.[10] The second and third models (see Fig. 11-4, B and C) are common strategies for evaluating quality improvement in the clinical setting. The clinical informatics strategies for assessing systems and process improvement are very useful for thinking about the application of informatics to population health.

Social and Political Challenges That Affect Public Health Informatics

Many aspects of public health are inherently governmental functions. As a result, the architecture of public health reflects the constitutional structure of the United States. The founding fathers of the United States did not envision a need for a national-level public health system. Such a vision was beyond the grasp of even our greatest thought leaders at the end of the eighteenth century. Further, the framers of the Bill of Rights saw the need to limit federal powers. The Tenth Amendment to the U.S. Constitution essentially states that any powers not reserved for the federal government or prohibited for the states are in the realm of the states' authority. Because of the limits on federal authority and the relatively late development of a national public health infrastructure, public health laws and functions evolved primarily as state and local government functions.

The lead government agency for public health, the Centers for Disease Control and Prevention (CDC), was not created until after World War II, long after the value of public health regulations for control of contagion were recognized. While the CDC evolved into its role as a national public health agency through its work in the 1950s and 1960s, its legislative authority is limited by the Tenth Amendment. Congress has not mandated, nor could it require, states to cooperate with the CDC except in situations where there is a threat to national security. So, how does the CDC get states and local governments to work with it toward national interests? It must use grants and contract vehicles to persuade states to work with the national government, including sharing of data. With respect to informatics this means that the CDC cannot require states to maintain specific kinds of information systems or even to send data to the CDC. Data exchange with the federal government is voluntary and driven by obligations and incentives embedded in grants and contracts administered by the CDC to states.

An example of voluntary cooperation between the states and the federal government is the National Notifiable Disease Surveillance System (NNDSS). While states have all agreed to contribute data to the NNDSS to allow the country to track infectious diseases, integration of these data is difficult due to each state being its own arbiter of the types of data it collects for each notifiable disease and even of the types of tests and findings considered relevant for reporting a condition. This immensely complicates the creation of a nationwide view of the impacts of disease.

In the same way that the national government has severe limitations on its authority in most matters of public health, many state governments have similar challenges with local authorities. In most states (Fig. 11-5), called Home Rule states, local governments have all necessary authorities not specifically claimed by the state or federal governments, which typically includes authority for public health functions. In Home Rule states, state governments can regulate many aspects of health. However, state governments may have little control over local (city or county) public health departments, which are free to adopt their own business practices for health investigations and use information systems that differ from those of state agencies. The issues are particularly problematic in large municipalities where local public health officials may wield greater resources than their state counterparts (e.g., Los Angeles County, New York City). In states without Home Rule, public health activities within the state tend to be more centralized and managed at the state level.

As a result of the history and structure of public health departments, public health authority and activity is largely a local function in the United States but the responsibility for planning and policy is largely at the state and federal levels. This creates a continuing series of problems with data standardization, data ownership, lack of willingness to share data across levels of government, complexities with data integration, and system planning and development. In contrast, in countries with a strong national authority for public health issues, such as Canada, Great Britain, or China, a single information system can be used across the country to manage specific public health issues or even the entire public health enterprise. In the United States, informatics solutions have to allow state and local governments to be the stewards of their own computational resources and data.

Sociological Context of Public Health

While public health, nursing, and medicine share a similar set of facts about disease, health, prevention, and treatment, each

States with Home Rule

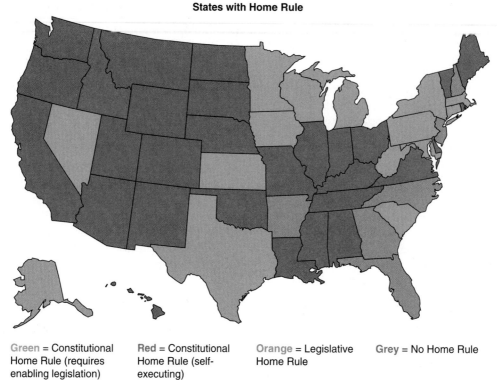

Green = Constitutional Home Rule (requires enabling legislation)   Red = Constitutional Home Rule (self-executing)   Orange = Legislative Home Rule   Grey = No Home Rule

FIG 11-5 Distribution of the status of Home Rule among the 50 U.S. states. (Data from Community Environmental Legal Defense Fund [CELDF]. Municipal Home Rule in the 50 states. CELDF. http://celdf.org/home-rule-in-the-states.)

has a different approach to these problems and a different world view. The world view of the practitioners is reflected in the knowledge artifacts they produce, including papers, books, and computer programs that are particularly relevant to this chapter. Public health software systems reflect the language and world view of the population health perspective. Systems are developed to serve specific operational needs and, as a result, focus on one type of public health activity or another. For example, public health departments might use one system to track patients with sexually transmitted diseases and another to track patients receiving immunizations.

Many of the tasks performed by public health workers do not require a patient-centered, comprehensive view but rather can be accomplished by determining the rate of events in a population, such as the changes in the infections occurring in a community or the vaccine coverage rate in a particular community. As a result, and in contrast to clinical systems, there is no patient-specific view in most public health systems. Data are typically captured about one event (disease, lead test result, immunization administered) at a time, often without the ability to link reports about an individual across different systems. The difference in the world view of public health and the design of public health information systems complicates the tasks associated with sharing data across systems and, in particular, complicates the task of integrating clinical systems with public health systems.

A second difference in world view concerns the sharing of information. In many public health practice circumstances,

clinical systems send data about an individual to a public health system without incurring any direct benefit for the patient or the healthcare provider. For example, information about patients is included in the hospital discharge datasets sent to public health but this sharing of information does not benefit the patient or healthcare provider directly. In contrast, in the clinical system data movement primarily occurs for patient benefit or reimbursement. The Health Insurance Portability and Accountability Act (HIPAA) Privacy Rule recognizes and supports these differences but sometimes clinicians are reluctant to share information because of their different world view and training.

In 2003 the CDC published the following guidance:

The Privacy Rule permits covered entities to disclose protected health information (PHI), without authorization, to public health authorities or other entities who are legally authorized to receive such reports for the purpose of preventing or controlling disease, injury, or disability. This includes the reporting of disease or injury; reporting vital events (e.g., births or deaths); conducting public health surveillance, investigations, or interventions; reporting child abuse and neglect; and monitoring adverse outcomes related to food (including dietary supplements), drugs, biological products, and medical devices [45 CFR 164.512(b)]. Covered entities may report adverse events related to FDA-regulated products or activities to public agencies and private entities that are subject to FDA jurisdiction [45 CFR 164.512(b)(1)(iii)].

To protect the health of the public, public health authorities might need to obtain information related to the individuals affected by a disease. In certain cases, they might need to contact those affected to determine the cause of the disease to allow for actions to prevent further illness. Also, covered entities may, at the direction of a public health authority, disclose protected health information to a foreign government agency that is acting in collaboration with a public health authority [45 CFR 164.512(b)(1)(i)].[11]

It is the job of the public health informaticist to develop tools or methods to translate the data representations generated by the public health and the clinical world views. This translation is necessary to enable interoperability and support the various uses of the information. For example, clinical records are usually patient centered whereas public health may request aggregated information such as the number of encounters for influenza-like illness during the week.

Two questions should be considered in the field of public health informatics:

- How can information and communication technologies improve the effectiveness of public health agencies?
- How can information and communication technologies improve the health of the American public?

It is important to understand that there is a difference between these questions. Improvements in population health will require addressing both of these questions and considering the goals, breadth of data quality, sources, needs, and the sociopolitical and governmental context in which informatics solutions are being applied. The Public Health Informatics Institute (PHII) has been instrumental in articulating the business processes within public health agencies to address the first question. A list of its resources is available at www.phii.org.

THE VALUE OF INFORMATICS FOR THE DOMAIN OF PUBLIC HEALTH

To demonstrate the value of informatics for the domain of public health, it is useful to explore current public health methods, applications, and processes. The descriptions will help the reader to understand the value of informatics and the challenges encountered in the real world. A single chapter on the topic of public health informatics cannot begin to describe the breadth of public health systems but examples will be instructive. The sections that follow describe surveillance as a public health method, immunization information systems as a public health application, and health information exchange and public health reporting as public health processes.

Surveillance

Public health surveillance is the ongoing collection, analysis, interpretation, and dissemination of data for a stated public health purpose.[12] The primary goal of surveillance is to provide actionable health information to public health staff, government leaders, and the public to guide public health policy and programs.[12] Hence surveillance activities and the information generated guide decisions and monitor progress. These are critical for meeting all three functions required of

a public health system: assessment, policy development, and assurance. It is important to note that surveillance is an activity that often requires partnerships with private and public entities in the community and legislation to enforce it. Surveillance is difficult to delegate to others in the community, so it has generally been a public health department activity.

While new technologies, health reforms, and national security concerns are affecting surveillance efforts in the twenty-first century, the following specific goals of surveillance have not changed over time:

- To recognize cases or clusters of disease or injury to (1) trigger investigations, (2) trigger interventions to prevent disease transmission or to reduce morbidity, and (3) help to ensure the adequacy of medical diagnosis, treatment, and infection control
- To measure trends; characterize diseases, injuries, and risk factors; and identify high-risk population groups or geographic areas toward which needed interventions can be targeted
- To monitor the effectiveness of public health programs, prevention and control measures, and intervention strategies, which includes providing information to determine when a public health program should be modified or discontinued
- To develop hypotheses leading to analytic studies about risk factors for disease and injury and disease propagation or progression
- To provide information both to the public to enable individuals to make informed decisions regarding personal behaviors and to healthcare providers to ensure that they base their care of individual patients on the most current surveillance information available[12]

Currently, surveillance of infectious diseases (through either case reporting or sentinel surveillance) is performed at the local level where control efforts are localized and may be urgent. Surveillance of noninfectious events is typically managed by state health agencies because the interventions involved are often statewide and long term (such as cancer screening and prevention campaigns) and there are more resources to support electronic systems for vital records, immunization and cancer registries, newborn screening for heritable disorders, electronic laboratory reporting, and so forth. In addition, state agencies usually manage the hospital discharge datasets, claims data, and other administrative data generated from clinical encounters and shared with public health. State agencies conduct surveys for the Behavioral Risk Factor Surveillance System (BRFSS) and the Pregnancy Risk Assessment Monitoring System (PRAMS). Finally, the CDC and other federal agencies, such as the FDA, EPA, and the U.S. Department of Agriculture (USDA), monitor national trends and support state activities, conduct national surveys (e.g., National Health and Nutrition Examination Survey, National Health Interview Survey, Bureau of Labor Statistics' annual survey of work-related injuries and illnesses, federal tracking of coal workers' pneumoconiosis), interface with the World Health Organization (WHO) on global health concerns, and use data to generate research hypotheses.[12]

The range of events under surveillance span the causal pathway of disease (Fig. 11-3), including environmental exposures (e.g., folate levels in fortified grains, fluoride levels in water, air and water quality, air lead levels in indoor firing ranges), hazards (e.g., leaded paint in older housing, toxic releases), behaviors and risk factors (e.g., smoking, cancer screening, use of sunscreen, use of helmets when biking), exposure (e.g., needlestick injuries, newborns of mothers infected with hepatitis B, children in households with smokers), presymptomatic phase (e.g., blood lead levels in children), apparent disease or injury (e.g., persons diagnosed with hepatitis, tuberculosis, traumatic brain injury), and death. In their blueprint for surveillance in the twenty-first century, public health epidemiologists note that surveillance methods should match surveillance goals, data should be collected in the least expensive manner possible, and data should flow in an efficient, timely, and secure manner as defined by local, state, and federal laws.[12] High-quality data are needed if surveillance information is to be relied on but data quality should match its use. Perfecting data can be costly and may not be necessary. With this in mind, the authors of the blueprint matched purposes for surveillance with methods commonly used (Table 11-1)[12] and noted that systems should be evaluated for efficiency and security as well as timeliness, sensitivity, positive predictive value, simplicity, and flexibility of the system for the level of public health agency using the data.[13] In the twenty-first century, surveillance systems should also be evaluated on their sustainability and scalability to meet other needs and interoperate with existing systems.

In an effort to improve the timeliness with which outbreaks are detected (influenza outbreaks in particular), informatics researchers have been testing new signals for event detection, evaluating statistical models for finding significant events

TABLE 11-1 EXAMPLES OF MATCHING SURVEILLANCE PURPOSES WITH METHODS	
PURPOSE	METHOD
Provide case management; notify exposed partners; provide prophylaxis to contacts; detect outbreaks; quarantine exposed contacts; isolate cases; take regulatory actions to prevent exposures by others; target interventions to remediate hazards to exposed persons	Case reporting to local and state health departments by clinicians, healthcare facilities, and laboratories
Monitor common diseases for which detection of every case is not needed (e.g., influenza, Lyme disease)	Sentinel surveillance (collection of detailed information about a subset of cases) or sampling of suspected cases for full investigation
Monitor population vital statistics	Birth and death certificate reporting to states
Monitor population cancer incidence	Case reporting to state health department cancer registries by clinicians, healthcare facilities, and pathology laboratories
Monitor prevalence of childhood vaccination rates	Reporting of all childhood vaccinations by clinicians to state immunization information systems
Monitor population prevalence of risk factors and health-related conditions	Public health telephone, school-based, community, or other self-report surveys; public health examination surveys; analysis of deidentified electronic health record data, hospital data, claims data, and other clinical encounter data
Measure population levels of environmental and occupational risk factors	Public health or community and worker surveys; environmental monitoring and modeling; biomonitoring
Monitor antibiotic resistance in communities	Electronic laboratory reporting
Monitor characteristics and quality of care for health events and conditions (e.g., myocardial infarction, stroke, cardiac arrest, diabetes)	Quality improvement registries (e.g., Paul Coverdell National Acute Stroke Registry)
Detect evidence for an unreported change in community health or track situational awareness during public health emergencies	Analysis of deidentified clinical data by public health to detect changes in population health (syndromic surveillance)
Evaluate effectiveness of public health programs and interventions; monitor health trends in a population	Trend analysis of vital statistics reports, case reports, vaccination prevalence, clinical and billing data, population survey data, worksite injury and death reports, law enforcement records, special surveys
Characterize the epidemiology of specific diseases or injuries and develop hypotheses about and target interventions toward their risk factors	Analysis of population data or case-based data to describe disease or injury characteristics and risk factors

Adapted from Smith PF, Hadler JL, Stanbury M, et al. "Blueprint version 2.0": updating public health surveillance for the 21st century. *J Public Health Man.* 2012 [epub ahead of print]. doi:10.1097/PHH.0b013e318262906e.

among normal variation, and devising new strategies for visualizing information and engaging a broader community. Table 11-2 illustrates the relationship between illness-related events and the variety of surveillance systems that may capture those events. The quest to identify early events must balance the potentially less predictive quality of the information with improved opportunities to identify infections and outbreaks and then implement control measures to prevent further spread. Events that occur earlier in the chain of illness-related events may be less specific and lead to false-positive signals. The quality of the detected signals must be evaluated before they are routinely used in public health practice.

Finally, there are new opportunities to use personal health records (PHRs) and social media to monitor indicators of health status and attitudes and beliefs in the community. For example, researchers at Harvard University have shown that online social networks may be an efficient platform for bidirectional communication with and data acquisition from populations with diseases, such as diabetes, that affect public health.[14] Unadjusted aggregate A1c levels reported by users from the United States closely resembled aggregate levels reported in the 2007–2008 National Health and Nutrition Examination Survey (respectively, 6.9% and 6.9%, $p = 0.85$).[14]

In a second example, researchers archived and analyzed more than 2 million Twitter posts containing keywords such as "swine flu" and "H1N1" during the 2009 outbreak and found that with the rise of participatory web and social media tools, the user-generated content has the potential to serve as a near real-time source of data to trigger a public health response and also serves as a vehicle for knowledge dissemination to the public.[15] These authors believe that "infodemiology" data can be collected and analyzed in near real time and have the potential for analysis of queries from Internet search engines to predict disease outbreaks (e.g., influenza); monitor people's status updates on microblogs, such as Twitter, for syndromic surveillance; detect and quantify disparities in health information availability; and identify and monitor public health–relevant publications on the Internet (e.g., antivaccination sites, news articles, expert-curated outbreak reports). Another example of this approach is included in Chapter 31 with the discussion of MappyHealth. Such automated tools may be useful for measuring information diffusion and knowledge translation and for tracking the effectiveness of health marketing campaigns.[16]

Immunization Information Systems

Immunization information systems (IISs) are confidential, population-based, computerized databases that record all immunization doses administered by participating healthcare providers to persons residing within a given geopolitical area.[17] As one of the best examples of a public health informatics application, they interact with both clinical and public health systems, have successfully implemented vocabulary and messaging standards, can be used to deliver public health decision support in a clinical setting, and provide information useful for making public health policy and

TABLE 11-2	RELEVANT SURVEILLANCE SYSTEMS FOR ILLNESS-RELATED EVENTS
ILLNESS-RELATED EVENT	**SURVEILLANCE SYSTEMS THAT CAPTURE THE EVENT**
Actions in the Home or Community	
Search for information about "flu" in Google	Google Flu Trends (www.google.org/flutrends/)
Stay home from school	School absenteeism surveillance
Buy over-the-counter cough medicine	National Retail Data Monitor (http://rods.health.pitt.edu/NRDM.htm)
Read news article about possible outbreak in the community	HealthMap (www.healthmap.org/en)
Healthcare Surveillance	
Visit an urgent or emergency care setting and report chief complaint	Syndromic surveillance of chief complaints from all or sentinel clinics
Have a medically attended visit for influenza-like illness	U.S. Outpatient Influenza-like Illness Surveillance Network (ILINet)
Be diagnosed with a reportable disease	National Electronic Disease Surveillance System
Be hospitalized with influenza	Influenza hospitalizations CDC's Flu Activity & Surveillance (www.cdc.gov/flu/weekly/fluactivitysurv.htm)
Get a laboratory test for a viral pathogen	Pathogen surveillance (GermWatch)
Receive positive lab result	Electronic laboratory reporting
Mortality Surveillance	
Succumb to illness and die	Death registration system (i.e., vital records)
Child less than 5 years	Influenza-associated pediatric mortality
Resident of a city included in the 122-city system	122 Cities Mortality Reporting System

CDC, Centers for Disease Control and Prevention.

programmatic decisions. IISs are an important tool for helping to achieve and maintain effective vaccination coverage levels greater than 90% for universally recommended vaccines among young children (Box 11-2).[18] IISs represent the successful blending of multiple standards (including data, messaging, policy, interface, privacy, and so forth) managed by multiple governing bodies (Box 11-3).

IISs are in routine use throughout the United States. In 2008, 75% of children under 6 years of age had two or more immunizations recorded in an IIS. The Healthy People goal is to reach 95% by 2020 because vaccines are among the most cost-effective clinical preventive services.[18] Childhood immunization programs provide a very high return on investment. For example, for each birth cohort vaccinated with the routine immunization schedule (this includes DTap, Td, Hib, Polio, MMR, Hep B, and varicella vaccines), society saves 33,000 lives, prevents 14 million cases of disease, reduces direct healthcare costs by $9.9 billion, and saves $33.4 billion in indirect costs.[18]

At the point of clinical care, an IIS can provide consolidated immunization histories for use by a vaccination provider in determining appropriate client vaccinations.[17] When children receive vaccines in a variety of clinical settings, which is common, missing records can lead to repeated vaccinations (overimmunization) and added costs. In addition,

an IIS can evaluate the consolidated record and provide recommendations based on the immunization schedules published and updated annually by the CDC.[19] Since the vaccine schedules are updated every year, students should access the CDC website to view the most current vaccine schedules and assess their structure and complexity for implementing in a decision-support application. The schedules represent rule-based logic that may initially appear simple because it is primarily based on age. However, the schedule quickly becomes more complicated when one reads the footnotes, considers the time that is required to elapse between vaccine doses, and determines whether a different schedule is required if a child or adult is overdue and needs "catch-up" vaccines. The embedded decision support can determine the vaccines due today and forecast the vaccines required in the future to inform scheduling appointments.

At the population level, an IIS provides aggregate data about vaccinations that are useful for surveillance and program operations and can guide public health action aiming to improve vaccination rates and reduce vaccine-preventable disease.[17] An IIS can also provide information for health plans and healthcare providers that need to track and report quality measures, such as the HEDIS measures.[20] Finally, IISs have also provided previously unrealized critical functionality in public health emergencies. For example, only

---

BOX 11-2   IMMUNIZATION INFORMATION SYSTEM (IIS) OBJECTIVES

- Primary objective: Reduce, eliminate, or maintain elimination of cases of vaccine-preventable diseases
- Sample of sub-objectives for Healthy People 2020:
  - Increase the percentage of children aged 19 to 35 months who receive the recommended doses of DTaP, polio, MMR, Hib, hepatitis B, varicella, and pneumococcal conjugate vaccine (PCV). (Baseline: 44 percent of children aged 19 to 35 months in 2009 received the recommended doses of DTaP, polio, MMR, Hib, hepatitis B, varicella, and PCV; Target: 80%)

- Maintain the vaccination coverage level of 2 doses of measles-mumps-rubella (MMR) vaccine for children in kindergarten (Baseline: 95 percent of children enrolled in kindergarten for the 2009–2010 school year received 2 or more doses of MMR vaccine; Target: 95%)
- Increase the percentage of noninstitutionalized adults aged 18 to 64 years who are vaccinated annually against seasonal influenza (Baseline: 27 percent of noninstitutionalized adults aged 18 to 64 years received influenza vaccine for the 2008–2009 influenza season; Target: 80%)

From The U.S. Department of Health and Human Services. Immunization and Infectious Diseases. http://www.healthypeople.gov/2020/topicsobjectives2020/overview.aspx?topicid=23.

BOX 11-3   GOVERNANCE: SAMPLE IMMUNIZATION INFORMATION SYSTEM STANDARDS AND GUIDELINES AND THE RELEVANT GOVERNING BODY

- Core Data Standards: National Vaccine Advisory Committee
- Minimum Functional Standards: National Immunization Program's Technical Working Group
- IIS Operational Best Practice Guidelines: American Immunization Registry Association
- Data Transaction Guideline for HL7 version 2.3.1: CDC Immunization Information Systems Support Branch

- Privacy and Confidentiality Resources: National Immunization Program
- A Guide to Indian Health Service and State IIS Interfaces: Indian Health Service
- Electronic Exchange of Public Health Data: Public Health Information Network

From Centers for Disease Control and Prevention (CDC). IIS web resources. CDC. http://www.cdc.gov/vaccines/programs/iis/resources-refs/web-resources.html. 2012.
CDC, Centers for Disease Control and Prevention; HL7, Health Level Seven; IIS, immunization information system.

days after Hurricane Katrina in September 2005, the Houston-Harris County Immunization Registry was connected to the Louisiana Immunization Network for Kids Statewide, which provided immediate access to the immunization records of children forced to evacuate the New Orleans, Louisiana, area.[19] One year later more than 18,900 immunization records were found by persons querying the system, representing avoided vaccinations.[19] The researchers estimated a cost savings of more than $1.6 million for vaccine alone and $3.04 million for vaccine plus administration fees.[19] Similarly, during a recent measles outbreak the registry was instrumental in helping to prioritize contact tracing efforts. Named contacts with no measles vaccination information in the registry could be prioritized for intensive phone calling efforts to ensure that appropriate control measures were implemented.

Health Information Exchange

To succeed in its mission and carry out core functions, public health entities rely on data and partnerships with healthcare and other settings in a community. Health information exchange (HIE) initiatives and organizations provide an infrastructure to improve the required communication between public health and community partners. In the past the primary aim of an HIE has been to bring unavailable clinical data from patients' disparate health records to the point of care where clinicians and their patients need it most. The motivation for exchanging health data has been to create a complete health record to address safety and quality concerns, gain efficiencies, reduce duplication of efforts and control costs, notify participants about problems and potential drug seekers, and perform research. Box 11-4 includes potential HIE applications for use in achieving these public health benefits. When public health agencies participate in an HIE, they can both provide *and* receive value from their participation. Public health benefits from particpating in an HIE include the following additional benefits:

BOX 11-4 POTENTIAL HIE APPLICATIONS FOR USE IN PUBLIC HEALTH

- Mandated reporting of lab findings
- Nonmandatory reporting of lab data
- Mandated reporting of physician diagnoses
- Nonmandatory reporting of clinical data
- Public health investigation
- Clinical care in public health clinics
- Population-level quality monitoring
- Mass casualty events
- Disaster medical response
- Public health alerting: patient level
- Public health alerting: population level

Adapted from Shapiro JS, Mostashari F, Hripcsak G, Soulakis N, Kuperman G. Using health information exchange to improve public health. *Am J Public Health.* 2011:101(4):616-623.

- More timely and complete receipt of disease reports
- Faster transmission of better information to public health case managers (for communicable disease control, newborn screening follow-up)
- Easier identification and analysis of gaps in preventive health services (immunization, Papanicolaou smears) and of patterns that could improve performance
- Easier identification and analysis of follow-up failures (treatment of sexually transmitted diseases, environmental evaluation of lead poisoning) and of patterns that could improve performance
- Analysis and display of geographic distribution of illness or injury to focus public health interventions or services
- Analysis and display of the temporal and geographic epidemic spread
- Improved ability to communicate with selected healthcare provider and patient populations.[21]

Public health also *provides* value to HIE partners.[21,22] Public health can provide patient information (e.g., immunization records, newborn screening results, tuberculosis clinical findings, child health clinic records) and epidemiologic information to improve diagnosis (e.g., distribution and incidence of Lyme disease to improve a clinician's estimation of pretest probability). A public health agency may serve as a trusted neutral party for confidential health information or may maintain a community master patient index that can support the HIE using identifiers generated by healthcare organizations, birth records, and other sources. Public health involvement in an HIE has the potential to reduce the cost and labor of reporting. Finally, public health can provide personalized patient care information available in the community and alert healthcare providers to urgent community health issues.

Public Health Reporting

In the U.S., public health reporting to perform surveillance and implement control measures has been going on since the eighteenth century when tavern owners were asked to report persons with illness to a local board of health. Today, public health reporting to recognize and control communicable disease in a community is a quintessential public health activity. The rules concerning what diseases should be reported and the actions to take if reporting is necessary vary among the 50 states and may vary among cities or counties within a state, vary by disease, and sometimes vary by reporting entity (i.e., whether the reporter is a laboratory or a clinician) and other factors. As shown in Figure 11-6, a local health department is often the agency responsible for (1) receiving reports from laboratories, clinicians, hospitals and other reporters (e.g., schools, daycare centers); (2) investigating the situation; and (3) implementing control measures. Information gathered during the investigation informs the public health response and helps to establish whether to count the event for surveillance purposes.

Local and state agencies may share a single web-based system or the two levels of governmental public health may have separate systems. Either way, more data are collected

Selected examples from Utah:
    Within 24 hrs, report anthrax, measles, hepatitis A, tuberculosis
    Within 3 days, report AIDS, influenza-associated hospitalization

Selected examples from Maryland:
    Immediately report botulism, hepatitis A, rabies, pertussis
    Within 1 working day, report AIDS, chlamydia, mumps, infectious meningitis

FIG 11-6 Overview of the current public health reporting process. (Copyright 2010 Catherine Staes. Reprinted with permission.)

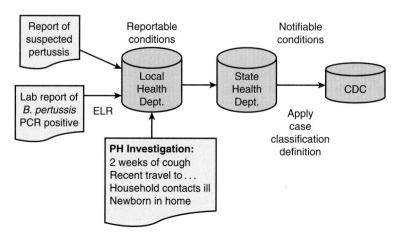

during an investigation than are needed for "notification" from the local to state health department. The information shared is often summary information ascertained after completing the investigation. Depending on the information available from the completed investigation, a disease report may be classified as either a "confirmed" or a "probable" case, for example. This classification is used when summarizing surveillance data in order to consistently report similar events over time while still quantifying the unconfirmed but relevant events.

The information used by the state health department for surveillance is a subset of the information gathered during an investigation. When information is sent to the CDC as a "notifiable report," the record is deidentified and filtered again to include only the data needed for national surveillance. Finally, the set of conditions included in NNDSS is not reported in every local and state jurisdiction and does not include all conditions reported everywhere.[23]

There are many complexities associated with the detailed processes of public health reporting but the high-level process shown in Figure 11-7 illustrates a set of activities that is commonly carried out across the U.S. Informatics solutions may be applied to each step in the process. For example, the first step in public health reporting concerns the publishing of reporting criteria (e.g., specifications). Currently, the guidance and regulations that laboratories and other reporters

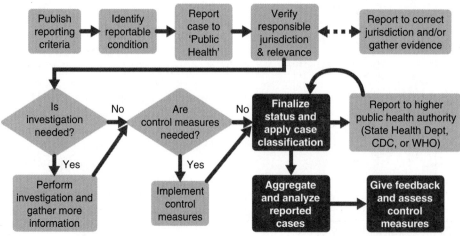

FIG 11-7 Process of public health case health reporting. (Copyright 2010 Catherine Staes. Reprinted with permission.)

need to follow are described on websites and posters.[24] The information cannot be processed by electronic systems; it changes periodically, especially during an outbreak; and it differs among states as well as between states and the CDC. Case reporters must interpret the criteria expected and maintain the reporting criteria in their systems. This situation could be improved using knowledge management strategies that allow public health authorities to author structured content and disseminate the laboratory and clinical reporting specifications in both a human-readable format and a structured format for use by automated laboratory and clinical systems.

Several factors make it difficult for clinicians, laboratories, and others to identify reportable conditions. Underreporting is common when manual processes are involved and reporting relies on clinicians to remember to report.[25] Studies have shown a lack of knowledge among clinicians about reporting requirements.[26] In addition, even as the use of detection logic is becoming more common in laboratory and clinical systems, the sensitivity and specificity of logic can vary by reportable condition. For example, a single lab test result is sufficient for detecting chlamydia while a clinical diagnosis is required for identifying culture-negative tuberculosis or suspected measles and a combination of laboratory and clinical findings is required to identify chronic hepatitis B infection.[27] There are informatics opportunities for defining and publishing detection logic (including codes such as ICD-9, LOINC, and SNOMED-CT) and using surrogate markers for reportable events, such as administration of hepatitis B immune globulin to a newborn as an indicator of an infected mother.

There are challenges with the process of reporting a case or lab result to public health agencies that result in delayed reporting, inefficient data gathering with incomplete reports, variable data collection, and nonstandard formats used to transfer the information (e.g., fax, phone, email, mail, web forms, electronic laboratory reports). Some of these challenges are being addressed by increased use of EHRs, Meaningful Use incentives, and Health Level Seven (HL7) standards.

While these factors improve the capabilities for the sender, there are also challenges on the receiving end of the transaction. Health departments must receive, sort, filter, deduplicate, and consolidate information that arrives "at their doorstep" via fax, phone, online web forms, and electronic messaging systems and from records routed from their state or other local health department colleagues using statewide electronic disease surveillance systems. Health departments often manage a large volume of reports using manual processes.

For example, in an observational study of workflow in a local health department, 3454 reportable conditions were manually entered into an electronic data system during an 18-month period of time.[28] In a prospective evaluation of the information being received, 18% of the reports were for other counties, 3% were not reportable, 16% were duplicates, and 18% were updates on previously reported cases.[28] Personnel resources are used to manage all of the paper arriving to find the new, relevant information among all incoming paper.

In an ideal world a health department would receive complete information in a timely manner only *once* and updates and duplicates would be managed automatically. There are numerous informatics opportunities to do the following:

- Enable the use of specifications (computable logic) to define where and how reports should be sent, the urgency of reporting, and the information to include in a report
- Automate information extraction of additional information in the EHR
- Improve standardization of message structure and content
- Enable secure information exchange
- Create public health information systems to receive case reports and allow access by local and state public health entities

Systems are being built to receive laboratory reports but this is only part of the information required to manage persons with communicable diseases in municipalities, counties, and states.

The processes associated with performing an investigation and implementing control measures (such as excluding a person with salmonella from food service or daycare or vaccinating contacts of a person with meningitis) can be complex. Decisions must be made on incomplete and evolving information, and guidelines are often ambiguous. The situation could be improved by the following:

- Automated linkage between clinical and electronic lab reports with information concerning updated or redundant reports
- Improved quality of the information in a report (e.g., include additional associated lab findings needed for investigation)
- Improved tools to explore the existing findings[29]
- Decision support tools that improve the management of new information and apply guidelines

The processes associated with aggregating information across jurisdictions and sharing subsets of information to a higher authority could be addressed using new strategies. Currently, aggregation occurs by copying information and sending it up the chain. However, "central" aggregation is defined differently among different stakeholders and does not adequately support sudden unanticipated needs. Currently, ad hoc queries must be initiated or informal communication and data aggregation may be required. A goal for future systems should be the ability to perform dynamic aggregation across jurisdictions and to access complete data in their native environments, with appropriate permissions (Fig. 11-8). In addition, future systems should allow surveillance data to be more accessible for decision support in near real time to healthcare systems and the community.

In summary, case reporting and management will benefit from computable knowledge managed and served by public health reporting standards about what, how, where, and when to report; automated event detection; electronic, standardized information exchange; improved systems for receiving and integrating case reports; and the ability to access disparate systems with appropriate permissions to dynamically aggregate data across jurisdictions and respond to new situations, data, and priorities.

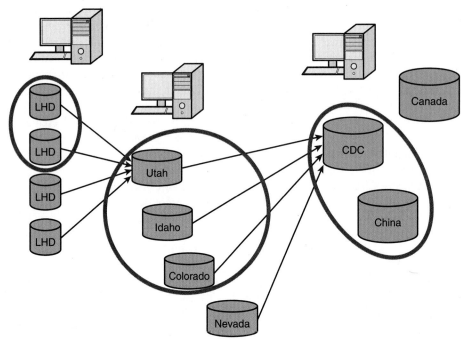

Goal:
- Dynamic aggregation across jurisdictions
- Access complete data in their native environments

FIG 11-8 An example of dynamic aggregation across local health departments (LHDs) and state and national departments of health. (Copyright 2010 Catherine Staes. Reprinted with permission.)

CONCLUSIONS AND FUTURE PUBLIC HEALTH INFORMATICS STRATEGIES

Transforming Practice with New Strategies

As discussed in this chapter, public health IT reflects the division of authority for population health between national, state, and local governments. In the past this division was less important because records systems were largely paper based. Each department could have its own approach to information management and the departments to which it reported or with which it shared information would have to manually convert information from one format to another. Given the complexities of data collection in the past, public health practitioners focused on information gathering to ensure the validity of the information supply chain for its own program. There was no way to reuse data across programs and it was not deemed highly important since the costs of reuse were almost as high as the costs of primary data collection and the validity of "reused" data could not be assured.

As public health practice moves into the future, the concept of the information supply chain needs to evolve toward an alternative model: an information ecology. Public health departments will receive data from a variety of sources that are *repurposed* for population health uses. Electronic data elements collected for one purpose (as part of one information supply chain) will be linked with other data to create an integrated environment. The old paradigm of public health programs setting up systems that measured specific factors, with primary data collection for surveillance, will be replaced by systems that network healthcare, environmental, and commerce data in order to collect data that are relevant to public health. Perhaps the biggest change for public health is the idea that public health systems need to "give to get." In the past, federal, state, and local governments used legislative authority to mandate reporting to public health. In the future, public health departments will need to be partners with other data producers, adding value for partners to the data received and republishing those data to contribute to the local information ecology.

An example of this approach is ongoing work with the CDC and General Electric (GE) Healthcare on public health alerting in EHRs. At the time of this writing the government efforts to implement syndromic surveillance have involved attempts to require healthcare providers to report emergency room data and other data to public health departments through the regulatory process of Meaningful Use.[30] However, efforts to require transmission of these data are controversial with both hospitals and provider organizations because of the cost involved and the lack of return for their efforts. Working with GE Healthcare, the CDC has developed an alternative approach based on a web services model that integrates syndromic surveillance in clinical workflows using decision support.[31] When a clinician sees a patient with a new complaint, he or she considers the following question: "Could this patient's symptoms be caused by an infectious disease?" Public health departments might answer this question by publishing "disease weather maps" for their local regions that clinicians could consult.[32] This type of decision support, whereby community-level information is summarized and displayed, is important but insufficient. Work can go further to create an interdependent system.

What would be most useful to clinicians is an individual specific interpretation of the current "epidemiologic weather." How could this be obtained? What if instead of merely sending data to local public health departments when required, information systems could harness the power of artificial intelligence to highlight patterns of data indicative of the types of symptoms a patient might be experiencing to assist the practitioner in determining whether they match the pattern of a known public health problem? At the public health department, data would be stored to track the nature of symptoms in a community and the individual data would be matched to public health alerts in the region. If the symptoms were consistent with a known problem, the sending electronic records system might receive an alert back from public health through secure messaging processes, and most appropriately after a review of data within an HIE, informing the clinician that the patient may be part of a public health outbreak. This type of cycle defines what is meant by information ecology: a public health department that integrates with clinical care and provides interpretations of the data generated by and sent from healthcare providers that justifies the provider's costs of extraction and transmission of information.

In addition to increasing access to data from healthcare systems, public health has the opportunity to use data from an increasingly connected environment to measure and affect health in the community. Mobile devices with global positioning system (GPS) locators are tools for people to find their way but also could be tools for governments to assess how active their citizens are in daily life. Do the regulations that try to make neighborhoods more walkable result in more people walking? In the past, observers would use clipboards and might sample streets or survey persons about how often they walk. But now a more efficient and accurate method for determining whether people are walking might be to see how many phones are moving around the community at walking speeds. Walkability might be defined by the patterns in which they move. Cellular phone companies have these data and they sell them for commercial use. Legislators and other policy-makers need to consider how private business can be incentivized (or regulated) to provide this information to public health.

Similarly, in the past, understanding dietary patterns of a community has required extensive in-person or mail surveys to ascertain food consumption. These methods are expensive and time consuming and limit the use of such data for public health purposes. An alternative approach that uses existing sources of data to inform population dietary habits would be to analyze shoppers' purchasing habits. Many stores use shopper cards to track purchasing decisions and behaviors. These same data could be used by public health officials to monitor consumption of fresh fruits and vegetables, salt, and sodas and to identify other dietary needs and risks. The use of such data raises many privacy issues at an individual level.

However, public health operations may not always need individual-level data. Many policy issues could be addressed by geocoding the data and anonymizing data clustering at a home or work location. If one can understand that a particular neighborhood is a "hot spot" for sugary beverage use or salt intake, then targeted efforts can be made to work within the community to change the community's values and habits to promote health. As described earlier, the population perspective assumes that individuals have levels of risk that are reflected in their community. Disease prevention strategies focused on a community do not require that public health officials know that Mrs. Jones drinks too much soda. Public health officials need to know where to conduct an education campaign in schools to reverse trends of students often preferring sugared beverages over healthier ones.

Advancing the Technical Infrastructure

The future of public health requires new advanced information technologies and infrastructures. However, public health departments, particularly local health departments, are resource-challenged environments. Departments often do not have the IT resources to take on new initiatives to connect themselves to clinical care systems or other sources of data, such as schools or occupational health entities that could provide the value-added capabilities discussed above. State governments may exploit the relative poverty of local public health, providing funding for IT for specific programs in order to capture very limited data. Likewise, federal public health programs provide their less-funded state colleagues with task-specific IT. The availability of such technology might provide secondary benefits to local and state public health departments, except that funding typically comes with contractual requirements that prevent technology resources from being used for other tasks. How can this problem be addressed and resolved? How can there be a future for public health informatics if resources are a continuing problem?

The CDC's first effort at helping the public health community to coordinate information management technologies was the Public Health Information Network (PHIN). This program proposed a set of communication and vocabulary standards for public health software designed to promote interoperability and to support reuse of information. The PHIN program had a number of elements, including standardized vocabulary based on the HL7 version 3.0 Reference Information Model (HL7 v3 RIM), solutions for composing value sets for applications (standard codes), an interoperability solution for transforming messages from one vocabulary to another, and a message transport solution called PHIN-MS for securely sending data from one public health department to another.[33] The success of the PHIN program was limited, except with regard to its transport solution, which was widely adopted. In general, the advantages of adopting one set of standards for vocabulary for public health systems were offset by the costs of implementation and the lack of fit between the HL7 v3 RIM vocabulary model and public health workflows. Public health departments found it easier and cheaper to continue to use their existing information management tools than to develop new tools based on the CDC standards or to convert existing tools to those specifications. PHIN continues to evolve as a program.[34] However, the question of whether a standards-based approach alone can achieve the ends of interoperability at reduced cost remains open.

Standards are critical but by themselves may not be adequate to provide the level of support needed to advance public health informatics. A flawed environment for acquiring systems results in agencies duplicating each other's efforts to develop and implement systems. Often jurisdictions implement proprietary, stand-alone systems that preclude data exchange, which is fundamentally important for surveillance and two-way communication. An alternative to individual jurisdictions creating the specifications for and purchasing software on their own, with inherent inefficiencies, may be the use of open source and collaborative development methods. Collaborative development can take many forms. In a project funded by the Robert Wood Johnson Foundation, state public health departments collaborated to develop a set of shared specifications of business processes for laboratory information systems. Through joint work at defining business processes a group of state laboratories was able to develop a shared specification for a laboratory information system.[35] These shared specifications were then used to guide shared open source development of a laboratory information system, where different jurisdictions assumed responsibility for different modules of the final product. This same group went on to work collaboratively to develop its own information exchange solutions, working as a group to modify the CDC's PHIN-MS software to support routing hubs (PHIN-MS initially was designed to support only point-to-point communications).

A service-oriented architecture (SOA), explained in Chapter 12, and open source methods may be useful in shared development. If a set of standard functions based on an enterprise architecture view can be developed to support public health applications, then these components could be reused to support a wide variety of additional public health applications. This concept is the foundation of the "service-oriented" systems approach. A critical issue is developing a set of modular programs designed to work together. These might include data transport tools like PHIN-MS, interoperability engines, standardized vocabularies, databases, master patient indexes, and other critical components. Importantly, this set of components should be open source, software available to potential developers at low or no cost. In an open source environment, public health departments with significant capabilities for developing software can work together to advance the field as a whole.

Currently the goal of many vendors of public health information systems (and other software systems as well) is to attempt to lock departments into proprietary systems, guaranteeing future revenue streams. Open source methodologies can help to prevent this. Some examples of successful open source software systems are as follows:

- The community version of the TriSano case management application

- OpenELS, which is the public health laboratory information system described above
- OpenMRS, an enterprise-level medical records application that is widely used in Africa for public health applications

Many public health departments, particularly local ones, have no significant capabilities to develop IT and typically lack the resources to hire vendors to support development or customization efforts. One approach to this lack of capability may be to move public health systems to the "cloud." As explained in Chapter 12, cloud computing systems migrate the location of software to a remote site where resources can be shared by different users. Examples of cloud-based software systems include Amazon.com, Facebook, and other web applications. These applications operate as "software as a service" (SaaS), where the developer attempts to present an integrated single application or a tightly integrated suite of applications.[36] BioSense 2.0[37] is an example of a SaaS application for public health. In this application each state can receive, parse, store, and analyze data streams from the EHR systems in hospital emergency departments, as required by the government's Meaningful Use program. Without this service each state is developing its own infrastructure to receive emergency department data. BioSense 2.0 allows states to rapidly develop procedures and use data sent in a prescribed format from the healthcare system, without the requirement to create their own infrastructure to manage the information. The system also allows states to share data across jurisdictions when necessary. For example, when a Super Bowl game draws large numbers of fans from one region of the country to another, this creates a need to link emergency room data from those cities to detect outbreaks that may occur after the event, when people have returned home.

The approach to computing that may be the most relevant to public health is platform as a service (PaaS).[38] PaaS architecture is based on virtualization of an entire computer operating system. For example, a PaaS system might allow a user to access a functional "PC" (entire version of Windows 8, for example) on a remote computer. This "PC" might have the entire library of relevant and most up-to-date public health programs on it. PaaS architecture would allow each public health department to select the applications it deems most relevant to its own workflows. These programs hopefully would and should draw on a public health SOA that would facilitate the creation of new public health applications. Applications could share databases and services for transforming and managing data. Because the operating system for each PC is identical, the task of configuring and managing software would be greatly simplified. A suite of applications could be created based on off-the-shelf components that work well together and in addition public health departments could access and use this suite from any location with high-speed Internet service. Moreover, the task of interoperability between users and jurisdictions would become greatly simplified as the network settings and application configurations would be known and standardized. Importantly, the degree of standardization afforded by PaaS architecture might help to create a market for public health applications that would rapidly foster improvement and expansion through competition among vendors. Lenert and Sundwall provide further discussion of issues related to the market and to SaaS versus PaaS systems for public health.[38]

In conclusion, this chapter described the importance and unique features of public health practice and differentiated public health practice from clinical practice. The social, technical, and political challenges of public health and public health informatics were highlighted. The value of informatics tools to support public health's unique needs and mission was highlighted by reviewing existing systems. Current major public health informatics applications, such as surveillance and immunization information systems, were described. The supporting workflows associated with these systems and the value of the information technology, decision support, and standards that are necessary to make the systems work were reviewed along with the strengths and challenges associated with developing an information ecology. This chapter then reviewed future strategies underpinning the public health information infrastructure. Increasing use of EHRs, standards to improve information exchange, social networking tools, and cloud-based and mobile computing methods will transform the way in which public health accesses and uses information to improve the health of populations.

REFERENCES

1. National Center for Health Statistics. *Health, United States, 2010: With Special Feature on Death and Dying.* Hyattsville, MD: Centers for Disease Control and Prevention; 2011.

2. Bunker JP, Frazier HS, Mosteller F. Improving health: measuring effects of medical care. *Milbank Q.* 1994;72:225-258.

3. Centers for Disease Control and Prevention. Ten great public health achievements—United States, 1900–1999. *MMWR Morb Mortal Wkly Rep.* 1999;48(12):241-243.

4. Centers for Disease Control and Prevention. Achievements in public health, 1900–1999: tobacco use—United States, 1900–1999. *MMWR Morb Mortal Wkly Rep.* 1999;48(43):986-993.

5. Schroeder SA. We can do better: improving the health of the American people. *N Engl J Med.* 2007;357(12):1221-1228.

6. Mokdad AH, Marks JS, Stroup DF, Gerberding JL. Actual causes of death in the United States, 2000. *J Amer Med Assoc.* 2004;291(10):1238-1245.

7. Public Health Data Standards Consortium. *White Paper: Building a Roadmap for Health Information Systems Interoperability for Public Health.* 2008.

8. Committee for the Study of the Future of Public Health. *The Future of Public Health.* Washington, DC: National Academy Press; 1988.

9. National Center for Health Statistics. Summary of NCHS surveys and data collection systems. Centers for Disease Control and Prevention. http://www.cdc.gov/nchs/data/factsheets/factsheet_summary.htm. 2012. Accessed October 10, 2012.

10. Committee on Assuring the Health of the Public in the 21st Century. *The Future of the Public's Health in the 21st Century.* Washington, DC: The National Academies Press. 2002.

11. Centers for Disease Control and Prevention. HIPAA privacy rule and public health: guidance from CDC and the U.S. Department of Health and Human Services. *MMWR Morb Mortal Wkly Rep.* 2003;52:1-12.

12. Smith PF, Hadler JL, Stanbury M, Rolfs RT, Hopkins RS. "Blueprint version 2.0": updating public health surveillance for the 21st century. J Public Health Man. 2012 [epub ahead of print]. doi:10.1097/PHH.0b013e318262906e.

13. Centers for Disease Control and Prevention. Updated guidelines for evaluating public health surveillance systems: recommendations from the Guidelines Working Group. *MMWR Recomm Rep.* 2001;50(RR-13):1-35.

14. Weitzman ER, Adida B, Kelemen S, Mandl KD. Sharing data for public health research by members of an international online diabetes social network. *PLoS One.* 2011;6(4):e19256.

15. Chew C, Eysenbach G. Pandemics in the age of Twitter: content analysis of tweets during the 2009 H1N1 outbreak. *PLoS ONE.* 2010;5(11).

16. Eysenbach G. Infodemiology and infoveillance: framework for an emerging set of public health informatics methods to analyze search, communication and publication behavior on the Internet. *J Med Internet Res.* 2009;11(1):e11.

17. Centers for Disease Control and Prevention (CDC). Immunization information systems. CDC. http://www.cdc.gov/vaccines/programs/iis/index.html. 2012. Accessed October 18, 2012.

18. Office of Disease Prevention and Health Promotion, National Center for Health Statistics. Immunization and infectious diseases. HealthyPeople.gov. http://www.healthypeople.gov/2020/topicsobjectives2020/default.aspx. 2012. Accessed October 12, 2012.

19. Boom JA, Dragsbaek AC, Nelson CS. The success of an immunization information system in the wake of Hurricane Katrina. *Pediatrics.* 2007;119(6):1213-1217.

20. National Committee for Quality Assurance (NCQA). HEDIS measures. NCQA. http://www.ncqa.org/HEDISQualityMeasurement/QualityMeasurementProducts.aspx. 2012. Accessed October 12, 2012.

21. Foldy S, Ross DA. *Public Health Opportunities in Health Information Exchange.* Atlanta, GA: Public Health Informatics Institute; 2005.

22. Shapiro JS. Using health information exchange to improve public health. *Am J Public Health.* 2011;101:616-623.

23. Centers for Disease Control and Prevention (CDC). National Notifiable Diseases Surveillance System (NNDSS). CDC. http://www.cdc.gov/nndss/. 2012. Accessed October 2012.

24. Council of State and Territorial Epidemiologists (CSTE). State reportable conditions websites. CSTE. http://www.cste.org/dnn/ProgramsandActivities/PublicHealthInformatics/PHIStateReportableWebsites/tabid/136/Default.aspx. 2011. Accessed March 10, 2011.

25. Overhage JM, Grannis S, McDonald CJ. Comparison of the completeness and timeliness of automated electronic laboratory reporting and spontaneous reporting of notifiable conditions. *Am J Public Health.* 2008;98(2):344-350.

26. Staes CJ, Gesteland P, Allison M, et al. Urgent care physician's knowledge and attitude about public health reporting and pertussis control measures: implications for informatics. *J Public Health Manag Pract.* 2009;15(6):1-8.

27. Klompas M, Haney G, Church D, Lazarus R, Hou X, Platt R. Automated identification of acute hepatitis B using electronic medical record data to facilitate public health surveillance. *PLoS One.* 2008;3(7):e2626.

28. Rajeev D, Staes C, Evans RS, et al. Evaluation of HL7 v2.5.1 electronic case reports transmitted from a healthcare enterprise to public health. *AMIA Annu Symp Proc.* 2001;2011:1144-1152.

29. Livnat Y, Gesteland P, Benuzillo J, et al. Epinome: a novel work-bench for epidemic investigation and analysis of search strategies in public health practice. *AMIA Annu Symp Proc. 2010;* 2010:647-651.

30. Centers for Medicare & Medicaid Services (CMS). Stage 2 overview tipsheet. CMS. https://http://www.cms.gov/Regulations-and-Guidance/Legislation/EHRIncentivePrograms/Downloads/Stage2Overview_Tipsheet.pdf. 2012. Accessed October 12, 2012.

31. Garrett NY, Mishra N, Nichols B, Staes CJ, Akin C, Safran C. Characterization of public health alerts and their suitability for alerting in electronic health record systems. *J Public Health Manag Pract.* 2011;17(1):77-83.

32. Gesteland PH, Livnat Y, Galli N, Samore MH, Gundlapalli AV. The EpiCanvas infectious disease weather map: an interactive visual exploration of temporal and spatial correlations. *J Am Med Inform Assoc.* 2012;19(6):954-959.

33. Loonsk JW, McGarvey SR, Conn LA, Johnson J. The Public Health Information Network (PHIN) Preparedness Initiative. *J Am Med Inform Assoc.* 2006;13(1):1-4.

34. Centers for Disease Control and Prevention (CDC). Public Health Information Network (PHIN) strategic plan: strategies to facilitate standards-based public health information exchange (2011–2016). CDC. http://www.cdc.gov/phin/library/documents/PHINStrategicPlan_v3_0.pdf. 2011.

35. Public Health Informatics Institute (PHII). The LIMS project: summary of evaluation findings. PHII. http://www.phii.org/sites/default/files/resource/pdfs/LIMS Evaluation-website-FINAL-2.pdf. 2007.

36. Mell P, Grace T. The NIST definition of cloud computing: recommendations of the National Institute of Standards and Technology. Division of Computer Security, National Institute of Standards and Technology, U.S. Department of Commerce. http://csrc.nist.gov/publications/nistpubs/800-145/SP800-145.pdf. 2011.

37. Kass-Hout TA, Gallagher K, Foldy S, Buehler JW. A functional public health surveillance system. *Am J Public Health.* 2012;102(9):e1-e2.

38. Lenert L, Sundwall DN. Public health surveillance and Meaningful Use regulations: a crisis of opportunity. *Am J Public Health.* 2012;102(3):e1-e7.

DISCUSSION QUESTIONS

1. How might you develop a data and information exchange between acute care, subacute care, and home health settings that would support the work of public health? Do such systems already exist?

2. Monitoring population health status is a central public health activity. A variety of survey systems, such as the CDC's National Health and Nutrition Examination Survey (NHANES) and National Health Interview Survey (NHIS), as well as state and national reporting systems, such as the Behavioral Risk Factor Surveillance System (BRFSS), Pregnancy Risk Assessment Monitoring System (PRAMS), and National Electronic Disease Surveillance System (NEDSS), provide public health practitioners with the ability to assess health trends, identify and respond to emerging health hazards, and guide development of interventions and policies that address serious health conditions such as obesity, smoking, and diabetes. With the proliferation of EHRs within acute and ambulatory care systems, how much of this survey activity do you think can be folded in under routine data collection and exchange activities?

3. The primary goal of public health is to affect population health and ensure a healthy community. How might you see public health nurses using web-based tools to reach, manage, and educate populations of patients residing in targeted communities?

4. It was stated in this chapter that part of the job of the public health informaticist is to develop the tools required to translate between the clinical and the public health world views as they relate to information system development and data sharing across the specialties. As a clinical leader, by what means would you advocate to enable this sharing?

5. Personal health records (PHRs) are technological tools that are being implemented within the acute care setting to enable data exchange with EHRs and to encourage patient activation in healthcare. How might you foresee the use of patient-entered data from a PHR as a public health surveillance tool?

CASE STUDY

You have been hired as an informaticist at a state health department. The health department is developing systems to receive laboratory and clinical case reports from clinical settings, such as hospitals and doctor's offices. Your state has had an immunization registry in operation for several years and has been successful in getting cooperation from healthcare settings to send data to the system.

Discussion Questions

1. Why is the system for reporting immunizations and receiving results at the health department so successful, particularly in comparison to the struggles you are observing as the health department sets up its laboratory and case reporting systems?

2. What is the difference between the set of information required to report an immunization administration and the set of information required to report a communicable disease?

3. What standard vocabulary is used to code a vaccine name and how is this vocabulary different from the LOINC or SNOMED-CT vocabularies required for laboratory and clinical case reporting?

4. What is the value proposition for a healthcare provider to participate in an immunization registry?

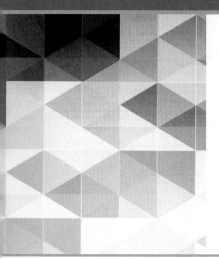

Technical Infrastructure to Support Healthcare

Scott P. Narus

No single off-the-shelf system today can support all needs of the healthcare environment. Therefore it is critical that the technical architecture be capable of supporting multiple system connections and data interoperability.

OBJECTIVES

At the completion of this chapter the reader will be prepared to:

1. Describe the key technical components of electronic health records and their interrelationships
2. Define interoperability and its major elements
3. Contrast networking arrangements such as regional health information organizations (RHIOs), health

information exchanges (HIEs), and health information organizations (HIOs)
4. Provide information about newer technical models such as cloud computing and application service providers (ASPs)
5. Synthesize current challenges for informatics infrastructure

KEY TERMS

ABSTRACT

This chapter introduces the technical aspects of electronic health records (EHRs) and the current infrastructure components. Complementing the functional components discussed elsewhere, this chapter introduces terms such as *clinical data repository*, *master person index*, *interface engine*, and *data dictionary* and other technical components necessary for EHRs to function. Recent material about national efforts related to the infrastructure and electronic data sharing, such as the Nationwide Health Information Network (NwHIN) and information exchange networks, is also reviewed.

INTRODUCTION

Understanding the information technology (IT) architecture underlying a healthcare organization's information systems is foundational to understanding how that system actually functions. Decisions about the technical infrastructure have important consequences for the overall system, in terms of both functional capabilities and support for clinical workflow. Many aspects of a clinical IT infrastructure are unique to the healthcare setting or have different properties or priorities. Understanding the needs of a clinical data repository or health data interface network as compared to their counterparts in other industries can mean the difference between successful and failed implementations.

EHR COMPONENT MODEL

The EHR may be thought of as a collection of several key components.[1] Each of these components contributes to the overall system functionality. In older EHRs these components were often bundled, making it difficult if not impossible to

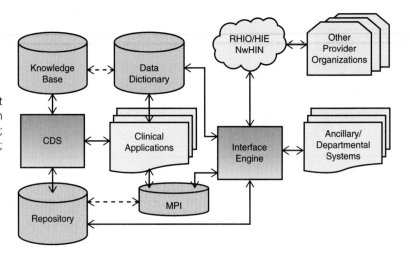

FIG 12-1 The electronic health record component model. *CDS*, Clinical decision support; *HIE*, health information exchange; *MPI*, master person index; *NwHIN*, nationwide health information network; *RHIO*, Regional Health Information Organization.

separate components from each other. In more modern technologies each of these components is often developed separately but may follow a common architectural design philosophy so that the components can be integrated easily. Each component could also be enhanced independent of the others as long as the component integration design was followed. Often the technical responsibility of the informaticist is to manage the component design and implementation life cycle, so understanding the component model and integration strategy is essential (Fig. 12-1). The following sections describe common EHR components and important considerations for each component.

Clinical Data Repository

The clinical data repository (CDR) is the storage component for all instance data of patient clinical records. By instance data we mean actual pieces of information collected by manual or automated means for a specific patient at a point in time. Data stored in a repository may be lab results, medication orders, vital signs, clinical documentation, etc. The data may be stored as free text or unstructured documents or as coded and structured elements (e.g., as columnar data in a relational database, as elements of a detailed model within an object-oriented database). The data within the repository are considered the most essential aspect of the EHR: without these data the other components of the EHR are meaningless. Therefore important aspects of the repository include accessibility, reliability, and security.

Accessibility means the ability to efficiently retrieve data stored within the repository. The repository must provide access methods that allow users of the repository (clinical applications, decision support rules, etc.) to find information using criteria that are meaningful to the users. For example, the repository should be able to distinguish data based on patient characteristics such as a patient identifier or encounter number. Data should also be classified by type to permit easy and quick retrieval of lab results versus radiology results. Other important data attributes that help with accessibility include dates (e.g., date recorded, date observed), data owners

and entry personnel (e.g., ordering physician, charting nurse, case manager), and location. The access methods for the repository should be robust enough to support current and future users' access needs.

Reliability refers to the dependability and consistency of access to the repository. In a critical healthcare setting a repository needs to support its users on a 24/7 basis. There is little tolerance for downtime. Inconsistent performance of the repository—for instance, longer wait times for data retrieval during high usage times of the day—also affects the reliability of the repository. Because of its importance to the functions of all EHR components, the reliability of the repository is the major factor in determining the perceived reliability of the EHR. Various architectural and procedural models may be employed to increase the reliability of the repository, including redundancy of storage hardware and access routes, system backup policies, and regular performance reviews and maintenance.

Security is essential to the repository because of both the sensitive nature of the data within and the critical role it plays in the healthcare environment. Various regulations, such as the Health Insurance Portability and Accountability Act (HIPAA),[2] as well as sound ethical practices demand that organizations provide a high level of confidentiality and privacy for the health information they handle. The repository must incorporate security measures in order to prevent, to the extent possible, inadvertent and intentionally inappropriate access to data. Data encryption, secure access paths, user authentication, user and role-based authorization, and physical security of the repository itself are typical methods employed. Some security methods may conflict with accessibility and reliability goals, and EHR implementers must weigh the benefits and costs of each, but good system design can mitigate conflicts while supporting the needs of the healthcare setting.

Repositories are distinguished along two axes that describe storage characteristics of the data: central versus distributed storage and encounter-based versus longitudinal-based storage.

Central versus Distributed Storage

In the central storage model, a single repository is used to store all (or most) clinical data and is used as the primary source for reviewing data. There may still be departmental or function-specific clinical information systems, as well as automated data collection devices, that are used to gather data. Some of these systems may even store copies of their information in their own repositories but these data are also forwarded to the central repository and stored there. In the case of a healthcare enterprise with multiple facilities, potentially consisting of inpatient and outpatient areas, the central model could store information from each of these facilities in one repository. This model improves the ability of a single application to display data from multiple original sources and locations and provides the capability to perform clinical decision support (CDS) more efficiently across multiple data types (e.g., combining lab results with medication administration and nutrition data to provide input for medication ordering). Central storage usually requires that data collected from secondary systems be transformed (mapped) to a common storage model and terminology before being stored in the repository. This model does not imply that data cannot be replicated to other locations for safety and disaster recovery purposes.

In the distributed storage model, each data collection application stores its information in its own repository and data are federated through a real-time data access methodology. In this case, a results review application may have to access separate repositories for lab, microbiology, radiology, etc., in order to provide a composite view of information. In the previous example of an enterprise with multiple facilities, each facility might store its own data in a facility-based repository. The distributed model provides some reliability to the EHR because, for example, if one repository goes down, the user may still be able to access information from the other repositories. It also allows the most efficient storage and access for particular data types and lessens the complexity of having to map data from one system to another. However, the distributed model produces many single points of failure for each repository, limits performance because of the multiple data access paths that may be required, and makes integrated tasks such as CDS much more difficult.

Encounter-Based versus Longitudinal-Based Storage

Encounter-based (or episodic) storage was typically used in older, hospital-based EHRs. In this model, data are collected according to the current patient encounter and then are usually purged or archived from the repository when the patient is discharged. If the patient has a future encounter with the facility, data may need to be collected completely anew, including patient history, allergies, and previous medications. Encounter-based storage is very efficient in terms of system performance for supporting the current encounter because the data in the repository are always the most current and reflect only what has been collected as relevant to the present circumstances. In this case, the repository's storage space can be quite small. However, since data are purged, some duplication of effort is inherent in this model since data collected during a previous visit may still be relevant and will need to be collected again. There is also a chance that pertinent information from a previous encounter may be lost if a clinician omits collecting it in a subsequent visit.

A longitudinal-based repository, on the other hand, stores data across all encounters. It is often referred to as a "cradle to grave" or "womb to tomb" repository because data may extend over the entire lifespan of an individual. The obvious advantages are that clinicians have access to all data collected on a patient from all clinical interventions and data that do not change and are relevant across all encounters, such as allergies, family medical history, and past procedures, do not need to be reentered at each visit. As with the central (versus distributed) storage model, the longitudinal record may contain data from multiple facilities and health enterprises as well. Access to historical data may be helpful in automated CDS. The disadvantage is that a patient's record (and therefore the entire repository) can grow tremendously large with data that become less relevant over time.

Master Person Index

The master person index (MPI) (also known as the master patient index or master member index) is the repository for the information used to uniquely identify each person, patient, or customer of a healthcare enterprise. One or more registration systems may be used at each visit to collect identifying information about the patient, which is then sent to the MPI in order to match against existing person records and resolve any conflicting information. The MPI stores demographic information about the patient, such as names, addresses, phone numbers, date of birth, and sex. Other organizational identifiers, such as social security number, driver's license number, and insurance identification, also may be stored. Identifiers from within the healthcare enterprise, such as individual facility medical record numbers, are also stored. (This is often a vestige of paper medical record systems that used facility-specific identifiers for each patient.)

As any of this information is updated or added to, the MPI record is updated. The MPI then serves as both the master of all information collected, forming what is often referred to as the "golden record" for a person, and the source for distinguishing a patient from all other patients in the system. The latter point is important because it helps to ensure that data are attributed to the correct patient during healthcare encounters. Each MPI record will have a unique patient identifier or number that is used in the repository to associate a clinical record with the appropriate patient and also is used by applications to properly retrieve and store information for the right patient. The MPI will typically support standard access methods for storing and retrieving data (e.g., Health Level Seven [HL7] Admit/Discharge/Transfer messages) so that systems that need to use the MPI can rely on a common interface mechanism. A user-facing patient selection application connected to the MPI is typically provided in the EHR so that EHR users can search for and find a particular patient for use in clinical documentation, review, and patient management applications.

Clinical Applications

Clinical applications provide the user-facing views of the EHR to clinicians. When clinicians think and talk about the EHR, they usually are referring to these applications. Applications are provided in a variety of technologies and user interface paradigms, including web-based applications, rich clients installed on a user's desktop, and mobile apps. A rich client (also called a fat, heavy, or thick client) is a client–server architecture or network that provides rich functionality independent of the central server. In contrast, a thin client refers to a client–server architecture that is heavily dependent on a server's applications.

When supplied by a single vendor, applications are typically "wrapped" inside a single desktop framework that provides global EHR functions such as user authentication and patient selection and then launches the individual applications as part of a clinical workflow. When supplied by different vendors, applications can still share user and patient context by using technologies such as Clinical Context Object Workgroup (CCOW), provided the vendor supports such functionality.[3,4] CCOW is an HL7 standard protocol designed to enable different applications to work together in real time at the user interface level. The CCOW standard exists to facilitate interoperability across disparate applications.

Clinical applications can be divided into four broad areas of functionality: review and reporting, data collection, patient management, and clinician productivity. For more information on individual applications in the patient care setting, refer to Chapter 6.

Review and Reporting

One of the most widely used functions of an EHR is review and reporting of clinical data in the repository. In general, a *review* application is typically focused on one area of clinical data (e.g., a lab results review application, a vital signs review module). On the other hand, a *reporting* application often has a broad range of clinical data that displays to the user (e.g., a 24-hour rounds report that combines lab, vitals, medications, intake and output (I/O), invasive line status, assessments, and plan in one view). A reporting application also typically allows much more user customization for selecting content and layout. A review and reporting application is optimized for display of data and does not necessarily allow direct data entry. However, to improve clinical workflow the application may provide a simple, one-click shortcut to a data collection application in order to edit or enter new data. A "smart" review and reporting application may also provide links from displayed data to more detailed information about that data, such as might be found with an *Infobutton*.[5-9] In more complex graphical user interface environments, the review and reporting application might provide functionality for graphing results, creating timeline associations between data points, and incorporating baseline, average, and goal parameters. The ability of the review and reporting application to support more advanced data display functions will depend

significantly on the granularity of data stored in the repository; primarily text-based storage will limit the amount of functionality while highly coded and structured data will allow increased possibilities. The performance and overall display capabilities of the applications are also affected by the repository's central versus distributed and encounter-based versus longitudinal-based storage characteristics.

Data Collection

The ability of clinical applications to collect data in the healthcare environment has improved dramatically as new technologies have become available. Older clinical information systems were typically text-based screens that required heavy use of a computer keyboard or 10-key pad for navigation and data entry. More modern graphical user interfaces allow a variety of input and screen navigation possibilities. Some systems may even allow direct collection of information from devices such as blood pressure monitors and weight scales. Data are usually collected one patient at a time and stored in the repository. Data may be collected in narrative form as unstructured notes or in a much more granular form as coded and structured data. For example, a vital signs assessment is typically collected in a structured format so that it may be used in a variety of reporting and CDS applications.

Data collection applications often are linked to review functions so that the clinician can see the current status of the patient and then add new or updated information. More advanced clinical workflows such as activity documentation (e.g., medication administration) may involve computerized decision support and computerized documentation flow processes to improve data collection. As with review and reporting applications, links to detailed information about the data to be collected (Infobuttons) may be provided to assist the clinician with evidence-based and regulatory and accreditation requirements for documentation. For example, in a medication administration application, an Infobutton linked to a particular drug might provide information on potential side effects, adverse effects, and therapeutic effects to assess for a particular patient.

Patient Management

Some clinical applications fit within a category that deals with clinician cognitive tasks, particularly around therapeutic and care delivery responsibilities. Ordering and care planning are examples of patient management responsibilities that are increasingly being supported by health information technology (health IT) applications. Each of these responsibilities requires an elevated cognitive load in order to process the amount of available patient information as well as the number of potential decisions a clinician can make. Successful EHRs will provide appropriate capabilities within patient management applications so as to support clinicians' ability to appropriately adopt these applications and support their cognitive tasks.[10] Quite often patient management applications will provide in-line access to review and reporting applications to improve the ordering and care planning process. The use of standard terminologies from a central data dictionary (discussed below) within these applications ensures that appropriate items are used by clinicians and communicated to other members of the care team. CDS systems and access to knowledge resources (discussed below) may also be employed to enhance decision making.

Clinician Productivity

EHRs often provide clinicians with functionality to assist with care process tasks that cut across many patients and address clinical workflow. Examples include care coordination and physician signature applications as well as interclinician messaging and notification functions. Point-of-care analytic applications that address quality issues are also becoming popular, particularly because of national health IT initiatives such as Meaningful Use.[11,12] These applications provide information on a clinician's patient population in order to monitor care and outcomes according to desired goals and can compare progress over time or against either standard criteria or other similar clinicians. For example, this type of application might report that one physician's patients with a specific diagnosis average an extra day in the hospital but also show a lower average readmission rate than other patients with the same diagnosis.

Data Dictionary

A key component of many modern EHRs is a data dictionary that contains the medical vocabulary terms used to store data within the repository. These same terms are used by the EHR applications to collect and display clinical data. In its simplest form the data dictionary can be viewed as a list of the health terms and their definitions needed by the EHR, usually stored in one or more database tables. The dictionary might contain terms for diagnoses, medications, lab tests, clinical exam measures, etc. Each of the terms may be assigned a specific code that is independent of how the term is represented to a user. For example, a diagnosis of dyspnea might be assigned a code of 1234. The actual representation for the term dyspnea (medical concept) could be "dyspnea" (English medical text representation), "shortness of breath" (English common text name), or "SOB" (English abbreviation of shortness of breath). In this case all of the representations would have the same definition and dictionary code because they are equivalent. Medical concepts from standard terminologies such as International Classification of Diseases (ICD)-9, ICD-10, or Systematized Nomenclature of Medicine (SNOMED) are also added to the data dictionary so that these terms can be used in applications and in the repository.

The data dictionary is particularly useful in the EHR because it is the central source for defining all terms and their corresponding codes used by the EHR. Instead of hard-coding these terms and codes within applications, the data dictionary allows more flexibility at application runtime to access new and updated terms as they become available over the lifetime of the EHR. For example, as new medications and diagnoses are created they can be added easily to the data dictionary and made accessible to all applications within the EHR. If these terms were hard-coded within an application instead, the programs would have to be updated and recompiled to make the terms available. In addition, all instances where the terms are used would potentially have to be updated (e.g., if two or more applications were exposing medication information). This leads to a greater maintenance burden for the EHR and can potentially lead to errors if term sources are not kept synchronized.

The data dictionary also provides the ability to create term relations. These relations take the form of hierarchical or associative relations. Hierarchical relations are the most common and can be used to describe domains and subdomains for terms. For example, a domain term for "diagnosis" can be created and then subdomains of "cardiovascular diagnosis," "respiratory diagnosis," and "endocrine diagnosis" could be defined. Within each of these subdomains, additional subdomains may be defined for more granular categorization but eventually the domains would list individual diagnosis terms, such as "hypertension" or "pneumonia." The domain relationships are useful in applications and decision support logic when, for example, a user wants to narrow a disease search in a problem list application to just cardiovascular diseases or when a decision support rule broadly defines an inclusion statement such as "IF Ordered_Drug Is_A Cardiovascular_Drug THEN . . . ," where "Ordered_Drug" is an instance of a drug ordered for a patient, "Cardiovascular_Drug" is defined as the domain for all cardiovascular drugs, and "Is_A" is the relationship used by the data dictionary to define hierarchical domain relationships between parent and child terms.

Associative relations can be used to define other useful, nonhierarchical relationships between terms. For example, we could associate the diagnosis term *hypertension* with the drug domain term *beta blocker* by creating a relationship called "can be treated by." In this case, since "beta blocker" is a domain, we can assume that all terms within this domain would inherit the "can be treated by" relationship with hypertension. Another example of an associative relationship is a link created between two different coding systems that might describe similar terms. For example, a local laboratory information system (LIS) might contain its own coding for all lab tests it performs. However, the EHR and other external systems might use a standard lab terminology such as Logical Observation Identifiers Names and Codes (LOINC).[13-15] In this case the dictionary could define a mapping relationship between the terms in each of the systems so that information could be shared between the systems and maintain the semantic meaning of the terms.

One final note about data dictionaries concerns the desire or need to provide a unique code for each term in the dictionary. The unique code is necessary because the same term representation might be used to describe different concepts. For example, the word *temperature* might be used by a patient to describe having a "high temperature" (chief complaint) while a nurse might use this word to chart a physical measurement of "body temperature" (observation). These are different concepts and the concept codes ensure that they remain distinct. Other reasons to use unique codes are because term representations may change over time or multiple representations for the same term may be allowed depending on the user or display context. In these cases the code would remain the same. Lastly, it is usually much faster to search for codes rather than representations within a repository when they follow a strict numeric or alphanumeric syntax. This makes the repository and thus applications more responsive to user access, although the overhead of translating stored codes to user-readable term representations must be considered.

Knowledge Base

A knowledge base (or knowledge repository) is a component within the EHR that stores and organizes a healthcare enterprise's information and knowledge used by the enterprise for clinical operations. This information might range from simple material such as lists of orderable items, available services, or policy documents, to richer content such as order sets and searchable medical subject matter, to highly complex knowledge such as clinical guidelines and decision support rule sets.

The content in the knowledge base is usually organized by attaching *metadata* (information describing the content) to content items, allowing categorization of the knowledge content based on contextual need. The content itself usually follows a defined *metadata model* (detailed data format description) so that it can be consumed easily by applications. In some cases the content may be human readable, such as content consisting of medical journal articles that are indexed by subject matter. In other cases the content may be machine consumable; that is, the content may be read by a computer program and used to automatically produce an output, such as a logic statement that might be executed by a decision support engine in order to produce a suggestion or alert from a clinical guideline. Often the data dictionary is used to supply coded content and index information within the knowledge base. This ensures that the knowledge base remains synchronized with the patient data repository and clinical applications.

The knowledge base's content (often known as knowledge "artifacts") allows an EHR to become a "content-driven" system as opposed to a system whose knowledge is hard-coded in software programs. When knowledge such as treatment protocols, drug–drug interaction rules and descriptive content is hard-coded in clinical applications it is much more difficult and costly to update those applications. By separating the knowledge artifacts from the software and providing access through linkage services, clinical programs can keep pace with the rapidly changing and expanding medical environment, as represented by approaches such as evidence-based practice.

One example of a knowledge-based environment is use of the Infobutton standard: the Infobutton allows clinical applications to link dynamically to contextually relevant content located either within or outside a provider system.[5] The content provider may update this content as newer information is discovered or produced but the applications that link to the content through the Infobutton do not need to be changed because the interface (link) remains the same, providing a more robust EHR. Content-driven systems can also use local knowledge about a healthcare enterprise's operations in order to optimize workflows and enhance clinician interactions with the EHR.

As the content within a knowledge base grows, knowledge management tools become necessary in order to maintain the information.[16] Authoring tools that allow knowledge content to be created and updated and then facilitate the review process are particularly useful.[17,18] In addition, governance policies and procedures must be instituted to ensure the integrity of and promote and coordinate the use of the knowledge within the repository.

Clinical Decision Support System

A CDS system provides the technical means to combine general medical and health knowledge with specific data about a patient and current clinical context in order to assist a clinician in making appropriate treatment choices and to alert healthcare providers about relevant information and important events. For example, during the ordering process a clinician might be alerted about a potential drug–drug interaction that was found by the CDS system when a newly submitted prescription was compared with the patient's current medications. The CDS system also might be used to advise a clinician on the preferred treatment actions for a diabetic patient, based on the institution's best practice guidelines and the patient's current medical state. In addition, a hospital staff member might be alerted about a critically abnormal lab result that could affect medical care.

The CDS system typically consists of an inference engine that runs rules or logic (programs), methods for receiving or pulling data from clinical sources, and a communication system for notifying users or other systems about decision support results. The CDS system may be tied to a knowledge base in order to receive its rules, in which case the rules can be updated as needed without having to change or recompile CDS code. The CDS system also may contain hard-coded rules that must be changed by recompiling code, or the logic may be based on machine-learning algorithms that dynamically update as new information is processed by the system.

Data services may be used by the CDS system to access clinical data in the repository. Sometimes these data are automatically sent to the CDS system by a "data drive" mechanism that automatically triggers a feed to the CDS system whenever data are stored in the repository. Clinical applications also may supply data directly to the CDS system for real-time decision support, for instance when a clinician is in the process of performing an action and needs assistance from the CDS system before making a final judgment. Quite often, even if data are automatically sent to the CDS system through a data drive mechanism or directly from an application, the rules to process the data require additional information from the repository. In this case the CDS system may use data access services to retrieve the needed repository data.

The CDS system may need a queuing mechanism in order to support rules that will be triggered at a later time. For example, a rule processed on a lab result might trigger an output that says to wait for a new lab value in 24 hours before making a final recommendation to the clinician. If another lab result is not found within 24 hours, the rule will provide a different output recommendation, such as "order a new lab X." Another use for the queue is to support "stateful" clinical protocols, that is, protocols that remember the state of the patient from a previous point in time and use this information to make recommendations at a later time.

Once a rule is run the output result must be communicated to the appropriate recipients. The CDS system might store a decision support result in the data repository if the rule was triggered without direct user input so that a clinician can see the result at a later time. There might also be a mechanism for notifying a specific user of a result through email, pager, or other communication device. When accessing the CDS system directly from a clinical application, the CDS system must have a method for communicating its results back to the application, usually through a service or application programming interface (API). CDS systems are explained in additional detail in Chapter 10.

SYSTEM INTEGRATION AND INTEROPERABILITY

The EHR is often only one piece of a larger health information system environment within a healthcare enterprise. In fact, it is common for larger institutions to run two or more EHRs. Because no single EHR today can provide all of the functionality needed in most healthcare facilities, the ability to share information between systems is necessary. Departmental and ancillary systems for lab, pharmacy, radiology, registration, billing, etc., must be able to pass information to and receive information from the EHR. Integrating these systems is typically the responsibility of an interface engine (see following section). The different methods for storing and communicating data used by health information systems today necessitate interoperability standards to ensure proper communication.

Interface Engine

Older intersystem communication methodologies used point-to-point connections to allow different systems to share data and information; that is, a specialized interface was created between one system (A) and another system (B). The interface between systems A and B only knew how to translate between these two systems and could not be used to talk to another system. This method is fine if there are few systems in the network. However, as the number of systems grows, the number of connections multiplies rapidly. For a network with N systems where all of the systems are interconnected, there are $N \times (N-1)/2$ connections; for example, a network with six systems would have $6 \times (6-1)/2 = 15$ connections. Each system in the network must individually expose $N-1$ interfaces in order to be fully interconnected with all other systems in the network. In practice this means that for a network with 6 systems and 15 connections a total of 30 interfaces must be maintained. If a system in the network is replaced, all of its $N-1$ interfaces must be replaced, too.

Because of the cost and complexity of point-to-point interfaces, modern information systems often employ an interface engine (IE). An IE allows each network data source to have one *outbound* interface that can then be connected to any receiving system on the network. The IE is able to queue the messages from a data source, transform the messages to the proper format for the receiving systems, and then transmit the messages to appropriate systems. Acknowledgment and return messages also can be routed appropriately by the IE.

IEs use proprietary software or standard programming languages such as Java to write routines for translating one system's data message model into another system's model. Most of today's IEs support standard messaging interfaces like HL7 and X12. The IE must also translate terminology between systems because quite often systems will use different vocabularies or coding methods to represent comparable concepts. Sophisticated interface engines will use external sources such as a standard data dictionary to provide the necessary terminology translation services. This allows the IE to remain up to date on the latest coding conventions and translations for the systems on the network.

The following scenario explains how an IE could be used to integrate an EHR with various ancillary systems. At the beginning of a clinical encounter the patient is registered in the facility's registration system. The collected demographic information and encounter identifiers are transmitted by the registration system to the IE, which then transforms and forwards this information to the EHR and the LIS. During the patient's visit the physician uses the EHR to order a laboratory test. The lab order message is appended with the correct patient identifiers and routed through the IE to the LIS. The EHR uses a proprietary coding system for lab tests that the physician orders; these are mapped to LOINC codes that the LIS uses. When the lab completes processing of the test, the lab results are returned by the LIS to the EHR via the IE. The IE also branches LIS administrative information for the test to the facility's billing system for reimbursement purposes.

This scenario describes a somewhat simple network of five interfaces. In reality, the registration system may be tied to many more systems that need demographic and patient identifier information. The EHR will provide order messages not only to an LIS, but also to departmental systems for radiology, pharmacy, nutrition, etc. Each department system's results may need to be routed to several receiving systems for storage, processing, and reporting; the EHR will typically need an inbound interface from each of these diagnostic systems. The impact when one or more of the systems on the network is replaced must be considered. An IE greatly improves the ability to address this complicated network environment in an efficient and usually less costly manner.

Interoperability Standards

System and data sharing or interoperability has long been a problem for EHRs. Most EHRs and departmental and ancillary systems have been written using proprietary programming and data storage schema. This has made it difficult to share data between systems. When trying to connect two systems, integrators must first agree on a common exchange mechanism and message format (called syntactic interoperability). Then, to ensure that the data passed between the two systems are understandable by the receiving system, the content of the message must be mapped to a comparable and comprehensible model and terminology in the receiving system (called semantic interoperability).

Some of the most widely used clinical messaging standards are produced by the HL7 organization.[19] The HL7 version 2.x message standard is supported by virtually all major clinical information systems in the U.S., providing a common method for connecting EHRs and departmental and ancillary systems. The version 2.x standard specifies the format for messages but does not specify a standard for the content. The HL7 version 3 standard uses a much more formal specification to define messages and is based on the Reference Information Model (RIM). RIM and the Clinical Document Architecture (CDA) can be used to ensure better semantic interoperability between systems. Version 3, initially published in 2005, is not as widely implemented in clinical information systems in the U.S. as version 2.x because of its added complexity and significant implementation costs. Most clinical interface engines support the HL7 standards.

Many national and international terminology standards have been developed to support the exchange of clinical data and promote semantic interoperability of systems. Most of these standards were started around a specific clinical domain but may have been expanded to cover additional domains as the terminology was adopted. For example, LOINC was originally developed to describe clinical laboratory data but has been expanded to cover other clinical observations such as vital signs. SNOMED CT was originally developed as a nomenclature for pathology. It has been extended to become a highly comprehensive terminology for use in a wide variety of applications, including EHRs. Other terminology standards include ICD-9 and ICD-10, Current Procedural Terminology (CPT), RxNorm, and nursing terminologies such as Nursing Interventions Classification (NIC), Nursing Outcomes Classification (NOC), and North American Nursing Diagnosis Association (NANDA). For additional information on terminology standards, refer to Chapter 22. Information on the Omaha System is included in Chapter 9, which deals with home and community-based health systems.

NETWORKING SYSTEMS

In the previous section we discussed system interoperability within the walls of a single institution. However, there is a growing desire and need to share patient information between institutions for quality, financial, and regulatory purposes. Sections of the Meaningful Use criteria in the 2009 Health Information Technology for Economic and Clinical Health (HITECH) Act specifically call for sharing of clinical data between healthcare providers and with public health.[11] Various organizational models for sharing data have been developed at the local, regional, and national level.

RHIOs, HIEs, and HIOs

One of the earliest models for a data sharing network was the Regional Health Information Organization (RHIO). A RHIO is typically characterized as a quasi-public, nonprofit organization whose goal is to share data within a region. RHIOs were quite often started with grant or public funding. Health information exchanges (HIEs) followed RHIOs and are differentiated from them by having an anchor provider organization and usually being started for financial incentives. The anchor organization often provides a data sharing mechanism with affiliated providers. In practice the operating characteristics of RHIOs and HIEs may be quite similar and the distinctions are only in the terminology used.

Health information organizations (HIOs) are the latest models and support the 2009 HITECH Act mandate for health information sharing between EHRs. The role of the HIO is to facilitate data exchange according to nationally recognized standards. This may mean that the HIO only provides guidance to the organizations in an information exchange network or that the HIO assumes the technical responsibility for providing the exchange mechanism.

To facilitate data sharing, the information exchange network is designed as either a centralized or a distributed data architecture (although hybrids of the two are also sometimes deployed). In the centralized model the participants on the networks push their data to a central repository housed in one location. Organizations then retrieve data from the repository as needed. In a distributed model the network participants keep their data and provide a mechanism to answer requests for specific data. In either model the network must provide the ability to correctly match patients between organizations. Without this matching functionality, the network participants are unable to share information accurately. The network may use a global MPI that can map patient identifiers between organizations. In addition, to provide syntactic and semantic interoperability of the data, the network participants must agree on standards for information exchange. These standards may be similar to those discussed in the previous section on interoperability standards. Lastly, the exchange network must provide appropriate security mechanisms to authenticate and authorize appropriate use, prevent unwanted access, and accommodate necessary auditing and logging policies.

To connect to the information exchange network, participants may simply treat the network as another interface on their local interface engines. This allows participants to use existing methods for sharing data, particularly if a centralized model is used and data are pushed to the central repository. In the case where a distributed model is used and participants must accept ad hoc, asynchronous data requests, some additional effort may be required to effect data sharing. Another model for linking to the exchange network is to provide a service layer that accepts ad hoc requests for data. The data request services are accessible by network participants, often in the same way that web pages are made available as URLs on the World Wide Web. This method is becoming more popular and is particularly advantageous in the distributed exchange model because it better supports pulling data from an organization as it is needed.

Nationwide Health Information Network (NwHIN)

The Office of the National Coordinator for Health Information Technology (ONC) is facilitating the development of a national "network of networks" that will enable health care provider organizations and consumers to share information across local information exchange networks. The Nationwide Health Information Network (NwHIN) is a set of policies and national standards that will allow trusted exchange of health information over the Internet.[20] An initial implementation of the NwHIN architecture called CONNECT was demonstrated in 2008, with participation by various public and private entities,[21] and includes components for core services (locating patients, requesting documents, authentication, etc.), enterprise services (MPI, consumer preferences management, audit log, etc.), and a client framework (application components for building test and user interfaces to CONNECT). A simplified implementation of the NwHIN architecture called Direct allows two organizations to share medical information through common methods, such as email-like protocols.[22] These methods require a provider directory to ensure secure, point-to-point routing of messages.

OTHER INFRASTRUCTURE MODELS

The previous sections on the EHR component model and system integration focused on technical infrastructure that may be deployed locally within an organization. Other models exist that can also supply this infrastructure, but from sources outside an organization's walls.

Application Service Provider

Rather than purchasing and installing an EHR, some institutions opt to partner with an application service provider (ASP) for their clinical application needs. An ASP is a company that hosts an EHR or departmental system solution for a healthcare enterprise and provides access to the application via a secure network. Users of the application are usually unaware that they are connecting to a vendor's offsite computing facilities. An ASP model relieves the healthcare enterprise from having to host and support the technical components of the EHR, which may lead to lower capital infrastructure costs. This obviously helps smaller facilities that lack funding for a complete IT shop but it may be financially beneficial for larger facilities as well because of the economies of scale that an ASP vendor can provide over many customers.

On the other hand, the ASP model implies some loss of control of the EHR. ASP customers must be content with their data being stored at the vendor's off-site location. They must also accept that versions of application software, functionality, configurations, and levels of support typically will be what the majority of the other ASP customers are using. Lastly, it may be more difficult to integrate with other IT systems at the local site since the ASP vendor may not support interfaces for a healthcare enterprise's entire portfolio of departmental and ancillary systems. Interfaces may be more difficult to develop and maintain since the ASP vendor controls its half of each interface and may not prioritize projects in sync with the facility's needs.

Cloud Computing

One of the growing trends in IT is the concept of cloud computing. Although the term *cloud computing* is somewhat new, the basic idea behind it goes back decades. It can be traced to early suggestions that computing would some day be like other public utilities and that IT consumers would plug in to networks of applications and physical resources in the same way that electricity and phone lines are accessed. Computing resources would be supplied by either public organizations or a few private enterprises and shared by the consumer community.

The term *cloud* was attached to this concept because early networking diagrams enclosed these "public" computing resources within a cloud figure in order to represent resources outside of an organization's physical walls and the ability for these resources to change location without affecting the consumer's ability to access them. While we often still consider clouds as being available in a public space (i.e., accessible by many consuming individuals and organizations), a cloud may also be private (i.e., deployed within the walls of single organization for use by that organization's various entities). Cloud computing can be separated into three models: software as a service (SaaS), infrastructure as a service (IaaS), and platform as a service (PaaS).[23]

In the SaaS model, service providers run applications (services) at one or more locations and make these available to consumers. Consumers connect to the services through a cloud client, often something as simple as a web browser. This eliminates the need for consumers to host and support the applications themselves. The SaaS provider can also use economies of scale to provide multiple servers and sites that host applications, potentially increasing the efficiency, performance, and reliability of the applications. SaaS applications may be as simple as a service that provides a single function, such as Google Maps, or an application that covers an entire set of workflow requirements. The ASP model described in the previous section may be considered a type of SaaS. In clinical computing SaaS might be used to provide an entire EHR or EHR function (e.g., scheduling, lab results review from a lab services provider) or more focused functions within an EHR application such as drug–drug interaction checking during the ordering process, information retrieval for clinical descriptions of diagnoses and abnormal lab results, or terminology mapping between coding systems.[24]

The most utility-like example of cloud computing is IaaS. In this model, the cloud provider makes computing machinery available to consumers from large pools of resources. The IaaS provider can scale the computing resources to the needs of the consumer. This practice has become simpler with the growing use of *virtual machines*, which can be installed as multiple instances on physical hardware and simulate most of the characteristics of an operating system and its environment. The consumer is responsible for deploying the operating system, applications, databases, tools, etc., and then supporting those installed assets. Users may connect to the assets deployed on the IaaS resources through the Internet or via a virtual private network. The IaaS provider can help organizations to lessen the cost of ownership of physical resources and offload the need to employ local technical personnel to maintain equipment.

The PaaS model is a simplification of the IaaS model in which the cloud provider deploys an entire platform for running the customer's computing needs. This may include the operating system, application server, web server, database, etc. The consumer then installs or develops software on the resources provided. The PaaS provider supports the computing resources supplied by its cloud while the cloud user supports the assets built on top of it.

CURRENT CHALLENGES

Even though most of the technologies discussed so far have existed for decades, many technical challenges and barriers remain for implementation in the clinical environment. For the EHR repository, primary challenges remain around the robustness of storage architectures. With transitions to patient-centered longitudinal records, the size and content scope of the repository has grown considerably. Additionally, as new data types are added to the EHR in order to capture more detailed information about clinical encounters and patient health (particularly to meet the expanding requirements of Meaningful Use), the repository must be able to handle new information that was not anticipated in its original design. These facts demand that the database and storage mechanisms be flexible.

Databases must be able to scale in size to accommodate large amounts of online data. As they grow in size, they must retain performance characteristics that do not slow down the workflow of the clinical environment. Some database architectures and their storage services require new designs and recompilations as new data types are added. Some are not designed for the volumes of information that may be stored, especially in the future. Careful consideration of repository architecture must be performed before system selection to ensure that the system will meet the ongoing needs of the healthcare organization. Consider that patient data will have a lifetime measured in decades, whereas the technology will be enhanced or replaced on a 5- to 10-year, or less, lifespan. There must be a graceful way to transition the data in the repository to new technology without loss of information.

Data integration and interoperability remain the most difficult challenges in health information systems. The lack of standards, or the lack of implementation of standards, is a significant barrier. Expanding federal requirements around data exchange are forcing EHR vendors to abandon proprietary data architectures and adopt accepted standards for many types of data, but considerable work still needs to be accomplished to ensure semantic interoperability of data. This issue, coupled with older, outdated repository architectures, may leave some health IT vendors, and therefore their customers, without a path forward for their systems.

Some underlying system architectures make the EHR component model described earlier in the chapter difficult, impractical, or impossible to implement. Component APIs and services may be inflexible and require considerable effort in order to add new components, particularly if a different development group or vendor supplies those components. This issue reflects a lack of system integration standards (to accompany the lack of data integration standards discussed previously). Because of this, quite often a health IT vendor must supply all pieces of the component model, locking customers into a single solution that may lack needed robustness in one or more of the components.

Lastly, one of the most vexing challenges for health IT has been the ability for clinical applications to integrate well with clinical workflow. Informatics professionals address these workflow issues during system analysis and usability activities to improve application adoption by clinicians. Additional information for understanding usability activities is included in Chapter 21. Still, a thorough analysis and usability assessment may not ensure acceptance in all environments. Some amount of application adaptability is often necessary to tailor the system to specific settings and for specific individuals. On the other hand, allowing for application customization at the facility, department, and user level may be quite difficult to accomplish and support (depending on the system architecture and technical abilities of the application support staff) and can lead to nonstandard implementations that may prove costly. Upgrades to nonstandard and highly tailored applications can also be extremely challenging. How well application providers support customization is an important consideration in system selection. It can have significant consequences on overall clinical IT systems infrastructure. Too little customization may mean that multiple applications must be added to the infrastructure to address the specific needs of each department or unit. More liberal customization, besides adding user complexity, may force larger manual and automated governance structures on the organization to ensure that individual solutions still support organizational policies and goals. In either case the underlying technology of the clinical applications has a profound effect on the ability of users to do customization. In some cases a programmer must change or add source code in order to make local adaptations. In other cases tools supplied with the application allow configuration changes that can be incorporated more easily and quickly in the application, but obviously with limits to the scope of customization.

CONCLUSION AND FUTURE DIRECTIONS

The technical infrastructure of a health information system includes several key components that are unique to the healthcare environment. A sound understanding of the attributes of these components and how they interact is essential for a successful system implementation that supports the needs of the clinician users. No single off-the-shelf system today can support all needs of the healthcare environment. Therefore it is critical that the technical architecture be capable of supporting multiple system connections and data interoperability. More functionality will also become available from third-party vendors and infrastructures should be designed to support linking these capabilities directly to the clinical workflow. It should also be expected that the desire, and requirement, to share data outside an institution's walls will expand. The informatics role will continue to grow as the need to understand new technologies and how they can be combined with existing systems and exploited in the healthcare environment gains heightened importance.

Many new technologies are being explored or contemplated for health IT infrastructure. Most of these technologies are not new to other industries; healthcare has been much slower to adopt IT in general. In some cases these technologies have been implemented in organizations that possess strong informatics experience but they have not been employed more widely. Certainly the increasingly technology-savvy clinicians practicing at healthcare institutions are demanding functionality that looks more like what they use daily in web-based applications, smartphones, and tablet computers.

Mobile Apps

The growing use of mobile electronic devices has resulted in an explosion of smarter technologies for operating systems, user interfaces, and applications. Apple advertised more than 500,000 apps available for its iPhone and iPad as of June 2012. Google advertises hundreds of thousands of apps for its Android operating system, which is used in smartphones and tablets. Several hundred of the mobile apps available can be categorized as medical or health related, and that number is growing. The apps range from medical reference materials, to radiology image and diagnostic results viewers, to fairly robust clinical documentation tools.

A valuable aspect of these apps is that they are easily installed on a user's device. They are typically much cheaper than applications that run on laptop and desktop computers. The ability to "carry" the app anywhere the user goes and remain connected to an institution's network (through a cellular or wireless network) is appealing to clinicians who roam to several locations throughout their workday. The volume, ease of installation, and inexpensiveness of apps can provide a much more "democratic" user voice in the selection of apps that are most useful or appealing to the user. The lightweight nature of mobile apps and the use of common user interface and application programming interface standards may make it easier for healthcare institutions to develop their own apps, customized to local needs.

There are challenges, however, to the use of mobile apps in the healthcare setting. First, the small screen factor of mobile devices limits the amount of information that may be displayed or collected. This can mean scrolling or paging through many screens to eventually get to the information needed by the clinician. It also may be easier to miss important information on the screen because of the smaller font and image sizes.

Wireless networking may be another challenge for healthcare institutions. The increasing number of mobile devices in a healthcare facility, coupled with the "chatty" nature of many mobile apps, may overwhelm a hospital or clinic network. Organizations may need to develop support for virtual private networks in order to accommodate users who wish to use their mobile devices and apps outside the institution's walls. IT departments also must be able to handle devices brought into a facility by clinicians who are not employed by the organization, leading to potentially significant support and security issues. Finally, while the "democratization" of apps referred to earlier may seem at first blush to be a positive trait, a healthcare institution must be concerned with the support, data, and process standardization issues that may ensue. If clinicians are free to choose any app (e.g., for charting vital signs or ordering), will those apps be able to access and store data in the institution's required format, run decision support rules required for patient safety and quality reporting, and share information with co-workers and referral partners?

Service-Oriented Architecture

There has been much hype for years in the IT industry in general about service-oriented architecture (SOA), and healthcare has certainly been an active topic area in the discussion. SOA can be described as an architecture design pattern in which services are business oriented, loosely coupled from other services and system components, vendor and platform independent, message based, and encapsulated with internal architecture and program flow that are hidden from the service user. SOA services are most evident today as web-based (URL) services that are accessed through Hypertext Transfer Protocol (HTTP). Extensible Markup Language (XML) is commonly used as the message format. The interface to a web service, including its allowed input parameters and return data, is often described using the Web Services Description Language (WSDL).[25] SOA fits in the SaaS category of cloud computing but it has much more highly defined design and implementation patterns.

What this means to IT is potentially a more decentralized approach to system design in which solution providers concentrate on specific aspects of a business need. System architects can pull together many business services to meet the larger application needs of the organization without having to worry about the complexity inside the service code. Reuse is a key benefit of SOA because services may be used by different consumers for a variety of applications. Because the services are loosely coupled from each other and from other aspects of the service user's system, service code may be changed and enhanced without necessarily having to change other aspects of the overall consuming system. Changes can easily be communicated to service users through updates in a service's WSDL.

The SOA design philosophy has been researched in healthcare for a number of years. A joint effort by HL7 and the Object Management Group (OMG) to develop standards for healthcare services has resulted in the Healthcare Services Specification Project (HSSP).[26,27] HSSP has been investigating several health IT functional areas that could become the building blocks for EHR services. One example is CDS.[28] By exposing CDS services over the web, users would be able to access CDS content from a variety of sources without having to maintain the content locally. Other areas being pursued by HSSP include services for terminology mediation and clinical data access and update.

Because no single vendor product can meet all needs of a healthcare enterprise, vendors and market segments (e.g., pharmacy fulfillment, HIE) are also incorporating SOA principles in their architectures in order to more easily and quickly provide functionality to users. Whether a major EHR product will ever be entirely composed of SOA services supplied by third-party providers is an open question, but it is likely that health IT infrastructures will provide increased support for services as standards continue to emerge and service providers become more numerous and relevant to the healthcare community.

Open Source Software

Open source software (OSS) can be defined as software whose source code is made available to users, who then may be able to examine, change, and even redistribute the code according to the software's open source license. OSS is often developed in a public forum in which many programmers from different organizations, or acting as independent agents, contribute to the code base. There is typically a central code repository where all contributors place their updates and where users can download latest versions of code or compiled objects. Users may also keep a list of bug reports and feature requests. Open source advocates believe that OSS may be more secure, bug-free, interoperable, and relevant to specific user needs than proprietary (vendor) software because a more heterogeneous group of individuals with varying uses for the software has direct access to the source code. Some noted examples of OSS are the Apache HTTP web server, the Linux and Android operating systems, the Eclipse software development platform, the Mozilla Firefox web browser, and the OpenOffice software suite.

Several examples of OSS exist in the healthcare arena. EHR applications include OpenMRS, a multiinstitution project led by the Regenstrief Institute and Partners In Health, a Boston-based philanthropic organization,[29] and OpenEHR, an ONC-certified ambulatory EHR.[30] The U.S. Department of Veterans Affairs is seeking to develop an open source version of its VistA EHR.[31] The openEHR Foundation is developing open clinical archetypes (standard data models) to promote sharable and computable information.[32] Open source, standards-based CDS tools and resources are being developed as part of OpenCDS.[33,34] Mirth Connect is an OSS interface engine that is built for HL7 integration.[35] Apelon provides its terminology engine, Distributed Terminology System (DTS), as an open source platform[36]; 3M Health Information Systems has announced that it will make its health data dictionary available through open source.[37,38] These examples, and the many more in development or production, point to a future health IT infrastructure environment with wider clinician collaboration and less expensive software licensing costs.

Organizations need to be aware that "open source" does not mean "free"; they must budget for local customization, implementation, training, support, and hardware costs.

SMART

Through its Strategic Health IT Advanced Research Projects (SHARP), the ONC has funded the Harvard-based Substitutable Medical Applications, Reusable Technologies (SMART) Platforms project.[39] The goal of SMART is to provide a health IT platform based on core services that allows apps to be substituted easily. Inspired by the boom in mobile apps for cellphones and tablets, researchers have developed an application ecosystem in which data can be accessed easily and presented to apps constructed for specific purposes. The apps can be bundled to provide an entire health IT solution. Institutions can decide which apps their "containers" will deploy for their clinicians based on local needs and specific app aspects such as security capabilities. The API is open source, allowing anyone to develop new applications, which can then be provided to the user community as open or closed source code. A government-funded effort initially, it will be interesting to see whether the SMART platform will be adopted widely by the healthcare provider and vendor community or a similar effort may compete with SMART.

REFERENCES

1. Clayton PD, Narus SP, Huff SM, et al. Building a comprehensive clinical information system from components: the approach at Intermountain Health Care. *Methods Inf Med.* 2003;42(1):1-7.
2. Gostin L. Health care information and the protection of personal privacy: ethical and legal considerations. *Ann Intern Med.* 1997;127(8 Pt 2):683-690.
3. Marietti C. The eyes have it: CCOW (Clinical Context Object Workgroup) brings both cooperation and competition together to tackle visual integration. *Healthc Inform.* 1998;15(6):39.
4. Berger RG, Baba J. The realities of implementation of Clinical Context Object Workgroup (CCOW) standards for integration of vendor disparate clinical software in a large medical center. *Int J Med Inform.* 2009;78(6):386-390.
5. Cimino JJ, Li J, Bakken S, Patel VL. Theoretical, empirical and practical approaches to resolving the unmet information needs of clinical information system users. *Proc AMIA Symp.* 2002:170-174.
6. Reichert JC, Glasgow M, Narus SP, Clayton PD. Using LOINC to link an EMR to the pertinent paragraph in a structured reference knowledge base. *Proc AMIA Symp.* 2002:652-656.
7. Cimino JJ, Li J. Sharing Infobuttons to resolve clinicians' information needs. *AMIA Annu Symp Proc.* 2003:815.
8. Collins S, Bakken S, Cimino JJ, Currie L. A methodology for meeting context-specific information needs related to nursing orders. *AMIA Annu Symp Proc.* 2007:155-159.
9. Del Fiol G, Huser V, Strasberg HR, Maviglia SM, Curtis C, Cimino JJ. Implementations of the HL7 Context-Aware Knowledge Retrieval ("Infobutton") Standard: challenges, strengths, limitations, and uptake. *J Biomed Inform.* 2012;45(4):726-735.
10. Weir CR, Nebeker JJ, Hicken BL, Campo R, Drews F, Lebar B. A cognitive task analysis of information management strategies in a computerized provider order entry environment. *J Am Med Inform Assoc.* 2007;14(1):65-75.

11. Centers for Medicare & Medicaid Services (CMS). Meaningful Use. CMS. http://www.cms.gov/Regulations-and-Guidance/Legislation/EHRIncentivePrograms/Meaningful_Use.html. 2012. Accessed September 17, 2012.

12. Anderson C, Sensmeier J. Alliance for nursing informatics provides key elements for "Meaningful Use" dialogue. *Comput Inform Nurs.* 2009;27(4):266-267.

13. Forrey AW, McDonald CJ, DeMoor G, et al. Logical Observation Identifier Names and Codes (LOINC) database: a public use set of codes and names for electronic reporting of clinical laboratory test results. *Clin Chem.* 1996;42(1):81-90.

14. Huff SM, Rocha RA, McDonald CJ, et al. Development of the Logical Observation Identifier Names and Codes (LOINC) vocabulary. *J Am Med Inform Assoc.* 1998;5(3):276-292.

15. Logical Observation Identifier Names and Codes (LOINC). Regenstrief Institute. http://loinc.org. 2012. Accessed September 17, 2012.

16. Sittig DF, Wright A, Simonaitis L, et al. The state of the art in clinical knowledge management: an inventory of tools and techniques. *Int J Med Inform.* 2010;79(1):44-57.

17. Hulse NC, Rocha RA, Del Fiol G, Bradshaw RL, Hanna TP, Roemer LK. KAT: a flexible XML-based knowledge authoring environment. *J Am Med Inform Assoc.* 2005;12(4):418-430.

18. Rocha RA, Bradshaw RL, Bigelow SM, et al. Towards ubiquitous peer review strategies to sustain and enhance a clinical knowledge management framework. *AMIA Annu Symp Proc.* 2006: 654-658.

19. Health Level Seven International (HL7). http://www.hl7.org. 2012. Accessed September 17, 2012.

20. The Office of the National Coordinator for Health Information Technology (ONC). Nationwide Health Information Network: overview. ONC. http://healthit.hhs.gov/portal/server.pt/community/healthit_hhs_gov__nationwide_health_information_network/1142. 2011. Accessed September 17, 2012.

21. CONNECT Community Portal. http://www.connectopensource.org/. 2012. Accessed September 17, 2012.

22. The Direct Project. http://wiki.directproject.org. 2012. Accessed September 18, 2012.

23. Glaser J. Cloud computing can simplify HIT infrastructure management. *Healthc Financ Manage.* 2011;65(8):52-55.

24. Paterno MD, Maviglia SM, Ramelson HZ, et al. Creating shareable decision support services: an interdisciplinary challenge. *AMIA Annu Symp Proc.* 2010:602-606.

25. Web Services Description Language (WSDL) 1.1. W3C. http://www.w3.org/TR/wsdl. 2001. Accessed September 17, 2012.

26. Kawamoto K, Honey A, Rubin K. The HL7-OMG Healthcare Services Specification Project: motivation, methodology, and deliverables for enabling a semantically interoperable service-oriented architecture for healthcare. *J Am Med Inform Assoc.* 2009;16(6):874-881.

27. Healthcare Services Specification Program. http://hssp.wikispaces.org. 2012. Accessed September 17, 2012.

28. Kawamoto K, Lobach DF. Proposal for fulfilling strategic objectives of the U.S. roadmap for national action on clinical decision support through a service-oriented architecture leveraging HL7 services. *J Am Med Inform Assoc.* 2007;14(2):146-155.

29. Mamlin BW, Biondich PG, Wolfe BA, et al. Cooking up an open source EMR for developing countries: OpenMRS—A recipe for successful collaboration. *AMIA Annu Symp Proc.* 2006: 529-533.

30. Kalra D, Beale T, Heard S. The openEHR Foundation. *Stud Health Technol Inform.* 2005;115:153-173.

31. Mosquera M. VA's VistA open source agent to launch in August. *Government Health IT* [serial online]. http://www.govhealthit.com/news/vas-vista-open-source-agent-launch-august. 2011. Accessed September 18, 2012.

32. Garde S, Hovenga E, Buck J, Knaup P. Expressing clinical data sets with openEHR archetypes: a solid basis for ubiquitous computing. *Int J Med Inform.* 2007;76(suppl 3):S334-S341.

33. Kawamoto K. OpenCDS. http://www.opencds.org/. 2012. Accessed September 17, 2012.

34. Kawamoto K, Del Fiol G, Strasberg HR, et al. Multi-national, multi-institutional analysis of clinical decision support data needs to inform development of the HL7 virtual medical record standard. *AMIA Annu Symp Proc.* 2010:377-381.

35. Mirth Corporation. Mirth Connect. Mirth Corporation. http://www.mirthcorp.com/products/mirth-connect. 2012. Accessed September 17, 2012.

36. Apelon. DTS—Distributed Terminology System. Apelon. http://www.apelon.com/Products/DTS/tabid/97/Default.aspx. Accessed September 17, 2012.

37. 3M Terminology Consulting Services. http://www.3mtcs.com. Accessed September 17, 2012.

38. Goedert J. 3M health data dictionary going open source. *HealthData Management* [serial online]. http://www.healthdatamanagement.com/news/3M-data-dictionary-open-source-interoperability-coding-44468-1.html. 2012. Accessed September 17, 2012.

39. Mandl KD, Mandel JC, Murphy SN, et al. The SMART Platform: early experience enabling substitutable applications for electronic health records. *J Am Med Inform Assoc.* 2012; 19(4):597-603.

DISCUSSION QUESTIONS

1. Describe the role of the informaticist in designing and implementing the EHR technical infrastructure as outlined by the component model discussed in the chapter.

2. How does a data dictionary influence the design and implementation of an EHR? How does the data dictionary enhance and restrict the EHR?

3. In what circumstances might a clinical infrastructure based on either third-party service providers or mobile applications be desirable? What cautions would we place on these technologies in the same circumstances?

4. How will incentive programs such as Meaningful Use affect, both positively and negatively, technical infrastructures in healthcare settings?

5. Assume that you are leading a group developing a CDS system for your organization. Choose a particular clinical environment and set of clinical problems you want to address and describe the types of interfaces you would

need with other components in the clinical infrastructure in order to be successful.

6. What would be potential areas of concern for an EHR that heavily used third-party services to supply critical clinical functionality, such as decision support or medical reference links?

7. Meaningful Use criteria mandate that healthcare organizations be able to share data with other healthcare providers and public health organizations. These mandates will likely continue to expand over time. Describe how you would design the technical infrastructure to support this expansion so that new data sharing criteria are easily incorporated into the system.

8. Vendors often design "closed" infrastructures in order to lock customers into their products. What would be positive and negative aspects, from the healthcare organization's viewpoint, of having such an infrastructure?

9. As opposed to the closed infrastructure of most vendor systems, open source systems may allow multiple sources to contribute to the underlying system code and architecture. Describe the positive and negative aspects of this approach for the healthcare organization.

10. The Infobutton standard for access to knowledge resources is receiving growing interest from health IT vendors and users. If more medical knowledge resources are made available through this standard, how might this change the nature of EHR applications, CDS systems, and local knowledge development and storage?

CASE STUDY

An integrated delivery network (IDN) serving a large urban and rural demographic area is using separate EHR systems in its inpatient and outpatient settings. Some of the specialty departments have also purchased their own systems for documentation. Unfortunately this means that information collected in the inpatient setting is not available when patients are seen in the IDN's outpatient clinics (and vice versa). The clinicians need this information to be better informed about their patients and to provide optimal care. In addition, new Meaningful Use requirements for problems, medications, and allergies as well as new chronic disease care initiatives that the IDN is implementing for its patient population are being hindered by the separate systems. The clinicians have been given accounts on both EHRs but this is cumbersome for the users because they must be trained on multiple systems, they use valuable time logging into different systems and navigating for information, and there is a potential safety issue if the user selects different patients on the two EHRs. A coordinated decision support environment has also been difficult to implement because the two EHRs use different coding systems and do not share most of their information. This means, for example, that admission rules for congestive heart failure patients are unable to use the ambulatory medication list and recent vital signs measurements in order to run the IDN's standard care process models.

The IDN realizes that it will not be able to replace either EHR in the near future and, even if it could, there will still be issues with integrating information from the specialty care systems. It decides on a strategic plan to create a clinical data repository (CDR) that is fed with high-value data from each of the clinical systems. The outpatient EHR's master person index already was being used as the master unique identifier for most of the IDN's systems, so it can be incorporated with the new CDR. A robust interface engine is implemented to supply data from the clinical systems to the CDR. To normalize the different terminologies used on their various systems,

the IDN engages a terminology services vendor to provide a central data dictionary for the CDR and map the concepts from the current systems to the central standard terminology. The interface engine uses the terminology services to normalize inbound data to the CDR from the other systems.

The second phase of the strategic plan is to build a CDS system on top of the CDR in order to develop and maintain enterprise patient care rules. As rules are fired, their results will be both sent through the interface engine to the existing EHRs and stored in the CDR; storing the decision support results in the CDR provides a link to supporting data from all clinical systems, which can help with rule triage and maintenance. Another effort in this phase is to provide clinician views into the CDR. The IDN plans to build data services that can be called by third-party EHRs in order to display longitudinal, enterprise-wide patient data from within the EHRs. Several simple web- and mobile-based viewing applications using the data services will also be developed and will be available in a stand-alone mode or as callable modules within the current EHRs. The IDN will use CCOW to provide the user and patient context from the EHR to these viewing apps so that the clinicians will not have to log in twice and find the patient.

Discussion Questions

1. Describe the advantages and disadvantages of the situation in the case study.

2. You are the chief medical informatics officer for the organization. You are asked to comment about how the technical plans will impact clinicians. Based upon the case study, how do you respond?

3. The organization receives a $3 million gift from an informatics benefactor. You are an informaticist in the organization. What would your technical priorities be to remedy the issues in the case study?

Participatory Healthcare Informatics and Healthcare on the Internet

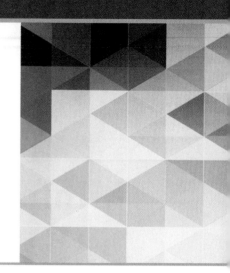

The Evolving ePatient

Sally Okun and Christine A. Caligtan

The epatient is and will continue to be a pivotal force in accelerating the healthcare system's adaptation to the ever-evolving world of technology, information management, and communication.

OBJECTIVES

At the completion of this chapter the reader will be prepared to:

1. List at least three "e" terms used to describe epatients
2. Explain the driving forces behind the emergence of the epatient movement
3. Discuss the characteristics of online healthcare consumers
4. Describe how the quantified selfer uses health-related data
5. Analyze the implications of epatients on clinical practice
6. Identify technological innovations likely to be used in routine practice by clinicians when caring for patients in the future

KEY TERMS

Crowdsourcing, 219
eHealth, 213
ePatient, 213
ePatient movement, 213
Guided discovery, 218
Health 1.0, 215
Health 2.0, 215
Health 3.0, 215

P4 Medicine, 222
Participatory healthcare, 218
Participatory medicine, 218
Quantified selfer, 217
Virtual communities, 221
Web 2.0, 215
Web 3.0, 215

ABSTRACT

The term *epatient* was coined long before the advent of the Internet to describe patients who take an active role in their health and healthcare by being equipped, enabled, empowered, and engaged. Today, epatients connect electronically to a vast array of online health information and resources, such as traditional chat rooms, support sites, health-related social media, and patient-to-patient research-based social networks. ePatients understand the value of engaging in a collaborative partnership with their healthcare providers and view the integration of participatory healthcare across the U.S. healthcare system as essential. The epatient is and will continue to be a pivotal force in accelerating the healthcare system's adaptation to the ever-evolving world of technology, information management, and communication.

HISTORICAL BACKGROUND AND DRIVERS OF THE EPATIENT EVOLUTION

ePatient as a Pioneering Concept

As early as the 1960s clinical researchers[1] used emerging technology to test computer-based patient-driven medical interviews. Slack's philosophical view of "patient power" coupled with his belief that computers had a place in medical practice were controversial at the time. Often asked, "Will your computer replace the doctor?" Slack's response then was as true then as it is today: "Any doctor who can be replaced by a computer deserves to be."[2(pS135)] Empowering patients with innovative tools should not be about removing power from healthcare providers. Empowerment helps individuals to lead more proactive and fulfilling lives.[3]

In 1975 another pioneering physician, author, and researcher, Thomas Ferguson, was interested in the empowered health consumer. Ferguson coined the term *epatient* and characterized epatients as people who are equipped, enabled, empowered, and engaged in decisions about their health and healthcare.[4] By the early 1990s, with the rapid emergence of personal computers and the World Wide Web, Ferguson recognized the power and potential for consumer use of online health resources. In *Looking Ahead: Online Health & the Search for Sustainable Healthcare*, Ferguson wrote:

> . . . the 21st Century will be the Age of the Net-empowered epatient, and . . . the health resources of today will evolve into even more robust and capable medical guidance systems which will allow growing numbers of epatients to play an increasingly important role in medical care. Online patients will increasingly manage their own healthcare and will contribute to the care of others. Medical professionals will increasingly be called upon to serve as coaches, supporters, and coordinators of self-managed care.[5]

Ferguson's work is largely seen as the impetus of the epatient movement and his early observations, ideas, and recommendations continue to resonate today.

The use of the term *epatient* predated the availability of online medical resources. However, today an epatient is characterized as one who uses technology to actively partake in his or her healthcare and manages the responsibility for his or her own health and wellness.[6] ePatients are online, seeking information, sharing their knowledge, and connecting with others. An epatient manages health decisions on a daily basis and uses the Internet to supplement his or her health journey. The collection of data and knowledge from online sources helps to organize and support epatients with contextual information and medical vocabulary necessary to converse with their healthcare providers.

The first evolutionary phase of the epatient movement occurred as access to health information and health-related services became increasingly available through electronic means. By late 1999 the term ehealth emerged in the lexicon as a way to describe electronic communication and information technology (IT) related to health information and processes accessible through online means.[7]

In 2001 ehealth was described as "the use of emerging information and communication technology, especially the Internet, to improve or enable health and health care."[8(p8)] Conceptually, the term *ehealth* was considered a bridge for both the clinical and the nonclinical sectors capable of supporting health-related tools for individuals and populations. For this potential to be fully realized, Eng believed that ehealth initiatives require integrated information systems that use common data elements and infrastructure standards that can serve multiple stakeholders.

Today, ehealth remains a broad concept used to describe Internet or web-based activities that relate to healthcare yet no consensus about the definition exists among researchers, policy-makers, clinicians, or patients.[9] Pagliaro et al. identified 36 different definitions of ehealth in publications and Internet sources.[10] In the final analysis they felt that the definition put forth by Eng, augmented by Eysenbach's definition, appropriately represented ehealth and captured the fluid nature of emergence as a defining characteristic.[11] Eysenbach defined ehealth as:

> . . . an emerging field of medical informatics, referring to the organization and delivery of health services and information using the internet and related technologies. In a broader sense, the term characterizes not only a technical development, but also a new way of working, an attitude, and a commitment for networked global thinking, to improve healthcare locally, regionally, and worldwide by using information and communication technology.[11]

Technology, Policy, and Legislative Influences

This transformation must be considered in the context of the emergence of the World Wide Web, now more commonly called the Internet. Traversing the twentieth and twenty-first centuries, the proliferation in the use of the Internet has had an unprecedented impact on access to information, sharing, and connectedness; moreover, it has been a driving force in the emergence of the twenty-first–century consumer.

Just as growth in the number of individuals using online resources is assured, disparities between Internet access "haves" and "have-nots" will always exist in large part due to cost, literacy, computer skills, language, and education. For some, the lack of access is intentional due to a conscious decision not to use the Internet. Nonetheless, the volume of Internet users is staggering. In 1995 there were an estimated 16 million users. By 1998, when search engine Google was launched, there were 147 million users. In 2001, just more than a decade after the graphic browser was conceived, 500 million users were online. As of the first quarter of 2012, approximately 2.3 billion people worldwide were on the Internet, with nearly eight new users added every second (Fig. 13-1).[12] Given the pace of growth across the globe (over two thirds of the world's population is not yet online), these numbers will soon be outdated.

The emergence of the Internet as a valuable tool for health and healthcare became better understood at the turn of the century. In *The Future of the Internet in Health Care: Five-Year Forecast*, Mittman and Cain declared, "Health care has discovered the internet and the internet has discovered health care!"[13(p1)] Between 1999 and 2001 the Institute of Medicine (IOM) issued two reports published by the Committee on the Quality of Health Care in America that shed light on significant safety and quality issues related to health and healthcare in the U.S. These reports continue to influence the emergence of a more patient-centered healthcare system. Patients and those close to them are being included as integral members of the healthcare team and technology is being highlighted as a critical component for improving safety and quality. The

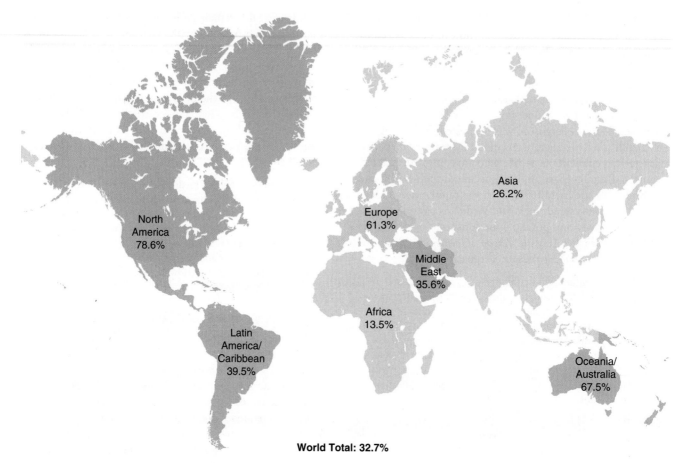

Asia
26.2%

Europe
61.3%

North
America
78.6%

Middle
East
35.6%

Africa
13.5%

Latin
America/
Caribbean
39.5%

Oceania/
Australia
67.5%

World Total: 32.7%

FIG 13-1 World Internet usage. (Data from Internet World Stats. Internet usage statistics. 2012. Copyright 2001–2012, Miniwatts Marketing Group. All rights reserved worldwide.)

IOM report, titled *Crossing the Quality Chasm: A New Health System for the 21st Century*, focused attention more broadly on the multiple dimensions of quality and safety concerns in need of fundamental change across the U.S. healthcare system.[14] To narrow the quality chasm, the report offered six specific areas that represent what healthcare ought to be for all Americans. Healthcare should be safe, effective, patient centered, timely, efficient, and equitable. In addition, the report provided "ten simple rules for the 21st century health care system" that describe what patients should expect from their healthcare (Box 13-1).

While the rules in the IOM report align well with the interests of epatients, the report's most important contribution to the epatient movement is the attention paid to using IT to improve the quality and safety of healthcare. This theme resonates throughout the report with recommendations that directly support the previously mentioned six aims. The report highlights the potential benefits of harnessing health-related applications for the Internet that include consumer health, clinical care, public health, professional education, research, and administrative and financial transactions. Since the report a number of health-related improvements have been initiated in both public and private sectors.

The recognition of safety and quality flaws in the U.S. healthcare system led many patients and those close to them to become vigilant advocates. Access to the Internet coupled with simplified search solutions such as Google made looking for health-related information online more feasible for an increasing number of people. Thus began the new generation of epatients who started searching online for health information, to learn more about their symptoms and conditions and to better understand the options available to treat and manage them.

An enduring source of rich data about the use of online resources is the Pew Research Center's Internet & American Life Project, which began to monitor basic online activities in 1999 to understand who was using the Internet and what people were doing while online. Susannah Fox of the Internet & American Life Project explored the impact of the Internet on families, communities, work and home, daily life, education, healthcare, and civic and political life.[15] Over the years, findings from Fox's reports have shown that health information remains a popular online pursuit. In fact, by February 2011 the report found that 8 in 10 Internet users look online for health information, making it the third most popular online activity, following email and using a search engine.[16,17]

For those interested in online health-related resources the Internet has proven to be much more than a unidirectional source of information. Web 1.0, as the early functionality is now known, provided information based on simplified search

BOX 13-1 WHAT PATIENTS SHOULD EXPECT FROM THEIR HEALTHCARE

1. Beyond patient visits: You will have the care you need when you need it . . . whenever you need it. You will find help in many forms, not just in face-to-face visits. You will find help on the Internet, on the telephone, from many sources, by many routes, in the form you want it.

2. Individualization: You will be known and respected as an individual. Your choices and preferences will be sought and honored. The usual system of care will meet most of your needs. When your needs are special, the care will adapt to meet you on your own terms.

3. Control: The care system will take control only if and when you freely give permission.

4. Information: You can know what you wish to know, when you wish to know it. Your medical record is yours to keep, to read, and to understand. The rule is: "Nothing about you without you."

5. Science: You will have care based on the best available scientific knowledge. The system promises you excellence as its standard. Your care will not vary illogically from doctor to doctor or from place to place. The system will promise you all the care that can help you, and will help you avoid care that cannot help you.

6. Safety: Errors in care will not harm you. You will be safe in the care system.

7. Transparency: Your care will be confidential, but the care system will not keep secrets from you. You can know whatever you wish to know about the care that affects you and your loved ones.

8. Anticipation: Your care will anticipate your needs and will help you find the help you need. You will experience proactive help, not just reactions, to help you restore and maintain your health.

9. Value: Your care will not waste your time or money. You will benefit from constant innovations, which will increase the value of care to you.

10. Cooperation: Those who provide care will cooperate and coordinate their work fully with each other and with you. The walls between professions and institutions will crumble, so that your experiences will become seamless. You will never feel lost.

From National Research Council. *Crossing the Quality Chasm: A New Health System for the 21st Century.* Washington, DC: The National Academies Press, Copyright 2001, National Academy of Sciences.

---

parameters; for healthcare resources it was known as Health 1.0. Since then, Web 2.0 has become available and is more sophisticated, with social engagement, interaction, and networking capabilities. The presence of social media platforms such as Myspace and later Facebook and Twitter has demonstrated the power of the Internet to support the formation of spontaneous social, commercial, and political groups rapidly and in real time. For epatients, Web 2.0 has brought about Health 2.0, allowing previously unavailable interactive communication with other patients and healthcare resources across the country and around the world. Online patient communities can range from traditional chat rooms and listservs to more formalized social networking platforms. Patient-to-patient communities such as PatientsLikeMe, CureTogether, and others have emerged as places where epatients can seek and find communities formed around common illnesses, treatments, or symptoms. Within these communities patients connect with each other for various reasons, including emotional support, ongoing learning, and advocacy. Today, Google and other online environments learn from user search behavior and other Internet activity to serve up predictive content, suggesting that Web 3.0 is emerging, within which Health 3.0 will surely follow.

Health-related resources on the Internet are constantly growing and becoming more innovative and complex. They provide epatients with access to incredible resources and data previously unavailable, such as personal genetic information. To appreciate the power of technology, consider the Human Genome Project. It took 13 years and nearly $3 billion to complete the identification and sequencing of genes within human DNA.[18] In contrast, 23andMe, an Internet company launched in 2007, made it possible for anyone to access his or her personal genetic information quickly, simply, and for less than $500. As of Dec 14, 2012, the price was as low as $99.[19]

Another area of explosive growth has been in mobile technology. Anyone with a smartphone can access thousands of health- and fitness-related applications. There is every expectation that the use of mobile health applications will continue to grow as technology becomes more sophisticated and increasingly connected to clinical aspects of the healthcare delivery system by patients and their clinicians.

The economics of healthcare influenced the evolution of epatients and their use of nontraditional sources for healthcare information. Patients with insurance have seen their out-of-pocket expenses, including deductibles and copayments, increase over the last decade, leading many to look for alternative ways to get answers and support for healthcare questions. The uninsured are often left to their own devices in managing their own and their family members' healthcare needs. Additionally, with changes in the healthcare reimbursement structure shifting care from the hospital to home, patients and caregivers are assuming more responsibility for increasingly complex care needs. The responsibilities of self-managing health and navigating the healthcare system motivated many to become epatients to find, connect with, and learn from others who may share similar experiences.

Policy and legislative actions in the U.S. have been important drivers in the epatient movement. In 2009 the American Recovery and Reinvestment Act was signed into law. A hallmark of this legislation destined to affect the next phase of the epatient movement is the requirement known as Meaningful Use. Stage 1 Meaningful Use objectives were created around five domains. Key to the epatient movement is the domain requiring the engagement of patients and families.

The focus on access to health information has fueled the development of patient portals within EHR systems of large health systems, hospitals, physician practices, and other eligible healthcare providers. Another mechanism for epatient health information access is personal health records (PHRs). PHR features may vary from one system to another but most support a menu of transactions including the ability to review test results, schedule appointments, refill prescriptions, and communicate via electronic messaging with healthcare providers. While widespread adoption of PHRs by patients has been slow, it is expected to increase as more healthcare providers comply with current policies on Meaningful Use from the Office of the National Coordinator for Health Information Technology (ONC). Additionally, other healthcare reform measures, including provisions in the Patient Protection and Affordable Care Act (PPACA) and the Health Care and Education Reconciliation Act of 2010, which amended the PPACA and became law on March 30, 2010, significantly affect healthcare coverage and care delivery. Patients and their healthcare providers will bear increasing responsibility for managing cost and care, leading to the need for more collaboration and engagement at the actual point of care.

Characteristics of Online Healthcare Consumers

In a report titled *Health e-People: The Online Consumer Experience*, Cain, Sarasohn-Kahn, and Wayne introduced three categories of online healthcare consumers: those who are *well*, those who are *newly diagnosed* with an illness, and those who are *chronically ill* and their caregivers.[20] The report suggests that people in each group behave in certain ways on the Internet and that their behavior is a reflection of their health status.

- *The well:* When the report was written, approximately 60% of consumers looking online for health and healthcare information were well. The online needs of the well are largely considered episodic and occasionally driven by the need to seek out specific information related to prevention and wellness. They tend to move across various resources both online and off-line for information and they typically place value on convenience over loyalty.
- *The newly diagnosed:* This group represented only 5% of the total number of online health consumers in 2009. The newly diagnosed are driven by a sense of urgency to understand, manage, and mitigate a recent change in their health status. Their presence and behavior online depend largely on the nature of the condition and its usual trajectory. Most newly diagnosed individuals are expected to spend large amounts of time online in the weeks following the news of their diagnosis. Those diagnosed with a condition amenable to intervention and eventual resolution have different needs than those moving from a state of wellness to a state of chronic illness. For the latter, the need for online resources is expected to evolve and change to reflect changes in their health over time.
- *The chronically ill:* This group represented about 35% of online health consumers in 2009. Chronically ill patients who use online sites often align their loyalty to sites with

resources, services, and support for their specific condition. According to the report, 51% of American adults living with chronic disease go online for health topics related to disease, medical procedures, medications, or health insurance information; 1 in 4 adults with a chronic illness have looked online for someone who shares the same condition.[21]

Caregivers and loved ones of those living with illness or disability often become active online. One early pioneer, Gilles Frydman, became involved in 1995 after looking online for information about his wife's diagnosis of breast cancer.[22] The wealth of knowledge, support, and information that he and his wife discovered in an online cancer support community inspired him to find ways to improve and expand the listserv for other cancer patients. Frydman learned much about online communication and that information was not being stored in a searchable database. He knew that the information he learned on a daily basis was helpful to him and his wife and that it could be helpful to others, too. With his skill and background in IT, he founded the Association of Cancer Online Resources (ACOR), a supportive online community rich in resources for cancer patients and for sharing valuable information about their experiences. The Internet opened the door and redefined the idea of community for Frydman and his family. He continues as a true epatient activist to this day.

As the evolution of the epatient continues, more prominent examples of contemporary epatients emerge. One emblematic epatient is Dave deBronkart, who in recent years has dedicated himself to being a patient activist, blogger, international speaker at health and social media conferences, and health policy advocate for the epatient movement.[23] His call to action came in 2007 when he received a diagnosis of Stage IV renal cell carcinoma that had spread to his muscles, bones, and lungs. He was told that his median survival time was about 24 weeks. With this prognosis deBronkart was highly motivated to find an effective treatment and scoured the Internet for viable options. With help from other patients on ACOR with a similar diagnosis, he learned about a promising clinical trial as well as tips on medications to avoid in order to not jeopardize his trial eligibility. Armed with this information he engaged in meaningful discussions with his clinician about his options. Fortunately, deBronkart had a favorable outcome and the treatment regimen from the clinical trial led to his successful recovery. One year after his treatment ended he began publicly sharing his story by blogging and participating in healthcare conferences and events. deBronkart believes that patients are the most underused resource within healthcare and champions the message of "Let Patients Help." His proactive research and engagement with his healthcare providers helped provide a favorable outcome. However, he is always quick to state that what actually saved him was phenomenal medical science provided by experts in their field in an institution well grounded in patient-centered care.

Other epatients are called to activism as a result of their experiences with the healthcare system. Regina Holliday chose art as the medium to express her family's difficult experiences during her husband's illness and untimely death.[24] Holliday shares her story in a powerful and provocative mural depicting the journey she and her family traveled through a fragmented and uncoordinated healthcare system. The journey was exemplified by her inability to access her husband's medical records in a timely way to ensure that he received needed care. The mural is titled *73 cents*, the price Holliday was told she would have to pay per page to make a copy of his medical record. Since completing the mural Holliday has continued to bring a voice to the patient and family experience through art. She frequently paints poignant and thematic paintings while on-site at healthcare conferences, events, and policy meetings, using them as an opportunity for public advocacy. Holliday has also started the Walking Gallery. She and other artists depict patients' stories or elements of medical advocacy on the back of jackets or lab coats for government employees, technology gurus, medical professionals, social media activists, executives of companies, and artists. These wearable images comprise the exhibits in the Walking Gallery. The purpose is to remind the public of the importance of patient advocacy. Roni Ziegler, MD, formerly Chief Health Strategist at Google, owns a Walking Gallery jacket and has been known to end presentations by turning his back to the audience and displaying his painted jacket as a reminder that all health data points lead back to individual patients.

Contemporary epatients, in general, seek information and data gatherers. They take personal responsibility to research online and off-line resources to improve their health and well-being. The *well* epatient is inclined to peruse online resources episodically to prepare for medical appointments, investigate intermittent family health questions, or search just out of curiosity. *Active* epatients, including those newly diagnosed and those with chronic illnesses and their caregivers, are more invested in gathering important data points by tracking their health with the use of online self-management tools and biosensors, such as heart rate monitors, seizure trackers, mood maps, sleep diaries, and glucose monitors. Tracking their health data in conjunction with online searches empowers epatients to gain a sense of participation and ownership of their well-being, treatment options, and health.

A new type of health consumer has emerged in the last few years. The quantified selfer refers to a person invested in using tools and data to quantify and monitor his or her daily experiences using personal metrics.[25] Quantified selfers measure a range of inputs such as food consumption, environmental factors, emotional and biophysical states, and mental and physical performance. These data collected at baseline and over time can encourage and promote healthy behaviors as well as provide signals for early detection of illness or changes from the baseline state of health. The real-time feedback from the wearable sensors provides awareness of one's own physiologic response.[26]

Semantically, quantified selfers may not consider themselves to be epatients but rather people whose goals are to achieve and maintain good health and who have an innate interest in tracking personal metrics. They capture health-related data such as blood pressure, exercise, activity, sleep, and dietary intake using personal informatics tools for self-monitoring so that they can monitor their progress toward their goals. This type of tracking has the potential to identify health changes more quickly and may affect outcomes favorably, especially in circumstances when a nuanced change leads to an early diagnosis. Further, aggregation of personal metrics has the potential to expand healthcare provider understanding of patient responses to wellness and illness, both behaviorally and physiologically.

Today a perfect, positive storm is brewing as technology, policy, legislation, patient-centered reform, and patients' interests in personal health data converge. Observing the evolution of the epatients from their earliest days to today is akin to watching a movie in slow motion. However, a shift to fast-forward is rapidly occurring; the impact of an increasing number of epatients on health and healthcare will result in disruptive innovation for healthcare providers and healthcare delivery systems. More importantly, epatients will continue to be a driving force in achieving improvements in the quality and safety of healthcare in the U.S.

CONVERGENCE OF EPATIENTS, CLINICIANS, PATIENT-CENTERED MODELS OF CARE, AND INFORMATICS

Participatory Patient-Centered Healthcare

The maxim of "doctors know best" is a statement of the past. Until the early twenty-first century, the old paradigm was a paternalistic model in which the healthcare provider was the exclusive source of medical knowledge. Deeply rooted cultural assumptions in this old medical model view the patient as the uninformed layperson and the medical professional as the keeper of all health knowledge. In a clinician-controlled environment the patient is the outsider with little ability to gather and access data about his or her condition and is expected to play the "good patient" role. This is changing with patient-centered care models.

As patient-centered care models rapidly evolve in the U.S., questions emerge about who should direct the care: the patient or the healthcare provider.[27] Patient-centeredness promulgates a model in which the patient is not only at the center of care but also a full member of the healthcare team. Patients know best when it comes to having the most intimate understanding of their personal circumstances, their preferences, and their bodies. Yet in most healthcare organizations, including patient-centered medical homes and primary care practice settings, provider-directed care remains the norm, perhaps for political, legal, and reimbursement reasons. Scherger suggests that the Internet will test this paradigm of provider-directed care in much the same way that online banking, travel services, and other previously brokered services have given way to consumer control.

The epatient movement does not support replacing physicians and other healthcare providers. On the contrary, epatients understand the value of collaborative patient–provider partnerships and seek healthcare providers who appreciate the value of allowing patients to participate. ePatients appreciate the need for provider-directed care for certain circumstances such as trauma, acute medical events, and surgical emergencies; however, the model of patient-centered care exists with the premise that patients are considered experts in their own care and self-management and must be allowed to exercise patient-driven controls. Patient-centered care is viewed as a critical component of achieving the Triple Aim of improving the experience of care, improving the health of populations, and reducing per capita costs of healthcare.[28] For patient-centered care to succeed, patients and their clinicians must have respectful partnerships within which patients and clinicians mutually determine how care will be directed and managed to meet needs.

An unprecedented opportunity exists to fundamentally change the experience of healthcare encounters for both patients and their clinicians. ePatients have the tools and are developing the skills to elevate discussions with their healthcare providers and use limited office visit time engaged in a more constructive dialog. This can result in greater satisfaction for both stakeholders. This meaningful collaboration between the epatient and the healthcare provider, known as participatory healthcare or participatory medicine is defined by the Society for Participatory Medicine as:

> a cooperative model of healthcare that encourages and expects active involvement by all connected parties, including patients, caregivers, and healthcare professionals, as integral to the full continuum of care. The "participatory" concept may also be applied to fitness, nutrition, mental health, end-of-life care, and all issues broadly related to an individual's health.[29]

The Society for Participatory Medicine was founded as a movement in which networked patients shift from being mere passengers to responsible drivers of their health. Healthcare providers encourage and value them as full partners.[28]

Participatory healthcare also requires epatients and clinicians to use a variety of data sources to genuinely collaborate on shared goals and decision making for improved health and outcomes. Iverson, Howard, and Penney found that gathering information online fosters more patient engagement in health maintenance and care.[30] The movement toward participatory patient-centered care requires that epatients, health professionals, and informatics systems align accordingly. Berwick offered three maxims that he finds useful when considering a participatory patient-centered model of care:

- The needs of the patient come first
- Every patient is the only patient
- Nothing about me without me[31]

The last maxim is often associated with epatients and calls for openness and transparency among all involved stakeholders, especially when it comes to their health data. deBronkart's notoriety flourished after his keynote presentation at the 2009 Medicine 2.0 conference titled "Gimme My Damn Data," which was picked up by Cable News Network (CNN) in a series on the empowered patient.[32]

While opportunities for health professionals' growth in participatory healthcare exist, it is equally important to acknowledge the challenges. Current care models may not be structured to support patient-centeredness and even well-intentioned clinicians may find it difficult to allocate sufficient time and resources to fully engage with epatients who come with a well-prepared agenda. However, there is no doubt that epatients will continue to push and advocate for their place in the healthcare system.

Many epatients seek to integrate empirical knowledge into their understanding of their health conditions. Therefore clinicians should engage these epatients in developing a shared hypothesis based on data and patient-reported experiences to help explain symptoms and other findings. This is in addition to including the epatient in creating a plan to manage care, thus initiating a process known as guided discovery. Guided discovery includes integrating open-ended questions into the medical encounter, preidentifying data collection parameters that have meaning to the epatient, planning time for analysis of collected information, completing an evaluation of outcomes, and recognizing that those results may require experimentation to achieve shared goals.[33]

The New Role of Clinicians and Informaticists in ePatient Care

Clinicians involved in informatics are uniquely positioned to participate in system changes that support epatients' desire for data openness and transparency by helping to build data collection models that support connection, partnership, and guided discovery.[34] Patients and healthcare providers need the right tools at the right time to collect data to support their need to investigate and hypothesize health issues to create a shared plan. Clinicians may need to learn new skills and gain new knowledge to serve as a "guide" for epatients as they integrate information and data from multiple sources while navigating their healthcare experience. It is within this culture of partnership that guided discovery of the epatient's health and well-being can be fully realized.[33] Healthcare providers must be flexible and open to the possibility that patients may be more intimately adept at the experience of their own illness and that clinicians should not be expected to have all of the answers. However, epatients expect their clinicians to use timely online sources to build on their own knowledge and expertise.

ePatients have inherent knowledge of their sense of self and are campaigning the healthcare field to recognize and support this notion. As deBronkart has been known to say, "Patients have more skin in the game." ePatients look to clinicians not only for their clinical expertise, but also for their willingness to support changing needs across the journey of an illness. Health professionals can demonstrate this willingness by understanding the value of online resources to epatients. Clinicians have the opportunity to research Internet sites that are relevant to their specialty, recommend those that provide value to both them and their patients, and be open to learning about and exploring other sites favored by their epatients.

There is no doubt that the integration of patient-centered care in the U.S. healthcare system will continue and that epatients will be integral participants in its realization. As with any change, resistance should be expected. However, initial resistance will not stem the tide that is occurring across the country to create a model of care that supports safety, efficiency, and health for all stakeholders.[35]

Health Informatics and ePatients

Disruptive communication technologies, such as the Internet, have drastically altered the way we communicate with one another. From electronic messaging and texting to tweeting and updating social networks, this cultural norm has increased our ability to share knowledge, communicate, and connect to each other. Online businesses are harnessing the power of communication and connection by researching buyer reviews and purchasing history data of customers to help drive sales. The idea of using buyer reviews can also be found within healthcare. One example is the Hospital Consumer Assessment of Healthcare Providers and Systems (HCAHPS), the first national, standardized, public report of patients' perspectives of their experiences with healthcare organizations and healthcare providers.[36]

The aggregation of data across similar experiences is known as crowdsourcing. Crowdsourcing is useful in recognizing patterns within the population and can also help to expand our knowledge for public health. The idea of crowdsourcing information and participatory healthcare is growing; one example is PatientsLikeMe. This research-based online platform was created for patients to share and learn from real-world experiences and to produce outcome-based health data for advancing the current pace of research.[37] Imagine a patient who has recorded data about his or her symptoms over time; the historical data not only can lead to productive encounters with healthcare providers but also may contribute to emerging knowledge about the experience of living with certain conditions. Crowdsourced data from real patients in real time expand and challenge how we view and study health.[38]

Despite the growing move toward participatory health and collaborative care, for most healthcare organizations the current health information technology (health IT) infrastructure does not foster the ability for both patients and healthcare providers to interact and communicate effectively and efficiently. Immediate electronic access to one's health records and electronic messaging with healthcare providers is not yet commonplace in most provider practices. Health informatics has been touted as one of the solutions to changing healthcare, by improving quality, efficiency, and safety of care while decreasing costs, but the delay in implementing systems is impeding the ability for healthcare to evolve more rapidly.

Informatics alone cannot build the learning health system as described in the IOM's Learning Health System Series and described in Chapter 26.[39] The vision of a learning health system aligns scientific knowledge, biomedical informatics, value-added incentives, and cultural norms to ensure that continuous improvement and innovation become natural by-products of the experience of healthcare. Consumer participation and collaboration are essential elements of a learning health system.

Personal Health Records, Transparency, and Access to Data

PHRs, discussed in Chapter 15, can be tools to facilitate the epatient phenomenon, although their development has been slow in the U.S. Other projects related to transparency, such as OpenNotes, show promise. The OpenNotes Project, which began in 2011, evaluated the impact of sharing clinical encounter notes for primary care providers and patients online. Participating providers believed in the tangible benefits of sharing notes with patients. Nonparticipating providers indicated worry over the increased demand on their time and lengthier visits as well as an inability to record their thoughts candidly about sensitive issues regarding mental health, obesity, cancer, and substance abuse. In addition, nonparticipating providers noted that the transparency of the notes would negatively affect their current practices and have minimal positive effect on patients. In contrast, patients reported positive interest in reading clinical notes and fewer than one in six patients expressed worry or confusion over reading the notes, regardless of demographic and health characteristics. Many patients in the study also indicated that they would consider sharing the notes with friends and family.[40]

Many epatient supporters are advocating transparency and challenging the question of who owns the data. Dave deBronkart has heavily advocated for transparency of data because of his experiences with inaccurate information in his health record and his family members' records that could have led to potentially fatal mistakes. For example, his mother's diagnosis of hyperthyroidism was transcribed incorrectly and treatment for hypothyroidism was prescribed. His wife's allergy to penicillin was not recorded and she was almost given the harmful medication. deBronkart reviewed his own health record and noted erroneous diagnoses.[41] Regina Holliday's advocacy work, mentioned earlier, is solidly in favor of access to the health record. She believes that no patient or family should ever have to struggle, as she did, to gain timely access to health records. Similar efforts in support of transparency and open access are occurring in the research realm. Interest has grown over the past several years and on June 4, 2012, a petition was signed by thousands of advocates urging the White House to make taxpayer-funded research available online to everyone. Since the petition received the required 25,000 signatures, the White House will issue a response.[42] The impetus for this is that epatients are attempting to access studies on their chronic illnesses but closed access to research papers constrains their efforts. In addition, closed access is prohibiting patients who participated in studies to be able to review study outcomes. Unfortunately, this common practice within the research and publishing world has created a roadblock for patients and an imbalanced dissemination of knowledge. Open access to research literature would give epatients the ability to critically evaluate their best course of

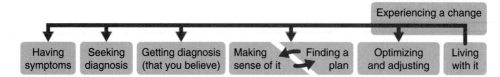

FIG 13-2   The patient and caregiver journey. (Copyright PatientsLikeMe. http://www.patientslikeme. com/patients/view/40?patient_page=1. 2012.)

action and allow a new voice in evaluating the science of their conditions.

EVOLUTION OF HEALTH 2.0 AND BEYOND

Health 2.0 Environment

Over the last decade the Internet has evolved from the static unidirectional experience of Web 1.0 to the dynamic and interactive environment of Web 2.0 within which collective intelligence is harnessed.[43] With this framework in mind, Van De Belt et al. identified definitions for the parallel evolution of Health 2.0 and Medicine 2.0, terms that are often used interchangeably.[9] They found 46 unique definitions from 44 resources, suggesting that the concept is continuing to develop. Seven recurrent themes indicated that a set of characteristics for Health 2.0 is emerging: Web 2.0 and technology, patients, professionals, social networking, health information and content, collaboration, and change of healthcare.

As Health 2.0 continues to mature, innovative environments will emerge in which collective intelligence and knowledge of multiple stakeholders is gathered, exchanged, and shared. ePatients participate across various health-related social media spaces: some blog; some tweet and retweet; some form patient-related pages on Facebook; some express their experiences through music and art; and some seek opportunities to communicate their messages at professional conferences, political gatherings, and citizen forums. ePatients influence the experiences of other patients on a global scale.

The viral capability of social media provides epatients with a powerful platform from which the experiences of even the most vulnerable can be collected, appreciated, and shared. Yet gaps exist in Internet accessibility despite the proliferation of technology across all aspects of society. This digital divide has both individual and public health implications since those lacking access are unable to benefit from the wisdom of collective knowledge to improve health outcomes, whether in real time or longitudinally. As Health 2.0 continues to mature it is essential to consider how to bridge the growing gap between the Internet "haves" and "have-nots."

Health 2.0 and the Creation of Virtual Patient Communities

In *Peer-to-Peer Healthcare*, Fox found that 18% of Internet users are going online to find others who may have similar health concerns.[44] Among those users living with chronic illnesses such as diabetes, heart, or lung conditions, 23% reported going online to look for others with similar experiences. The report also highlights that 71% of adults seek information, care, or support from a health professional during an acute moment of need. This important point reinforces the notion that epatients want a partnership with healthcare providers to collaborate and share in decision making. ePatients seeking health information and support are increasingly turning to innovative Health 2.0, tools that include mobile health-related applications, comprehensive web-based content, and interactive and robust social networks. These online spaces provide the opportunity to reframe one's experience from "Why me?" to "Oh, you too? Tell me more." The interactions that occur provide support, validation, and a place to share ideas about how to live as well as possible with illness. This journey is depicted in Figure 13-2.

One of the most transformative developments for epatients has been the emergence of patient-focused virtual communities in which patients interact, freely share health-related data, and learn from each other's experiences while being unbounded by geographic limitations, social stigma, or other limiting characteristics. Eysenbach et al. defined virtual community:

> . . . as a group of individuals with similar or common health related interests and predominately non-professional backgrounds (patients, healthy consumers, or informal caregivers) who interact and communicate publicly through a computer communication such as the internet, or through any other computer based tool (including non-text based systems such as voice bulletin board systems), allowing social networks to build over a distance.[45(p1)]

In an online environment epatients exchange information, compare notes, learn about treatment options, and engage in discussions that may seem superfluous and deemed not within the purview of the medical professional. For example, they can exchange tips on where to purchase wigs in preparation for chemotherapy, advice on raising children, or advice on working while managing a chronic illness. Online communities can also function as a lifeline for those trying to manage the fear and uncertainty associated with illness. For the uninsured, underinsured, and those with high-deductible plans, spending time online to explore ideas with others may be a reasonable first step in deciding what to do next about a health concern. Patients with rare diseases can search for specialists, researchers, and new discovery information for their rare disease. Schweizer, Leimeister, and Kremat found that among cancer patients virtual communities play an important role in helping patients to cope with their situation.[46] Establishing social relationships with other cancer patients complements and supplements their off-line social relationships. While emotional support is a benefit, evidence also exists that patients derive physical and quality-of-life benefits as well.[47]

ePatients are looking for more than social support from their interactions with online communities. Nambisan found that patients participating in online health communities experienced enhanced perceived empathy when their information seeking was supported by relevant tools and data displays similar to those used by PatientsLikeMe (on this site epatients have access to a variety of tools to share data about their health conditions, symptoms, treatments, and side effects).[48] In a user survey conducted in 2010, PatientsLikeMe members reported improved understanding of how their treatments worked, feeling more involved in decisions regarding their treatments, and better communication with members of the healthcare team.[49]

Health-related social networking sites have become a rich source of support, information, and advocacy for epatients and their caregivers. However, as with all activities on the Internet, users should review the terms of use and privacy and data sharing policies to ensure that they are well informed. Reputable sites display links to their privacy policies on every page of the site (Table 13-1).

Virtual communities share many of the characteristics of any social group and these characteristics may evolve and change as the community grows and matures. For the most part virtual communities can afford the user some degree of anonymity since engagement is not typically face to face. This can be both a benefit and a risk. Patients may feel more comfortable sharing sensitive information anonymously than they would in person. Among 1267 members of PatientsLikeMe polled, 41% said that they have withheld information from their doctors about certain symptoms and 39% did not share information about lifestyle habits such as exercise, diet, and alcohol use. Reasons for withholding this information from their doctors included not wanting to be lectured, feeling too embarrassed, not thinking the information was important or the doctor's business, forgetting to bring it up, and fearing that the treatment they wanted would not be provided.

A survey conducted in 2011 by iVillage, an online community for women, found that women placed more trust in and value on information obtained from online women's communities than from other social networks.[50] The respondents believed that sites such as iVillage, CafeMom, and BabyCenter offered more expertise to understand and meet their needs.

Virtual communities may also carry risks, especially for epatients who may feel uncertain or vulnerable in this new environment. Many patient communities incorporate moderators as part of the experience yet there is an inconsistent approach to moderating these communities. Research is needed in this area. Organizations that create and support online communities should measure user input to gauge the perceived benefits, risks, and social health of the community from the patient's perspective.

Online communities can be important sources of patient experience data that could be harnessed by researchers. The growing interest in patient-reported outcomes (PROs) includes academic and clinical researchers, government agencies, policy institutes, and patients themselves. Information collected within virtual patient communities offers a novel source of PRO data.

CONCLUSION AND FUTURE DIRECTIONS
Moving toward Health 3.0

As we look to the future for epatients, consider the Google generation, a generation of computer users born after 1993. They have grown up with immediate access to information and knowledge sources that were previously unavailable. This generation is called the Net generation, the Google generation, digital natives, and millennials. They are very skilled at navigating Internet resources and are accustomed to sharing data in real time in online environments.[51] Insight into this generation of users is important because they have little or no recollection of life without the Internet. These are the epatients of the future and their appetite for immediacy and responsiveness from online and digital tools will drive innovation across all consumer interactions including healthcare.

As the Google generation enters the workforce and health IT continues to innovate, the phenomenon of the epatient will no longer be a novelty. The evolution of the web might be summed up this way: Web 1.0 was akin to a library where you could access loads of information but you could not contribute anything. Web 2.0 has more of a community feel; it is a place where groups can gather, where you can exchange information, and where your contribution can be included

TABLE 13-1	PATIENT VIRTUAL COMMUNITIES: USER AND PRIVACY POLICIES	
PATIENT VIRTUAL COMMUNITY	**USER TERMS**	**PRIVACY POLICY**
CureTogether	http://curetogether.com/terms.php	http://curetogether.com/privacy.php
PatientsLikeMe	www.patientslikeme.com/about/user_agreement	www.patientslikeme.com/about/privacy www.patientslikeme.com/about/openness
Inspire	www.inspire.com/about/terms/	www.inspire.com/about/privacy/
Army of Women	www.armyofwomen.org/termsofuse	www.armyofwomen.org/privacypolicy
Association of Cancer Online Resources (ACOR)	www2.acor.org/pages/termsAndConditions	www2.acor.org/pages/privacyPolicy

and even judged by others for its value. So what might Web 3.0 bring about? Some speculate that browsers will act more like a personal assistant, much like an improved iPhone 4S's Siri. Search capabilities on the Internet are already showing signs of increasing intelligence. Google uses past searches to display content of interest to include personally tailored advertising. Some suggest that Web 3.0 will use previous data to place searches into context and deliver information to meet your needs and interests.

What does this mean for health and healthcare? Technological advances in medical devices and other diagnostic tools are already emerging in practice.[52] Research institutes such as P4 Medicine Institute think that systems biology, digital and information technology, clinicians, and patients will collaborate to form P4 Medicine, medicine that is predictive, preventive, personalized, and participatory.[53]

As the vision of a learning health system is realized, patients and those close to them need to have opportunities to contribute. In May 2012 a summit was convened in Washington, D.C., bringing together representatives from government, industry, nonprofits, and patients to build consensus on the core values and principles needed to support a national-scale, person-centered, continuous learning health system. Regina Holliday, the artist-in-residence for the 2-day summit, painted *Chaordic*, depicting powerful images of multiple stakeholders navigating the fine line between the chaos and order of our current healthcare environment as they converge to achieve the vision of a learning health system (Fig. 13-3).[54]

The time will come when the term *epatient* becomes irrelevant. The future of healthcare will include patients that are equipped, enabled, empowered, and engaged as full members of their healthcare team and supported by an electronically sophisticated patient-centered healthcare system that promotes participatory medicine and shared decision making.

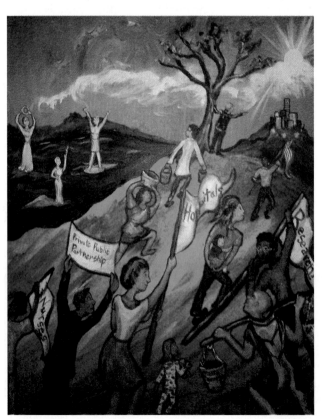

FIG 13-3 *Chaordic.* (Copyright Regina Holliday, 2012.)

REFERENCES

1. Slack W, Hicks G, Reed C, Van Cura L. A computer-based medical-history system. *N Engl J Med.* 1966;274(4):194-198.
2. Slack W. The patient online. *Am J Prev Med.* 1999;16(1):43-45.
3. Patient empowerment—Who empowers whom? *The Lancet.* 2012;379(9827):1677. doi:10.1016/S0140-6736(12)60699-1670.
4. Ferguson T. ePatients: how they can help us heal healthcare [white paper]. e-patients.net. http://epatients.net/. 2007.
5. Ferguson T. Looking ahead: online health & the search for sustainable healthcare [online exclusive]. *Ferguson Report.* 2002;9. http://www.fergusonreport.com/articles/fr00901.htm.
6. Gee P, Greenwood D, Kim K, Perez S, Staggers N, Devon H. Exploration of the epatient phenomenon in nursing informatics. *Nursing Outlook.* 2012;60(4):e9-e16.
7. Della Mea V. What is ehealth (2): the death of telemedicine? *J Med Internet Res.* 2001;3(2):e22. http://www.jmir.org/2001/2/e22/. doi:10.2196/jmir.3.2.e22.
8. Eng T. *The eHealth Landscape—A Terrain Map of Emerging Information and Communication Technologies in Health and Health Care.* Princeton, NJ: The Robert Wood Johnson Foundation; 2001. http://www.hetinitiative.org/media/pdf/eHealth.pdf.
9. Van De Belt T, Engelen L, Berben S, Schoonhoven L. Definition of Health 2.0 and Medicine 2.0: a systematic review. *J Med Internet Res.* 2010;12(2):e18. doi:10.2196/jmir.1350.
10. Pagliaro C, Sloan D, Gregor P, et al. What is ehealth (4): a scoping exercise to map the field. *J Med Internet Res.* 2005;7(1):e9. doi:10.2196/jmir.7.1.e9.
11. Eysenbach G. What is ehealth? *J Med Internet Res.* 2001;3(2):e20. http://www.jmir.org/2001/2/e20/.
12. Internet World Stats. Internet usage statistics. Internet World Stats. http://internetworldstats.com/stats.htm. 2012.
13. Mittman R, Cain M. The future of the internet in health care: five-year forecast [white paper]. California HealthCare Foundation. http://www.chcf.org/publications/1999/01/the-future-of-the-internet-in-health-care-fiveyear-forecast. 1999.
14. National Research Council. *Crossing the Quality Chasm: A New Health System for the 21st Century.* Washington, DC: The National Academies Press; 2001.
15. Fox S, Jones S. *The Social Life of Health Information: Americans' Pursuit of Health Takes Place within a Widening Network of Both Online and Offline Sources.* Washington, DC: Pew Internet & American Life Project; 2009. http://www.pewinternet.org/Reports/2009/8-The-Social-Life-of-Health-Information.aspx.
16. Fox S. *The Social Life of Health Information.* Washington, DC: Pew Internet & American Life Project; 2011. http://www.pewinternet.org/Reports/2011/Social-Life-of-Health-Info.aspx.
17. Fox S. *Health Topics.* Washington, DC: Pew Internet & American Life Project; 2011. http://pewinternet.org/Reports/2011/Health Topics.aspx.
18. National Human Genome Research Institute. The Human Genome Project completion: frequently asked questions. National Human

Genome Research Institute. http://www.genome.gov/11006943. 2003.

19. 23andMe; n.d. https://www.23andme.com/.

20. Cain M, Sarasohn-Kahn J, Wayne J. Health e-people: the online consumer experience. [white paper]. California HealthCare Foundation. http://www.chcf.org/publications/2000/08/health-epeople-the-online-consumer-experience. 2000.

21. Fox S, Purcell K. Chronic disease and the internet. Pew Internet & American Life Project. http://pewinternet.org/Reports/2010/Chronic-Disease.aspx. 2010.

22. Keene N. Meet activist Gilles Frydman [online exclusive]. onconurse.com. http://www.onconurse.com/news/activist_gilles.html. 2001. Accessed May 3, 2012.

23. deBronkart D. About Dave. e-Patient Dave. http://epatient dave.com/about-dave/. 2012.

24. Holliday R. The Walking Gallery. Regina Holliday's Medical Advocacy Blog. http://reginaholliday.blogspot.com/2011/04/walking-gallery.html. 2011.

25. Technology Quarterly. The quantified self, counting every moment, technology and health: measuring your everyday activities can help improve your quality of life, according to aficionados of "self-tracking." *The Economist*. 2012. http://www.economist.com/node/21548493

26. Singer E. The measured life: do you know how much REM sleep you got last night? New types of devices that monitor activity, sleep, diet, and even mood could make us healthier and more productive [online exclusive]. *Technology Review*. http://www.technologyreview.com/biomedicine/37784/. 2011. Accessed April 30, 2012.

27. Scherger J. Future vision: is family medicine ready for patient-directed care? *Family Medicine*. 2009;41(4):285-288.

28. Berwick D, Nolan T, Whittington J. The triple aim: care, health and cost. *Health Affairs*. 2008;27(3):759-769.

29. Society of Participatory Medicine. http://participatorymedicine.org/. 2009.

30. Iverson S, Howard K, Penney B. Impact of internet use on health-related behaviors and the patient-physician relationship: a survey-based study and review. *J Am Osteopath Assoc*. 2008;108(12):699-711. http://www.jaoa.org/content/108/12/699.full.pdf.

31. Berwick D. What "patient-centeredness" should mean: confessions of an extremist. *Health Affairs*. 2009;28(4):555-565.

32. deBronkart D. Gimme my damn data. Keynote speech at: World Congress on Social Networking and Web 2.0 Applications in Medicine, Health, Health Care, and Biomedical Research; September 17, 2009; Toronto. http://www.medicine20congress.com/ocs/index.php/med/med2009/paper/view/267.

33. Dill D, Gumpert P. What is the heart of health care? Advocating for and defining the clinical relationship in patient-centered care [online exclusive]. *J Particip Med*. 2012;4. http://www.jopm.org/evidence/reviews/2012/04/25/what-is-the-heart-of-health-care-advocating-for-and-defining-the-clinical-relationship-in-patient-centered-care/#footnote_82.

34. Sarasohn-Kahn J. The wisdom of patients: health care meets online social media. California HealthCare Foundation. http://www.chcf.org/publications/2008/04/the-wisdom-of-patients-health-care-meets-online-social-media. 2008.

35. Sarasohn-Kahn J. Participatory health: online and mobile tools help chronically ill manage their care. California HealthCare Foundation. http://www.chcf.org/~/media/MEDIA%20LIBRARY%20Files/PDF/P/PDF%20ParticipatoryHealthTools.pdf. 2009.

36. Hospital Consumer Assessment of Healthcare Providers and Systems (HCAHPS). HCAHPS fact sheet. HCAHPS. http://www.hcahpsonline.org/files/HCAHPS%20Fact%20Sheet%20May%202012.pdf. 2012. Accessed May 6, 2012.

37. PatientsLikeMe. http://www.patientslikeme.com/patients/view/40?patient_page=1. 2012.

38. Swan M. Crowdsourced health research studies: an important emerging complement to clinical trials in the public health research ecosystem. *J Med Internet Res*. 2012;14(2):e46. http://www.jmir.org/2012/2/e46/.

39. Institute of Medicine. *The Learning Health System Series*. Washington, DC: The National Academies Press; 2011.

40. Delbanco T, Walker J, Darer J, et al. Open notes: doctors and patients signing on. *Ann Intern Med*. 2010;153(2):121-125. http://annals.org/article.aspx?volume=153&issue=2&page=121.

41. deBronkart D. The magic incantation (for rich products). e-Patient Dave. http://epatientdave.com/. 2012.

42. Higginbotham A. 25,000 advocates urge White House to open taxpayer-funded research to everyone. Scholarly Publishing and Academic Resources Coalition. http://www.arl.org/sparc/media/25000-advocates-urge-white-house-to-open-tax payer-.shtml. June 4, 2012.

43. O'Reilly T. What is Web 2.0: design patterns and business models for the next generation of software. O'Reilly. http://oreilly.com/web2/archive/what-is-web-20.html. 2005.

44. Fox S. Peer-to-peer healthcare. Pew Internet & American Life Project. http://www.pewinternet.org/~/media//Files/Reports/2011/Pew_P2PHealthcare_2011.pdf. 2011.

45. Eysenbach G, Powell J, Englesakis M, Rizo C, Stern A. Health related virtual communities and electronic support groups: systematic review of the effects of online peer to peer interactions. *BMJ*. 2004;328(7449):1166.

46. Schweizer K, Leimeister J, Kremat H. The role of virtual communities for the social network of cancer patients. Paper presented at: 12th Americas Conference on Information Systems; August 4-6, 2006; Acapulco, Mexico. http://www.uni-kassel.de/fb7/ibwl/leimeister/pub/06-33.pdf.

47. Frost J, Massagli M. Social uses of personal health information within PatientsLikeMe, an online patient community: what can happen when patients have access to one another's data. *J Med Internet Res*. 2008;10(3):e15. doi:10.2196/jmir.1053.

48. Nambisan P. Health information seeking and social support in online health communities: impact on patients' perceived empathy. *J Am Med Inform Assoc*. 2011;18(3):298-304.

49. Wicks P, Massagli M, Frost J, et al. *J Med Internet Res*. 2010;12(2):e1. doi:10.2196/jmir.1549.

50. Goudreau J. Online, women more likely to trust each other. *Forbes*. http://www.forbes.com/sites/jennagoudreau/2011/01/20/online-women-more-likely-to-trust-each-other-facebook-yahoo-twitter-myspace-marketing/. January 20, 2011.

51. British Library and the Joint Information Systems Committee. Information behaviour of the researcher of the future. http://www.jisc.ac.uk/media/documents/programmes/reppres/gg_final_keynote_11012008.pdf. 2008.

52. Topol E. *The Creative Destruction of Medicine: How the Digital Revolution Will Create Better Health Care*. New York, NY: Perseus Books Group; 2011.

53. P4 Medicine Institute. http://p4mi.org/. 2012.

54. Holliday R. The word of the day is "Chaordic." Regina Holliday's Health Advocacy Blog. http://reginaholliday.blogspot.com/2012/05/word-of-day-is.html. 2012.

■ DISCUSSION QUESTIONS

1. Discuss reasons why clinicians may be reluctant to change their current practice to accommodate the principles of participatory medicine.
2. What ethical concerns do you have about the sharing of health data online?
3. Considering today's privacy rules, how can you be expected to maintain confidentiality when patients are sharing data so freely? How might privacy rules evolve?
4. Defend or refute the following: Patients should have real-time access to all information in their health records, including narrative notes.
5. How can we narrow the gap between technology "haves" and "have-nots"?
6. Develop strategies for working with epatients in your personal practice and consider if those would be acceptable in your work setting.

7. Debate this statement: Employers who contribute to the cost of employee health insurance can require employees to monitor certain health parameters to maintain coverage.
8. If you believe that participatory healthcare should become the standard of care, what policy and legislative changes are needed to make that a reality?
9. Create a vision for the model of healthcare you want in place by 2020. What is the single most important characteristic of your vision on which you're unwilling to compromise?
10. In the interest of public health shouldn't all patients be expected to monitor their health using accessible tools? What, if any, are the unintended consequences of that expectation?

■ CASE STUDY

A few weeks ago you were hired as the Director of Patient Education for a regional medical center located in the Midwest. The medical center includes three community hospitals ranging from 175 to 321 beds, four outpatient clinics, and five centers of excellence. The five centers of excellence are located at two of the hospitals and focus on heart disease, cancer care, care of the aging, neuromuscular disorders, and women's health.

In your position you are responsible for coordinating patient education across the medical center, including all programs and print materials. Your staff includes three BSN-prepared nurses, one located at each of the hospitals. As one of your initial steps in this new position you have completed an assessment of the current educational offerings and staff satisfaction with the quality of the current programs. One area of need stands out: The professional staff

report that a growing number of patients have been joining online social networking sites. One staff member said, "I think they are all helping each other get online." These patients are now raising new and sometimes difficult questions about treatment options. None of the staff has explored any of the online sites, and they are afraid to join for fear that they could become involved in some sort of violation of the Health Insurance Portability and Accountability Act (HIPAA).

Discussion Questions
1. Describe how you would develop a staff education program and create an outline of key points that you would include.
2. Develop a patient handout that the staff can use to educate patients on the effective use of online social media materials.

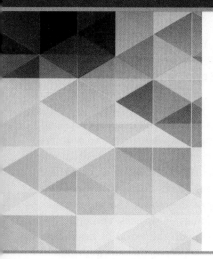

Social Networking and Other Web-Based Applications in Healthcare

Diane J. Skiba, Paul Guillory, and Elizabeth S. Dickson

Peer-to-peer healthcare is a way for people to do what they have always done—lend a hand, lend an ear, lend advice—but at internet speed and at internet scale. It is the evolution of internet use that the Pew Internet Project has been tracking in other industries, and it is just finally having an impact on healthcare.

Susannah Fox

OBJECTIVES

At the completion of this chapter the reader will be prepared to:
1. Describe social media tools and their benefits
2. Explore the current and potential use of social media in healthcare
3. Analyze the issues and challenges associated with the use of social media in healthcare
4. Provide guidance for writing social media policies

KEY TERMS

Microblogging, 227
Social media, 225

Social networking, 226

ABSTRACT

The concept of social media is new to healthcare professionals and to informatics specialists. To better understand the concept of social media, this chapter starts with the definition of social media and describes the various tools included under this concept. Current and potential ways that both healthcare professionals and patients/consumers can use social media tools are also highlighted. The challenges of social media in healthcare also are examined within the context of privacy, confidentiality, inappropriate behavior, security, regulatory issues, and market pressure. To address some of these challenges, the chapter provides extensive information about the development of social media policies for organizations.

WHAT IS SOCIAL MEDIA?

Social media can be defined in a myriad of ways. Merriam-Webster provides a comprehensive definition of social media as "forms of electronic communication (Web sites for social networking and microblogging) through which users create online communities to share information, ideas, personal messages, and other content."[1] Social media offers an interactive facet to the Internet.[2] As noted by Kaplan and Haenlein, "Social media is a group of Internet-based applications that build on the ideological and technological foundations of Web 2.0, and that allow the creation and exchange of user generated content."[3(p61)] Anthony Bradley of the Gartner Blog Network identified six core principles that differentiate social media from other forms of communication and collaboration:
1. Participation
2. Collective
3. Transparency
4. Independence
5. Persistence
6. Emergence[4]

These characteristics collectively define social media as "an on-line environment established for the purpose of mass collaboration."[5]

Social media tools are undeniably transforming how groups and individuals acquire and disperse information, communicate with others, and connect to those with similar interests. It is of no surprise that consumers and businesses have gravitated toward these powerful tools. The healthcare field has not been isolated from this phenomenon and has recognized the potential of social media to increase awareness of healthcare services, disseminate health promotion and preventative education, recruit new clients, connect patients to others with similar experiences, and increase access to health services. Social media steps away from traditional print, radio, and one-way Internet methods of mass communication and offers heathcare a new venue for fast, efficient means of sharing information on new services, health promotion programs, and advances in patient care.[6] For many, long gone are the days of waiting for a response from a physician to find the answer to a healthcare question.

The Healthcare Information and Management Systems Society (HIMSS) Social Media Work Group speculated that in the long term social media will become ubiquitous and be considered part of routine healthcare operations as well as consumers' everyday lives. The group referred to the concept of "health care + social media = 'social health.'"[7(p3)] Several reports examining the future transformation of healthcare touted the use of social media as a viable method to meet the widespread needs of patient populations. The Bipartisan Policy Center,[8] in particular, asserted social media platforms can facilitate the promotion of health and wellness.

SOCIAL MEDIA TOOLS

There are various ways to classify social media tools. One method is a classification[3] system based on social theories (social presence[9] and media richness[10]) and two key social processes elements (self-presentation and self-disclosure). This system is particularly useful for researchers examining the impact of social media tools. Assumptions that follow from this classification system include:

- The higher the social presence (awareness of the communication partners), the more communication partners can influence each other's behavior.[3]
- In terms of media richness, the more information that is shared, the less likelihood there is of ambiguity.
- Self-presentation focuses on how someone depicts his or her image.
- Self-disclosure in the social media world involves the amount of personal information, including feelings and thoughts, that is shared.

Another way to categorize the use of social media tools is to understand that the structure of a social media site is dependent on its purpose and the exchange of information (Box 14-1).[7] A fairly simple method of organizing social media is to classify by the types of tools. For example, these tools can be commonly divided into five categories:

- Social networking (Facebook)
- Blogging and wikis
- Microblogging (Twitter)
- Social bookmarking (Delicious) and social sharing news (Digg, reddit)
- User-generated content (YouTube, Flickr, Pinterest)

This last method will be used to illustrate how consumers and healthcare professionals are using social media tools.

Social Networking

Social networks are online platforms that enable groups and individuals to connect with others who share similar interests. They transcend time and geographic restrictions, opening lines of communication and allowing users to share text, photographs, and videos. The notion is that social networks build on the wisdom of the crowd.[11] Social networks are changing the way individuals, businesses, and organizations experience and interact with the world of healthcare. Services provided by social networks include information sharing, social support, and the ability for people to access clinical trials and monitor their health data.[12]

Seemingly an infinite number of social networking sites exist, created by not-for-profit groups, healthcare institutions, and most of all, consumers. CaringBridge (www.caringbridge.org), a nonprofit organization, allows users to create their own private and personal websites,

---

BOX 14-1   SOCIAL MEDIA STRUCTURE

- *Provider–Consumer:* Information exchange between a medical provider or institution and patients or others in the healthcare community. A good example is the Mayo Clinic's Facebook page.
- *Consumer–Consumer:* The use of social media by patients, families, or caregivers (consumers) to lend support or gather and share information relating to their diagnosis, treatments, or healthcare providers. A good example is the PatientsLikeMe community where patients not only share information but their healthcare data on various outcomes.
- *Companies (Life Sciences) connections with consumers:* Pharmaceutical and medical device companies use of social media to engage patients and providers, research use and side effects, market products, support or oppose legislation, and facilitate notification of recalls. An example is AstraZeneca's use of Facebook and Twitter.
- *Advocacy Group–Consumer:* Engagement between consumers and advocacy organizations such as the American Heart Association or Autism Speaks.
- *Provider–Provider:* Connection between medical providers for the purposes of clinical information and experience exchange. Good examples are SERMO for MDs and ANA's NurseSpace.
- *Public Health–Provider/Consumer:* Release of public health messages to promote safety and prevention. A good example is the CDC's campaign for H1N1.

Adapted from Healthcare Information and Management Systems Society (HIMSS) Social Media Work Group. HIMSS white paper: Health care "friending" social media: what is it, how is it used, and what should I do? HIMSS. http://www.himss.org/ASP/ContentRedirector.asp?ContentID=79496. February 10, 2012. Accessed April 5, 2012.

facilitates health status information exchange, and encourages support between friends and family members during a health crisis. Other networks such as PatientsLikeMe, CureTogether, and Inspire link patients with each other and facilitate data and information sharing among patients with similar diagnoses. Facebook, one of the more popular and well-known social networking sites, is also one of the most commonly accessed sites. Individuals, businesses, interest groups, and organizations are able to maintain Facebook pages. Although not exclusively designed as a forum for healthcare, these types of Facebook pages are often accessed to gather healthcare information[13] and to market practices or institutions to patients.[14]

Blogging and Wikis

Blogs represent a web-based, chronological journal of an individual author's thoughts. They allow for asynchronous conversations and invite readers to comment and join in conversation.[15] Blogs contain a variety of media types beyond simple text, including links to other websites, video, and images. "The popularity of a blog hinges on its ability to draw together disparate individuals interested in a specialized topic, creating a community of ideas, interest, and expertise."[16(p512)] Medical journals, healthcare facilities, nursing organizations, healthcare provider networks, and educational institutions commonly maintain blogs to relay the latest information and facilitate discussion.

Wikis represent a collaborative, web-based effort to compile information on a particular topic. These sites contain search functions and links to other articles and could be compared to an online encyclopedia. Wikis create a flexible document, allowing many authors to add and edit content. Wikis may be devoted to specific professional sectors. Examples include Medpedia (www.medpedia.com) and ganfyd (www.ganfyd.org), developed by medical providers and researchers to generate healthcare-specific documents. Clinfowiki (www.clinfowiki.org) is another example focused specifically on clinical informatics.

Microblogging (Twitter)

Microblogging is a form of blogging in which entries are kept brief using character limitations. Twitter, a popular microblogging site, restricts blog threads known as "tweets" to 140 characters. These posts are delineated with a hashtag (#) symbol to organize "tweets" of a particular topic. Twitter is emerging as an increasingly popular site for public health research and is used in many studies to track trends and behaviors related to illnesses and conditions.[17] It has also been a useful tool for instant communication of vital information during crises or disasters.[15] For a multipurpose overview of different healthcare uses of Twitter, see Phil Baumann's "140 Health Care Uses for Twitter" at http://philbaumann.com/2009/01/16/140-health-care-uses-for-twitter/.

Social Bookmarking

Social bookmarking is a way to organize and store online resources. Unlike saving bookmarks to your individual computer browser, the bookmarks are tagged on a third-party website such as Delicious, Connotea, or Digg. Connotea allows saving website bookmarks and also journal articles, a great advantage for researchers. There are three advantages to social bookmarking: "availability, tagging and collaboration."[18(p236)] Availability means that your bookmarks are accessible from any computer. The bookmarks are no longer tied to a particular computer; instead, the social bookmarking service allows connecting and accessing all saved bookmarks. Second, tagging allows the creation of established tags that are meaningful to the user and not just those established by a computer algorithm. Users can share their tags with others in their network or join other networks to view their tags. In the spirit of social media these tools facilitate collaboration within specific or general networks. The downsides of tagging are "no standardization with taxonomies such as MeSH [Medical Subject Headings] terms, no hierarchical associations, [and] mis-tagging due to spelling errors and highly personalized tags."[18(p236)]

User-Generated Content

Another method for sharing health information is through the video-sharing website YouTube. This social media channel allows visitors to view and share videos posted by individuals, businesses, and organizations. Content has been developed by professional and amateur videographers and can be "liked" or "disliked." This site can serve as a useful source of education for patients and healthcare providers, as it offers useful visual instruction for hands-on skills such as how to change a tracheotomy dressing and how to give an insulin injection. Readily available content includes health-promoting exercise instructions, computer-generated depictions of how a condition such as diabetes affects internal organs, and general educational content on diseases. Along with videos, there are podcasts, asynchronous recordings designed to also provide healthcare information, and current events announcements. Flickr is a public photo-sharing site that offers a forum for sharing photos and encouraging conversation and dialog. Medical facilities are actively using these social media tools to interact with clients, promote facility activities, and open alternate means of communication.

Foursquare, a social media tool designed specifically for mobile applications, allows users to "check in" at various venues, instantly communicating with friends and at times receiving discounts at "checked-in" locations (http://foursquare.com). Medical facilities that use mobile platforms are creating the opportunity for visitors to comment on their hospital experience.

Other healthcare sectors are turning to Second Life, a multi-user virtual environment (MUVE) or virtual world, which allows users to create a three-dimensional arena with graphics and sound simulation for education and socialization purposes.[15] The disability community has embraced Second Life and has created the Virtual Ability Island[19]; several schools of nursing use this tool for educational purposes.[20] This use of Second Life is further explored in Chapter 28.

SOCIAL MEDIA STATISTICS

According to the International Telecommunication Union, "the number of active social media users surpassed the first billion in 2011, many of whom connect to social media using their mobile devices."[21(p5)] In the United States nearly 4 in 5 active Internet users visit blogs and social networks daily, spending approximately 23% of their Internet time at these sites.[22]

According to National Research Corporation's Ticker survey,[13] 1 in 5 Americans use social media to obtain health-care information. The Pew Research Center, in describing the social life of health information, revealed that 59% of U.S. adults have used the Internet to obtain health information while 46% of adults use social media.[23] Only 15% of those users (or 7% of all adults) have sought health information from a social media site.[23] Eleven percent of all adults have followed a friend's health experiences on social network sites and 17% of social network site users have used social networks to memorialize someone.[23] Twenty-four percent of Internet users have sought drug reviews online.[23] Caregivers and those living with chronic conditions are most likely to seek information from social network sites.[23]

Health-related social network use is expanding rapidly. Specific social networks, such as PatientsLikeMe, MedHelp, and Inspire, present membership and daily usage statistics on their web pages and demonstrate an impressive number of members. Social media is also being used by hospitals throughout the United States. As of September 2012 there were 1264 hospitals using social networking tools, with a combined 6370 hospital social networking sites.[24]

A majority of physicians are using social media for personal use,[14] including 28% using online professional physician communities, mainly for educational purposes but also to communicate with colleagues, socially and professionally. However, use by physicians to communicate with patients is rare.[14] Professional workforce sites such as LinkedIn allow healthcare professionals to connect with others in their field. Doc2doc, Sermo, and Student Doctor Network all offer forums designated specifically for physician collaboration and networking. Sermo is designed exclusively for physicians and can be used to hold "closed door" consultations with colleagues and access experts in the field.[16] Nurses and other healthcare specialists maintain their own profession-specific social networking sites to communicate field-relevant information such as American Nurses Association's (ANA's) Nurse Space and NurseGroups.com.

Many major healthcare systems have realized the positive influence of social media and committed to the use of social networking tools to support the delivery of healthcare information, describe their services, recruit employees, and communicate their mission.[6] The U.S. Department of Veterans Affairs (VA) recognized the power of social media and is aggressively incorporating social media tools into its agenda. In December 2011 the VA announced Facebook pages for all of its 151 facilities with more than 352,000 subscribers. While the Facebook sites restrict specific discussion of individual veterans, the staff members monitoring the site have at times intervened to lend support in mental health crisis situations.[25] The VA has its own YouTube channel, 64 Twitter feeds, a Flickr page for photos, and a veteran-run blog. The VA's *Directive 6515: Use of Web-Based Collaboration Technologies* not only highly encourages the use of social media, but also "endorses the secure use of Web-based collaboration and social media tools to enhance communication, stakeholder outreach collaboration, and information exchange; streamline processes; and foster productivity improvements to achieve seamless access to information."[26(p1)] The VA believes that the use of social media technologies will support the organization's mission effectiveness through the benefits of speed, broad reach, targeted reach, collaboration, a medium for dialog, and expansion of real-time, sensitive communications.[26]

The Mayo Clinic has also embraced social media, pioneering a first-of-its-kind social media center. The Mayo Clinic Center for Social Media "exists to improve health globally by accelerating effective application of social media tools throughout Mayo Clinic and spurring broader and deeper engagement in social media by hospitals, medical professionals and patients."[27] The Mayo Clinic Center for Social Media's mission to "lead the social media revolution in health care"[27] is driven by a philosophy of improved health through patient empowerment and collaboration among healthcare providers. To facilitate the growth of social media in healthcare, the Mayo Clinic offers a residency training program that provides advanced intensive training in the use of social media.

Healthcare insurance companies are also joining the trend of using social media tools to promote well-being. Blue Cross and Blue Shield (BCBS) maintains a social media site for its members that allows individual profiles, blogs, discussion threads, and access to experts in nutrition, cooking, and health coaching. Pharmaceutical companies are using social media tools to provide customers and physicians with educational materials.[14] Input from physicians facilitates a relationship with pharmaceutical companies to "collaborate for adherence solutions" for improved patient outcomes.[14] These sites also offer customer and patient services, opening channels for medication users to discuss experiences and needs.[14]

BENEFITS OF SOCIAL MEDIA

There are several benefits associated with social media. One of the first benefits is in the area of research. A growing number of descriptive studies are describing potential benefits of social media. These studies can be divided into three general areas of research in social media: (1) description of the content on social media sites, (2) the use of social media, and (3) potential use of social networks for research. The first area examined the content of social media being disseminated through social networks and the microblogging tool Twitter. Content analyses and text mining techniques were used to assess the nature and quality of the content. Findings from this research include the following:

- The most common health conditions on social media are diabetes, cancer, pregnancy, mental health, and neurologic conditions.[28]
- Social networks are places where information, including personal experiences and personal stories, can be shared with the intended community.[29-32]
- The majority of the information is valid, although this can vary from network to network.[30,33-35]
- Twitter messages produce valuable public health information about the public's knowledge of antibiotics,[34] H1N1,[33,35] seizures[36] and "validated Twitter as a real-time content, sentiment[37] and public attention trend-tracking tool."[35(pe14118)]
- "Twitter might also be a promising platform for leveraging social support to motivate health behavior change"[38 (p1159)] and promoting healthy behaviors.[39]

The second area of studies examined how specific patient populations used social media. PatientsLikeMe[40-42] is the most studied network to date. Other studies examined specific patient populations (oncology,[43-46] depression,[47] traumatic brain injury,[48] and asthma[49]). Highlighted findings are as follows:

- Benefits noted by patients included finding others with similar health conditions[40-44] and seeking information related to symptom management and treatments.[40-42]
- Patients used various techniques to search for other patients' video stories[43] and used them for encouragement[44] and social support.[45,47]
- Facebook had the largest number of social networks for breast cancer but most were for increasing public awareness and fundraising.[46]

The final area examined two major uses of social networks in the research process. First, researchers are recruiting potential clinical trial subjects from within disease-specific web and social networking sites that then provide this information to pharmaceutical companies, universities, and research labs.[12,15,50,51] Second, researchers are using social networks to accelerate clinical discoveries[12,52,53] and provide "a low-cost and scalable model of citizen science"[54(pe19256)] for data sharing and bidirectional communication within a disease population. "Self-run clinical trials and structured self-experimentation are emerging as patients no longer have to wait for formal research findings and pharmaceutical company-sponsored clinical trials. These efforts may fill the gap for orphan diseases and other conditions that do not make good business cases in the existing pharmaceutical model."[12(p500)]

Additional benefits of social media include access to information and social support. Facebook, YouTube, and Twitter are the most common social media sites used by patients to obtain healthcare information or interact with other patients with similar diseases or health and wellness interests. "Social media platforms for online dialogue and support among individuals with common conditions, needs or interests support prevention, wellness, and healthy behaviors."[8(p14)] Social media sites[2] not only foster social support but also enable patients to manage their own health conditions, typically at no cost.

Two predominant forces are "driving online health conversation: 1) the availability of social tools and 2) the motivation, especially among people living with chronic conditions, to connect with each other."[21(p3)] The most popular social media sites, specifically geared toward patients (PatientsLikeMe, CureTogether, MedHelp, and Inspire), offer venues for dialog and also shift the power of achieving health and well-being into patients' own hands. As healthcare evolves from paternalistic to partnership models,[12] these two forces will continue to fuel the growth of social media in healthcare. The development of social media arenas has created a community of epatients engaged in their health and healthcare decisions (http://e-patients.net/about-e-patientsnet). Many of these individuals will take part in quantified self-tracking (online data entry of condition, symptom, treatment, and other biological information to monitor personal progress) and search for "patients like me."[12]

There is no doubt that the active role of the patients or consumers in their healthcare will continue to dramatically change the landscape of the healthcare arena over the next decade. The emergence of upcoming generations born into a world immersed in social media will result in consumers taking control of their personal health and will foster a community of both collaboration and independence to achieve an optimal state of well-being. The growing number of baby boomers already immersed in the social media space may also contribute to the changing healthcare landscape.[55] Despite the promise of social media in healthcare, this area is not without its challenges and risks.

CHALLENGES OF SOCIAL MEDIA

Social media can enhance the consumer's healthcare experience but also has the potential to undermine the healthcare profession.[56] Thus the strengths of social media's open platform and networking capabilities are also its greatest weaknesses. Health professionals should be aware of the dangers associated with social media use prior to engaging in its activities.[56,57] The primary principle influencing the use of social media in healthcare is the obligation to serve the best needs of the public; however, clinicians are bound by laws, practice ethics, and professional codes of conduct governing how and when to use social media applications. The digital environment is not isolated from the real world[58] and professional standards that exist in one realm should carry over to the other. Moreover, naive and negligent social media practices bring about security vulnerabilities that can compromise professional integrity and consumer confidence.[56] Fortunately, private and professional organizations recognizing these issues have begun to provide guidance regarding appropriate social media practices. Each of these issues will be explored in more detail in the sections that follow.

Privacy and Confidentiality

The most significant challenge for healthcare providers who use social media is to maintain privacy and confidentiality. Social media applications tout the ability for users to establish "many-to-many" relationships. As promising as that may sound, these open forums provide the opportunity for clinicians to inadvertently divulge consumer information to a vast number of people. A valuable mindset to have is to equate a social media application to the circumstances inside a hospital elevator;[59] any number of people can ride in an elevator and all can hear the conversations taking place within them. Further, healthcare providers are "dual citizens" in the social media arena[60] because they have professional and private uses for social media–generated content. This dual role increases the chance that professional boundaries may blur and may encourage clinicians to inadvertently communicate too openly.[61-67]

Healthcare providers are accountable to federal laws and professional standards that protect the privacy of patients' protected health information (PHI).[56,68] The Health Insurance Portability and Accountability Act (HIPAA) of 1996 defined the appropriate handling of PHI.[68] Government agencies and employees are further restricted by the Privacy Act passed in 1974.[69] Both require that a patient must provide authorization before healthcare professionals and organizations can release any part of the patient's record.[65,70] PHI refers to individually identifiable information that is related to delivery of healthcare[71] and does not always mean obvious identifiers such as name, social security number, and date of birth.[72] Additional information about the privacy and security rules within the HIPAA legislation is included in Chapter 19, and additional information about the legal protections of PHI is presented in Chapter 24. Even without explicit representation of such individually identifiable information, social media applications are rich with other details that could identify a particular consumer.[73] Social media profiles displaying a consumer's hometown, personal interests, and family photographs may be pieced together to reveal the consumer's identity. Consequently, healthcare providers may inadvertently reveal certain key facts that could lead others to recognize a specific patient.[72]

In addition to federal regulation, healthcare providers are bound by their professional codes of conduct, which regard privacy and confidentiality as compulsory. For example, the ANA's *Code of Ethics* states that the "nurse has a duty to maintain confidentiality of all patient information."[74(p6)] Further, according to ANA's *Principles of Social Networking and the Nurse*, "patient privacy is a fundamental ethical and legal obligation of nurses."[56(p4)] Physicians are also obligated to keep patient information private. According to the American Medical Association's (AMA's) *Code of Ethics*,[75] physicians should not share confidential information without prior consent of the patient. In addition, the AMA has established a social media policy for physicians.[76] These standards apply even when healthcare providers are not physically in their clinical roles.[56]

Conscious awareness and diligent adherence to laws and professional standards may not be enough. Healthcare providers acting in good faith may still unwittingly expose consumers to privacy and confidentiality risks. The primary reason lies in the naive trust they may have in the privacy settings of the social media application itself.[65] Risks often arise because clinicians fail to invoke certain privacy settings in their social media accounts.[65] Further, social networking sites such as Facebook often push privacy barriers and wait until consumers complain before tightening privacy restrictions.[77] "Friending" is one example of a less conspicuous means of breaching privacy. A healthcare provider may "friend" a patient in hopes of keeping in better contact but fail to realize that the other "friends" on his or her account may also be able to view the patient's name and information.[63,78] Another critical point to consider is the consumers' own account settings, as they may not share the same level of social media literacy.[15] For instance, a patient may not realize that adding a healthcare provider as a friend may expose the patient to unwanted scrutiny from other friends. Although this is entirely the patient's choice, healthcare providers are responsible for advocating for the best interests of their patients.[74,75]

Another naive assumption about the use of social media is believing that consumers are who they claim to be.[79] Healthcare providers unaware of identity impersonation or hacking may unknowingly be divulging private information to someone other than the intended consumer. Just because consumer social media pages may have images and some recognizable data does not quantifiably identify them as those individuals. Unless clinicians have a means to authenticate the consumer's identity, there is no way to guarantee that any social media contact, no matter how secure or confidential, involves the intended individuals. The relative permanence of online activity[56] adds an even greater degree of harm when sharing information with consumers who are not validated.

Inappropriate Behaviors

In addition to the risk of jeopardizing patient privacy and confidentiality, healthcare providers are also in danger of openly engaging in inappropriate behaviors. The danger arises from a healthcare provider's "dual citizenship" in the social arena.[58] This dichotomous role can blur the personal and professional boundaries that exist more clearly in the physical world.[63,64,66,67,80] In some cases the information a healthcare provider shares with his family and friends may be inappropriate for the general public to see. Consequently, healthcare providers must maintain the same level of professionalism online as they would in a clinic.[56,61,68]

Inappropriate behaviors can include questionable blog and photo postings, unprofessional commenting, and projecting attitudes unbecoming of respectable healthcare personnel.[81] Not only does such behavior tarnish the clinician's reputation, it can also result in disciplinary action. For example, physicians have been reprimanded for misrepresenting their credentials, improper Internet prescribing, and sexual misconduct.[82] Moreover, news agencies from various countries around the world have reported incidences of clinician improprieties, including nursing students posting images of organs (e.g., displaying a photograph of a placenta), medical students being vulgar or sexually suggestive, and doctors engaging in unprofessional social "games" online.[83-85]

Although these behaviors reflect a lack of personal accountability,[80] other professional indiscretions can be even more profound. Healthcare providers may find themselves endorsing drug products or third-party businesses by joining their online groups or "friending" one of their employees.[61] Such activities, without the appropriate declaration of conflict of interest,[66] could give consumers false impressions.

Another indiscretion involves clinicians actively seeking out patient information online. In particular, behavioral healthcare providers face professional dilemmas when determining whether to view a client's social media site to gain further clinical insight.[86] Although intended to facilitate clinical evaluations, such actions could be viewed as a violation of the patient's trust.[86] Behavioral healthcare providers are also particularly challenged when gauging the appropriate amount of client contact: too much contact through social media could encourage client transference and too little could lead to patients feeling rejected or abandoned.[64] Further, nurses who are excessively passionate about social media use for consumer advocacy may also be vulnerable to crossing boundaries.[87] Patient advocacy is a professional obligation for nurses;[74] however, social media applications enable nurses to overstep their boundaries. In an effort to connect with patients and win patient approval, some nurses can end up disclosing too much of their own personal information and come across as flirtatious or self-centered and misrepresent their profession.[87] Healthcare providers can falter in attempts at appropriate online behavior if they do not keep the patients' best interests in mind and advocate for patient well-being.[61,87]

Healthcare providers who use social media must consider who might view their postings and what impact those postings could have on their individual careers as well as their profession.[56,88] They must always consider social media platforms to be public domain and open to others who are unintended participants.[61] Failure to recognize these truths can have untoward consequences. Organizations and academic programs have taken punitive steps to address inappropriate behaviors, including expulsion of students and suspension or termination of employees.[80,84,89,90] Licensing boards have held disciplinary hearings in response to member misconduct.[82] Employers have also passed over applicants that have questionable content on their social media sites. Insurance companies likewise use social media platforms to validate claims or check on beneficiaries.[91,92] Thus inappropriate behaviors could lead to loss of coverage or cancellation of insurance payments.[93] These consequences can be mitigated if healthcare professionals maintain an expected code of conduct when engaging with social media applications.

Security

Social media applications reside on the Internet, which is characteristically and notoriously unsecure.[94,95] This high-risk environment is one of the principal reasons why healthcare organizations often restrict employee access to social media sites.[80,96,97] Although there are few reports of social media–related security breaches in healthcare, organizations do not have to look far to comprehend the risk that social media use can bring. Even with strict security settings, healthcare information systems are still susceptible to viruses, spyware, phishing, and other Internet threats.[94,97] The primary reasons for these vulnerabilities are the personnel themselves[98,99] who succumb to social engineering deceptions and can inadvertently allow the social media site to be a vector for malicious behavior.[79,98] Social engineering is the use of tactics to lure or deceive people into doing something they would not normally do. Social media applications have made it easier for dishonest individuals to attack others by enabling contact with numerous people at relatively little or no cost and with virtually complete anonymity.[100] These deceptions can be carried out through the social media site's electronic mail, which can contain deleterious software or an infected link on someone's blog. The social media user's interaction with these malicious attacks enables harmful applications to bypass electronic defenses and enter an organization's previously secure network.[98]

Another avenue for perpetrators to infiltrate another computer network is by "malicious friending."[98] This occurs when a person who is accepted as a friend changes his or her profile to include malicious code or unwanted content.[98] Malicious friending can also happen through distal extensions, or friends of friends. Users who open up their privacy settings to friends may inadvertently allow extended friends into their personal sites and subsequently make themselves vulnerable to attack.[100] These vulnerabilities are considered a type of social engineering that thrives in the social media arena where users are quick to assume trust in the social media platform as well as in other users.[99,101]

Even with sound judgment and scrupulous navigation, social media users may engender security vulnerabilities by placing too much trust in the social media platform they are using.[99] Hackers, or those who infiltrate websites for malicious purposes, can implant malicious code into the social media site itself.[99] This is often done through advertisements[99] or by deceiving users into accessing an alternate log-in screen.[102] There is also free software that allows anyone to access another's social media account when both are on an unsecured wireless network.[79] Further, sites like Twitter, which enable broadcasting of microblogs, can also promulgate the spread of malicious activity by disseminating abbreviated links to websites that appear safe but are in fact gateways that lead the recipient to a harmful Internet location.[99,103]

The means of accessing social media platforms has also elevated security risks. In particular, more and more users engage in social media via mobile devices[99,101,104] such as laptops, notepads, and smartphones. These increase social media use and have also made users more vulnerable.[105-107] The ease of social media use on these platforms encourages users to divulge too much personal information.[108] Unwitting consumers who post their location and activity on their social networking site may, for instance, actually invite thieves to rob their homes.[106] Social media use on a mobile device is also subject to additional threats from other third-party applications on the device itself.[99,106] These remote access Trojans (RATs) can appear harmless but may allow third parties to access the user's personal information.[99,107,109] These apps can then share the information with others, destroy it outright, or use it to impersonate the content owner.[99,109] Moreover, apps often operate in the background, unnoticed by the user, and can steal passwords, personal account data, and other private information.[94] Finally, storing personal information, such as details of a social media profile, on a mobile device increases security vulnerabilities if the device is lost or stolen.[103,107]

Security breaches from any of these vulnerabilities can result in loss of data and varying degrees of criminal activity.[96] Hackers could obtain clinician passwords and gain access to a hospital's vast database of PHI, leading to privacy breaches and financial damages. While loss of financial data is damaging, access to PHI could lead to identity theft and cyberbullying or cyberstalking, all of which may cause significant emotional and mental turmoil. Identity theft has been labeled as one of the top five social networking scams.[102] Moreover, identity theft was one of the most frequent consumer complaints regarding Internet use in 2010, second only to nondelivery of goods.[110] Identity theft is also the number one consumer complaint category, according to the Federal Trade Commission (FTC), and these grievances continue to grow.[111]

Social media application use can contribute to the threat of identity theft by expanding the user's digital footprint, described as lingering electronic information that can be linked back to the user who provided it.[112,113] The bits of information disseminated across the Internet can be combined to form a more detailed profile of the individual.[113] Social media users' naive efforts to become visible to friends and relatives actually may make them "knowable" to others who may have malicious inclinations.[111] Thus the open and trusted sharing of personal information can turn on the user and be employed for purposes other than what the user intended.[114,115]

Cyberharassment and cyberstalking are also increasing.[110] These terms are synonymous with cyberbullying but refer to adult behavior, whereas cyberbullying generally refers to underage harassment.[116] Regardless of the terminology, these are all considered social threats and are described as the stigmatizing, bullying, and threatening of others. This intimidation can pose significant danger to the recipients and their affiliates or friends.[72] Cyberstalking is not limited to threats or intimidation of specific individuals; it can be targeted at organizations as well.[79] Discrimination can be toward an individual's or organization's religious affiliation, political views, sexual orientation, or group association[73]; it can even include an individual's medical diagnosis or hospitalizations. Cyberharassment, sometimes called digital abuse, includes online threats or aggression toward individuals or groups with the objective of intimidating or coercing others who are perceived as being unable to retaliate.[117,118] Social media platforms, which enable anonymous activity, have propagated these behaviors in the Internet environment.[118] In addition to

practicing these behaviors in relative anonymity, cyberstalkers may also impersonate another individual, thus causing further harm while displacing the blame.[102] Healthcare providers are not immune to such behavior, as was seen when a British surgeon's identity was stolen and used to create a Facebook page that slandered an Olympic swimmer.[119]

Regulatory Issues

Many of the challenges and risks discussed here exist because social media sites and the Internet as a whole are not regulated.[56,120] The Federal Communications Commission (FCC)[121] is the U.S. government body responsible for regulating communication through various media, including those employed for Internet use. In 2010 the FCC voted to maintain "net neutrality," thereby safeguarding consumers' rights to view what they choose on the Internet.[122] Although websites themselves may not have government oversight, the content on these sites is considered to be under some degree of regulation.

One of the key agencies in healthcare with legal authority to control who may contribute social media content is the U.S. Food and Drug Administration (FDA).[123] The FDA regulates the distribution of drugs and medical devices.[123,124] Pharmaceutical companies often engage in social media to promote consumer interaction and adverse events reporting.[124] Although their intentions seem benign, these companies must be cautious and avoid posting anything that could be viewed as off-label promotion.[125] They must also be careful when using social media to respond to unsolicited requests for drug information, as this avenue reaches a broader audience and remains viewable for an indefinite period of time.[123] Consequently, pharmaceutical and device manufacturing companies must respond according to FDA guidance to not appear to be promoting their products for unapproved purposes.[123]

Further, as discussed earlier, healthcare provider behavior is governed by laws limiting the kinds of information to be disclosed and to whom. This is directly related to the appropriate use of consumers' PHI. In addition to patient content restrictions, healthcare providers must be aware of the medical information they post and the advice, if any, they provide. This information should be appropriate and reliable and avoid any copyright infringement.[126] Misinformation can be detrimental as well as dangerous to the individual and organization.[56,127] It is also critical that healthcare providers avoid engaging in behavior that might be regarded as fraudulent or an abuse of their position. Certain social media information exchanges could be construed as kickbacks or inappropriate in the medical-legal environment.[126,128] If healthcare providers use social media with the intention of providing care, they are using telehealth, allowing for the provision of care over a distance using telecommunication technology.[129] Accordingly, social media used as a form of telecommunication could be regulated by the clinician's state and local agencies overseeing telehealth licensing and scope of practice.[130] Additional information about these regulations can be found in Chapter 8.

In light of the absence of more definitive regulation of social media sites, some have pushed the need for federal government to intervene.[131] The risk to the public regarding privacy, confidentiality, and information security would seem to endorse that sentiment. Still, others have suggested that social media sites engender crowd wisdom and can engage in their own self-regulation.[104]

Market Pressure

The myriad risks associated with social media use has caused some healthcare providers to avoid using these applications.[132] Yet market pressure and consumer demand for social media applications are growing. Healthcare providers who rely on advertising to increase clientele may have no other choice but to enter the social media arena.[132,133,134] One of the great risks of social media is not knowing what information, whether good or bad, is being shared.[135] Social media has become a driving force for corporate marketing as well as consumer ratings.[133,135] In addition, more and more social media resources are emerging to provide public opinion on goods and services.[136] The fact is that consumers are the primary driving force for using social media in healthcare and increasing numbers of consumers seek health information online.[137] Their resource of choice for health information is a healthcare provider.[138] Consequently, consumers may expect to learn more about their healthcare questions from clinicians using these sites. As more and more private practice physicians join accountable care organizations (ACOs), marketing and consumer ratings will become more significant. The push to provide patient-centered care[139] in ACOs will add pressure to those organizations and physicians who are currently reluctant to use social media as one option to connect with their patients.

Many organizations and individual clinicians have recognized these trends and the value that social media tools can bring, such as ease of use, information sharing, and timely updates.[140,141] From a business perspective, healthcare providers find the low cost of use of social media an economical means to market their resources,[142] educate patients, and engender client loyalty.[143] The increase in clientele gained from social media use[7, 89] could counter the lack of financial reimbursement[132,144] as well as the time and effort needed to stay involved.[127,145] This, in fact, may be the case. The number of participating organizations and clinicians is expected to grow, adding to the expanding use of social media to market healthcare goods and services. Nonparticipating individuals and groups may feel pressured to opt in just so that they too may gain market exposure.

Consumers are more frequently posting their opinions online as to whether or not they like a particular service or experience.[136] Consequently, consumers often seek ratings or rankings from others before making a decision about purchasing goods and services, including healthcare.[138] Numerous websites allow patients to rate their physician or hospital experiences (e.g., Vitals.com, DoctorScorecard.com). General business websites such as Yelp also allow consumers to rate and post comments on various hospitals and healthcare

service organizations. With the growing number of sites and consumer interest in them, healthcare organizations and clinicians may feel compelled to create a social media site to promote their strengths and perhaps counter any negative ratings.[133] Contributing to this urgency is the fact that organization rankings have been posted on hospital scoring websites such as Healthgrades, Hospital Compare (operated by the U.S. Department of Health & Human Services), and ConsumerReports.org.

Another compelling reason to enter the social media arena is to dispel misinformation and bridge the digital divide. Consumers have unprecedented access to health information on the Internet but may encounter inaccurate data.[125,137,144,146] Social media enables the creation and propagation of inaccurate and misleading information.[56,88,120,147-149] Largely due to lack of oversight,[149] web-based information can be created by anyone[120] and be disseminated far too easily.[125] Just about anyone can enter, alter, edit, and even sabotage social media applications.[142] Moreover, authors of social media content do not need to identify themselves[148] or provide any credentials.[88] Site association can also perpetuate inaccuracies. Authors of blog content who are not members of the health profession may associate themselves with reputable sites in order to seem as though they are in the field.[88] Consumers may also be misled by inaccuracies or opinions that dominate a particular site.[145,150] For example, an overabundance of opposition to child vaccinations on certain sites[145,150] could dissuade parents from immunizing their children, even though vaccines are valuable and could even save a child's life.[151] Information, even when accurately presented, can be reviewed out of context in the social media arena[152] and subjective healthcare material can be easily accessed, circumventing any disclaimers or warnings.[153]

Healthcare providers are in a position to counter inaccuracies by sponsoring a social media site themselves or guiding consumers to reputable sites.[147] By choosing the latter strategy, healthcare professionals can become apomediaries.[146] Apomediation involves standing by to direct consumers to high-quality information on the Internet rather than standing between the consumer and the information, as has been the usual practice in the past.[146] Clinicians may do this in person by interpreting web-based healthcare information that patients bring to their office visits.[150,154] Clinicians could also perform outreach via social media applications to contact and guide consumers who post questions or concerns regarding health conditions or services. Caution in these situations is necessary, as clinicians do not control the content of the referred site and there is a chance that a healthcare provider could recommend an unreliable source.[146]

The final incentive to clinician adoption of social media use is to facilitate the bridging of the "digital divide." Since the inception of the Internet there has been a disparate representation of users across those who have the means and knowledge to use it and those who lack either the means or the wherewithal to navigate the web.[155,156] Social media emerged as a means to bridge this divide because there is relative uniformity of use of social media across cultural and economic groups.[137,156-158] More disabled consumers can be reached through social media use.[56] Consumers in the older age demographic are about the only ones that have been identified as underrepresented in the social media arena.[138,157-159] Nevertheless, clinicians could accommodate older consumers via the usual methods, including in-person visits, telephone calls, and written media, while expanding their impact to others via social media.

POLICY

Social media has the potential to enable healthcare providers to foster professional relationships while facilitating interpersonal communication and consumer education.[160] However, healthcare providers who use social media are subject to increased security vulnerabilities,[98,161] blurred professional boundaries,[60,62,66,158,162] and confidentiality breaches.[160,161] For these and other reasons, policies are needed to help guide organizations and clinicians through recommended social media practices.[163,164] In addition to risk avoidance, social media policies can also illuminate professional expectations and establish definitions for acceptable behavior. The three critical elements that a well-constructed social media policy could mitigate are information disclosure, professional integrity, and productivity.[81]

A social media policy should limit information disclosure. It must illuminate the behaviors that increase the potential for breaches of patient privacy and confidentiality as well as how such violations conflict with privacy laws and professional ethical standards.[68,74,75] Social media policies should also engender professional integrity by discouraging clinicians from divulging too much of their own personal information in addition to discouraging them from creating or disseminating inaccurate or potentially harmful information.[56] Written guidelines could also require healthcare providers to create separate accounts for private and professional use when choosing to use social media for consumer engagement.[165] A social media policy should define acceptable limits for social media use and consequences for overuse.[164,166] It may further delineate the organization's definition of overuse, repercussions for loss in productivity, and ramifications if social media indulgence creates an impression among customers that clinicians are not paying attention to their work.[89]

The final consideration regarding social media policy creation is to determine which level of development would best serve the needs of the public as well as the industry. Health-related public policies are created at the national or state level and establish authoritative oversight by the executive, judicial, or legislative branches of government.[167] These types of policies tend to protect the interests of certain groups of people, such as the elderly or underserved, or types of organizations, such as healthcare plans or employers.[167] Although some have argued for government oversight,[131] social media use remains accessible to nearly everyone and extends beyond cultural and economic boundaries.[138,157-159] Since government entities like the FTC have decided to keep the Internet open,[122] public policy may not be the avenue of choice when seeking to regulate social media.[168] Further, encouraging government oversight of Internet activity, no matter how loosely defined, could lead to undesirable restrictions through fragmented and gradual policy changes that often produce limited results or benefits.[169]

Organizational-level social media policies, if well written, should be the primary means of mitigating risks associated with social media use.[170] They can also promote social media engagement by helping healthcare providers to overcome knowledge barriers and issues of mistrust with social media applications.[125] Policies can establish appropriate boundaries between healthcare provider authority and consumer vulnerability,[87] foster user accountability,[171] and define appropriate consumer engagement.[172] Entering the realm of social media use without strategic planning, including sound policies, could result in unexpected consequences and security threats.[161,172] Healthcare providers have a responsibility to promote patient health and protect consumers.[75,173] Social policies can help healthcare providers to positively affect the quality of the consumers' online and real-life social environment.[167]

Guidelines for Writing Policies

Policy development requires careful planning and implementation. Too lenient a policy would be ineffective; however, too stringent a policy becomes counterproductive and unenforceable.[60] It is also important to not enter the realm of social media policy too hastily[170] and to develop a strategy to make social media work for the organization.[170,174,175] There are no international standards guiding social media so it is imperative that policies are carefully created to define appropriate social media behavior.[79] Healthcare organizations and providers should understand the reason they wish to engage in social media before attempting to create a policy.[174] Once this purpose has been realized, guidelines can be crafted to protect the organization and employees[176] and to circumvent draconian rules that might stymie social media use.[170,174]

Of equal importance to the content of a social media policy is the process used to create it.[166] The first step in constructing a sound policy is to form a project team. By bringing key stakeholders together, the organization can be sure that essential elements will be included in the policy.[79,140] The project team should consist of representatives from public relations, marketing, information technology (IT), legal, administration, representative healthcare and staff members, as well as the community.[172,176-178] These individuals should have a varying range of technological aptitude and experience with social media.[166] Invariably, staff member representation should include nurses.[56,62] Not only do healthcare professionals advocate on behalf of patient interests, but they are able to help define and adhere to professional boundaries.[62] Healthcare professionals can also harness their commitment to ethics and scope of practice when providing recommendations for policy development.[56,179]

Subsequently, an assessment of the organization environment should be performed.[180] The outcomes of an assessment will enable the team to establish the intent and scope of the policy. It will also help the project team to determine which social media platform to adopt: internally or externally hosted applications. Internally hosted applications are developed and operated by the organization using them.[79] Although more resource intensive, this type of application enables the organization to control the security of the site as well as the data generated from it.[79] Externally hosted platforms, such as Twitter and YouTube, have vendors that administer the application but also control the sites' security protocols.[79] Operating in the social media arena without complete control over site security can be an added risk for healthcare providers and organizations.

The outcomes of the environmental assessment and platform appraisal enable the project team to establish its objectives for the policy and to generate its content. Content will need to be concise, consistent, use simple vernacular,[166,170,176] be specific, and include the owner of the policy and responsibilities of the various departments involved,[79] the organization's attitude regarding social media, and the organization's view on acceptable behavior and consequences for misuse.[79,164,181] Content should also include relevant security, regulatory, and safety implications.[175]

Additionally, the policy should set a framework for appropriate social media etiquette.[176] As each application has different features, guidance should be written for each application, whether it is blogs, social networking, or content communities such as YouTube.[15] For instance, when posting blogs, employees may be able to state where they work but should never say that they speak on behalf of the organization unless they are in an official position to do so.[161,176] Also, when engaging in social networking, healthcare providers should not "friend" a current or former patient.[62,66] Further, regarding content communities, employees may not be allowed to "favorite" objectionable material that could be discovered by consumers and associated with the organization. Lastly, employees may be expected to review each application's privacy policy and to enact specific privacy settings. Box 14-2 provides an example of the material covered in a social media policy.

A sound institutional policy can help to address social media security needs[176] but its mere creation should not be the end of the process. Organizations are obligated to educate their employees about the policy.[79,176,182-185] Clinicians should understand that a primary objective of social media use is a positive consumer experience[186] and that the policy is designed to guide and protect everyone involved, from the consumers to the staff.[176] As the project team carries out the training they will need to adjust their tactics according to the varying degree of social media experience among the staff.[176] One potentially successful method would be to train key individuals in each area of the organization and establish them as social media experts.[176] These individuals could be the resource for their respective areas to help monitor for appropriate usage, train staff, and continuously update the ever-evolving nature of the social media landscape.

RESOURCES FOR POLICY DEVELOPMENT

Creating policy does not have to be resource intensive or performed in isolation. Healthcare organizations may find internal and external resources to assist them with social media policy development. One option is the institution's existing information security policy, which may be adapted to meet identified needs; it could provide foundation guidance to minimize threats, ensure privacy, and secure company data and could be modified to include expected rules of behavior.[160,187] Healthcare organizations can also find useful guidance from other institutions, government bodies, and professional organizations.[89,159,178,184,188] One valuable resource containing examples of existing healthcare policies is Ed Bennett's website, titled "Found in Cache," located at http://ebennett.org. The website contains examples of different policies from major healthcare providers across the country, including trendsetting organizations, such as the Mayo Clinic. The Mayo Clinic has established its own medical director[189] and created a Center for Social Media dedicated to helping its clients connect with clinicians and make healthy choices.[27]

CONCLUSION AND FUTURE DIRECTIONS

If Healthcare + Social media = Social health (today)

Then Social health (today) = Health (future)[7(p3)]

As discussed in this chapter, healthcare is discovering the opportunities and challenges offered by social media. By changing the media of communication, social media is changing the conversation and in turn the professional relationship between consumers and patients, healthcare providers, and healthcare institutions. The number and types of social media tools are expanding as the current tools are meshed and new tools are evolving. The use of social media by all ages and social and cultural groups is growing rapidly and can be expected to continue.

The use of social media is woven into the tapestry of healthcare; therefore the statement above by HIMSS Social Media Work Group[7] may in fact predict the future. Consumers and patients will lead the movement toward social health and healthcare professionals and the healthcare delivery system will eventually join the social health movement. Federal initiatives such as the Health Information Technology Pledge (www.healthit.gov/pledge/) encourage healthcare professionals to educate consumers about being active participants in their healthcare and may increase the number of healthcare professionals and consumers using social media. Rannie and Wellman[190] described the phenomenon of people connected to social media as networked individualism; it is the new "operating system" because it describes the ways in which people connect, communicate, and exchange information. The near-term future will likely determine the fate of this new operating system.

BOX 14-2 SAMPLE OUTLINE OF A SOCIAL MEDIA POLICY

Introduction
- Definition of social media, including what is included under its umbrella (i.e., blogging, social networking, content sharing, etc.)
- Intent of the policy, including how social media coincides with the organization's mission and values

Purpose
- Define the purpose of the policy
- Define the scope of the policy and whom it covers
- Identify the policy's goals, including promotion of ethical and professional use of the various forms of social media
- Link policy to any other company policies that may have overlapping guidance, such as an information security policy
- Link policy to comply with any applicable regulations and laws, including the Health Insurance Portability and Accountability Act (HIPAA), the Privacy Act, U.S. Food and Drug Administration (FDA) regulations, and others

Responsibility
- Identify the policy owners who created it and will do periodic updates
- Identify the responsibilities of the organization's leadership, including their exemplary use of social media tools
- Identify the responsibility of the information technology department and information security officer, including security and system monitoring issues (if any)
- Identify the responsibility of the marketing and public relations departments, including any monitoring of social media content
- Identify the responsibility of all employees, including following company policy for employee conduct as well as the rules of behavior outlined within the policy

Rules of Behavior (General)
Provide guidelines for acceptable and unacceptable use. Consider the following:
- Appropriate and inappropriate tone and content
- Content management: whether organization has authority to remove or censor postings and other activity
- Company representation: employees may identify with the company but not speak on its behalf
- Promote ethical behavior: to coincide with professional standards organizations (i.e., American Nurses Association, American Medical Association, etc.)
- Promote legal behavior: avoidance of copyright infringement, defamation, conflicts of interest, and plagiarism
- Expect privacy and confidentiality of patient and company information

- Expect everyone to review each social media site's privacy policy
- Expect a minimum level of privacy settings for each social media site used
- Require that everyone create separate social media accounts for professional and personal activities
- Describe reasonable usage amounts, including avoidance of excessive use
- Consider having employees sign the "rules of behavior" and "etiquette" guidelines
- Describe the consequences for violation of policy guidelines
- Establish an environment of open communication, including reporting policy violations by other staff

References
- Cite all sources for the content of the policy, including other company policies
- Include any professional organization guidance

Supplemental Guidelines on Social Media Etiquette
- Social networking
  - Define it and identify its uses or objectives for use
  - Expect staff to create separate personal and professional accounts (to dissociate their "two lives")
  - Set guidelines for managing vendor contacts and "friending"
  - Provide guidelines for configuring site privacy settings
  - Set guidelines for managing patient contact and "friending"
  - Set guidelines for managing negative comments
- Blogging and microblogging
  - Define it and identify its uses or objectives for use
  - Address the practice of link-shortening
  - Consider providing guidelines for user profile names
  - Address the approval process (if any) for blogging on, or from, the company site
- Content sharing
  - Define it and identify its uses or objectives for use
  - Identify appropriate and inappropriate content
  - Provide guidelines for configuring site privacy settings
  - Describe the process when inappropriate content is discovered and how it will be retracted
- Other: add any other forms of social media within the organization's purview
  - Define it and include its uses or objectives for use
  - Provide guidelines for configuring site privacy settings
  - Set guidelines for managing etiquette according to the functionality of the application

Adapted from Bahadur G, Inasi J, de Carvalho A. *Securing the Clicks: Network Security in the Age of Social Media.* OH: McGraw-Hill Osborne Media; 2011; Barton A, Skiba D. Creating social media policies for education and practice. In: Abbott PA, Hullin C, Ramirez C, Newbold C, Nagle L, eds. *Studies in Informatics: Advancing Global Health through Informatics. Proceedings of the NI2012. The 11th International Congress of Nursing Informatics.* Bethesda, MD: AMIA 2012:16-20; Centers for Disease Control and Prevention (CDC). CDC social media tools, guidelines & best practices. CDC. http://www.cdc.gov/SocialMedia/Tools/guidelines/?s_cid=tw_eh_78. July 17, 2012; and Mayo Clinic. For Mayo Clinic employees. Mayo Clinic. http://sharing.mayoclinic.org/guidelines/for-mayo-clinic-employees.

REFERENCES

1. Social media. Merriam-Webster Dictionary. http://www. merriam-webster.com/dictionary/social%20media. Accessed October 10, 2012.

2. Fox S. Medicine 2.0: peer-to-peer health care. Paper presented at: Medicine 2.0 Congress; September 11, 2011; Stanford, CA. http://pewinternet.org/Reports/2011/Medicine-20.aspx. Accessed April 3, 2012.

3. Kaplan AJ, Haenlein M. Users of the world, unite! the challenges and opportunities of social media. *Business Horizons.* 2010;53:59-68.

4. Bradley A. A New Definition of Social Media. Gartner Blog Network. http://blogs.gartner.com/anthony_bradley/2010/01/07/a-new-definition-of-social-media/. January 11, 2010. Accessed April 2, 2012.

5. Bradley A. A new definition of social media. Gartner Blog Network. http://blogs.gartner.com/anthony_bradley/2010/01/07/a-new-definition-of-social-media/. January 7, 2010. Accessed April 5, 2012.

6. Backman C, Dolack S, Dunyak D, Lutz L, Tegen A, Warner, D. Social media + health care. *J AHIMA.* 2011;82(3):20-25.

7. Healthcare Information and Management Systems Society (HIMSS) Social Media Work Group. HIMSS white paper: health care "friending" social media: what is it, how is it used, and what should I do? HIMSS. http://www.himss.org/ASP/ContentRedirector.asp?ContentID=79496. February 10, 2012. Accessed April 5, 2012.

8. Bipartisan Policy Center. Transforming health care: the role of health IT. Bipartisan Policy Center. http://www.bipartisanpolicy.org/sites/default/files/Transforming%20Health%20Care.pdf. January 2012. Accessed April 5, 2012.

9. Short J, Williams E, Christie, B. *The Social Psychology of Telecommunications.* Hoboken, NJ: John Wiley & Sons Ltd; 1976.

10. Daft RL, Lengel RH. Organizational information requirements, media richness, and structural design. *Mgmt Sci.* 1986;32(5):554-571.

11. Surowiecki J. *The Wisdom of Crowds.* New York, NY: Anchor Books; 2005.

12. Swan M. Emerging patient-driven health care models: an examination of health social networks, consumer personalized medicine and quantified self-tracking. *Int J Environ Res Publ Health.* 2009;6:492-525. doi:10.3390/jerph6020492.

13. National Research Corporation. 1 in 5 Americans use social media for health care information. National Research Corporation. http://hcmg.nationalresearch.com/public/News.aspx?ID=9. February 28, 2011. Accessed April 5, 2012.

14. Modahl M, Tompsett L, Moorhead T. Doctors, patients, and social media. QuantiaMD. Care Continuum Alliance. http://www.quantiamd.com/q-qcp/DoctorsPatientSocialMedia.pdf. September 2011. Accessed April 5, 2012.

15. Bacigalupe G. Is there a role for social technologies in collaborative health care? *Fam Sys Health.* 2011;29(1):1-14. doi:10.1037/a0022093.

16. Sparks MA, O'Seaghdha CM, Sethi SK, Jhaveri KD. Embracing the internet as a means of enhancing medial education in nephrology. *Am J Kidney Dis.* 2011;58(4):512-518.

17. Paul M, Dredze M. You are what you tweet: analyzing Twitter for public health. Johns Hopkins University, Department of Computer Science. http://www.cs.jhu.edu/~mdredze/publications/twitter_health_icwsm_11.pdf. 2011. Accessed April 5, 2012.

18. Barton A. Social bookmarking: what every clinical nurse specialist should know. *Clin Nurse Spec.* 2009;23(5):236-237.

19. Skiba D. Nursing education 2.0: second Life. *Nurs Ed Persp.* 2007;28(3):156-157.

20. Skiba D. Nursing education 2.0: a second look at Second Life. *Nurs Ed Persp.* 2009;30(2):129-131.

21. International Telecommunication Union. *Trends in Telecommunication Reform 2012: Smart Regulation for a Broadband World.* Geneva, Switzerland: International Telecommunication Union; 2012. http://www.itu.int/ITU-D/treg/publications/trends12.html. Accessed May 20, 2012.

22. Nielson and NM Incite. State of the media: the social media report Q3 2011. http://blog.nielsen.com/nielsenwire/social/. 2011.

23. Fox S. The social life of health information. Pew Internet & American Life Project. http://pewinternet.org/Reports/2011/Social-Life-of-Health-Info.aspx. 2011. Accessed April 5, 2012.

24. Mayo Clinic Center for Social Media. Health care social media list. Mayo Clinic. http://network.socialmedia.mayoclinic.org/hcsml-grid/. Accessed September 22, 2012.

25. Brewin B. Looking for friends in all the right places: VA expands its Facebook presence. Nextgov-Technology and the Business of Government. http://www.nextgov.com/nextgov/ng_20111222_5947.php. December 22, 2011. Accessed April 5, 2012.

26. Department of Veterans Affairs (VA). Use of web-based collaborative technologies: VA Directive 6515. http://www.va.gov/vapubs/viewpublication.asp?pub_id=551. June 28, 2011. Accessed March 25, 2012.

27. Mayo Clinic Center for Social Media. About. Mayo Clinic. http://socialmedia.mayoclinic.org/. Accessed April 4, 2012.

28. Orizio G, Schulz P, Gasparotti C, Caimi L, Gelatti U. The world of e-patients: a content analysis of online social networks focusing on diseases. *Telemed J E Health.* 2010;16(10):1060-1066.

29. Gallant LM, Irizarry C, Boone G, Kreps G. Promoting participatory medicine with social media: new media applications on hospital websites that enhance health education and e-patients' voices. *J Partic Med.* 2011;3:e49. http://www.jopm.org/evidence/research/2011/10/31/promoting-participatory-medicine-with-social-media-new-media-applications-on-hospital-websites-that-enhance-health-education-and-e-patients-voices/. Accessed April 5, 2012.

30. Sajadi KP, Goldman HB. Social networks lack useful content for incontinence. *Uro.* 2011;78(4):764-767. doi:10.1016/j.urology.2011.04.074.

31. Ahmed OH, Sullivan SJ, Schneiders AG, McCrory P. iSupport: do social networking sites have a role to play in concussion awareness? *Disabil Rehabil.* 2010;32(22):1877-1883. doi:10.3109/09638281003734409.

32. Greene JA, Choudhry N, Kilabuk E, Shrank WH. Online social networking by patients with diabetes: a qualitative evaluation of communication with Facebook. *J Gen Int Med.* 2011;26(3):287-292. doi:10.1007/s11606-010-1526-3.

33. Kim S, Pinkerton T, Ganesh N. Assessment of H1N1 questions and answers posted on the web. *Amer J Infect Control.* 2012;40(3):211-217. doi:10.1016/j.ajic.2011.03.028.

34. Scanfeld D, Scanfeld V, Larson EL. Dissemination of health information through social networks: Twitter and antibiotics. *Amer J Infect Control.* 2010;38(3):182-188. doi:10.1016/j.ajic.2009.11.004.

35. Chew C, Eysenbach G. Pandemics in the age of Twitter: content analysis of tweets during the 2009 H1N1 outbreak. *PLoS ONE.* 2010;5(11):e14118. doi:10.1371/journal.pone.0014118.

36. McNeil K, Brna PM, Gordon KE. Epilepsy in the Twitter era: a need to re-tweet the way we think about seizures. *Epilepsy Behav.* 2012;23(2):127-130. doi:10.1016/j.yebeh.2011.10.

37. Keelan J, Pavri V, Balakrishnan R, Wilson K. An analysis of the human papilloma virus vaccine debate on MySpace blogs. *Vaccine.* 2010;28(6):1535-1540. doi:10.1016/j.vaccine.2009.11.060/.

38. Kendall L, Hartzler A, Klasnja P, Pratt W. Descriptive analysis of physical activity conversation on Twitter. *Proceedings of the 2011 Annual Conference on Human Factors in Computing Systems.* New York, NY: Association of Computing Machinery; 2011. doi:10.1145/1979742.1979807.

39. Gold J, Pedrana AE, Sacks-Davis R, et al. A systematic examination of the use of online social networking sites for sexual health promotion. *BMC Pub Health.* 2011;11:583. http://www.biomedcentral.com/1471-2458/11/583. Accessed April 5, 2012.

40. Frost JH, Massagli MP. Social uses of personal health information within PatientsLikeMe, an online patient community: what can happen when patients have access to one another's data. *J Med Internet Res.* 2008;10(3):e15. doi:10.2196/jmir.1053.

41. Wicks P, Massagli M, Frost J, et al. Sharing health data for better outcomes on PatientsLikeMe. *J Med Internet Res.* 2010;12(2):e19. doi:10.2196/jmir.1549.

42. Wicks O, Keininger D, Massagli M, et al. Perceived benefits of sharing health data between people with epilepsy on an online platform. *Epilepsy Behav.* 2012;23:16-23. doi:10.1016/j.yebeh.2011.09.026.

43. Overberg R, Otten W, de Man A, Toussaint P, Westenbrink J, Zwetsloot-Schonk B. How breast cancer patients want to search for and retrieve information from stories of other patients on the internet: an online randomized controlled experiment. *J Med Internet Res.* 2010;12(1):e7. doi:10.2196/jmir.1215.

44. Chou WYS, Hunt Y, Folkers A, Augustson E. Cancer survivorship in the age of YouTube and social media: a narrative analysis. *J Med Internet Res.* 2011;13(1):e7. doi:10.2196/jmir.1569.

45. McLaughlin M, Nam Y, Gould J, et al. A videosharing social networking intervention for young adult cancer survivors. *Comput Hum Behav.* 2012;28:631-641. doi:10.1016/j.chb.2011.11.009.

46. Bender JL, Jimenez-Marroquin MC, Jadad AR. Seeking support on Facebook: a content analysis of breast cancer groups. *J Med Internet Res.* 2011;13(1):e16. doi:10.2196/jmir.1560.

47. Takahashi Y, Uchida C, Miyaki K, Sakai M, Shimbo T, Nakayama T. Potential benefits and harms of a peer support social network service on the internet for people with depressive tendencies: qualitative content analysis and social network analysis. *J Med Internet Res.* 2009;11(3):e29. doi:10.2196/jmir.1142.

48. Tsaousides T, Matsuzawa Y, Lebowitz M. Familiarity and prevalence of Facebook use for social networking among individuals with traumatic brain injury. *Brain Injury.* 2011;25(12):1155-1162. doi:10.3109/02699052.2011.613086.

49. Baptist AP, Thompson M, Grossman KS, Mohammed L, Sy A, Sanders GM. Social media, text messaging, and email-preferences of asthma patients between 12 and 40 years old. *J Asthma.* 2011;48(8):824-830. doi: 10.3109/02770903.2011.608460.

50. Atkinson NL, Saperstein SL, Massett HA, Leonard CR, Grama L, Manrow R. Using the internet to search for cancer clinical trials: a comparative audit of clinical trial search tools. *Contemp Clin Trials.* 2008;29(4):555-564.

51. Allison M. Can Web 2.0 reboot clinical trials? *Nat Biotech.* 2009;27(10):895-902. [Erratum appears in *Nat Biotech.* 2010;28(2):178].

52. Frost J, Okun S, Vaughan T, Heywood J, Wicks P. Patient-reported outcomes as a source of evidence in off-label prescribing: analysis of data from PatientsLikeMe. *J Med Internet Res.* 2011;13(1):e6. doi:10.2196/jmir.1643.

53. Wicks P, Vaughan TE, Massagli MP, Heywood J. Accelerated clinical discovery using self-reported patient data collected online and a patient-matching algorithm. *Nature Biotech.* 2011;29(5):411-416. doi:10.1038/nbt.1837.

54. Weitzman ER, Adida B, Kelemen S, Mandl KD. Sharing data for public health research by members of an international online diabetes social network. *PLoS ONE.* 2011;6(4):e19256. doi:10.1371/journal.pone.0019256.

55. Zickuhr K, Smith A. Digital differences report. Pew Internet & American Life Study 2012. http://pewinternet.org/Reports/2012/Digital-differences/Overview.aspx. April 13, 2012. Accessed April 5, 2012.

56. American Nurses Association. *Principles of Social Networking and the Nurse.* Silver Spring, MD: American Nurses Association; 2011.

57. Kappel D. ANA and NCSBN unite to provide guidelines on social media and networking for nurses. National Council of State Boards of Nursing. https://www.ncsbn.org/2927.htm. October 19, 2011. Accessed March 15, 2012.

58. Baker SA. From the criminal crowd to the "mediated crowd": the impact of social media on the 2011 English riots. *Safer Communities.* 2012;11(1):40-49. doi:10.1108/17578041211200100.

59. Strategies for Nurse Managers. Social media: patient friend or foe? Strategies for Nurse Managers. http://www.strategiesfornursemanagers.com/ce_detail/272966.cfm. 2012. Accessed March 17, 2012.

60. Mostaghimi A, Crotty B. Professionalism in the digital age. *Ann Intern Med.* 2011;154:560-562.

61. Snyder L. American College of Physicians ethics manual sixth edition. *Ann Intern Med.* 2012;156(1):73-101.

62. Cole L. Professional boundaries and social media. *New Hampshire Nursing News.* 2012; January–March:7.

63. Jain SH. Practicing medicine in the age of Facebook. *N Engl J Med.* 2009;361:649-651. http://www.nejm.org/doi/full/10.1056/NEJMp0901277. Accessed March 17, 2012.

64. Luo J. Social media link you in but raise thorny patient issues. *Psychiatric News.* 2011;46(11):12-22. http://psychnews.psychiatryonline.org/newsArticle.aspx?articleid=108689. Accessed March 17, 2012.

65. MacDonald J, Sohn S, Ellis P. Privacy, professionalism and Facebook: a dilemma for young doctors. *Med Educ.* 2010;44:805-813. doi:10.1111/j.1365-2923.2010.03720.x.

66. British Medical Association. *Using Social Media: Practical and Ethical Guidance for Doctors and Medical Students.* London, England: British Medical Association; 2011. http://www.bma.org.uk/images/socialmediaguidance_tcm41-206859.pdf. Accessed March 15, 2012.

67. Davies M, Brannan S, Chrispin E, et al. New guidance on social media for medical professionals. *J Med Ethics.* 2011;37(9):577-579.

68. Centers for Medicare & Medicaid Services (CMS). HIPAA security series. CMS. http://www.hhs.gov/ocr/privacy/hipaa/administrative/securityrule/securityruleguidance.html. September 17, 2009. Accessed March 15, 2012.

69. Federal Trade Commission (FTC). Privacy Act of 1974, as amended. FTC. http://www.ftc.gov/foia/privacy_act.shtm. November 3, 2010. Accessed March 16, 2012.

70. Department of Health and Human Services (HHS). The Privacy Act. HHS. http://www.hhs.gov/foia/privacy/index.html. April 17, 2007. Accessed March 17, 2012.

71. Department of Health and Human Services Office for Civil Rights. OCR privacy brief: summary of the HIPAA privacy rule. Department of Health and Human Services. http://www.hhs.gov/ocr/privacy/hipaa/understanding/summary/privacy.html. May 2003. Accessed March 15, 2012.

72. Nosko A, Wood E, Molema S. All about me: disclosure in online social networking profiles: the case of Facebook. *Comput Hum Behav.* 2010;26:406-418.

73. Duffy M. Patient privacy and company policy in online life. *Am J Nurs.* 2011;111(9):65-69.

74. American Nurses Association. *Code of Ethics.* Silver Spring, MD: American Nurses Association; 2001.

75. American Medical Association (AMA). AMA code of ethics. AMA. http://www.ama-assn.org/ama/pub/physician-resources/medical-ethics/code-medical-ethics.page#. December 13, 2011. Accessed March 15, 2012.

76. American Medical Association (AMA). AMA policy: professionalism in the use of social media. AMA. http://www.ama-assn.org/ama/pub/meeting/professionalism-social-media_print.html. February 24, 2012. Accessed March 25, 2012.

77. Terry K. Why you could—but shouldn't—use Facebook to coordinate care. FierceHealthIT. http://www.fiercehealthit.com/story/why-facebook-shouldnt-be-used-care-coordination/2011-04-11. April 11, 2011. Accessed March 17, 2012.

78. Dimick C. Privacy policies for social media. *Journal of AHIMA.* http://journal.ahima.org/2010/01/06/social-media-policies/. January 6, 2010. Accessed March 16, 2012.

79. Bahadur G, Inasi J, de Carvalho A. *Securing the Clicks: Network Security in the Age of Social Media.* OH: McGraw-Hill Osborne Media; 2011.

80. Balog EK, Warwick AB, Randall VF, Kieling C. Medical professionalism and social media: the responsibility of military medical personnel. *Mil Med.* 2012;177(2):123-124.

81. Cain J. Social media in health care: the case for organizational policy and employee education. *Am J Health Syst Pharm.* 2011;68:1036-1040.

82. Greysen SR, Chretien KC, Kind T, Young A, Gross CP. Physician violations of online professionalism and disciplinary actions: a national survey of state medical boards. *JAMA.* 2012;307(11):1141-1142.

83. Press Association. Hospital staff suspended for playing Facebook "lying down game." *The Guardian.* 2009;September 9. http://www.guardian.co.uk/uk/2009/sep/09/hospital-lying-down-game?INTCMP=SRCH. Accessed March 17, 2012.

84. Huckabee C. Judge orders college to reinstate student who posted a placenta photo online. Chronicle of Higher Education. http://chronicle.com/blogs/ticker/judge-orders-college-to-reinstate-student-who-posted-a-placenta-photo-online/29555. January 6, 2011. Accessed April 7, 2012.

85. Emery C. Medical students using Facebook and Twitter can get expelled. KevinMD. http://www.kevinmd.com/blog/2009/09/medical-students-facebook-twitter-expelled.html. September 2009. Accessed March 16, 2012.

86. Tunick RA, Mednick L, Conroy C. A snapshot of child psychologists' social media activity: professional and ethical practice implications and recommendations. *Prof Psychol-Res Pr.* 2011;42(6):440-447.

87. National Council of State Boards of Nursing. *A Nurse's Guide to Professional Boundaries.* Chicago, IL: National Council of State Boards of Nursing; 2011.

88. Lagu T, Kaufman EJ, Asch DA, Armstrong K. Content of weblogs written by health professionals. *J Gen Intern Med.* 2008;23(10):1642-1646. doi:10.1007/s11606-008-0726-6.

89. Baldwin G. Social media: friend or foe? Health Data Management. http://www.healthdatamanagement.com/issues/19_9/social-media-friend-or-foe-43067-1.html. September 1, 2011. Accessed March 17, 2012.

90. Doctors suspended after playing Facebook lying down game. *The Telegraph.* 2009;September 9. http://www.telegraph.co.uk/technology/facebook/6161853/Doctors-suspended-after-playing-Facebook-Lying-Down-Game.html. Accessed March 17, 2012.

91. Nance-Nash S. What insurers could do with your "social media score." Daily Finance. http://www.dailyfinance.com/2011/12/12/what-insurers-could-do-with-your-social-media-score/. December 12, 2011. Accessed March 17, 2012.

92. National Insurance Commission. The use of social media in insurance (draft). National Association of Insurance Commissioners. http://www.naic.org/documents/committees_d_social_media_exposures_111201_whitepaper_draft_social_media.pdf. December 1, 2011. Accessed March 17, 2012.

93. Ewing SM. Insurance companies using social media to catch fraud. WUSA9.com. http://www.wusa9.com/news/article/170054/373/Social-Media-Mining-By-Insurance-Companies. October 6, 2011. Accessed March 16, 2012.

94. Acoca B. Scoping paper on online identity theft. Organisation for Economic Co-operation and Development. http://www.oecd.org/dataoecd/35/24/40644196.pdf. January 9, 2008. Accessed March 15, 2012.

95. LaRose R, Rifon N. Your privacy is assured—of being invaded: websites with and without privacy seals. *New Media and Society.* 2006;8:1009-1029.

96. Fraser M, Dutta S. Web 2.0: security threat to your company? *SC Magazine.* 2009;February 17. http://www.scmagazine.com/web-20-security-threat-to-your-company/article/127417/. Accessed March 16, 2012.

97. Webroot. New Webroot survey shows Web 2.0 is top security threat to SMBs in 2010. Webroot. http://www.webroot.com/En_US/pr/threat-research/ent/web-2-security-survey-170210.html. February 17, 2010. Accessed March 17, 2012.

98. Centers for Disease Control and Prevention (CDC). Social media security mitigations. CDC. http://www.cdc.gov/SocialMedia/Tools/guidelines/pdf/securitymitigations.pdf. December 3, 2009. Accessed March 15, 2012.

99. Nemey C. Five top social media security threats. Network World. http://www.networkworld.com/news/2011/053111-social-media-security.html. May 31, 2011. Accessed March 17, 2012.

100. Investor.gov. Investor alert: social media and investing—Avoiding fraud. U.S. Securities and Exchange Commission. http://investor.gov/news-alerts/investor-alerts/investor-alert-social-media-investing-avoiding-fraud. January 4, 2012. Accessed March 17, 2012.

101. Haley K. 2011 internet security threat report identifies increased risks for SMBs. Symantec. http://www.symantec.com/connect/2011_Internet_Security_Threat_Report_Identifies_Risks_For_SMBs. April 6, 2011. Accessed March 16, 2012.

102. Scambusters.org. The 5 most common social networking scams. Scambusters.org. http://www.scambusters.org/socialnetworking.html. Accessed March 17, 2012.

103. Barwick H. Virtualisation, mobile devices pose largest security risks: Symantec, security industry leaders weigh in on 2011 security trends. Computerworld. http://www.computerworld.com.au/article/375028/virtualisation_mobile_devices_pose_largest_security_risks_symantec/. February 1, 2011. Accessed March 15, 2012.

104. Sarasohn-Kahn J. *The Wisdom of Patients: Health Care Meets Online Social Media*. Oakland, CA: California HealthCare Foundation; 2008. http://www.chcf.org/topics/chronicdisease/index.cfm?itemID=133631. Accessed March 17, 2012.

105. Hamada J. Attempts to spread mobile malware in tweets. Symantec. http://www.symantec.com/connect/blogs/attempts-spread-mobile-malware-tweets. March 11, 2012. Accessed March 17, 2012.

106. Symantec. Symantec report finds cyber threats skyrocket in volume and sophistication. Symantec. http://www.symantec.com/about/news/release/article.jsp?prid=20110404_03. April 5, 2011. Accessed March 17, 2012.

107. Verizon. Mobile devices and organizational security risk. Verizon. http://www.verizonbusiness.com/resources/whitepapers/wp_mobile-devices-and-organizational-security-risk_en_xg.pdf. October 2010. Accessed March 17, 2012.

108. Symantec. Norton study reveals "over-sharing" of holiday cheer puts consumers at risk. Symantec. http://www.symantec.com/about/news/release/article.jsp?prid=20101216_01. December 16, 2010. Accessed March 17, 2012.

109. SearchSecurity. RAT (remote access Trojan). http://searchsecurity.techtarget.com/definition/RAT-remote-access-Trojan. October 2009. Accessed March 25, 2012.

110. Internet Crime Complaint Center. 2010 internet crime report. National White Collar Crime Center. http://www.ic3.gov/media/annualreport/2010_IC3Report.pdf. 2011. Accessed March 17, 2012.

111. Federal Trade Commission (FTC). Consumer sentinel network databook for January–December 2011. FTC. http://www.ftc.gov/sentinel/reports/sentinel-annual-reports/sentinel-cy2011.pdf. February 2012. Accessed March 16, 2012.

112. Greysen SR, Kind T, Chretien KC. Online professionalism and the mirror of social media. *J Gen Intern Med*. 2010;25 (11):1227-1229.

113. Madden M, Fox S, Smith A, Vitak J. Digital footprints: online identity management and search in the age of transparency. Pew Internet & American Life Project. http://pewresearch.org/pubs/663/digital-footprints. December 16, 2007. Accessed March 17, 2012.

114. Lee DH, Im S, Taylor CR. Voluntary self-disclosure of information on the internet: a multi-method study of the motivations and consequences of disclosing information on blogs. *Psychol Market*. 2008;25:692-710.

115. Marx G. Ethics for the new surveillance. *Inform Soc*. 1998;14:171-185.

116. Aftab P. Understanding cyberbullying & cyberharassment. Wired Safety. http://www.wiredsafety.org/index.php?option=com_content&view=article&id=193:cyberbullying-and-cyberstalking-and-harassment&catid=96:cyberbullying–stalking-a-harassment-&Itemid=41. June 2, 2008. Accessed March 15, 2012.

117. Dooley JJ, Pyzalski J, Cross D. Cyberbullying versus face-to-face bullying, a theoretical and conceptual review. *J Psychol*. 2009;217(4):182-188. http://icbtt.arizona.edu/sites/default/files/cross_set_al_cyber_vs_face-to-face.pdf. Accessed March 16, 2012.

118. Spears B, Slee P, Owens L, Johnson B. Behind the scenes and screens: insights into the human dimension of covert and cyberbullying. *J Psychol*. 2009;217(4):189-196.

119. Daily Mail Reporter. Brain surgeon's identity stolen for fake Facebook slur on Olympic gold medalist. MailOnline. http://www.dailymail.co.uk/news/article-1044714/Brain-surgeons-identity-stolen-fake-Facebook-slur-Olympic-gold-medallist.html#ixzz1pLDshJtb. August 14, 2008. Accessed March 16, 2012.

120. Schmidt CW. Trending now, using social media to predict and track disease outbreaks. *Environ Health Persp*. 2012;120 (1):A30-A33.

121. Federal Communications Commission (FCC). About the FCC. FCC. http://transition.fcc.gov/aboutus.html. November 28, 2011. Accessed March 16, 2012.

122. Schatz A, Raice S. Internet gets new rules of the road. *The Wall Street Journal*. 2010;December 22. http://online.wsj.com/article/SB10001424052748703581204576033513990668654.html. Accessed March 17, 2012.

123. Food and Drug Administration (FDA). Guidance for industry responding to unsolicited requests for off-label information about prescription drugs and medical devices. FDA. http://www.fda.gov/downloads/Drugs/GuidanceComplianceRegulatoryInformation/Guidances/UCM285145.pdf. December 2011. Accessed March 16, 2012.

124. TNS Media. Connecting with patients, overcoming uncertainty. TNS Media. http://www.seyfarth.com/dir_docs/news_item/1d21aaf1-4ad5-4e22-af28-af3feea533e6_documentupload.pdf. September 2007. Accessed March 17, 2012.

125. Baldwin M, Spong A, Doward L, Gnanasakthy A. Patient-reported outcomes, patient-reported information from randomized controlled trials to the social web and beyond. *Patient*. 2011;4(1):11-17. doi:10.2165/11585530-000000000-00000.

126. Lawry TC. Recognizing and managing website risks. *Health Progress*. 2001;82(6):12-13, 74.

127. Sharp J. Social media in health care: barriers and future trends. iHealthBeat. http://www.ihealthbeat.org/perspectives/2010/social-media-in-health-care-barriers-and-future-trends.aspx. May 6, 2010. Accessed March 17, 2012.

128. Goldman D. Legal issues (part 2): unique issues in health care social media. Mayo Clinic. http://socialmedia.mayoclinic.org/2010/08/02/legal-issues-part-2-unique-issues-in-healthcare-social-media/. August 2, 2010. Accessed March 25, 2012.

129. National Council of State Boards of Nursing (NCSBN). Position paper on telenursing: a challenge to regulation. NCSBN. https://www.ncsbn.org/TelenursingPaper.pdf. 1997. Accessed March 17, 2012.

130. American Telemedicine Association (ATA). Telehealth nursing, a white paper developed and accepted by the Telehealth Nursing Special Interest Group. ATA. http://www.americantelemed.org/files/public/membergroups/nursing/TelenursingWhitePaper_4.7.2008.pdf. April 7, 2008. Accessed March 15, 2012.

131. Noyes K. Social nets need new privacy rule, says senator. E-Commerce Times. http://www.ecommercetimes.com/story/Social-Nets-Need-New-Privacy-Rule-Book-Says-Senator-69862.html. April 26, 2010. Accessed March 17, 2012.

132. Hawn C. Take two aspirin and tweet me in the morning: how Twitter, Facebook, and other social media are reshaping health care. *Health Affair.* 2009;28(2):361-368.

133. Fluss D. Using social media for customer service is a strategic imperative: protect and enhance your company's image. *Customer Relationship Management.* 2011;December.

134. Vartabedian B. Are physicians obligated to participate in social media? 33charts. http://33charts.com/2009/10/are-physicians-obligated-to-participate-in-social-media.html. October 20, 2009. Accessed March 17, 2012.

135. Scott DM. Be an agent of change. *EContent.* http://www.econtentmag.com/Articles/Column/After-Thought/Be-an-Agent-of-Change-79113.htm. December 29, 2011. Accessed March 17, 2012.

136. O'Donnell O. DataContent 2011: make room for data. *Information Today.* 2012;January:18.

137. Powell JA, Darvell M, Gray JA. The doctor, the patient and the World Wide Web: how the internet is changing health care. *J Roy Soc Med.* 2003;96:74-76.

138. Fox S, Jones S. The social life of health information. Pew Internet & American Life Project. http://www.pewinternet.org/Reports/2009/8-The-Social-Life-of-Health-Information/01-Summary-of-Findings.aspx. June 11, 2009. Accessed March 17, 2012.

139. Centers for Medicare & Medicaid Services (CMS). Accountable care organizations overview. CMS. https://www.cms.gov/ACO/. February 2, 2012. Accessed March 15, 2012.

140. Ajjan H, Hartshorne R. Investigating faculty decisions to adopt Web 2.0 technologies: theory and empirical tests. *The Internet and Higher Education.* 2008;11(2):71e80.

141. Mejias U. Nomad's guide to learning and social software. Australian Flexible Learning Framework. http://knowledgetree.flexiblelearning.net.au/edition07/download/la_mejias.pdf. 2005. Accessed March 17, 2012.

142. Boulos MNK, Maramba I, Wheeler S. Wikis, blogs and podcasts: a new generation of web-virtual collaborative clinical practice and education. *BMC Medical Education.* 2006;6:41. doi:10.1186/1472-6920-6-41.

143. Chaiken BP. Social networking: a new tool to engage the clinical community. *Patient Safety and Quality Healthcare.* 2009; 6(2):6-7.

144. Crampton K. Social networking and health information: an emerging consumer health resource? What librarians need to know! La Crosse, WI: Gundersen Lutheran; 2010. http://www.caphis.mlanet.org/chis/Social-Networking-and-Health-Information.ppt. Accessed March 15, 2012.

145. Robinson MA. Navigating the world of social media. *Alberta RN.* 2012;67(6):42.

146. Eysenbach G. Medicine 2.0: social networking, collaboration, participation, apomediation, and openness. *J Med Internet Res.* 2008;10(3):e22.

147. Young SD. Recommendations for using online social networking technologies to reduce inaccurate online health information. *J Health Allied Sci.* 2011;10(2):2. http://www.ncbi.nlm.nih.gov/pmc/articles/PMC3196338/. Accessed March 17, 2012.

148. Myers SB, Endres MA, Ruddy ME, Zelikovsky N. Psychology graduate training in the era of online social networking. *Training and Education in Professional Psychology.* 2012; 6(1):28-36.

149. Kaslow FW, Patterson T. Ethical dilemmas in psychologists accessing internet data: is it justified? *Prof Psychol.* 2011; 42(2):105-112.

150. Keelan J, Pavri-Garcia V, Tomlinson G, Wilson K. YouTube as a source of information on immunization: a content analysis. *J Amer Med Assoc.* 2007;298(21):2482-2484.

151. Centers for Disease Control and Prevention (CDC). Five important reasons to vaccinate your child. CDC. http://www.cdc.gov/media/matte/2011/04_childvaccination.pdf. 2011. Accessed March 15, 2012.

152. Edwards IR, Lindquist M. Social media and networks in pharmacovigilance: boon or bane? *Drug Saf.* 2011;34(4):267-271. doi:10.2165/11590720-000000000-00000.

153. Eysenbach G, Diepgen TL. Towards quality management of medical information on the internet: evaluation, labeling, and filtering of information. *BMJ.* 1998;317. doi:10.1136/bmj.317.7171.1496.

154. Rodrigues RJ. Ethical and legal issues in interactive health communication: a call for international cooperation. *J Med Internet Res.* 2000;2(1):e8. http://www.jmir.org/2000/1/e8/. Accessed March 17, 2012.

155. Baur C, Kanaan S. *Expanding the Reach and Impact of Consumer E-Health Tools.* Washington, DC: U.S. Department of Health and Human Services; 2006. http://www.health.gov/communication/ehealth/ehealthTools/default.htm. Accessed March 15, 2012.

156. Cashen MS, Dykes P, Gerber B. eHealth technology and internet resources: barriers for vulnerable populations. *J Cardiovasc Nurs.* 2004;19(3):209-214.

157. Mazman SG, Usluel YK. Modeling educational usage of Facebook. *Comput Educ.* 2010;55(2010):444-453.

158. Chou WS, Hunt YM, Beckjord EB, Moser RP, Hesse BW. Social media use in the United States: implications for health communication. *J Med Internet Res.* 2009;11(4):e48. doi:10.2196/jmir.1249.

159. Chu LF, Young C, Zamora A, Kurup V, Macario A. Anesthesia 2.0: internet-based information resources and Web 2.0 applications in anesthesia education. *Curr Opin Anaesthesiol.* 2010; 23:218-227.

160. National Council of State Boards of Nursing (NCSBN). White paper: a nurse's guide to the use of social media. https://www.ncsbn.org/Social_Media.pdf. August 17, 2011. Accessed March 17, 2012.

161. Chi M. Security policy and social media use. Sans Institute. http://www.sans.org/reading_room/whitepapers/policyissues/reducing-risks-social-media-organization_33749. March 16, 2011. Accessed March 25, 2012.

162. Goldman D. Legal issues (part 4): specific suggestions when drafting your policies. Mayo Clinic. http://socialmedia.mayoclinic.org/2010/08/09/legal-issues-part-4-specific-suggestions-when-drafting-your-policies/. August 9, 2010. Accessed March 25, 2012.

163. Boudreaux C. Policy database. Social Media Governance. http://socialmediagovernance.com/policies.php#axzz1pjfBq4VE. 2011. Accessed March 26, 2012.

164. Shinder DL. 10 things you should cover in your social networking policy. Tech Republic. http://www.techrepublic.com/downloads/10-things-you-should-cover-in-your-social-networking-policy/1088217?tag=content;siu-container. July 14, 2009. Accessed March 25, 2012.

165. Lagu T, Greysen SR. Physician, monitor thyself: professionalism and accountability in the use of social media. *J Clin Ethics.* 2011;22(2):187-190.

166. Junco R. The need for student social media policies. *Educause Review.* 2011;46(1). http://www.educause.edu/EDUCAUSE+Re

view/EDUCAUSEReviewMagazineVolume46/TheNeedfor StudentSocialMediaPo/222666. Accessed March 25, 2012.

167. Longest B. *Health Policy Making in the United States.* 5th ed. Washington, DC: Health Administration Press; 2010.

168. Thierer A. *The Perils of Classifying Social Media Platforms as Public Utilities.* Fairfax, VA: George Mason University; 2012. http://www.insideronline.org/summary.cfm?id=17127. Accessed March 28, 2012.

169. Berkowitz B. The policy process. In: Mason D, Leavitt J, Chafee M, eds. *Policy & Politics in Nursing and Health Care.* St. Louis, MO: Elsevier; 2011:49-64.

170. Dryer L, Grant M, White LT. Social media, risk, and policies for associations. Social Fish & Croydon Consulting. http://www.socialfish.org/wp-content/downloads/socialfish-policies-whitepaper.pdf. 2009. Accessed March 25, 2012.

171. Chretien KC, Azar J, Kind T. Physicians on Twitter. *JAMA.* 2011;305(6):566-568.

172. Scott PR, Jacka JM. *Auditing Social Media: A Governance and Risk Guide.* Hoboken, NJ: John Wiley & Sons; 2011.

173. American Nurses Association. *Social Policy Statement.* Silver Spring, MD: American Nurses Association; 2010.

174. Strom D. Who owns your followers? time to revise your social media policy. Readwrite Web. http://www.readwriteweb.com/enterprise/2011/12/time-to-revise-you-social-medi.php. December 27, 2011. Accessed March 25, 2012.

175. Wolfe I. Before you write that social media policy . . . stop, look & listen. Toolbox.com. http://hr.toolbox.com/blogs/ira-wolfe/before-you-write-that-social-media-policystop-look-listen-45660. April 20, 2011. Accessed March 25, 2012.

176. Barger C. *The Social Media Strategist: Build a Successful Program from the Inside Out.* Ashland, OH: McGraw-Hill; 2011.

177. Ohio State Medical Association. Social networking and the medical practice. Ohio State Medical Association. http://www.osma.org/files/documents/tools-and-resources/running-a-practice/social-media-policy.pdf. September 22, 2010. Accessed March 25, 2012.

178. Barton A, Skiba D. Creating social media policies for education and practice. In: Abbott PA, Hullin C, Ramirez C, Newbold C, Nagle L, eds. *Studies in Informatics: Advancing Global Health through Informatics. Proceedings of the NI2012. The 11th International Congress of Nursing Informatics.* Bethesda, MD: AMIA; 2012:16-20.

179. Bard R. CEO outlook: embracing social media. *Canadian Nurse.* http://www.canadian-nurse.com/index.php?option=com_

content&view=article&id=586&Itemid=32&lang=en. January 2012. Accessed March 25, 2012.

180. Malone RE. Assessing the policy environment. *Policy Politics Nursing Practice.* 2005;6(2):135-143.

181. Guiness A. 7 (More) must-haves for your social media policy. Social Media Policy Templates. http://socialmediapolicytemplates.wordpress.com/. November 7, 2010.

182. Mayo Clinic. For Mayo Clinic employees. Mayo Clinic. http://sharing.mayoclinic.org/guidelines/for-mayo-clinic-employees/. 2012. Accessed March 25, 2012.

183. American Council for Technology–Industry Advisory Council (ACT-IAC), Collaboration & Transformation (C&T) Shared Interest Group (SIG). *Best Practices Study of Social Media Records Policies.* Fairfax, VA: American Council for Technology; 2011.

184. Black T. How to write a social media policy. *Inc.* http://www.inc.com/guides/2010/05/writing-a-social-media-policy.html. May 27, 2010. Accessed March 25, 2012.

185. Goldman D. Legal issues (part 3): general thoughts on developing your social media policy. Mayo Clinic. http://socialmedia.mayoclinic.org/2010/08/04/legal-issues-part-3-general-thoughts-on-developing-your-social-media-policy/. August 4, 2010. Accessed March 25, 2012.

186. AstraZeneca. White paper: social media in the pharmaceutical industry. AstraZeneca. http://www.astrazeneca.us.com/_mshost795281/content/media/AZ_Social_Media_White_Paper.pdf. 2011. Accessed March 25, 2012.

187. Photopoulos C. *Managing Catastrophic Loss of Sensitive Data: A Guide for IT and Security Professionals.* Rockland, MA: Syngress Publishing; 2008.

188. Goodchild J. 4 Tips for writing a great social media security policy. http://www.csoonline.com/article/505593/4-tips-for-writing-a-great-social-media-security-policy. October 21, 2009. Accessed March 25, 2012.

189. Aase L. Center names new medical director. Mayo Clinic Center for Social Media. http://socialmedia.mayoclinic.org/2011/12/19/center-names-new-medical-director/. December 19, 2011. Accessed March 25, 2012.

190. Rannie L, Wellman B. Networked individualism: what in the world is that? Pew Internet & American Life Project. http://networked.pewinternet.org/2012/05/24/networked-individualism-what-in-the-world-is-that-2/. May 24, 2012. Accessed May 20, 2012.

DISCUSSION QUESTIONS

1. What are the strengths of using social media in healthcare?

2. What are the challenges of using social media in healthcare?

3. Why are healthcare professionals slow to adopt social media as a tool in healthcare?

4. Is social media a fad?

5. In a hospital setting, what are the key questions that the C-suite (CEO, CFO, CNO, CIO) should ask about using social media?

6. How does social media affect the relationship between patients and their healthcare providers?

7. Is social media a part of patient-centric care?

8. How can health professional schools prepare future healthcare providers in the area of social media?

9. Describe the meaning of the following statement:
   If Healthcare + Social media = Social health (today)
   Then Social health (today) = Health (future)[7]

10. Describe networked individualism and the benefits for one's healthcare.

CASE STUDY

Social Media in Education and Healthcare

Grace Speak is a fourth-year student at Best University. She and her fellow classmates are working hard in their final courses and preparing for exams. Inspired by the teamwork that the healthcare profession espouses, Grace gets an idea for a study group. She thinks it will really help to share case experiences, course notes, and study tips. Unfortunately, several members of her peer group live out of town, which makes it difficult for them to participate fully. Grace is torn, as she does not want to exclude them from the study group. When she voices her concerns to a classmate, her friend suggests using social media tools as the primary medium for sharing information.

Discussion Questions

1. What types of social media tools could Grace's study group use?
2. How would those tools facilitate the objectives of the study group?
3. What are some of the risks associated with using social media for such purposes?
4. What might Grace need to do from the outset when she forms the study group?

Personal Health Records (PHRs)

Bryan Gibson

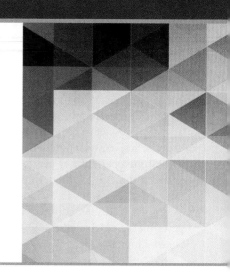

If the desire for personal health records (PHRs) persists, and trends in adoption continue, PHRs have the potential to become the platform for a more efficient, effective, and personalized healthcare system.

OBJECTIVES

At the completion of this chapter the reader will be prepared to:

1. Analyze trends and events leading to the development and adoption of electronic personal health records
2. Describe the ideal personal health record (PHR) and its proposed benefits
3. Explain the different types of PHRs and the pros and cons of each type of PHR.
4. Provide examples of existing PHRs, including their function and usage
5. Evaluate current research and other evidence regarding the effectiveness of PHRs as an approach to improving healthcare
6. Explore issues affecting the adoption and function of current PHRs
7. Examine the future of PHRs

KEY TERMS

ABSTRACT

This chapter begins with a definition of the electronic personal health record (PHR) and a description of the historical trends contributing to the development and adoption of PHRs. Attributes of an ideal PHR and proposed benefits are outlined. Types of PHRs, the pros and cons of each type, and examples of current PHRs and their use are discussed. The small but increasing body of evidence supporting the benefits of PHRs is discussed in terms of the Triple Aim for healthcare (improving the patient's experience of care, improving health, and reducing costs). Issues in improving the adoption of PHRs are outlined. The chapter concludes with a brief discussion of the future of PHRs.

DEFINITIONS OF THE PERSONAL HEALTH RECORD

Although no single definition is universally agreed upon, several organizations have attempted to define the personal health record (PHR). A joint PHR Task Force of the Medical Library Association and the National Library of Medicine[1(p244)] states:

> Electronic personal health record [is]: a private, secure application through which an individual may access, manage and share his or her health information. The PHR can include information that is entered by the consumer and/or data from other sources such as pharmacies, labs, and healthcare providers. The PHR may or may not include information from

the electronic health record (EHR) that is maintained by the healthcare provider and is not synonymous with the EHR. PHR sponsors include vendors who may or may not charge a fee, healthcare organizations such as hospitals, health insurance companies, or employers.

In *Connecting for Health*, the Personal Health Working Group of the Markle Foundation[2] defined the PHR as:

An electronic tool that enables individuals or their authorized representatives to control personal health information, supports them in managing their health and ill-being, and enhances their interactions with healthcare professionals.

The Office of the National Coordinator for Health Information Technology (ONC)[3] defined a PHR as:

An electronic application through which individuals can maintain and manage their health information (and that of others for whom they are authorized) in a private, secure, and confidential environment.

These definitions emphasize two essential aspects of the PHR. The first is that the PHR serves as an information aggregator and storage system. The second is that the PHR is a tool, or suite of tools, that individuals may use to manage their health.

THE DEVELOPMENT OF THE ELECTRONIC PERSONAL HEALTH RECORD

Individuals have long kept paper records of their healthcare as an adjunct to their medical record. Common examples include paper records of immunizations and lists of prescription medications or medical problems that individuals may carry in their wallets. A 2004 Harris Interactive poll conducted online found that most people thought it a good idea to keep personal health records, 46 percent of those surveyed actually kept records, and 86 percent of those who kept records did so using paper.[4] One of the primary reasons that most PHRs have been maintained in a paper format is that much of this type of information has been provided in a paper format. Paper records serve several important functions: they are persistent and minimize the need for individuals to remember the details of their medical history, they are portable, and they are shareable. An electronic PHR is proposed to improve on these functions and to provide unique functions. A California HealthCare Foundation survey[5] conducted in 2010 found that "Americans who have access to their health information through personal health records (PHRs) report that they know more about their health, ask more questions, and take better care of themselves than when their health information was less accessible to them in paper records." While paper records likely remain the most common form of PHR, subsequent references to the PHR in this chapter will refer to an electronic personal health record.

The development and adoption of the PHR in the United States is the result of several converging historical trends:

- The rise of personal computing devices and the Internet
- The development of EHRs

- Governmental policies related to health information technology (health IT)
- Consumer demands for the functions provided by a PHR

The personal computing revolution began when desktop computers became affordable in the 1980s and continues today with the increasing adoption of mobile devices. Concurrent with the increase in adoption of personal computing devices was the development of the Internet, which in 2012 an estimated 80% of Americans use.[6] Figure 15-1 presents the trends in the percentage of U.S. households owning common electronic devices from 2006 to 2012. As is evident in the figure, most Americans now own at least one type of personal computing device, with cellular phones being the most prevalent. A recent survey found that approximately 46% of U.S. adults own smartphones and that this percentage is increasing steadily.[7] As will be discussed later, mobile computing offers tremendous possibilities to expand the scope and functionality of PHRs.

While the widespread adoption and use of personal computing devices and the Internet provide the infrastructure that make PHRs possible, EHRs serve as the primary source of data populating the PHR. Large-scale implementation of EHRs became more prevalent in the early 1990s at several integrated health systems, such as the Veterans Health Administration (VHA),[8] Intermountain Healthcare in Utah, and the Regenstrief Institute in Indiana.[9] One of the first electronic PHRs, the VHA's My HealtheVet (MHV) pilot program in 1999, was made feasible by the presence of the VHA's EHR.[10]

In recent years the United States government has implemented policies specifically intended to increase the adoption of both EHRs and PHRs. See Chapters 24 and 25 for additional information on these policies as well as their legal implications. The Health Insurance Portability and Accountability Act (HIPAA) of 1996 requires that individuals be granted access to their health records upon request. In addition, the law requires that individuals be provided with an audit trail describing who has accessed their health information and why.[11] HIPAA did not require that this information be provided or monitored electronically; however, since these provisions are most easily addressed with an electronic record, HIPAA could be seen as a first step in encouraging the adoption of EHRs.

Subsequent policy has had a more direct effect on electronic records adoption. In April 2004 President George W. Bush set a goal that most Americans would have their medical information maintained in electronic records by 2014.[12] To facilitate this goal the Office of the National Coordinator for Health Information Technology (ONC) was created and later funded by the Health Information Technology for Economic and Clinical Health (HITECH) Act of 2009. ONC is the "principal Federal entity charged with coordination of nationwide efforts to implement and use the most advanced health information technology and the electronic exchange of health information."[2] In the same year the American Reinvestment and Recovery Act of 2009 authorized the Centers for Medicare & Medicaid Services (CMS) to provide financial incentives for adoption and Meaningful Use of the EHR.

Percentage of American adults who own each device

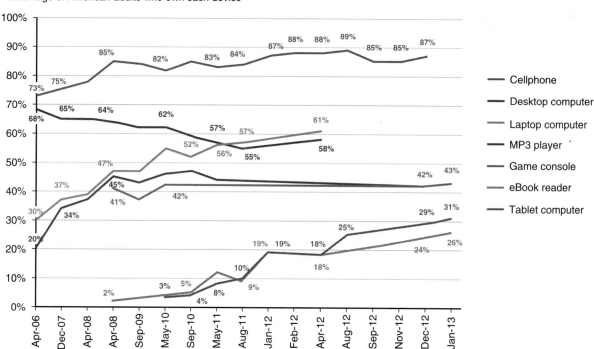

Source: Pew Internet surveys, 2006–2012.

FIG 15-1 Adult gadget ownership over time (2006 to 2013). (From http://www.pewinternet. org/Static-Pages/Trend-Data-%28Adults%29/Device-Ownership.aspx.)

ONC has proposed three stages of Meaningful Use, with each stage characterized by a group of requirements necessary for certification.

In 2010 the CMS began to certify healthcare information system products for compliance with Stage 1 Meaningful Use. Eligible healthcare providers and eligible hospitals who use these products and meet other specific criteria are eligible for financial incentives.[13] The incentives appear to be driving adoption: the prevalence of hospitals in the United States with EHRs increased from 16% in 2009 to 35% in 2011.[14] The ONC solicited public comments on Stage 2 Meaningful Use requirements and the final rule was published in September 2012. Some of the Stage 2 requirements directly tie the Meaningful Use of the EHR and PHR adoption together. Specifically, there is a requirement about implementing secure messaging and that at least 5% of patients must actually use this function. In addition, there are requirements that patients visiting a certified healthcare provider can access their EHR data electronically and that at least 5% of patients will actually use this function. Finally, the rule requires that patients could view their data within 4 days of the data becoming available to the healthcare provider and could transmit the health data if they desire. These rules will become requirements for certification in 2014[15] and will likely increase the adoption of both EHRs and PHRs, as it is anticipated the requirements related to patient access to their data will increase with Meaningful Use Stages 3 and 4.

The final and possibly most important trend leading to adoption of PHRs is individuals' desire for the functions that PHRs provide. In 1998 Tang and Newcomb conducted focus groups to explore patients' information needs and desires. They found that patients wanted to receive personalized, physician-endorsed health information summarizing recent healthcare encounters and the next steps in their care. Focus group participants reported that being better informed would increase their understanding of their treatment plan, increase their motivation to comply with the plan, and improve their satisfaction with the office visit.[16] A 2005 survey by the Markle Foundation found that 60% of those surveyed supported the creation of a PHR service they could use to refill prescriptions, email with their doctor, and get results over the Internet. In addition, more than 70% supported the use of such a system to allow healthcare providers to review their medical records when needed.[17] A 2006 Harris Interactive poll reported similar findings: most people wanted to be able to email with their doctors and schedule visits via the Internet and wanted reminders for medical visits. About half of respondents wanted a system that could transfer self-monitoring data (such as blood pressure at home) to their doctors. While individuals wanted functions provided by a PHR, less than 8% of respondents reported having these services available to them.[18] Interest in a fully functioning PHR continues to grow. A national survey conducted in 2010 by the California HealthCare Foundation found that of those who do not have a PHR, 40% express interest in using one.[5]

PRINCIPLES OF AN IDEAL PERSONAL HEALTH RECORD

The following is a list of principles for an ideal PHR aggregated from several publications and reports.[2,19,20,21] No current system fully implements all of these principles; however, examples of ideal functions are available from current systems that partially address these principles.

- *Comprehensive, longitudinal data storage:* The PHR should serve as a persistent longitudinal record of individuals' health and healthcare over their lifespan. Fully implementing this principle requires data integration from multiple sources (e.g., EHRs, pharmacies, and patient-entered data). Developing these kinds of interoperable records is one of the missions of the ONC and one of the primary reasons for the Meaningful Use criteria discussed above.
- *Data ownership, control, and privacy:* Individual users (patients) should be considered the "owner" of data in PHRs. This principle has several corollaries: users should control access to the PHR, be able to annotate data created by others (e.g., data from the EHR), be able to create entirely new data fields, and be able to assign a proxy who can control and use the system on their behalf. The Markle Foundation's report titled *Connecting for Health* focused on this principle of users' ownership and control of the data in PHRs. Table 15-1 provides a summary of the core principles for PHR design delineated in the *Connecting for Health* report. These core principles reflect the Fair

Information Practice Principles.[22] Additional information related to these principles is included in Chapter 19.

- *Portability:* The system should be available to the user regardless of physical location. For example, several PHR developers have recently deployed mobile phone–based access to their systems.
- *Data sharing:* The system should allow users to share all or parts of the PHR with others. The shared data should be provided in a format that allows for electronic representation and manipulation of the data. This principle is based on the premise of interoperable records.
- *Technology independence:* Access to the data within the PHR should not require a specific device such as a smartphone or specific software such as a proprietary PHR application. This will require a "plug and play" culture implemented via national standards.
- *Access:* The system should provide a convenient means for users to access health-related information and services. This information or service may improve on or augment existing processes. Examples include the capability for secure messaging between patients and healthcare providers, the possibility of e-visits (e.g., web-based video or text consultations between patient and provider), online medication refills, and administrative functions such as scheduling of appointments.[23]
- *Unique and desired services:* The system should provide users with unique services that are otherwise unavailable. Current PHRs provide functions that improve on existing

TABLE 15-1	CORE PRINCIPLES OF PERSONAL HEALTH RECORD DESIGN FROM *CONNECTING FOR HEALTH*
1. Openness and transparency	Consumers should know what information has been collected about them, the purpose of its use, who can access and use it, and where it resides. They should also be informed about how they may obtain access to information collected about them and how they may control who has access to it.
2. Purpose specification	The purposes for which personal data are collected should be specified at the time of collection and the subsequent use should be limited to those purposes, or to others that are specified on each occasion of change of purpose.
3. Collection limitation and data minimization	Personal health information should be collected only for specified purposes and obtained by lawful and fair means. The collection and storage of personal health data should be limited to that information necessary to carry out the specified purpose. Where possible, consumers should have knowledge of or provide consent for collection of their personal health information.
4. Use limitation	Personal data should not be disclosed, made available, or otherwise used for purposes other than those specified.
5. Individual participation and control	Consumers should be able to control access to their personal information. They should know who is storing what information on them and how that information is being used. They should also be able to review the way their information is being used or stored.
6. Data quality and integrity	All personal data collected should be relevant to the purposes for which they are to be used and should be accurate, complete, and up to date.
7. Security safeguards and controls	Reasonable safeguards should protect personal data against such risks as loss or unauthorized access, use, destruction, modification, or disclosure.
8. Accountability and oversight	Entities in control of personal health information must be held accountable for implementing these principles.
9. Remedies	Remedies must exist to address security breaches or privacy violations.

healthcare processes. However, several authors have suggested that PHRs could provide a wider array of functions not currently available. For example, PHRs could provide decision aids to assist patients with complex therapeutic decisions or provide personalized motivational health promotion messages to facilitate healthy behaviors. These kinds of functions are needed if PHRs are to make a significant impact on users' behaviors and health.

- *Customization:* PHRs should allow content customization to address individual users' needs. As an example, the system might provide a translation service to help individuals understand clinical notes imported from their EHR or information could be tailored to the user's knowledge and health literacy. Tailoring content in PHRs has yet to be implemented.

Proposed Benefits of an Ideal PHR

An ideal PHR has multiple proposed benefits. For instance, by serving as a single comprehensive record an ideal PHR could facilitate improved care coordination between healthcare providers and improve patient safety.[20] Similarly, a function allowing users to assign a delegate or proxy to access and control their record might result in improved care by their informal caregivers (e.g., adults taking care of elderly parents).[24] Finally, a system that is ubiquitously available and provides individuals with customized health education and promotion could improve individuals' health self-management.[19,25]

TYPES OF PERSONAL HEALTH RECORDS

PHRs are often grouped into four main types: *stand-alone, untethered, tethered,*[26] and *networked.*[20,27,28] Each type is discussed below.

Stand-alone personal health records store health information on an individual's computer or USB device. While these systems might be of use in particular cases (e.g., the capacity for emergency medical providers to access the USB-stored data), they have not been widely adopted. This is likely because they require manual data entry by the user.[28]

Untethered personal health records are web-based systems separated from an EHR. The advantage of these systems over stand-alone PHRs is that they can automatically aggregate data from multiple sources. The drawback is that they do not link to healthcare providers; thus users cannot email their doctors, request medication refills, or schedule appointments. Proponents of untethered and stand-alone systems indicate that these formats offer individuals maximum control over the content and access to information included in the PHR.[29]

A tethered personal health record is linked to a single entity or healthcare system. Because these systems allow the user to view EHR data via the PHR, they are sometimes called a *patient portal* (i.e., the system provides a portal into the person's medical information within the EHR). The advantages of these systems are several: they provide direct access to functions such as secure messaging with healthcare

providers, medication refills, and appointment scheduling and they require much less manual entry of data than untethered PHRs since the PHR is automatically populated with EHR data. The main disadvantage is that the information is linked only to a specific healthcare provider or system. This creates a problem for individuals with multiple healthcare providers in different healthcare systems because only the information from the linked system is represented in the PHR.

While stand-alone and tethered systems each have strengths and limitations, neither provides all of the desired functions of the ideal PHR described above. Networked PHRs may address these deficits.[20,27,30] In a networked personal health record patients can access data from multiple locations (e.g., different healthcare providers, health plans, or laboratories). The data are integrated through use of access services that conduct user authentication before allowing patient or proxy access to data in the system. Ideally, patients sign on once and gain access to comprehensive, integrated data. As with EHRs, the development of comprehensive, integrated PHRs is dependent on the wide implementation of data representation and exchange standards needed to create interoperable records. Figure 15-2 depicts the differences in information flow between current processes and a networked PHR.

EXAMPLES OF EXISTING PERSONAL HEALTH RECORDS

Several approaches have been used in developing PHRs (Fig. 15-3). Selected examples are presented in this section. Additional examples of existing PHRs are available in recommended websites on the Evolve website.

The VHA launched its PHR called My HealtheVet (MHV) in 2003. This system has two levels of use. The first level allows anyone to create an account online and use the system as an untethered web-based PHR. The second level is for individuals receiving care through the VHA. These users can take full advantage of MHV's functionality by completing an in-person authentication process at their nearest VHA clinic or hospital. Once individuals are authenticated they can use the system as a tethered PHR to exchange secure emails with their healthcare providers, view portions of their EHRs, view upcoming appointments, and receive wellness reminders.[31] As of February 2012 MHV had more than 64 million visits, more than 1.6 million individuals had registered on it, and more than 570,000 veterans (roughly 10% of individuals who use the VHA for healthcare) were authenticated users.[32] The majority of system adopters (75%) use the system to order prescription refills, with more than 27.5 million refills requested online by February 2012. In January 2010 the VHA began a rollout of secure messaging within MHV. Secure messaging was available in primary care clinics as of March 2012. Expansion to specialty ambulatory clinics was planned for rollout beginning in September 2012.[32]

Kaiser Permanente (KP) is an integrated nonprofit provider of both health insurance and healthcare in the U.S.

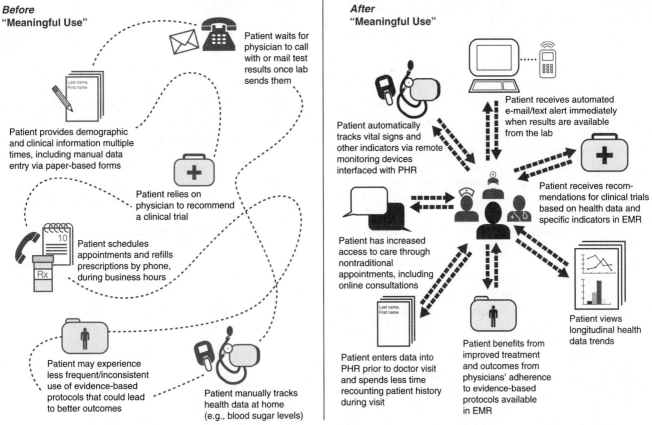

FIG 15-2 How Meaningful Use changes the healthcare experience for patients and families. *EMR*, Electronic medical record; *PHR*, personal health record. (From Health Research Institute. Putting patients into Meaningful Use. PricewaterhouseCoopers. http://www.pwc.com/us/en/health-industries/publications/putting-patients-into-meaningful-use.jhtml. Page 2.)

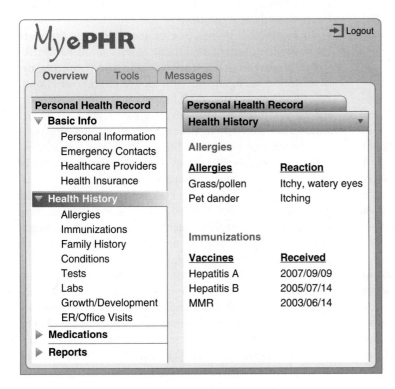

FIG 15-3 Example of a personal health record. *MMR*, Measles, mumps, and rubella.

Between 2004 and 2010 KP implemented a system-wide EHR called KP Health Connect with its tethered PHR called My Health Manager.[33] The PHR provides secure messaging with healthcare providers, online appointment scheduling, and prescription refills. Currently 3.9 million Kaiser Permanente members are registered for My Health Manager (63% of eligible members), more than 12 million secure messages have been sent to healthcare providers, and more than 68 million lab test results have been viewed online. In addition, the system allows individuals to assign a proxy who can access and control the PHR on their behalf. In January 2012 KP launched a mobile-optimized kp.org website and Android app to allow individuals to use the functions described above from their mobile devices.

Microsoft launched its web-based PHR platform, Health-Vault, in 2007. The system integrates data from multiple sources: individuals can upload documents and images, have their records added directly to HealthVault via fax from their healthcare providers, or pay a service to collect their records and digitize their medical information. HealthVault serves as an application platform. When an individual uses a Health-Vault application for the first time, he or she authorizes the application to access a specific set of data types from their record and the application exchanges those data with the platform. One of the strengths of the platform is the ability to use compatible self-monitoring devices such as pedometers, glucometers, and blood pressure monitors to automatically capture data. If the individual's healthcare provider, lab, or pharmacy is partnered with HealthVault, electronic data exchange is possible. HealthVault can therefore function as an untethered, tethered, or networked PHR depending on the number of data sources connected to the platform. For example, if all data sources for a specific patient were Health-Vault partners, the patient's PHR would be an integrated, comprehensive record and could be considered a networked PHR.

CURRENT EVIDENCE OF BENEFITS OF PHR USE

Available evidence regarding the positive impact of PHR use on (1) individuals' experience of care, (2) quality of care, and (3) costs of care has continued to grow as use of PHRs has increased. The goal of improving these three dimensions of healthcare was developed by the Institute for Healthcare Improvement and is referred to as the "IHI triple aim for health care."[34] Each dimension should be considered when evaluating an intervention or healthcare process because these aims are interdependent and can at times be at odds with each other.[35] For example, an intervention that improves quality of care might also increase costs. Similarly, a system that reduces costs might also degrade a person's experience of care. Several key studies with common themes provide evidence demonstrating the impact of PHRs. For example, reviews of the impact of patient portals in general and in the specific case of care of individuals with diabetes have been published recently.[36,37]

Experience of Care

Currently evidence regarding the effect of a PHR on individuals' experience of healthcare is limited to user satisfaction surveys. Ralston et al. surveyed users of an integrated PHR and found that most users report high satisfaction (>86% were either satisfied or very satisfied) with functions such as online medication refills, secure messaging, and the ability to view lab test results.[38] Similarly, Liederman et al. found that patients from an integrated academic medical system reported high satisfaction with secure messaging. They also reported that patients' levels of satisfaction with the system decreased as response times to their secure messages increased from 1 to 3 days.[39] The decrease in satisfaction suggests that increased access to information and communication with healthcare providers may affect patients' expectations and, in turn, demands.

The flexibility offered by PHRs may improve individuals' experience of care. This is suggested by the results of a survey of PHR users at the Geisinger Health System, patients preferred email communication for some interactions (e.g., requesting prescription renewals, obtaining general medical information) and preferred in-person communication for others (e.g., receiving treatment instructions).[40]

Quality of Care

Since the PHR is a relatively new phenomenon, evidence about PHR use on the quality of healthcare is limited and data on the effect of PHRs on long-term health outcomes (e.g., mortality) are not yet available. The available evidence comes from two types of studies. The first type is association studies that have examined the relation between an individuals' use of the PHR (usually secure messaging in particular) and their intermediate health outcomes. The second type is a set of randomized trials with the PHR as a component of a larger clinical intervention.

In association studies, use of the PHR was related to improved intermediate health outcomes.[41,42,43] At KP Northwest a positive association was found between patients' use of secure messaging and the likelihood of meeting the Healthcare Effectiveness Data and Information Set (HEDIS) performance measures for diabetes and blood pressure quality care.[42] This effect was significant even after comparing users to nonusers matched on baseline HEDIS scores, age, sex, and healthcare provider. Similarly, a cross-sectional analysis of individuals with diabetes found that the use of secure messaging in the MyGroupHealth PHR was associated with better glycemic control.[43] While these results are encouraging, these studies did not control for potential confounding factors such as the patient's self-efficacy, attitudes toward medical care, race, socioeconomic status, and health literacy.[43]

Several trials have been conducted using the PHR as a component of a larger intervention. Two trials have compared the effect of PHR use and an automated blood pressure cuff on subsequent blood pressure. The first was reported by Green et al. and was conducted in the Group Health integrated healthcare system in Washington state. In this trial the investigators compared three interventions: the PHR alone

(UC); a home blood pressure monitor and the PHR (eBP); or a home blood pressure monitor, the PHR, and a pharmacist who engaged with the patient regularly via secure messaging (eBP-Pharm). The outcome of interest was the percentage of subjects whose blood pressure was controlled (<140/90 mm Hg) at the 1-year follow-up. Results were as follows: 56% of individuals in the eBP-Pharm group, 36% in the eBP group, and 31% in the UC group had controlled blood pressure at the end of the trial.[44] More recently Wagner et al. reported on a cluster randomized with either a PHR or none and automated blood pressure cuff or none for 1 year. Of 1686 patients approached, only 453 patients agreed to participate. The authors found no association between adoption of the PHR and blood pressure over 1 year. However, in a subgroup analysis they found that patients who used the PHR more than twice a month reduced their blood pressure by 5 mm Hg. They also reported that increased PHR usage was associated with patients' perception of the usefulness of the system.[45] Similar trials in individuals with diabetes showed that PHR-based care management modules are useful in affecting physiologic outcomes[46] and reducing diabetes-related distress.[47]

While most work on the efficacy of PHRs in affecting users' health focused on individuals with chronic disease, Lau et al. reported on a trial comparing the effect of a PHR educational module on flu vaccination rates among university students. This module included the capacity to schedule appointments online, which may account for its success,[48] in contrast to a similar system that had failed to demonstrate an effect of PHR use on immunization rates.[49]

Cost and Utilization

Evidence regarding the effect of use of a PHR on healthcare costs is not yet available.[36] However, several studies measured the association between PHR use and healthcare utilization. The assumption behind these studies is that shifting use away from in-person encounters will lead to decreased costs.

Zhou et al. compared users of KP's My Health Manager PHR with a nonuser group matched for age and disease and found that PHR use was associated with reduced telephone calls to the clinic and a reduced number of outpatient visits per year.[50] Other investigators have found an opposite association. Harris et al. reported that increased use of secure messaging by individuals with diabetes was associated with increased outpatient visits.[43] The limitations of these two studies are that they are cross-sectional studies and the authors did not discuss whether or not the change in use was appropriate. For instance, in the Harris study, use of the PHR's secure messaging function may have helped individuals to realize that they needed to seek out care more regularly and therefore the increased clinic visits may have been appropriate.

In summary, the available evidence suggests that PHRs may improve the quality of care and patients' satisfaction with their care. PHRs also seem to change utilization patterns. The effects of this change on costs remain to be seen. Two facts qualify these statements. First, virtually all of the evidence discussed above comes from studies of tethered PHRs in integrated healthcare systems. More evidence from a more diverse sample is needed. Second, a common finding across these studies is that regular use of the PHR by patients is necessary to see improvements; therefore more research on engagement of patients with the PHR over time is needed.

CURRENT PHR USE

Some authors found that early adopters of the PHR tended to be younger and more affluent with fewer medical problems than nonenrollees.[51] Other more recent studies have found that PHR users are more likely to have multiple medical problems than nonusers.[50,52] Even among individuals with the same disease, individuals with a higher disease burden may use the PHR more frequently than those who are less ill. As an example, Weppner et al. reported that among older individuals with diabetes, higher morbidity was associated with increased usage of secure messaging.[53]

Data on the frequency of log-ins to PHRs has been reported for several systems. Among VHA patients using MHV, approximately half report using the PHR monthly and 30% say that they use it weekly.[54,55] Thirty percent of respondents in a California HealthCare Foundation survey about PHRs reported using their PHR monthly.[56] New enrollees logged in most frequently in the first month but about half of respondents continued to access the portal at least monthly. They most often examined laboratory and radiology results and sent secure messages to their healthcare providers.

Ralston et al. reported that the following PHR functions were the most commonly used (in order of decreasing usage): medical test results review, medication refills, secure messaging, after-visit summary review, medical condition review, appointment requests, immunization review, and allergy review.[57]

BARRIERS TO PHR ADOPTION

Self-reported adoption of PHRs has increased from 3% of the population in 2008 to 10% in 2011.[58] While this trend is encouraging, several barriers must be considered and dealt with before PHRs will affect the population at large. These include patient and healthcare provider awareness of PHRs, the usability of PHRs, individuals' concerns over privacy, and the digital divide. In addition, the lack of interoperability in current systems and legal and regulatory barriers may limit the functionality and use of PHRs.

Awareness

A national survey by the California HealthCare Foundation in 2010 asked, "How much have you heard about websites where people can get, keep, and update their health information like test results and prescriptions?" More than half of respondents answered "not sure/not heard." A full 76% of respondents indicated that they had not heard about cellphone programs to track their own health information.[56] In 2008 Fuji et al. examined rural physicians' awareness of PHRs and use of them by their patients. They found that more than 25% of physicians had no awareness of PHR functions and 59% did not know whether their patients had or used PHRs.[59]

Weitzman et al. conducted interviews and focus groups with administrators, clinicians, and community members as a component of a formative evaluation of a PHR. They found that many individuals had limited awareness of PHRs yet held high expectations of what such a system should do. Common expectations were that the PHR would allow searching and linking within the record, that the system would include tailored communications, and that linkages would exist between self-report and clinical data. The authors commented that these high expectations create a risk of disappointment when individuals encounter existing PHRs.[60]

The studies discussed above indicate the most significant barrier to widespread PHR adoption: lack of awareness about PHRs and their benefits and risks. To address this problem several governmental and nongovernmental organizations have launched websites to educate the public about PHRs (see the Evolve website for a representative list). On an encouraging note, two studies reported that aggressive marketing campaigns of tethered PHRs were successful in improving adoption of PHRs. In the first study a total of 16 techniques were employed, including automated greetings on the practice's telephone system, posters in waiting areas and examination rooms, postcard and letter mailings, staff speaking to the patient in the office or over the telephone, and onsite enrollment with a computer kiosk. Authors reported nearly threefold greater likelihood of PHR adoption among patients of practices employing five or more of these techniques.[61] At the Mayo clinic, North et al. compared the use of a promotional video to a paper instruction sheet and to a no-attention control group to promote PHR adoption and use. In the following 45 days individuals' PHR adoption was 11.7% among individuals who saw the video, 7.1% among those who received the paper instructions, and 2.5% among the control group. The superiority of the video intervention persisted when the authors measured whether users went on to use the PHR to initiate secure messaging with their healthcare providers.[62]

Usability

Poor PHR usability may also hinder adoption. For example, in a test of the usability of the My HealtheVet PHR, only 25% of users successfully completed registration with the system.[63] In 2007 the National Health Service in the United Kingdom implemented a PHR called HealthSpace and found that adoption and use was much less than expected. Interviews with users suggested that users perceived it as neither useful nor easy to use. They were disappointed with the amount and type of data available, the need to enter data themselves, and the limited options for sharing these data with their clinicians.[64]

Privacy Concerns

A 1999 study at the University of California, San Diego found that when properly designed, PHRs can securely exchange health information over the Internet.[65] However, a 2010 survey found that 63% of PHR users and 68% of PHR nonusers are "somewhat or very concerned" about the privacy of their health information.[56] This discrepancy suggests that despite available security precautions, individuals remain concerned about the privacy of PHRs and more work may be needed to allay these fears.

The Digital Divide

Research suggests that a digital divide exists in the United States resulting in individuals of lower socioeconomic status, ethnic minorities, and older individuals being less likely to adopt a PHR.[61,66-68] For example, Yamin et al. found that among patients in the Partners HealthCare system, African-Americans were half as likely as Caucasians to adopt a PHR and individuals of lower income were about a third less likely than individuals of higher income to adopt a PHR (OR 0.64, 95% CI 0.57–0.73).[61] Similarly, limited access to high-speed Internet among veterans living in rural communities was identified as a barrier to adoption of the My HealtheVet PHR.[68]

Interoperability

As described earlier, PHR data and functions are constrained by the systems to which the PHR is linked. Current PHRs are integrated with a limited number of systems and therefore represent only a subset of the data and services that an ideal PHR should include. It is likely that a comprehensive, ideal PHR would be more attractive than current PHRs and would be adopted at a higher rate than current PHRs. In principle, all that is required to address the data requirements of an ideal PHR is for all healthcare data systems in the U.S. to agree to use the same data representation and exchange standards.

Several data representation and exchange standards have been developed and proposed, including Continuity of Care Record (CCR), Clinical Document Architecture (CDA), and Continuity of Care Document (CCD). For additional information about standards, see Chapter 22. As an example standard, CCR was developed by a consortium of medical societies and adopted by the American Society for Testing and Materials (ASTM).[69] By describing the exact format of the information to be exchanged, this and other standards provide the possibility for portable and syntactically interoperable PHRs. To achieve true semantic interoperability (in which the *meaning* of exchanged information is understood throughout exchanges between parties) constraint of the number of vocabularies is required.[70] Recent laws and policies, such as the promotion of Nationwide Health Information Exchange by the ONC[71] and the development of accountable care organizations created in the recent Patient Protection and Affordable Care Act, are intended to promote and use interoperable records and should facilitate PHR adoption.

Law and Policy

Current laws, regulations, and policies affect patients' access to their data and the ability of healthcare providers to use PHRs to provide remote healthcare services. For example, a

California law superseding HIPAA requires additional physician and patient consent before patients can access their information electronically. Certain results may not be released electronically for any reason, regardless of a patient's request.[72] In addition, current laws limit healthcare providers delivering care across state lines. This limits the capacity for PHR-based delivery of healthcare.[73]

While the Federal Communications Commission estimates that 90% of Americans will have Internet access by 2020[74] and the adoption of mobile devices appears to be decreasing the digital divide,[7] only 10% of the U.S. population had adopted PHRs by 2011.[58] Perhaps many patients are simply unaware of PHRs and their functions and potential benefits, or it may be that patients are concerned about privacy and the poor usability of existing PHRs. Finally, the interoperability and functionality of PHRs, while steadily improving, is limited by nationwide adoption of relevant standards and policies.

CONCLUSION AND FUTURE DIRECTIONS

Though early in their evolution, currently available PHRs appear to have positive effects on patients' experience of care, healthcare outcomes, and healthcare use. If the desire for PHR functions persists and trends in adoption continue, PHRs have the potential to become the platform for a more efficient, effective, and personalized healthcare system. To achieve this promise, improvements in current systems as well an expansion of the scope and functionality of PHRs are needed.

The available evidence for current PHRs is generally positive. However, most PHR evaluations have been limited to primary care settings in a small number of integrated healthcare systems. Evidence is needed regarding the adoption, use, and efficacy of current systems in larger and more diverse groups of healthcare settings and among users of varying age, ethnicity, race, socioeconomic level, and disease status. Similarly, current efforts to promote adoption of PHRs (e.g., marketing campaigns to increase awareness) and governmental policy changes to promote adoption need to be evaluated and may need to be refined for specific subpopulations.

As pointed out at the beginning of this chapter, PHRs serve two main functions: as data storage systems and as a suite of tools intended to improve both professional and health self-management. Both of these functions need to be expanded in future PHRs.

In terms of data storage, the ultimate goal is to develop PHRs that are comprehensive, longitudinal records of individuals' health. To move toward this goal, systems will need to be interoperable and networked.[20] As discussed, the barriers to interoperability are not technical but primarily political and economic. Recent governmental policy has begun to address this problem by shifting the incentives in the U.S. healthcare system from rewarding waste to promoting cost effectiveness; time will tell if these policies are effective.

In terms of functionality, Krist and others have argued that current PHRs are just the beginning and that the functionality of these systems should evolve to become more personalized and effective over time.[19] The first step in making PHRs more patient centered is to include services such as allowing proxies to access PHRs, PHR access for minors, viewing EHR notes, viewing a full list of diagnoses, patient control over information access, inclusion of an emergency "break the glass" function, and clinician response to emails in less than 24 hours.[75] PHRs could also be used to collect patient-reported behaviors and outcomes.[76] This kind of patient-generated data could then be integrated into care. For example, EHRs are commonly missing information on individuals' occupational and family medical history[77]; these data could be captured via the PHR. Similarly, mobile systems could be used to capture "observations of daily living," such as measures of dietary behaviors or self-report of symptoms, and presented back to patients as personalized real-time feedback.[78] Finally, research on PHRs as "persuasive technologies" (technologies intended to change people's attitudes and behaviors)[79,80] is in its infancy but holds great promise. A mobile phone–based PHR, for example, could serve as an individualized tool to promote health across the population.

In summary, PHRs are an evolving concept with great potential to facilitate improvement in the health of individuals and the efficiency of healthcare. While current trends are encouraging and substantial progress has been made in recent years, significant work remains to be done if PHRs are to reach their full potential.

REFERENCES

1. Jones DA, Shipman JP, Plaut DA, Selden CR. Characteristics of personal health records: findings of the Medical Library Association National Library of Medicine Joint Electronic Personal Health Record Task Force. *J Med Libr Assoc.* 2010; 98(3):243-249.

2. Connecting for Health Work Group. *Connecting for Health Common Framework for Networked Personal Health Information.* Markle Foundation. http://www.markle.org/sites/default/files/Overview_Consumers.pdf. 2008.

3. Office of the National Coordinator for Health Information Technology. Glossary Health IT terms. HealthIT.gov. http://www.healthit.gov/policy-researchers-implementers/glossary. Accessed December 10, 2012.

4. Harris Interactive. Two in five adults keep personal or family health records and almost everybody thinks this is a good idea. *Health Care News.* 2004;4(13). http://www.zweenahealth.com/PDF/HI_HealthCareNews2004Vol4_Iss13.pdf. Accessed December 12, 2012.

5. Sherman SA. New national survey finds personal health records motivate consumers to improve their health. California HealthCare Foundation. http://www.chcf.org/media/press-releases/2010/new-national-survey-finds-personal-health-records-motivate-consumers-to-improve-their-health. 2010.

6. Pew Internet & American Life Project. Demographics in internet users. Pew Internet & American Life Project. http://www.pewinternet.org/Static-Pages/Trend-Data/Whos-Online.aspx. 2012.

7. Smith A. Nearly half of American adults are smartphone owners. Pew Internet & American Life Project. http://pewinternet.org/Reports/2012/Smartphone-Update-2012.aspx. 2012.

8. Timson G. The history of the hardhats. Hardhats.org. http://www.hardhats.org/history/hardhats.html. Accessed December 10, 2012.

9. McDonald C. The Regenstrief medical record system: a quarter century experience. *Int J Med Inform*. 1999;54:225-253.

10. Nazi, KM. Presentation to Institute of Medicine. My HealtheVet. http://iom.edu/~/media/Files/Activity%20Files/PublicHealth/HealthLiteracy/NaziVAMyHealtheVet.pdf. 2008.

11. U.S. Department of Health & Human Services (HHS). Understanding health information privacy. HHS. http://www.hhs.gov/ocr/privacy/hipaa/understanding/index.html. Accessed December 10, 2012.

12. The Office of the President. Executive Order 13335. *Federal Register*. 2004;April 30.

13. Office of the National Coordinator for Health Information Technology. Electronic health records and Meaningful Use. HealthIT.gov. http://healthit.hhs.gov/portal/server.pt?open=512&objID=2996&mode=2.

14. U.S. Department of Health & Human Services (HHS). HHS Secretary Kathleen Sebelius announces major progress in doctors, hospital use of health information technology. HHS. http://www.hhs.gov/news/press/2012pres/02/20120217a.html. 2011.

15. U.S. Department of Health & Human Services. Health information technology: standards, implementation specifications, and certification criteria for electronic health record technology, 2014 edition; Revisions to the Permanent Certification Program for Health Information Technology. *Federal Register*. 2012;77(45).

16. Tang P, Newcomb C. Informing patients: a guide for providing patient health information. *J Am Med Inform Assoc*. 1998;5(6):563-570.

17. Markle Foundation. Attitudes of Americans regarding personal health records and nationwide electronic health information exchange. Markle Foundation. http://www.markle.org/publications/951-attitudes-americans-regarding-personal-health-records-and-nationwide-electronic-hea. 2005.

18. Harris Interactive. Few patients use or have access to online services for communicating with their doctors, but most would like to. *Wall Street Journal Online*. 2006;5(16).

19. Krist A, Woolf S. A vision for patient-centered health information systems. *JAMA*. 2011;305(3):300-301.

20. Detmer D, Bloomrosen M, Raymond B, Tang P. Integrated personal health records: transformative tools for consumer-centric care. *BMC Med Inform Decis Mak*. 2008;8(45).

21. Johnston D, Kaelber D, Pan E, et al. A framework and approach for assessing the value of personal health records (PHRs). *AMIA Annu Symp Proc*. 2007:374-379.

22. Federal Trade Commission (FTC). Fair information practice principles. FTC. http://www.ftc.gov/reports/privacy3/fairinfo.shtm. Published September 23, 2012.

23. Ahern D, Woods S, Lightowler M, Finley S, Houston T. Promise of and potential for patient-facing technologies to enable Meaningful Use. *Am J Prev Med*. 2011;40(5S2):s162-s172.

24. Zulman D, Nazi K, Turvey C, Wagner T, Woods SS, An L. Patient interest in sharing personal health record information: a web-based survey. *Ann Intern Med*. 2011;155:805-810.

25. Archer N, Fevrier-Thomas U, Lokker C, McKibbon K, Straus S. Personal health records: a scoping review. *J Am Med Inform Assoc*. 2011;18:515-522.

26. Endsley S, Kibbe D, Linares A, Colorafi K. An introduction to personal health records. *Fam Pract Manag*. 2006;13(5):58-62.

27. Woods S, Weppner W, McInnes D. Personal health records. In: Hebda T, Czar P, eds. *Handbook of Informatics for Nurses and Health Care Professionals*. Upper Saddle River, NJ: Prentice Hall; 2012.

28. Vincent A, Kaelber D, Pan E, Shah S, Johnston D, Middleton B. A patient-centric taxonomy for personal health records (PHRs). *AMIA Annu Symp Proc*. 2008:763-767.

29. Simons W, Mandl K, Kohane I. Model formulation: the PING personally controlled electronic medical record system: technical architecture. *J Am Med Inform Assoc*. 2005;12:47-54.

30. Health Research Institute. Putting patients into Meaningful Use. PricewaterhouseCoopers. http://www.pwc.com/us/en/health-industries/publications/putting-patients-into-meaningful-use.jhtml. 2012.

31. Veterans Health Administration. My HealtheVet. U.S. Department of Veterans Affairs https://www.myhealth.va.gov/index.html. 2012.

32. My HealtheVet product intranet website: statistics. 2011; Vaww://myhealth.va.gov.

33. Christensen K, Silvestre A. Making health personal. In: Liang L, ed. *Connected for Health: Using Electronic Health Records to Transform Care Delivery*. Hoboken, NJ: Jossey-Bass; 2010.

34. Institute for Healthcare Improvement (IHI). The IHI Triple Aim. IHI. http://www.ihi.org/offerings/Initiatives/TripleAim/Pages/default.aspx. Accessed December 10, 2012.

35. Berwick D, Nolan T, Whittington J. The Triple Aim: care, health, and cost. *Health Affair*. 2008;27(3):759-769.

36. Emont S. Measuring the impact of patient portals. California HealthCare Foundation. Available from: http://www.chcf.org/publications/2011/05/measuring-impact-patient-portals. 2011.

37. Osborn C, Mayberry L, Mulvaney S, Hess R. Patient web portals to improve diabetes outcomes: a systematic review. *Curr Diab Rep*. 2009;10(6):422-435.

38. Ralston J, Carrell D, Reid R, Anderson M, Moran M, Hereford J. Patient web services integrated with a shared medical record: patient use and satisfaction. *J Am Med Inform Assoc*. 2007;14:798-806.

39. Liederman E, Lee J, Baquero V, Seites P. Patient-physician web messaging: the impact on message volume and satisfaction. *J Gen Intern Med*. 2005;20:52-57.

40. Hassol A, Walker J, Kidder D, et al. Patient experiences and attitudes about access to a patient electronic health care record and linked web messaging. *J Am Med Inform Assoc*. 2004;11(6):505-512.

41. Shaw R, Ferranti J. Patient-provider internet portals: patient outcomes and use. *Comput Inform Nurs*. 2011;29(12):714-718.

42. Zhou Y, Kanter M, Wang J, Garrido T. Improved quality at Kaiser Permanente through e-mail between physicians and patients. *Health Affair*. 2010;29(7):1370-1375.

43. Harris L, Haneuse S, Martin D, Ralston JD. Diabetes quality of care and outpatient utilization associated with electronic patient-provider messaging: a cross-sectional analysis. *Diabetes Care*. 2009;32:1182-1187.

44. Green B, Cook A, Ralston J, et al. Effectiveness of home blood pressure monitoring, web communication, and pharmacist care on hypertension control. *JAMA*. 2008;299(24):2857-2867.

45. Wagner P, Dias J, Howard S, et al. Personal health records and hypertension control: a randomized trial. *J Am Med Inform Assoc*. 2012;19(4):626-634.

46. McMahon G, Gomes HE, Hohne S, Hu TM, Levine B, Conlin PR. Web-based care management in patients with poorly controlled diabetes. *Diabetes Care*. 2005;28(7):1624-1629.

47. Fonda S, McMahon G, Gomes HE, Hickson S, Conlin C. Changes in diabetes distress related to participation in an internet-based diabetes care management program and glycemic control. *J Diabetes Sci Technol*. 2009;3(1):117-124.

48. Lau A, Sintchenko V, Crimmins J, Magrabi F, Gallego B, Coiera E. Impact of a personally controlled health management system on influenza vaccination and health services utilization rates: a randomized controlled trial. *J Am Med Inform Assoc.* 2012;19(5):719-727.

49. Bourgeois F, Simons W, Olson K. Evaluation of influenza prevention in the workplace using a personally controlled health record: randomized controlled trial. *J Med Internet Res.* 2008;10(e5).

50. Zhou Y, Garrido T, Chin H, Wiesenthal A, Liang L. Patient access to an electronic health record with secure messaging: impact on primary care utilization. *Am J Manag Care.* 2007;13:418-424.

51. Weingart S, Rind D, Tofias Z, Sands D. Who uses the patient internet portal? The PatientSite experience. *J Am Med Inform Assoc.* 2006;13(1):91-95.

52. Ralston J, Rutter C, Carrell D, Hecht J, Rubanowice D, Simon G. Patient use of secure electronic messaging within a shared medical record: a cross-sectional study. *J Gen Intern Med.* 2009;24(3):349-355.

53. Weppner W, Ralston J, Koepsell T, et al. Use of a shared medical record with secure messaging by older patients with diabetes. *Diabetes Care.* 2010;33(11):2314-2319.

54. Nazi K, Woods S. My HealtheVet PHR: a description of users and patient portal use. *AMIA Annu Symp Proc.* 2008;6:1162.

55. Nazi K. Veterans' voices: use of the American Customer Satisfaction Index (ACSI) Survey to identify My HealtheVet personal health record users' characteristics, needs, and preferences. *J Am Med Inform Assoc.* 2010;17:203-211.

56. Lake Research Partners. Consumers and health information technology: a national survey. California HealthCare Foundation. http://www.chcf.org/publications/2010/04/consumers-and-health-information-technology-a-national-survey#ixzz1razHRCuv. 2010.

57. Ralston J, Hereford J, Carrell D. Use and satisfaction of a patient web portal with a shared medical record between patients and providers. *AMIA Annu Symp Proc.* 2006;1070.

58. *PHR Adoption on the Rise.* Markle Foundation. 2011. http://www.markle.org/health/publications-briefs-health/1440-phr-adoption-rise. Accessed December 12, 2012.

59. Fuji K, Galt K, Serocca A. Personal health record use by patients as perceived by ambulatory care physicians in Nebraska and South Dakota: a cross-sectional study. *Perspect Health Inf Manag.* 2008;5:15.

60. Weitzman E, Kaci L, Mandl K. Acceptability of a personally controlled health record in a community-based setting: implications for policy and design. *J Med Internet Res.* 2009;11(2):e14.

61. Yamin C, Emani S, Williams D, et al. The digital divide in adoption and use of a personal health record. *Arch Int Med.* 2011;171(6):568-574.

62. North F, Hanna B, Crane S, Smith S, Tulledge-Scheitel S, Stroebel R. Patient portal doldrums: does an exam room promotional video during an office visit increase patient portal registrations and portal use? *J Am Med Inform Assoc.* 2012;18:i24-i27.

63. Haggstrom D, Saleem J, Russ A, Jones J, Russell S, Chumbler N. Lessons learned from usability testing of the VA's personal health record. *J Am Med Inform Assoc.* 2011;18:i13-i17.

64. Greenhalgh T, Hinder S, Stramer K, Bratan T, Russell J. Adoption, non-adoption, and abandonment of a personal electronic health record: case study of HealthSpace. *BMJ.* 2010;341:5814-5825.

65. Baker D. PCASSO: a model for safe use of the internet in health care. *Journal of AHIMA.* 2000;3:33-36.

66. Roblin D, Houston TK, Allison J, Joski PJ, Becker ER. Disparities in use of a personal health record in a managed care organization. *J Am Med Inform Assoc.* 2009;16(5):683-690.

67. Goel MS, Brown TL, Williams A, Cooper AJ, Hasnain-Wynia R, Baker DW. Patient reported barriers to enrolling in a patient portal. *J Am Med Inform Assoc.* 2011;18(suppl 1):i8-i12.

68. Schooley B, Horan T, Lee P, West P. Rural veteran access to health care services: investigating the role of information and communication technologies in overcoming spatial barriers. *Persp Health Inform Manag.* 2010;Spring:1-10.

69. International. E2369-05e2 standard specification for continuity of care record. ASTM International. http://enterprise.astm.org/filtrexx40.cgi?+REDLINE_PAGES/E2369.htm. Accessed December 10, 2012.

70. Essential similarities and differences between the HL7 CDA/CRS and ASTM CCR. Center for Health IT. http://www.centerforhit.org/PreBuilt/chit_ccrhl7.pdf. 2005.

71. Office of the National Coordinator for Health Information Technology. Nationwide Health Information Network: overview. U.S. Department of Health & Human Services http://healthit.hhs.gov/portal/server.pt?open=512&objID=1142&parentname=CommunityPage&parentid=25&mode=2&in_hi_userid=11113&cached=true. Accessed May 15, 2012.

72. Tang P, Lansky D. The missing link: bridging the patient–provider health information gap. *Health Affair.* 2005;24(5):1290-1295.

73. American Telemedicine Association (ATA). Removing medical licensure barriers: increasing consumer choice, improving safety and cutting costs for patients across America. ATA. http://media.americantelemed.org/licensurewebsite/. 2012.

74. Federal Communications Commission. National broadband plan. Broadband.gov. http://www.broadband.gov/download-plan/. 2010.

75. Reti S, Feldman H, Ross S, Safran C. Improving personal health records for patient centered care. *J Am Med Inform Assoc.* 2010;17:192-195.

76. Glasgow R, Kaplan R, Ockene J, Fisher E, Emmons K. Patient-reported measures of psychosocial issues and health behavior should be added to electronic health records. *Health Affair.* 2012;31(3):497-504.

77. Institute of Medicine Committee on Patient Safety and Health Information Technology. Health IT and patient safety: building safer systems for better care. Institute of Medicine. http://www.iom.edu/Reports/2011/Health-IT-and-Patient-Safety-Building-Safer-Systems-for-Better-Care/Report-Brief.aspx. 2011.

78. Robert Wood Johnson Foundation. Project Health Design. http://www.projecthealthdesign.org/.

79. Fogg B. *Persuasive Technology: Using Computers to Change What We Think and Do.* San Francisco, CA: Morgan Kaufmann; 2003.

80. Chatterjee S, Price A. Healthy living with persuasive technologies: framework, issues, and challenges. *J Am Med Inform Assoc.* 2009;16(2):171-179.

DISCUSSION QUESTIONS

1. In addition to those trends discussed in the chapter, what societal and technological trends do you see that might promote increased adoption and use of PHRs?

2. What specific types of data or functions do you think would draw people who are not current PHR users to adopt and use the PHR? How do you think this might vary by user attributes (e.g., age, disease status, health literacy)?

3. Examine information on the web about PHRs and current health policies. What new information did you discover and how will this information affect the adoption and use of PHRs?

4. In your health organization, what are the main barriers to PHR adoption and use?

5. What is the nurse's role in engaging populations to understand information about their health and understand how to access health information resources?

6. In thinking about a PHR that patients can use to annotate their EHR data (e.g., comment on the problem list), what steps do you think patients will likely take to correct their data? What do you think the advantages and disadvantages of such a system would be?

7. Examine the PHRs that are available to you; what are their relative benefits and disadvantages?

CASE STUDY

An academic medical center in the western U.S. recently adopted a commercial EHR and plans to adopt and integrate a PHR with its EHR. The hospital CEO drafts a vision statement that states: "By using the latest technology, University Hospital will improve how our patients experience healthcare. Instead of patients coming to us for help, we will be there wherever and whenever they need us, asking, "How can we help you?" This initiative will make healthcare easier to access and more convenient to use, improve patients' health, and reduce the rising cost of healthcare in our area."

The CEO convenes a meeting of the chief technology officer, the chief nursing informatics officer, the chief medical officer, and a liaison from the EHR vendor to develop a strategic plan for the PHR. This meeting includes a specific list of functionalities, a timeline for their implementation, and considerations regarding the effects of the PHR on current workflows and revenue streams.

Discussion Questions

1. Based on your reading in this chapter, what else should be considered in the CEO's vision statement? Which parts are supported by evidence and which are less supported? How does this vision compare to your organization's view of PHRs?

2. As this group moves forward in developing and implementing the vision, who else should be involved in this discussion?

3. Imagine that you are the chief technology officer for the hospital. What PHR functionalities will you recommend be implemented first? Why?

4. Imagine that you are the chief nursing informatics officer. What concerns might you have about implementing a PHR?

5. If you were the chief technology officer, what questions would you need to ask the liaison from the EHR vendor to plan for this PHR development and implementation?

Project Management: Tools and Procedures

Identifying and Selecting an Information System Solution

Cynthia M. Mascara and Mical DeBrow

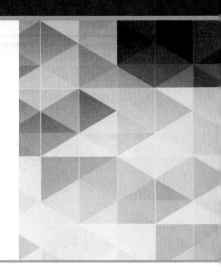

The pace of change in healthcare is anticipated to only accelerate and both the organization and the vendor must be able to adapt quickly.

OBJECTIVES

At the completion of this chapter the reader will be prepared to:

1. Use an institution's vision and strategic plan as a guide in selecting a new or upgraded healthcare information system

2. Organize and implement a system selection process using the initial phases of the systems development life cycle

3. Prepare a request for information (RFI) and a request for proposal (RFP)

KEY TERMS

ABSTRACT

This chapter is designed to provide guidance in the identification and selection of a healthcare information system. The most critical factor in a selection process is strategic alignment with both the organization and the information technology department. Understanding the systems development life cycle and performing an assessment of an organization's requirements are essential to a successful selection process. The chapter describes the requirements of both a request for information and a request for proposal. Evaluation criteria for system selection are also explored. Appraisal of vendors and their capabilities to meet current and future needs are outlined.

INTRODUCTION

When the decision has been made to identify and select a new or first healthcare information system, an initial search will soon identify more than 200 companies marketing healthcare information systems. This large number of choices must be narrowed to a reasonable number of systems that can meet the organization's unique needs by considering factors such as the size, type, complexity, and unique cultural aspects of the organization. Although the natural inclination of an organization is to reach out to well-known companies or those used in the local community in selecting a system, a systematic process involving a thorough review of available information systems is recommended. However, selecting a new system or upgrading a current system is doomed to failure if that process is not based on a careful analysis of the institution's current status and desired future. This chapter provides the framework for that process.

STRATEGIC VISION AND ALIGNMENT

A strategic vision is the desired future state. Strategic alignment involves matching two or more organizational strategies to ensure that they synergistically support the organization's goals and vision. Before beginning the system selection process for any new or updated system the institution must develop and implement a strategic vision and plan. In addition, the information technology (IT) department must develop its own strategic vision and plan in alignment with and guided by the organization's strategic vision and plan. It is essential that these plans consider the multiple internal and external stakeholders, including users of the patient's healthcare information such as physicians, nurses, ancillary healthcare staff, payers, regulatory groups, and finally, the patient.

The strategic vision and plan for an organization provides a long-term road map for the organization and is critical in light of economic, regulatory, and market pressures. Strategic planning in healthcare is used to determine the desired future of the organization. It involves a variety of organizational processes including, for example, external and internal scans. The strategic plan sets the goals, objectives, assignments, and measures based on the community's needs and provides the direction for the organization when planning how it will achieve its clinical and financial goals and objectives. The plan will provide guidance in selecting the information systems that most closely align with the desired future of the organization, stakeholder buy-in, engagement, productivity, and efficiency. The strategic vision and plan should also create a sense of urgency that begins with the vision of the organization. Strategic plans typically do not address issues or problems but rather chart the direction of the organization.

The IT plan should strategically align with the organization's mission, vision, and overall strategic plan. Strategic planning for both the organization and the IT department is not a linear process; rather, it is iterative in nature and requires consideration of multiple variables, including future goals and directions.

Key factors in identifying and selecting information systems are the business plans for the organization and the IT department. It makes little sense to consider $20 million systems when the business plan states a maximum of $10 million. However, cost is not the only consideration. System selection teams must review key objectives of the organization and the IT department to ensure that the objectives of the selection team are in alignment with the institution and the IT department before proceeding with selection of potential information systems. Once objectives are aligned, the team identifies and selects the systems that will most closely align with the economic, operational, and clinical objectives of the organization. The stakeholders in each of those three areas must be heard, considered, and educated about what systems can and cannot do to support the objectives of different stakeholders within the organization. No system in isolation supports the practices of medicine or nursing, improves financial reporting of outcomes, and changes the operation of the organization. Rather, systems support the decision makers and stimulate process changes in these areas in order to realize institutional objectives. A thorough review and understanding of the clinical objectives as well as the

financial and operational objectives of the organization and the IT department are essential, as this should guide the ongoing evaluation and system selection process.

Once the alignment of objectives has been completed, the IT department should review and update the inventory of existing systems. All of the current systems in place in the organization should be identified, including independent departmental systems as well as large integrated systems and those buried in areas outside IT. A review of the inventory allows the organization to identify overlapping functionality as well as gaps among systems. It is not unusual for multiple systems that accomplish the same task or goal to be in place. This happens when individual departments have implemented systems they need without addressing the organization's overall plan. Within the objectives of the IT department, clinical, financial, and operational goals of the organization are considered in identifying which systems are to be replaced and why.[1]

Answering a series of questions provides a straightforward approach for the institution to determine which systems may be replaced or updated:

1. *Need for the system.* What are the functions that the system addresses and how frequently do those functions occur? In addition, are there some tasks or functions that are not addressed by the system? Is current staff using the system? Have work processes been developed to accomplish tasks or functions that the system does not address or that the staff find difficult to accomplish using the system?

2. *Development process.* Which information systems are in development and what is the nature of the development team and its methodology? New is not always better but neither is what is familiar and comfortable. Are the requirements of the stakeholders being met, including management, financial, clinical, and operational stakeholders as well as the largest group of stakeholders, patients and their families?

3. *Basic structure.* What parts or functions can be observed? Are these items working to meet today's requirements or tomorrow's desired function? Does the current system work as designed and to meet future needs?

4. *Functionality.* What are the system response times, accuracy, reliability, and ease of use for end-users? What are the plans to continue development of the system to meet new and ongoing requirements? How are the new and ongoing requirements determined?

5. *Impact.* How does the system affect providers, patients, processes, and the organization's users in nonpatient care areas? Does the system support data collection and reporting?

6. *Integration.* How does this system interface with other systems in the institution from a technical perspective as well as from a workflow perspective?

The following key areas are important in detailing and documenting this institutional analysis:

1. Mission critical requirements
2. Regulatory and accreditation requirements
3. Financial and increased net revenue requirements

4. End-user demands and functionality requirements that are "must have"
5. End-user demands and functionality requirements that are "nice to have"

This assessment of the institution's current status and needs will form the basis for the search and initial requests for information (RFIs) for specific health information systems. The systems analysis is an internal document and is best done in comparative format (such as a spreadsheet) that is easy for technical and nontechnical readers to evaluate. An additional approach is to document the strengths and weaknesses of each system. Using the data and information from this assessment the institution should carefully document system requirements from both an institutional and a department perspective. These requirements will then be used to develop key criteria to use during the system identification and selection process.

SYSTEMS DEVELOPMENT LIFE CYCLE

Knowledge about the life cycle of an information system will help in understanding the importance of a carefully designed system selection process in obtaining overall success in meeting an organization's needs. The systems life cycle (SLC) is a framework for understanding the process of developing or configuring, implementing, and using an information system. This process is described in a series of sequential logical steps or phases listed below. These phases are based on the Staggers and Nelson SLC model discussed in Chapter 2 and depicted in Figure 2-6.

1. Analyze
2. Plan
3. Develop or purchase
4. Test
5. Implement or go-live
6. Maintain and evolve
7. Evaluate
8. Return to analyze

System selection, the focus of this chapter, involves the first three phases of the SLC model: analyze, plan, and develop or purchase. The remaining phases of the SLC model are discussed in Chapter 17.

Analysis and Requirements Definition

The project planning and analysis phases often occur concomitantly in a recursive process. In this section, for the purposes of discussion, analysis is presented first, although others may decide that the planning step is first. The decision to purchase and implement a new information system usually begins with the realization that the systems currently in place do not meet the needs of the organization and its users. At this point the selection team should identify specifically which type of information system needs to be replaced or added by the organization by completing the analysis described in the previous section. However, this initial understanding of needs does not provide enough information to begin a formal search process, as one cannot determine

if a system meets the organization's needs without a thorough evaluation and understanding of those needs or requirements.

Requirements definition is the process of determining the specific needs that the organization has for an information system and the specific functionality that is desired. This analysis is built upon the institutional inventory and analysis discussed in the previous section. However, at this point in the system selection process the analysis is focused on the specific system being selected and the specifications are much more detailed. Therefore a detailed plan for data gathering is essential to effectively determining system requirements. Some components of the requirements definition plan include:

1. *Review and if necessary update the inventory of current information systems and functionality.* The focus at this point is on these systems that will interface with or be directly affected by the new system. This evaluation should include a list of the components and functions of each system, listing the tasks that can be performed as well as any supporting information to better describe the functionality. An understanding of the general data flow between systems is also important in determining system requirements.

2. *Inventory paper documents and forms.* It is also important to obtain samples of all paper forms currently in use as well as reports from current information systems. Including paper forms in the inventory as opportunities for additional automation may drive the development of additional requirements for a new information system. A review of the paper chart and forms that it could contain should be evaluated to determine if any additional opportunities for automation can be identified and added to the list of system requirements. Importantly, the paper process should not be replicated; however, forms are used to understand requirements, especially for subspecialties and linkages between departments.

3. *Interview and observe staff.* The selection team should plan to interview hospital staff in various departments and roles regarding their work. One goal of the interviews is a determination of which functions are currently supported by an information system as well as functions and documentation that are not yet supported by an information system. Interview questions should also be used to gain an understanding of the decisions that staff will need to make as they perform their job functions and which data are needed for these decisions. Management and front-line staff can provide valuable information about the work that is actually performed and how data are collected and used while observations of the staff at work may uncover additional requirements and provide an increased understanding of the use of data.

Members of the selection team should include interview questions for key stakeholders and front-line staff to elicit their opinions and experience with the current information system. The SWOT strategic analysis tool is useful in guiding these questions. SWOT is an acronym that represents the identification of strengths, weaknesses, opportunities, and threats.[2] Box 16-1 contains several sample interview questions to consider.

4. *Collect samples of system and manual reports.* The selection team should collect samples of reports that are provided by existing information systems as well as reports that are generated manually. In addition, front-line staff, management, and hospital administration should provide information about their specific data needs, including other desired reports that are not currently available. Consideration should be given to data and reports that would support the hospital in determining how well they are meeting regulatory and accreditation requirements defined by organizations such as The Joint Commission (TJC) and Centers for Medicare & Medicaid Services (CMS).

5. *Develop process and dataflow maps.* Developing process and dataflow maps for each function or role will also clearly document the data needs of various groups of users.[3] Process maps illustrate an organization's workflow, which is a series of steps representing work activities and resources that follow a path to produce desired outcomes or outputs.[4] A thorough analysis of the workflow of future users of the new information system will help to identify system requirements that may not have been identified during the interview process. Dataflow diagrams are often used to document this type of information. See Figures 16-1 and 16-2 for examples of how this type of information may be documented.

6. *Identify hospital standards and policies and regulatory and accreditation requirements.* Hospital standards of care and policies as well as evidence-based practice must be supported by the information system that is selected. In

addition, regulations established by state and federal governments and requirements of accreditation groups such as TJC must be considered. A recent example of legislation that has had a great impact on clinical information system functionality is the Health Information Technology for Economic and Clinical Health (HITECH) Act, signed in 2009. The goal of this legislation is to promote the adoption and Meaningful Use of health information technology (health IT). More information about the HITECH Act and Meaningful Use can be found at www.hhs.gov and in Chapters 24 and 25. The selection team should identify specific system requirements related to how the information system might support the organization in meeting these standards.

Following these various methods of information collection regarding system requirements, the selection team should develop a comprehensive list of requirements that it will evaluate as each potential information system is reviewed. This thorough list of requirements will guide the selection team as it develops the request for information (RFI) and the request for proposal (RFP). When developing the list, an effective strategy is to list the objectives related to each requirement without specific decisions or details about how the software will meet this objective. By listing requirements as objectives instead of specific descriptions of how these objectives are to be met, the team will not limit potential vendor solutions before it has had a chance to evaluate them.

Objectives can be logically grouped into several categories that will facilitate organization of the requirements list:

1. *Patient care objectives.* Determine the types of patient data that should be entered as well as any specific patient care areas that may require special processes, such as the emergency department, critical care units, or labor and delivery areas. Example patient care objectives are listed in Box 16-2.

2. *Usability.* Usability is the extent to which a product can be used by specific users in a specific context to achieve specific goals with effectiveness, efficiency, and satisfaction.[5] The information system that is selected should be easy to use and intuitive. A variety of methods for testing usability are described in detail in Chapter 21. Improved usability reduces user frustration as well as the time needed for education about the system. Efficiency examples follow. The user should be able to easily find a patient in the system and then proceed to view or enter patient data. System reports providing summarized patient data for management and administration can also greatly improve efficiency. See Box 16-3 for examples of efficiency objectives.

3. *IT department objectives.* The IT department will also be able to list some requirements for a new information system. These may be related to the degree of customization allowed as well as the ease of customization. These factors will affect the IT resources needed to implement and maintain the system. Information regarding hardware and third-party software requirements should also be included in the IT objectives, as this will affect both the

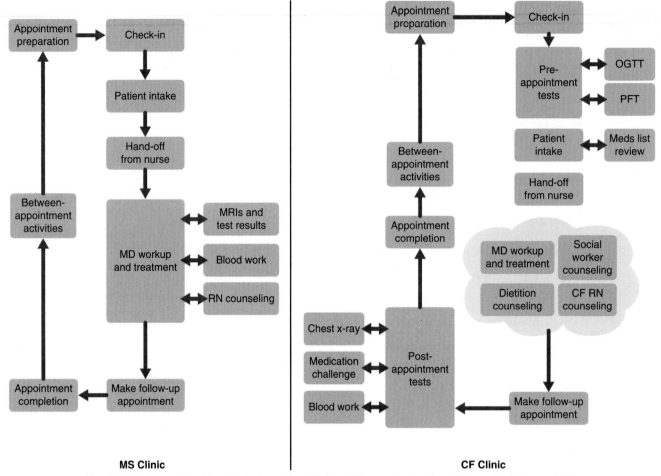

FIG 16-1 Information Flow in MS and CF Clinics. *CF*, Cystic fibrosis; *MD*, medical doctor; *MRI*, magnetic resonance imaging; *MS*, multiple sclerosis; *OGTT*, oral glucose tolerance test; *PFT*, pulmonary function test; *RN*, registered nurse. (Modified from Unertl KM, Weinger MB, Johnson KB, Lorenzi NM. Describing and modeling workflow and information flow in chronic disease care. *J Am Med Inform Assoc.* 2009;16:830. With permission from BMJ Publishing Group Ltd.)

BOX 16-2   EXAMPLE REQUIREMENTS FOR A HOSPITAL INFORMATION SYSTEM: PATIENT CARE OBJECTIVES

1. Patient care documentation (assessments and notes) by clinical users
   - Nursing
   - Physician
   - Social work and case managers
   - Nutrition
   - Wound care
   - Respiratory therapy
   - Pharmacy
   - Occupational therapy and physical therapy
   - Other ancillary users
2. Orders management
   - Order entry, including order sets by stakeholder groups
   - Order selection menu based on physician clinician specialty
3. Care plan and problem list
4. Patient data displays
   - Summary view of patient data
   - View longitudinal data across visits
5. Clinical decision support and alerts
6. Medication reconciliation
7. Patient discharge processes
   - Instructions and prescriptions
   - Continuity of care document, summary of care
8. Requirements for special care areas
   - Medical and surgical units
   - Critical care units
   - Step-down units
   - Ambulatory services
   - Psychiatry
   - Rehabilitation
   - Long-term care
   - Labor and delivery
   - Oncology

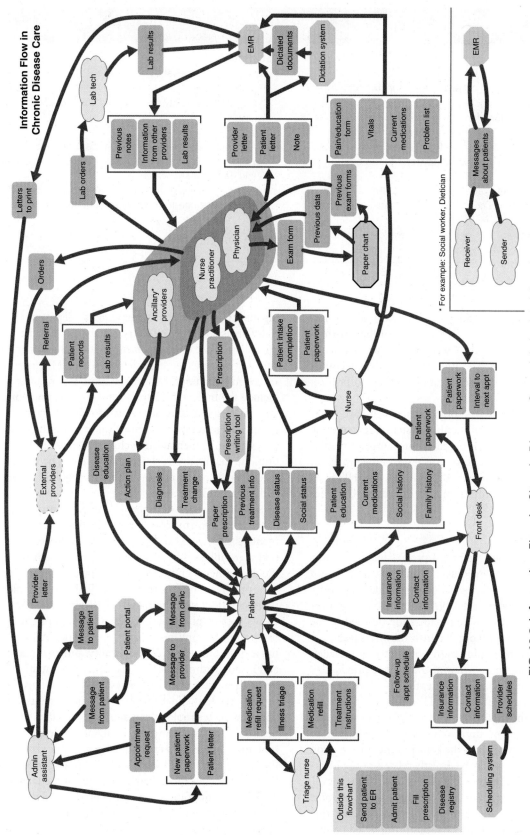

FIG 16-2 Information Flow in Chronic Disease Care. *Admin,* Administration; *appt,* appointment; *EMR,* electronic medical record; *ER,* emergency room. (From Unertl KM, Weinger MB, Johnson KB, Lorenzi NM. Describing and modeling workflow and information flow in chronic disease care. *J Am Med Inform Assoc.* 2009;16:832. With permission from BMJ Publishing Group Ltd.)

BOX 16-3   EXAMPLE REQUIREMENTS FOR A HOSPITAL INFORMATION SYSTEM: EFFICIENCY OBJECTIVES

Data Collection
- Ease of data entry by end-users
  - Does the orders management system support customization for different categories of users?
  - How long does it take for an end-user (pharmacy, nurses, physicians) to enter a complex medication order?
  - Does the system support difficult orders such as total parenteral nutrition, chemotherapy, and future orders?
- Integration
  - Is integration or interface with other systems supported, allowing bidirectional communication of data and information?
  - Does the system support point-of-care data collection device integration, such as vital signs monitors?

Data Retrieval
- Ease of data retrieval by end-users
  - Is the process for viewing results easy to use while providing flexibility for the end-user to choose what is needed?
- Reports
  - Are reports available to supply data needed to users at various levels, including the front-line staff, management, and administration?
  - Is the creation of customized reports possible and does the skill set needed for this exist within the organization?

---

initial cost of implementation and the cost of maintenance. Another key objective is the ability of the information system to support data security and protection of patient confidentiality. The importance of this factor is highlighted as an objective of Meaningful Use certification as outlined by the HITECH Act.

4. *Organization objectives.* The organization will have additional objectives for the information system. Some of these may be related to how the organization can meet regulatory and payer requirements such as those of the American Recovery and Reinvestment Act (ARRA), the HITECH Act, and the Patient Protection and Affordable Care Act (PPACA).

Project Planning

Because of the importance of solid project planning, project management has emerged as a formal specialty within and outside health IT. University courses and even entire university-level majors are available on the topic. The Project Management Institute is an organization devoted to the topic. Available at www.pmi.org, the Institute offers resources for those interested in learning more about project management. In this section, an overview of the topic is provided.

During the project planning phase, the high-level project goals are identified and established. The goals for the system should be in alignment with the strategic vision of the organization. Any change or improvement in an information system should directly support the ability of the organization to meets its goals. Goals may be directly related to the information system, such as ease of data entry and data retrieval. Systems that support accurate and easy data access support improved decisions during care. In addition, systems that allow easy and accurate data entry support improved patient care and can be designed to provide information about patient outcomes.[6]

When selecting an information system it is also important to consider whether the system functionality is appropriate for the type of patients cared for by the facility, including inpatients, outpatients, and emergency department and specialty areas such as psychiatry. Goals may also be related to the ability of the system to facilitate the achievement of regulatory goals such as compliance with CMS measures and successful Meaningful Use attestation. Financial goals might include the budget guidelines for purchase, implementation, and ongoing maintenance related to the information system. Finally, the selection team must understand the goals related to system implementation, including the ease of implementation, the degree to which the software can be customized to meet specific needs, and the resources required to implement and maintain the system.

Another important aspect of project planning is the creation of the information system selection team and development of their roles and responsibilities. System selection is best accomplished by a multidisciplinary team representing the departments and roles that will be affected by the system to be purchased by the organization. This team should include representation from nursing; physicians; ancillary departments such as pharmacy, occupational and physical therapy, respiratory therapy, nutrition, social work and case management, infection control, and quality and risk management; and hospital administration. Clinical representatives must be involved in every step of the system selection process. Their input is key to the identification of requirements and system selection, as technology can support clinicians in providing better patient care. However, many of the department representatives on the team may not have previous experience with the system selection process. The system selection process will be more effective if the initial meetings of the team include a clear statement of the scope of the project and an orientation to the system selection process. The IT department must also be included in the system selection team. Ideally there are clinical and IT representatives who have had previous experience with the system selection process. The organization should consider carefully the goals of this group as well as the leadership. Requirements of users as well as the IT staff who will be supporting the system are important to consider.

For more information about informatics governance and its role in the system selection process, see Chapter 23.

Develop or Purchase

Once analysis and planning are completed the institution must decide if it will develop a new system, reconfigure or upgrade the current system, or select a new system. For the purposes of discussion this chapter is presented with the assumption that a decision has been made to select a new system. Reconfiguring or upgrading a current system is discussed in Chapter 17.

Developing, Obtaining, and Evaluating Requests for Information (RFIs) and Requests for Proposals (RFPs)

Once the selection team has been established and oriented to the system selection process its first job is to develop a request for information (RFI). The RFI will determine who should be encouraged to submit a request for proposal (RFP). Understanding the essentials of RFIs and RFPs facilitates decision making and selection processes. Basically, the RFI is an information step in vendor evaluation. The organization prepares a list of system goals and high-level requirements and asks vendors to respond to them with specific information such as projected costs. Larger institutions often have a template with sections, such as a description of the institution already provided. Common sections often found in an RFI can be seen in Box 16-4.

The response to an RFI describes the vendor's experience and product and how it communicates with clients. Any vendor that cannot meet the RFI expectations or omits requested information may not remain on the evaluation list. An RFI is requested from potential vendors to determine which of their products and services are potentially available in the marketplace to meet the institution's needs. The response also lets organizations know the capability of the vendor in terms of strengths and offerings. For example, if the vendor has consistently installed in small community hospitals and the institution is a large academic medical center, this may not be a vendor worth further investigation.

RFIs are commonly used on major procurements, such as hospital information systems, but they are not an invitation to bid so some vendors will not respond, even if they have systems that meet requirements. An RFI is not binding on either party and may or may not lead to an RFP. An RFI should inform the vendor of the organization's goals and how they will be achieved. An RFI should be specific enough to foster clear collection and evaluation of responses that enable a comparison of vendors to determine from whom more detailed responses (e.g., including price, quality of delivery, guarantees, and other considerations) to an RFP should be requested. This is not an insignificant step, as the organization will be investing large dollar amounts and committing resources to a new information system.

For financial considerations (actual bids for a health IT product), organizations should submit an RFP. An RFP is an invitation for vendors to submit back to an organization a

---

| BOX 16-4 | SECTIONS OF A REQUEST FOR INFORMATION |

Purpose of Request
A brief statement describing the type of information system that the institution is planning to select. For example, is it searching for an electronic health record for use in physician offices or a classification and staffing system for use in the outpatient clinics?

Background
The description of the institution, including mission size and number and type of patients treated.

Qualifications
Any specific qualifications required by the vendor. For example, does it need to have been in business for 5 or more years?

Information Requested
A list of specific elements that should be answered, for example:
- Size, history, and financial status of the company
- Basic system architecture and software configuration
- Number of installations and selected names of customers

Time and Type of Response
This section includes the due date for the response, where the response should be sent, and who the vendor should contact if the vendor has any questions. The vendor should be discouraged from contacting anyone else at the institution.

---

formal proposal that clearly spells out what system (including functionality and capability) can be delivered and at what price. The RFP gives the vendor a very clear and detailed understanding of what the organization is looking for in a system and starts the negotiation process based on price and quality of delivery. An RFP requires much more effort and is done at the stage where the organization clarifies its expectations and receives assurances from the vendor that it can deliver the system on the organization's timetable and terms. The RFP is a more complete and formal step, with the vendor response often translating directly into the formal contract.

The RFP is the organization's way of soliciting competitive bids to supply a specific information system. An RFP should include detailed information about the organization as well as questions that elicit differences among competing vendors. An RFP should solicit cost quotes for installation and implementation and security standards, as well as delivery time (and estimated completion time) and resource requirements. Resource requirements should be spelled out for both the organization and the vendor in the response. The best RFP also seeks information on total cost of ownership (TCO) over the expected lifetime of the system. The RFP should require information such as corporate information on the vendor as well as its history with this kind of system. Customer references that can and should be validated must be part of the response from the vendor.

Prior to issuing an RFP, an organization should establish certain items:

1. The organization's needs as outlined in the organizational and IT vision and strategic plan and the specific needs.
2. The organization's evaluation criteria. These should include vendor experience, vendor staff strength, market and industry understanding, and differential advantages such as usability or available functionality and cost.

When responses are received, they should be evaluated in total—not just on cost or any other single criteria. Following that, the organization should interview the vendors that have live, working systems and distinguish between available functions and future capability or functionality. Healthcare systems or hospitals will be using this information system for years, even decades, to come. Organizations want to ensure that available functionality is real today and will continue to grow with the needs of the health system or hospital.[7]

As much as everyone dislikes deadlines, organizations need to set a time limit for responses to both RFIs and RFPs; 6 to 8 weeks should be the outside limit of the timeline, although very complex organizations such as the Department of Defense may allow 60 to 90 days. Also, allow a sufficient time for the organization to evaluate responses adequately; healthcare today moves at a very fast pace but ensure that the organization has carefully measured the responses and interviewed those who can deliver.

Evaluating Vendors

There are some basic characteristics to look for when finding an information system vendor. A fundamental element is the fit between the organization and the vendor. For example, is the organization small and more informal? Is the vendor large and bureaucratic? Does the organization make change rapidly? Can the vendor do the same? Does the vendor come across as professional? Also, a vendor should be expected to have a great deal of experience in the same type of facility or organization that is seeking an information system.[8] Information system support (24/7) and help desk, as well as education and training, are key areas to examine when deciding on the vendor for a product. New or replacement systems without proper installation and implementation can be doomed from the start. For additional information on vendors check the data available from the major information technology research groups: Forrester, Gartner, and KLAS. These major research firms provide clear, unambiguous analysis of vendors and systems. Table 16-1 gives additional information about these research groups.

Additionally, valuable information is available from the Healthcare Information and Management Systems Society (HIMSS) at www.himss.org. A detailed analysis of vendor

TABLE 16-1	MAJOR HEALTHCARE INFORMATION TECHNOLOGY RESEARCH FIRMS IN THE UNITED STATES
FIRM AND LOCATION	**OVERVIEW**
Forrester Research, Inc. Cambridge, Mass. www.forrester.com	Forrester is a global research and advisory group. Forrester serves clients as they face increasingly complex business and technology decisions on a daily basis. To help them understand, strategize, and act on opportunities brought about by change, Forrester provides proprietary research, consumer and business data, custom consulting, events and online communities, and peer-to-peer executive programs. Forrester guides leaders in IT, marketing, and strategy and the technology industry through independent, fact-based insight, ensuring their business success today and tomorrow.
Gartner, Inc. Stamford, Conn. www.gartner.com	Gartner, Inc. is an IT research and advisory company. Gartner delivers the technology-related insight necessary for its clients to make the right decisions every day. From CIOs and senior IT leaders in corporations and government agencies, to business leaders in high-tech and telecom enterprises and professional services firms, to technology investors, Gartner is a partner to clients in 12,000 distinct organizations. Through the resources of Gartner Research, Gartner Executive Programs, Gartner Consulting, and Gartner Events, it works with every client to research, analyze, and interpret the business of IT within the context of its individual role. Gartner is headquartered in Stamford, Conn., and has 5000 associates, including 1280 research analysts and consultants, and clients in 85 countries.
KLAS Research Orem, Utah www.klasresearch.com	KLAS conducts over 1900 healthcare provider interviews per month, working with over 4500 hospitals and over 3000 doctor's offices and clinics. KLAS is independently owned and operated. KLAS has ratings on over 250 healthcare technology vendors and over 900 products and services. KLAS publishes approximately 40 performance and perception reports per year. KLAS is headquartered in Orem, Utah, with independent researchers working throughout North America. The name KLAS is an acronym comprising a letter from each of the founders' names.

Information is adapted from the appropriate company's website.
CIO, Chief information officer; *IT*, information technology.
Adapted from Forrester Research Inc. at www.forrester.com, Gartner Inc. at www.gartner.com, and KLAS Enterprises LLC at www.klasresearch.com.

research should include visiting the vendor's website. Also, a number of Internet blogs have comments, both positive and negative, about vendors. An example is HIStalk at http://histalk2.com/. Organizations should also validate information with peers in other hospitals and health systems.

Selecting the System

Now that the selection team has defined objectives and requirements for the new system, developed an RFI and RFP, and completed research about various vendors, the team must have a plan for how it will select an information system. The team must take steps to develop specific system evaluation criteria and a process for recording its individual and group decisions. This should be done before actually reviewing the RFI and RFP responses so that each team member can begin to evaluate and score the various information systems as soon as information is obtained. One effective approach is to develop a scoring system, where all of the system requirements are listed and each requirement is given a numeric score or weighted numeric score based on the degree to which it meets each objective. By using numeric ratings, organizations are able to obtain an overall score for each vendor's system. It may help to classify the requirements as "must have" or "nice to have," as this information will be useful as findings are evaluated. As team members complete the scoring document for systems, it is essential that they be open-minded and broadly explore all options presented by various vendors. The software that vendors present may meet the requirements but in a manner that is different from what was anticipated.

During the evaluation process it is important to evaluate potential software products very rigorously since the amount of time and money invested in purchasing and implementing an information system is quite large. The impact of a new health information system on an organization's users cannot be minimized, so the task of evaluating and selecting a system should be given adequate attention and resources. Vendors responding to an RFP will provide presentations and demonstrations aimed at showing how the system can meet or exceed the requirements. In the past, organizations have found it helpful to script scenarios for the vendors to follow during the demonstrations. In this way the organization can tailor the scenarios to its own patient populations and highlight the patient flow across modules. For example, a script may be developed following a patient from outpatient to the operating room, postanesthesia recovery, intensive care, and surgical unit, then back to outpatient.

During this process, clinicians, IT, and hospital leaders should remember to focus on deployed, working systems only, as this is what will be delivered once the system is purchased. Vendors will spend some time explaining what their plans are for future development but it is important for all to know what can actually be configured and implemented when receiving the software. Plans for future development by the vendor can be considered. There is no guarantee when new functions will be available, if at all, or how they will actually work if delivered.

After initial presentations by various vendors, the selection team will have good ideas about the top contenders for the organization. Once the group has narrowed down the list to a handful of vendors, it will make arrangements with the different vendors for site visits to actual customers using the information system. There is an advantage to not giving a vendor complete control in selecting the site. The selection team should also determine if the site selected for the visit will receive direct or indirect remuneration from the vendor for providing a site visit.

The site visit team should be interdisciplinary and use specific evaluation criteria to guide the visit. This will allow the team to see how this organization has configured the system to work at its site. The biggest advantage of a site visit is the opportunity to talk with people at various levels to obtain their opinions and information about their experiences with the system. In planning for the visit, ask for sessions or opportunities where all can talk with various clinical users of the system such as nurses, physicians, and ancillary users. IT staff will also want to talk with IT representatives to get their opinions and perspective. Some of these frank discussions will be most effective if the vendor representative is not present, allowing the staff at the hospital site to be more open and honest. After the visit there are often additional questions. The selection team should obtain the names and contact information for individuals they may want to contact after the site visit with follow-up questions.

As the group evaluates various information systems keep in mind the total cost of ownership (TCO). This is a financial estimate of the cost of implementing and maintaining the information system over the life of the project, also known as life cycle costing.[9] This estimate should include all hardware, software, and resource costs associated with all phases of the project, including design, implementation, testing, and ongoing support over the entire lifespan of the system. Typical life cycles are about 11 years but can run much longer. During the evaluation phase make sure that the group obtains this type of information from the vendor. Include discussions about the frequency of software updates and upgrades and the IT resources needed to test and implement these changes. Ask how specific change requests from one organization are prioritized and what the average time lapse is from request to delivery. Include discussions about the frequency and duration of planned downtimes to accomplish updates.

Once the information systems have been reviewed and the vendors offering these systems have been evaluated, the selection task force makes a recommendation. If possible the recommendation should include two or three potential options with a ranking and rationale statement for each option. The rationale should include the pros and cons of each option. Usually the decision on which product to recommend is made at the next-to-last meeting of the task force. The meeting should start with a general summary of the findings for each vendor and its product. Plenty of time should be given for discussion. If there are any major disagreements on which product to select, it is helpful if key administrative personnel such as the chief information officer (CIO) and the vice-president for the department most affected by the new system join the discussion.

At the final meeting of the task force, members should agree on the items to be placed in the contract and recommendations for the implemention of the product, including whether a pilot unit or the entire hospital should be undertaken. The final job of the IT staff for this product selection task force is to summarize the process and findings in a report for senior management. The final report includes the recommended products and vendors as well as the rationale for each recommendation. The report should also include any recommendations for the contract and implementation process.

Negotiating the Contract

For major purchases, contract negotiations are usually performed by the CIO with approval by the chief executive officer (CEO), the chief financial officer (CFO), and attorneys. The negotiations will be based on the final report from the selection committee. This report may include specific recommendations for items to be placed in the contract. Examples of such items are specific training programs to be offered by the vendor or the stipulation that the hospital or clinic will be a test site for new functionality that is very important to the hospital or clinic. Other items that might be included are an agreement on the arbitration process and the placement of the actual programming code in a guarded location for the agency to access in the event that the vendor firm fails as a business. Also, it is wise to request a detailed explanation of line items in the pricing schedule, especially those items that might be misinterpreted. All third-party software should be defined with a clear reason as to why it is required. It is also beneficial to require that the vendor define all vendor-specific terms and concepts referred to in the contract at the very beginning of the contract.[10] The chair of the selection committee should be available if there are questions but once formal negotiations begin the vendor should deal only with the CIO, the purchasing agent, or others who have been selected by the CIO to speak with the vendor.

Establishing a Working Relationship with the Vendor

From the day the RFI is mailed, the institution will begin managing its vendor relationship. The toll and nature of these relationships can be expected to change through the life cycle. However, an effective open and professional relationship can be key to the success of the project throughout the total project. Managing a vendor relationship requires skilled and careful leadership and a level of personal finesse. Vendor managers are usually experts in their own subject matter area. In many cases they also have project management and business skills. But not every vendor manager has leadership expertise. Therefore communicating with the vendor is as important as communicating with an organization's stakeholders. Establishing communication channels and information flow between local clinicians, IT, and leaders and the vendor can lead to increased efficiency, reduced costs, and

better service. The vendor will play a key role in local success. Building mutually strong relationships with a chosen vendor is critical and can ultimately strengthen overall performance. Vendor management is more than getting a lower price or better service. Properly managed vendor relationships can give the vendor and local setting a significant competitive advantage. A successful vendor relationship shares local priorities and mutually agrees upon factors such as:

- The definition of a quality implementation
- Metrics for successful adoption of the system
- Elements of the vendor's quality assurance program, including measurable outcome metrics—not just response times and limits to unplanned downtime and upgrades but the real outcome to end-users

A good vendor must understand and share priorities but the organization must first communicate those priorities. If a vendor cannot help with stated priorities, a good vendor will disclose this limitation or weakness up front. Thus it is absolutely essential that the chosen vendor becomes a partner in the implementation, optimization, and ongoing use and upgrades of the organization's information system. There is a concrete need to drive contract terms and obligations but in the end no contract will adequately cover all long-term goals and expectations. A solid, true collaborative partnership with a vendor will provide for such needs. When some things go bad, as they most assuredly will at some point, the organization will be better served to have a partner at the table, not just a vendor. Early on, demand proof of concept. If an organization is seeking value, then the group needs to see it first-hand. A good vendor will prove it can be done.

The International Organization for Standardization (ISO) has developed a set of minimum standards, practices, terminologies, and requirements that, when adopted, demonstrates a vendor's products and services have achieved a minimum level of quality. ISO certification demonstrates a vendor's commitment to quality and service. These standards are outlined on the ISO website (www.iso.org) but since clinical practice varies around the world, students will need to adapt minimum standards to their country's requirements.

CONCLUSION AND FUTURE DIRECTIONS

When selecting an information system, clinicians, IT, and leaders need to understand the vendor's plan for responding to changes in the market and regulatory environments. The pace of change in healthcare is anticipated to only accelerate, and both the organization and the vendor must be able to adapt quickly. The group may wish to review the selected vendor's history with response to changes such as these, including the timeliness of software changes and compliance. In the future, the vendor model may erode from full-service or monolithic health IT products such as electronic health records (EHRs) to commodity or component providers. For example, organizations may choose their pharmacy applications from one vendor and clinical documentation from another. The interoperability requirements being promulgated today would then allow organizations to compile functions using off-site cloud computing versus installing huge systems on-site. However, with this more futuristic notion the phases and concepts listed in this chapter are still needed.

REFERENCES

1. Sittig D, Hazelhurst BL, Palen T, Hsu J, Jimison H, Hornbrook MC. A clinical information system research landscape. *The Permanente Journal.* 2002;2(6):1-6.
2. Helms MM, Moore R, Ahmadi M. Information technology (IT) and the healthcare industry: a SWOT analysis. *Int J Healthc Inf Syst Inform.* 2008;3(1):75-92. doi:10.4018/jhisi.2008010105.
3. Staccini PM, Joubert M, Quaranta JF, Fieschi M. Towards elicitation of users requirements for hospital information system: from a care process modeling technique to a web based collaborative tool. *Proc AMIA Symp.* 2002;732-736.
4. Damelio R. *Basics of Process Mapping.* 2nd ed. Boca Raton, FL: CRC Press; 2011.
5. International Organization of Standards. ISO 9241-11: guidance on usability. UsabilityNet. http://www.usabilitynet.org/tools/r_international.htm#9241-11. 1998. Accessed February 7, 2012.
6. Nurse leaders discuss the nurse's role in driving technology decisions. *American Nurse Today.* 2010;1(5):16-19. http://www.americannursetoday.com/Article.aspx?id=6142&fid=6116. Accessed May 1, 2012.
7. Adler KG. How to select an electronic health record system. *Fam Pract Manag.* 2005;12(2):55-62.
8. Gortzis LG. Selecting healthcare information systems provided by third-party vendors: a mind map beyond the manuals. *Inform Health Soc Ca.* 2010;35(1):1-9.
9. Cellucci F. What is the true TCO for information technology projects? ConnectivITy. http://www.docutech.com/blog/bid/54338/What-Is-The-True-TCO-For-Information-Technology-Projects. 2011. Accessed May 20, 2012.
10. Craig JB. Life cycle of a health care information system. In: Englebardt S, Nelson R, eds. *Health Care Informatics: An Interdisciplinary Approach.* St. Louis, MO: Mosby-Year Book, Inc; 2002:181-208.

DISCUSSION QUESTIONS

1. How do strategic vision and alignment affect decisions made in your organization?
2. What is the role of healthcare providers in the identification and selection of a healthcare information system?
3. The selection team should be an interdisciplinary team but how should the chair of the committee be selected?
4. What is the impact of a well-defined and complete RFI and RFP process on identification and selection of a healthcare information system?
5. What are the key roles and functions in identification of system requirements?
6. Why are vendor relationships with management essential? Brainstorm ideas for maintaining good site–vendor relationships.

CASE STUDY

You have been chosen to participate in the selection team for a new clinical information system to be purchased and implemented at the community hospital where you are a staff nurse. The selection team has been asked to develop an initial list of requirements that they would like to use for the evaluation of potential systems in relation to documentation of assessments for interprofessional use, including nursing, physicians, and some other departments such as physical therapy and occupational therapy.

The selection team has decided to group the requirements that they identify into the following categories:

- Patient Care Objectives
- Usability
- Information Technology Department Objectives
- Organization Objectives

Your task for this case study is to use the key considerations listed below to develop a list of system requirements for electronic documentation in a clinical information system, grouping the requirements into the four categories listed above. The key considerations include information that the selection team has gathered in anticipation of developing system requirements.

Key Considerations for System Selection

Findings from inventory of current systems and functionality:

- Electronic laboratory and radiology report results are produced by ancillary information systems.
- The intensive care units have an ICU information system where some documentation is done electronically, including vital signs, intake and output, and some interfaced data from monitoring systems.

Findings from inventory of paper documents and forms:

- Nursing notes and care planning currently are documented only in the paper chart on medical/surgical units.
- Physician progress notes and orders currently are documented only in the paper chart.
- There are numerous paper forms and various versions of forms in use with no consistency across the organization.
- Paper order sets are in use. Some order sets are physician specific, with multiple versions for the same diagnosis or procedure. None appear to be evidence based.

Findings from staff interviews and observations:

Direct observation studies were conducted in the ICU, medical/surgical units, and pediatric unit. Observations and interviews also were conducted in various other clinical departments including PT, OT, and wound care. The study revealed that there are similarities in the types and needs of data collection in all of these areas. Key findings included:

- Need to be able to document using structured data such as predefined drop-down boxes.
- Need to be able to enter free-text comments.
- Entry of an electronic assessment must include the user's electronic signature and the current date and time.
- All entries must have the capability to be edited, and changes to the document must be tracked by the system.

SWOT Analysis

A SWOT analysis of the current documentation was conducted with the following findings:

Strengths: Structured electronic data in the ICU facilitates accurate and timely data collection.

Weaknesses: Lack of standardization may result in inconsistent patient care.

Opportunities: An electronic order management and documentation system could support evidence-based practice methodology.

Threats: Paper documentation is difficult to read and could result in patient safety issues.

Implementing and Upgrading an Information System Solution

Christine D. Meyer

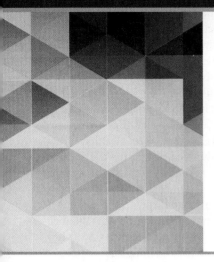

No matter whether the electronic health record (EHR) is new or an upgrade, the ultimate goal in implementations is to provide the highest level of care at the lowest cost with the least risk.

OBJECTIVES

At the completion of this chapter the reader will be prepared to:

1. Discuss the regulatory and nonregulatory reasons for implementing or upgrading an electronic information system
2. Compare the advantages and disadvantages of the "best of breed" and integrated system approaches in selecting healthcare information system architecture
3. Explain each step in developing an implementation plan for a healthcare information system
4. Develop strategies for the successful management of each step in the implementation of a healthcare information system
5. Analyze the benefits of an electronic information system with an integrated clinical decision support system
6. Explain the implications of unintended consequences or e-iatrogenesis as it relates to implementing an electronic health record (EHR)

KEY TERMS

ABSTRACT

The decision to implement a new electronic health record (EHR) or to upgrade a current system is based on several factors, including providing safe and up-to-date patient care, meeting federal mandates and Meaningful Use requirements, and leveraging advanced levels of clinical decision support. Implementing EHRs entails multilayered decisions at each stage of the implementation. Major decisions include evaluating vendor and system selection, determining go-live options, redesigning workflow, and developing procedures and policies. The timeline and scope of the project is primarily dictated by expenses, staff, resources, and the drop-dead date for go-live. Success depends on variables such as a well-thought-out and detailed project plan with regular review and updating of the critical milestones, unwavering support from the organization's leadership, input from users during the design and build phases, mitigation of identified risk factors, and control of scope creep. The implementation of an EHR is never finished. Medication orders, nonmedication orders, and documentation screens or fields will continuously need to be added, modified, or inactivated; patches will be installed and tweaks to workflows and functionality will be ongoing.

INTRODUCTION

This chapter focuses on the implementation of healthcare information systems. Of course, many different types of applications are used within a healthcare information system. The general principles for implementing these many different applications are the same; however, for the purposes of discussion this chapter will focus mainly on the implementation of an electronic health record (EHR) to demonstrate these general principles. In 2004 President George W. Bush promoted the idea of a fully functional electronic medical record (EMR) for Americans within 10 years.[1] This proposal officially initiated the massive changes that we are now witnessing in health informatics. Healthcare information systems are widely used today in many diverse settings. Small hospitals, ambulatory clinics, and small physician practices generally implement a simple and streamlined system with limited features but tailored for quicker implementation and easier long-term maintenance. Large medical centers, multifacility enterprises, and multiphysician practices with more complex needs typically opt to install a more robust system that allows for customizations. However, there are still hospitals and physician practices without an EHR or that have an outdated system that cannot accommodate recent regulatory mandates. An outdated system may be one reason to implement or upgrade a health information technology (health IT) solution, but there are others.

Reasons to Implement or Upgrade a Healthcare Information System

There are several reasons why a health organization (hospital organization, physician office, or clinic) may decide that a major change is needed. A careful review of the reasons for the change will start the process of deciding whether to install a new information system or upgrade the current system. One of the primary reasons for making such a major change is changing government regulations.

The American Recovery and Reinvestment Act (ARRA)

The American Recovery and Reinvestment Act (ARRA), enacted in 2009, spawned the Health Information Technology for Economic and Clinical Health (HITECH) Act. One of its primary goals is that each person in the United States would have a certified health record by 2014, including the electronic exchange of health information across healthcare institutions to improve quality of healthcare. As discussed in detail in Chapters 24 and 25, the HITECH Act created a $27 billion federally funded incentive program providing Medicare and Medicaid payments over 5 to 10 years to three groups: (1) eligible providers (EP), (2) eligible hospitals (EH), and (3) Critical Access Hospitals (CAH). CAH are defined as rural hospitals certified to receive cost-based reimbursement from Medicare. Within the HITECH Act there are two EHR incentive programs: the Medicare EHR Incentive Program administered by the Centers for Medicare & Medicaid Services (CMS) and the Medicaid EHR Incentive Program, which is governed by individual states and territories.

It is important to note that these incentive programs were not established to cover the cost of implementing an EHR system but to encourage or "incentivize" healthcare organizations and healthcare providers to use an EHR in a meaningful way, called Meaningful Use (MU), and to foster much-needed faster adoption across the nation.[2] Additional requirements include the submission of detailed and timely reports to CMS and the states demonstrating MU adoption. Other terms often used for this incentive program are "stimulus funds," "stimulus package," or simply "ARRA funds."[3]

To meet these MU requirements an EHR should be a "certified complete EHR" or have individual modules that are "certified EHR Modules." This means that they are certified by the Office of the National Coordinator for Health Information Technology (ONC) Authorized Testing and Certification Body. Complete EHR certification means that the system has the functionality, required data elements, and logic to support ambulatory, emergency room, outpatient, and inpatient MU requirements. EHR module certification means that the ancillary application meets one or more requirements. Most hospitals and physician offices purchase a commercial system that is deemed certified, meaning that the vendor incorporated these essential capabilities. A search engine providing a list of certified products can be found at http://oncchpl.force.com/ehrcert?q=chpl and each product has links to other pages that include information about that product.

MU criteria do not require purchasing a commercial, certified product. Hospitals and eligible providers may have developed their own "homegrown" EHRs that may or may not include commercial components, and have no need to purchase a new product. For example, legacy systems at Intermountain Healthcare and the Regenstrief Institute are accepted systems developed over decades.[4] CMS welcomes organizations to certify their systems using the three-step EHR Alternative Certification for Healthcare Providers (EACH) program established by the Certification Commission for Health Information Technology (CCHIT). The three-step process provides a mechanism to determine whether the system measures up to U.S. Department of Health & Human Services (HHS) requirements to support MU and to obtain certification for an existing EHR system that is not already covered by a vendor certification. Major medical centers that successfully opted for this alternative include Health Management Associates, New York University, Langone Medical Center, Northwestern University, Tenet Health System, and Medical University of North Carolina.[4]

A 2011 survey conducted by the American Hospital Association found that the percentage of U.S. hospitals that had adopted EHRs more than doubled from 16% to 35% between 2009 and 2011. Moreover, 85 percent of hospitals report that they intend to take advantage of the incentive payments made available through the Medicare and Medicaid EHR Incentive Programs by 2015.[5]

The Transition from ICD-9-CM to ICD-10-CM Codes and from HIPAA Version 4010 to HIPAA Version 5010

Complicating implementation of the MU criteria is the change in the International Classification of Diseases (ICD) coding. ICD-10-CM is a U.S. modification of the tenth revision of the International Classification of Diseases, which is used to report medical care and cause of deaths, process payments, calculate trends, and perform statistical analyses. Older versions of healthcare information systems cannot adopt the new ICD-10-CM codes because they were configured to accept the old ICD-9-CM codes consisting of three to five numeric-only characters. The ICD-10-CM codes have three to seven characters. Making things even more complex, the first and third characters are always alpha characters, the second character is always numeric, and characters four through seven can be either alpha or numeric.[6] The ICD-9-CM system has 17,000 codes to define diagnoses and procedures. In contrast, the ICD-10-CM version contains 155,000 codes, which allows for a more detailed definition and better reporting for reimbursement and biosurveillance (Tables 17-1 and 17-2).[7] The United States lags behind other countries in implementation of ICD-10 codes. Already, 138 other countries are using ICD-10 codes to track mortality and 99 countries are using these codes to track morbidity (Table 17-3).[6] The original deadline for adopting ICD-10-CM codes was October 1, 2011. However, the Secretary of Health & Human Services delayed the mandatory adoption of ICD-10-CM until October 1, 2014.

In addition, all health plans, healthcare providers, and clearinghouses that conduct business electronically were required to convert to the Health Insurance Portability and Accountability Act (HIPAA) standard for electronic transactions: Version 5010. Failure to comply means that any electronic transactions using the old Version 4010 standard form that were submitted to CMS as of June 30, 2012, were rejected. The upgrade to Version 5010 is also important because the new version is able to accommodate the forthcoming and mandatory ICD-10-CM and ICD-10-PCS code sets.

Best Practices: Evidence-Based Content and Clinical Decision Support (CDS) Systems

With each new release, information systems are more robust, enabling them to incorporate evidence-based content (called evidenced-based practice or EBP) and to use clinical decision support (CDS) features in the system. Detailed information is included in Chapter 3; however, one of the most frequently quoted definitions for EBP is one proposed by Sackett, Rosenberg, Gray, Haynes, and Richardson: EBP is "the conscientious, explicit, and judicious use of current best evidence in making decisions about the care of individual patients. The practice of evidence based medicine means integrating individual clinical expertise with the best available external clinical evidence from systematic research."[8(p71)] EBP involves making decisions for clinical care based on the most current recommended treatments for specific diagnoses. These recommendations are derived from an ongoing review and analysis of high-caliber, peer-reviewed scientific studies in the literature. While entering orders from an EBP order set, the practitioner may override any of the recommended

TABLE 17-1	COMPARISON OF ICD-9-CM AND ICD-10-CM CODES	
CHARACTERISTIC	**ICD-9-CM**	**ICD-10-CM**
Field Length	3-5 characters	3-7 characters
Available Codes	Approximately 13,000 codes	Approximately 68,000 codes
Code Composition (i.e., Numeric, Alpha)	Digit 1 = alpha or numeric Digits 2-5 = num	Digit 1 = alpha Digit 2 = numeric Digits 3-7 = alpha or numeric
Character Position within Code	Characters 1-3 = Category Characters 4-5 = Anatomic site, etiology, manifestation*	Characters 1-3 = Category Characters 4-6 = Anatomic site, etiology, severity, or clinical detail† Character 7 = Extension
Available Space for New Codes	Limited	Flexible
Overall Detail Embedded within Codes	Ambiguous	Very Specific
Laterality	Does not identify right vs. left	Often identifies right versus left
Sample Code	438.11, Late effect of cerebrovascular disease, speech and language deficits, aphasia	I69.320, Speech and language deficits following cerebral infarction, aphasia following cerebral infarction

From ICD-10 State Medicaid Readiness Medicaid ICD10 Implementation Handbook.docx. Retrieved January 14, 2013 from http://www.medicaid.gov/Medicaid-CHIP-Program-Information/By-Topics/Data-and-Systems/ICD-Coding/Downloads/icd-10-implementation-assistance-handbook.pdf.
ICD, International Classification of Diseases.
*Not always the case for ICD-9-CM.
†Not always the case for ICD-10.

TABLE 17-2	COMPARISON OF ICD-9-CM AND ICD-10-PCS CODES	
CHARACTERISTIC	**ICD-9-CM**	**ICD-10-PCS**
Field Length	3-4 characters	7 alpha-numeric characters; all are required
Available Codes	Approximately 3,000	Approximately 72,081
Technology	Based on outdated systems	Consistent with current medical technology and advances
Available Space for New Codes	Limited	Flexible
Overall Detail Embedded within Codes	Ambiguous	Very Specific Precisely defines procedures with detail regarding anatomic site, approach, device used, and qualifying information
Laterality	Code does *not* identify right vs. left	Code identifies right versus left
Terminology for Body Parts	Generic description	Detailed description
Procedure Description	Lacks description of approach for procedures	Detailed description of approach for procedures. Precisely defines procedures with detail regarding anatomic site, approach, device used, and qualifying information
Character Position within Code	N/A	There are 16 PCS sections that identify procedures in a variety of classifications (e.g., medical surgical, mental health, etc.). Between these sections, there may be variations in the meaning of various character positions, though the meaning is consistent within each section. For example, in the Medical Surgical section, Character 1 = Name of Section* Character 2 = Body System* Character 3 = Root Operation* Character 4 = Body Part* Character 5 = Approach* Character 6 = Device* Character 7 = Qualifier*
Example Code Laparoscopic Appendectomy	47.01	0DTJ4ZZ

From ICD-10 State Medicaid Readiness Medicaid ICD10 Implementation Handbook.docx. Retrieved January 14, 2013 from http://www.medicaid.gov/Medicaid-CHIP-Program-Information/By-Topics/Data-and-Systems/ICD-Coding/Downloads/icd-10-implementation-assistance-handbook.pdf.
ICD, International Classification of Diseases.
*For the "Medical Surgical" codes.

TABLE 17-3	COUNTRIES THAT USE ICD-10 CODES
YEAR ADOPTED	**COUNTRY**
1994 to 1997	Scandinavian countries (Denmark, Finland, Iceland, Norway, Sweden)
1995	United Kingdom
1997	France
1998	Australia
1999	Belgium
2000	Germany
2001	Canada
2014 or 2015 (projected)	United States • Original compliance date was October 1, 2013 • AMA and HHS requested delay to October 1, 2014, but this will probably be extended to 2015

Adapted from Brooks P (2010) ICD-10 Overview. http://www.cms.gov/Medicare/Medicare-Contracting/ContractorLearningResources/downloads/ICD-10_Overview_Presentation.pdf, slide 15. 2010.

diagnostic or treatment options based on the individual needs of the patient. Some healthcare providers strongly object to a preconfigured EBP order set, referring to it as "cookbook medicine," and resist incorporating it into practice. Berner offers an analogy of CDS including EBP similar to the nursing process of the traditional "five rights" for medication administration: "The clinical delivery system should provide the *Right* information to the *Right* person in the *Right* format through the *Right* channel at the *Right* time."[9(p7)]

A major stumbling block to EBP is the continuous discovery of new knowledge and the resulting changes to the recommended best practices guidelines embedded in EHRs. Commercial products can assist organizations in updating protocols by providing current EBP clinical solutions, such as order sets and care plans. Most major EHRs have been upgraded with common CDS features that help to meet some of the specific MU mandates, such as alerts for critical lab results or a history of MRSA (methicillin-resistant *Staphylococcus aureus*) on new admissions, pregnancy warnings on select medications and diagnostic tests, drug allergies, drug–drug interactions, drug–diagnosis warnings, dosage range limits, the capture of specific data such as smoking status and advance directives, and immunization reminders.

The advantages of using a system that incorporates evidence-based content and CDS include the following:

- Defines standardized, appropriate care and reduces variability of care for common diagnoses.
- Defines local or facility-owned orderables (elements that can be ordered using computerized provider order entry, or CPOE) available at that setting.
- Triggers alerts and other CDS features based on locally built logic (rules). For instance, an alert may be triggered if (1) blood products are ordered on patients who request no blood products be administered, (2) pregnancy category teratogenic medications are ordered on patients of child-bearing age with an unknown pregnancy status, or (3) the potassium level is below a preset level on patients receiving digoxin medications.
- Collects detailed metrics for specific reports required to demonstrate meeting MU criteria. These reports address a variety of MU requirements such as patient education, smoking status assessment, native language, discharge instructions, deep vein thrombosis prophylaxis in select patient populations, and the use of thrombolytic and antithrombotic medications in stroke patients.
- Enables a more timely update of treatment plans based on best practices. The study Translating Research Into Practice (TRIP), conducted by researchers sponsored by the Agency for Healthcare Research and Quality (AHRQ) in 1999, concluded that it took an average of 10 to 20 years to incorporate new clinical findings into general clinical practice.[10] This time lag between the discovery of new treatment options and the use of this new knowledge at the point of care is sometimes call the "fatal lag." CDS and EBP are likely to accelerate the incorporation of new findings into clinical practice.

Patient Safety and Improved Quality of Care

Before MU rules were initiated most healthcare leadership and professionals cited patient safety as the primary reason for implementing an EHR, but it now may seem to some that the sole reason for implementing an EHR is to qualify for the incentive package. In response to this concern, leadership needs to communicate to staff that the primary deciding factors for implementing or upgrading an EHR include patient safety, improved quality of patient care, and efficiency. ARRA is not the reason for the implementation or upgrade but rather is the match that has ignited the process. Reinforcing this message on a regular basis through all the stages of the implementation cycle helps to counteract resistance to using the system due to major changes in workflows.

For example, EHRs help to decrease medication errors, especially if closed-loop bedside bar-coding medication administration is an integral piece of the system. Quality of care and outcomes improve when decision support mechanisms, standardized order sets, and care plans based on best practices are incorporated in the EHR. Besides being aware of all of the positive functionalities and advantages of the EHR, staff also need to be well informed on what the EHR cannot do.

Major implementations can include major pushbacks from hospital staff for a variety of reasons. A primary reason is that a major implementation often involves changes in workflows and processes. This will result in a temporary decrease in productivity, particularly in the early stages when clinicians are still learning the system. In addition, while the new system may offer significant advantages to the institution, the individual practitioner may be more aware of the disadvantages for them as individuals. For example, with initial implementations that move processes from paper to computer, clinicians accustomed to writing orders quickly or checking off boxes on a preprinted order set often resist spending their time entering orders on a computer. Although more time is needed to enter orders electronically, other gains are made, such as a decrease in medication errors, reduced time between order entry and delivery of services, and a dramatic decrease in telephone calls from nursing and pharmacy to physicians about illegible or questionable orders.

In a paper world, some healthcare providers created their own personal order sets for their practice and titled them using their own name, such as Dr. Smith's Routine Admission Orders for Surgery. Once records become electronic, personalized order sets are discouraged. Each specialty should collaborate to create a single order set for each of its common procedures, diagnoses, surgeries, and admissions, incorporating EBP. This approach minimizes wide variances in care and avoids an IT maintenance nightmare to keep individual physicians' order sets up to date. One of the most important success factors in the implementation of an electronic health system is to involve as many users as possible in the design and planning of that system and discuss the inevitable changes to workflows, processes, policies, and procedures.[11]

The number of unnecessary verbal or telephone orders has long been a major patient safety issue even though certifying organizations voice strong warnings against using them too often for convenience reasons. The Joint Commission (TJC) has a standard requiring that all verbal and telephone orders be recorded and "read back" to the ordering healthcare provider.[12] This scenario exemplifies another source of clinician frustration because the clinician must remain on the telephone while the person recording the verbal order retrieves the electronic record, enters it into the system, goes through all prompts, and reads the order back to the ordering practitioner. One study examined the number of verbal and telephone orders pre-CPOE and post-CPOE and reported a 12% reduction in the number of verbal orders and a 34% decrease in unsigned verbal orders after implementation.[13]

Using the EHR to perform a task for which it is not designed or using a poorly designed system may produce poor results or outcomes. Published studies report a variety of unintended consequences for EHRs. Ash, Sittig, Dykstra, Campbell, and Guappone identified nine types of unintended consequences and corresponding interventions to minimize each of these risks.[14] A few of the unintended consequences are associated with human error, such as selecting the wrong patient or the wrong medication from a list. They refer to this type of error as a juxtaposition error. Recommended strategies to decrease unintended consequences are very similar to best practices for a successful implementation discussed below.[15] Weiner, Kfuri, Chan, and Fowles coined a new term, *e-iatrogenesis*, to describe the most critical of the new type of errors seen in EHRs.[16] Other types of errors include users who fail to validate or read the list of all orders entered during a session before final acceptance or who accept the defaults for select orders without review.

The EHR may use Tall Man lettering (i.e., the use of mixed-case lettering) for look-alike names of medications recommended by the Institute for Safe Medication Practices (ISMP). Studies indicate that using mixed-case lettering in similar drug names helps to decrease medication errors during order entry, medication dispensing, and medication administration by highlighting the differences in the drug names. A few examples of medication names using Tall Man lettering are NiFEDipine versus niCARdipine, DOBUTamine versus DOPamine, and CISplatin versus CARBOplatin.[17]

Another safety benefit associated with the implementation of an EHR is that it can enforce the use of CMS-approved abbreviations. In addition, EHRs can incorporate real-time updates or revisions to the order item master (a master list of orderable items) and electronic order sets. For example, Darvon and Darvocet were recalled in 2010 because of serious cardiac arrhythmias. Institutions with EHRs were able to quickly remove these medications from the pharmacy formulary, automatically inactivating Darvon and Darvon equivalents on all electronic order sets in their EHRs.

NEW IMPLEMENTATION VERSUS AN UPGRADE

Once the decision has been made that a major change is needed in the current information system, the next question is whether to upgrade or implement a new system. Answering the question "do we need to make a change?" begins to answer the follow-up question: "What specific changes are needed?" The institution or healthcare provider should begin by determining what level or degree of change is needed to achieve MU. If there already is a well-established homegrown system, it usually is wiser to upgrade. However, this can best be determined by using the EACH process.

Decision Factors to Implement or Upgrade a System

Many competing factors must be evaluated in deciding whether to implement a new system or upgrade the current system.

Sufficient Resources

The three major resources that will have the most impact on this decision are staff, budget, and physical or environmental constraints. Having a sufficient number of available and knowledgeable staff with the specific skill sets needed for each step in the process is imperative to the success of the project. The needed skill sets relate to the following:

- Installing and testing new hardware, software, and wireless networks
- Designing, building, and modifying applications
- Testing new applications and interfaces
- Providing staff education and support
- Maintaining hardware, software, and wireless networks.

The project manager will usually create a grid of all resource assignments for easy tracking and reference. Regardless of the type of project, informatics projects are expensive and often incur unexpected costs for unexpected items such as adding computer memory, upgrading wireless systems, and developing new interfaces. Funds must be allocated for staff, servers, hardware such as new computers, scanners, printers, wiring, antennas, training rooms, software, and postlive vendor support. Physical requirements may include creating additional space in the clinical units, patient rooms, dictation areas, doctor lounges, etc.

Risk Factors

A good project plan identifies all probable and possible risk factors that may interfere with achieving a successful project completed on time, with sufficient quality, and within budget. A risk management plan lists corresponding reasonable strategies to mitigate the identified risks. Some risk factors can be anticipated with plans to minimize their effect, such as an upcoming accreditation inspection, the possibility of a strike by workers, new construction, and remodeling. Unexpected risk factors may be a loss of key project players, a publicized sentinel event, or a natural disaster in the area.

Scope Creep

Scope creep is one of the most frequent causes of project delays. Scope creep occurs when requirements are added after the initial project is defined and those added requirements are substantial enough to affect the project timeline.

Well-defined objectives for the parameters of the project and strong project management can help to minimize scope creep. However, even with the best planning some informatics projects must be expanded for valid yet unanticipated reasons. There are several reasons for scope creep. Sometimes users do not understand the product until they interact with it. They then realize that the system will not meet their needs, creating an impetus to incorporate changes in the product and project plan. Likewise, the extent of workflow changes may not be apparent until the EHR is piloted. Sometimes projects that begin as an upgrade shift to the implementation of a totally new system due to changes in leadership and management, new regulations, and new enhancements or options that are now viewed as critical.

Best of Breed versus an Integrated Health System

There are two approaches to implementing an EHR: (1) best of breed and (2) monolithic or fully integrated EHR. The best of breed approach involves reviewing several vendors for their "best" module or application, such as an admission, discharge, and transfer (ADT) system or emergency department module. Then multiple modules are purchased from different vendors to create a full suite of functions. Purchase decisions are based on each module's or application's most desired or robust features and connectivity capabilities. This approach typically provides the customer with tools to customize the application according to local, specialized needs. Vendors typically incorporate enhancement requests more quickly in a hot fix (fast fix), through software patches (fixes), or in the next version. Both of these advantages can be important to large medical or research-intensive university centers. The disadvantages to this approach are the need for multiple complex interfaces to integrate all of the products; the need for highly skilled and specialized IT staff to support the different interfaces; and the existence of various hardware platforms and operating systems that may be on different versions of software and therefore complicate integration. Lastly, each module may have a different user interface, meaning that each application looks and acts differently to the end users. All of these factors make the best of breed approach more expensive and resource intensive but it is frequently selected by large medical, university, and research medical centers.

A monolithic or fully integrated health information system is an electronic health record system that includes a suite of modules to support care. It is typically easier to install and easier to support and usually has a similar-looking user interface across modules, which helps users to learn the EHR more quickly. Because all applications share a common database, the information exchange among the modules is quicker. The initial installation is frequently faster and less expensive because a scaled-down IT department is required at the local site. Smaller medical facilities and those not wanting large IT departments tend to favor this approach. The downside is that the system may not have specific features that the health facility needs and vendors often have applications that are excellent for some areas and less optimal for others. In addition, the customer cannot easily customize the system without assistance from the vendor, which may involve a work order and additional cost. System changes can incur long delays from large vendors as they prioritize changes across many clients. For example, orders for TPN (total parenteral nutrition) are generally customized to the patient's needs and are difficult to construct for CPOE (computerized provider order entry). Thus TPN orders may remain on paper and be faxed to the Pharmacy department. Of course, having both paper and electronic orders creates a fragmented health record, potential safety issues, and issues with workflow.

Opportunities for Improvement

The decision to implement a new system or to upgrade an existing one provides an opportunity to increase patient safety and quality of care, enhance communication, increase EBP, and create more efficient workflows and processes. A new system allows the organization to thoroughly evaluate, correct, and clean up a current database to address common issues such as misspellings, order names that do not comply with established naming conventions, and the addition of helpful aliases for orders. In most scenarios multiple analysts will build the EHR system, especially in a multifacility enterprise. The IT team, which includes members with technical and clinical expertise, must emphasize that all analysts use the same style, such as a specified naming convention and uniform data assays (or elements), so that all orders or charting screens have a consistent look and feel. Defining a naming convention includes decisions about details such as building applications using all capitals or mixed case and commas versus dashes, colon or a space, and an understanding to not use specific special characters, such as semi-colons, ampersands, or backward slashes, in order names that may be misinterpreted as a part of a Health Level Seven (HL7) message. Sometimes order names were originally built in an ancillary system such as a laboratory or radiology system and abbreviated with archaic or cryptic acronyms that are understood only by that department but are not meaningful to the clinician. These department-specific systems were likely standalone applications that did not interface with other applications. Once they are integrated, older department-specific orders need to be reviewed and renamed to be more user-friendly to clinicians. When different builders are constructing new orders and not adhering to a naming convention over the lifespan of the CPOE application, the orderables cannot be found easily by clinicians. For example, radiology may have orders that start with a modality like "CT Head w Cont." Other computed tomography (CT) orders may start with the body part, as in "Head CT w/o Cont." Some orders may spell out "with" or abbreviate it using "w" or "w/." This lack of standardization can result in alphabetized lists that clinicians do not understand, long search times by clinicians, and sending incorrect orders to radiology. This issue is very important in CPOE applications because orders will not line up alphabetically when a clinician searches for "CT HEAD" if dashes, colons, or spaces are used inconsistently.

A common mistake in the implementation of a new EHR is replacing a legacy system but designing the new system with old workflows and processes. Organizations should resist building a new system to imitate the current system or current workflows; rather, they should evaluate the system and transform to more updated evidence-based efficient processes. If this is ignored, a risk exists that the new EHR will merely automate and magnify broken processes that exist in the current organization and system.

Another improvement that often accompanies a new implementation or an upgrade is the introduction of more advanced decision support features not available in the older system. Features not available in older EHRs typically are duplicate order checking; codified (coded) allergies; allergy checking against medication and diet orders; drug–drug, drug–food, and drug–diagnosis interactions; dose checking; weight-based medication dosages; suggested drug level monitoring; automatic discontinuation of controlled substances; and the display of critical lab values *during* order entry before orders are placed. Older pharmacy systems performed these checks *after* order entry, requiring the pharmacist to contact the ordering healthcare provider when alerts were displayed, thereby delaying the first medication dose to the patient. More recent EHRs employ logic, allowing the institution to create rule-based logic for specific scenarios or variables, such as patient gender, age, weight, diagnosis, patient location, active order list, and other miscellaneous attributes. Examples of rule-based logic follow:

- Patient allergies and the patient's height and weight must be entered in the system before orders on a patient are entered but can be overridden in emergencies
- An alert is triggered when a provider orders a blood product be administered to a patient who is a Jehovah's Witness
- An alert is triggered when a clinician orders a radiology test that requires contrast on a patient with a documented allergy to iodine

IMPLEMENTATION AND THE SYSTEMS LIFE CYCLE

Successful implementations follow the systems life cycle introduced in Chapter 2. To summarize, the main phases of the systems life cycle are as follows:

- *Analyze:* The existing environment and systems are evaluated. Major problems and deficiencies are identified using informal or formal methods. A needs assessment is developed. Gaps are noted and current capabilities and limitations are outlined. Initial user and system requirements are formulated.
- *Plan:* The proposed system is planned comprehensively. Planning includes strategic levels, such as whether the system will be developed internally, purchased and tailored, or designed and developed jointly with a vendor.
- *Develop or purchase:* At this stage either the system is purchased or the new system development begins. New

components and programs are obtained and installed. For vendor-supported solutions, extensive tailoring occurs.

- *Test:* At this stage extensive testing occurs just before Stage 5 and "go" or "no go" decisions are made about deadlines. Toward the end of this phase, marketing and communication efforts are accelerated to make users aware of the impending change.
- *Implement or go-live:* The system is implemented using a selected method best suited to the organization and its tolerance for risk. User training is completed.
- *Maintain and evolve:* Once the system has been formally acknowledged as passing user acceptance testing, typically at 90 or 120 days after go-live, it enters a maintenance phase.
- *Evaluate:* Activities in each phase are assessed for their quality and effectiveness.

For purposes of discussion, Chapter 16 assumes that the institution would purchase a new system. This chapter follows up after that point by presenting reasons to upgrade. Once an option is selected, the institution will move forward to the implementation phase of the systems life cycle.

Project Planning

The process of project planning occurs throughout the systems life cycle. Two key points in the life cycle when planning becomes more intense are (1) the planning required for system selection and (2) the planning required for system implementation. Chapter 16 discusses planning related to system selection. In this chapter the discussion focuses on the process of project planning as it relates to system implementation. Students interested in more information about project planning and project management principles can consult the Project Management Institute (www.pmi.org) or a project management text. Large organizations typically employ a project manager certified in project management techniques.

Defining Success

One of the first planning steps includes defining the project and its success factors. Before an implementation can be called a success, the term *success* must be defined using measurable terms or goals. An example might be reducing medication errors by 15% by installing medication and bar-coding applications. Any required baseline metrics should be determined and measured before implementation if post go-live comparisons are required (Box 17-1). Other examples are pre and post statistics for the number of pharmacy callbacks to physicians; the volume of nonformulary medications; and the time between order entry and first medication dose, especially for critical medications such as tissue plasminogen activator (tPA); the time between "stat" order entry and order completion; the percentage of suspected acute myocardial infarction patients who receive aspirin within 24 hours before or after arrival at the emergency department; the number of duplicate laboratory or radiology orders; and the number of verbal or telephone orders with a documented read-back.[18]

- Project team defines a clear scope of the project.
- Senior leadership, clinical leaders, and EHR champions provide enthusiastic and unwavering support for the project.
- Employ a health IT professional to lead the project and be sure to have adequate resources.
- Solicit input from representatives from each discipline at every stage of the initiative.
- Have default clinical information and responses to order prompts on orders and fill in as much as possible on order sets.
- Consider mandatory use of computerized provider order entry (CPOE).
- Educate users, particularly physicians, on the trade-off of initial reduced productivity and time to perform ordinary tasks such as order entry with long-term positive gains of reduced callbacks, reduced time between order entry and first dose medications and "stat" orders, and "everywhere" access to the chart. If clinicians understand and are educated on why the change was made, they tend to be accepting of the change.
- Examine and develop collaborative detailed plans for the anticipated changes in current workflows early in the project with a sign-off from each user group.
- Provide one-on-one education to physicians and a dedicated physician liaison.
- TEST, TEST, TEST the system from every user's perspective.
- TRAIN, TRAIN, TRAIN: Provide ample education to IT staff and end-users.
- Use the "train the trainer" approach for maximum mileage.
- Use superusers for go-live and post go-live support.
- Provide abundant support during go-live and 7 to 10 days following go-live.
- Anticipate user resistance and plan for it.
- Possess an understanding that there is no finish line for EHR maintenance.
- Have a strong resolve, knowing that the project will be difficult.

Whether undertaking a new implementation or an upgrade, organizations will want to adhere to solid project management principles, such as the use of a project plan. It is essential that the implementation team creates a comprehensive and detailed project plan that includes all of the critical milestones, assumptions, and tasks with target dates and assigned resources. The project plan can be created using Microsoft Office Excel but most facilities use more sophisticated applications specifically designed for project planning, such as Microsoft Office Project (Fig. 17-1). The project plan includes resources across the organization in IT and clinical and the use of superusers. Superusers are selected staff who receive extra training and help to provide additional support during the go-live process.

Facilities should develop a go-live theme, such as giving the implementation project an official name and a slogan, reference the project name each time the implementation is discussed, and start early with a slogan and use it continuously throughout the project for activities such as project marketing with pamphlets, posters, flyers, and announcements. Some organizations will also select a color scheme and use it for all publicity, communications, updates, banners, posters, table tents, and T-shirts or buttons that support staff may wear during the go-live. Large facilities will have a marketing plan for the project, especially closer to go-live.

Executive Management Support

A second planning step includes eliciting the support of organization executives. One of the key factors for a successful implementation or upgrade is public attestation and repeated unwavering support for the project by the executive team. This kind of support is needed from the project's kickoff day to after go-live. Leaders need to communicate this message to the organization at every possible opportunity and on a regular basis.[19,20] This commitment is especially critical when users, particularly physicians, repeatedly escalate EHR issues, such as difficulties with CPOE, to the executive suite with requests that could undermine the project. Regarding issues with CPOE, some healthcare organizations mandate that physicians enter orders into CPOE modules with a few well-defined exceptions. Organizations that have more success with such mandates include those that employ a large percentage of physicians, such as the military and Veterans Health Administration. Other tactics used to deal with CPOE resistance include policies that instruct nurses and unit secretaries to inform physicians that they are not allowed to enter orders on a physician's behalf. However, if the physician submits a complaint against a staff member as a result, executive management must support this policy when challenged.

Engage Stakeholders

Another important factor in planning is to solicit input from representatives in every discipline from the beginning and continue to inform them of the progress of the project.[21] Informatics governance structures discussed in Chapter 10 provide representation for stakeholder groups. Savvy implementers will ensure that voices from each group are heard. One of the most effective methods for engaging stakeholders is to involve them in the analysis of current workflow processes and the redesign of those processes.

Redesigned Workflows

As mentioned earlier, a new system will change the current workflows, processes, and policies. Redesigned workflows require preparation so that professional practice processes match the available EHR functions. This early work is imperative to preclude modified workflows or negative workarounds (a method used to circumvent a problem without solving it). New policies need to be adopted for new

COMPUTERIZED ORDER ENTRY (CPOE) PLAN

PART I. SYSTEM SELECTION	RESOURCE(S)	DECEMBER 6	13	20	27	JANUARY 3	10	17	24	31
RESPONSIBLE GROUPS/INDIVIDUALS IDENTIFIED		▓								
Establish CPOE Steering Committee										
Establish CPOE Advisory Committee										
INITIAL DATA COLLECTION		▓	▓	▓	▓					
Identify all current and overlapping projects related to CPOE										
Review literature with focus on real installations										
Obtain CPOE related guidelines/regulations										
Develop list of vendors that offer CPOE										
Develop list of institutions/contacts with CPOE experience										
Identify all upstream and downstream information systems that will interface with CPOE										
DEVELOPMENT OF GOALS AND BENEFITS						▓	▓	▓		
Prepare draft of goals and benefits										
Present draft goals to Steering Committee										
Finalize CPOE goals and benefits										
Develop feasibility statement										
Send requests for information (RFI) to potential vendors										
RFP DRAFT DEVELOPMENT AND DISTRIBUTION							▓	▓	▓	▓
Conduct site visits										
Define and prioritize system requirements										
Review and revise the Request for Proposal (RFP)										
Develop criteria and mechanisms for response evaluation										
Prepare draft RFP and present to Steering Committee										
Finalize and distribute RFP to potential vendors										
RECEIPT OF VENDOR RESPONSES										
VENDOR PROPOSAL ANALYSIS AND SELECTION										
Evaluate responses to RFP										
Conduct vendor demonstrations and site visits										
Develop system proposal and recommendations										
Present options to Steering Committee										
Select option										

FIG 17-1 Sample timeline. The timeline in its entirety is posted with the Evolve resources for this chapter. *CPOE,* Computerized provider order entry. (Copyright McKesson Corporation.)

workflows. All current workflows and processes need to be assessed in successful implementations. The best approach to obtaining this information is to schedule separate meetings with representatives from each department, being certain to include unit secretaries, who frequently know the unofficial workarounds. Actual end-users are important to include in the process. While department or unit managers can easily provide the organization's approved workflows and processes, they may not be aware of the unofficial workarounds used by the staff. In short, the goals of scheduled meetings with each department are to identify all current official and unofficial workflows and processes and to plan the future workflows and processes using the EHR's new functionalities so that users can anticipate how their jobs will change. At these separate meetings the areas of overlap or instances where workflow moves from one department to another should be noted.

These can be critical and sometimes difficult points in planning a redesigned workflow. Redesigned workflows and planned changes must be included and thoroughly reviewed in all end-user training classes.

Building or Tailoring the Product

Once the current workflow is understood and redesigned, teams work to build or tailor the EHR to match the new workflow. Typically, clinical analysts work with vendor analysts to tailor a product for the current environment or actual end-users may be involved in the process. At a minimum, once a module is initially tailored analysts have end-users assess the module in an iterative fashion. The following tips can be useful in this design process:

- Design and build the system to keep the number of clicks and amount of scrolling to an absolute minimum. Physicians in particular will calculate the time it takes to perform common tasks. Excess clicking can be a huge user dissatisfier and can discourage users. To avoid excessive clicks, implementation analysts often use what is commonly referred to as the 80/20 rule. The term *80/20* refers to a mathematical formula proposed by an Italian economist in 1906 that states that 80% of our results or outcomes are derived from 20% of our efforts or causes.[22] An example of applying the 80/20 rule in health informatics is to assign default responses when a specific response is selected 80% of the time. For instance, builders will prefill as many of the fields as possible in order entry with prompts such as "Routine" for the priority and "Once" for the frequency for all laboratory and radiology orders to facilitate faster order entry. The underlying rule is to minimize all keystrokes and excessive scrolling whenever possible. Default settings can be especially useful in saving time but they also need to be evaluated carefully to ensure that they do not increase safety issues.

- Do not ask clinicians to respond to prompts that they cannot answer. For example, most radiology systems have a mandatory prompt for "Method of Transportation." Physicians most likely do not know if the patient requires a gurney or a wheelchair, and will typically select the first option to place the order. Some organizations now use a default of "Wheelchair" or a term such as "Call Unit" for the "Method of Transportation." Avoid the overuse of alerts in order to minimize alert fatigue. Alert fatigue occurs when a user becomes desensitized to pop-ups or alerts if too many are triggered during an average session. Set the level of sensitivity so that only critical medical alerts fire and those with marginal clinical significance are suppressed.

- Maintain a consistent look and feel to the screens so the same information is always found in the same place and color coding is consistent on every screen. Ideally this consistency should extend across vendors and institutional departments.

Testing

Implementing or upgrading an electronic health system involves extensive testing. The different types of testing must be carefully planned and conducted throughout the project. These include hardware, software, and functional testing. Functional testing is used to determine whether the system functions as designed and works effectively with the newly structured work processes. All testing should be done first within a module. Once all modules are functioning correctly, integrated testing across modules is performed using patient flow scenarios. Table 17-4 outlines several different types of testing that are often part of the testing protocol.

A test plan is often created in a spreadsheet format. The plan should include fields for the name of the test, date of the test, name of the tester, log-in used for the test, role of the

TABLE 17-4	DIFFERENT TYPES OF TESTING DURING AN IMPLEMENTATION AND POST GO-LIVE	
TESTING TYPE	**DESCRIPTION**	**EXAMPLES**
ADT testing (see Fig. 17-2)	ADT testing involves testing for every possible type of ADT transaction used in the organization for inpatients, outpatients, serial patients, and preadmits. These transactions include admit; discharge; transfer; cancel admit; cancel discharge; cancel transfer; change beds, rooms, or departments; merge accounts; etc.	The tester will ask registration to admit several new patients. Tester will verify that patient is in correct department, room, and bed and all data entered during admission are correct. Admissions then will cycle through the various transactions with the tester validating each change.
Unit testing and functional testing	Unit testing is a very basic type of testing where the tester runs through the basic functionalities and features of an application. It is a high-level cursory walk-through of the application. The goal is to identify deviations from the expectations and to correct these unexpected results. The tester will not test every order or documentation field but will need to test every possible scenario.	For a CPOE application the tester will enter interfaced and noninterfaced orders in the application and follow them through. The tester will verify that order details display appropriately and that orders are received in the ancillary system.

Continued

TABLE 17-4	DIFFERENT TYPES OF TESTING DURING AN IMPLEMENTATION AND POST GO-LIVE—cont'd	
TESTING TYPE	**DESCRIPTION**	**EXAMPLES**
Integrated testing	Integrated testing tests the transmission of messages between all systems such as the healthcare information system, laboratory, radiology, pharmacy, dietary, cardiology, etc. This test includes testing all bidirectional order messages and results going across the interface(s).	The tester will enter different kinds of orders in the CPOE system to interfaced ancillary applications like laboratory, radiology, pharmacy, dietary, and cardiology and then cycle through all actions that are permitted per user role, including canceling the order, discontinuing the order, modifying the order, holding the order, etc. This also includes testing "unsolicited" orders, orders that originate in an ancillary system. An example of an unsolicited order is when the laboratory system initiates an order in response to the result of a previous order such as performing an HIV Western blot if HIV antibody is positive.
Hardware testing	Hardware testing includes the capability of hardware interfacing with the EHR such as computers, printers, label printers, bar code printers, tablets, scanners, modems, etc.	The IT team will test that diet requisitions print in the dietary department but dietitian consults print to the dietitian's office at the specific times based on table settings. Another example is that lab labels print in the patient departments for specimens that are collected by the nurse but print in the lab for specimens that are collected by lab personnel.
Volume testing	Volume testing is sometimes called "stress testing." Systems are built to accommodate the largest number of users accessing the system at the same time with no or minimal reduction in overall performance.	Early morning physician rounding and early afternoons are typically peak times for accessing the EHR. This type of testing may include asking a large group of students to log on and perform a variety of tasks simultaneously.
Security testing	Different staff members will have different reasons to access an EHR and their roles will define what they can and cannot do in the system. Security testing checks that each provider type is able to perform functionalities specific to the role (entering orders, vital signs, nursing documentation, viewing results, medication reconciliation, etc.) but is prohibited from unauthorized actions, viewing, or access.	The IT department will validate that nursing assistants have the security to document vital signs, height, weight, I&O, and percentage of meals consumed but not be able to review the chart or enter orders. Another example is that a physician or RN can perform medication reconciliation with a change in the level of care but a nursing assistant cannot.
ARRA-related Meaningful Use testing	With the introduction of Meaningful Use, eligible providers, hospital organizations, and Critical Access Hospitals (CAH) must test their ability to collect required information and demonstrate that they meet Meaningful Use criteria.	A few of the CMS requirements for MU Stage 1 include: • Assessing all patients for VTE prophylaxis • Recording smoking status on more than 50% of patients 13 years and older • Recording advance directives for more than 50% of patients 65 years and older • Providing more than 50% of patients with an electronic copy of their discharge instructions at time of discharge, upon request • Reporting hospital clinical quality measures to CMS or the states

ADT, Admission, discharge, and transfer; *ARRA,* American Recovery and Reinvestment Act; *CMS,* Centers for Medicare & Medicaid Services; *CPOE,* computerized provider order entry; *EHR,* electronic health record; *I&O,* intake and output; *IT,* information technology; *RN,* registered nurse; *VTE,* venous thromboembolism.

tester (MD, NP, RN, RT, US, etc.), test objective, and test instructions. An example of such a test plan is shown in Figure 17-2.

The testing process requires that a testing environment be created within the organization's electronic system. Box 17-2

lists the different environments that are usually created in order to install and maintain a healthcare information system. These environments can be conceptualized as copies of the same application. Using the test environment to execute test plans, the implementation team will develop detailed test

Date:			Tester Ext:
Tester Name:			**Tester Dept.**

Application:
ABC Clinical System
Test Title:
ADT Test PLAN
Test Objective:
To test each inbound and outbound ADT interface planned for the system
Test Conditions:
Only test message types relevant to customer site

Test Instructions:

1. Review the test steps defined below and execute the steps as they are written. Please attempt to execute all steps of the test.
2. Review the expected results for each step.
3. If the result is achieved, select PASS in the Status column.
4. If a different result is achieved, select FAIL in the Status column.
5. If the result is Fail, describe the actual outcome in the Actual Outcome/Exception Description column.
6. If you are unable to execute a step because of a defect or an error, try to navigate to a point where you can resume the steps and indicate what you did in the Actual Outcome column.
7. If it is not possible to continue with the test, indicate what happens in the Actual Outcome column.

Test Execution & Results:

Step #	Step Description	Test Data	Expected Results	Date Executed	Status	Actual Outcome/ Exception Description	Issue ID	Pass	Fail
			ADT						
1			**(A01) Admit Pt**						
1.01	Admit a patient in the HIS system. Assign a station, room, and bed.		Interface receives an ADT A01 message. Message posts successfully. Patient visit accessible in HealthView.					0	0
1.02								0	0
1.03								0	0
2			**(A02) Transfer Pt**						
2.01	Transfer a patient in the HIS system to a different station, room, or bed.		Interface receives an ADT A02 message. Message posts successfully. Patient visit accessible in Healthview, with correct location.					0	0
2.02								0	0
2.03								0	0
3			**(A03) Discharge Pt**						
3.01	Discharge a patient in the HIS system.		Interface receives an ADT A03 message. Message posts successfully. Patient visit accessible in Healthview with discharge date.					0	0
3.02								0	0
3.03								0	0
4			**(A04) Register Pt**						
4.01	Register a patient in the HIS system.		Interface receives an ADT A04 message. Message posts successfully. Patient visit accessible in Healthview.					0	0
4.02								0	0
4.03								0	0
5			**(A05) Pre-Admit Pt**						
5.01	Pre-admit a patient in the HIS system.		Interface receives an ADT A05 message. Message posts successfully. Pre-admit patient visit accessible in Healthview.					0	0
5.02								0	0
5.03								0	0
6			**(A06) Transfer O/P to I/P**						
6.01	Transfer an outpatient visit to inpatient status. Assign to a station.		Interface receives an ADT A06 message. Message posts successfully. Patient visit accessible in Healthview in correct location.					0	0
6.02								0	0
6.03								0	0
7			**(A07) Transfer I/P to O/P**						
7.01	Transfer an inpatient visit to outpatient status.		Interface receives an ADT A07 message. Message posts successfully. Outpatient visit accessible in Healthview.					0	0
7.02								0	0
7.03								0	0
8			**(A08) Update Pt Info**						

FIG 17-2 Sample test plan. The plan in its entirety is posted with the Evolve resources for this chapter. *ADT*, Admission, discharge, and transfer; *HIS*, healthcare information system; *Pt*, patient. (Copyright McKesson Corporation.)

BOX 17-2   **HEALTHCARE INFORMATION SYSTEM ONLINE ENVIRONMENTS**

- *Live or Production* environment refers to the healthcare information system application's actual use with patient and hospital data. Testing and teaching should not be done using this environmnet since changes are very likely to affect patient care.
- *Build* environment refers to a copy of a healthcare information system application that is used to configure and customize an application. Building usually occurs at the module level. Once a module is designed it is moved to the test environment.
- *Test* environment refers to a copy of the healthcare information system application that is used to test the application. It should be a complete copy of the most recent version of the actual application. The test version of the software should not be an empty shell but should reflect the actual

type and amount of data one would expect to see in the live environment.
- *Teaching* environment refers to a copy of the healthcare information system application that is used for teaching users. Like the test version of the software, this version should not be an empty shell but should reflect the actual type and amount of data one would expect to see in the live environment.
- *Teaching/testing* environment refers to the combined use of a healthcare information system application for both testing and teaching activities. This does require careful scheduling since testing should not occur at the same time that a class is using the environment for teaching. However, the advantages are that this approach saves resources and using the test environment for teaching provides additional testing for the application.

---

plans for each staff group such as healthcare providers (physicians and mid-level providers such as physician assistants and advanced practice registered nurses), staff nurses, pharmacists, unit secretaries, and ancillary personnel for each application. Test plans evaluate information and data flow throughout the application including, for example, messages, allergies, orders, test and other diagnostic results, automatic and manually demanded reports, and archiving of the patient's record postdischarge. If this is an upgrade implementation, medical facilities often have ready-made test plans that they use with each upgrade but modify to accommodate changed or new functionalities, improved features, and fixes to previous defects. An upgrade test plan differs from a new implementation test plan in that the upgrade test plan typically has a short list of test items or orders for each department versus a new implementation that involves testing every item in the order item dictionary as well as every prompt and combination of prompt responses on each order. Testing includes all devices such as computers, printers, handheld devices, bar code scanners, etc.

PREPARING FOR GO-LIVE

Preparing for go-live involves deciding on the go-live approach, developing the go-live plan and schedule, and preparing the end-users.

Big Bang or Incremental Go-Lives

There are two approaches to a go-live: big bang or incremental (also called a phased or a staged approach). The big bang approach occurs when all applications or modules are implemented at once. This approach is favored by vendors and facilities conducting large upgrades. With a phased go-live approach, both paper and electronic environments exist at the same time within the healthcare institution; however, the existence of both paper and electronic environments forces the clinician to use different work flows in patient units that have implemented the system than in units that have not,

potentially creating safety concerns. The advantages of the big bang approach are that it is usually less expensive and implementation time is shorter, allowing staff to return to a new normal and see early improvements in the project metrics more quickly. The negatives associated with the big bang approach are the significant reductions in productivity seen immediately at go-live and for a short time afterwards due to users' unfamiliarity with the new system and a large influx of requests to tweak the system (Box 17-3).

The incremental approach is usually selected when a facility has limited resources that cannot support a housewide implementation or when the facility has a low tolerance for or ability to respond to institutional changes. There are a variety of ways to employ this method. Some facilities may decide to go-live with specific staff groups such as nurses, unit secretaries, and ancillary staff, including laboratory, pharmacy, radiology, respiratory therapy, physical therapy, occupational therapy, speech therapy, and dietary, followed by physicians and other clinicians a short time later. Others may choose to go-live with select clinical departments or product lines (e.g., patient flow within a specialty such as surgery). Reasons for selecting the first units to go-live may be based on their perceived support and enthusiasm for the project or their low number of admissions, transfers, and discharges. Advantages of the incremental approach are that it allows time to make changes to the build or the workflows and does not decrease productivity housewide while creating constant change for end-users. The early adopters or the new users of the initial departments normally will share their experiences, perceptions, and satisfaction with others. However, this communication can either support or speak against the project. The disadvantages include the potential for errors due to multiple systems and the possibility that the project can be protracted and workflow disruptions will occur over a longer period, although on a smaller scale. Another factor to consider with the incremental approach is the availability of support for each successive unit. Most vendors typically like to transition from their implementation or services team to

BOX 17-3   ADVANTAGES AND DISADVANTAGES OF THE BIG BANG APPROACH

ADVANTAGES	DISADVANTAGES
Eliminates staff having to use two systems or processes in different departments, which decreases the number of errors	Significant decrease in productivity in the initial days and immediately after go-live with a gradual return to baseline
Total cost of entire implementation is lower	Less time to make changes to the build or workflows
Project is less likely to stall and is more likely to fully implement the system	Changes in workflows and processes are turned on housewide with everyone on same learning curve, making implementation pain and anxiety greater
Shorter implementation cycle and shorter implementation pain	
Quicker improvements in electronic health record–related metrics (decreased use of nonformulary medications, decreased pharmacy callbacks)	Must plan for large number of support personnel in the information technology department and roaming superusers to all departments
Immediate compliance with American Recovery and Reinvestment Act–mandated requirements for Meaningful Use to receive "stimulus" funds	
On-site and remote support personnel and implementation consultants from the vendor are available for the initial days of the go-live	

BOX 17-4   ADVANTAGES AND DISADVANTAGES OF THE INCREMENTAL APPROACH

ADVANTAGES	DISADVANTAGES
Allows time to make changes to build and workflows with each new batch of users	Staff that circulate through the organization must use two workflows, which can increase the number of errors
Early reports of success breed enthusiastic support for the upcoming departments	Project may stall due to users' dislike of using different processes or workflows in different departments and changes that are made after each mini go-live
Less impact on productivity	
Restricts implementation pain to a smaller number of select users or departments	Total cost of entire implementation is higher due to extended support and training
	Longer implementation time with feelings that system is "not ready for prime time" and will not end soon enough
	Delays compliance with American Recovery and Reinvestment Act–mandated requirements for Meaningful Use to receive "stimulus" funds
	Most vendors transition customers to their support division within 2 to 4 weeks post go-live
	Early reports of dissatisfaction may dissuade others from embracing the system

the support team 2 to 4 weeks after initial go-live. Continued support can be expensive for organizations. This also means that the organization will be calling vendor employees who may not be familiar with the build, workflows, and customizations when issues arise with each new mini go-live. Repetitive go-lives also tax the IT department and the superusers and delay the deployment of fixes and physician requests from the initial go-live departments. Sometimes the rollout is more prolonged than originally planned or it may even stall indefinitely due to user dissatisfaction. The early go-live users who do not see quick resolution of easily fixed issues will complain because the support staff is too busy with the next go-live unit (Box 17-4).

Detailed Go-Live Plan

A detailed go-live plan includes each planned activity as a line item assigned to a specific individual or team with a completion date for each task. The go-live plan should include critical tasks that are scheduled to be completed a few days to a few weeks before the go-live date. Some project managers may break down the immediate days before go-live to the number of hours before go-live, marking tasks that must precede other tasks.

Education and Training

A common mistake in an implementation or upgrade is not planning sufficient time to thoroughly train end-users or failure to allot a sufficient budget to conduct training.[23] Education of all end-users is a mini project and is best assigned to a person or facility education department that can coordinate or oversee all of its components. In fact, training is complex enough that software support in the form of a learning management system (LMS) is often used. An LMS includes planning and tracking the end-users trained and the results of any competency tests. A training plan must address the development of teaching plans, training manuals, and job aids that provide instructions on common tasks and can be used during training and on the job. Different types of training must be developed for the different groups of end-users, including physicians, nurses, pharmacists, unit secretaries, students, and ancillary personnel such as respiratory therapy, rehabilitative services, clergy, quality control, etc. For example, physicians will need instruction on using CPOE, viewing test results, viewing charting, and performing medication reconciliation, while nurses will need education related to order entry, nursing documentation, and medication administration.

Questions to consider in planning education hours are the number of users to be educated, education methodology, the timing and length of the classes for each user group, the number of training rooms and training devices available, the training schedule, and trainers for each group. The content of the course should reflect the scope and standards for practice with role-specific processes, decisions, tasks, and supportive EHR functions for each group of users. During training, common user errors or system quirks should be highlighted to help the users to avoid them. MU-related tasks such as assessing smoking status, advance directives, and immunization status should also be addressed so that users understand the importance of completing those data fields. Privacy and security policies, including not sharing one's log-in and password and accessing only those medical records the user needs to review, should be emphasized in every class. The consequences for violating privacy and security policies and practices should also be stated clearly.

Trainers

Depending on the organization's structure, the trainers might be in-house staff, vendor educators, temporary consultants, superusers or power users, or a mix of these. If the organization is using a big bang approach, it will often need to bring in temporary trainers in order to get all users trained and then revert to in-house educators or superusers following go-live for new hires, system upgrades, and remediation training. The advantages of using in-house educators are that they are familiar with the organization's policies and usually have a background in adult education. Vendor educators and consultants frequently know the application very well but are not familiar with the organization's future workflows and policies. Superusers who can spend time with students who are having difficulties are valuable as assistants in the classroom. Training is an ongoing process that will continue after go-live to orient new hires and to address new responsibilities or changes in staff roles that consequently cause changing workflows.

Training Methodology

Most organizations use a combination of different training methods. One of the most popular methods is an instructor-led class in a classroom that contains all of the equipment needed to demonstrate essential functionalities, including printers, bar code scanners, identification bands, medication labels, etc. The advantages of instructor-led training are the ability for end-users to ask questions, quick clarification of complex concepts, and easy identification of users who may need additional help. The primary disadvantages are the expense and resources needed to have multiple instructor-led classes. In addition, the number of students per session is limited and no-shows are common among nurses and physicians since training competes with patient care needs. Another common training method includes a blended approach in which end-users complete an "anytime/anywhere" online module about EHR basics and then attend a brief instructor-led session. These are also used as mini-refreshers or primers during upgrades.[24] A major drawback to using a variety of approaches is the constant need to update all of the training materials with the introduction of new functionalities. No matter the approach, the use of competency tests to assess proficiency is recommended.

With a CPOE implementation, most organizations create a new position for CPOE liaisons who are dedicated to clinician training 24 hours a day, 7 days a week. Physicians may be unable or unwilling to attend scheduled classes and prefer just-in-time or one-on-one education.[25] Some organizations employ physician liaisons who are dedicated exclusively to assisting physicians. Even though this is a labor-intensive strategy, physicians quickly become adept at their new workflows, report greater user satisfaction, and have a greater likelihood of using and being satisfied with the new system.

Length of Class and Class Schedule

Depending on the EHR functions needed, class time will vary. For example, CPOE classes for unit secretaries in an organization where prescribers will be expected to use CPOE may be 2 to 3 hours whereas the same classes for nurses may require 6 to 8 hours. Once the total number of users and the number of hours for each learning module are determined a training schedule is developed, often using the LMS mentioned earlier. With a housewide go-live, training will need to be provided around the clock. If users must attend class during their off-duty time, organizations will have to consider paying overtime. Alternately, if user education is incorporated into the 40-hour workweek, replacement staff may be required. End users should not be expected to attend class immediately after a shift when they are most likely tired and may not be able to leave their department when planned. Education should be conducted as close to the go-live date as possible to facilitate retention of the new knowledge and skills with a goal of no more than 4 weeks prelive. Once a majority of employees has completed the training, the institution is ready for go-live.

GO-LIVE

During the initial weeks of the go-live, organizations must plan to provide close support ("elbow-to-elbow" support) for end-users. Many institutions will provide 24/7 support for a week or two and a few may offer it for several weeks. Assigning superusers wearing easily identifiable apparel to roam departments offering assistance to users is an excellent tactic that is well received by the end users. Issues, questions, and misunderstandings should be reported to the project team, which then catalogues, prioritizes, and tracks them for resolution and future reference.[16] Additional tips include the following:

- Avoid a go-live date that falls on a weekend, a Monday or Friday, or close to a major holiday when vendor support personnel may be less available. Two exceptions to this guideline are the implementation of a new financial system that must start at midnight on the first day of the month for billing purposes and a big-bang implementation, which is typically scheduled to start on a weekend to minimally affect surgery and procedure services.
- Set up an organized and well-equipped command center for the go-live that includes:
  - A highly publicized hotline number for assistance; incoming calls need to roll over to a bank of well-staffed phones.
  - A system for reporting, cataloging, assigning criticality, and assigning skilled resources to identified issues and problems.
- A hotline number is one communication method, but urgent issues need to be addressed and, if necessary, escalated immediately to the vendor or IT department for resolution. Stock the command center with supplies such as whiteboards, poster boards, phones with outside access, preprinted "Issue Reporting'" forms, printers, office supplies, meals, snacks, and water. Devices must be loaded with new software and integrated with upstream (ADT) and downstream (laboratory, radiology, pharmacy, dietary, electrocardiography, etc.) systems for immediate troubleshooting.
- Devise several different mechanisms to obtain and give user feedback in a timely manner.
- Include clearly identified people associated with the command center and project. For example, roaming superusers could wear an identifying T-shirt, vest, or large easy-to-read badge in the project 'color.'

Other go-live tactics include the following:
- Give small gifts to units (donuts or bakery items, boxes of candy, popcorn tins, balloons for desks).
- Use posters or banners in main lobbies, atriums, and waiting rooms.
- Provide a well-publicized process for end-users to communicate with the implementation team and change-control committee (which collects and prioritizes system changes).
  - Generic email address for users to ask questions, request a change or new item, or make suggestions, with prompt feedback to users' questions and requests.
  - Suggestion box that allows anonymous input and has scheduled collections.
  - Notebooks in staff lounges with scheduled pickups and returns.
  - Emails to all users that include FAQs and "Tips and Tricks."

POSTLIVE MAINTENANCE

A vendor-supported implementation is officially over when the system formally transitions from the vendor's services team to its support division. With in-house development, the project leader announces when the go-live is over. Maintenance is an ongoing process that involves a variety of tasks such as applications updates, patches for identified defects, and a continuous revision of the system in response to users' requests. This includes revising documentation screens, adding new content, creating new orders such as new medications, and inactivating obsolete content such as outdated interventions and medications that are no longer in the hospital formulary. The change control committee receives input for new content, such as newly defined order sets, as well as requests for revisions to current order sets so that they align with updated best practices. Users may discover system flaws that were not detected during testing and these need to be submitted to the change control committee and vendor. IT departments may conduct regularly scheduled rounds to the clinical units to solicit input from the users.

As mentioned earlier, major reasons to implement EHRs are patient safety, improved patient care, and clinical outcomes. One of the final tasks in the implementation plan is to evaluate whether and how the system made a difference according to the metrics identified and collected during the preimplementation phase. This collection of data is typically performed approximately 3 to 6 months after the go-live to allow users to become more proficient with the EHR. Implementing a new EHR or upgrading an older version is a process without a definitive end point. After installation an EHR will require software upgrades, new hardware, ongoing training of staff, and education of IT staff.[23]

CONCLUSION AND FUTURE DIRECTIONS

Meeting MU for Stage 2, expected to begin in 2014, and Stage 3 in 2016 will continue to spur growth of EHRs. In the future patients will likely interact with their healthcare providers more frequently via electronic means to set up appointments; send questions and requests for prescription refills; and be able to retrieve and review their health record, including test results. There will be movement away from stand-alone outpatient EHR systems and toward integrated systems. Mobile devices such as smartphones and iPads will play a larger role in patient–clinician relationships and nurse–patient–family relationships in the home. Health-related apps that allow for home monitoring of vital signs, blood glucose levels, electrocardiography monitoring, and fetal monitoring will become more commonplace.

In the future the U.S. may develop a registry to track EHR-related safety issues. The registry could be used to monitor safety and adverse issues and initiate timely notifications to medical providers and patients.[26] In a similar vein, the Institute of Medicine advocates the creation of a new federal agency or National EHR Safety Board under the auspices of HHS to oversee EHR safety. Presently there is no formal national or global process through which organizations or individual users can report possible EHR-related safety issues. The IOM also recommends that the federal agency have the authority to (1) require IT vendors to register their products and communicate negative events associated with their applications, (2) establish mandatory IT safety criteria, and (3) publish an annual report on identified safety issues and strategies in an effort to minimize or eliminate them.[27-29]

No matter whether the EHR is new or an upgrade, the ultimate goal in implementations is to provide the highest level of care at the lowest cost with the least risk.

REFERENCES

1. The White House. Promoting innovation and competitiveness: President Bush's technology agenda. The White House. http://www.whitehouse.gov/infocus/technology/economic policy2004 04/innovation.pdf. 2004.
2. One Hundred Eleventh Congress of the United States of America. The American Recovery and Reinvestment Act of 2009, Title XIII, Heath Information Technology. http://www.gpo.gov/fdsys/pkg/BILLS-111hr1enr/pdf/BILLS-111hr1enr.pdf. 2009.
3. Healthcare Information Technology Standards Panel (HITSP). HITSP quality measures technical note ED, VTE, and stroke examples for implementation of the HITSP quality interoperability specification: HITSP/TN906. HITSP. http://www.hitsp.org/ConstructSet Details.aspx?&PrefixAlpha=5&PrefixNumeric=906. 2011.
4. Manos D. CCHIT certification for homegrown EHRs proves worthwhile. Healthcare IT News. http://www.healthcareitnews.com/news/cchit-certification-homegrown-ehrs-proves-worthwhile. 2011. Accessed February 19, 2012.
5. American Hospital Association (AHA). AHA survey on hospitals' ability to meet Meaningful Use requirements of the Medicare and Medicaid electronic health records incentive programs. AHA. http://www.aha.org/content/11/11EHRsurveyresults.pdf; 2011.
6. Centers for Medicare & Medicaid Services (CMS). ICD-10 overview. CMS. http://www.cms.gov/ContractorLearningResources/Downloads/ICD-10 Overview Presentation.pdf. 2012.
7. Department of Health & Human Services (HHS). HHS proposes adoption of ICD-10 code sets and updated electronic transaction standards. HHS. http://www.dhhs.gov/news/press/2008pres/08/20080815a.html; 2008 Accessed April 1, 2012.
8. Sackett DL, Rosenberg WM, Gray JA, Haynes RB, Richardson WS. Evidence based medicine: what it is and what it isn't. *Brit Med J*. 1996;312(7023):71-72.
9. Berner ES. Clinical decision support systems: state of the art. Agency for Healthcare Research and Quality. http://healthit.ahrq.gov/images/jun09cdsreview/09 0069 ef.html. 2009 Accessed April 1, 2012.
10. Agency for Healthcare Research and Quality (AHRQ). Translating research into practice (TRIP)-II: fact sheet. AHRQ. http://www.ahrq.gov/research/trip2fac.htm. 2001.
11. Menachemi N, Collum T. Benefits and drawbacks of electronic health record systems. *Risk Manag Healthc Policy*. 2011;4:47-55 doi:10.2147/RMHP.S12985.
12. Joint Commission of Accreditation of Healthcare Organizations. Hospitals' national patient safety goals. The Joint Commission.

http://www.jointcommission.org/PatientSafety/NationalPatientSafetyGoals/04 npsgs.htm. 2004 Accessed April 1, 2012.
13. Kaplan JM, Ancheta R, Jacobs BR. Clinical informatics outcomes research group: inpatient verbal orders and the impact of computerized provider order entry. *J Pediatr*. 2006;149:461-467.
14. Ash JA, Sittig DF, Dykstra R, Campbell E, Guappone K. The unintended consequences of computerized provider order entry: findings from a mixed methods exploration. *Int J Med Inform*. 2009;78:S69-S76 doi:10.1016/j.ijminf2008.07.15.
15. Ash JA, Stavri Z, Kuperman GJ. A consensus statement on considerations for a successful CPOE implementation. *J Am Med Inform Assn*. 2003;10:229-234 doi:10.1197/jamia.M1204.
16. Weiner JP, Kfuri T, Chan K, Fowles JB. e-Iatrogenesis: the most critical unintended consequence of CPOE and other HIT. *J Am Med Inform Assn*. 2007;14:387-388 doi:10.1197/jamia.M2338.
17. Institute for Safe Medication Practices (ISMP). FDA and ISMP lists of look-alike drug names with recommended Tall Man letters. ISMP. http://www.ismp.org/tools/tallmanletters.pdf. 2011.
18. Agency for Healthcare Research and Quality (AHRQ). Percentage of verbal orders: 2009. AHRQ. http://healthit.ahrq.gov/portal/server.pt/gateway/PTARGS 0 3882 868890 0 0 18/Percent of Verbal Orders.pdf.
19. Ash JA, Fournier L, Zoë Stavri P, Dykstra R. Principles for a successful computerized physician order entry implementation. *AMIA Annu Symp Proc*. 2003;36-40. http://www.ncbi.nlm.nih.gov/pmc/articles/PMC1480169/pdf/amia2003_0036.pdf.
20. Sklardin NT, Granovsky SJ, Hagerty-Paglia J. Electronic health record implementation at an academic cancer center: lessons learned and strategies for success. *American Society of Clinical Oncology 2011 Educational Book*. http://www.asco.org/ASCOv2/Home/Education%20&%20Training/Educational%20Book/PDF%20Files/2011/zds00111000411.PDF. Accessed January 2, 2013.
21. McGonigle D, Mastrain K. *Nursing Informatics and the Foundation of Knowledge*. Sudbury, MA: Jones and Bartlett Publishers; 2009.
22. Hafner AW. Pareto's principle: the 80-20 rule. Ball State University. http://www.bsu.edu/libraries/ahafner/awh-th-math-pareto.html. 2003 Accessed July 28, 2012.
23. Grant JT. Allow time to implement EHR. *Ophthalmology Times*. 2010;35(7):54-56.
24. Jain V. Evaluating EHR systems. *Health Manag Technol*. 2010;31(8):22-24.
25. Classen DC. Leading patient safety expert speaks on CPOE implementation strategy and success factors. *J Healthc Inf Manag*. 2004;18:15-17.
26. Consumer Reports. Dangerous devices. *Consumer Reports*. 2012;77(5):24-28.
27. Goedert J. New report echoes call for national EHR safety board. *HealthData Management*. 2011.
28. Institute of Medicine (IOM). Health IT and patient safety: building safer systems for better care. IOM. http://www.iom.edu/hitsafety. 2011 Accessed April 7, 2012.
29. Sittig DF. Safe electronic health record use requires a comprehensive monitoring and evaluation framework. *J Amer Med Assoc*. 2010;303(5):450-451. doi:10.1001/jama.2010.61.

DISCUSSION QUESTIONS

1. Discuss why some healthcare providers continue to use a paper medical record.
2. What effects will a fully implemented EHR have on patients? How might it change the cost of care?
3. Why did the ONC elect to use the term electronic health record (EHR) and not electronic medical record (EMR)?
4. If EHRs significantly reduce medication errors and increase the quality of care through the use of evidence-based protocols, should insurers and certifying organizations such as The Joint Commission require healthcare providers and organizations to implement a certified EHR as a standard practice of good medicine?
5. Should insurers offer incentives to patients to select healthcare providers who have an EHR?
6. Review the EMR Adoption Model (EMRAM), an eight-step scale developed by the Healthcare Information and Management Systems Society (HIMSS) to monitor hospitals' and health systems' EHR progress toward a paperless or near paperless system, at www.himssanalytics.org/home/index.aspx. What are the characteristics of the organizations who have successfully achieved Stage 7 status?
7. What are the advantages and disadvantages of a Healthcare Information Technology Standards Panel (HITSP)–certified health IT system versus a homegrown IT system that meets certification standards?
8. What do you anticipate will be barriers to meeting the requirements for Meaningful Use Stage 2?
9. Identify creative strategies to encourage physicians and other clinicians to participate in the implementation of a new health IT system.
10. Discuss ramifications and causes regarding interoperability issues among electronic health systems and applications.

CASE STUDY

Middleville Hospital, located in a small rural town, is a 58-bed acute care facility with both inpatient and outpatient services. The hospital consists of more than 600 employees and more than 300 volunteers. It is a community owned, not-for-profit hospital dedicated to providing compassionate, accessible healthcare close to home. The facility primarily serves one major county and nine surrounding counties.

The hospital has a homegrown electronic health record (EHR) system but it has the functionality to allow the hospital to barely meet Meaningful Use Stage 1. The hospital's primary goal is to implement a certified EHR but the leaders are weighing the benefits of two options: recruiting a skilled professional to rebuild the current system or purchasing a commercial system. There is pressure to make a decision as soon as possible.

What are the musts, constraints, and barriers?

- The new system must be fully implemented and operational no later than June 2014.
- The EHR must be able to meet MU Stages 2 and 3.
- The EHR must be capable of accepting new ICD-10 codes.
- The hospital has a very small IT department and a modest budget.
- Physicians do not enter orders in the current system. Nurses, unit secretaries, and ancillary personnel enter orders in the EHR from written orders on a paper chart.
- The new EHR requires larger servers, new devices, central monitors, printers, and tablets.
- The wireless infrastructure must be upgraded to eliminate known dead spots in areas of the facility.
- The hospital wants to take advantage of select features such as clinical decision support and incorporate best practices or evidence-based medicine.

Discussion Questions

1. Based on what you read in this chapter and the case study, compile an initial list of functional requirements (functions needed) for the new EHR.
2. Create a brief evaluation plan by developing five or six criteria for evaluating vendors' products.

Case Study Follow-Up

The hospital made a list of all pros and cons of rebuilding a homegrown system or buying a commercial product. Realizing that regulations governing healthcare and reimbursement will only become more complicated, the hospital decided to go with a vendor-supplied EHR. Ultimately, it decided to purchase a fully integrated electronic health system that shares a common database to eliminate the issues often seen with interfaces.

Fourteen months later the EHR went live housewide for all staff, including housekeeping and pastoral services. The implementation included the functionality to meet MU and the installation of new servers and hardware in addition to an upgrade of the wireless network. All staff can even view a large monitor showing occupied, clean, and dirty beds that is updated by housekeeping.

The new EHR benefits are many. Initially the physicians grumbled about having to do "secretaries' work" in CPOE but they gradually came to realize the benefits for their patients. Pharmacy reports a 55% decrease in nonformulary medications and a 73% reduction in physician callbacks. The time between a "stat" medication order and administration of the medication and the time between a "stat" lab test order and posting of the lab results have also decreased significantly. Due to the introduction of order sets based on best practices and evidence-based medicine, the hospital has seen a dramatic decrease in its 30-day readmission rates for heart attack, heart failure, and pneumonia patients compared to the U.S. national average and has the lowest rate in the county.

Discussion Question

1. Brainstorm two additional factors you would evaluate for this installation.

Health Information Systems: Downtime and Disaster Recovery

Nancy C. Brazelton and Ann Lyons

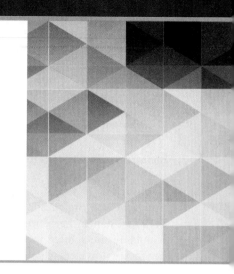

The primary objective for downtime and disaster planning is to protect the organization and the patients who are served by that organization by minimizing disruption to the operations.

OBJECTIVES

At the completion of this chapter the reader will be prepared to:

1. Explain downtime risk assessment
2. Analyze considerations for a health system inventory
3. Describe an assessment tool for evaluating a downtime event
4. Summarize the clinician's role in system downtime planning
5. Summarize information technology's role in system downtime planning
6. Establish key components of a business continuity plan for an organization
7. Formulate communication strategies for downtime in an organization

KEY TERMS

ABSTRACT

Healthcare entities are complex operations that are becoming increasingly dependent on computerization. This chapter identifies tactics related to planning for and responding to computer downtime events and disasters. Focus areas include the clinical impact, the information technology (IT) impact, business continuity, and communications. A model for assessing the level of downtime response is provided.

INTRODUCTION

Healthcare entities, no matter how small or large, are extremely complex businesses that are becoming increasingly dependent on computerization in their quest to provide exceptional healthcare. The employees of these healthcare organizations move through a unique labyrinth of systems, machines, workflows, regulatory requirements, business rules, and tools to provide the best care for patients and their families and to keep the business intact.

Given the importance of information systems within a healthcare entity, these institutions and their employees must be prepared for the many variations of downtime including human errors, software and hardware failures, power cables that get severed, software viruses that invade the firewall, and disruptions caused by Mother Nature. The bulk of literature around the topic of downtime is in white papers, blogs, and industry group publications found via Internet searches and there are very few research articles. The impetus to write is often spurred by a downtime event experienced by the author, who admonishes the reader to get plans in place.[1-3] Anderson reports a study conducted by AC Group that determined that each hour of downtime can cost $488 per physician per hour.[4] In their time and motion study, the authors determined that a physician spends 2.15 minutes during recovery for each minute the system was unavailable. The costs are staggering when translated to a large healthcare enterprise. Given the cost and the risk to patient care, working to prevent downtime and recovering quickly if an incident occurs are priorities for every healthcare institution.

This chapter focuses on practical, tactical ways to put plans in place for managing health system downtime and disaster recovery. Tips and tools for downtime risk assessments, downtime and disaster response planning, clinical and IT system recovery, and business continuity are provided. The chapter also provides information on developing a communication strategy and ideas for keeping patients safe and the business functioning because downtime does happen.

DOWNTIME RISK ASSESSMENT

Planning for downtime can and should occur from project inception through system maturity and must include all existing systems and infrastructure. The complexity and criticality of the organization will determine how extensive an exercise this must be. Potential types of downtime and their impacts on the systems should be anticipated, with mitigation plans put in place.

Downtimes can be classified by the root cause and the degree of impact. Thus if the root cause is network related this is different than power outage downtimes or planned software upgrades. A single noncritical software application may be unavailable, which would have a different impact than the admission, discharge, and transfer (ADT) system being unavailable or a third-party ancillary system (i.e., radiology and imaging, anesthesiology, respiratory therapy) or bedside physiologic monitors being down.

Determining the root cause of a downtime is not always straightforward. Determining what is and is not functioning can be a first step but not the final answer. For example, a network downtime may be diagnosed easily by asking the following questions: Can you access the Internet *and* the intranet? How about the computer next to you? What about the computer on the unit downstairs? If the answer to these questions is "no," suspect an entire network downtime. However, networks in many healthcare enterprises are now segmented for security purposes and include a series of switches, firewalls with coded rules, as well as the actual fiber network, cable pulls, and other components. This makes diagnosis of the specific network problem or the location of the problem complex, potentially increasing the length of the network downtime. Also, external factors may exist, such as telecommunication fiber vendors that may be having problems as well as the millions of miles of fiber infrastructure vulnerable to physical damage, commonly referred to as a "backhoe outage."

Thus, the first step in preventing or managing a downtime is to determine what might cause a downtime and then to perform a risk assessment of the impact for each potential downtime. This step can be iterative with step three discussed below, which is compiling an inventory of existing applications and systems. Classifying all potential downtimes and putting them into mutually exclusive categories can be difficult. It is usually best to start by identifying the most common technology source of downtimes and document these. A systematic approach starting with infrastructure is more likely to ensure a comprehensive list. Begin by dividing the infrastructure into IT infrastructure and physical infrastructure.

IT infrastructure can include the network and application delivery systems, such as those listed in Box 18-1. Examples of physical structures include those listed in Box 18-2. Some overlap exists between the IT infrastructure and the physical infrastructure. Also, this model does not address partial versus complete downtimes. Box 18-3 includes examples of

---

BOX 18-1 SAMPLE ELEMENTS OF INFORMATION TECHNOLOGY INFRASTRUCTURE

- Electronic health record software
- Clinical and ancillary system software (e.g., physiologic monitoring, endoscopy, registry databases)
- Picture archiving and communication system (PACS)
- Laboratory applications
- Cardiology applications
- Radiology applications
- Anesthesia systems
- Surgical processing systems
- Revenue cycle software
- Interfaces or the interface engine
- Enterprise data warehouse

BOX 18-2 EXAMPLES OF INFORMATION TECHNOLOGY PHYSICAL STRUCTURE

- Hardware related to the chillers that keep the data center cool
- Storage (physical hardware that stores the electronic health record, email, and other third-party systems)
- Electrical power
- Network switches and hubs
- Biomedical devices
- Any component of the buildings themselves

BOX 18-3   INFORMATION TECHNOLOGY (IT) AND PHYSICAL INFRASTRUCTURE

IT INFRASTRUCTURE	PHYSICAL INFRASTRUCTURE
Application delivery system (e.g., Citrix)	Biomedical devices
Asset management	Buildings and facilities (list most likely maintained by an
Biomedical devices with software components or	environment of care committee per requirements of
network requirements	The Joint Commission and other regulatory agencies)
Databases	Cabling
Email, other communications	Chillers for data center
Enterprise data warehouse	Generators and fuel supply
Help desk and computer support	Help desk and computer support
Identity management (e.g., active directory)	Inventory (think broadly; replacement computer
Interface engine	hardware to patient care supplies and paper forms)
Interfaces	Medical record (paper) storage
Keyless entry systems or other security software	Network cables and other physical components
Middleware servers	Operator switchboard
Network	Pneumatic tube systems
Scanning software	Physical security of buildings
Security systems	Storage area network, other storage
Software or applications (should have a complete list	Scanners
with interdependencies identified)	Servers
Telecommunication systems (hospital operators, paging,	Switches and hubs
cellphone, analog, voice over Internet Protocol)	Utilities: power, heating, cooling, water
Web services	

IT infrastructure and physical infrastructure. The order of the elements does not reflect their priority. Priority will be unique for each organization. Networks include both hardware and software components and therefore need to be examined from both aspects.

The second step is to identify the most common potential causes of a downtime in the facility, areas of vulnerability, and the most likely scenarios of natural disasters or human-made disasters in the geographic area. Is the facility or data center on an old or outdated power grid? Is the building only rated to withstand a 6.5 magnitude earthquake in an area where experts predict one much stronger? Is the facility's generator located in an area that is vulnerable to flooding? Common disasters are noted in Table 18-1; these lists are not mutually exclusive but instead provide a starting point for planning at a specific organization.

The third step is to complete an inventory of all systems and document them. All systems in use at the organization should be inventoried because each is important to some aspect of the business. A sample inventory is located in Table 18-2.

An inventory list can be surprisingly difficult to compile and may involve doing walk-throughs of departments or units to observe systems and devices that end-users are actually using in their day-to-day workflow. This is especially critical if the institution has a hybrid system (i.e., a system using multiple vendors for specific functionality). For instance, often the ancillary systems within a hospital have a limited amount of data requirements but highly specific ones. These unique systems are added on to the main electronic health record (EHR) because of the need for specific functionality or perhaps because the ancillary application was built and implemented prior to the EHR. Table 18-3 lists

areas that may have special considerations within an acute care setting.

To locate applications, consider functional operations, type of personnel, data and information being processed or consumed, how and where vital records are housed, and policies and procedures that guide the business or practice.[5] This compilation will involve persistently reaching out to all members of the IT team or others who host applications or provide some component of infrastructure for input. The more specific and complete the inventory, the more useful and helpful it will be for planning purposes in the event of an actual planned or unplanned downtime. Due to the difficulty of getting a very complete inventory, it is best to start with the most critical applications and work on less critical ones later. Minimally, the inventory should include the items listed in Box 18-4.

Other data useful for general system support and downtime planning should be carefully documented as well. These items may be part of the application inventory or they may be housed in a separate document, including those listed in Box 18-5.

System dependencies, configuration diagrams, and interface data should also be documented and stored in a place that is easily accessible and backed up on a routine basis as the final step. Best practices for maintaining this inventory and documentation from an Information Technology Infrastructure Library (ITIL) perspective is a configuration management database (CMDB) that has configuration items unique to the organization. However, many tools or combinations of tools are available for this purpose, such as shared drives and folders, spreadsheets, databases, vendor-supplied tools, wiki sites, collaboration software, document management systems repositories, or even simple paper notebooks.

TABLE 18-1	DOWNTIME VULNERABILITIES AND COMMON HUMAN-MADE AND NATURAL DISASTERS		
MOST SIGNIFICANT DOWNTIME VULNERABILITIES		**HUMAN-MADE DISASTERS**	**NATURAL DISASTERS**
Buildings or data center not to current code or vulnerable to natural or human-made disasters		Biologic: intentional	Biologic
Cyber attack		Cyber attack	Dam failure
Lack of recovery site		Explosion: intentional (bomb)	Drought
Lack of disaster planning or business continuity planning		Explosion: unintentional (natural gas line rupture)	Earthquake
Lack of backups or inability to recover from backups		Fire	Fire
Lack of high availability or failover for critical systems or applications		Hazmat incident	Flood
Lack of downtime planning		Nuclear incident	Hurricane
Outdated or aging physical infrastructure		Pandemic	Landslide, mudslide, debris flow
Outdated or aging technology (i.e., not on current or supported level of code or servers that are no longer supported)		Terrorist attack	Pandemic
Power grid and supply		Workforce violence, shootings, loss of life of key personnel	Snowstorm, blizzard
System resources at or near capacity (disk space, database, storage, etc.)			Space weather, geomagnetic storm Tornado Tsunami

TABLE 18-2	SYSTEM INVENTORY CONSIDERATIONS*
TYPE OF SYSTEM	**EXAMPLES**
Core clinical applications	Electronic medical record (EMR), electronic health record (EHR), emergency department, computerized provider order entry (CPOE), clinical documentation, medication administration record (MAR), surgical services and anesthesia information system
Ancillary service and procedure area information services	Pharmacy, radiology and imaging, laboratory, arterial blood gas, cardiology, endoscopy, respiratory, neurology, nutrition care, dictation, health information management, biomedical devices (physiologic monitors, vital sign machines, intravenous pumps, ventilators, pneumatic tube systems, etc.)
Online reference databases	Drug information references; patient education; policies and procedures; disease, diagnosis, and interventional protocol databases; formulas or health-related calculators
Revenue cycle	Admission, discharge, and transfer; enterprise scheduling; preauthorization; facility and technical billing; coding; professional and physician billing; claim scrubbers; print vendors; address verification; electronic data interchange (EDI) transactions; benefit checking
Business, finance, and personnel	Email, office software, cash collections, credit card transactions, banking, business intelligence, reports and reporting, supply chain and enterprise resource planning (ERP), budgeting, human resources, payroll, staff scheduling, keyless entry, facilities and engineering, telephone systems and wiring, telephone operators, paging systems, wireless communication devices
Miscellaneous	Printers, Bluetooth devices (scanners, label printers), reports, data warehouse, scanning, print vendor, Internet-based public web pages, Intranet and related internal web sites, wikis, clinical health information exchanges, retail outlets (retail pharmacies, gift shops, food service)

*Not a complete list.

TABLE 18-3	CONSIDERATIONS BY AREA FOR ACUTE CARE SETTING
AREA	**SPECIALTY REQUIREMENTS**
Anesthesia	Ventilators, anesthetic gases, frequent vital signs
Automated charge capture	Can be from many systems
Cardiac catheterization lab	Hemodynamic monitors, image capture, documentation for registries
Emergency department	Tracking patients in the waiting room and through the department
Endoscopy	Image capture and specific discreet documentation for registries or billing
Health information	Coding, release of information, maintenance of the legal medical record, legal cases, insurance queries, scanning solutions
Medicine	Computerized provider order entry (CPOE), clinical decision support systems, diagnostic test results, dictation
Newborn intensive care	Bedside monitoring and extracorporeal membrane oxygenation devices, ventilators, intravenous pumps
Nursing	Care planning, CPOE, Bar Code Medication Administration or electronic medication administration record, telemetry, patient communication systems with nurses, clinical decision support reminders, nursing databases (e.g., patient education resources)
Obstetrics	Fetal monitoring, mother and baby monitoring and documentation during the labor period, preterm wave forms, information from mother's record that needs to be available on newborn's record for continuity of care
Pharmacy	Medication dispensing machines (Pyxis and Omnicell), robots, inpatient versus retail pharmacy ordering systems, intravenous pumps that contain drug-specific information (Alaris, etc.), pharmacy ordering system often interfaces with the medication supplier
Physical, occupational, and speech therapies	Therapy systems have specific patient education content
Physiologic monitoring	Often supported by biomedical engineering and has vendor-specific content
Radiology, imaging, and picture archiving and communication system	Image and procedure capture, multiple modalities, questionnaires
Respiratory therapy	Contains respiratory measures like ventilator settings, ventilator weaning parameters, respiratory treatments and measurements

BOX 18-4   INVENTORY ITEMS

- Vendor name
  - If developed in-house, where is source code and other documentation?
  - Date of contract and its current location
- Application or module name
  - Date of original go-live
- Current version
  - Date of upgrade
- Categorization (site defined): major/minor, Tier I/II/III, other
- Host model (where the application or service is located): in-house or remote
  - If remote, supported by whom?
- Interfaces, both inbound and outbound
- Third-party bolt-on systems
- Other key dependencies
- Primary use
- Primary users and number of users
- Business owners
- IT contacts
- Notes and comments

BOX 18-5   ELEMENTS FOR GENERAL SYSTEMS SUPPORT

- A checklist for the team to follow when a planned or unplanned downtime occurs
- Known system vulnerabilities
- Frequent error messages
- Patterns of error messages indicating known problems or pending system failure
- Knowledge objects used in supporting or maintaining system
- Contact information with phone numbers for vendors and the teams supporting the application
- Service level agreements (SLAs) with key users of the application
- Preferred user communication plan for planned and unplanned downtimes
- Unit- or department-based workflow diagrams
- Unit or department blueprints that document all electronic devices connected to the wired or wireless network
- Agreed-upon time for planned changes and maintenance work, also known as a change window
- Policies, procedures, rules, or standards from information technology or the broader organization applying to the particular application

With the appropriate data collected, IT should work very closely with the organization's emergency preparedness and disaster planning groups in planning for disasters. Having some component of IT downtime as a part of disaster drills is a very effective way for IT and staff to practice disaster response and hone plans. The Federal Emergency Management Agency (FEMA) website at www.ready.gov is extremely helpful for planning at an institutional and personal level and is full of information in the event of an actual disaster.

DOWNTIME AND RESPONSE PLANNING

Once the system documentation has been developed and the risks are understood, the healthcare institution is ready to define the different types of potential downtimes on a continuum indicating the degree of significance for each potential downtime. The significance of the different downtimes will depend on the level of complexity and the installed base of the institution. For example, if the organization has results review implemented and a single results feed is down, the response will be very different than if the organizations has a mature EHR and the network is unavailable. Is this a physician's office with a single provider and a very experienced staff or a huge integrated delivery network (IDN) spread across multiple states or geographic regions? Consider both planned and unplanned downtimes. If a downtime has been scheduled, there should be ample time to plan; however, if the downtime is unexpected, there may be no contingency plans in place. A worst-case scenario of an unplanned downtime could be a total loss of the network occurring midweek at the start of the business day when the hospital and clinic schedules are full, all operating rooms are in use, and the emergency department is busy and expecting two traumas (one via flight service) on a snowy winter day when 20% of staff is late due to road conditions.

Table 18-4 identifies a number of elements that will influence the impact of an individual downtime. The list in Table 18-4 is not intended to be followed linearly. Different scenarios or error messages will lead down different paths just as different symptoms might lead to different diagnoses in patient care. One would take different actions if a patient's temperature increased by a half-degree Celsius and the heart rate increased by 10 beats per minute over the last 45 minutes as opposed to if a patient had a detached intravenous. The same process occurs when managing EHRs or other systems. Being able to quickly translate error messages and recognize patterns are keys to reducing the length of the downtime and restoring clinician and staff workflow.

Once the organization has clear definitions for downtimes and has methods of assessing the significance of potential events,[2] the emergency preparedness and disaster planning team can develop the response and recovery plans. A comprehensive and accurate assessment will provide a reliable starting point for the team responding to the downtime,

TABLE 18-4 **IMPACT CONSIDERATIONS**	
ATTRIBUTE	**CONTINUUM**
Expected or actual duration	≤1 hour to >4 hours; should also plan for a catastrophic event where network or systems will have to be rebuilt, which will be weeks to months
Time of day	Middle of the slowest night of the week to middle of the day on the busiest day of the week
Number of users affected and scope and breadth of downtime or outage	Single user or department to the entire facility; partial to full; single system or infrastructure component to complete loss of application, network, or building
Information technology (IT) infrastructure	Intact to completely damaged and replacement parts need to be ordered
Impact on workflow	Users are able to carry on activities with minimal disruption to complete change in workflow reverting to inefficient manual systems
Complexity of IT installs and criticality of applications	Single system with review-only functionality to an organization that is >90% electronic and paperless with multiple systems for all business and healthcare requirements
Planned or unplanned	Downtime is scheduled during agreed-upon service level agreement and system comes back up as promised to an unexpected systemwide downtime with no estimated time to recovery
Complexity of health system or complexity and criticality of unit or department affected	Single office to multistate integrated delivery network; office that still keeps paper records to a fully electronic intensive care unit with patients on multiple assistive devices
Communication methods and mechanisms	All communication mechanisms except word of mouth are unavailable to multiple different mechanisms that account for multiple different scenarios
Redundancy of infrastructure and the ability to recover	No redundant systems or infrastructure to fully redundant, highly available system in a colocated data center
Maturity of downtime plans, policies, and procedures and availability of backup supplies	No plans or supplies to mature and tested policy, procedure, and plans with stocked supplies and staff aware of them

thereby decreasing chaos and saving critical time at the start of an event. The downtime plan will include different levels of interventions for different events. For example, a downtime event with a simple application may be managed with a decision tool. An example of a simple decision tree is shown in Figure 18-1. However, this same approach may become too cumbersome when dealing with multiple systems. In these cases an organization may use a "level" system such as the one shown in Table 18-5.

With a multiple systems downtime event, the use of a tool to quickly assess the significance of the downtime event will help the IT team and users to determine which of the

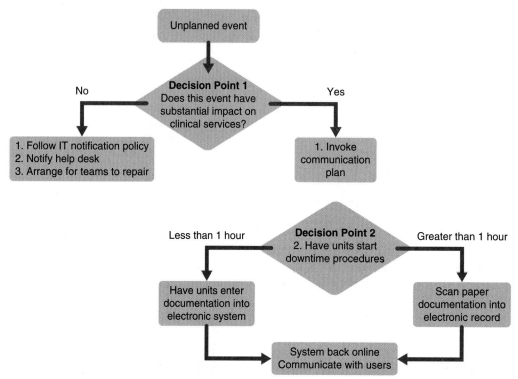

FIG 18-1 Simple downtime decision tree. *IT,* Information technology.

TABLE 18-5	DOWNTIME LEVELS	
	DEFINITION	**RESPONSE EXAMPLES**
Level 1	Part of a system down or unavailable but minimal impact and no loss of content or data integrity. Expected time to recovery less than 1 hour.	Information technology (IT) team and targeted users only are involved per standard service level agreement (SLA).
Level 2	Complete system unavailable, data may be unavailable, and data will have to be entered into the system to maintain integrity. Expected time to recovery up to 4 hours.	IT team and targeted users are involved per standard SLA. Unit-based downtime plans invoked. May require additional communication to stakeholders and plans for reentry of data.
Level 3	Multiple systems unavailable, big impact on workflow, and content may be unavailable and will have to be entered into the system to maintain integrity. Expected time to recovery greater than 4 hours.	IT incident response team involved along with multiple teams. Downtime plans invoked. Broad communication to the organization. Notification to key stakeholders and administration. Plan for reentry of data.
Level 4	All systems and network unavailable but root cause is known and recovery is possible. Users must complete downtime plans. Estimated time to recovery greater than 4 hours.	IT incident response team involved along with multiple teams. Downtime plans invoked. Broad communication to the organization. Notification to key stakeholders and administration. Plan for reentry of data. May involve emergency response team and opening of command center.
Level 5	All systems and network unavailable. Major catastrophic event and facility structure may be compromised. Systems and infrastructure need to be rebuilt. Systemwide emergency plans and response invoked.	All hands on deck and event directed per emergency response team or administration. May require communication to the wider community.

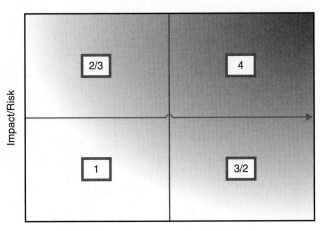

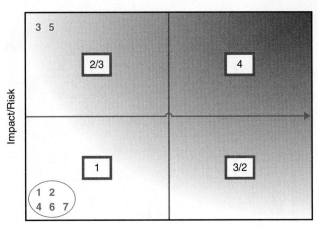

Plot each component in one of the four quadrants to
determine where the items cluster

1. Time of day/number of users
2. IT infrastructure affected
3. System criticality
4. Planned versus unplanned
5. Health system complexity
6. Communication: Amount required and are methods affected?
7. Ability to recover

FIG 18-2 Downtime Determinator model. *IT,* Information
technology.

Plot each component in one of the four quadrants to
determine where the items cluster

1. Time of day/number of users
2. IT infrastructure affected
3. System criticality
4. Planned versus unplanned
5. Health system complexity
6. Communication: Amount required and are methods affected?
7. Ability to recover

FIG 18-3 Downtime Determinator quadrant 1 example. *IT,*
Information technology.

predefined responses should be invoked. One example of
such a tool is the Downtime Determinator© depicted in
Figure 18-2. The *x*-axis is the length of downtime (or time to
recovery) and the *y*-axis is the impact and risk. Each of the
seven risk attributes is plotted on the Downtime Determinator tool in one of the four quadrants and a pattern or cluster
of numbers will start to emerge. The pattern of numbers
becomes the basis for evaluating the event.

Using the risk attributes described above, quadrant responses would be defined by the organization and might be
similar to the earlier examples provided with the levels. For
example, when the majority of numbers cluster in the lower
left quadrant, this should invoke a quadrant 1 response;
numbers clustered in the upper right quadrant should invoke
a quadrant 4 response. The lower left quadrant represents the
least critical events and the upper right quadrant represents
the most critical events. The Downtime Determinator displays the numbers 2/3 and 3/2 in the upper left and lower
right quadrants, respectively. Each organization will need to
assign quadrants 2 and 3 based on its assessment of each
individual downtime event, after considering the impact and
risk versus time. There may be times when the length of the
downtime is so long that the event warrants a quadrant 3
(more intense) response. There may be other times when the
event is so massive that even though the downtime is scheduled for 30 minutes, the impact to the organization is so great
that it warrants a quadrant 3 response.

The Downtime Determinator is similar to the "level" system
mentioned earlier, as both have four categories. However, the
Downtime Determinator allows for more specificity and

nuances in responses because each of the attributes can be considered separately and responded to in relation to other attributes. When using a tool such as the Downtime Determinator,
each organization should customize the tool by defining each
attribute and delineating time along the *x*-axis that is significant
to the organization. Four scenarios are outlined below using the
Downtime Determinator, ranging from least to most impact.

- Scenario 1: Level I trauma and teaching hospital. Planned
  EHR downtime from 0200 to 0500 on a Wednesday night.
  IT infrastructure and communications intact (Fig. 18-3).
- Scenario 2: Community hospital. Unplanned downtime of
  the hospital billing system at 1530 on a Monday. Multiple
  staff unable to do work but patient care is not affected.
  Recovery expected in 3 hours. System requires replacement of a hard drive; the hard drive is available locally and
  it should be delivered to the data center by the vendor
  shortly. Communications intact (Fig. 18-4).
- Scenario 3: Acute care hospital with multiple intensive care
  units (ICUs) with a physiologic monitoring system interfaced to the EHR via bedside medical device integration
  (BMDI). The vendor-specific server is damaged due to a
  water spill in the communication closet and the BMDI
  unexpectedly quits working at 0800 on a Saturday
  morning. The vendor indicates a 2-week lag until a replacement server will be available (Fig. 18-5).
- Scenario 4: An F-16 military airplane crashes into the data
  center of an academic medical center at 1900 on a Friday
  night during training exercises. The data center is destroyed
  physically, a large fuel spill covers the area, and there is
  complete IT system downtime. The hospital and campus

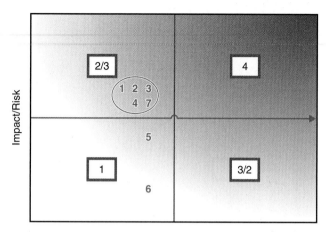

Plot each component in one of the four quadrants to
determine where the items cluster

**Plot each component in one of the four quadrants to
determine where the items cluster**

1. Time of day/number of users
2. IT infrastructure affected
3. System criticality
4. Planned versus unplanned
5. Health system complexity
6. Communication: Amount required and are methods affected?
7. Ability to recover

FIG 18-4 Downtime Determinator quadrant 2 example. *IT,*
Information technology.

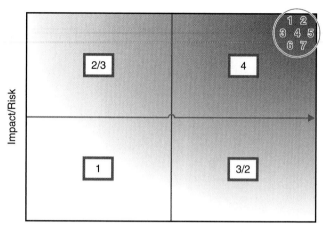

**Plot each component in one of the four quadrants to
determine where the items cluster**

1. Time of day/number of users
2. IT infrastructure affected
3. System criticality
4. Planned versus unplanned
5. Health system complexity
6. Communication: Amount required and are methods affected?
7. Ability to recover

FIG 18-6 Downtime Determinator quadrant 4 example. *IT,*
Information technology.

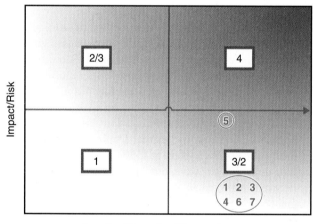

**Plot each component in one of the four quadrants to
determine where the items cluster**

1. Time of day/number of users
2. IT infrastructure affected
3. System criticality
4. Planned versus unplanned
5. Health system complexity
6. Communication: Amount required and are methods affected?
7. Ability to recover

FIG 18-5 Downtime Determinator quadrant 3 example. *IT,*
Information technology.

are otherwise intact. The academic medical center has a
hot site that can host approximately 30% of critical
systems and a cold site that has capacity to host the
remainder of the systems. The critical hot site applications
can be available in 24 hours but the remaining 70% of
applications to be built in the cold site will take 30 days
for complete recovery (Fig. 18-6).

As seen with these scenarios, the clustering of numbers
helps to guide the response of the organization in managing
the event or disaster. A quadrant 1 event (scenario 1) should
be a routine event that is managed with standard processes,
communications, and service level agreements (SLAs) that
are already in place. With a quadrant 4 major disaster (scenario 4), the response should be massive and system- and
organization-wide. Such a disaster would have a significant
impact on the ability of the organization to carry on the business of healthcare. Taking time to plan and put realistic processes into place previous to the event will determine whether
the organization will continue to care for patients safely and
have the business remain intact.

Clinical Impact and Planning: Acute Care Focus

With the increased use of technology at the point of care
and in the clinical environment, healthcare organizations
must now determine their response when this technology is
unavailable. How do clinicians find historical data, including
recent vital signs, the first of three troponin results, the history
and physical prior to surgery, and the last time the PRN (as

needed) pain medication was given and the patient's response to it? How do healthcare providers document new events, medications, and treatments? How does the pharmacy dispense a medication and keep track of the dispensing? Do the automated supply cabinets have programming that permits overriding the system and, if so, how are charges captured after the fact? These are the potential problems that may arise at institutions in the event of EHR unavailability. Each addition to the technology in use can produce unintended consequences and in turn affect the initial assessment and resulting plan. For example, a 4-year analysis of the unintended consequences of computerized provider order entry (CPOE) identified nine types of unintended consequences.[6] A list of these unintended consequences is included in Box 18-6.

Logically, the more electronic components in the organization, the more complex troubleshooting becomes. The elements that need to be considered include inpatient and outpatient venues, networks, intranets, printers, databases, interfaces, storage hardware, published applications, and layering software used to manage the myriad devices in an institution. Failure at any of these points may result in some sort of downtime for clinicians. Reducing the risk of a downtime can be accomplished by using the approaches outlined in the following sections.

Redundant Systems

Redundant systems, also known as backup systems, provide clinicians the ability to access some if not all patient data during an electronic downtime. If clinicians can recover just enough information to carry on with patient care from the point at which the downtime begins, care can proceed safely.[7] Therefore a subset of critical data must always be available, even during downtime. Each individual organization should define the required subset of data according to applications and services. Suggestions are basic demographics, orders, medication administration records (MARs), most recent vitals, laboratory values, imaging reports, and physician and provider progress notes.

BOX 18-6   UNINTENDED CONSEQUENCES OF THE IMPACT OF COMPUTERIZED PROVIDER ORDER ENTRY

- Increased workload
- Workflow issues with mismatch of order entry and related activities
- Never-ending demands
- Paper persistence
- Communication issues with changes in communication patterns
- Emotional reactions to issues and problems
- New kinds of errors introduced by use of a computer
- Changes in the power structure
- Overdependence on technology

Vendors are increasingly responding to the need for improved downtime solutions. As an example, a vendor might install one to four stand-alone machines in each patient care area depending on the average patient census and geographic layout of the unit. Each machine might be designed to store a subset of historical patient data up to 30 days. During a downtime, staff access these machines to retrieve the previous 30 days of patient-related data. Once the downtime begins, these systems will no longer be updated. New patient data that are generated as patient care continues must be maintained manually during the downtime event. Because healthcare providers may need printed data during the downtime event, each machine should be directly connected by cable to a printer so it is not dependent on the down network connection for printing services. Another benefit of these machines is that they can be portable. In the event of a hospital evacuation, these machines can be removed from the premises and data from these machines can be used until a recovery plan is in place.

However, this particular downtime solution has limitations. One concept that is difficult for clinical and IT staff to understand is that once the network becomes unavailable, these downtime machines are no longer updated with patient information. This requires the healthcare providers to check the new manually recorded data as well as the historical data maintained in the temporary system when providing care. Another limitation is that the data may be organized differently than in the EHR and as a result information may be displayed or print in a different format. This can cause confusion and even errors in patient care.

The downtime solution using temporary machines must meet Health Insurance Portability and Accountability Act (HIPAA) requirements for security, privacy, and confidentiality. As a result, these machines require an extra layer of encryption to prevent information theft in the event that the machine is removed from the hospital. However, these encryption systems typically are add-ons that slow down the response time of patient care applications running on the machines.

Other terms used to describe redundant systems are *shadow*, *mirror*, or *read-only systems*. The downtime system described above is a shadow or mirror system that is able to be only read by clinicians. Clinicians cannot add any patient data to this type of system. Some shadow or mirror systems duplicate the EHR. In the event that the primary system crashes, the secondary system automatically, and hopefully seamlessly, transitions the clinician to the secondary system. The clinician continues to document orders, medications, or care. Generally these systems reside on separate hardware that "mirrors" the configuration of the primary system. These systems are generally more robust than the redundant downtime solution described above, encompassing a similar look and feel and often read and write capability. These systems are beneficial because clinicians use their current log-in and password to access the system, the look and feel of the system are almost identical to the EHR, and printing can be available.

Redundant systems often resemble the configuration of the existing EHR, requiring a substantial financial investment with the vendor. The financial investment can be an obstacle, therefore, a business case should be made with and for the clinicians on behalf of patients. The more mature the EHR, the more dependent the clinicians are on the system to get information to provide patient care. Investing in a backup system of this caliber is arguably a necessity after institutions have reached a certain level of EHR maturity and organizations should assess this requirement frequently.

In addition to the above solutions, homegrown web-based solutions are available for use by clinicians prior to a planned downtime. For example, a web-based solution may be configured so that clinicians can print an MAR or all current patient orders. These have proven helpful during planned upgrades because they provide clinicians with enough information to weather the upgrade as well as provide a place to begin the manual documentation of patient care in the immediate period following the downtime.

DOWNTIME POLICIES AND PROCEDURES

Approved downtime policies and procedures are needed to guide the clinical team. These policies should be prescriptive, include roles and responsibilities, and define workarounds or manual procedures that allow for the continuity of critical functions. They should include specific instructions about required data entry to the legal and permanent EHR record at the conclusion of the downtime. Examples of downtime policies are available in the literature and on the Internet.[7-10]

A best practice is for patient units to have up-to-date "downtime" boxes.[11] Each box contains documentation specific to the patient care area. For example, ICUs may revert to traditional six-panel paper flow sheets. Other patient care areas have screenshots of the electronic "patient admission" form or other forms directly from the EHR. When no pre-printed forms are available, blank or lined pieces of paper are used and work as long as healthcare providers are aware of documentation requirements. Each downtime box should be stocked to last at least 24 hours and have a documented plan in the event of a catastrophic event. Each patient care area is expected to maintain and customize the contents of its "downtime" box.[11] Informaticists can partner closely with clinicians to create downtime policies and procedures to ensure that clinical requirements are matched with available IT solutions.

IT IMPACT AND PLANNING

The IT impact and downtime risk can be reduced by following a systematic process when applying changes to the "production" or "live" system. One approach is to organize a service management program to organize a risk assessment and downtime planning document. Service management is a discipline for managing IT systems that focuses on the customer and the business and its operations as opposed to simply being technology-centric. The service life cycle

includes service strategy, service design, service transition, service operation, and continual service improvement.[12] Interestingly, this life cycle is similar to both the system development life cycle used to implement computer systems[13] and the nursing process.[14] Various process-based systems exist to assist the IT team in instituting a service management program, including ITIL,[12,15] Six Sigma, and total quality management (TQM). These systems require standardized terminology, problem identification and management, change control measures, and communication patterns. The benefits of using these systems are agreed-upon, realistic service levels; predictable and consistent processes; metrics; and alignment with business needs.

Implementing a service management program requires financial and time commitments from the organization, the IT executive, and all members of the IT team but is well worth the investment. Commitments are needed from the IT staff to fill roles on committees such as the change advisory board, incident response team (IRT), and IT service management. The benefits of a service management program include a framework with clear rules and processes to structure IT activities so there are fewer unplanned events. The disadvantages of a service management program include that the new program will invariably increase the time to implementation for some new code or new functionality. However, waiting reduces knee-jerk reaction time and gives the IT team more time to test the new functionality and discover any dependencies. Waiting also benefits clinicians because they can negotiate a standard change time and reduce unnecessary downtimes.

DISASTER PLANNING

Organizations are obligated to have contingency and disaster plans to be compliant with the HIPAA security rule of 1996, the U.S. Department of Health & Human Services, and The Joint Commission. A separate set of IT policies should exist to supplement the organization's overall disaster plan and include security and privacy components. Senior leadership of the IT department, the security and privacy office, the emergency preparedness group, and senior leadership from the broader organization should review and approve the plans.[5] These plans should be frequently reviewed, tested, and revised as needed. Staff need to be updated on a consistent basis so they are prepared to implement a contingency and disaster plan with minimum effort. Considerations for the IT components of an IT disaster plan are listed in Table 18-6.

Once contingency and disaster plans have been implemented and at the point when the institution is converting back to its standard systems the organization needs to be prepared to test the clinical system rapidly to ensure that all aspects of the system are functioning as planned. Having up-to-date test plans for all clinical systems is an integral part of turning around a downtime quickly once hardware and database issues have been resolved. Software upgrades can take place every 6 months. If the test plans are not current,

TABLE 18-6	INFORMATION TECHNOLOGY (IT) CONTINGENCY AND DISASTER RECOVERY PLAN CONSIDERATIONS
ELEMENT	**ACTIVITIES**
Staff competencies	• Identify and agree on roles and responsibilities • Document and make accessible system documentation • Demand "knowledge transfers"; all members to avoid SPOFs (single points of failure) • Develop stakeholder relationships • Update emergency contacts for vendors and IT staff
Data backups are completed with the intent to prevent data loss and provide the ability to recover data if they are lost or corrupt. Scheduled daily or as needed, determined by the business. There are hardware and software components for storage and backup. Backups should be stored with the same care and level of security as the production data.	• Preserve all critical data associated with the patient, the business, finances, payroll, and personnel • Be knowledgeable about retention policies of medical records and business documents for the organization and state • Duplicate data on tapes, disks, and optical disks • Store data in one of the clouds and/or across multiple servers
Off-site storage of removable media	• Include a secure plan for transporting the media to an offsite location • Encrypt data
Ensuring that there is adequate storage for the production systems	• Evaluate storage capacity and procedures proactively
Having development and test domains for all systems	• Test all changes to production prior to promoting the code to production using a formal process
System monitoring and notifications	• Keep a spreadsheet of common errors to help speed up diagnostics • Introduce various types of downtimes to a test (nonproduction) system and evaluate the error messages or system issues; for example, in the nonproduction system, turn off the interfaces to see what types of errors or alerts you receive in the monitoring • Work with the database team to mimic at-capacity database tables and carefully monitor system errors that are displayed
Plan for relocation of equipment for continuity of operations. All contracts signed with vendors should have a disaster recovery component based on the organization's requirements.	• Design systems are highly available and redundant • Archive source code with a reputable third-party company • Complete negotiations are completed up front for replacement hardware with commitments on days to ship and configure • Arrange, with vender, colocation sites with adequate network bandwidth and dual network pathways • Have reciprocal agreements or consortium arrangements
An organization that has a data center should also have internal plans for colocation sites, which may be hot sites, warm sites, or cold sites	• Ensure that there is adequate network bandwidth
Be disciplined with postevent review and complete revisions of processes and policy as appropriate	• Have formal process for the review, including documentation • Complete and document event review as near to the event as possible

Data from Hoong LL, Marthandan G. Factors influencing the success of the disaster recovery planning process: a conceptual paper. *Research and Innovation in Information Systems (ICRIIS), 2011 International Conference.* 2011;1-6, 23-24. doi:10.1109/ICRIIS.2011.6125683; and Federal Emergency Management Agency (FEMA). IT disaster recovery plan. FEMA. http://www.ready.gov/business/implementation/IT; 2012.

the testing process may not be reliable. In addition, without systematic preplanned processes in place it is difficult to enlist the help of non-IT people. Keeping test plans up to date ensures that people external to the recovery team can assist with testing and getting the system online sooner.

Disaster Recovery

Preparedness and planning are the keys to disaster recovery following either a simple incident or a catastrophic event. In fact, the process of planning can be as beneficial to an organization as the final written plan. Recovery should include all components identified as crucial: network, servers, connectivity, data, telecommunications, hardware, software, desktops, security, wireless, and any other specific items.

The goal of disaster recovery is to recover the business fully and completely. Depending on the severity of the event or disaster, it may be necessary to do an incremental recovery. Key administrative leaders, with input from the staff, should be involved in the decisions about the sequence of recovery of systems or applications. All employees in an organization will likely have changed workflows during the disaster and it is important that they understand their roles during the disaster or downtime and during the recovery period. The steps to actual recovery will be different for each event and for each organization. Because of this complexity and the time involved to develop a comprehensive disaster recovery plan, an organization may choose to hire outside consultants instead of using internal resources.[16,17]

Business Continuity

Business continuity management is a complementary process to disaster recovery. Business continuity has a larger scope than recovering only IT systems. It also includes determining which administrative and healthcare services must be available using a defined timeline and identifies which systems can be excluded from initial recovery. Business continuity management outlines the functions, processes, and systems needed to allow the core business of providing health services to continue.

A tier system works well for this purpose and each organization will have unique requirements. For example, Tier I applications would be identified as critical and they are recovered first. The organization defines the expected time to recovery based on the requirement for service and available resources. As a general rule, the faster the recovery must occur, the more expensive the recovery process will be. The cost should also be evaluated in comparison with the cost of the downtime. For a Tier I application to be recovered in 24 hours or less, it is likely that a hot site would be required with hardware standing by. Tier II applications would come next and may be identified as needing to be available within 72 hours. Finally, Tier III and Tier IV may be identified as requiring recovery within 1 week and 1 month, respectively. For healthcare, business continuity includes providing care of both patients and the revenue cycle. Defining business continuity should be a formal process that includes the following:

- A business impact analysis that takes into consideration the institution's business needs and the needs of the community for healthcare services
- Definition of recovery strategies
- Development of a formal plan
- Planned exercises to test the plan

As with other elements discussed above, this process will need resources (both human and financial) from the organization's senior leadership.[18,19]

Downtime boxes were mentioned earlier in this chapter. Every business unit needs to have a downtime box that includes items such as registration forms, charge sheets, fax forms, and other commonly used forms for that business area. In addition, it is a good idea to have these documents stored on a portable media device to be kept in the downtime box. In the event of a disaster, these forms can be stored on another portable device and kept in a secure location. Organizations should make specific assignments to ensure that these are kept up to date.

Communication

Communication is an integral part of any downtime. Five components of communication plans are needed to determine the following:

- Who needs to know the details
- What details are needed
- What media or modes of communication will be used
- Who will communicate what information
- The systems or workflow processes that are affected

Of course, the more complex the downtime is, the more people need to be notified and the more information needs to be communicated. For example, if the bedside monitoring device is not transmitting data to the EHR, only the ICU staff need to be notified. If the EHR database becomes corrupt, then all clinicians who use the system will need to be notified as well as all IT teams and possibly hospital administration and the risk management department.

Fahrenholz et al.[9] compiled a downtime communication template useful to readers. Their questions are as follows:

- What system will be down?
- When will the downtime begin?
- How long will the system be unavailable?
- Why will the system be down?
- What changes are being made to the system?
- Who will be affected and what can the end-user expect?
- What procedures should be followed during the downtime?

These guidelines can be adapted for any facility's use during an unexpected downtime.

If the hospital or facility uses a tool for IT service management such as ITIL, the procedures discussed here will be used. If the facility does not use one of these systems, policies and procedures are needed to ensure that communication occurs properly. Communication occurs most predictably and reliably when the responsibility belongs to one consistent team or group of people. A service management or equivalent team works well to manage the communications. Whoever is designated as the primary communication team must work very closely with the incident response team (IRT) and the help desk. Communications are coordinated and the help desk is kept informed of the event and of the information it should supply to end-users as inquiries are made about the event. The help desk is critical to communications. In most cases, when the staff are experiencing technical problems they will contact the help desk first. The help desk staff are on-site and on-call agents available 24 hours a day. Training the help desk staff to manage these communications allows the infrastructure and application teams to work on resolving the problems. Some tools that might be used in addition to managing the trouble ticket queue are continuous or intermittent conference calls, individual and group paging for the IT department, individual and group instant messaging, webcasts, updated web pages, group email updates, recorded phone messages, and coordination with hospital operators. Multiple means of communication need to be considered when planning for an event. The technical problems causing the downtime or the disaster event may also eliminate certain communication modes. For example, if the network is down, an email with information about managing the downtime cannot be sent to the clinical units.

The hospital telecommunications operators can manage many aspects of the communication plan, including individual and group pagers, cellphones, tablets, and other communication devices for clinicians and the operational areas. Sending information to these communication devices may help to manage information distribution during sudden or extended downtimes. A best practice in the age of Internet-based phone systems is to have some analog phones available in key hospital areas because they function during network and electrical downtimes. These phones can be identified by using a different color of phone, such as red. Hospital telecommunications operators can also use the overhead paging system in the hospital to distribute information. The point is to be sure to include these hospital operators in the downtime communication plans.

In the event of a major disaster, satellite radios and phones can be used. Satellite phones and radios are network independent but require electricity to recharge their batteries. The local emergency management office in the organization will have more information about these capabilities.

Responsibilities

The IT staff is responsible for communicating the necessary information to the help desk agents. In addition, some electronic systems contain notification alert capability. For example, planned downtimes can be communicated using the notification system in the facility's EHR. Obviously this method would not be available during an EHR downtime, but it can be used to announce a planned downtime or when any of the ancillary systems are off-line.

IT leaders are responsible for communicating with the organization's senior leadership and the public relations department so they can manage media relations with the community. Social media applications can also be used to manage information with the media and to distribute information to staff in the event of a downtime (assuming that staff members have subscribed to the service and the service can provide the appropriate level of security and privacy).

Other mechanisms may be in place depending on the institution and the setting. For example, if the institution is affiliated with a university, a "campus alert" system may be available. Using this system, notifications can be sent via email, cellphone, work phone, home phone, or a combination of these. This communication strategy can be very helpful during disaster drills as well as unexpected events.

There are numerous ways to communicate with hospital employees and leadership, IT staff, news media, and the public. Finding the right combination for the facility's budget and staff and formalizing the ownership of specific communication will facilitate the workflow transitions during EHR downtimes at the facility.

CONCLUSION AND FUTURE DIRECTIONS

This chapter identifies tactics for health system downtime planning and disaster recovery. It challenges clinicians and informaticists to assess, plan for, respond to, recover from, communicate about, continue business during, and prevent downtimes and disasters when possible. The primary objective for downtime and disaster planning is to protect the organization and the patients who are served by that organization by minimizing disruption to the operations. This includes minimizing economic loss; ensuring organizational stability; protecting critical assets of the organization; ensuring safety for personnel, patients, and other customers; reducing variability in decision making during a disaster; and hopefully minimizing legal liability.[5] In healthcare and health information technology, the single most important reason to carry out the activities described in the chapter carefully and methodically is the ability to provide uninterrupted, exceptional service and safe care to all patients.

Going forward, the potential impact of downtimes and disasters will continue to grow as healthcare entities become more dependent on technology and as individual healthcare institutions continue to become part of a larger network. This should drive administrators to invest additional human and material resources in assessing and planning to minimize the impact of potential threats. Advances in technology can be expected to offer better solutions than currently exist. These solutions may be less costly as new and improved technology eventually reduces the potential for downtimes. Additional research is very much needed to help clinicians and health systems understand the experience of downtime workflow interruptions, the patient safety implications, and the operational impacts. In addition, research to drive a health system standard approach to downtime planning, disaster recovery, and business continuity efforts should be initiated. There are many focus areas along the continuum of disaster planning to business continuity where research could have a very positive impact for the health system and its clients.

REFERENCES

1. Polaneczky M. When the electronic medical record goes down. The Blog that Ate Manhattan. http://www.tbtam.com/2007/03/when-the-electronic-medical-record-goes-down.html. 2007.
2. Getz L. Dealing with downtime: how to survive if your EHR system fails. *For the Record.* 2009;21(21):16. http://www.fortherecordmag.com/archives/110909p16.shtml.
3. Capital One. Business continuity and disaster recovery checklist for small business owners. Continuity Central. http://www.continuitycentral.com/feature0501.htm. 2011.
4. Anderson M. The costs and implications of EMR system downtime on physician practices. XML Journal. http://xml.sys-con.com/node/1900855. 2011.
5. Wold GH. Disaster recovery planning process. Disaster Recovery Journal. http://www.drj.com/new2dr/w2_002.htm. 2011.
6. Ash JS, Sittig DF, Poon EG, Guappone K, Campbell E, Dykstra RH. The extent and importance of unintended consequences related to computerized provider order entry. *J Am Med Inform Assn.* 2007;14(4):415-423.
7. Nelson, N. Downtime procedures for a clinical information system: a critical issue. *J Crit Care.* 2007;22:45-50.
8. Zodum MA. Practice management and electronic medical record implementation best practices: guide to successful implementation for primary care and federally qualified health centers. Eastern Shore Rural Health System, Inc. http://www.himss.org/content/files/Code%2067%20Practice%20Mgmt%20And%20EMR%20Best%20Practices_2008.pdf. November 2008.
9. Fahrenholz CG, Smith LJ, Tucker K, Warner D. A practical approach to downtime planning in medical practices. American Health Information Management Association. http://library.ahima.org/xpedio/groups/public/documents/ahima/bok1_045486.hcsp?dDocN. 2009.
10. The University of Kentucky. Department of Pharmacy policy: computer down time procedures (unplanned). The University of Kentucky. http://www.hosp.uky.edu/policy/pharmacy/depart policy/PH18-04.pdf. 2010.
11. Vaughn S. Planning for system downtimes. *Comput Nurs.* 2011;29(4):201-203.
12. Arraj V. ITIL: the basics. *Best Management Practice.* White Paper. 2010. www.best-management-practice.com/gempdf/itil_the_basics.pdf.
13. Whitten J, Bentley L. *System Analysis and Design Methods.* 7th ed. New York, NY: McGraw-Hill Higher Education; 2007.
14. American Nurses Association. The nursing process. *Nursing World.* http://nursingworld.org/EspeciallyForYou/What-is-Nursing/Tools-You-Need/Thenursingprocess.html. 2012.
15. Hoerbst A, Hackl WO, Blomer R, Ammenwerth E. The status of IT service management in health care: ITIL in selected European countries. *BMC Med Inform Decis Mak.* 2011;11:76.
16. Hoong LL, Marthandan G. Factors influencing the success of the disaster recovery planning process: a conceptual paper. *Research and Innovation in Information Systems (ICRIIS), 2011 International Conference.* 2011;1-6, 23-24. doi:10.1109/ICRIIS.2011.6125683.
17. Federal Emergency Management Agency (FEMA). IT disaster recovery plan. FEMA. http://www.ready.gov/business/implementation/IT. 2012.
18. Federal Emergency Management Agency (FEMA). Business continuity plan. FEMA. http://ready.gov/business/implementation/continuity. 2012.
19. Nickolette C. Business continuity planning description and framework. Comprehensive Consulting Solutions, Inc. http://www.comp-soln.com/BCP_whitepaper.pdf. 2001.

DISCUSSION QUESTIONS

1. Explain the importance of an organization-specific downtime risk assessment.
2. Describe the pros and cons of different assessment tools for evaluating downtime events and discuss scenarios in which they might be used to their best advantage.
3. Compare and contrast the roles of the informaticist, the clinician, and IT personnel in system downtime planning.
4. Describe key components of a business continuity plan and (a) how they might differ for different types of organizations and (b) how they might differ depending on EHR maturity level.
5. Contrast different communication methods for system downtime events and summarize the pros and cons of each.

CASE STUDY

At your Level 2 trauma center an unplanned EHR downtime occurs at 1700 on a Tuesday. After 1 hour of troubleshooting and working with the vendor's help desk, the IT team attempts a system reboot, which is unsuccessful. The vendor is in a different time zone so specialists have to be called in from home to respond to this incident. The initial assessment is that the downtime is due to database corruption and the system will have to be recovered from backup systems. Unfortunately the system is not configured with high availability techniques nor is it redundant. The IT department estimates that it will take 8 hours to recover the system for a total downtime of 10 hours.

Discussion Questions

1. Plot each component on the Downtime Determinator for both part 1 and part 2 of the scenario as it unfolded and document your IT response, end-user response, and communication plans.
2. Make changes to the assessment and plans to account for changes to the scenario.

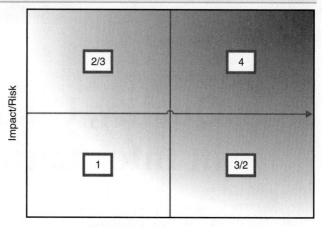

Length of Downtime/Time to Recover

Plot each component in one of the four quadrants to determine where the items cluster

1. Time of day/number of users
2. IT infrastructure affected
3. System criticality
4. Planned versus unplanned
5. Health system complexity
6. Communication: Amount required and are methods affected?
7. Ability to recover

Quality, Usability, and Standards in Informatics

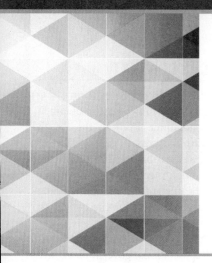

Privacy, Confidentiality, Security, and Data Integrity

Nancy Staggers, Lisa Gallagher, Luciana Schleder Gonçalves, and Ramona Nelson

> *Neither patients nor healthcare providers will fully accept electronic healthcare systems unless they can trust that private patient data are held in confidence through effective policies and procedures and secure information systems.*

OBJECTIVES

At the completion of this chapter the reader will be prepared to:
1. Distinguish among common concepts related to this area of informatics: privacy, confidentiality, security, covered entity, and data integrity
2. Analyze current federal and state laws and regulations and their implications for privacy and security practices and procedures

3. Use appropriate resources in establishing and implementing security- and privacy-related policies and procedures
4. Apply common procedures for securing sensitive health information

KEY TERMS

Availability, 318
Confidentiality, 308
Covered entity, 322
Data integrity, 318
Informed consent, 320
Privacy, 308
Protected health information (PHI), 317

Risk, 318
Risk assessment (risk analysis), 318
Security, 308
Threat, 318
Transparency, 309
Vulnerability, 318

ABSTRACT

This chapter provides an overview of definitions and concepts related to privacy and security of electronic health data and information. International, national, and local security and privacy related practices, guidelines, principles, laws, and regulations are outlined. To avoid overlap with other chapters, the discussion in this chapter of laws and regulations such as HIPAA and HITECH related to health information technology (health IT) is focused on security only. The chapter concludes with an examination of security concepts and procedures to ensure the safety and integrity of electronic health data.

INTRODUCTION

Unless healthcare providers and the general public can be assured that health data in any and all formats are held in confidence, the benefits of computerized health information will be compromised. The importance of privacy, confidentiality, and security has grown exponentially as the number of electronic health records (EHRs), health devices, and health data transmissions have expanded. With increased numbers of users, types of use, and volumes of health IT–based data come increased opportunities for privacy breaches. Both patients and healthcare providers are concerned about health IT privacy and security, especially as health data are used for secondary purposes such as research. Both groups generally support the concept of electronic health data storage and communication but concerns about security persist.[1]

This chapter provides an overview of definitions and concepts related to privacy and security of electronic health data. International, national, and local guidelines, principles, laws, and regulations concerning security and privacy practices are outlined. To avoid overlap with other chapters the discussion of HITECH and HIPAA and related regulations is focused on the security of healthcare information systems and the privacy of health information only.

DEFINITIONS AND CONCEPTS

In general, privacy is concerned with the rights of individuals to control access to their person (body privacy) or information about themselves (information privacy).[2] In informatics the concern is focused primarily on privacy of information. Designing systems that ensure information privacy is one of the most difficult challenges in the digital age.[3] Health records can contain information on any or all aspects of an individual's life and as a result are a source of highly sensitive information. They must be protected from misuse by nonauthorized personnel (i.e., privacy). Health data and information must be kept private if such data are to be considered trusted information and a primary resource for building new knowledge. Moreover, specific policies and procedures must be implemented to prevent disclosures or breaches that encroach on the privacy of the data's primary owner—the patient.[4]

The difference between privacy, confidentiality, and security can be confusing. Terms central to these concepts are defined in Table 19-1. Privacy concerns who has access to information, a patient's rights to confidentiality, and what constitutes inappropriate access. Confidentiality concerns protecting information from inappropriate access.

Security is the means to ensure health record privacy and confidentiality.

LEGAL AND HISTORICAL CONTEXT

Today's focus on health information security is built on a long history of concern with the privacy of information obtained during a caregiver–patient encounter. Even in the fourth century the Hippocratic Oath addressed the privacy of communications between patients and their healthcare providers.[2,5] In 1860 Florence Nightingale's *Notes on Nursing* addressed various uses of health information, including the importance of its proper acquisition for the benefit of the patient first and foremost, a concern that exists today. Privacy and confidentiality continue as concerns of healthcare providers, professional associations, governments, and civil rights commissions in many countries. After all, the information that individuals share with their caregivers as part of that trusted relationship may not have been shared with even their families or close friends.[6]

Caregiver Requirements

Healthcare providers are knowledge workers. This means that they focus on the data they collect and analyze how these data are processed to create information and then knowledge. One of the key competencies expected of knowledge workers in healthcare is the capability to protect patients' privacy, particularly in information-related areas such as EHRs. Ensuring a patient's privacy and confidentiality is not just a healthcare provider's prerogative but a requirement.

Patient Rights

In healthcare, consumers' rights must be preserved. These include the rights to choose how their health data might be used, to access their own health data, and to contest inaccuracies. In addition, consumers must have available to them a

TABLE 19-1	DISTINCTIONS AMONG TERMS
TERMS	**DEFINITIONS**
Confidentiality	Information is kept secret or is accessed by or disclosed to only those with a need to know, i.e., authorized users.
Integrity	Information has all its original features as established by the data owner in all phases of its lifecycle.
Availability	Information is always available for use to authorized users.
Accountability	Information related to an unambiguous identification of users.
Authenticity	Assures that the information source is actually what it is declared to be, and it is trusted.
Patient data safety	Actions undertaken to maintain data integrity, meaning that data will not be lost or modified by someone not authorized to do so.
Privacy	Restricting access to subscriber or relying party information in accordance with federal law and agency policy.
Security	The administrative, technical, and physical safeguards in an information system to prevent privacy breaches.

From Kissel R, ed. *Glossary of Key Information Security Terms* (NIST IR 7298, revision 1). Washington, DC: U.S. Department of Commerce & National Institute of Standards and Technology; 2011.

TABLE 19-2	DEFINITIONS OF FAIR INFORMATION PRACTICE PRINCIPLES
PRINCIPLE	**DESCRIPTION**
Individual access	Individuals should be provided with a simple and timely means to access and obtain their individually identifiable health information in a readable form and format.
Correction	Individuals should be provided with a timely means to dispute the accuracy or integrity of their individually identifiable health information and to have erroneous information corrected or to have a dispute documented if their requests are denied.
Openness and transparency	There should be openness and transparency about policies, procedures, and technologies that directly affect individuals and their individually identifiable health information.
Individual choice	Individuals should be provided a reasonable opportunity and capability to make informed decisions about the collection, use, and disclosure of their individually identifiable health information.
Collection, use, and disclosure limitation	Individually identifiable health information should be collected, used, and disclosed only to the extent necessary to accomplish specified purposes and never to discriminate inappropriately.
Data quality and integrity	Persons and entities should take reasonable steps to ensure that individually identifiable health information is complete, accurate, and up to date to the extent necessary for the person's or entity's intended purposes and has not been altered or destroyed in an unauthorized manner.
Safeguards	Individually identifiable health information should be protected with reasonable administrative, technical, and physical safeguards to ensure its confidentiality, integrity, and availability and to prevent unauthorized or inappropriate access, use, or disclosure.
Accountability	Appropriate monitoring and other means and methods should be in place to report and mitigate nonadherence and breaches.

process of redress when these rights are violated as well as information on how their rights can be exercised.[7]

Fair Information Practice Principles

Fair Information Practice Principles (FIPPs), also referred to as the Code of Fair Information Practices, are a set of internationally recognized practices for addressing privacy of information. The principles are the result of joint work by U.S., Canadian, and European government agencies over time and are available in reports, guidelines, and legal codes that ensure that information practices are fair and provide adequate privacy protection to individuals.[7] Although these statements can vary according to the source, typical FIPPs are included in Table 19-2.

Since the late 1970s many government agencies have addressed the impact of computerization of health records. Some industrialized countries have codified FIPPs into a privacy law at the federal level, although this has not yet occurred in the United States. Instead, in the U.S. the FIPPs are the basis of many individual laws at federal and state levels. The value of the FIPPs is that they provide a framework for privacy laws and also can form the foundation for an organization's or an industry's privacy policy. For example, although the Health Insurance Portability and Accountability Act of 1996 (HIPAA) does not formally codify FIPPs in the legislation, it implements all FIPPs in some way.[8] Table 19-3 outlines the use of FIPPs in various U.S. organizations to illustrate the varying nature of regulations on privacy.

Code of Ethics for Health Informatics Professionals

In 2002 the International Medical Informatics Association (IMIA) published a Code of Ethics for Health Informatics

Professionals that is closely related to the FIPPs.[9] This code has two major sections. The first addresses fundamental ethical principles: autonomy, equality and justice, beneficence, nonmalfeasance, impossibility, and integrity as applied to informatics (Table 19-4). The second section concerns the rules of ethical conduct for health informatics professionals. As this code demonstrates, FIPPs are now an integral aspect of ethical practices in health informatics.

PRINCIPLES, LAWS, AND REGULATIONS GUIDING PRACTICE

Over the centuries health professionals have used a combination of ethical codes, guiding principles, laws, and regulations to meet the responsibility of maintaining patients' privacy. The introduction of computers to managing healthcare information did not change the basic rights of patients or the responsibility of health professionals but it did offer new challenges and opportunities for securing health-related data and protecting patient privacy.

Early evidence is available that the federal government recognized the need for legislation to protect privacy in an electronic environment: the passage of the Privacy Act in 1974. This Act protects certain personal information held by federal agencies in computerized databases.[10] It includes three important factors. First, privacy of health data is considered within the larger context of privacy in general. The Privacy Act is not specific to the protection of health data but provides for protection of health-related data in federal agencies with health-related databases such as the Veterans Health Administration (VHA) or Medicare.

Second, this legislation was clearly molded to reflect the Code of Fair Information Practices described earlier in this

TABLE 19-3   SUMMARY OF FAIR INFORMATION PRACTICE PRINCIPLES AND SOME OF THEIR SOURCES

SOURCE	PRINCIPLES			
	ACCESS/ PARTICIPATION	NOTICE/ AWARENESS	CHOICE/CONSENT	INTEGRITY/ SECURITY
Federal Trade Commission, November 2012	Access/ Participation	Notice/ Awareness	Choice/Consent	Integrity/Security
U.S. Department of Health & Human Services, 2012; Nationwide Privacy and Security Framework for Electronic Exchange of Individually Identifiable Health Information	Individual access Correction	Openness and transparency	Individual choice Collection, use, and disclosure limitation	Data quality and integrity Safeguards Accountability
Organisation for Economic Co-operation and Development, 2008; Guidelines on the Protection of Privacy and Transborder Flows of Personal Data	Individual participation principle Correction limitation	Openness principle	Purpose specification Use limitation principle	Data quality Security safeguards principle Accountability principle
Canadian Standards Association, 1995; Model Code for the Protection of Personal Information	Individual access	Openness	Identifying purposes/ consent Limiting collection/ limiting use, disclosure, and retention	Accuracy Safeguards Accountability Challenging compliance
U.S. Department of Health, Education and Welfare, 1973	Record correction		Collection limitation Disclosure/secondary usage	Security

Data from Gellman R. *Fair information practices: a basic history.* BobGellman.com. http://bobgellman.com/rg-docs/rg-FIPShistory.pdf. November 12, 2012. Accessed December 3, 2012.

TABLE 19-4   GENERAL PRINCIPLES OF INFORMATIC ETHICS INCLUDED IN THE IMIA CODE OF ETHICS FOR HEALTH INFORMATICS PROFESSIONALS

PRINCIPLE	DESCRIPTION
1. Information—privacy and disposition	All persons have a fundamental right to privacy, and hence to control over the collection, storage, access, use, communication, manipulation, and disposition of data about themselves.
2. Openness	The collection, storage, access, use, communication, manipulation, and disposition of personal data must be disclosed in an appropriate and timely fashion to the subject of those data.
3. Security	Data that have been legitimately collected about a person should be protected by all reasonable and appropriate measures against loss, degradation, unauthorized destruction, access, use, manipulation, modification, or communication.
4. Access	The subject of an electronic record has the right of access to that record and the right to correct the record with respect to its accurateness, completeness, and relevance.
5. Legitimate infringement	The fundamental right of control over the collection, storage, access, use, manipulation, communication, and disposition of personal data is conditioned only by the legitimate, appropriate, and relevant data-needs of a free, responsible, and democratic society, and by the equal and competing rights of other persons.
6. Least intrusive alternative	Any infringement of the privacy rights of the individual person, and of the individual's right to control over person-relative data as mandated under Principle 1, may only occur in the least intrusive fashion and with a minimum of interference with the rights of the affected person.
7. Accountability	Any infringement of the privacy rights of the individual person, and of the right to control over person-relative data, must be justified to the affected person in good time and in an appropriate fashion.

From International Medical Informatics Association (IMIA). IMIA Code of Ethics for Health Information Professionals. *IMIA*. http://www.imia-medinfo.org/new2/pubdocs/Ethics_Eng.pdf. 2002.
IMIA, International Medical Informatics Association.

chapter. While the code is not specific to health data it has become a set of foundational principles used in the development of international and national guidelines, laws, and regulations designed to protect health privacy. Third, the Privacy Act included specific legislation on the mixing and matching of databases across agencies. Any one database may not contain data that could be considered private. However, combining databases can create new information that may more clearly identify individuals and in turn may include protected private data. Informatics professionals play a key role in understanding these complexities and developing policies and procedures to protect patient privacy within and across health-related databases.

The use of federal legislation to protect health data began in narrowly defined areas. For example, in 1975 the Department of Health, Education, and Welfare published rules and regulations governing the confidentiality of patient records that contained information on alcohol and drug abuse.[11] In 1996 the Privacy and Security Rules developed under HIPAA were the first federal regulations to broadly address the privacy and security of health data.[12]

National Privacy and Security Framework for Health Information

Neither individuals nor healthcare providers are willing to share complete and accurate health-related data unless they can trust that these data are secured in a protected, private environment. "Clear, understandable, uniform principles are a first step in developing a consistent and coordinated approach to privacy and security and a key component to building the trust required to realize the potential benefits of electronic health information exchange."[12] To meet this need the Office of the National Coordinator for Health Information Technology (ONC) developed a set of principles to guide the actions of healthcare personnel and entities involved in the electronic exchange of individually identifiable health information. These principles are listed in Table 19-3 and are consistent with the FIPPs seen elsewhere. These principles are designed to complement and work with existing federal, state, and local laws.

Laws and Regulations

Numerous principles, guidelines, laws, and regulations deal with privacy and are important when considering the privacy of health data maintained in electronic format. Therefore this section focuses on guidelines, laws, and regulations related to privacy of health data.

International

Since individuals, health-related problems, and institutions offering healthcare services do not stay within national borders, comprehensive electronic healthcare systems providing the full benefits of computerization require that countries, institutions, and individuals are able to share data safely across borders. Sharing such data requires privacy standards, legislation, and rules. While there are differences between countries and cultures in how privacy is conceived and in the value placed on privacy of health data, privacy of health data is increasingly being recognized as an international value.[13] Understanding these differences and building health information systems that can share data across national borders requires first an understanding of the current status of privacy and security across nations.

The World Health Organization (WHO), recognizing the potential of IT to strengthen health systems and to improve care, has encouraged its member states to incorporate ehealth in health systems and services. To support this effort WHO established an ehealth program and defined ehealth as "the use of information and communication technologies (ICT) for health."[14] In 2005, the same year in which the ehealth program was established, WHO established the Global Observatory for eHealth (GOe). GOe is an initiative dedicated to the study of ehealth with the goal of providing member states with strategic information and guidance on effective practices and standards in ehealth. In meeting its goal GOe conducted an ehealth survey in 2005 and again in 2009. As of 2012 a third survey was in the planning stages. The 2009 survey included 114 WHO member states representing more than 80% of the world's population.[15] The results of this survey were reported in six volumes, which can be accessed at www.who.int/goe/publications/en/.

The survey questionnaire included questions dealing specifically with privacy and legislation. The first two of these questions focused on the existence of legislation protecting the privacy of personal and health-related data. Seventy percent of the reporting countries indicated that they had legislation ensuring privacy of personal health information; however, only 30% had legislation protecting personal identifiable data in an EHR. The survey went on to ask about legislation dealing with sharing health-related data between healthcare staff via an EHR. Twenty-six percent of the reporting countries indicated that they had legislation dealing with sharing data within a network of healthcare providers; 23% had legislation dealing with sharing data between healthcare entities within the country and 11% had legislation dealing with sharing data with other countries.

As this survey demonstrated, selected countries have created agreements and legislation supporting the transfer of health data across their borders. One of the earliest and best recognized agreements was created by the European Union (EU) in 1995 when it passed a comprehensive data privacy law titled the EU Directive on the Protection of Individuals with Regard to the Processing of Personal Data and on the Free Movement of such Data. The EU selected a "directive" approach that required each EU member state to enact its own law based on the fair principles outlined in the directive. Health data are discussed under Article 8, Section III of the directive titled Special Categories of Processing:

> Member States shall prohibit the processing of personal data revealing racial or ethnic origin, political opinions, religious or philosophical beliefs, trade-union membership, and the processing of data concerning health or sex life.[16]

Needed exceptions are included in paragraph 3:

> Paragraph 1 shall not apply where processing of the data is required for the purposes of preventive medicine, medical diagnosis, the provision of care or treatment or the management of health-care services, and where those data are processed by a health professional subject under national law or rules established by national competent bodies to the obligation of professional secrecy or by another person also subject to an equivalent obligation of secrecy.[16]

However, Article 24 of the directive prohibits sending personal data to any country that does not meet the EU standards of data protection. To enforce this article the directive imposes tight limits on transmitting personal data outside of Europe. Health data related to European individuals can be transmitted only to countries with data protection laws that the European Commission considers adequately safeguard Europeans.[17]

As each EU member state developed and implemented its legislation, it implemented the 1995 rules differently, resulting in divergences in enforcement and a number of related problems. In January 2012 a comprehensive reform of the directive was proposed. Key changes include a single set of rules on data protection, valid across all of the EU, and a streamlined approach for applying EU rules if personal data are handled abroad by companies that are active in the EU market and offer their services to EU citizens.[18] Additional information about the proposed directive and what it will mean for international businesses, including healthcare organizations, can be found at http://ec.europa.eu/justice/data-protection/document/review2012/factsheets/5_en.pdf.

A number of other countries, in addition to those in the EU, have developed international agreements and legislation related to privacy of personal data. What does not exist at this point is a single set of standards, rules, or legislation that could be used in designing information systems that store health-related data. Therefore informaticists must approach each international situation on an individual basis. Both the Electronic Frontier Foundation (EFF) (www.eff.org/issues/international-privacy-standards) and the Electronic Privacy Information Center (https://epic.org/privacy/intl/) maintain websites listing privacy-related international accords and agreements. Neither list is comprehensive but these can be used as a starting point in exploring international privacy agreements pertinent to the privacy of health-related data.

Federal

U.S. Federal efforts to ensure the security and privacy of health-related data include federal legislation and collaborative state–federal initiatives. A list of related laws and regulations is provided in Box 19-1. The primary federal legislation dealing with privacy is HIPAA, which is discussed in detail in Chapter 24. In this chapter the discussion of HIPAA is limited to its importance in designing and implementing health information systems.

Congress incorporated in HIPAA provisions that mandate the adoption of federal privacy protections for individually identifiable health information by requiring that the U.S.

Department of Health & Human Services (HHS) adopt national standards for security. HHS published a modified final Privacy Rule in August 2002. This rule set national standards for the protection of individually identifiable health information by three types of covered entities: health plans, healthcare clearinghouses, and healthcare providers who conduct standard healthcare transactions electronically. The final Security Rule was published in February 2003. This rule set national standards for protecting the confidentiality, integrity, and availability of electronic protected health information. Basically, the Privacy Rule focuses on what protections are provided and the Security Rule specifies how data must be protected. Both rules are administered and enforced by the HHS Office for Civil Rights. The Health Information Technology for Economic and Clinical Health (HITECH) Act widened the scope of privacy and security protections provided under HIPAA. A list of the provisions affected by the HITECH Act is provided in Box 19-2. These laws and the

---

BOX 19-1 HEALTHCARE-RELATED PRIVACY AND SECURITY LAWS AND REGULATIONS*

- Health Insurance Portability and Accountability Act (HIPAA)
- CMS Security Standard
- Confidentiality of Alcohol and Drug Abuse Patient Records
- The Privacy Act of 1974
- Family Educational Rights and Privacy Act (FERPA)
- Gramm-Leach-Bliley Act

From Brown GD, Patrick TB, Pasupathy K. *Health Informatics: A Systems Perspective.* Chicago, IL: Health Administration Press; 2012.
CMS, Centers for Medicare & Medicaid Services.
*Additional information on each of these laws and regulations is located at http://healthit.hhs.gov/portal/server.pt/community/healthit_hhs_gov__federal_laws_and_regulations/1178.

BOX 19-2 PROVISIONS OF HIPAA EXPANDED BY THE HITECH ACT

- Application of privacy provisions and penalties to business associates of covered entities
- Application of security provisions and penalties to business associates of covered entities; annual guidance on security provisions
- Notification in the case of breach
- Education on health information privacy
- Limitations on certain contacts as part of healthcare operations
- Breach notification requirement for vendors of personal health records and other non-HIPAA covered entities
- Expanded use of business associate contracts
- Application of wrongful disclosures criminal penalties
- Required audits

HIPAA, Health Insurance Portability and Accountability Act; *HITECH Act,* Health Information Technology for Economic and Clinical Health Act.

related rules define what data are protected, under what conditions and how that protection must be provided. Each healthcare institution is required to interpret and apply these rules within its own environment. For example, HIPAA does not refer to cybersecurity; however,

> Meaningful Use criteria make it virtually certain that eligible providers will have to have an Internet connection. To exchange patient data, submit claims electronically, generate electronic records for patients' requests, or e-prescribe, an Internet connection is a necessity, not an option. To protect the confidentiality, integrity, and availability of electronic health record systems, regardless of how they are delivered; whether installed in a physician's office, accessed over the Internet, basic cybersecurity practices are needed.[19]

In January of 2013 HHS announced the final omnibus rule based on statutory changes under the HITECH Act and the Genetic Information Nondiscrimination Act of 2008 (GINA). As can be seen in Box 19-3 "the final omnibus rule greatly

---

BOX 19-3   OVERVIEW OF THE HIPAA FINAL RULES

Final HIPAA Rule Overview. The omnibus final rule strengthens and expands patient rights as well as enforcement and is comprised of the following four components:

1. **HIPAA Privacy, Security, and Enforcement Rules and HITECH Act.** The final rule modifies the Privacy, Security, and Enforcement Rules. These modifications include:
   - changes regarding business associates;
   - limitations on the use and disclosure of PHI for marketing and fundraising;
   - prohibition on the sale of PHI without authorization;
   - expanded rights to receive electronic copies of health information and to restrict disclosures to a health plan concerning treatment paid out of pocket in full;
   - requirement to modify and redistribute notice of privacy practices;
   - modified the individual authorization and other requirements to facilitate research, disclose child immunization proof to schools, and access decedent information by family members/others.
2. **Enforcement Rule.** Final rule adopts changes to the HIPAA Enforcement Rule to incorporate the increased and tiered civil money penalty structure provided by the HITECH Act.
3. **Breach Notification Rule.** Final rule adopts the Breach Notification for Unsecured PHI created under the HITECH Act, and replaces the Breach Notification Rule's "harm" threshold with a more objective standard.
4. **HIPAA Privacy Rule as It Relates to Genetic Information.** Final rule modifies the HIPAA Privacy Rule as required by the Genetic Information Nondiscrimination Act (GINA) to increase privacy protections for genetic information by prohibiting most health plans from using or disclosing genetic information for underwriting purposes.

From eHealth Initiative. New HIPAA Rules and Implications for the Industry. (PDF document). January 29, 2013. Retrieved from http://www.ehealthinitiative.org/complimentary-webinars/viewdownload/118/641.html.

---

enhances a patient's privacy protections, provides individuals new rights to their health information, and strengthens the government's ability to enforce the law."[20] Health plans, healthcare clearinghouses, and healthcare providers must follow state laws and regulations in addition to federal laws and regulations. This requirement is further complicated when health services and institutions cross state lines.

Federal–State Collaboration

The Health Information Security and Privacy Collaboration (HISPC) consisting of 34 states and territories was established in 2006 and charged with:
- Assessing variations in privacy- and security-related organization-level business policies and state laws that affect health information exchange
- Identifying and proposing solutions while preserving the privacy and security requirements of applicable federal and state laws
- Developing detailed plans to implement the proposed solutions

In 2008 HISPC moved into its third phase, with 42 states and territories addressing the privacy and security challenges presented by electronic health information exchange through multistate collaboration. Phase 3 projects included:
- Studying intrastate and interstate consent policies
- Developing tools to help harmonize state privacy laws
- Developing tools and strategies to educate and engage consumers
- Developing a toolkit to educate healthcare providers
- Recommending basic security policy requirements
- Developing interorganizational agreements[21]

Each project was designed to develop common, replicable multistate solutions for reducing variation in and harmonizing privacy and security practices, policies, and laws. A number of products and reports have been produced as a result of these efforts and can be accessed at www.healthit.gov/policy-researchers-implementers/health-information-security-privacy-collaboration-hispc.

In addition to being used in the provision of healthcare, protected health data can be used for a number of other activities. This is referred to as the secondary use of health data and it presents its own special privacy and security issues when dealing with electronic health data.

Secondary Uses of Electronic Health Data

The three most common secondary uses of personal health information are public health monitoring or surveillance, research, and marketing.

Public Health Monitoring or Surveillance

Public health agencies, which frequently must work within states and across state lines, are required to follow both federal and relevant state laws and regulations. In addition to HISPC, discussed above, the Public Health Data Standards Consortium (PHDSC) provides information, education, and tools for protecting the privacy of personal health data. PHDSC is a national nonprofit membership-based organization of federal, state, and local health agencies; professional associations; academia; public and private sector organizations; international members; and individuals. Its mission focuses on promoting health IT standards to empower health communities to improve individual and community health. Its Privacy, Security, and Data Exchange Committee addresses individual and organizational privacy and security standards related to maintaining and sharing health information, in electronic form, for public sector health programs and health services research purposes. The goals include the following:

- To represent and educate broad public sector health and health services research interests on privacy and security issues
- To focus on priorities related to privacy, security, and data standardization
- To balance the need for individual privacy, confidentiality, and security with the need for use of data for public health and research activities

PHDSC used the data in the state survey conducted by HISPC to complete a systematic analysis of the public health domain with the goal of identifying all privacy-related variations, solutions, and implementation plans reported by states that directly involved or affected public health practice. Two reports were issued. The first report summarizes the variations in privacy and security policies, practices, and state laws affecting the interoperability of public health information exchanges. The second report focuses on the analysis of solutions and implementation plans proposed by states and aimed at addressing barriers to public health information exchanges. These two reports are available from PHDSC at www.phdsc.org.

With the information in these reports PHDSC developed a Privacy Toolkit for Public Health Professionals (PRISM). PRISM consists of a series of tables that outline different types and purposes of information use and disclosure and the general legal requirements relevant to each type of use or disclosure. The tables describe the baseline privacy requirements for disclosure of health information using HIPAA, other federal laws affecting health privacy, and common state privacy laws and related requirements. The PRISM tables can be accessed at http://phdsc.org/privacy_security/prismtool.asp.

Deidentification Data

Health data used for marketing are almost always deidentified; deidentified health information neither identifies nor provides a reasonable basis to identify an individual. HIPAA includes no restrictions on the use or disclosure of deidentified health information.[22] However, there are regulations concerning the specific procedures that can be used to deidentify protected data.[23] These two procedures, the safe harbor method and the expert determination method, are outlined in Figure 19-1.

THE IMPORTANCE OF INFORMATION SECURITY

While privacy and confidentiality are the goals, they are not the main issues when dealing with health IT. The primary

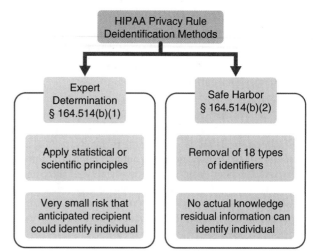

FIG 19-1 Two methods to achieve deidentification in accordance with the Health Insurance Portability and Accountability Act's (HIPAA's) Privacy Rule. (Copyright The U.S. Department of Health & Human Services. http://www.hhs.gov/ocr/privacy/hipaa/understanding/coveredentities/De-identification/guidance.html#standard. Accessed December 5, 2012.)

issue is information security. Privacy is assured through adequate security measures.[24] Four areas emphasize the importance of health information security today: the public trust, legal requirements and fines, increasing security threats to healthcare data, and recent changes in health data practices.

Patients' requirements for privacy and society's need for improving efficiency and reducing costs must be balanced.[25] With increased connectivity comes the sharing of highly sensitive data as well as social and political pressure to avoid inappropriate sharing.

The Public Trust

Healthcare providers earn patients' trust by guaranteeing the privacy of their health information. Patients entrust their most intimate information to healthcare providers and they do not expect either their health information or their identities to be exposed publicly.[26] Thus breaches of privacy and security undermine patients' confidence in their healthcare providers. On the other hand, adequate security measures can bolster the public trust and perhaps boost EHR adoption rates.[24]

Legal Requirements and Fines

Legal requirements and potential fines make information security critical to organizations. The largest fine to date was $4.3 million for an organization that refused to release health records to several patients and then did not cooperate with the government's investigation of the matter.[24] Penalties under HIPAA can be as large as $68 million if an organization has no information security measures in place.[24] Additional examples of HIPAA-related fines and other penalties are provided in Table 19-5.

TABLE 19-5	**EXAMPLES OF HIPAA VIOLATIONS AND RELATED FINES**			
NEWS RELEASE DATE	INSTITUTION OR COMPANY	REPORTED BY	VIOLATIONS	SETTLEMENT AGREEMENT
September 17, 2012	Massachusetts Eye and Ear Infirmary and Massachusetts Eye and Ear Associates Inc. (MEEI)	MEEI	• Theft of an unencrypted personal laptop containing the ePHI (included patient prescriptions and clinical information) of MEEI patients and research subjects. • MEEI failed to conduct a thorough analysis of the risk to the confidentiality of ePHI maintained on portable devices and failed to implement security measures to ensure the confidentiality of ePHI when using portable devices, policies and procedures to restrict access to ePHI to authorized users of portable devices, and policies and procedures to address security incident identification, reporting, and response.	Pay a $1.5 million fine and adhere to a corrective action plan to ensure compliance with the Security Rule.
June 26, 2012	Alaska Department of Health and Social Services (DHSS)	DHSS	• A USB hard drive possibly containing ePHI was stolen from the vehicle of a DHSS employee. • DHSS did not have adequate safeguard policies and procedures in place. • DHSS had not completed a risk analysis, implemented sufficient risk management measures, completed security training for its workforce, implemented device and media controls, or addressed device and media encryption.	Pay a $1.7 million fine and take corrective action to ensure compliance with the Security Rule.
April 17, 2012	Phoenix Cardiac Surgery (PC)	Unknown	• Staff were posting clinical and surgical appointments for patients on an Internet-based calendar that was publicly accessible. • PC failed to implement adequate policies and procedures to safeguard patient information • PC failed to document that it trained any employees on policies and procedures. • PC failed to identify a security official and conduct a risk analysis. • PC failed to obtain business associate agreements with Internet-based email and calendar services where the provision of the service included storage of and access to its ePHI.	Pay a $100,000 fine and develop a corrective action plan to ensure compliance with the Security Rule.
March 13, 2012	Blue Cross Blue Shield of Tennessee (BCBST)	BCBST	• Fifty-seven unencrypted computer hard drives were stolen from a leased facility. The drives contained the ePHI of more than 1 million individuals, including member names, Social Security numbers, diagnosis codes, dates of birth, and health plan identification numbers. • BCBST failed to implement appropriate administrative safeguards by not performing the required security evaluation. • BCBST failed to implement appropriate physical safeguards.	Pay a $1.5 million fine and implement a corrective action plan to address gaps in its HIPAA compliance program.

Data from U.S. Department of Health & Human Services (HHS). Health information privacy: case examples and resolution agreements. HHS. http://www.hhs.gov/ocr/privacy/hipaa/enforcement/examples/index.html.
ePHI, Electronic protected health information; *HIPAA*, Health Insurance Portability and Accountability Act.

As can be seen in Table 19-5, security breaches are costly to organizations. The average cost of a health record breach in 2010 was $301 per compromised record.[27] Considering that a single breach can include thousands of records, even one breach is costly. Any breach costs organizations in lost productivity and damage to the public trust. Also, total costs for security breaches may be less visible. Fines are certainly noticeable but remediation costs are less so because they are absorbed as redirected priorities, time-consuming forensic analyses, and productivity losses.[27] For example, under HIPAA physicians and organizations must notify each person affected by a breach, set up a call center for victims, pay legal fees of about $1000 per victim, and pay fines and penalties for each breach incidence.[28]

Increasing Security Threats to Healthcare Data

In 2010 there were 221 major security breaches and 30,000 smaller breaches.[27] A single one of these breaches in the U.S. involved 4.9 million health records, with the total number of affected records at 10 million for 2009 and 2010 combined. In addition, healthcare is no longer exempt from hackers and malicious cyberattacks. One in six cyberattacks in 2009 were in healthcare.[27,29] By 2011 an Internet security report by Symantec identified healthcare as the top target of cyberattacks.[24] These attacks will only increase as availability of electronic health data increases.

Security threats are not limited to the exposure of health information but also include personal identity theft and fraud.[28] In fact, health identity theft is growing quickly because Social Security numbers and Medicaid and Medicare information do not change as credit card numbers do. These data, once stolen, can be sold or used to file fraudulent claims over time for large sums. For example, a worker in Florida used stolen data to file for $2.8 million in false Medicare claims.[28]

Recent Changes in Health Data Practices

Recent health practices, including increased electronic health data access and transmission due to the use of mobile devices and expanded health data sharing within and across health organizations, increase the risk of a security breach. Mobile devices are attractive to healthcare providers because they support increased health data access and increased individual productivity. However, these devices also increase opportunities for interception of health data and, in turn, data loss.

Health data are being increasingly shared. EHR information is no longer tied to one institution and traditional stakeholders are changing to include patients inputting information in their own records.[30] Health information exchange, by design, is meant to allow data sharing within a region. Population-based research is growing and, with it, the need for increased security for "big data."[1] Authors are now publishing material about how to share health data nationally and internationally.[31] Each of these levels has security implications and opportunities for breaches.

CURRENT SECURITY VULNERABILITIES

Current security vulnerabilities can be classified into three types of events: natural events such as floods or hurricanes, external events such as malicious messages or hacking, and events internal to an organization.[32] Obviously natural events such as lightning strikes can disable whole systems, networks, or security servers. In one example, a health organization abandoned a building but left clinical data in a locked closet. A power loss unlocked the door; nine servers containing clinical data were stolen.[24] Although natural events are

dramatic, these events account for only a few of the reported security events.

External Events

Examples of external security events include outside attempts to access an organization's network (hacking), intrusions though a firewall, and installing malicious code or sending malicious messages via email. Recent security conferences such as DefCon and BlackHat featured sessions about hacking into health systems.[24]

Large health systems have long protected their information systems and data using security controls described later in this chapter. Small organizations are more vulnerable[27] because they may lack the knowledge and resources necessary to implement security measures and information security may not be a high priority for them. For example, the network for a surgeons' group in California was hacked and data were stolen and encrypted to prevent access. Subsequently, the hackers sent a ransom note to the surgeons for return of their data; the surgeons refused to pay and lost all of their patients' data.[24]

Internal Vulnerabilities

Most security events are internal and can be unintentional or intentional.[27,32] Security policies and procedures may be lacking in some organizations or HIPAA compliance may not be a high priority,[25] especially in smaller organizations. Even if internal policies exist, current practices may not comply with either internal or external policies. Although security risk assessments or risk analyses are required under HIPAA, some organizations have never completed one and others do not complete them regularly.[27] In the latest available annual survey of professionals in health organizations, only 75% of respondents indicated that their organizations completed required risk analyses. This number was constant over the previous 4 years of surveys.[3] Thus 25% of respondents were in organizations that do not complete risk assessments. Since the 326 respondents do not represent all U.S. health organizations, the number of noncompliant organizations is likely much higher. Also, third party organizations may not be using due diligence even if main health organizations are compliant. The largest threat to security is insider abuse of privileges.[24] Leaders indicate that insider mistakes and abuse are their number one security concern.[27]

Many breaches are lapses in judgment and involve IT personnel. For example, in Utah a system administrator installed a new server on the local area network but did not configure it using recommended methods (instead using a simple password like "admin admin"). Hackers gained access to the server on March 10, 2012, and downloaded information on March 30, stealing more than 280,000 Social Security numbers and less sensitive information about 500,000 other people. The breach was not detected until April 2, 2012.[34]

Medical Devices

Medical devices as basic as intravenous (IV) pumps represent a special area of vulnerability. Medical devices are proliferating and are being used for (1) monitoring (e.g., glucometers, oximetry, home blood pressure devices), (2) resuscitating (e.g., defibrillator, IV pumps), (3) surgical procedures (e.g., lasers, robotics such as da Vinci), (4) imaging (e.g., computed tomography, magnetic resonance imaging, echograms), and (5) diagnostic procedures (e.g., ultrasound, endoscopy). Many of these devices have the capability to connect and share data through networks or even operate remotely through wireless or cellular networks.

Because these devices can connect to a network and share data, they also can be hacked. The U.S. General Accountability Office was asked to examine security issues of medical devices after a computer security professional hacked his own insulin pump at a BlackHat security conference in 2012. He showed how he could remotely alter his own pump settings to change insulin dosages and even indicate to the user that sufficient insulin was being delivered when, in fact, it was not.[35] In another example, security researchers showed that pacemakers and defibrillators could be hacked wirelessly, allowing an attacker to, for example, send a fatal shock to a patient with an implanted cardiac defibrillator or simply stop the defibrillator altogether.[36]

The medical device itself can store sensitive data, including protected health information (PHI), that are often not encrypted.[29] Many medical devices are sold without common security controls such as antivirus software. In health organizations medical devices are typically deployed and managed by biomedical or clinical engineering staff who may operate separately from the IT department. This can create issues about the number and kinds of devices deployed as well as confusion about which are connected to the IT network.

CURRENT SECURITY CHALLENGES

Challenges to health data security can be grouped into the following three main areas:
- Competing goals of access to support patient care and limiting access to support security
- Competing priorities and adequate resources
- Multiple and evolving regulations

Health information access and security constitutes a balancing act. Healthcare organizations involve activities such as communications in shared workspace, work under time constraints, and the need to transmit sensitive data quickly across settings. These kinds of needs can conflict with security goals. Even with privacy and security training, care goals or productivity losses may discourage clinicians from adhering to security-related procedures and policies. Fernando and Dawson examined how clinicians worked with existing privacy and security policies in tertiary care settings in Australia.[37] Among other factors, they found that these hampered compliance with security policies: poor-quality training on identifying confidential information, security measures on EHRs took time away from patient care, usability errors increased security avoidance techniques, and clinicians were skeptical about the value of privacy and security implementations on EHRs. The overall conclusion was that clinicians

could not completely control the security of health information due to the nature of the clinical setting.

As an industry, healthcare allocates only about 3% of fiscal resources on security while other industries typically spend 6% to 12%.[33] While HIPAA requires that a security officer be appointed, many organizations do not have a person dedicated to security. Healthcare Information and Management Systems Society (HIMSS) survey respondents in 2011 indicated that about half of their organizations had a full-time person; more commonly security may be just one of many responsibilities assigned to an individual.[24] Perhaps for these reasons and due to only recent HIPAA compliance audits, the adoption of security technologies has been slow.

Multiple regulations exist. HIPAA has been in place since 1996. The HITECH Act introduced a breach notification rule in 2009 but each state can have separate and unique breach requirements. For example, California requires notification of the state's attorney general if a fax with protected data is sent to the wrong recipient. In Minnesota this same event would constitute a security breach.[27] Also, Meaningful Use requirements are evolving with each stage. Meaningful Use Stage 2 security requires automated security monitoring for systems as well as automatic log-off and encryption. Meaningful Use Stage 3 security requirements are now being developed.

MANAGING SECURITY RISKS WITH SECURITY CONTROLS

All methods to manage security risks revolve around the following common security goals:
- Confidentiality. In addition to the notions about access to sensitive information, this concept also refers to an individual's obligation to safeguard PHI.
- Data integrity. This includes accuracy and completeness of health information. An example of data integrity concerns identifying and linking disparate patient records, such as merging duplicate records for the same patient.
- Availability. Obviously it is important that electronic patient data be available when needed at the point of care. Availability is increased when system redundancy, resiliency, and robust backup capabilities are implemented and these are considered components for security.[30,32]

Most solutions to security are simple and not costly.[24] Security controls are typically grouped into three areas: administrative, technical, and physical.

Administrative

Administrative controls include establishing and adhering to security policies and procedures as well as dedicating resources to security. Formal policies and procedures set internal rules about how an organization and its employees will protect PHI. These should be based on federal guidelines for HIPAA and the HITECH Act. In addition to these, the National Institute of Standards and Technology (NIST) has published a series of security guidelines called the "800 series," available at http://csrc.nist.gov/publications/PubsSPs.html. These are documents of interest to the security community and include current topics such as security measures for cloud computing and mobile devices. Although the health community is not mandated to adhere to these guidelines, they can be used for HIPAA compliance.[24]

Internal policies should include processes such as installing software service packs, installing antivirus software, and testing. While most organizations do install service packs, the issue may be timing. Installation of required software patches can be delayed in lieu of other priorities. Instead, these need daily monitoring and updating.[27] Organizations should also have policies and procedures in place for intrusion protection to avoid malware and malicious attacks. Finally, policies need to be in place to encrypt mobile devices used for PHI. Encrypting a laptop with clinical data costs only about $150.[24] Wireless handheld devices should also be encrypted, as they are vulnerable to loss.[26] Given the increased attention to the vulnerabilities of medical devices, organizations will want to assess the security capabilities of these devices before purchase. Probably most important, health organizations need to have policies and procedures in place to conduct security risk assessments.

Conducting Risk Assessments or Risk Analysis

Risk assessment also called risk analysis is required by the HIPAA Security Rule and by Meaningful Use.[27] The purpose of these assessments is to identify gaps or weaknesses that could lead to security breaches. These also assist in prioritizing risk remediation efforts.[24] More formally, security risks are assessed by examining vulnerabilities and threats, where:

- Risk is the likelihood that something adverse will happen to cause harm to an informational asset (or its loss)
- Vulnerability is a weakness in the information system, device, or environment that could endanger or cause harm to an informational asset
- Threat is a human act or an act of nature that has the potential to cause harm to an informational asset[38]

Risk assessments should be conducted regularly with at least one complete assessment done annually. A comprehensive risk assessment can cost between $10,000 and $100,000 depending on the complexity of the environment.[27] Risk assessments include an evaluation of how and where PHI is stored within the organization, who is managing these data, how these data are being used, and where data are transmitted. A risk assessment includes a review of the security measures and technical architecture.[24,27]

A number of toolkits are available for conducting risk assessments in a healthcare setting. A suite of toolkits is available from the HIMSS Security Task Force as well as the Agency for Healthcare Research and Quality (AHRQ) website (URLs are available at the end of the chapter). These toolkits include, for example, risk assessments for small practices, mobile devices, and cybersecurity. An application risk assessment tool examines areas such as:

- Access management (passwords)
- Audit capabilities (audit logs)
- Security for remote access to clinical data

- Protection from malicious code
- Configuration management and change control (updates to software)
- Data export and transfer capabilities (PHI transmission)

Risk assessments should include an assessment of high-risk medical devices, especially those storing PHI. Not all of these devices have security controls and only some allow connectivity to the local network, meaning that PHI data storage exists within the devices, outside more common access control, and PHI can exist in multiple areas.[29]

Technical

Technical security procedures and technologies are implemented using technology that protects against inappropriate access to PHI. Common technical security controls include access management and control, encryption, and privacy enhancing technologies.

Access Management and Control

Access management and control is achieved through authentication, where authentication is defined as the technology and techniques for verifying the identity of human users of an information or computer system.[38] Authenticating a person means verifying that the person is who he or she claims to be. This is typically accomplished by verifying something the user *has* (e.g., an employee number) and something the user *knows* (e.g., a password). Common examples of authentication include the following:

- *User name and password.* The most widely used form of authentication is entering a user name and associated password. Once entered, these are then verified against information stored in the computer system by a person with responsibility for managing the system users (e.g., a system administrator). Password requirements have increased in complexity to avoid unauthorized access. A combination of letters, numbers, and symbols is common, with periodic required changes to an individual's stored password.
- *Biometrics.* Biometrics refers to technology that can identify humans by their characteristics or traits (e.g., fingerprint, voice, or retinal pattern).[38] Using one of these traits to authenticate a person verifies something the user *is* or *does.* The benefits of biometrics over traditional methods such as passwords are that they are more secure, nearly impossible to reproduce or defraud, and reliable.[39] They can be used for authentication, identifying patients, or encrypting clinical data in EHRs. Their disadvantages include technical and usability issues. Obtaining a good initial biometric template can be problematic and biometric features can be affected by temperature, humidity, age, skin color, and degradation or damage to the feature. Also, some environments are not conducive to biometric use (e.g., using fingerprints in areas where gloves are worn).[39]

Role-based access is a typical access control model currently but it can be uneven by allowing excessive access for some roles.[40] That is, nurses may be restricted to access to patients on a specific patient care unit while any physician, including those in research, may be allowed access to all patients' data anywhere in the institution. Newer models are being explored that match a person with the resource being accessed, the requested action, and the environment.[41]

Encryption

Encryption is defined as the conversion of data into a form, called ciphertext, that cannot be easily understood by unauthorized people.[38] This technical method protects PHI against unauthorized access. To be able to access the data an authorized person has to decrypt the data, that is, change the ciphertext into understandable data. This is accomplished through the use of a security key such as a password. Encryption is a primary method of rendering PHI unusable, unreadable, or indecipherable to unauthorized individuals.

Encryption technology is available for use on many technology platforms (e.g., EHRs, desktop computers, laptops, etc.). Facilities can also encrypt PHI on mobile devices, email, and files. This technology is not currently available for all platforms; for example, not all cellphone devices contain encryption capability. However, users can purchase encryption software separately and download it for use on devices. In some cases the software is free for individual users but not for enterprise contracts. When cellphones are used to store PHI, use of encryption capability is critical.

While encryption is helpful to control access to PHI, it is not a panacea. It still relies on specific security controls, processes, and human interaction (humans must actively encrypt data) for the technique to be successful.[24] Also, PHI such as digital images can be encrypted but still be intercepted during transmission.[42]

Privacy Enhancing Technologies

Privacy enhancing technologies (PETs) are viewed as technologies that:

- Reduce the risk of bypassing privacy and security policy and principles
- Minimize the amount of data held about individuals
- Allow individuals to retain control of information about themselves at all times[38]

PETs are designed to safeguard the data owner's privacy and rights by protecting personal data and preventing its unnecessary or undesired processing.[38] PETs are relatively new technologies being targeted and marketed to individuals. Although encryption can be considered a type of PET, other methods include the following:

- *Communication anonymizers.* These methods hide the real online identity of a person (email address, IP or Internet Protocol address, etc.) and replace it with a nontraceable identity such as a disposable or one-time email address, random IP address of hosts participating in an anonymizing network, or pseudonym. These can be used for email, web browsing, point-to-point networking arrangements, voice over Internet Protocol (VoIP), and instant messaging.
- *Shared bogus online accounts.* In this method users create an account on Microsoft Network (MSN) but provide bogus data for their names, addresses, phone numbers, preferences, and life situation. A user then publishes the user identification and password on the Internet. Anyone can use this account and the original user is assured that there are no personal data in the account profile.

These techniques have uses as well as drawbacks. Encryption prevents unauthorized access to primary data but it also prevents secondary data uses such as research. Data encryption is also time consuming. Anonymization, on the other hand, is a technique amenable for secondary data uses such as research but it cannot be reversed, preventing the use of full primary health records. Also, if anonymization is used for secondary data uses such as research, then patients do not benefit because their identity cannot be known.

One set of authors describes a newer technique to avoid both of these disadvantages.[25] Called pseudonymization, this technique allows data to be associated with a patient only under specific and controlled circumstances. Two data tables are needed, one with personal data and one with pseudonymized clinical data. The relationship between these tables can be restored using a secret key stored on a device such as a smart card held by a patient. A centralized list of linkages is also stored in case of smart card loss. Obviously the centralized list can be a target but it can operate off-line to preclude unauthorized access.

Physical

The third category of security controls is physical control. This involves physical methods to protect inappropriate access to PHI.[38] Examples are controlled access to buildings, workstation security and use, and securing portable devices such as medical devices or laptops with a cable and locking them to a desk.[29] Defined by administrative controls, actual physical devices or measures are put into place for improved security.

RESOURCES

A number of resources are available to guide organizations in the administrative, technical, and physical aspects of information security. Examples include the following:

- AHRQ security toolkits available at http://healthit.ahrq. gov/portal/server.pt/community/health_it_tools_and_ resources/919/the_health_information_security_and_ privacy_collaboration_toolkit/27877
- HIMSS Privacy and Security Task Force website at www. himss.org/ASP/topics_privacy_committees.asp?faid=83& tid=4
- HIMSS Privacy and Security Task Force toolkits—risk assessments, small provider privacy and security guides, and mobile devices cloud computing security—available at www.himss.org/ASP/topics_pstoolkitsDirectory.asp? faid=569&tid=4
- HIPAA Security 101 for Covered Entities from HHS available at www.hhs.gov/ocr/privacy/hipaa/administrative/ securityrule/security101.pdf

- NIST Computer Security Resource Center (CSRC) website at http://csrc.nist.gov/
- NIST security guidelines available at http://csrc.nist.gov/publications/PubsSPs.html

CONCLUSION AND FUTURE DIRECTIONS

Neither patients nor healthcare providers will fully accept electronic healthcare systems unless they can trust that private patient data are held in confidence through effective policies, procedures, and secure information systems. This chapter discussed the underlying principles for designing and implementing secure systems. Legislation, rules, and regulations were reviewed. Using these as a basis, specific security measures were explored.

The need for information security will continue to expand in the future. Newer models for security are being developed in lieu of current role-based models. For example, one model being developed places information control and release in the hands of patients.[30] These kinds of security frameworks allow patients to give informed consent for access to any data. Every piece of data is tagged with a unique identification code to prevent linking to unauthorized data. The framework provides a link to access control with a device such as a smart card and traceable information flow through the use of data on a central server should the mobile device be lost. This is more flexible than HIPAA security, where blanket consent is given.

In summary, privacy and security have been and will continue to be concerns for patients and healthcare providers. Health informaticists need a solid grounding in the concepts and solutions for these important principles.

REFERENCES

1. Stevenson F, Lloyd N, Harrington L, Wallace P. Use of electronic patient records for research: views of patients and staff in general practice. *Fam Pract.* 2012;[epub ahead of print].
2. Soares NV, Dall'Agnol CM. Patient privacy: an ethical question for nursing care management. *Acta paul enferm.* 2011;24(5):683-688. http://www.scielo.br/scielo.php?pid=S0103-21002011000500014&script=sci_arttext.
3. Hartzog W. Information privacy: chain-link confidentiality. *Ga L Rev.* 2012;46(3):657-704.
4. Neuhaus C, Polze A, Chowdhuryy M. *Survey on Healthcare IT Systems: Standards, Regulation and Security.* Potsdam, NY: Potsdam University; 2011.5. Rothstein MA. The Hippocratic bargain and health information technology. *J Law Med Ethics.* 2010;38(1):7-13.
5. Rothstein MA. The Hippocratic bargain and health information technology. *J Law Med Ethics.* 2010;38(1):7-13.
6. Olsen DP, Dixon JK, Grey M, Deshefy-Longhi T, Demarest JC. Privacy concerns of patients and nurse practitioners in primary care: an APRNet study. *J Am Acad Nurse Prac.* 2005;17(12):527-534.
7. Federal Trade Commission (FTC). Fair information practice principles. FTC. http://www.ftc.gov/reports/privacy3/fairinfo.shtm. 2012. Accessed December 3, 2012.
8. Gellman R. Fair information practices: a basic history. BobGellman.com. http://bobgellman.com/rg-docs/rg-FIPShistory.pdf. 2012. Accessed December 3, 2012.
9. International Medical Informatics Association (IMIA). IMIA code of ethics for health information professionals. IMIA. http://www.imia-medinfo.org/new2/pubdocs/Ethics_Eng.pdf. 2002. Accessed December 5, 2012.
10. The Privacy Act of 1974 5 U.S.C. § 552a. U.S. Department of Justice. http://www.justice.gov/opcl/privstat.htm. 1974.
11. Department of Health, Education and Welfare. Confidentiality of alcohol and drug abuse patient records. *Federal Register.* 1974;40(127). http://www.hhs.gov/ohrp/archive/documents/19750701.pdf.
12. Office of the National Coordinator for Health Information Technology. National privacy and security framework for the electronic exchange of identifiable health information. U.S. Department of Health & Human Services. http://healthit.hhs.gov/portal/server.pt/community/healthit_hhs_gov__privacy___security_framework/1173. 2008.
13. Kay M, Santos J, Takane M. *Global Observatory for eHealth Series: Legal Frameworks for eHealth.* Vol 5. Geneva, Switzerland: World Health Organization; 2012.
14. World Health Organization (WHO). eHealth. WHO. http://www.who.int/ehealth/en/. 2012.
15. Kay M, Santos J, Takane M. *Global Observatory for eHealth Series: Atlas eHealth Country Profiles.* Vol 1. Geneva, Switzerland: World Health Organization; 2011.
16. European Parliament and the Council of 24 October. Directive 95/46/EC of the European Parliament and of the Council of 24 October 1995 on the protection of individuals with regard to the processing of personal data and on the free movement of such data. EUR-LEX Access to European Union Law. http://eur-lex.europa.eu/LexUriServ/LexUriServ.do?uri=CELEX:31995L0046:en:NOT. October 24, 1995.
17. Mittman JM, Dowling JDC. International data protection and privacy law. In: Basri CL, ed. *International Corporate Practice.* New York, NY: Practising Law Institute; 1996–2012:24-3-24-83.
18. European Commission. Commission proposes a comprehensive reform of data protection rules to increase users' control of their data and to cut costs for businesses. EUROPA: Press Releases Rapid. http://europa.eu/rapid/press-release_IP-12-46_en.htm?locale=en. 2012. Accessed January 2012.
19. HealthIT.gov. Cybersecurity: 10 best practices for the small healthcare environment. HealthIT.gov. http://www.healthit.gov/sites/default/files/basic-security-for-the-small-healthcare-practice-checklists.pdf. 2010.
20. HSS. News release: new rule protects patient privacy, secures health information. http://www.hhs.gov/news/press/2013pres/01/20130117b.html. 2013.
21. HealthIT.gov. Federal-state privacy & security collaboration (HISPC).(nd). HealthIT.gov. http://www.healthit.gov/policy-researchers-implementers/federal-state-privacy-security-collaboration-hispc.
22. U.S. Department of Health & Human Services (HHS) Office for Civil Rights. Summary of the HIPAA Privacy Rule. *Health Information Privacy.* http://www.hhs.gov/ocr/privacy/hipaa/understanding/summary/index.html.(nd).
23. U.S. Department of Health & Human Services (HHS) Office for Civil Rights. Guidance regarding methods for de-identification of protected health information in accordance with the Health Insurance Portability and Accountability Act (HIPAA)

Privacy Rule. HHS. http://www.hhs.gov/ocr/privacy/hipaa/understanding/coveredentities/De-identification/guidance.html. 2012.

24. McMillan M. A national perspective on helping IT play a meaningful role in healthcare reform. Paper presented at: Summer Insight Educational Session; August 16, 2012; Salt Lake City, UT.

25. Neubauer T, Heurix J. A methodology for the pseudonymization of medical data. *Int J Med Inform.* 2011;80(3):190-204.

26. Huang C, Lee H, Lee DH. A privacy-strengthened scheme for E-healthcare monitoring system. *J Med Syst.* 2012;36(5):2959-2971.

27. McMillan M. HITECH security mandates for healthcare organizations. *Healthc Financ Manage.* 2011;65(11):118-122, 124.

28. Civelek AC. Patient safety and privacy in the electronic health information era: medical and beyond. *Clin Biochem.* 2009;42(4-5):298-299.

29. Swim R. Keeping data secure: protected health information and medical equipment. *Biomed Instrum Technol.* 2012;46(4):278-280.

30. Haas S, Wohlgemuth S, Echizen I, Sonehara N, Muller G. Aspects of privacy for electronic health records. *Int J Med Inform.* 2011;80(2):e26-e31.

31. Li JS, Zhou TS, Chu J, Araki K, Yoshihara H. Design and development of an international clinical data exchange system: the international layer function of the Dolphin Project. *J Am Med Inform Assn.* 2011;18(5):683-689.

32. Liu CH, Chung YF, Chen TS, Wang SD. The enhancement of security in healthcare information systems. *J Med Syst.* 2012;36(3):1673-1688.

33. Healthcare Information and Management Systems Society (HIMSS). HIMSS Security Survey. Chicago, IL: HIMSS; 2011.

34. Utah Department of Health. Utah Data Breach. Utah Department of Health. http://www.health.utah.gov/databreach/common-questions.html. 2012. Accessed November 30, 2012.

35. Zetter K. Lawmakers call for probe of medical devices after researcher hacks insulin pump. Wired.com. http://www.wired.com/threatlevel/2011/08/medical-device-security/. 2011.

36. Timmer J. Hacking implanted defibrillators: shockingly easy. Ars Technica. http://arstechnica.com/science/2008/03/hacking-implanted-defibrillators-shockingly-easy/. 2008. Accessed November 30, 2012.

37. Fernando JI, Dawson LL. The health information system security threat lifecycle: an informatics theory. *Int J Med Inform.* 2009;78(12):815-826.

38. Brown GD, Patrick TB, Pasupathy K. *Health Informatics: A Systems Perspective.* Chicago, IL: Health Administration Press; 2012.

39. Flores Zuniga AE, Win KT, Susilo W. Biometrics for electronic health records. *J Med Syst.* 2010;34(5):975-983.

40. Malin B, Nyemba S, Paulett J. Learning relational policies from electronic health record access logs. *J Biomed Inform.* 2011;44(2):333-342.

41. McGraw D. Privacy and health information technology. *J Law Med Ethics.* 2009;37(Suppl 2):121-149.

42. McGraw D, Dempsey JX, Harris L, Goldman J. Privacy as an enabler, not an impediment: building trust into health information exchange. *Health Affair.* 2009;28(2):416.

DISCUSSION QUESTIONS

1. Hospitals usually have a policy and related procedure for responding when patients request a copy of their records. Select a procedure from your current place of employment or a local hospital. Compare and contrast the selected procedure with the principles of fair information practice (FIPPs).

2. Country profiles of the 114 WHO member states that participated in the 2009 global survey on eHealth can be found at www.who.int/goe/publications/atlas/en/index.html. Select two countries, one that is of interest to you and your country of origin. Compare the survey results for these two countries. What are the challenges and resources for creating an agreement to share health data across the borders of these two countries?

3. The following websites include toolkits for completing a risk assessment:
   a. www.himss.org/ASP/topics_pstoolkitsDirectory.asp?faid=569&tid=4
   b. http://healthit.ahrq.gov/portal/server.pt/community/health_it_tools_and_resources/919/the_health_information_security_and_privacy_collaboration_toolkit/27877#Scenarios Guide

   Review the risk assessment guides available at these sites and then answer the following question. Since HIPAA requires that a covered entity appoint a security officer, what is the role of the health informatics specialist in working with the security officer to complete a risk assessment? In your discussion consider who has access to the information required to complete the assessment and how the information should be collected.

4. Providing access to healthcare providers and securing a system from inappropriate access can be a difficult balancing act. In many cases the more secure a system is, the more restricted access to that system becomes. Discuss situations where this balancing act has created conflict within the clinical area and how that conflict was managed.

5. Increasingly patients are creating and maintaining personal health records (PHRs) with data from a variety of healthcare providers as well as data they have generated about their health. What provisions should be included in a model privacy and security policy that patients might use in making decisions related to their privacy and the security of their PHRs?

CASE STUDY

Last month you were hired with the title Chief Health Informatics Specialist at an independent community care hospital with 350 beds. The hospital includes a comprehensive outpatient clinic, a rehabilitation center with both inpatient and outpatient services, a cardiac care center, and an emergency room. In addition, four family health centers are located throughout the community. More than 930 primary care and specialty physicians are associated with the hospital, which has a staff of just over 2000 employees. The hospital is moving ahead with installing an EHR system following the Meaningful Use criteria.

The hospital has a working relationship with a major academic medical center located 23 miles away. Acute care patients who need more extensive treatment are usually transferred to the medical center. These are often emergency situations and data are freely shared between institutions with the best interests of the patient in mind.

Located directly beside the hospital is a 194-bed skilled nursing home. While the nursing home has its own medical staff consisting of a physician and two nurse practitioners, patients needing consults or additional care are usually seen at the hospital with follow-up at physicians' offices. While the nursing home, most of the physicians' offices, and the hospital are independent institutions, there is a long history of sharing health-related data when treating patients who live at the nursing home and are seen at the hospital or in the physicians' offices. This coordination has been a general benefit for a number of patients. It appears that most patients have signed a form giving the hospital permission to send information to the nursing home. However, these forms have been stored in individual offices so it is difficult to determine who has signed what forms and what permission has or has not been given to share information between the nursing home, hospital, and independent medical practices.

Discussion Questions

1. What additional information is needed to clarify what problems may exist and what changes may be needed in terms of shared data between the institutions?

2. Can the EHR system currently being installed be used to share data between these different institutions more effectively and securely? If yes, how would this be done? For example, what agreements, policies, and procedures might need to be developed?

3. In your position as Chief Health Informatics Specialist how would you go about determining whether there are other potential security issues that now need to be managed by the hospital?

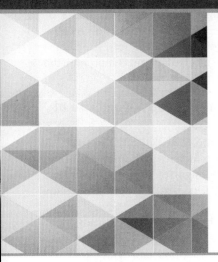

20

Patient Safety and Quality Initiatives in Informatics

Patricia C. Dykes and Kumiko Ohashi

Because of the complexity of the errors in healthcare, multifaceted strategies including health information technology tools are needed to realize improvement in clinical processes and patient outcomes when striving to improve quality and safety.

OBJECTIVES

At the completion of this chapter the reader will be prepared to:
1. Define patient safety and quality of care and describe the role of health IT in advancing the quality and safety of healthcare in the United States
2. Review three national initiatives driving adoption and use of health IT in the United States

3. Review two national initiatives related to promoting quality data standards in the United States
4. Discuss the components of the Framework for Patient Safety and Quality Research Design and describe how this framework can be used to evaluate quality and patient safety interventions and research.

KEY TERMS

Adverse event, 328
Health information technology (health IT), 323
Meaningful Use, 323

Patient safety, 324
Pay for performance, 329
Quality of care, 324

The chapter begins by defining quality of care and patient safety and by discussing key regulatory initiatives that drive a focus on quality and safety in the United States. The Framework for Patient Safety and Quality Research Design is then introduced as a means to classify and to evaluate adverse patient safety and quality events with a focus on medication safety, chronic illness screening and management, and nursing sensitive quality outcomes. The chapter ends with a discussion of success factors, lessons learned, and future directions for using the Framework for Patient Safety and Quality Research Design as a guide for both informatics research and practice.

INTRODUCTION

For more than a decade a series of Institute of Medicine (IOM) reports on the quality of healthcare have led to widespread recognition that errors occur far too often and

that the quality of patient care is variable across the U.S. healthcare system.[1-5] Evidence suggests that the use of health information technology (health IT) supports better communication and error reduction.[6,7] Widespread adoption of health IT is a recommended strategy to facilitate effective, high-quality, and safe patient care.[8]

The passage of the American Recovery and Reinvestment Act (ARRA) of 2009 is expected to improve the quality of care by promoting adoption and supporting Meaningful Use of electronic health records (EHRs)[9] and through widespread improvement in the ability to detect and reduce clinical errors.[10] ARRA requires that hospitals demonstrate Meaningful Use of EHRs through the following mechanisms:
1. Use of a certified EHR
2. Facilitation of care coordination and quality by participating in the exchange of electronic health information
3. Submission of data for quality reporting

In this chapter the use of health IT to improve quality of care and patient safety is examined. First, the concepts "quality of care" and "patient safety" are defined and some of the key regulatory initiatives that are driving a focus on quality of care and patient safety in the U.S. are discussed. Next, the Framework for Patient Safety and Quality Research Design[11] is introduced and used to classify adverse patient safety and quality events, discuss key success factors and lessons learned, and then make recommendations for implementation and future research.

Definitions

Inconsistent use of language is a barrier to understanding quality and patient safety and to benchmarking beyond the organizational level.[12] To provide a foundation, the definitions of *quality of care* and *patient safety* put forth by the IOM and the World Health Organization (WHO) World Alliance for Patient Safety are presented.

Quality of Care

In its 1990 report titled *Medicare: A Strategy for Quality Assurance* the IOM defined quality of care as "the degree to which health services for individuals and populations increase the likelihood of desired health outcomes and are consistent with current professional knowledge."[4(p21)] In 2001, in its report titled *Crossing the Quality Chasm*, the IOM proposed six aims as a means to narrow the quality chasm that exists in the U.S. healthcare system.[2] It proposed that healthcare should be:

- *Safe:* prevents injury or other adverse outcomes
- *Effective:* ensures that evidence-based interventions are used, with patients always receiving the treatments most likely to be beneficial
- *Patient-centered:* ensures that patient preferences, needs, and values are front and center in the process of clinical decision making
- *Timely:* delivered when needed and without harmful delays
- *Efficient:* prevents the waste of valuable human and material resources
- *Equitable:* provided to all individuals without regard for ethnic, racial, socioeconomic, or other personal characteristics

The WHO World Alliance for Patient Safety adopted the IOM definition of quality of care in its International Classification for Patient Safety (ICPS) released in 2009.[12]

Patient Safety

The IOM defined patient safety as "freedom from accidental injury due to medical care, or medical errors" where error is defined as "the failure of a planned action to be completed as intended or the use of a wrong plan to achieve an aim."[3(p4)]

The ICPS defined safety as "the reduction of risk and unnecessary harm to an acceptable minimum" and patient safety as "the reduction of risk of unnecessary harm associated with healthcare to an acceptable minimum."[12(p21)] The ICPS defined error as "failure to carry out a planned action as intended or application of an incorrect plan" and healthcare-associated harm as "harm arising from or associated with plans or actions taken during the provision of healthcare, rather than an underlying disease or injury."[12(pp19,21)]

These definitions highlight the multifaceted nature of quality and safety and the notion that failures of both omission (e.g., failure to provide evidence-based care) and commission (e.g., providing care incorrectly) can compromise the quality and safety of healthcare.

National Initiatives Driving Adoption and Use of Health IT

A key lesson learned from the IOM's *Quality Chasm Series* is that achievement of higher quality and safer care in the U.S. requires systemic redesign of established clinical processes and that health IT is needed to support and maintain the transition to best practices.[1-3,5,8,13] Several initiatives on the national level have maintained a steady focus on quality and patient safety. Recent U.S. policy is aligning incentives with the goal of adoption and widespread use of health IT to ensure a healthcare system characterized by uniform high quality and safe patient care.[14] In 2011 the Office of the National Coordinator for Health Information Technology (ONC) published a report titled *Federal Health Information Technology Strategic Plan: 2011–2015.*[15] This report defines the ONC's plan for working with the private and public sectors to achieve the nation's health IT agenda. Specific examples of accreditation and policy efforts designed to achieve the six quality aims defined by the IOM through a focus on redesign of clinical processes and adoption and Meaningful Use of health IT are included in Table 20-1.

Key areas of focus for ongoing accreditation and policy efforts include improving the quality of care and preventing adverse events. Evidence suggests that the U.S. may be making progress in the quest for higher quality and safer care but there is much room for improvement. Downey, Hernandez-Boussard, Banka, and Morton evaluated national trends in patient safety indicators (PSI) such as postoperative pulmonary embolism, deep vein thrombosis, and pressure ulcers. They found significant PSI trends for the decade 1998 to 2007. PSIs with the greatest levels of improvement during that period included birth trauma injury to neonates, postoperative physiologic and metabolic derangements, and iatrogenic pneumothorax. The PSIs with the greatest increase in incidence included pressure ulcers, postoperative sepsis, and infections due to medical care. Downey and colleagues noted that health IT holds potential for decreasing PSIs through standard reporting requirements and by supporting evidence-based practices through decision support and the use of order sets.[16]

National Efforts Related to Quality Data Standards

As mentioned in the previous section, the Meaningful Use initiative aims to improve the quality of care in the U.S. through routine exchange of electronic health information for care delivery and quality reporting purposes. However, much work is needed to build the informatics infrastructure required to support the interoperability of systems and routine data exchange. An important component of the

TABLE 20-1	ACCREDITATION AND POLICY INITIATIVES FOCUSING ON IMPROVING QUALITY OF CARE AND PATIENT SAFETY THROUGH HEALTH INFORMATION TECHNOLOGY (HEALTH IT)
INITIATIVE	**DESCRIPTION**
The Joint Commission National Patient Safety Goals (NSPG)[17]	Program established in 2002 by The Joint Commission to assist accredited organizations in addressing patient safety concerns.[17] Examples of 2012 NPSG facilitated by health IT include the following: • Reduce the likelihood of patient harm associated with the use of anticoagulant therapy (NPSG.03.05.01). (1) EMR-based clinical decision support to alert and manage potential food and drug interactions, (2) use of "smart pumps" to provide consistent and accurate dosing, and (3) use of MedlinePlus to educate patients about the importance of follow-up monitoring, compliance, drug–food interactions, and the potential for adverse drug reactions and interactions. • Maintain and communicate accurate patient medication information (NPSG.03.06.01). (1) Use of an electronic medication reconciliation system to obtain information on the medications the patient is currently taking at all care transitions and (2) use of MedlinePlus to provide the patient (or family) with written information about the medications prescribed.
The Leapfrog Group[18]	Initiative led by healthcare purchasers designed to improve the quality, safety, and affordability of healthcare by reducing preventable medical mistakes.[18] Examples of 2012 Leapfrog goals facilitated by health IT include the following: • Prevent medication errors: Use of CPOE • Steps to avoid harm: Use of clinical decision support in EMR decision support to prevent medical mistakes • Reduce pressure ulcers: Electronic assessment and plan of care application to link areas of risk with tailored interventions to prevent pressure ulcers from occurring • Reduce in-hospital injuries: Electronic assessment and plan of care application to link areas of risk with tailored interventions to prevent falls and related injury
CMS Hospital-Acquired Conditions[9]	In response to the Deficit Reduction Act of 2006, CMS identified a list of preventable hospital-acquired conditions for which hospitals would no longer receive additional payment.[9] Examples of hospital-acquired conditions that could be prevented through use of health IT include the following: • Pressure ulcers: Electronic assessment and plan of care application to link areas of risk with tailored interventions to prevent pressure ulcers from occurring • Patient falls with injury: Electronic assessment and plan of care application to link areas of risk with tailored interventions to prevent falls and related injury • Manifestations of poor glycemic control: Use of clinical decision support in EMR for postoperative insulin dosing
Pay for Performance (P4P)[19]	Medicare initiative designed to improve quality of care in all healthcare settings through collaboration with providers and other stakeholders, to ensure that valid reliable measures of quality determine levels of reimbursement for care provided.[19] Examples of P4P measures facilitated by health IT include the following: • Cholesterol management–LDL control <100: Patient use of self-management tools through patient portal • HbA1c control <7.0%: Patient use of self-management tools through patient portal • Implement drug–drug and drug–allergy interaction checks: Use of clinical decision support in EMR for automated interaction checking
Meaningful Use[20]	American Recovery and Reinvestment Act (ARRA) of 2009 initiative designed to provide incentives for providers and healthcare organizations to improve quality of care through Meaningful Use of EHRs. Examples of Meaningful Use of health IT performance measures include the following: • Use CPOE • Use eMAR • Provide online access to health information to patients[20]
National Committee for Quality Assurance (NCQA)	A nonprofit organization established in 1990 by the Robert Wood Johnson Foundation to improve the consumer's ability to evaluate health plans through voluntary public reporting.[21] The Healthcare Effectiveness Data and Information Set (HEDIS) was developed and is maintained by NCQA.
Utilization Review Accreditation Commission (URAC)	An independent, nonprofit organization that aims to promote continuous improvement in the quality and efficiency of healthcare management through processes of accreditation and education.[22]

CMS, Centers for Medicare & Medicaid Services; *CPOE,* computerized provider order entry; *EHR,* electronic health record; *eMAR,* Electronic Medication Administration Record; *EMR,* electronic medical record; *LDL,* low-density lipoprotein.

informatics infrastructure is the establishment and adoption of standards at multiple levels to support semantic interoperability. Semantic interoperability means that data are exchanged without a loss of context or meaning. Semantic interoperability is only possible when all organizations adopt the same standards for quality measurement and reporting and use those standards in their electronic systems. The ultimate goal is to capture data for quality reporting in the context of existing documentation workflows. This requires that standard clinical content is adopted and used in electronic systems, standard taxonomies or vocabularies are used to encode that content, and messaging standards are used to transfer information from one healthcare organization to another.

To automatically track the quality of care, standard quality measures are needed to ensure that all organizations are using consistent metrics for benchmarking and that organizations are using the same types of data to populate the quality metrics. For data to be collected as a by-product of documentation, the standard quality metrics must define standard value sets (allowed values), taxonomies (standard terminologies), concept codes (codes assigned by the terminology developer), attributes (characteristics that provide context), and data structures and these same standards must also be used to encode the content in the electronic record.

Currently, work aimed at mapping (linking) specific quality concepts to recommended terminologies is ongoing for 16 Center for Medicare & Medicaid Services (CMS) and The Joint Commission (TJC) inpatient measures in the domains of Stroke, Venous Thromboembolism, and Emergency Department as part of a quality measure retooling effort. The resulting work is published in the Healthcare Information Technology Standards Panel (HITSP) Quality Measures Technical Note (version 1.2), providing a detailed use case for applying existing standards to specify measures electronically.

Defined standards to support Meaningful Use are included in Table 20-2.[23] As mentioned above, representation of the complete data element set (e.g., the entire question-answer pair) by standardized terminologies and codes within an EHR system is required for full automation of quality reporting. Adoption and use of the same standards by all organizations are required for quality reporting and benchmarking beyond the organizational level. Many of these standards are included in the Stage 2 Meaningful Use initiative that aims to provide incentives for their use in EHR systems and subsequently to provide the informatics infrastructure needed across the U.S. to collect and report quality data as a by-product of documentation.

TABLE 20-2	CATEGORIES AND TYPES OF DATA ELEMENTS COMMON TO HIGH-PRIORITY MEASURES AND ADOPTED TERMINOLOGIES		
DATA CATEGORIES	**DATA TYPES**		**ADOPTED VOCABULARY STANDARDS TO SUPPORT MEANINGFUL USE STAGE 1/STAGE 2**
Adverse drug event	Allergy	Intolerance	NA/Unique Ingredient Identifier (UNII)
Communication	Provider–provider	Provider–patient	
Diagnostic study	Order	Result	ICD-9 CM, CPT 4/ICD-10 CM, CPT 4
Diagnosis	Outpatient (billing) Outpatient (problem list)	Inpatient	ICD-9 CM, SNOMED CT/ICD-10 CM, SNOMED CT
History	Behavioral (smoking) Birth Care classification Death Enrollment trial Ethnicity/race	Language Payment source Primary care provider Sex Symptoms	
Laboratory	Order	Result	LOINC
Location	Source/current/target	Transfer type	
Medication	Discontinue order Inpatient administered Inpatient ordered	Outpatient duration Outpatient order Outpatient filled	RxNorm
Opt out	Other reason		
Physical exam	Vitals		
Procedure	Inpatient end Inpatient start Order	Outpatient Past history Consult results	ICD-9 CM, CPT 4/ICD-10 CM, CPT 4

Adapted with permission from American Medical Informatics Association and based on Dykes PC, Caligtan C, Novack A, et al. Development of automated quality reporting: aligning local efforts with national standards. *AMIA Annu Symp Proc.* 2010; 2010:187-191.
CPT, Current Procedural Terminology; *ICD,* International Classification of Diseases; *LOINC,* Logical Observation Identifier Names and Codes; *SNOMED,* Systematized Nomenclature of Medicine.

EVALUATING QUALITY AND PATIENT SAFETY

The foundation for the approach used to evaluate quality and patient safety in healthcare organizations in the U.S. is based on the work of Avedis Donabedian, who developed a framework for measuring quality based on organizational structure, processes, and their linkages to patient outcomes.[24] Donabedian's model provides the underpinnings for the framework for patient safety and quality research design (PSQRD) (Fig. 20-1).[11]

- *Structure:* The setting and its attributes (e.g., the physical structure of buildings, staffing ratios, the equipment available within an organization, and the budget to support care provision) are all part of its structure. Exogenous factors that may not be completely under the local control of a hospital or healthcare organization are also part of the structure. Examples include TJC accreditation standards, Meaningful Use requirements, and other accreditation, licensing, and payment directives.
- *Process:* The managerial (human resource policies, training practices, management practices) and clinical (use of evidence-based interventions to promote quality and safety, communication practices at the bedside) processes in place to support the provision of care are all included under the process component. Managerial processes have a latent effect on outcomes, as they influence communication and care practices that aim to affect patient care

delivery. Interventions aimed at clinical processes may have an immediate effect on patient outcomes.
- *Outcomes:* The outcomes or end result of the structures and processes in place. These may include both clinical outcomes (e.g., improved health status, decreased mortality) and throughput (i.e., the number of patients treated). The outcomes are often the aim of health IT and other interventions implemented to improve patient status.

Conceptual Framework for Patient Safety and Quality

The framework for PSQRD builds on Donabedian's structure-process-outcome model to support evaluation of an intervention from the preimplementation testing phase through implementation and evaluation.[11] In the case of a health IT intervention, the expanded framework supports understanding where the health IT intervention is most likely to have an effect, within the organizational causal chain of quality and safety events (see Fig. 20-1). The PSQRD framework provides a means to categorize interventions according to areas of the causal chain targeted (e.g., the structure, the management or clinical processes, and the patient outcomes or throughput targeted by the intervention or that drive adoption and use of the intervention in clinical practice).

The PSQRD framework is pertinent to evaluating the effect of health IT interventions on quality and patient safety, as it provides a means to better explain why a health IT intervention was successful (or not). There are many reasons why

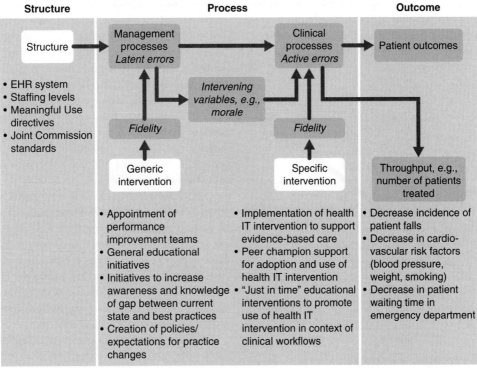

FIG 20-1 A framework for patient safety and quality research design. *EHR,* Electronic health record. (Modified from Brown C, Hofer T, Johal A, et al. An epistemology of patient safety research: a framework for study design and interpretation. Part 1. Conceptualising and developing interventions. *Qual Saf Health Care.* 2008;17[3]:160.)

health IT interventions are not adopted in practice.[25,26] Health IT tools not widely adopted and used will have a limited effect on patient outcomes. In the sections below we use the PSQRD framework to first evaluate health IT interventions designed to improve quality and patient safety. We then use it to make some recommendations to improve the implementation and evaluation of health IT interventions aimed at enhancing quality and patient safety.

Within the PSQRD framework, quality and safety issues are not mutually exclusive entities but exist on a "vector of egregiousness" (Fig. 20-2). Quality is at one end of the vector, representing frequent events with lower levels of immediacy. Causality and patient safety are at the opposite end of the vector, encompassing more immediate events with high levels of causality. Errors or events that do not fall on or close to the vector are included within the quality–safety continuum and classified as having components of both. The PSQRD framework defines causality as "the confidence with which a bad outcome, if it occurs, can be attributed to an error" and defines immediacy as "immediate or rapid."[11(pp158-159)] For example, there is good evidence on the population level that screening mammography decreases breast cancer mortality in women.[27] When an unscreened woman develops end-stage breast cancer, the adverse outcome was preventable. However, the causal link is low and the time over which breast cancer occurs is typically not immediate or rapid.

Using this model as a framework, a hospital-acquired infection from poor handwashing practices has a high degree of causality and a low to moderate degree of immediacy. Patient falls and pressure ulcers are located midway up the vector of egregiousness with lack of tailored interventions to mitigate risk, placing patients at risk for injury with moderate degrees of causality and immediacy. Serious medication errors are higher on the vector, as they may occur due to

inadequate adherence to the "5 rights" for medication safety (right patient, right time, right drug, right dose, and right route). Medication errors are the most common adverse event (an unintended and unfavorable effect of medical care or treatment) in hospital settings and are largely preventable through use of health IT systems with decision support at the bedside (i.e., closed loop bar-coding, medication administration, and smart pumps).[28] Medication errors are high on the vector of egregiousness toward safety because these types of errors are preventable through adherence to the "5 rights" and, when they occur, have the potential to cause immediate and significant patient harm.

Medication Safety

Health IT systems hold promise for improving the quality and safety of care, particularly in the area of medication safety. To date, computerized provider order entry (CPOE) and clinical decision support (CDS) systems have been used successfully in clinical practice to reduce errors during the process of ordering medications.[7,29] In addition, Bar Code Medication Administration (BCMA) and Electronic Medication Administration Record (eMAR) systems have been adopted in a number of hospitals to improve patient safety and streamline clinical workflow, focusing in particular on improving administration processes at the point of care.[30-32] These systems leverage bar-coding applications, with bar code labels placed on patient wristbands and on medications. The systems can ensure adherence to the "5 rights" to reduce medication errors and to document administration of drugs in real time. BCMA and eMAR systems are effective when implemented and used properly.[33-35] For example, after BCMA system implementation, the scanning compliance rate is often suboptimal for scanning both drugs and patient IDs.[36,37] One study found that compliance with scanning medications was only 55.3%.[36] Another study revealed that nurses may bypass scanning processes and create workarounds to reduce workloads or prevent delay of medication administrations.[35] Workarounds are defined as any use of an operating system outside its designed protocol.[35] This problem occurs most often in the system implementation stage and may create potential new paths to medical errors or other negative effects, such as inefficiency.[34,38]

The IOM reports, the TJC Standards, and the National Patient Safety Goals (NPSG) represent structural incentives for use of health IT to improve medication safety.[8,17] TJC is an international nonprofit organization that aims to inspire healthcare organizations to excel in providing safe and effective care of the highest quality and value. The NPSG and TJC Standards relevant to medication administrations (Table 20-3) are requirements for institutions in the U.S. and other countries that seek TJC accreditation.

Published studies suggest that successful implementation of BCMA and eMAR systems that improve patient safety depends on several factors, including the following:

1. A positive workplace culture (leadership, teamwork, and clinician ownership)
2. Training and support

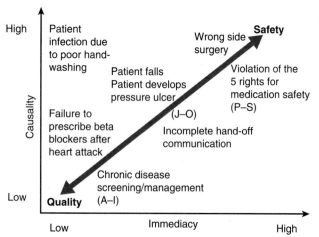

FIG 20-2 The quality–safety continuum. (Modified from Brown C, Hofer T, Johal A, et al. An epistemology of patient safety research: a framework for study design and interpretation. Part 1. Conceptualising and developing interventions. *Qual Saf Health Care.* 2008;17(3):159.)

TABLE 20-3	THE JOINT COMMISSION STANDARDS AND NATIONAL PATIENT SAFETY GOALS	
	REQUIREMENTS	**ELEMENTS OF PERFORMANCE**
National Patient Safety Goals (NPSG): NPSG.01.01.01	Use at least two patient identifiers when providing care, treatment, and services	Use at least two patient identifiers when administering medications, blood, or blood components; when collecting blood samples and other specimens for clinical testing; and when providing treatments or procedures. The patient's room number or physical location is not used as an identifier.
NPSG.03.04.01	Label all medications, medication containers, and other solutions on and off the sterile field in perioperative and other procedural settings*	All medications and solutions both on and off the sterile field and their labels are reviewed by entering and exiting staff responsible for the management of medications.
Medication Management: MM.06.01.01	The hospital safely administers medications	Before administration, the individual administering the medication does the following: • Verifies that the medication selected matches the medication order and product label • Verifies that the medication has not expired • Verifies that no contraindications exist • Verifies that the medication is being administered at the proper time, in the prescribed dose, and by the correct route

Data from The Joint Commission (TJC). Facts about Joint Commission accreditation standards. *TJC.* http://www.jointcommission.org/assets/1/18/Standards1.PDF. 2011. Accessed April 12, 2012; TJC. Facts about the National Patient Safety Goals. *TJC.* http://www.jointcommission.org/assets/1/18/National_Patient_Safety_Goals_6_3_111.PDF. 2012. Accessed April 12, 2012.
*Medication containers include syringes, medicine cups, and basins.

3. Acceptance of the major impact of work practices by all team staff
4. A usable system with adequate decision support[30-32]

Systems implemented using these principles can meet TJC Standards and NPSG and are likely to improve patient safety.

Chronic Illness Screening and Management

Health IT has demonstrated potential in improving the quality of care with regard to chronic illness screening and management.[39-46] As noted in Figure 20-2, health IT interventions that target chronic illness screening and management fall on the quality end of the vector of egregiousness, with lower levels of causality and immediacy.

Examples of structural incentives for use of health IT to improve clinical processes include practice guidelines such as the U.S. Preventive Services Task Force (USPSTF) recommendations on screening for breast cancer[47] and depression,[48] pay for performance measures,[49] and CMS core measures.[50] Analysis of these types of external programs on process improvement and patients' outcomes suggests that the long-term effect is limited and that tailoring quality improvement programs (e.g., the management and clinical processes) based on organization-specific situations is recommended.[49]

One strategy that is successful in improving quality outcomes is the use of health IT interventions that target patients to improve access to treatment,[44] adherence with medication, diet and exercise regimens,[42] adherence with recommended screening guidelines,[41] and engagement in symptom management.[40] Involvement of patients using health IT is a successful strategy for improving adherence with screening and best practices management of chronic illness and improved quality outcomes.

Nursing Sensitive Quality Outcomes: Patient Falls and Pressure Ulcers

Health IT interventions are also effective for improving quality of care and patient safety related to fall and pressure ulcer prevention.[51-55] The patient characteristics and factors related to risks for falls and pressure ulcers are multifaceted. For example, the patient's risks increase or decrease when skin surveillance is inadequate or when fall prevention interventions are not ordered and taught to the patient and family. As noted previously and in Figure 20-2, patient falls and pressure ulcers are located midway on the vector of egregiousness between quality and safety, with moderate levels of causality (failure to consistently implement tailored interventions) and immediacy (time to patient fall or development of pressure ulcer). An important structural component present for hospitals in the U.S. was the Deficit Reduction Act of 2006, through which CMS identified a list of preventable, hospital-acquired conditions for which hospitals would no longer receive additional payment.[9] The regulations regarding nonpayment for hospital-acquired conditions included both patient falls and pressure ulcers.[9] The regulations provided an external directive (e.g., structure) that created a sense of urgency within organizations to eliminate preventable patient falls and pressure ulcers.

Management processes including an administrative focus on fall and pressure ulcer prevention are key factors in improving the quality of care related to fall and pressure ulcer prevention. At the organizational level interventions such as training, the use of health IT systems for decision support, and involvement of peer champions in identifying and implementing interventions that are both feasible and effective, provide an environment conducive to fall and pressure ulcer prevention.[53,55] The use of clinical experts to improve the knowledge base of nurses and other healthcare providers[51] and the use of a peer champion model[51,53,55] support fidelity of both management processes (e.g., communication, importance of behavior change, advocacy for fall and pressure ulcer prevention initiatives) and clinical processes (e.g., end-user training, support, modeling the intervention set on patient care units).

When implementing complex practice change, as required for fall and pressure ulcer prevention, health IT is often a single component of a multifaceted performance improvement intervention and leadership support for the practice change is essential. Health IT interventions are most effective when both clinical and management processes are addressed and where organizational leadership demonstrates strong support for improvement strategies.[51,53,55]

SUCCESS FACTORS AND LESSONS LEARNED

The effects of health IT interventions aimed at improving quality and patient safety using the PSQRD framework have been evaluated to identify key success factors and to provide a foundation for making recommendations for health IT implementation and future research. The PSQRD framework is useful for exploring the relationships between the organization's structural forces (e.g., setting attributes, exogenous factors) that support organizational change, including adoption and use of health IT as a tool to improve clinical processes and patient outcomes. External accreditation or regulatory requirements provide structural incentives for the changes in clinical processes that are supported by health IT interventions. The PSQRD framework expands the process component of the Donabedian model to include both management and clinical processes. The expanded process components underscore the relationship between managerial interventions, improved clinical processes, and patient outcomes. Management interventions are effective in maximizing stakeholder support for a project. An example of a management intervention is the appointment of a task force to address poor adherence with best practice guidelines. The task force is charged by management with identifying and overcoming barriers to best practice. These types of interventions improve overall adherence to practice changes and improve fidelity with health IT interventions. In addition, the PSQRD framework includes a focus on intervening variables that improve staff commitment to process changes such as incentive payments and morale.[56] Additional examples of management strategies to improve fidelity with the intervention include the use of peer champion support networks[51,57,58] and end-user education.[55,56,58]

CONCLUSION AND FUTURE DIRECTIONS

Because of the complexity of the errors in healthcare, multifaceted strategies including health IT tools are needed to realize improvement in clinical processes and patient outcomes when striving to improve the quality and safety of healthcare.[30-32,45,46,51-53,57,59]

Prerequisites for health IT systems that will improve quality and patient safety include an informatics infrastructure where standards are adopted and used by all healthcare organizations. In addition to standardized measures and benchmarks, standard clinical content used in electronic systems, standard taxonomies or vocabularies to encode that content, and messaging standards to transfer information from one healthcare organization to another are needed. The Meaningful Use initiative puts forth a set of standards that, if adopted, will begin to build an informatics infrastructure to support quality and patient safety across the U.S. However, standards are often the minimum required and much more than minimum is necessary to advance best practices in each setting. Standards are a place to ensure quality and safety at a very basic level but patients often define (and expect) quality at a much higher level. Many organizations strive to meet and exceed patient expectations of quality and safety through the adoption and use of health IT.

The PSQRD framework provides a means to plan for and evaluate health IT interventions designed to improve quality and patient safety. Characteristics of successful health IT implementation projects include the following:

1. Leadership support for adoption and use of health IT to improve patient care and facilitate practice changes
2. A comprehensive approach to implementation and adoption of health IT, including attention to both management and clinical processes to promote fidelity with the intervention
3. Health IT applications considered a tool or a single component of a multifaceted intervention to improve the underlying clinical processes and, ultimately, patient outcomes
4. Patients engaged in clinical process changes to deliver guideline-based care and to improve patient outcomes using health IT as a tool
5. Involvement of end-users in iterative development and implementation of health IT interventions to improve quality and safety
6. The use of peer support to facilitate adoption and proper use of health IT applications within clinical workflows

The PSQRD framework is a useful guide for development of a comprehensive implementation and evaluation plan that addresses the above success factors and provides an effective strategy for evaluating the effect of health IT on quality of care and patient safety outcomes.

The PSQRD framework is recommended as a guide for implementation and evaluation of health IT interventions. The PSQRD framework provides a means to introduce health IT interventions in a systematic way, and it serves as a reminder to incorporate measures of success across the causal chain. This approach supports implementation, performance improvement, and research projects with an appreciation for the effects and the limitations of health IT and other intervention components. Adoption of the PSQRD framework for both research and organizational implementations will provide a means to plan for successful implementation and to collect data on the structural and process factors that may affect adoption and use of health IT interventions and ultimately patient outcomes. This type of measurement is appropriate for both research-based and operational implementations of health IT.

Even well-designed health IT interventions require a comprehensive plan that includes a focus on structure; management and clinical processes; and intervening variables to address fidelity with the intervention. Failure to address these factors may prevent adoption and use of health IT tools and serve as a barrier to patient safety and quality in clinical practice. For example, Schnipper et al. describe a Smartforms application, a clinical documentation tool designed to facilitate real-time, documentation-based decision support to capture structured, coded data in the context of documentation.[60] A randomized controlled trial demonstrated a limited impact of the Smartforms on patient outcomes because only 5.6% of eligible healthcare providers used the application.[59] Investigators summarized their lessons learned, stating that in addition to well-designed health IT tools, improvements in chronic disease management require a comprehensive approach that includes the following:

- Financial incentives (structure)
- Multifaceted quality improvement efforts (management processes including interventions to promote fidelity with the intervention)
- Reorganization of patient care activities (clinical processes) across care team members[59]

This is one example where the PSQRD framework used during project planning could have highlighted strategies to promote adoption and use of the health IT intervention and potentially led to a more significant outcome. While many frameworks exist, this chapter introduced one framework that has been successfully used; however, others are available and deserve consideration. A process of thoughtful consideration of each setting and its characteristics is needed to identify what frameworks, models, and techniques should be considered to improve the quality and safety of patient care.

REFERENCES

1. Adams K, Corrigan J. *Priority Areas for National Action: Transforming Health Care Quality.* Washington, DC: Institute of Medicine; 2003.
2. Institute of Medicine. *Crossing the Quality Chasm: A New Health System for the 21st Century.* Washington, DC: Institute of Medicine; 2001.
3. Kohn L, Corrigan J, Donaldson M. *To Err Is Human: Building a Safer Health System.* Washington, DC: Institute of Medicine; 1999.
4. Lohr K, Committee to Design a Strategy for Quality Review and Assurance in Medicare, eds. *Medicare: A Strategy for Quality Assurance,* Vol. 1. Washington, DC: Institute of Medicine; 1990.
5. Page A. *Keeping Patients Safe: Transforming the Work Environment of Nurses.* Washington, DC: Institute of Medicine; 2004.
6. Bates DW, Gawande AA. Improving safety with information technology. *N Engl J Med.* 2003;348(25):2526-2534.
7. Kaushal R, Shojania KG, Bates DW. Effects of computerized physician order entry and clinical decision support systems on medication safety: a systematic review. *Arch Intern Med.* 2003;163(12):1409-1416.
8. The Joint Commission (TJC). Facts about Joint Commission accreditation standards. TJC. http://www.jointcommission.org/assets/1/18/Standards1.PDF. 2011. Accessed April 12, 2012.
9. Centers for Medicare & Medicaid Services (CMS). Hospital-acquired conditions (present on admission indicator). CMS. http://www.cms.hhs.gov/HospitalAcqCond/01_Overview.asp#TopOfPage. 2009.
10. Bradley R, Pratt R, Thrasher E, Byrd T, Thomas C. An examination of the relationships among IT capability intentions, IT infrastructure integration and quality of care: a study in U.S. hospitals. Paper presented at: 45th Hawaii International Conference on System Sciences; January 4-7 2012; Hawaii.
11. Brown C, Hofer T, Johal A, et al. An epistemology of patient safety research: a framework for study design and interpretation. Part 1. Conceptualising and developing interventions. *Qual Saf Health Care.* 2008;17(3):158-162.
12. Runciman W, Hibbert P, Thomson R, Van Der Schaaf T, Sherman H, Lewalle P. Towards an international classification for patient safety: key concepts and terms. *Int J Qual Health Care.* 2009;21(1):18-26.
13. Aspden P, Wolcott J, Bootman J, Cronenwett L, eds. *Preventing Medication Errors: Quality Chasm Series.* Washington, DC: National Academies Press; 2007.
14. Centers for Medicare & Medicaid Services. Medicare and Medicaid programs: electronic health record incentive program: final rule. *Federal Register.* 2010;75(144).
15. Office of the National Coordinator for Health Information Technology (ONC). *Federal Health Information Technology Strategic Plan 2011–2015.* Washington, DC: ONC; 2011.
16. Downey JR, Hernandez-Boussard T, Banka G, Morton JM. Is patient safety improving? National trends in patient safety indicators: 1998–2007. *Health Serv Res.* 2012;47(1 Pt 2):414-430.
17. The Joint Commission (TJC). Facts about the National Patient Safety Goals. TJC. http://www.jointcommission.org/assets/1/18/National_Patient_Safety_Goals_6_3_111.PDF. 2012. Accessed April 12, 2012.
18. The Leapfrog Group. http://www.leapfroggroup.org/home. 2012. Accessed April 12, 2012.
19. Centers for Medicare & Medicaid Services (CMS). Medicare "pay for performance (P4P)" initiatives. CMS. http://www.cms.hhs.gov/apps/media/. 2012. Accessed April 12, 2012.
20. Centers for Medicare & Medicaid Services (CMS). The official web site for the Medicare and Medicaid electronic health records (EHR) incentive programs. CMS. http://www.cms.gov/Regulations-and-Guidance/Legislation/EHRIncentivePrograms/index.html?redirect=/EHRIncentivePrograms/. 2012. Accessed April 12, 2012.
21. National Committee for Quality Assurance (NCQA). http://www.ncqa.org/. 2011. Accessed July 30, 2012.
22. Utilization Review Accreditation Commission (URAC). http://www.urac.org. 2012. Accessed July 30, 2012.

23. Department of Health and Human Services. Health information technology: initial set of standards, implementation specifications, and certification criteria for electronic health record technology. *Federal Register*. 2010;75(44).

24. Donabedian A. The quality of care: how can it be assessed? [Review]. *JAMA*. 1988;260(12):1743-1748.

25. Jha AK, Bates DW, Jenter C, et al. Electronic health records: use, barriers and satisfaction among physicians who care for black and Hispanic patients. *J Eval Clin Pract*. 2009;15(1):158-163.

26. Jha AK, DesRoches CM, Campbell EG, et al. Use of electronic health records in U.S. hospitals. *N Engl J Med*. 2009;360(16): 1628-1638.

27. Moss SM, Cuckle H, Evans A, Johns L, Waller M, Bobrow L. Effect of mammographic screening from age 40 years on breast cancer mortality at 10 years' follow-up: a randomised controlled trial. *Lancet*. 2006;368(9552):2053-2060.

28. Garrouste-Orgeas M, Philippart F, Bruel C, Max A, Lau N, Misset B. Overview of medical errors and adverse events. *Ann Intensive Care*. 2012;2(1):2.

29. Bates DW, Leape LL, Cullen DJ, et al. Effect of computerized physician order entry and a team intervention on prevention of serious medication errors. *JAMA*. 1998;280(15):1311-1316.

30. Paoletti RD, Suess TM, Lesko MG, et al. Using bar-code technology and medication observation methodology for safer medication administration. *Am J Health Syst Pharm*. 2007;64(5): 536-543.

31. Sakowski J, Leonard T, Colburn S, et al. Using a bar-coded medication administration system to prevent medication errors in a community hospital network. *Am J Health Syst Pharm*. 2005;62(24):2619-2625.

32. Yates C. Implementing a bar-coded bedside medication administration system. *Crit Care Nurs Q*. 2007;30(2):189-195.

33. Mills PD, Neily J, Mims E, Burkhardt ME, Bagian J. Improving the bar-coded medication administration system at the Department of Veterans Affairs. *Am J Health Syst Pharm*. 2006;63(15): 1442-1447.

34. Patterson ES, Cook RI, Render ML. Improving patient safety by identifying side effects from introducing bar coding in medication administration. *J Am Med Inform Assoc*. 2002;9(5): 540-553.

35. van Onzenoort HA, van de Plas A, Kessels AG, Veldhorst-Janssen NM, van der Kuy PH, Neef C. Factors influencing bar-code verification by nurses during medication administration in a Dutch hospital. *Am J Health Syst Pharm*. 2008;65(7):644-648.

36. Franklin BD, O'Grady K, Donyai P, Jacklin A, Barber N. The impact of a closed-loop electronic prescribing and administration system on prescribing errors, administration errors and staff time: a before-and-after study. *Qual Saf Health Care*. 2007;16(4):279-284.

37. Koppel R, Wetterneck T, Telles JL, Karsh BT. Workarounds to barcode medication administration systems: their occurrences, causes, and threats to patient safety. *J Am Med Inform Assoc*. 2008;15(4):408-423.

38. Patterson ES, Rogers ML, Chapman RJ, Render ML. Compliance with intended use of Bar Code Medication Administration in acute and long-term care: an observational study. *Hum Factors*. 2006;48(1):15-22.

39. Kwok R, Dinh M, Dinh D, Chu M. Improving adherence to asthma clinical guidelines and discharge documentation from emergency departments: implementation of a dynamic and integrated electronic decision support system. *Emerg Med Australas*. 2009;21(1):31-37.

40. Ruland CM, Andersen T, Jeneson A, et al. Effects of an internet support system to assist cancer patients in reducing symptom distress: a randomized controlled trial. *Cancer Nurs*. 2012. [Epub ahead of print].

41. Atlas SJ, Grant RW, Lester WT, et al. A cluster-randomized trial of a primary care informatics-based system for breast cancer screening. *J Gen Intern Med*. 2011;26(2):154-161.

42. Park MJ, Kim HS. Evaluation of mobile phone and internet intervention on waist circumference and blood pressure in post-menopausal women with abdominal obesity. *Int J Med Inform*. 2012. [Epub ahead of print].

43. Cebul RD, Love TE, Jain AK, Hebert CJ. Electronic health records and quality of diabetes care. *N Engl J Med*. 2011;365(9): 825-833.

44. Knaevelsrud C, Maercker A. Long-term effects of an internet-based treatment for posttraumatic stress. *Cogn Behav Ther*. 2010;39(1):72-77.

45. Simon GE, Ralston JD, Savarino J, Pabiniak C, Wentzel C, Operskalski BH. Randomized trial of depression follow-up care by online messaging. *J Gen Intern Med*. 2011;26(7): 698-704.

46. Saposnik G, Teasell R, Mamdani M, et al. Effectiveness of virtual reality using Wii gaming technology in stroke rehabilitation: a pilot randomized clinical trial and proof of principle. *Stroke*. 2010;41(7):1477-1484.

47. U.S. Preventive Services Task Force (USPSTF). Screening for breast cancer. USPSTF. http://www.uspreventiveservicestaskforce.org/uspstf/uspsbrca.htm. 2009. Accessed April 20, 2012.

48. U.S. Preventive Services Task Force (USPSTF). Screening for depression in adults. USPSTF. http://www.uspreventiveservicestaskforce.org/uspstf/uspsaddepr.htm. 2009. Accessed April 20, 2012.

49. Werner RM, Kolstad JT, Stuart EA, Polsky D. The effect of pay-for-performance in hospitals: lessons for quality improvement. *Health Aff (Millwood)*. 2011;30(4):690-698.

50. Chassin MR, Loeb JM, Schmaltz SP, Wachter RM. Accountability measures—Using measurement to promote quality improvement. *N Engl J Med*. 2010;363(7):683-688.

51. Carson D, Emmons K, Falone W, Preston AM. Development of pressure ulcer program across a university health system. *J Nurs Care Qual*. 2012;27(1):20-27.

52. Dowding DW, Turley M, Garrido T. The impact of an electronic health record on nurse sensitive patient outcomes: an interrupted time series analysis. *J Am Med Inform Assoc*. 2011. [Epub ahead of print].

53. Dykes PC, Carroll DL, Hurley A, et al. Fall prevention in acute care hospitals: a randomized trial. *JAMA*. 2010;304(17): 1912-1918.

54. Fossum M, Alexander GL, Ehnfors M, Ehrenberg A. Effects of a computerized decision support system on pressure ulcers and malnutrition in nursing homes for the elderly. *Int J Med Inform*. 2011;80(9):607-617.

55. Garrett J, Wheeler H, Goetz K, Majewski M, Langlois P, Payson C. Implementing an "always practice" to redefine skin care management. *J Nurs Adm*. 2009;39(9):382-387.

56. Riggio JM, Sorokin R, Moxey ED, Mather P, Gould S, Kane GC. Effectiveness of a clinical-decision-support system in improving compliance with cardiac-care quality measures and supporting resident training. *Acad Med*. 2009;84(12):1719-1726.

57. Day RO, Roffe DJ, Richardson KL, et al. Implementing electronic medication management at an Australian teaching hospital. *Med J Aust*. 2011;195(9):498-502.

58. Dykes PC, Carroll DL, Hurley A, et al. Fall TIPS: strategies to promote adoption and use of a fall prevention toolkit. *AMIA Annu Symp Proc 2009.* 2009;153-157.
59. Schnipper JL, Linder JA, Palchuk MB, et al. Effects of documentation-based decision support on chronic disease management. *Am J Manag Care.* 2010;16(12 suppl HIT):SP72-SP81.
60. Schnipper JL, McColgan KE, Linder JA, et al. Improving management of chronic diseases with documentation-based clinical decision support: results of a pilot study. *AMIA Annu Symp Proc.* 2008;1050.

DISCUSSION QUESTIONS

1. Describe the information architecture requirements of a health IT system that supports capture of data and information needed for quality reporting and benchmarking as a by-product of routine clinical documentation.
2. What is the utility of Donabedian's structure-process-outcome model as the basis for evaluating quality of care and patient safety associated with a health IT application? Describe two limitations. Discuss how the framework for patient safety and research design can be used to overcome these limitations.
3. Use the framework for patient safety and quality research design to create a comprehensive plan to support successful implementation of Bar Code Medication Administration.
4. Use the framework for patient safety and quality research design to evaluate a health IT intervention in a quality and patient safety research study (provide an example based on your research or from one of the articles reviewed in this chapter).

CASE STUDY

Western Heights Hospital (WHH) is a 1125-bed, 5-hospital academic healthcare system servicing central and western Massachusetts. WHH is the only designated Level I Trauma Center for adults and children in the area and is home to New England's first hospital-based air ambulance and the region's only Level III Neonatal Intensive Care Center. WHH launched a 5-year strategic plan with a fundamental goal of a system-wide move from a predominately paper environment to an electronic one. Phase I included implementation of an EHR system consisting of order entry for all laboratory, radiology, and patient care orders. Additionally, clinical documentation was implemented, including admission assessments and all nursing flow sheets. The nursing informatics counsel, a 25-member group of nurses representing all disciplines, developed the clinical content. The clinical content was custom built using both free text and structured data entry fields within the application.

Three months after go-live, hospital leadership is reporting that it is unable to report on various state and federally mandated quality measures. These measures track healthcare quality based on national standards, are compared to nationally accepted benchmarks, and are used to plan ways to improve quality. Leadership has communicated that the reports generated by the system are incomplete and are putting the hospital at financial risk due to lower reimbursement rates.

Clinicians are eager and excited to continue to develop content in the application. However, the project's program manager is proposing a stabilization and optimization approach and does not want to go forward with content development until the issue of reporting has been assessed and addressed.

Discussion Questions

1. Assuming that you are the clinical content manager and lead all reporting efforts, what approach would you take to address the reporting problem?
2. Preadmission testing data are currently collected on paper. The chief of surgery has identified an opportunity to have these data collected in the new EHR system by the preadmission testing area in the outpatient setting. Many of the collected data elements are shared with the current admission assessment. Describe how this effort can be approached. What methods can be used to implement the process?
3. Using the PSQRD methodology, identify an area of quality improvement in the hospital setting, develop a process plan, and identify the expected outcomes.

Improving the User Experience for Health Information Technology Products

Nancy Staggers

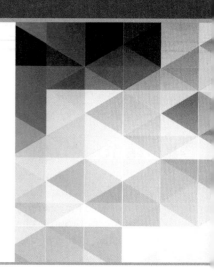

Usability has a strong, often direct relationship with clinical productivity, error rates, user fatigue and user satisfaction—critical factors for EMR adoption.

Healthcare Information and Management Systems Society, 2009

OBJECTIVES

At the completion of this chapter the reader will be prepared to:

1. Compare and contrast the terms *user experience, human factors, ergonomics, human–computer interaction,* and *usability*
2. Describe the goals of usability and user-centered design
3. Identify the major components to consider in human–computer interaction and usability studies
4. Analyze methods for conducting usability studies and relate them to a specific purpose of a usability study
5. Outline components of four different usability tests related to their position in the systems life cycle
6. Explain the basic steps in conducting a usability test on a healthcare product

KEY TERMS

ABSTRACT

Many health information technology (health IT) products are not designed for their intended users and are inefficient and even dangerous. Federal agencies are responding to this challenge by developing regulations and reports to guide improved usability. Clinicians and informaticists require a suite of skills to understand concepts about the user experience and to conduct usability tests. This chapter provides the knowledge and skills to meet those needs. First, the chapter outlines the need for attention to the user experience and how it might benefit individuals and organizations. Terms are defined, the concepts of usability goals are presented, and user-centered design precepts are discussed. Available human–computer interaction (HCI) frameworks are listed; one framework is explained in detail and traditional usability methods are offered. Then types of usability tests are discussed and linked to the systems life cycle using the HCI framework. Examples of actual usability studies in health settings are provided. After reading this chapter students will be able to design and conduct usability tests to determine the effectiveness and efficiency of and satisfaction with health IT products.

INTRODUCTION TO IMPROVING THE USER EXPERIENCE

While most students may be able to describe their own frustrations with poorly designed products, the systematic study of human factors and usability, plus the wide variety of resources supporting the development of usable systems, is likely new information. This section of the chapter begins by outlining users' current experience with health IT as well as the benefits that improved usability can provide to users and organizations as documented in the literature. This content is followed by the definitions of common terms and an explanation of their interrelationships.

The Current User Experience with Health IT Products

Issues with the usability of health IT products are now a critical national concern, especially because of the vast expansion of funding for and implementation of electronic health records (EHRs) in the U.S. Health IT involves complex interactions among multiple users, products, and environments, all with varying characteristics, commonly called a sociotechnical system. The language for Meaningful Use Stage 2 now includes usability assessments yet suboptimal user experience with current health IT products is well documented. Stead and Lin evaluated premier EHRs in the U.S. in 2009 and found that even the best EHRs had symptoms of poor usability. Physicians had difficulty finding critical information and developing the "big picture" of the patient. These authors claimed that health IT could decrease the quality of healthcare unless steps were taken to improve health IT support for clinicians' work and thought processes.[1] Although their study concentrated on physicians, the results can be extrapolated to the entire health team's interactions with health IT.

The professional literature is rich with evidence demonstrating poor and even dangerous user experience with health IT products. For example, unintended consequences occurred because of EHR usability issues.[2,3] In 2011 hospital staff transplanted an infected kidney after failing in at least 12 opportunities to discover a donor's positive hepatitis C result buried in the EHR.[4] Potential patient safety issues occurred with an Electronic Medication Administration Record (eMAR) because nurses could not view patients' medications easily to determine missed and due medications.[5] New errors emerged when computerized provider order entry (CPOE) facilitated 22 types of medication error risks.[6] An ambulatory application serving more than 9 million patients failed to support clinicians during patient encounters, did not allow them to obtain situation awareness of the patient (the "big picture" of the patient), promoted workarounds with nonintegrated systems, and greatly increased frustrations because of required structured documentation.[7] This application affected healthcare provider productivity and effectiveness, decreasing patient access worldwide.[8,9] These issues could be prevented by incorporating known usability principles and processes to improve the user experience with health IT.

Potential Benefits of Improving the User Experience

A white paper from the Healthcare Information Management and Systems Society (HIMSS), co-led by this author, describes methods for incorporating usability in health organizations.[10] This publicly available white paper includes a section on the benefits of usability to healthcare that is summarized here. The return on investment (ROI) was addressed largely outside healthcare in earlier publications as that community documented benefits and then moved on to address them.

Usability can add value to organizations across a range of areas. Usability ROI material is available from (1) nonhealthcare projects such as Bias and Mayhew[11] and Nielsen,[12] (2) the Usability Professionals' Association website,[13] and (3) Dey Alexander Consulting.[14] To the author's knowledge no research is yet available about ROI or cost savings for usability efforts in healthcare projects. Thus material is cited from nonhealthcare applications. However, findings from nonhealthcare IT projects are very likely to extend to healthcare because of the often dramatic changes that usability can create. Figure 21-1 outlines potential areas of value when the user experience is improved in health organizations.

Increased Individual Effectiveness

Usability can positively affect at least three areas of particular interest in health IT:
1. Increased user productivity and efficiency
2. Decreased user errors and increased safety
3. Improved cognitive support

Increased User Productivity and Efficiency. One of the most prevalent complaints about health IT in general and EHRs specifically is that the technology impedes users' productivity. For example, outpatient visits were reduced from four to three per hour after an ambulatory EHR was fielded.[8] A cognitive work analysis of the same system in a laboratory setting showed a large number of average steps to complete common tasks, a high average execution time, and a large percentage of required mental operators.[15]

Employing usability processes helps to improve productivity and efficiency. The Nielsen Norman Group estimated that "productivity gains from redesigning an intranet to improve usability are eight times larger than costs for a company with 1,000 employees; 20 times larger for a company with 10,000 employees; and 50 times larger for a company with 100,000 employees."[12(p5)] Website redesign statistics for the 42 cases collected by Nielsen Norman yielded an average increase in user productivity of 161%. After testing intranets for low and high usability, these authors projected a savings of 48 hours per employee if intranets were redesigned for high usability. Souza cited usability research showing that two thirds of buyers failed in shopping attempts on well-known sites.[16] Thus poor usability on intranets means poor employee productivity.

Decreased User Errors and Increased Safety. One of the major reasons why health IT is installed is to reduce errors in healthcare.[17,18] While clearly some classes of errors such as

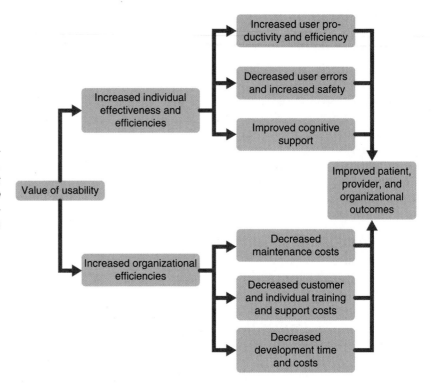

FIG 21-1 The value of usability to health organizations. (From HIMSS Usability Task Force. *Promoting Usability in Health Organizations: Initial Steps and Progress toward a Healthcare Usability Maturity Model.* Chicago, IL: Healthcare Information and Management Systems Society; 2011.)

medication errors can be reduced with health IT, technology can create unintended consequences and new errors due to usability.[3,19,20] For example, Kushniruk and colleagues were able to identify how certain types of usability problems were related to errors as physicians entered prescriptions into handheld devices.[21]

Nielsen and Levy collected case studies and found a decrease in user error rates in 46 redesign projects measuring user error.[22] A study showed a 25% decrease in user errors after screen redesign.[23] Users found needed information only 42% of the time on 15 large commercial websites, even when they were directed to the correct home page; 62% gave up looking for desired items on websites.[12] Redesigns could prevent errors in these types of interactions; thus incorporating usability can potentially decrease errors in health IT products.

Improved Cognitive Support. Stead and Lin concluded that the premier systems in the U.S. did not provide the required cognitive support for clinicians (i.e., tools for thinking about and solving health problems).[1] Cognitive support may include designs to provide an overview or summary of the patient, information "at a glance," intuitive designs, and tailored support for clinicians in specific contexts. An example of how usability can provide cognitive support is the work on novel physiologic monitoring designs. Researchers employed user-centered design and usability testing techniques to create novel designs integrating physiologic data in a graphic object.[24,25,26] The new design provided integrated, "at a glance" pictorial data to show changes to clinicians. These graphic objects are now being incorporated in vendors' products as an adjunct to numeric data displays.

Increased Organizational Efficiencies

Well-designed user interfaces and systems translate into organizational efficiencies, including the following:

1. Decreased maintenance costs
2. Decreased customer and individual training and support costs
3. Decreased development time and costs

Decreased Maintenance Costs. Eighty percent of software life cycle costs occur in the maintenance phase and are related to unmet user requirements and similar usability problems.[27] Usability experts estimated that by correcting usability problems early in the design phase of a project, two different American airlines projects reduced the cost of those fixes by 60% and 90%.[28] At IBM, researchers concluded that it is more economical to consider users' needs early in the design cycle than to solve them later.[29]

Decreased Customer and Individual Training and Support Costs. A study by Microsoft showed that time for support calls "dropped dramatically" after a redesign of the print merge function in Word.[28] Business analysts found that a well-designed user interface had an internal rate of return of 32%, realized through a 35% reduction in training, a 30% reduction in supervisory time, and improved productivity.[30] Logically, a well-designed user interface will require fewer resources to support, less time and effort in training, and decreased time on support calls. Souza also cited a web redesign at lucy.com that resulted in a 20% reduction in support calls.[16]

Decreased Development Time and Costs. According to Marcus, the rule of thumb in many usability-aware organizations is that the cost–benefit ratio for usability is $1:$10:$100.[31]

Once a system is in development, correcting a problem costs 10 times as much as fixing the same problem during design. If the system has been released, it costs 100 times as much relative to fixing the problem in design. This estimate is frequently quoted and while it may be overly optimistic, its main point is clear: It is far more expensive in time, costs, and effort to correct issues later in the development life cycle than to complete an informed design at the beginning of a project.

Best practices in usability engineering could alleviate major reasons for inaccurate cost estimates by managers in these areas: frequent requests for changes by users, overlooked tasks, users' lack of understanding of their own tasks, and insufficient communication and understanding between users and analysts.[28] By including usability techniques, two companies reduced time spent on development, one by 40%[28] and another by 33% to 50%.[32] An ROI analysis by Karat indicated a $10 return on each dollar invested in usability.[33] According to Landauer, when usability is factored in at the beginning of a project, efficiency improvements can be greater than 700%.[34] On a national level Landauer estimated in 1995 that the inadequate use of usability engineering methods in software development projects cost the U.S. economy about $30 billion per year in lost productivity. Of course, the cost would be even more substantial now.

Incorporating usability into health IT provides significant value to all such projects; therefore it is essential that healthcare team members, informaticists, and IT staff understand and apply usability principles and processes in their work. This chapter provides students with an understanding of the critical nature of usability as well as the knowledge and skills to conduct usability tests.

DEFINITIONS OF TERMS AND THEIR RELATIONSHIPS

Despite discussion in the literature for more than 30 years, precise definitions for user experience terms are a source of debate and overlapping concepts. The relationship of terms is depicted in Figure 21-2. As demonstrated in the figure, user experience is the most inclusive of these terms, with human factors, ergonomics, human–computer interaction (HCI), and usability embedded within it. Usability and ergonomics overlap and intersect human factors and HCI. These terms overlap in conceptual definitions and also because the physical attributes of ergonomics may be combined with software, which is more the purview of usability and HCI.

User Experience

The term *user experience* encompasses all aspects of users' interactions.[35] International Organization for Standardization (ISO) 9241-11 defines the term as "a person's perceptions and responses that result from the use or anticipated use of a product, system or service."[36] Schaffer indicates that user experience is concerned with a range of experiences from walking into a bank to designs that fit into complex ecosystems with many users interacting.[37] To achieve a

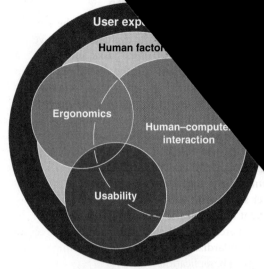

FIG 21-2 Terms and their relationships. (Adapted and expanded from Staggers N. Human factors: imperative concepts for information systems in critical care. *AACN Clin Issues.* 2003;14(3):310-319; quiz 397-318.)

high-quality user experience a seamless merging must occur from the talents of multiple disciplines, such as engineering, graphic and industrial design, interface design, psychology, and domain experts in the discipline at hand.[10,38]

Human Factors

According to the Human Factors and Ergonomics Society (HFES), human factors is "the scientific discipline concerned with the understanding of interactions among humans and other elements of a system, and the profession that applies theory, principles, data and methods to design in order to optimize human well-being and overall system performance."[39] Simple examples include how to open a door efficiently, how to turn on the lighting for one area of a room from a bank of light switches, and how to safely operate the controls to drive a car. In healthcare, human factors might concern the design of a new operating room to better support teamwork and patient flow. For additional information on this concept, see Donald Norman's classic book about the design of everyday objects.[40]

Ergonomics

The term ergonomics is used interchangeably with human factors by the HFES in Europe but in the U.S. and other countries its focus is on human performance with physical characteristics of tools, systems, and machines.[41] For example, ergonomics issues might address the design of a power drill to fit a human hand or the design of chairs to promote comfort and safety. In healthcare the number, types, and locations of workstations are typically the purview of ergonomics. The design of a surgical instrument to fit the human hand and perform desired functions effectively and efficiently deals with ergonomics.

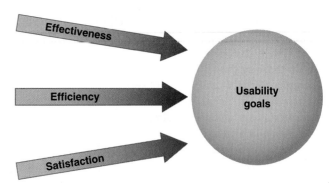

FIG 21-3 Usability goals. (From HIMSS Usability Task Force. *Promoting Usability in Health Organizations: Initial Steps and Progress toward a Healthcare Usability Maturity Model.* Chicago, IL: Healthcare Information and Management Systems Society; 2011.)

study of how
ve computer
k.[42] As with
psychology
, and infor-
hand. HCI
to include
and eval-
llowing:
ravenous
ation records
(or not) and meaning of icons on a
web application

- Principles of effective screen design, including mobile application design
- Issues with social media websites, such as the implications of "defriending" a person
- Analysis of the capabilities and limitations of users

Usability

The term usability is often used interchangeably with HCI when the product is a computer but usability also concerns products beyond computers. Usability is also more focused on interactions within a specific context or environment for a specific product. Formally, the ISO defines usability as the extent to which a product can be used by specific users in a specific context to achieve specific goals with effectiveness, efficiency, and satisfaction.[36] A product with good usability allows users in a particular context to achieve their goals when interacting with a product.[42] Usability is, however, fundamentally concerned with human performance rather than only subjective data. Usability can include the following dimensions:

- Speed and accuracy with a product
- Ease of learning a product and remembering interactions after time has elapsed
- User satisfaction or perceptions about the interactions with a product
- Efficiency and accuracy of interactions
- Designs to promote error-free or error-forgiving products
- Seamless fit of an information system to the tasks and goals of users

THE GOALS OF USABILITY

The overall goals of usability have been established by the ISO. Figure 21-3 depicts the ISO usability goals.

Effectiveness is the accuracy and completeness with which specified users achieve specified goals in particular environments, including worker and consumer or patient safety (ISO 9126-1).

Efficiency includes the resources expended in relation to the accuracy and completeness of goals achieved.

Satisfaction is the comfort and acceptability of users and other people to the product or work system and deals with users' perceptions.[10] Dimensions of usability correlate to elements depicted in Figure 21-1 to include improvements for individuals or groups of individuals: productivity and efficiency, effectiveness in product use, safety, and cognitive support (an aspect of effectiveness).

USER-CENTERED DESIGN

User experience experts insist on a process of user-centered design that comprises the following three axioms:

- An early and central focus on users in the design and development of products
- Iterative design
- Systematic measures of the interactions between users and products[41,42]

These principles were derived nearly 30 years ago by Gould and Lewis and are more salient than ever because contemporary environments are filled with an array of complex tools. An early and central focus on users means understanding users in depth (i.e., their characteristics, environment, and tasks).[42] Direct contact with users is needed early and often throughout a design or redesign process. Iterative design means having rounds of design and allowing key users to evaluate product prototypes to determine their effectiveness and efficiency in the care process and health decisions. One design is never adequate and typically three rounds are necessary. Once a design is available, even on paper or in PowerPoint, designers or informaticists work with users to determine any issues by having them interact with the initial design. Specific methods to accomplish this are explained in subsequent sections. The important point is that major usability issues are identified and corrected early in the process. Design and evaluation then occur in a cycle until all major usability issues are corrected. This dynamic, iterative process, which includes the three axioms listed above, is known as user-centered design. Importantly, structured and systematic observations, including identified measures, are necessary. Usability goals and axioms apply not only to developing products but also to the selection, purchase, customization, and redesign of products.

This kind of design allows us to integrate health data, information, and knowledge into health IT products. For example, a well-designed eMAR would filter medication routes to match the particular medication, eliminating options not appropriate (e.g., charting an antacid as an intravenous medication). Although this sounds like common sense, current designs in major EHRs often do not accommodate this kind of filtering.

HUMAN–COMPUTER INTERACTION FRAMEWORKS FOR HEALTH INFORMATICS

Frameworks provide guidance for understanding essential components that improve the user experience. They are helpful in completing user-centered design processes, usability tests, IT adoption evaluations, and usability research. This section of the chapter provides an overview of existing frameworks and describes in detail the Health Human–Computer Interaction Framework.

Human–Computer Interaction Frameworks

Various HCI frameworks and models with different foci are available.[43-50]

- FITT (Fit between Individuals, Task, and Technology), with the elements connected by interactions and influences[43]
- UFuRT (User, Function, Representation, and Task analyses). System knowledge is distributed across multiple users who have differences in expertise and cognitive characteristics. It includes a task analysis portion to describe steps in tasks and interactions.[50] Recently this framework was renamed TURF.
- A framework for employing usability methods to redesign a fielded system[47]
- Framework for technology-induced error[44]
- A combined health IT adoption and HCI model[45]
- Joint cognitive systems[46]

The last item bears more discussion. Hollnagel and Woods coined the term *cognitive systems engineering*, acknowledging that sociotechnical systems, or complex technologies embedded within social systems, are increasingly prevalent yet have frequent system failures.[46] The authors devised a cyclic model called contextual control model, or CoCom, with the following elements: event, modifies, constructs, determines, acts, and produces. Users and context are major components of the model. Importantly, joint cognitive systems imply that information is shared or distributed among humans and technology. This framework is useful for examining teamwork in healthcare where team members work together on patient care.

An analysis of the existing frameworks found each helpful but inadequate for health usability studies. Missing elements across frameworks included (1) interactions among disparate users, (2) characteristics and actions of products and users, (3) context, and (4) a developmental timeline. Context is critical in particular because it defines the kinds of users, tasks, and work design.[45,48] A developmental time element is also necessary because it accounts for users changing (maturing) in their interactions over time.[45,48] Therefore a new framework was created.

The Health Human–Computer Interaction Framework

The Health Human–Computer Interaction (HHCI) Framework is described here. The current framework builds on early work by Staggers and Parks describing nurse–computer interaction.[51,52] It was expanded in 2001 to include groups of healthcare providers and interactions with patients.[48,53] The framework is adapted further here to acknowledge that IT may be only one example of an available health IT product (e.g., physiologic monitors or intravenous pumps).

The elements of the framework are outlined in Figure 21-4. Information (e.g., patient care, administrative or educational information) is the exchange mechanism. Interactions occur in a system of mutual influences where elements (e.g., individuals, health IT) act and respond based on specific characteristics. Context is paramount, with all interactions embedded within a context. This means that any outcomes of interactions are distinct, as they are defined by a context. The developmental timeline indicates that interactions change over time. Thus the outcomes of interactions are different based on when an interaction occurs in time.

Humans or products can initiate interactions. The information is processed through either the product or the humans according to characteristics. The recipient then reacts to the information; for example, a healthcare provider could read and respond to email from a patient or a product might process interactions after the "enter" key is pressed. Iterative cycles continue as humans behave and products act according to defined characteristics. Goals and planning are implicit within the tasks displayed in the framework.

Essential Components for Improving the User Experience

The important point in this section is that using a framework or model can greatly assist students to think comprehensively about health IT adoption and usability and the conduct of usability studies. Choose a framework to match the need at hand. Usability methods can then be applied as appropriate while ensuring that critical elements are under consideration. This idea is expanded in later sections to illustrate how the framework assists usability testing. In summary, product interactions are a complex part of a sociotechnical system. Critical elements to consider are as follows:

- A user or users and their characteristics
- Interactions
- Tasks (goals of tasks)
- Information
- Products and their characteristics
- Context
- How interactions mature over time (developmental timeline)

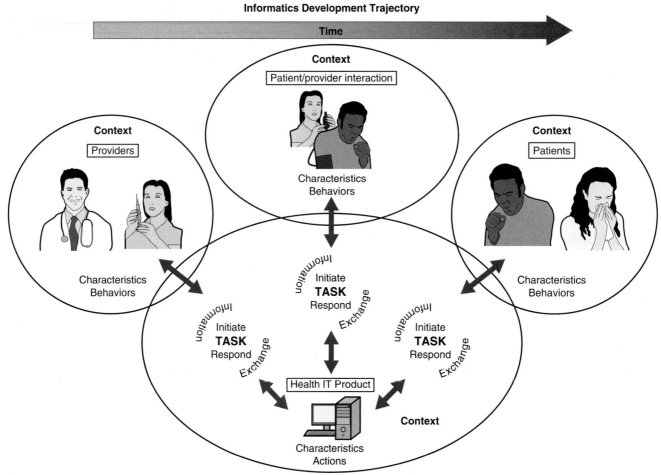

FIG 21-4 Health Human–Computer Interaction Framework. (Copyright Nancy Staggers. Reprinted with permission.)

SELECTING METHODS TO IMPROVE THE USER EXPERIENCE

Techniques to improve the user experience can be informal or formal, simple or complex, and employ a few individuals or a wide range of users. Students or researchers can design small projects or sophisticated studies by combining usability precepts with usability-specific or traditional research designs and methods such as quantitative, qualitative, or mixed methods. The type of usability study is dependent on the purpose of the project; when the assessment is targeted within the systems life cycle; the desired outcome of the project; and available resources, including time, people, and money. However, it uses the elements from the HHCI framework.

Usability projects can be done at any point in the systems life cycle from initial work (to identify usability issues; clarify requirements; and assess initial designs, technical prototypes, or simple computerized applications) to iterative development, product selection, product customization, or evaluation of the impact of a system after installation.[54] The important point is that user experience experts recommend usability tests early and often.

User experience methods were developed over decades of work and are robust. This section of the chapter concentrates on proven methods to choose and apply. These include discount usability methods and the more traditional usability methods described below.

Discount Usability Methods

Nielsen developed techniques he called discount usability methods to reduce the number of required users in usability projects and to use early design prototypes. Initially meant for user experience experts, these methods have proven useful for others involved in designing projects.[55,56] These methods offer economies of time, effort, and cost and can be completed at any point in the systems life cycle. Two common techniques are heuristic evaluation and think-aloud protocol.

Heuristic Evaluation

The definition of a heuristic is a "rule of thumb" or guideline. Heuristic evaluations compare products against accepted usability guidelines to reveal major and minor usability issues. It is a commonly employed technique and students can complete a heuristic evaluation after only a modest amount of training.

A number of usability heuristics are available to evaluate applications:

- Nielsen[57]
- Zhang et al.'s 14 heuristics[58]
- Dix et al.'s 10 heuristics[41]
- Shneiderman's "eight golden rules"[59]
- HIMSS's nine usability principles[60]

Zhang et al.'s guidelines have been used more extensively in health applications and devices. These authors combined Nielsen's and Shneiderman's heuristics and applied them to a project evaluating two infusion pumps, finding 192 and 121 heuristic violations, respectively, categorized into 89 and 52 usability problems. Using this technique they concluded that pump 1 might contribute to more medical errors than pump 2.[58] Zhang et al.'s 14 adapted heuristics and definitions are outlined in Table 21-1. Once students understand the meaning of each heuristic, they can evaluate a health IT product against the heuristics as in the following example.

An Example of a Heuristic Evaluation Project. Guo and colleagues used Zhang's heuristics to evaluate a vendor's eMAR installed at a tertiary care center.[5] The authors received training on the eMAR, defined typical tasks that nurses complete using the product, and also modified Zhang's heuristics to include concepts about patient safety. The authors independently completed the defined tasks and compared their interactions to the heuristics, synthesized results, and found 233 violations for 60 usability problems. Problems included having to manually update the screen by clicking an "as of" button to ensure that the most current medication orders were being viewed and nurses' difficulty in determining medications given "at a glance." The results have implications across all three usability goals of effectiveness, efficiency, and satisfaction as well as point to potential patient safety issues.

Think-Aloud Protocol

Think-aloud protocol also involves a small number of users and has them talk aloud while they interact with a product. Users voice what they are trying to do, indicate where interactions are confusing, and provide other thoughts about the product during interactions. This allows a detailed examination of the specified tasks, in particular to uncover major effectiveness issues. This method may be used in the design, redesign, development, or evaluation of applications at any time in the systems life cycle. Think-aloud methods are often used in conjunction with other techniques.

With this technique researchers first determine a specific set of tasks for users to complete, such as tasks to operate an infusion pump. Defining tasks ahead of time provides structure and consistency across participants and guides users through the procedure. Participants are asked to complete the tasks and talk aloud during the session. Methods to capture the session can include observation with notes, audiotaping or videotaping, automatic capture of keystrokes using software such as Morae, and user and evaluator paper-and-pencil

diaries or logs.[41] The resulting material is then analyzed. Be aware that the analysis portion of this method can be time consuming depending on the complexity of the product, the number of users tested, and the number of tasks. However, the information gained by using this method is robust and helpful.

Traditional Usability Methods

A large suite of methods is available to guide examination of the user experience of health products and processes. The HHCI framework elements will guide assessments (thinking about different user skills levels, different contexts, etc.). Two of these methods, task analysis and focused ethnographies, are presented here.

Task Analysis

Task analysis is a generic term for a set of more than 100 techniques that range from a focus on cognitive tasks and processes (called cognitive task analysis) to observable user interactions with an application (e.g., a systematic mapping of team interactions during a patient code). Task analyses are systematic methods that are used to understand what users are doing or required to do with a product by focusing on tasks and behavioral actions of the users and products. These methods provide a process for learning about and documenting how ordinary users complete actions in a specific context.[55,61,62] Task analyses are helpful to identify task completeness, the correct or existing incorrect sequencing of tasks, accuracy of actions, error recovery, and task allocation between humans and products. Task analysis can be used throughout the systems life cycle to determine user requirements for design and redesign or to identify usability issues for complex products. One type of analysis, cognitive task analysis, is particularly useful for understanding users' goals while interacting with products. These methods can be used, for example, to determine who is attending to patients' preventive health alerts in a clinic because alerts are seen by a variety of healthcare providers.

Methods of task analysis include the following:

- Interviews
- Observations
- Shadowing users at their actual work sites
- Observing users doing tasks
- Conducting ethnographic studies or interviews[63]

A critique of techniques is available for students who want to find the right method for their project.[64] References on performing task analyses are available.[61,65]

Sample output from task analyses is listed in Table 21-2. After observations and interviews students will record user actions (e.g., a flow chart with task descriptions). Students might videotape users as they interact with an EHR, asking users to perform specific tasks and use a think-aloud protocol to uncover tasks (especially cognitive tasks) and requirements.

Example of a Task Analysis. Staggers and Kobus videotaped nurses as they interacted with an existing eMAR in a military inpatient application.[20] They then observed nurses'

TABLE 21-1   NIELSEN-SHNEIDERMAN HEURISTICS AND A SEVERITY RATING SCHEME

HEURISTIC CATEGORY	DEFINITION
Consistency and standards	Consistency across all aspects of the product: methods of navigation, messages and actions, meaning of buttons, terms and icons. Congruence with known screen design principles for color and screen layout. Consistency with ISO usability guidelines.
Visibility of system state	Users understand what the system is doing and what they can do with the product from the system messages, information, and displays.
Match between system and world	The technology matches the way users think and do work, uses appropriate information flow, has typical options that users need, and includes expected actions by the system.
Minimalist	No superfluous information. System and screen design targeted to primary information users' need. Use of progressive disclosure to display details of a category of information only when needed. The exception can be designs for expert users where screen density is preferred.
Minimize memory load	Minimizing the amount of information and tasks users have to memorize to adequately use the technology. Product makes use of sample formats for data input such as a calendar for date format.
Informative feedback	The technology provides prompt and useful feedback about users' interactions and actions (e.g., feedback that orders were placed).
Flexibility and efficiency	The ability to tailor and customize to suit individuals' needs. Includes novice and expert capabilities (e.g., string searches).
Good error messages	Tell users what error occurred and how users can recover from the error. Not abstract or general such as "Forbidden!" Need to be precise and polite and not blame the user.
Prevent errors	Catastrophic errors must be prevented (e.g., pediatric medication order dosing mixed between kilograms and pounds, delivering a radiation dose with the device leaves wide open instead of being tailored to tumor size).
Clear closure	Users should know when a task is completed and all information is accepted. Displays should include progress toward 100% completion versus using a series of bars.
Reversible actions	Whenever possible, actions and interactions should be able to be undone within legal limits in electronic health records. If actions cannot be reversed, there is a consistent procedure for documenting the correction of any misinformation in the system.
Use the users' language	The technology uses language and terms the targeted users can comprehend and expect. Health terms are used appropriately.
Users in control	Users initiate actions versus having the perception that the technology is in control. Avoid surprising actions, ending up in unexpected places, and loud sounds with errors.
Help and documentation	Provide help for users within the context the actions occur (context-sensitive). Embed help functions throughout the application.

SEVERITY SCALE RATING ELEMENT	DEFINITION
0—No usability problem	No need to correct the issue.
1—Cosmetic problem	Correct the issue only if extra time and fiscal resources allow. Lowest priority.
2—Minor problem	Annoying issue with minor impact. Low priority to fix.
3—Major usability problem	Issue with major impact to use or training or both. Important to fix. Considerations are the numbers and kinds of users affected by a persistent problem.
4—Usability catastrophe	Severe issue that must be corrected before product release, especially those related to patient safety.

Data from Staggers N. The impact of screen density on clinical nurses' computer task performance and subjective screen satisfaction. *Int J Man Mach Stud.* 1993;39:775-792; Staggers N. Improving the usability of health informatics applications. In: Hebda T, Czar P, eds. *Handbook of Informatics for Nurses and Health Professionals.* Upper Saddle River, NJ: Pearson Education; 2012:170-193; and Zhang J, Johnson TR, Patel VL, Paige DL, Kubose T. Using usability heuristics to evaluate patient safety of medical devices. *J Biomed Inform.* 2003;36(1-2):23-30. *ISO*, International Organization for Standardization.

medication management tasks in the actual setting in a variety of acute care units. The researchers created a task flow diagram of medication tasks (including cognitive tasks) and delineated deficiencies with the current application. Using the researchers' findings, a novel and more effective eMAR was then developed.

Focused Ethnographies

Ethnography methods are borrowed from anthropology and sociology where fieldwork and analyses of people in cultural and social settings are completed. Focused ethnographies concentrate on individuals' points of view, their experiences and interactions in social settings, rather than on just the

TABLE 21-2	SAMPLE OUTPUT FROM TASK ANALYSES
TYPE OF TASK ANALYSIS OUTPUT	**DESCRIPTION**
Profiles of users	Short narrative, visual descriptions, and/or summaries about the characteristics of users
Workflow diagrams	A flow diagram of tasks or cognitive processes performed by users
Task sequences or hierarchies	Lists of tasks order by sequence or arranged to show interrelationships
Task scenarios	Detailed descriptions of events or incidents, including how users handle situations
Usability issues	A list and classification of usability problems with a product
Affinity diagrams	Bottom-up groupings of facts and issues about users, tasks, and environments to generate design ideas
Video and audiotape highlights	Clips that illustrate particular observations about users and tasks in a context

Adapted from Staggers N. Human–computer interaction. In: Englebardt S, Nelson R, eds. *Information Technology in Health Care: An Interdisciplinary Approach*. Philadelphia, PA: Harcourt Health Science Company; 2001:321-345.

actions of those individuals.[66] The researcher is an observer rather than a part of the society. During observations, detailed descriptions are generated with an emphasis on social relationships and their impact on work. Ethnographies have become important in understanding the user experience and to describe the impact of complex products.

Example of a Focused Ethnography. Ash and colleagues used this method to research the impact of CPOE on users in acute care facilities in the United States.[3,67,68,69] They completed interviews, focus groups, and observations and found unintended consequences for CPOE: new and more work, workflow issues, unusual system demands, disruptions in routine communications, extreme user emotions, and over-dependence on the technology.

USABILITY MEASURES AND TESTS

Usability measurements are to user interface design what physical exams are to patient care.[70]

A critical aspect of conducting a usability study is measuring human performance. To assist students, a taxonomy of usability measures is presented in Table 21-3. This table is adapted from Sweeney, Maguire, and Shackel and from Staggers and expanded here.[48,53,71] The taxonomy includes measures from three perspectives: users, experts, and organizations. The important points are that usability is measurable and that a suite of measures is available. In addition to the objective measures in Table 21-3, questionnaires are available to measure users' perceptions of or satisfaction with their product interactions.

Usability Questionnaires

At least four questionnaires are available to measure user interaction or interface satisfaction:
- System Usability Scale (SUS)[72,73]
- Questionnaire for User Interaction Satisfaction (QUIS)[74]
- Purdue Usability Testing Questionnaire[75]
- Software Usability Measurement Inventory (SUMI)[76]

The SUS is considered an industry standard among user experience professionals and has been used widely on a variety of products outside health.[72,73] The SUS is a publicly available, 10-item scale developed in 1986 by John Brooke at Digital Equipment Corporation.[65]

The QUIS has been used in numerous health informatics studies. Typically a computer system or application is assessed. Developed in the late 1990s, QUIS addresses users' overall perceptions of a product, including overall reaction, terminology, screen layout, learning, system capabilities, and other subscales such as multimedia applications. QUIS subscales can be mixed and matched to fit the application at hand. Participants can complete the QUIS in about 5 to 10 minutes. Reliability and validity assessments are available for this tool.

The Purdue Usability Testing Questionnaire has 100 open-ended questions about how features adhere to accepted guidelines. Students would need to be familiar with design guidelines before using this questionnaire. However, reliability and validity assessments of the questionnaire are not reported.

Less information is available about the SUMI, including its assessed reliability and validity. The instrument has three components: an overall assessment, a usability profile, and an item consensus analysis. The usability profile examines areas such as efficiency, helpfulness, control, and learnability. The consensus component addresses adherence to well-known design alternatives such as categorical ordering of data in a simple search task.

SELECTING A TYPE OF USABILITY TEST

A key decision before beginning a usability assessment is determining the type of usability study to conduct in a specific case. This section expands on work by Rubin and Chisnell and uses the systems life cycle to organize the types of tests available.[42]

Determining User Needs and Requirements

At the beginning of the systems life cycle, during initial design or redesign process, informaticists determine user needs and requirements from the following:
- Users' characteristics
- Tasks (including cognitive tasks)
- Work design
- Interactions among workers and tasks and products

TABLE 21-3 SAMPLE USABILITY MEASURES

USABILITY FOCUS	USABILITY MEASURES
User behaviors (performance)	Task times (speed, reaction times) Percentage of tasks completed Number, kinds of errors Percentage of tasks completed accurately Time, frequency spent on any one option Number of hits and/or amount of time spent on a website Training time Eye tracking Facial expressions Breadth and depth of application usage in actual settings Quality of completed tasks (e.g., quality of decisions) Users' comments (think-aloud) as they interact with technology System set-up or installation time, complexity of set-up Model of tasks and user behaviors Description of problems when interacting with an application
User behaviors (cognitive)	Description of or systems fit with cognitive information processing Retention of application knowledge over time Comprehension of system Fit with workflow
User behaviors (perceptions)	Usability ratings of products Perceptions about any aspect of technology (speed, effectiveness) Comments during interviews Questionnaires and rating responses (workload, satisfaction)
User behaviors (physiologic)	Heart rate EEG Galvanic skin response Brain-evoked potentials
User behaviors (perceptions about physiologic reactions)	Perceptions about anxiety, stress
User behaviors (motivation)	Willingness to use system Enthusiasm
Expert evaluations (performance)	Model predictions for task performance times, learning, ease of understanding Observations of users as they use applications in a setting to determine fit with work
Expert evaluations (conformance to guidelines)	Level of adherence to guidelines, design criteria, usability principles (heuristic evaluation)
Expert evaluations (perception)	Ratings of technology, informal or formal comments
Context (organization)	Economic costs (increased FTEs for the help desk for a new application) Number of support staff, time needed to support product Number of training staff, time needed to support product Costs (for support, training, loss of productivity) Observations about the fit with work design and workflow in departments, organizations, networks of institutions
Combined	Videotaping and audiotaping users as they interact with an application and capturing keystrokes. Can capture any combination of the above.

Adapted from Staggers N. Human–computer interaction. In: Englebardt S, Nelson R, eds. *Information Technology in Health Care: An Interdisciplinary Approach*. Philadelphia, PA: Harcourt Health Science Company; 2001:321-345; and Staggers N. Improving the usability of health informatics applications. In: Hebda T, Czar P, eds. *Handbook of Informatics for Nurses and Health Professionals*. Upper Saddle River, NJ: Pearson Education; 2012:170-193.
EEG, Electroencephalography; *FTE*, full-time equivalent.

• Requirements about the specific environments and particular needs related to the context of interactions

Studies can be conducted with limited resources if the scope of the investigation is focused. As the complexity increases, resource consumption increases concomitantly. Assessments early in the systems life cycle seek to answer the following questions:

• Who are the users and what are their characteristics?
• What are basic activities and tasks in this context?
• How do users cognitively process information?

- What information processing can be supported by products?
- What special considerations should be made for users in this environment?
- What attributes need to be in place for an initial design?

Task analysis and think-aloud protocol, both discussed above, can be used to determine users' needs and requirements and answer the questions listed here.

Example of a Requirements Determination Usability Study

Staggers and colleagues completed two studies focused on nurses' acute care hand-offs or change of shift reports to determine the current state of the activity and to develop requirements to support hand-off tasks.[77,78] Hand-offs are highly complex and cognitively intensive periods where nurses going off shift synthesize information about patients and communicate it to nurses coming on shift. Methods that would generate rich details about the process, such as observation, field notes, and interviews, were selected. The HHCI framework guided the thinking about requirements for different aspects of the hand-off process to be studied. For example, nurses (expertise levels, regular versus travel nurses), types of units (critical care, emergency department, medical and surgical), and types of product support in place (EHRs, CPOE, eMAR) were identified using this framework. Hand-off tasks can be completed in a variety of ways, including audiorecorded, face-to-face, and bedside reports. The researchers completed a focused ethnography across available medical and surgical units in different facilities. They observed change of shift reports, audiotaped nurses, photographed nurses' tools, and took field notes about nurses' interactions with the existing EHRs in the facilities. From the findings the researchers were able to derive detailed information about requirements for computerized support for change of shift activities.[79]

Exploratory Test

An exploratory test is conducted early in the systems life cycle after requirements are determined. These tests are conducted on very basic or preliminary designs or redesigns where few resources have been committed to programming the product. The objective of an exploratory test is to assess the effectiveness of emerging design concepts by asking the following:

- Is the basic functionality of value to users?
- Is basic navigation and information flow intuitive?
- Is fundamental content missing?
- How much computer experience does a user need to use this module?[42]

Exploratory tests are more informal, with extensive interaction between testers and users. The usability focus is on the goal of effectiveness. Users are asked to perform common tasks with the prototype or step through paper mockups of the application using a think-aloud protocol. Researchers strive to understand *why* users are behaving as they do with the application rather than how quickly they perform.[79] To assess effectiveness the researcher or informaticist is interested in finding cognitive disconnects with basic functions,

missing information or steps and assessing how easily users understand the task at hand.

Nielsen recommends having five users talk aloud or "think aloud" as an observer watches them and records any issues. This number of users can detect as much as 60% to 80% of design errors.[56] Later research confirms that as few as five to eight users are sufficient for most usability tests.[80-81]

Example of an Exploratory Test

A public health researcher wanted to develop an application to display reportable patient conditions across jurisdictions. After researching available applications and conducting a requirements determination, she developed a prototype using PowerPoint to meet initial requirements and assess usability for the following sample tasks: find out whether chlamydia is a reportable condition in Utah, Colorado, or Washington; determine the time frame for reporting the condition; and ascertain whether a specimen must be submitted and the location for the submission. She selected key public health, clinical, and laboratory users. These users were asked to think aloud as they completed common tasks. The researcher took notes to record the data related to their responses. Using these data several iterations of the prototype were designed to improve the user experience in completing the tasks.[82]

Assessment Test

An assessment test is conducted early in or midway through the development of a product application.[42] After the organization and general design are determined, this kind of test assesses lower-level operations of the application, stressing the efficiency goals of the product (versus effectiveness) and how well the task is presented to users. Questions during this test might include the following:

- How quickly and accurately can users perform selected tasks?
- Are the terms in the system consistent across modules?
- Are operations displayed in a manner that allows quick detection of critical information?

Users perform common tasks with a product that is partially developed. Usability measures (see Table 21-3) such as performance time and errors are selected. Users can perform tasks silently or researchers can use think-aloud methods to elicit issues. Again, designers use the results to craft a redesigned prototype to correct issues. Iterative development typically takes three rounds of design to eliminate major usability issues.

Example of an Assessment Test

The researcher in the exploratory test example above assessed a later version of the public health application. She asked the same key users to use the same tasks but now participants commented on operations, icons, and the arrangement of the radio buttons.

Validation Test

A validation test is completed later in the systems life cycle using a more mature product. This type of test assesses how this particular product compares to a predetermined standard, benchmark, or performance measure. A second purpose might be to assess how all modules in a technology application work as an integrated whole. A validation test can also be useful in a system selection process to decide how a new vendor supports critical tasks such as medication bar-coding or medication reconciliation. Questions for a validation test might include the following:

- Can 80% of users retrieve the correct complete blood count (CBC) test results within 10 seconds of interacting with the system?
- How many heuristic violations are identified for this product?
- Can users complete admission orders for a trauma patient with no errors?

This kind of test is more structured so it precludes extensive interactions between testers and users. The specific methods are carefully structured similar to the processes used in an experimental study.

Example of a Validation Test

A nurse researcher wanted to ensure that a new mobile device for rural care in Tanzania mirrored the established algorithms on paper. The goal was to assess whether the algorithms used with the mobile device were 100% accurate. She enlisted key users and informaticists to interact with each pathway in the device. Deviations from the established algorithms were documented and corrected.[83]

Comparison Study

Students can conduct comparison studies at any point in the systems life cycle but they are more commonly done to compare an existing design with a redesign or an early prototype with a more mature product. The major objective of this usability test is to determine which application, design, or product is more effective, efficient, and satisfying.[42] The study design can range from an informal side-by-side comparison with structured tasks or a classic experimental study. Results, however, are more dramatic if the designs are substantially different.

Examples of a Comparison Study

The purpose of this study was to determine whether a new user interface for orders management was different than an older interface in terms of performance times, errors, and user satisfaction.[84] The tasks and interactions were planned to minimize the amount of time that nurses would be away from patient care. The informaticists used an HCI framework, similar to the HHCI framework, to guide elements in the study. Identical computers were used to test both interfaces. Tasks were "real-world" nursing orders and the same across the two designs. The environment was a computer training room, a quiet room away from patient care units and distractions. The developmental trajectory was considered in this study to ensure that results were not affected by practice time. Therefore 40 tasks for each interface allowed nurses to become practiced at each user interface. The number of tasks

was determined in pilot work. Tasks, keystrokes, and errors were captured by the computer. The QUIS was administered after each interface. Each nurse interacted with both interfaces but the order in which they were presented was randomized. The results showed a significant difference on all three variables: performance times, errors, and user satisfaction.

In a second study a nurse researcher wanted to compare the traditional design of physiologic monitors and other products to a new design that integrated data across physiologic parameters, medication management, and communication. His target population was intensive care unit (ICU) nurses. The tasks were designed so that the study could be completed in about 20 to 30 minutes over two sessions. Paper prototypes were used to assess effectiveness, efficiency, and satisfaction before resources were expended to code bidirectional interfaces to the devices. Tasks were defined and nurses interacted with the prototypes. Findings included faster task times, higher detection of potential medication interactions, lower perceived mental workload, and higher satisfaction with the integrated monitoring view.[85,86]

Identifying Usability Issues with Fielded Products

As organizations begin to understand the importance of the user experience, leaders may be unsure where to begin identifying usability issues in their current environments. The following list includes symptoms of potential strategic usability issues and provides a framework for determining where initial energy and resources could be focused:

- Products or applications requiring long training times
- Support calls categorized by product or application
- Adverse events related to product interactions
- Lists of requested system change requests typically tracked in a database of system change requests across users and products
- User group requests for updates or changes
- Users' descriptions of their most vexing applications and interactions
- Users' identified delays or errors when they interact with complex applications, especially any requiring information synthesis such as eMARs, clinical summaries, and hand-offs

Once a usability problem is suspected, researchers or students begin assessing the issue more systematically using the techniques described above.

Steps for Conducting Usability Tests

At some point in their careers, students will likely be expected to or will want to conduct a usability project. Step-by-step guides are available.[42,60] The texts by Beth Crandell,[87] Rubin and Chisnell,[42] and Tom Tullis and Bill Albert[65] are easy to understand. HIMSS[60] and the National Institute of Standards and Technology (NIST)[88] have also published guides for conducting usability tests on EHRs. The basic steps for conducting usability tests can be summarized as follows:

1. *Define a clear purpose.* The specific purpose guides testers to determine the type of study, methods, and users

required. For example, if the purpose relates to assessment of a redesign of a CPOE module for an intraoperative surgical team, an exploratory test may be indicated.

2. *Assess constraints.* Testers are always mindful of study constraints: time; resources; availability of the software to be evaluated; and availability of other equipment such as video cameras, testing labs, or users, especially if the users are specialists. These constraints may drive the type of usability test. For example, if the tester's goal is to evaluate an application to support anesthesiologists, these time-constrained physicians may not be willing to spend more than 15 to 20 minutes participating in a usability test. Tasks, methods, and products are defined to work within this constraint.

3. *Use an HCI framework to define pertinent components.* Use a framework to assess each component against the planned study. Who are the key users? What are typical tasks? What information needs to be exchanged? What product characteristics and which actions are needed? What is the setting or context? Will it be a naturalistic setting to determine exactly how an application will be used or a laboratory setting to control interruptions? What is a representative time in the developmental trajectory? How much practice time needs to be considered, especially if the design is new? Be sure to examine the latter component carefully to ensure a valid comparison between users' interaction with a new product and a current one by including practice time in the study.

4. *Match methods to the purpose, constraints, and framework assessment.* Methods that produce rich results such as a think-aloud protocol will match a purpose of understanding key user requirements while a more structured method will allow a comparison of new and old designs. Long training and practice times for complex devices may constrain the number of tasks testers can offer. Other basic methodological steps are as follows:

   - Select representative end-users
   - Select a usability test appropriate to the purpose and point in the systems life cycle
   - Define and validate tasks
   - Measure key elements and control for others (e.g., measure performance time but control interruptions unless the effect of interruptions is the focus)
   - Define the context to be used
   - Consider training and practice for new products
   - Pilot test methods before running the main study to smooth out procedures and bugs

Once the methods are defined, all of these pieces can be put into action and the study can be conducted.

CONCLUSION AND FUTURE DIRECTIONS

In the U.S., federal agencies are now engaging in activities to improve the user experience for health IT products (e.g., NIST, the regulations crafted by the Office of the National Coordinator for Health Information Technology). The Food and Drug Administration has required usability testing for the last decade but EHR vendors and other health organizations are only beginning to employ the principles and processes for improving the user experience. The most immediate future direction concerns user-experience education and understanding of action steps to be taken. The current federal requirements will continue to expand. Organizations need to increase their knowledge and skills related to improving the user experience. One way is to use the material outlined by the HIMSS Usability Task Force in 2011 on a Health Usability Maturity Model.[10] The material can guide organizations in assessing their current level of user experience, selling usability to the organization, and increasing the user experience to reach a strategic level.

Future usability methods might include automated methods to ensure that designs conform to known standards, especially basic screen designs. Clearly, the future includes a focus on health IT products that support the way users think and do work in health settings.

This chapter described current issues with technology and the potential benefits of improving the user experience in health organizations. After definitions of terms, the axioms of usability were defined: an early and central focus on users in the design and development of systems, iterative design of applications, and systematic usability measures. Across HCI frameworks these major elements exist: users, products, contexts, tasks, information, interactions, and a developmental trajectory. Common usability methods and tests were discussed. Students are now prepared to conduct discount usability tests and four different types of usability tests: exploratory, assessment, validation, and comparison. Usability measures are available and four steps were outlined for planning and conducting usability tests.

REFERENCES

1. Stead W, Lin H. *Computational Technology for Effective Health Care: Immediate Steps and Strategic Directions.* Washington, DC: National Academies Press; 2009.
2. Ash JS, Berg M, Coiera E. Some unintended consequences of information technology in health care: the nature of patient care information system-related errors. *J Am Med Inform Assn.* 2004;11(2):104-112. doi:10.1197/jamia.M1471.
3. Ash JS, Sittig DF, Dykstra R, Campbell E, Guappone K. The unintended consequences of computerized provider order entry: findings from a mixed methods exploration. *Int J Med Inform.* 2009;78(suppl 1):S69-S76. doi:10.1016/j.ijmedinf.2008.07.015.
4. Silver JD, Hammil SD. Doctor, nurse disciplined by UPMC in kidney transplant case: failed to detect hepatitis C in kidney donated for transplant. *Pittsburg Post Gazette.* http://www.post-gazette.com/pg/11147/1149429-114-0.stm. 2011. Accessed March 1, 2012.
5. Guo J, Irdbarren S, Kapsandoy S, Perri S, Staggers N. eMAR user interfaces: a call for ubiquitous usability evaluations and product redesign. *Applied Clinical Informatics.* 2011;2(2):202-224.
6. Koppel R, Metlay JP, Cohen A, et al. Role of computerized physician order entry systems in facilitating medication errors. *J Amer Med Assoc.* 2005;293(10):1197-1203. doi:10.1001/jama.293.10.1197.

7. Staggers N, Jennings BM, Lasome CE. A usability assessment of AHLTA in ambulatory clinics at a military medical center. *Mil Med.* 2010;175(7):518-524.

8. Philpott T. Military access drops. Today in the Military. http://www.military.com. 2006. Accessed April 30, 2012.

9. Philpott T. Doctors see bigger role in electronic health record reform. Stars and Stripes. http://www.stripes.com. 2009. Accessed April 30, 2012.

10. Healthcare Information and Management Systems Society. *Promoting Usability in Health Organizations: Initial Steps and Progress toward a Healthcare Usability Maturity Model.* Chicago, IL: Health Information and Management Systems Society; 2011.

11. Bias RG, Mayhew DJ. *Cost-Justifying Usability: An Update for the Internet Age.* San Francisco, CA: Morgan Kaufman; 2005.

12. Nielsen J, Gilutz S. *Usability Return on Investment.* Fremont, CA: Nielsen Norman Group; 2003.

13. Usability Professionals' Association. http://www.upassoc.org/. 2012. Accessed April 4, 2012.

14. Dey Alexander Consulting. Return on Investment (ROI) discussion articles. Dey Alexander Consulting. http://www.deyalexander.com.au/resources/uxd/roi.html. 2009. Accessed April 4, 2012.

15. Saitwal H, Feng X, Walji M, Patel V, Zhang J. Assessing performance of an electronic health record (EHR) using cognitive task analysis. *Int J Med Inform.* 2010;79(7):501-506. doi:10.1016/j.ijmedinf.2010.04.001.

16. Souza R, Sonderegger P, Roshan S, Dorsey M. Get ROI from Design. Cambridge, MA: Forrester Research; 2001.

17. Institute of Medicine. *Crossing the Quality Chasm: A New Health System for the 21st Century.* Washington, DC: National Academy of Sciences; 2001.

18. World Health Organization. *Communication during Patient Hand-Overs.* Geneva, Switzerland: World Health Organization; 2007.

19. Ash JS, Sittig DF, Campbell EM, Guappone KP, Dykstra RH. Some unintended consequences of clinical decision support systems. *AMIA Annu Symp Proc.* 2007;26-30.

20. Staggers N, Kobus D, Brown C. Nurses' evaluations of a novel design for an electronic medication administration record. *Comput Inform Nurs.* 2007;25(2):67-75.

21. Kushniruk A, Triola M, Stein B, Borycki E, Kannry J. The relationship of usability to medical error: an evaluation of errors associated with usability problems in the use of a handheld application for prescribing medications. *St Heal T.* 2004;107(Pt 2):1073-1076. doi:D040004885 [pii].

22. Nielsen J, Levy J. Measuring usability: preference vs performance. *Communications of the ACM.* 1994;37(4):66-75.

23. Dray SM. The importance of designing usable systems. *Interactions.* 1995;2(1):17-20.

24. Drews FA, Westenskow DR. The right picture is worth a thousand numbers: data displays in anesthesia. *Hum Factors.* 2006;48(1):59-71.

25. Syroid ND, Agutter J, Drews FA, et al. Development and evaluation of a graphical anesthesia drug display. *Anesthesiology.* 2002;96(3):565-575. doi:00000542-200203000-00010 [pii].

26. Wachter SB, Agutter J, Syroid N, Drews F, Weinger MB, Westenskow D. The employment of an iterative design process to develop a pulmonary graphical display. *J Am Med Inform Assn.* 2003;10(4):363-372. doi:10.1197/jamia.M1207 [pii].

27. Pressman RS. *Software Engineering: A Practitioner's Approach.* New York, NY: McGraw-Hill; 1992.

28. Bias RG, Mayhew DJ. *Cost-Justifying Usability.* San Francisco, CA: Morgan Kaufmann Publishers; 1994.

29. IBM. Cost justifying ease of use: complex solutions are problems. http://www-01.ibm.com/software/ucd/ucd.html 2001. Accessed December 11, 2012.

30. Dray SM, Karat C. Human factors cost justification for an internal development project. In: Bias RG, Mayhew DJ, eds. *Cost-Justifying Usability.* San Francisco, CA: Morgan Kauffman Publishers; 1994:111-122.

31. Marcus A. *Return on Investment for Usable User-Interface Design: Examples and Statistics.* Berkeley, CA: Experience Intelligent Design, AM+A White Paper; 2004.

32. Bosert JL. *Quality Function Deployment: A Practitioner's Approach.* New York, NY: ASQC Quality Press; 1991.

33. Karat C. Iterative testing of a security application. Paper presented at: Proceedings of the Human Factors Society; 1989; Denver, CO.

34. Landauer TK. *The Trouble with Computers: Usefulness, Usability and Productivity.* Cambridge, MA: MIT Press; 1995.

35. Kuniavsky M. *Observing the User Experience: A Practioner's Guide to User Research.* San Francisco, CA: Morgan Kaufmann Publishers; 2003.

36. International Organization for Standardization (ISO). ISO 9241-9211. Usability Net. http://www.usabilitynet.org/tools/r_international.htm#9241-11. 1998. Accessed February 7, 2011.

37. Schaffer E. Is usability different than the user experience? HFI Connect.http://connect.humanfactors.com/profiles/blogs/is-user-experience-different. 2010. Accessed February 7, 2011.

38. Nielsen Norman Group. User experience: our definition. Nielsen Norman Group. http://www.nngroup.com/about/user experience.html. 2007. Accessed February 7, 2011.

39. Definitions of human factors and ergonomics. Human Factors and Ergonomics Society. http://www.hfes.org/Web/Educational Resources/HFEdefinitionsmain.html#govagencies. 2012. Accessed April 4, 2012.

40. Norman D. *The Psychology of Everyday Things.* New York, NY: Basic Books; 1988.

41. Dix A, Finlay JE, Abowd GD, Beale R. Human–Computer Interaction. 3rd ed. Essex, England: Prentice Hall; 2004.

42. Rubin J, Chisnell D. *Handbook of Usability Testing: How to Plan, Design and Conduct Effective Tests.* 2nd ed. New York, NY: John Wiley & Sons; 2008.

43. Ammenwerth E, Iller C, Mahler C. IT-adoption and the interaction of task, technology and individuals: a FIT framework and a case study. *BioMed Central.* 2006;6(3):1-13.

44. Borycki EM, Kushniruk AW, Bellwood P, Brender J. Technology-induced errors: the current use of frameworks and models from the biomedical and life sciences literatures. *Methods of Informatics in Medicine.* 2012;51(2):95-103. doi:10.3414/ME11-02-0009.

45. Despont-Gros C, Mueller H, Lovis C. Evaluating user interactions with clinical information systems: a model based on human–computer interaction models. *J Biomed Inform.* 2005;38(3):244-255. doi:10.1016/j.jbi.2004.12.004.

46. Hollnagel E, Woods D. *Joint Cognitive Systems: Foundations of Cognitive Systems Engineering.* Boca Raton, FL: Yaylor & Francis; 2005.

47. Johnson CM, Johnson TR, Zhang J. A user-centered framework for redesigning health care interfaces. *J Biomed Inform.* 2005;38(1):75-87. doi:10.1016/j.jbi.2004.11.005.

48. Staggers N. Human–computer interaction. In: Englebardt S, Nelson R, eds. *Information Technology in Health Care: An*

Interdisciplinary Approach. Philadelphia, PA: Harcourt Health Science Company; 2001:321-345.

49. Yusof MM, Stergioulas L, Zugic J. Health information systems adoption: findings from a systematic review. *Stud Health Technol Inform*. 2007;129(Pt 1):262-266.

50. Zhang J, Butler KA. UFuRT: a work-centered framework and process for design and evaluation of information systems. Paper presented at: Proceedings of HCI International; 2007; Beijing, China.

51. Staggers N, Parks PL. Collaboration between unlikely disciplines in the creation of a conceptual framework for nurse–computer interactions. *Proc Annu Symp Comput Appl Med Care*. 1992;661-665.

52. Staggers N, Parks PL. Description and initial applications of the Staggers & Parks Nurse–computer Interaction Framework. *Comput Nurs*. 1993;11(6):282-290.

53. Staggers N. Improving the usability of health informatics applications. In: Hebda T, Czar P, eds. *Handbook of Informatics for Nurses and Health Professionals*. Upper Saddle River, NJ: Pearson Education; 2013:170-193.

54. Thompson CB, Snyder-Halpern R, Staggers N. Analysis, processes, and techniques: case study. *Comput Nurs*. 1999;17(5):203-206.

55. Nielsen J. *Usability Engineering*. Cambridge, MA: AP Professional; 1993.

56. Nielsen J. Heuristic evaluation. In: Nielsen J, Mack RL, eds. *Usability Inspection Methods*. New York, NY: John Wiley & Sons, Inc; 1994.

57. Nielsen J. Severity ratings for usability problems. Useit.com. http://www.useit.com/papers/heuristic/severityrating.html. 1994. Accessed April 30, 2012.

58. Zhang J, Johnson TR, Patel VL, Paige DL, Kubose T. Using usability heuristics to evaluate patient safety of medical devices. *J Biomed Inform*. 2003;36(1-2):23-30.

59. Shneiderman B, Plaisant K. *Designing the User Interface: Strategies for Effective Human–Computer Interaction*. 4th ed. Boston, MA: Pearson/Addison-Wesley; 2005.

60. HIMSS EHR Usability Task Force. Defining and testing EMR usability: principles and proposed methods of EMR usability evaluation and rating. Healthcare Information and Management Systems Society. http://www.himss.org/content/files/HIMSS_DefiningandTestingEMRUsability.pdf. 2009. Accessed April 12, 2012.

61. Hackos JT, Redish JC. *User and Task Analysis for Interface Design*. New York, NY: John Wiley & Sons; 1998.

62. Mayhew D. Requirements specifications within the usability engineering lifecycle. In: Sears A, Jacko J, eds. *The Human–Computer Interaction Handbook*. New York, NY: Lawrence Erlbaum Association; 2008:917-927.

63. Courage C, Redish J, Wixon D. Task analysis. In: Sears A, Jacko J, eds. *The Human–Computer Interaction Handbook*. New York, NY: Lawrence Erlbaum Associates; 2008:928-937.

64. Wei J, Salvendy G. The cognitive task analysis methods for job and task design: review and reappraisal. *Behav Inform Technol*. 2004;23(4):273-299.

65. Tullis T, Albert B. *Measuring the User Experience: Collecting, Analyzing and Presenting Usability Metrics*. New York, NY: Elseiver; 2008.

66. Hammersley M, Atkinson P. *Ethnography: Principles in Practice*. 3rd ed. London, England: Routledge; 2007.

67. Ash JS, Sittig DF, Dykstra R, Campbell E, Guappone K. Exploring the unintended consequences of computerized physician order entry. *Stud Health Technol Inform*. 2007;129(Pt 1):198-202.

68. Ash JS, Sittig DF, Dykstra RH, Guappone K, Carpenter JD, Seshadri V. Categorizing the unintended sociotechnical consequences of computerized provider order entry. *Int J Med Inform*. 2007;76(suppl. 1):S21-S27. doi:10.1016/j.ijmedinf.2006.05.017.

69. Ash JS, Sittig DF, Poon EG, Guappone K, Campbell E, Dykstra RH. The extent and importance of unintended consequences related to computerized provider order entry. *J Am Med Inform Assn*. 2007;14(4):415-423. doi:10.1197/jamia.M2373.

70. Staggers, N. Invited testimony about EHR Usability. Washington, DC April 21, 2011: Office of the National Coordinator for Health Information Technology, Hearing on EHR Usability; 2011.

71. Sweeney M, Maguire M, Shackel B. Evaluating user–computer interaction: a framework. *Int J Man Mach Stud*. 1993;38:689-711.

72. Bangor A, Kortum P, Miller JT. An empirical evaluation of the System Usability Scale. *Int J Hum-Comput Int*. 2008;24(6).

73. Sauro J. Measuring usability with the System Usability Scale (SUS). Measuring Usability. http://www.measuringusability.com/sus.php. 2011. Accessed April 30, 2012.

74. Norman K, Shneiderman B, Harper B, Slaughter L. Questionnaire for user interaction satisfaction, version 7.0. http://lap.umd.edu/quis/. 1998. Accessed February 16, 2012.

75. Lin H, Choong Y, Salvendy G. A proposed index of usability: a method for comparing the relative usability of different software systems. *Behav Inform Technol*. 1997;16(4/5):267-278.

76. Kirakowski J, Corbett M. SUMI: the software measurement inventory. *Brit J Educ Technol*. 1993;24:210-212.

77. Staggers N, Clark L, Blaz JW, Kapsandoy S. Nurses' information management and use of electronic tools during acute care handoffs. *Western J Nurs Res*. 2012;34(2):153-173. doi:10.1177/0193945911407089.

78. Staggers N, Jennings BM. The content and context of change of shift report on medical and surgical units. *J Nurs Admin*. 2009;39(9):393-398. doi:10.1097/NNA.0b013e3181b3b63a00005110-200909000-00009 [pii].

79. Staggers N, Clark L, Blaz JW, Kapsandoy S. Why patient summaries in electronic health records do not provide the cognitive support necessary for nurses' handoffs on medical and surgical units: insights from interviews and observations. *Health Informatics J*. 2011;17(3):209-223. doi:10.1177/1460458211405809.

80. Shneiderman B, Plaisant C, Cohen M, Jacobs S. *Designing the User Interface: Strategies for Effective Human–Computer Interaction*. 5th ed. Reading, MA: Addison-Wesley; 2010.

81. Dumas JS, Fox JE. Usability testing: current practice and future directions. In: Sears A, Jacko J, eds. *The Human–Computer Interaction Handbook: Fundamentals, Evolving Technologies and Emerging Applications*. 2nd ed. New York, NY: Lawrence Erlbaum; 2008.

82. Rajeev D. Development and Evaluation of New Strategies to Enhance Public Health Reporting. [dissertation]. Salt Lake City, UT: Biomedical Informatics, University of Utah; 2012.

83. Perri S. Using Electronic Decision Support to Enhance Provider–Caretaker Communication for Treatment of Children Under Five in Tanzania. [dissertation]. Salt Lake City, UT: College of Nursing, University of Utah; 2012.

84. Staggers N, Kobus D. Comparing response time, errors, and satisfaction between text-based and graphical user interfaces during nursing order tasks. *J Am Med Inform Assn*. 2000;7(2):164-176.

85. Koch S, Westenskow D, Weir C, et al. ICU nurses' evaluations of integrated information integration in displays for ICU nurses

on user satisfaction and perceived mental workload. Paper presented at: Medical Informatics Europe; 2012; Pisa, Italy.

86. Koch SH, Weir C, Westenskow D, et al. Evaluation of the effect of information integration in displays for ICU nurses on situation awareness and task completion time: a prospective randomized controlled study. *Int J Med Inform.* epublication January 25, 2013.

87. Crandell B, Klein G, Hoffman R. *Working Minds: A Practioner's Guide to Cognitive Task Analysis.* Boston, MA: Massachusetts Institute of Technology; 2006.

88. National Institute of Standards and Technology (NIST). Technical evaluation, testing and validation of electronic health records. NIST. http://www.nist.gov/itl/iad/ehr-032012.cfm. 2011. Accessed April 30, 2012.

DISCUSSION QUESTIONS

1. Assess critical user experience issues in your own organization. Describe one example and apply the heuristic evaluation technique to analyze where the major violations exist.

2. Search the Internet for current policies on the user experience in health IT by searching the Office of the National Coordinator for Health Information Technology and the National Institute of Standards and Technology. Analyze how one of these current policies will affect your organization.

3. Outline a usability test for your current eMAR. Include the elements discussed in the chapter in your proposed usability test. Describe why you chose the methods you did.

4. Your organization is planning to purchase new physiologic monitors for the adult ICUs. You are the informatics person assigned to this project. Describe how you would include usability in the purchase process. Outline participants, methods, and tasks to be tested.

CASE STUDY

A tertiary care center in the western U.S. has an installed base of electronic health records supported by Cerner Corporation for inpatient areas and by Epic for outpatient areas. Other technology includes a suite of about 300 different applications supported by the IT department. The current environment, while including robust capabilities such as computerized provider order entry, is "siloed" with information. Healthcare providers complain that they have difficulty obtaining the "big picture" of the patient across systems and they have to remember information located in disparate systems. They are burdened with integrating information themselves. Not only is this time consuming, it is potentially prone to error. Providers have developed numerous work-arounds to the different systems in ambulatory and inpatient areas, including "shadow" files for patients they see frequently. Nurses complain that they have to "jump around" the inpatient system to find information they need for activities such as patient hand-offs.

The organization responds by developing a vision for the future that centered on the concept of knowledge management (KM). This concept is defined as the systematic process of identifying, capturing, and transferring information and knowledge that people can use to create, compete (with other organizations), and improve. A crucial aspect of KM is improving the user experience. As the leaders in the organization begin to address KM and improve the user experience, they are employing the same tactics described in this chapter.

Discussion Questions

1. Assume that you are the leader of the KM effort. Where would you start to improve the user experience?

2. Pharmacists supporting the ICUs are asking for your help to improve their situation (their user experience) because they are forced to use nonintegrated systems. What methods would you use to examine this issue?

3. The institution is in the process of purchasing new physiologic monitors for their step-down unit. Describe how usability should be incorporated as part of the purchasing process. Design a brief usability test to support the purchasing process.

Standards

Tae Youn Kim and Susan A. Matney

As personal health records become popular in the twenty-first century, the health practitioner also needs to be involved in the development of consumer health vocabulary. With standardized clinical terminology, patient data will be available across the full spectrum of healthcare settings.

OBJECTIVES

At the completion of this chapter the reader will be prepared to:

1. Use basic terms and resources available to health professionals regarding data standardization and health information exchange
2. Explain the difference between a standardized reference terminology and an interface terminology
3. Apply adopted evaluation criteria in assessing the quality of different standard terminologies
4. Compare and contrast the similarities and differences among standardized healthcare terminologies relevant to patient care

5. Examine how the adoption of standardardized terminologies can assist in the implementation of Meaningful Use criteria of electronic health records
6. Describe the importance of data exchange across settings and the role of standardized terminologies in the development process of data exchange
7. Discuss the areas of future research and development in relation to data standardization and exchange from a nursing perspective

KEY TERMS

Classification, 352
Data exchange, 363
Data standards, 363
Harmonization, 363
Interface terminology, 352
Interoperability, 363

Ontology, 352
Reference terminology, 352
Standardized terminology, 352
Terminology cross-mapping, 363
Terminology harmonization, 363

ABSTRACT

The current health information technology (health IT) environment is rapidly changing worldwide. There is increasing evidence that the adoption of health IT will ensure the use of best practices and improve quality of care in a cost-efficient manner. Using standardized terminologies is a fundamental component of health IT adoption. These terminologies facilitate coherent communication as well as the collection and aggregation of healthcare data across settings. This chapter introduces data standards relevant to the health professions. The advantages of adopting standard terminologies in practice include (1) an enhanced user interface in electronic health records, (2) effective data retrieval and exchange, (3) improved monitoring of quality of care, and (4) discovered knowledge through clinical research. The role of standardized terminologies in the process of exchanging healthcare data across systems is also discussed. The chapter concludes with a discussion of topics for future research and development, including data summarization and mining, knowledge management and decision support, linkage of professional vocabulary and consumer vocabulary, and clinical translational and comparative effectiveness research.

INTRODUCTION

The Institute of Medicine (IOM) identified health IT as critical to closing the quality chasm and shaping a better healthcare delivery system in the twenty-first century.[1] The use of health IT, including electronic health records (EHRs), has become a component of a funded national agenda in the U.S., as it is considered a tool to support patient-centered care and improve quality and safety of treatments during the last decade.[2] Of the various health IT products, EHRs are lauded as a means to collect longitudinal data, provide best evidence for practice, support efficient care delivery, and promote electronic access by authorized users for quality care, research, and policy development.[3] To make EHRs optimally beneficial, however, data standardization and data exchange are needed as fundamental components in that they facilitate clear, concise communication as well as the collection and aggregation of healthcare data across settings.

The Centers for Medicare & Medicaid Services (CMS) established an incentive program for the use of a certified EHR system to meet the standards and criteria of Meaningful Use.[4,5] EHRs should, for example, support eprescribing, maintaining patient problems and medication lists, and care management and demonstrate interoperability according to the Health Information Technology for Economic and Clinical Health (HITECH) Act.[5] Standards that facilitate data capture and data sharing play a key role toward fulfilling Meaningful Use of healthcare data. This chapter first examines current healthcare data standardization and exchange efforts. Applications of standardized health terminologies are further discussed along with future directions. Additional information concerning Meaningful Use and HITECH Act regulations is available in Chapters 24 and 25.

HEALTHCARE DATA STANDARDIZATION

Definitions

Patient records contain words, terms, and concepts that are used in a variety of ways. A *word* is a unit of language while a *term* is a linguistic label used to represent a particular concept.[6] A *concept* is defined as a construct representing the unique meaning for one or multiple terms. For example, *sudden pain in lower back* is composed of five words and the term *sudden pain* is identical to the term *acute onset pain* consisting of three words. In this case, both terms can be denoted with the concept *acute pain*. Also, the concept *pressure ulcer* can be represented with diverse terms such as *bedsore, decubitus, pressure sore, decubitus ulcer, pressure ulcer,* etc. These examples indicate that various expressions (including abbreviations) used with identical meanings can be characterized using a representative concept in patient records.

When a list of words or phrases is organized alphabetically, such a collection is called a *vocabulary*.[7] In contrast, a collection of representative concepts in a specified domain of interest is defined as a *terminology*, which is often organized in a hierarchical or tree structure according to semantic relationships among concepts. In other words, the concept *acute pain* is a type of *pain* and presents a narrower meaning than the parent concept *pain* in a terminology.

Identifying a representative concept for terms with the same meaning is particularly important when communicating healthcare data. Natural language, with its diverse expressions of terms with equivalent meanings, cannot be used to share information within or across systems in a consistent way. Incongruent descriptions of patient care contribute to poor quality care as well as hinder the Meaningful Use of EHRs. Accordingly, a number of healthcare terminologies have been developed by different disciplines and specialties. When a terminology meets specific requirements established by standards development organizations, it is referred to as standardized terminology. A reference terminology serves as a resource to represent domain knowledge of interest and thus facilitate data collection, processing, and aggregation. Such a terminology, however, may not be sufficient to design and structure documentation forms that are used by healthcare providers in daily practice.[8] Task-oriented terms with abundant synonyms can assist documentation practice of healthcare providers by enhancing expressivity and usability of standard concepts. An interface terminology is a collection of task-oriented terms considered to support data entry and display in EHRs.[8]

A terminology is often called a classification when concepts or expressions are organized according to their conceptual similarities rather than semantic (meaning) resemblances. For example, a set of concepts related to the human body could be arranged by physiologic function or body structure. In other words, *chest pain* and *growing pain* are semantically close in that both are considered a type of *pain*. In this sense, both terms can be categorized as a finding of the sensory nervous system. They, however, also could be classified by the location of pain (i.e., body structure); *chest pain* can be categorized as a finding of trunk structure and *growing pain* can be categorized as a finding of limb structure.

A concept refers to a class in ontology where the meaning of a concept is formally specified using properties and its relationships with other concepts through inheritance.[9] While a terminology often presents only a broad–narrow relationship between two adjacent concepts, an ontology contains multiple subsumptions or subclass relationships of a concept based on its formal definition. A reasoner or classification software can be used to assist in this process by automatically determining logical placements of asserted concepts and creating an inferred hierarchy.[10] An example of how ontology is structured is demonstrated by the BioPortal sponsored by the National Center for Biomedical Ontology, which houses 330 terminologies, classifications, and ontologies maintained by various organizations and individuals.[11] Figure 22-1 presents a hierarchical organization of sample concepts (or classes) related to human anatomy and a graphic view of the hierarchy in BioPortal.[11]

Foundational Model of Anatomy

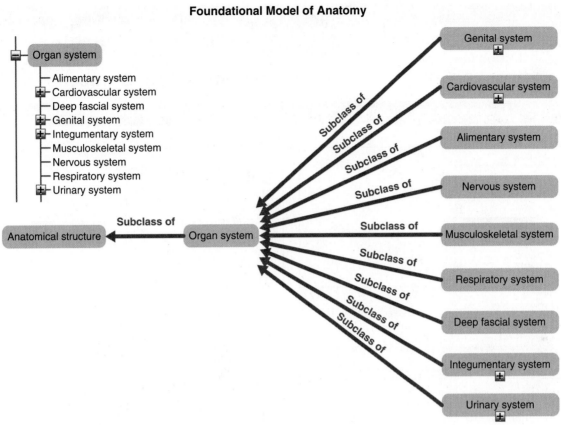

FIG 22-1 An example ontology. (From the Foundational Model of Anatomy in BioPortal. available at http://bioportal.bioontology.org/ontologies/44507?p=terms.)

Evaluation of the Quality of Terminology

Healthcare terminologies have a long history of research and development. Currently, the Unified Medical Language System (UMLS), the largest metathesaurus, contains more than 160 terminologies, classifications, and ontologies used in the healthcare domain.[12] Regardless of the structure of a source terminology, the UMLS consolidates all source concepts in a unified framework so that it is possible to examine lexical and semantic relations within and across source terminologies.[13] The UMLS is distributed by the National Library of Medicine (NLM) every 6 months and includes more than 2.8 million concepts and 11.2 million unique concept names, available for browsing through UMLS Terminology Services.[12] Any source concepts with semantically equivalent meanings are assigned to the same concept unique identifier in the UMLS.[13] Figure 22-2 displays a search result for the keyword "comfort alteration" in the UMLS browser.

Given the complexity of the healthcare delivery system in the twenty-first century, the health IT industry demands a comprehensive solution to promote data standardization and exchange. One terminology is unlikely to meet the needs of the wide range of disciplines within healthcare yet adopting quality terminologies is crucial for Meaningful Use of EHRs. Assessing the quality of a terminology is not a simple task, as each terminology evolves according to its *terminology life cycle* linked to structural and development processes.[14-17]

A terminology life cycle contains three major phases: change requests, terminology editing, and terminology publication.[17] A *terminology change request* is a formal mechanism for users to submit requests for any changes or additions with respect to a given terminology.[16,18-20] *Terminology editing* begins with the activation of a new concept, revision of an existing concept, or inactivation of a concept and follows formal concept change and version management guidelines. When terminology editing is completed with subsequent documentation, a series of tasks is performed throughout the *terminology publication* phase to release a new version of terminology for public use. Any products (such as terminologies, cross-maps, translations, subsets, and educational materials) generated through the terminology life cycle should be easily accessible, usable, and interoperable in EHRs.[17]

Requirements for maintaining the quality of a healthcare terminology address the terminology structure, content, mapping, and process management in alignment with the terminology life cycle.[17] Extensive research and development conducted during the past 2 decades has led to the development of international terminology standards under the auspices of the International Organization for Standardization (ISO).[21-27] Specifically, ISO/TS 17117:2002, Health Informatics—Controlled Health Terminology—Structure and High-Level Indicators, describes technical specifications to evaluate a controlled health terminology at a high level.

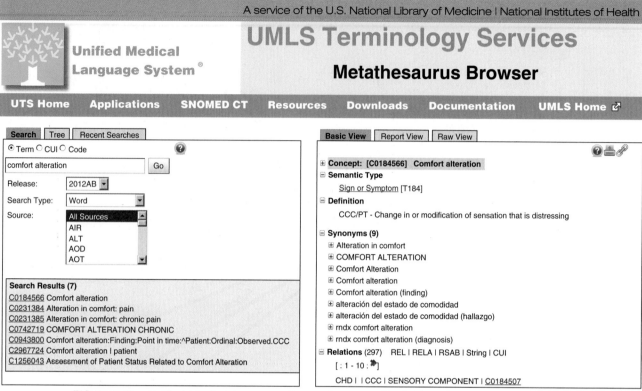

FIG 22-2 The Unified Medical Language System browser. (Available at https://uts.nlm.nih.gov/home.html.)

According to the specifications, the purpose, scope, and content coverage of a terminology should be explicitly stated for a specified domain of use. Each concept should be clearly defined with a unique identifier in a given terminology; hence there should be no redundancy, ambiguity, or vagueness.[28]

Further, ISO/TS 18104:2003, Health Informatics—Integration of a Reference Terminology Model for Nursing, describes high-level constituents and their semantic relations required to communicate nursing diagnoses and interventions across healthcare settings. This standard requires that a nursing diagnostic concept be composed of a focus concept and a judgment concept presenting potentiality, degree, acuity, or timing.[29,30] For example, the nursing diagnosis *acute pain* meets this standard, as it consists of the focus concept *pain* and the judgment concept *acute*. The ISO standard also requires that a nursing intervention be composed of at least one target concept and one action concept.[29] For example, the nursing intervention *teaching about acute pain management* comprises a nurse's *teaching* (action) on *acute pain management* (target).

Building on these standards that are required for terminology development and maintenance, the American Nurses Association (ANA), through the Committee for Nursing Practice Information Infrastructure (CNPII), has recognized 10 interface terminologies appropriate for use in nursing.[31,32] Of these, seven were designed specifically for nursing and the other three are considered multidisciplinary terminologies (Table 22-1). The ANA also recognized two minimum datasets: the Nursing Minimum Data Set (NMDS), as a

framework for collecting nursing care data, and the Nursing Management Minimum Data Set (NMMDS), as a framework for collecting nursing service data elements. That is, the NMDS requires patient demographics, nursing process data (i.e., assessments, diagnoses, interventions, and outcomes), and service elements (e.g., agency and admission and discharge dates) to assess the quality of care.[33] The NMMDS focuses on collecting 18 variables associated with nursing environment, nurse resources, and financial resources to support administrative analysis and decision making of nurse executives.[34-36]

Multidisciplinary Terminologies

Terminologies are essential to communicate and document patient care data in alignment with the care process. Various types of data are critical to clinical care, such as lab results, medications, medical diagnoses and procedures, and billing information. Accordingly, multidisciplinary terminologies as described in this section are essential.

Logical Observation Identifiers Names and Codes (LOINC)

Logical Observation Identifiers Names and Codes (LOINC), established in 1994 by the Regenstrief Institute, is a standardized coding system for laboratory and clinical test results or observations.[37] Each LOINC observation, measurement, or test is created using the following six axes:

1. Component: the name of the observation (or analyte)
2. Property (e.g., substance concentration, mass, volume)

TABLE 22-1   **AN OVERVIEW OF STANDARDIZED TERMINOLOGIES RELEVANT TO NURSING PRACTICE**

TERMINOLOGY OR CLASSIFICATION*	DEVELOPER	DISCIPLINE OR SPECIALTY	RELEASE TIME (CURRENT VERSION)	ANA RECOG-NIZED	CROSS-MAPS AVAILABLE	WEB-BASED TERMINOLOGY BROWSER† (LANGUAGE)
Clinical Care Classification (CCC)	SabaCare	Nursing	As needed (Version 2.5)	Yes	ICNP SNOMED CT	http://sabacare.com/ (English)
International Classification for Nursing Practice (ICNP)	International Council of Nurses (ICN)	Nursing	Every other May in ICN conference (2013)	Yes	CCC, ICF PNDS SNOMED CT	http://www.icn.ch/ pillarsprograms/ icnp-2011-download/ (Multilingual)
NANDA International (NANDA-I)	NANDA-I	Nursing	Every 2 years (2012–2014)	Yes	SNOMED CT	Not publicly available (member only)
Nursing Interventions Classification (NIC)	University of Iowa	Nursing	Every 4 years (2012; 6th ed.)	Yes	SNOMED CT	Not publicly available (member only)
Nursing Outcomes Classification (NOC)	University of Iowa	Nursing	Every 4 years (2012; 5th ed.)	Yes	SNOMED CT	Not publicly available (member only)
Omaha System (OS)	Martin, K.S.	Nursing	As needed (2005; 2nd ed.)	Yes	SNOMED CT	www.omahasystem.org (English)
Perioperative Nursing Data Set (PNDS)	Association of Perioperative Registered Nurses (AORN)	Perioperative nursing	As needed (2011; 3rd ed.)	Yes	SNOMED CT	Not publicly available (member only)
Logical Observation Identifiers Names and Codes (LOINC)	Regenstrief Institute, Inc.	Multidiscipline	Biannual (Version 2.42)	Yes	CPT HL7	http://loinc.org/ downloads/relma (Multilingual; note that it can be browsed after installing RELMA)
Systematized Nomenclature of Medicine— Clinical Terms (SNOMED CT)	International Health Terminology Standards Development Organisation (IHTSDO)	Multidiscipline	Biannual (Jan 2013)	Yes	ICD-10 ICD-9-CM Nursing terminologies	www.cliniclue.com/ (Multilingual; note that it can be browsed after installing CliniClue)
ABC Codes	ABC Coding Solutions	Multidiscipline	Annual (2012)	Yes	–	Not publicly available (member only)
Current Procedural Terminology (CPT)	American Medical Association (AMA)	Medicine	Annual (2013)	–	LOINC	Not publicly available (member only)

Continued

TABLE 22-1	AN OVERVIEW OF STANDARDIZED TERMINOLOGIES RELEVANT TO NURSING PRACTICE—cont'd					
TERMINOLOGY OR CLASSIFICATION*	DEVELOPER	DISCIPLINE OR SPECIALTY	RELEASE TIME (CURRENT VERSION)	ANA RECOG- NIZED	CROSS-MAPS AVAILABLE	WEB-BASED TERMINOLOGY BROWSER† (LANGUAGE)
International Classification of Diseases (ICD)	World Health Organization (WHO)	Medicine	As needed (10th ed.)	–	SNOMED CT	http://apps.who.int/ classifications/icd10/ browse/2010/en (English)
International Classification of Functioning, Disability and Health (ICF)	WHO	Multidiscipline	As needed (2008)	–	–	http://apps.who.int/ classifications/ icfbrowser/ (Multilingual)
RxNorm	National Library of Medicine (NLM)	Multidiscipline (drug)	Monthly (Jan 2013)	–	–	http://rxnav.nlm.nih.gov/ (English)

HL7, Health Level Seven; *RELMA*, Regenstrief LOINC Mapping Assistant.

*All terminologies and classifications are accessible through the Unified Medical Language System (UMLS) released every 6 months by the National Library of Medicine (NLM). Available at https://uts.nlm.nih.gov/home.html.

†All of the web browsers listed are publicly available at no cost. Also, personal digital assistant (PDA) versions of terminology browsers may be available as knowledge resources.

3. Timing of the measurement
4. System: the type of system or sample (e.g., serum, urine, patient, family)
5. Scale (e.g., qualitative, quantitative)
6. The method used to make the observation (optional)[38]

All LOINC names are case sensitive. Table 22-2 presents an example of blood glucose tests coded using the LOINC system. Actual values of observations and test results need to be documented using numeric values or other standardized terms.

LOINC contains 71,464 terms (as of 2013) and has been widely adopted for ordering and exchanging laboratory and clinical observations in the communication protocol called Health Level Seven International (HL7).[38] The laboratory portion of the LOINC database contains the usual laboratory categories such as chemistry, hematology, and microbiology. The domain and scope of clinical LOINC is extremely broad. Some of the sections include terms for vital signs, obstetric measurements, clinical assessment scales, outcomes from standardized nursing terminologies, and research instruments.[39] LOINC is also used for document and section names.[40] Nursing content is one of the scientific domains with a special focus on clinical LOINC.[41] Because of LOINC's early focus on laboratory testing, the breadth of nursing terms and nursing observations is not yet well represented.

Systematized Nomenclature of Medicine—Clinical Terms (SNOMED CT)

Systematized Nomenclature of Medicine—Clinical Terms (SNOMED CT) is the most comprehensive clinical terminology developed using description logics.[42] Originally developed as the Systematized Nomenclature of Pathology (SNOP) by the U.S. College of American Pathologists (CAP), SNOMED CT evolved upon the incorporation of additional content from the U.K. Clinical Terms Version 3 (CTV3).[43] SNOMED CT was acquired by the International Health Terminology Standards Development Organisation (IHTSDO) in 2007 and became an international standard for coding healthcare data.[43]

The IHTSDO has developed a set of principles to guide SNOMED CT development and quality improvement. SNOMED CT is continually updated to meet users' needs and is released every 6 months. Since the governments of member countries fund IHTSDO, healthcare institutions in IHTSDO member countries are able to use SNOMED CT without additional costs. For example, there are no fees for use in the U.S., whose national release center is responsible for managing concept requests and distributing and supporting IHTSDO products. The NLM, which also maintains and distributes the UMLS, is the U.S. member of the IHTSDO.

Each release of SNOMED CT includes core terminology (concept names and codes, descriptions, and relationships among the concepts) together with products to support the implementation of the terminology.[44] Each SNOMED CT concept code consists of six to nine numeric characters. Concept descriptions include a fully specified name, a preferred term, and synonyms if any (Fig. 22-3). SNOMED CT concepts are organized in a hierarchical tree structure in which parent–child relationships exist. Concepts lower in the hierarchy are more specific in meaning than those higher in the hierarchy, creating multiple levels of granularity. Defining attribute relationships further details the meaning of a

TABLE 22-2 CODING STRUCTURE AND APPLICATION OF LOINC

	DESCRIPTION
Code	Length: 3 to 7 characters The last digit (ranging from 0 to 9) of the LOINC code preceded by a hyphen is required to avoid errors in transcription of the code.
Fully specified name	<component/analyte>:<kind of property>:<time aspect>:<system/sample type>:<scale>:<method>
Example coding of laboratory tests	2339-0:Glucose:MCnc:Pt:Bld:Qn This example includes a LOINC code and four attributes: 1. Code = 2339-0 2. Name of component = Glucose 3. Property = Mass concentration (MCnc*) 4. Type of system/sample = Patient's blood (Pt:Bld*) 5. Measurement scale = Quantitative (Qn*)	2341-6:Glucose:MCnc:Pt:Bld:Qn:Test strip manual This example includes a LOINC code and five attributes: 1. Code = 2341-6 2. Name of component = Glucose 3. Property = Mass concentration (MCnc*) 4. Type of system/sample = Patient's blood (Pt:Bld*) 5. Measurement scale = Quantitative (Qn*) 6. Method = Test strip manual

LOINC, Logical Observation Identifiers Names and Codes.

*Details on the abbreviations can be found in McDonald C, Huff S, Mercer K, Hernandez J, Vreeman DJ, eds. *Logical Observation Identifiers Names and Codes (LOINC) Users' Guide*. Indianapolis, IN: Regenstrief Institute, Inc.; 2012. http://loinc.org/downloads/files/LOINCManual.pdf.

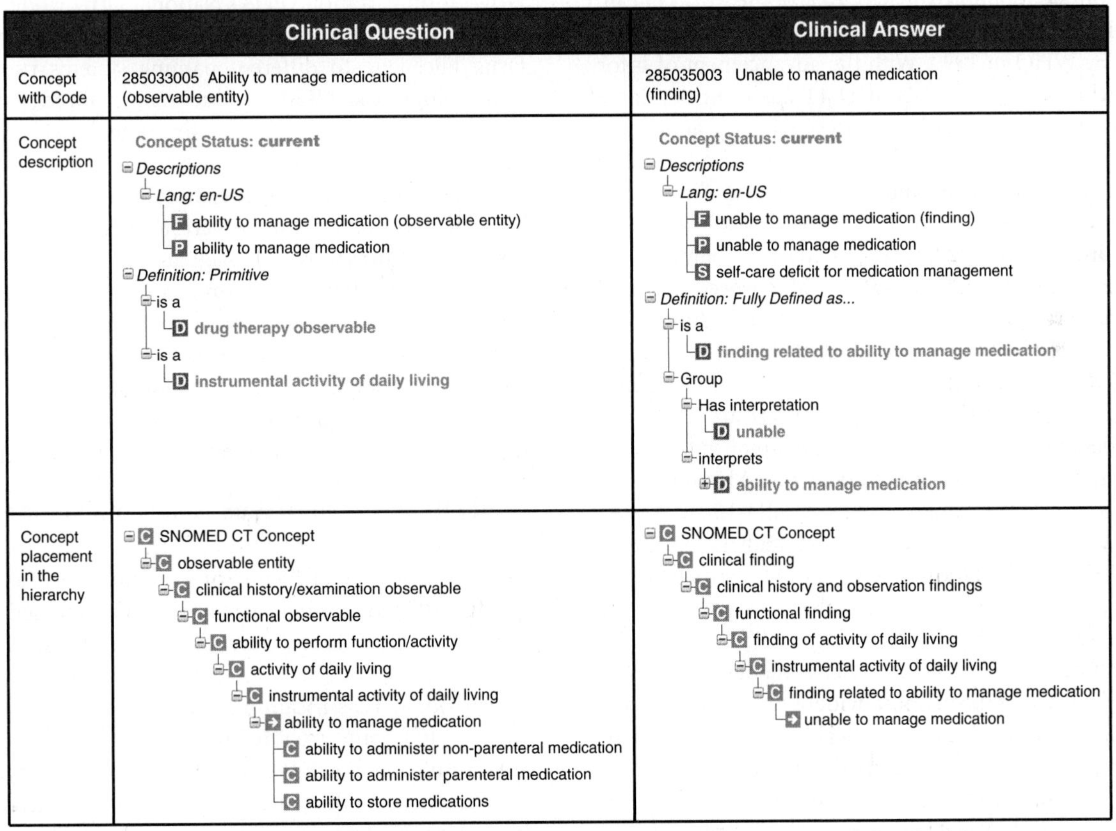

FIG 22-3 The structure and application of SNOMED CT. (Retrieved from the CliniClue browser. Available at http://www.cliniclue.com/.)

concept by relating all necessary and sufficient conditions. Figure 22-3 presents descriptions of example concepts and their placement in the SNOMED CT hierarchy.

SNOMED CT contains more than 300,000 preferred terms and 150,000 synonyms (including Spanish translations of preferred terms) organized under 19 top-level concepts such as body structure, clinical finding (e.g., diseases, disorders, drug actions), event, observable entity, procedure (e.g., treatment or therapy, surgical procedure, laboratory procedure), specimen, and substance.[44] In general, clinical questions for assessment and measureable outcomes (e.g., pain level) can be coded using concepts placed under *observable entity*. Most nursing diagnoses and outcomes can be found under *clinical finding* and *event* while nursing interventions and actions are found under *procedure*. An example code set of clinical question (*ability to manage medication*) and answer (*unable to manage medication*) is presented in Figure 22-3. Clinical observations and laboratory tests can be considered questions and coded using the LOINC system while findings (i.e., answers) of observations and tests can be coded using SNOMED CT.[37] Then, a set of questions and answers coded using standardized terminologies is ready for data exchange using messaging standards.

Classifications Used for Reimbursement

Since the release of its first edition in 1893, the International Classification of Diseases (ICD) has been used to report mortality and morbidity data worldwide and to compare statistics across settings, regions, or countries over time.[45] Further, ICD, copyrighted by the World Health Organization (WHO), is used for billing, reimbursement, and allocation of health service resources for approximately 70% of the world's health expenditures.[45] The current version is ICD-10 (10th edition), endorsed by WHO in 1990. With the advancement of information technology and EHRs, ICD-11 has been developed and currently is in a revision process with an anticipated release in 2015. ICD-11 provides more detailed information (such as definitions, signs, and symptoms) on disease in a structured way.

ICD Clinical Modification (ICD-CM) is a coding system developed to encode medical diagnoses and procedures (such as surgical, diagnostic, and therapeutic procedures) performed in U.S. hospital settings.[46] ICD-9-CM, a modified version of ICD-9, is updated annually by the National Center for Health Statistics (NCHS) and CMS. There are a few laboratory codes in ICD-9-CM for use in hospital billing only. The transition from ICD-9-CM to ICD-10-CM is under way in the U.S. given the enhancement of ICD-10 in content coverage and specificity for ambulatory and managed care service. The implementation of ICD-10-CM is anticipated by October 1, 2014.[47]

The Current Procedural Terminology (CPT) classification system, first developed by the American Medical Association (AMA) in 1966, has been most widely used for ordering, billing, and reimbursement of medical procedures and diagnostic services.[48] CPT has been used extensively in the U.S. since CMS mandated its use for reporting outpatient hospital surgical procedures in 1987 as part of the Omnibus Budget Reconciliation Act.[48] Each CPT item consists of a five-digit code and descriptor.

Diagnosis Related Groups (DRG) is a patient classification scheme designed to cluster similar cases using ICD and CPT codes as well as patient characteristics for reimbursement purposes according to the inpatient prospective payment system (IPPS).[49]

Other healthcare providers may use a different coding system for ordering, billing, and reimbursement for care delivered. For example, the *Diagnostic and Statistical Manual of Mental Disorders*, Fourth Edition (DSM-IV), developed by the American Psychiatric Association, has been widely used by clinicians to code mental and behavioral health–related conditions. All DSM-IV diagnostic codes have been integrated into ICD-9-CM but there are some differences between the two coding systems because of the annual change occurring in ICD-9-CM.[50] Another example is the ABC Coding Solutions, which provides more than 4500 codes for integrative healthcare services and products.[51] In other words, the ABC coding system covers clinical services related to nursing, behavioral health, alternative medicine, ethnic and minority care, midwifery, and spiritual care. An ABC code consists of five characters representing types of services, remedies, supplies, and practitioners.[51]

RxNorm

RxNorm is a normalized drug-naming system derived from 11 drug terminologies containing drug names, ingredient, strength, and dose form.[52] Example source terminologies within RxNorm include Micromedex RED BOOK, Food and Drug Administration (FDA) National Drug Code Directory, SNOMED CT, and Veterans Health Administration National Drug File. Due to different naming systems used in each terminology, the NLM produces normalized generic and brand names of prescription drugs and over-the-counter drugs available in the U.S.[52] The NLM uses the UMLS framework to maintain and distribute RxNorm, allowing consistent communication among various hospital and pharmacy systems. RxNorm preserves original drug names as synonyms and semantic relationships among drugs. It also serves as a knowledge resource to advance eprescribing systems with decision support functionality, as RxNorm contains pharmacologic knowledge such as drug interactions.[53] RxNorm is released every month by the NLM but is also accessible through the UMLS released every 6 months.

World Health Organization Family of International Classifications (WHO-FIC)

The WHO formed a Family of International Classifications (WHO-FIC) containing a suite of WHO-endorsed classifications, including three reference classifications, five derived classifications, and five related classifications.[54] ICD and International Classification of Functioning, Disability and Health (ICF) are core reference classification systems in WHO-FIC.[54] While the ICD system provides a set of diagnosis codes to encode causes of death and health conditions, ICF (formerly known as the International Classification of Impairments, Disabilities, and Handicaps) is a classification system that focuses on functional status as a consequence of disease or health conditions.[55] Although ICF has been used mainly in physical therapy and rehabilitation professions, previous studies demonstrated the usefulness of ICF in documenting nursing practice in acute care hospitals and early postacute rehabilitation settings.[56-59] Knowing that these core classifications lack in covering other specialty areas, the WHO recognizes an additional 10 classifications or terminologies in

WHO-FIC.[60] For example, ICD-10 Classification of Mental and Behavioral Disorders and ICF Version for Children and Youth are derived from the core classification systems (i.e., ICD and ICF). International Classification of Primary Care and International Classification for Nursing Practice (ICNP) are considered related classifications in WHO-FIC.

Nursing Terminologies

As shown in Table 22-1, the ANA recognized seven nursing terminologies or classifications supporting nursing practice as they conform to the terminology development standards.[61] All of the ANA-approved nursing terminologies have been integrated into the UMLS and widely adopted nationally and internationally. This section briefly introduces the nursing terminologies and describes their purpose, scope, content coverage, and structure.

Clinical Care Classification (CCC)

Clinical Care Classification (CCC) has been used for more than 20 years in nursing across the care continuum since its development as the Home Health Care Classification System in 1991.[62] CCC is a classification system of nursing diagnoses and interventions organized under 21 care components to support documentation of the nursing process.[63] In this classification a nursing care component is a navigation or high-level abstract concept clustering the nursing practice with similar patterns. These care components are further aggregated into four healthcare patterns of patient care: Functional, Health Behavioral, Physiological, and Psychological.

CCC Version 2.5 includes 176 nursing diagnoses (60 major categories and 116 subcategories) from which 528 nursing outcomes can be derived using three modifiers: (1) improve(d), (2) stabilize(d), and (3) deteriorate(d).[64] As such, 201 nursing interventions (77 major categories and 124 subcategories) can be expanded to as many as 804 nursing actions by combining four action types: (1) monitor/assess/evaluate/

observe, (2) perform/direct care/provide/assist, (3) teach/educate/instruct/supervise, and (4) manage/refer/contact/notify. This compositional ability of CCC allows users to express nursing care in any care setting while maintaining a simple classification structure (Table 22-3). Each nursing diagnosis, intervention, and outcome is assigned to a code with four or five alphanumeric characters.

International Classification for Nursing Practice (ICNP)

International Classification for Nursing Practice (ICNP) is a nursing terminology designed to represent nursing diagnoses and outcomes and interventions capturing the delivery of nursing care across settings.[19] The ICNP is an entity of the International Council of Nurses (ICN) eHealth Programme that was launched to transform nursing through information and communication technology.[65] The ICN is a federation of more than 130 national nurses associations that represent millions of nurses worldwide. Since 1989 the ICNP has evolved from a collection of nursing-related concepts to a logic-based nursing terminology system maintained in an ontology development environment.[19]

Since 2005 the ICNP has been developed using a sophisticated language (i.e., Web Ontology Language, or OWL) to ensure the sustainability of the ever-expanding terminology and maintain the quality of the terminology.[66] In conformance with the ISO standards (ISO/TS 18104:2003), nursing diagnosis, outcome, and intervention statements are precoordinated with primitive concepts such as focus, judgment, and action concepts.[66] Each precoordinated concept is assigned a unique identifier and it is possible for practitioners to postcoordinate primitive concepts to meet their needs. For example, as shown in Box 22-1, the nursing diagnosis *acute pain* is a precoordinated concept with an assigned code (10000454) but *acute abdomen pain* does not exist in ICNP, meaning that the concept could be postcoordinated with two

TABLE 22-3	STRUCTURE AND APPLICATION OF CCC IN RELATION TO THE NURSING PROCESS FOR PRESSURE ULCER	
NURSING PROCESS	**CCC STRUCTURE**	**EXAMPLE CONCEPTS**
Assessment	Healthcare pattern	Physiologic
	Care component	R. Skin Integrity
Diagnosis	Nursing diagnosis	
	• major category	R.46.0 Skin Integrity Alteration
	• subcategory	R.46.2 Skin Integrity Impairment
Outcome	Expected outcome	R.46.2.1 Skin Integrity Impairment Improved
Planning	Nursing intervention	
	• major category	R.51.0 Pressure Ulcer Care
	• subcategory	R.51.1 Pressure Ulcer Stage 1 Care
Implementation	Nursing action type	R.51.1.2 Perform/Direct Care/Provide/Assist Pressure Ulcer Stage 1 Care
Evaluation	Actual outcome	R.46.2.1 Skin Integrity Impairment Improved

CCC, Clinical Care Classification.

BOX 22-1   STRUCTURE AND APPLICATION OF ICNP

ICNP STRUCTURE: ASSERTED HIERARCHY	EXAMPLE CONCEPTS

• Process
  • Body process
    • Nervous system process
      • Perception
        • Impaired perception
          • Pain
            • **Acute pain***
            • Chronic pain
            • Labor pain
            • Musculoskeletal pain
	1. The concept *Acute pain* is a precoordinated nursing diagnosis composed of the primitive concepts *pain*, *acute*, and *actual*.
	10000454 Acute pain
	= has focus "10013950 pain" +
	  has onset "10001739 acute" +
	  has potentiality "10000420 actual"
	2. The concept *Acute abdominal pain* can be postcoordinated if needed by selecting the nursing diagnosis *Acute pain* and the body location *Abdomen*.
	Acute abdominal pain
	= 10000454 Acute pain +
	  10000023 Abdomen

ICNP, International Classification for Nursing Practice.
*This example shows the placement of the nursing diagnosis *Acute pain* in the ICNP asserted hierarchy.

---

concepts: *acute pain* (10000454) in *abdomen* (10000023). All ICNP primitive and precoordinated concepts are organized in a hierarchical tree structure.

A new version of ICNP is released every 2 years in conjunction with the ICN conference. The number of concepts included in each version has increased from 1994 in Version 1 to 3894 in the 2013 release. Version 2013 contains 2302 primitive concepts, 783 nursing diagnoses and outcomes, and 809 interventions. Due to the size and complexity of ICNP, subsets are created to promote the utility of ICNP in practice.[67] That is, ICNP Catalogues or subsets with select nursing diagnoses and interventions have been developed and distributed in collaboration with national nurses associations, health ministries and governments, and expert nurses worldwide. Example catalogs include Promoting Adherence to Treatment,[68] Palliative Care,[69] Nursing Outcome Indicators,[70] Community Nursing,[71] and Pediatric Acute Pain Management.

NANDA International (NANDA-I) Nursing Diagnoses

The North American Nursing Diagnosis Association (NANDA) dates back to 1970 and its terminology was the first to be recognized by the ANA.[72] The membership organization was renamed to NANDA-I in 2002 to reflect worldwide use of the terminology and has established network teams in Latin America, Europe, Asia, and Africa.[73] In NANDA-I a nursing diagnosis is defined as "a clinical judgment about actual or potential individual, family, or community experiences/responses to health problems/life processes."[73(p134)] The purpose of NANDA-I is to ensure consistent, accurate documentation of nurses by clinical reasoning judgments based on definitions, defining characteristics, and related or risk factors. Nurses' clinical judgments would drive nursing interventions and outcome evaluations.

The first taxonomic structure of NANDA was an alphabetical listing of nursing diagnoses with the evidence to support knowledge-based diagnostic decisions. As the terminology continued to grow in size, the Diagnoses Development Committee and Taxonomy Committee developed a new three-level structure to place diagnoses according to conceptual similarities.[73] As shown in Table 22-4, a nursing diagnosis (Level 3) is located in a class (Level 2) according to its definition, defining characteristics and related factors, or risk factors. A class is further clustered into a domain (Level 1). The NANDA-I 2012–2014 release includes 206 nursing diagnoses organized in 47 classes and 13 domains. Each diagnosis has a five-digit code constructed with values from seven axes conforming to the ISO standards (ISO/TS 18104:2003).

Nursing Interventions Classification (NIC)

Nursing Interventions Classification (NIC) is a funded research-based standardized classification of interventions describing nursing activities performed directly or indirectly. An intervention is defined as "any treatment, based upon clinical judgment and knowledge that a nurse performs to enhance patient/client outcomes."[74(p3)] This means that choosing a nursing intervention is based on the characteristics of nursing diagnosis and expected patient outcomes. The NIC was first published in 1992 and interventions have been designed to support the communication and documentation of nurses and other healthcare providers with the exception of physicians.[74]

The most current release (2008) includes 542 interventions clustered into 30 classes and 7 domains. Each intervention is assigned a unique four-digit code and may appear in more than one class. An intervention concept includes a definition and a list of detailed activities associated with the intervention, ranging from 10 to 30 activities. As a result, more than 12,000 narrative activity statements without a unique code exist.[74]

Nursing Outcomes Classification (NOC)

Nursing Outcomes Classification (NOC) is also a funded research-based standardized classification of patient and caregiver outcomes that can be used in the course of care delivery for any specialty and setting. An outcome is "a measurable individual, family, or community state, behavior or perception that is measured along a continuum and is responsive to

TABLE 22-4	STRUCTURE AND APPLICATION OF NANDA-I WITH KNOWLEDGE CONTENT TO REFERENCE
NANDA-I STRUCTURE	**EXAMPLE NURSING DIAGNOSIS**
Domain (Level 1)	11. Safety/Protection
Class (Level 2)	2. Physical Injury
Nursing Diagnosis Label (Level 3):	00045. Impaired Oral Mucous Membrane
Axis 1: Diagnostic concept (i.e., root of the diagnostic statement)	Axis 1: Mucous membrane
Axis 2: Subject of the diagnosis	Axis 2: Individual
Axis 3: Judgment (i.e., modifier specifying the meaning)	Axis 3: Impaired
Axis 4: Location (i.e., body parts or their functions)	Axis 4: Oral
Axis 5: Age	Axis 5: Adult
Axis 6: Time (i.e., duration)	Axis 6: Acute
Axis 7: Status of the diagnosis (i.e., potentiality, wellness/health promotion)	Axis 7: Actual
Definition	Disruption of the lips and/or soft tissue of the oral cavity
Defining characteristics	bleeding, coated tongue, fissures, gingival pallor, halitosis, oral lesions, white patches, etc.

NANDA-I, North American Nursing Diagnosis Association International.

nursing interventions."[75(p35)] Since 1997 the NOC has been expanded continuously. The most current release (2012) includes 490 outcomes clustered into 32 classes and 7 domains. Each outcome concept consists of a definition, a list of indicators, and five-point Likert-type scales. The scales, ranging from 1 to 5, are used to measure the existing level, patients' preferred level, and subsequent evaluation longitudinally to determine change scores in patients. A four-digit identifier is used to code each outcome while a six-digit identifier codes the descriptive indicator associated with the outcome.

The initial development of NIC and NOC was accomplished through initially NIH research and now the Center for Nursing Classification and Clinical Effectiveness (CNC) at the University of Iowa, College of Nursing.[74,75] The CNC also has ongoing collaboration and an alliance with NANDA-I to establish linkages among the three nursing classification

systems. Since the first publication of the linkages in 2006, research efforts were made to link NANDA-I, NIC, and NOC. A team of researchers continue to update the relationships and linkages for use in EHRs.[75] An example linkage of the three classifications is presented in Table 22-5.

Omaha System (OS)

Omaha System (OS) is a standardized classification designed to document nursing practice across the continuum of care. The work on OS began in the 1970s and was further expanded with the release of Version 2 in 2005.[76] The OS supports documenting and communicating the nursing process through the following three schemes:
1. Problem classification scheme (i.e., assessment)
2. Intervention scheme (i.e., care plans and services)
3. Problem measurement with a rating scale (i.e., evaluation)

TABLE 22-5	STRUCTURE AND LINKAGE OF NANDA-I, NIC, AND NOC		
STRUCTURE	**EXAMPLE NURSING DIAGNOSIS**	**EXAMPLE NURSING INTERVENTION**	**EXAMPLE NURSING OUTCOME**
Domain (Level 1)	11. Safety/Protection	1. Physiological: Basic care that supports physical functioning	II. Physiologic Health
Class (Level 2)	2. Physical Injury	F. Self-Care Facilitation	L. Tissue Integrity
Label (Level 3)	00045. Impaired Oral Mucous Membrane	1710. Oral Health Maintenance	1100. Oral Hygiene
NANDA-I description, NIC activity, or NOC indicator	Defining characteristics: bleeding, coated tongue, fissures, gingival pallor, halitosis, oral lesions, white patches	• Establish a mouth care routine. • Apply lubricant to moisten lips and oral mucosa as needed.	110011. Color of mucous membranes 110012. Oral mucosa integrity

NANDA-I, North American Nursing Diagnosis Association International; *NIC,* Nursing Interventions Classification; *NOC,* Nursing Outcomes Classification.

The problem classification scheme consists of four components: domains, problem statements, modifiers, and signs and symptoms (Table 22-6). Forty-two problem statements are neutral until two modifiers are attached to the problems. One set of modifiers is related to potentiality (i.e., actual and potential) and health promotion; the other set of modifiers is related to health problems (i.e., individual, family, and community). A problem is considered actual if related signs and symptoms associated with the problem have been selected from a predefined list. All problems are grouped into one of four domains: environmental, psychosocial, physiological, or health-related behaviors.

In the OS a nursing intervention is composed with a target intervention and an action type in accordance with ISO/TS 18104:2003.[76] Currently there are 75 target interventions and 4 action categories: (1) teaching/guidance/counseling, (2) treatments/procedures, (3) case management, and (4) surveillance. Patient problems are evaluated throughout the course of care using a Likert-style measurement scale ranging from 1 to 5 in the areas of client knowledge, behavior, and status. The OS is described in additional detail in Chapter 9.

Perioperative Nursing Data Set (PNDS)

Perioperative Nursing Data Set (PNDS) is a standardized classification system designed specifically to support the perioperative nursing process in documenting patient experience from preadmission to discharge.[77] The PNDS (2011) is composed of 74 nursing diagnoses, 153 nursing interventions, and 38 nurse-sensitive patient outcomes. The PNDS nursing diagnoses are adopted from NANDA-I. All nursing interventions consist of three different types of actions: assessment, implementation, and evaluation. These statements are clustered into one of four domains: safety, physiologic responses, behavioral responses (of family and individual), and health system (which is not directly related to nursing process).[77,78]

The classification system was constructed based on a conceptual framework called the Perioperative Patient Focused Model in which patients and their families are the focus for nursing practice.[77] The PNDS provides a systematic approach for identifying the contributions of perioperative nursing care by reporting and benchmarking. Table 22-7 shows example statements extracted from the PNDS in relation to the nursing process.

TABLE 22-6 STRUCTURE AND APPLICATION OF OMAHA SYSTEM

STRUCTURE	PROBLEM	INTERVENTION	OUTCOME
	EXAMPLE LINKAGE		
Level 1	Domain: 02 Physiological		Knowledge (1~5): • did not recognize worsening condition
Level 2	Problem: 29 Circulation	07 Cardiac care	
Level 3	Modifiers: • Actual • Individual	Category: 01 Teaching, guidance, and counseling	Behavior (1~5): • not taking daily weights and elevating legs
Level 4	Signs & Symptoms: • Edema • Abnormal cardiac laboratory results	Specific actions: • Relief of edema • Elevate legs • Schedule fluid intake	Status (1~5): • significant fatigue, edema in lower extremities, and dyspnea

TABLE 22-7 STRUCTURE AND APPLICATION OF PNDS IN RELATION TO THE NURSING PROCESS

NURSING PROCESS	EXAMPLE STATEMENTS	
Assessment	Domain: A.350	Safety Assesses susceptibility for infection
Diagnosis	00004	Risk for Infection (from NANDA-I)
Implementation	Im.300 Im.300.1 Im.360	Implements aseptic technique Protects from cross-contamination Monitors for signs and symptoms of infection
Evaluation	E.330	Evaluates for signs and symptoms of infection through 30 days following the perioperative procedure
Outcome	O.280	Patient is free from signs and symptoms of infection

NANDA-I, North American Nursing Diagnosis Association International; *PNDS,* Perioperative Nursing Data Set.

DATA EXCHANGE EFFORTS

Health terminologies keep evolving to incorporate changes in clinical practice and health policy and advances in science. It is unlikely that in the future any one standard language will be able to support all clinical practices within the different disciplines functioning within the healthcare system. A key concern is how to communicate and exchange data collected through the various clinical practices across settings while preserving terminology-related standards. HL7 standards have been established to regulate data exchange and integration using standardized terminologies and other terminology harmonization efforts.

HL7 Standards

Since 1987, HL7 has served as a standards-developing organization to promote data retrieval, exchange, and integration across different health information systems.[79] HL7 provides a comprehensive framework and the standards necessary to foster interoperability (or exchange) of healthcare data. Of the various standards developed, document markup standards and messaging standards are most commonly used in clinical practice. Document markup standards specify the structure of clinical documents and semantic relations among the subcomponents of clinical documents. For instance, HL7 created a document markup standard, Clinical Document Architecture (CDA), that is used to exchange documents such as patient assessments, discharge summaries, imaging reports, and quality reports.[80] The HL7 Continuity of Care Document (CCD) is an implementation guide for sharing patient summary data (e.g., advanced directive, diagnostic test results, problem list, medications, allergies, immunizations, vital signs, and plan of care) between healthcare providers using CDA.[81]

While the HL7 CDA specifies structural components, HL7 messaging standards address rules to communicate detailed information about patient care. Regardless of coding rules employed in individual departments or organizations, messaging specifications prevent any misclassification of data communicated between senders and receivers of clinical data.[79] The messaging standards thus ensure consistent descriptions of patient care among disparate systems. Standardized terminologies reviewed earlier in this chapter are the basic elements of the messaging standards.

Terminology Harmonization

Interoperability is defined as "the ability of health information systems to work together within and across organizational boundaries in order to advance the effective delivery of health care for individuals and communities."[82(p2)] The U.S. Department of Health & Human Services (HHS) recommends the implementation of a health IT infrastructure to enhance interoperability of healthcare data.[83] The Healthcare Information Technology Standards Panel (HITSP), founded in 2005 through a contract with the HHS, has contributed to enabling interoperability among EHRs through the development of technical specifications.[84]

Harmonization between standardized terminologies is an effort to complement each other to enhance the coverage of domain knowledge of interest. Terminology harmonization is regarded as one way to support interoperability considering variations in terminology adoption in practice. Cross-mapping healthcare terminologies is essential to preserve the meaning of exchanged information and facilitate integration of clinical data in a disparate information system so that the comprehensive picture of healthcare delivery can be understood.

As described above, numerous health and nursing terminologies exist, resulting in various harmonization activities within and across disciplines. The scope of these harmonization activities ranges from a simple survey designed to understand the characteristics of terminologies adopted in clinical practice to harmonization agreements between two standards organizations. Harmonization of the multidisciplinary terminologies includes maps of SNOMED CT and ICD-10, SNOMED CT and ICD-9-CM, and LOINC and HL7 vocabulary. These cross-maps are publicly available through the NLM. A draft cross-map of LOINC Version 2.15 and CPT Version 2005 is also available in the UMLS.[85]

Since LOINC and SNOMED CT are widely adopted and considered data standards nationally and internationally, nursing has participated actively in harmonization efforts through cross-mapping and integration of nursing terminologies into SNOMED CT and LOINC. All ANA-recognized nursing terminologies with the exception of ICNP have been mapped to SNOMED CT.[73,86,87] This means that nursing diagnoses, interventions, and outcomes have been modeled in SNOMED CT and assigned to a unique identifier according to the SNOMED CT development guidelines. The resulting products are available for purchase currently through CAP.[87] Terminology cross-mapping of ICNP to SNOMED CT is under way after the harmonization agreement between ICN and IHTSDO in 2009.[88] A cross-map table between ICNP and SNOMED CT is distributed through UMLS as interterminology maps are completed by the terminology developers. Table 22-8 presents examples of nursing concepts integrated into SNOMED CT.

ICNP has been mapped to CCC, ICF, and other local terminologies to enhance data capture and sharing and to develop national nursing datasets.[89-93] Harmonization agreements also have been established between ICN and SabaCare and between ICN and the Association of Perioperative Registered Nurses (AORN). The ICNP 2013 release reflects the integration of PNDS and CCC. Cross-maps between PNDS and ICNP can be acquired through AORN. ICNP and these two terminologies provide different yet complementary solutions to advance standardization of nursing process data across specialties and settings (Table 22-9). Tables 22-8 and 22-9 show a potential opportunity for collaboration in harmonizing all of the nursing terminologies and SNOMED CT.

APPLICATION OF STANDARDIZED TERMINOLOGIES

There are multiple ways of communicating and recording patient care data in EHRs. Many nursing records (e.g., physical

TABLE 22-8	**INTEGRATION OF NURSING CONCEPTS INTO SNOMED CT**	
SOURCE TERMINOLOGY	**EXAMPLE CONCEPTS IN SOURCE TERMINOLOGY**	**SNOMED CT (TYPE)**
CCC	K25.5 Infection risk	78648007 At risk for infection (finding)
	K30.0.1 Teach infection control	385820004 Teach infection control (procedure)
NANDA-I	00004 Risk for infection	78648007 At risk for infection (finding)
NIC	6540 Infection control	77248004 Infection control procedure (procedure)
NOC	1807 Knowledge: Infection control	405111006 Knowledge: Infection control (observable entity)
Omaha System	71 Infection precautions (Qualifier: Treatment/procedure)	77248004 Infection control procedure (procedure)
PNDS	A.350 Assesses susceptibility for infection	370782005 Assessment of susceptibility for infection (procedure)
	O.280 Patient is free from signs and symptoms of infection	397680002 Absence of signs and symptoms of infection (situation)

CCC, Clinical Care Classification; *NANDA-I*, North American Nursing Diagnosis Association International; *NIC*, Nursing Interventions Classification; *NOC*, Nursing Outcomes Classification; *PNDS*, Perioperative Nursing Data Set; *SNOMED CT*, Systematized Nomenclature of Medicine—Clinical Terms.

TABLE 22-9	**INTEGRATION OF NURSING CONCEPTS INTO ICNP**	
SOURCE TERMINOLOGY	**EXAMPLE CONCEPTS IN SOURCE TERMINOLOGY**	**ICNP**
CCC	Q45.0 Comfort alteration	10023066 Discomfort
	K25.5 Infection risk	10015133 Risk for infection
PNDS	A.350 Assesses susceptibility for infection	10002821 Assessing susceptibility to infection
	O.280 Patient is free from signs and symptoms of infection	10028945 No infection

CCC, Clinical Care Classification; *ICNP*, International Classification for Nursing Practice; *PNDS*, Perioperative Nursing Data Set.

assessments) are documented using prestructured clinical templates with discrete data elements and predefined value sets. Yet massive volumes of narrative text data (e.g., clinical notes from various disciplines, progress notes, discharge notes) are also documented in free-text forms in EHRs. Developing quality terminologies and classifications to cover domain-specific content is of critical importance for system design, data retrieval and exchange, quality improvement, and clinical research.[94-101]

Designing User Interface Using Terminologies

The comprehensiveness and completeness of a standardized health terminology vary depending on the domain of interest and the facility. When designing prestructured clinical templates for clinical documentation, interface terminologies can be used to facilitate data entry and storage of clinical data at the point of care. An interface terminology is considered a solution to enhance the user interface in EHRs because of its ability to cover clinicians' preferred terms with rich synonyms and conceptual relations among the terms.[8] An interface terminology either can be derived from standardized reference terminologies and classifications reviewed in this chapter or can be developed locally to support the documentation practice. However, if not careful, local systems might result in numerous duplicate and ambiguous concepts without development guidelines.[8] Accordingly, a

systematic approach should be undertaken to map any local interface terminology to standardized reference terminologies. Otherwise, clinical data cannot be communicated as intended.

Supporting Data Retrieval and Exchange

Storing clinical data using standardized terminologies means that data are encoded using concept unique identifiers or alphanumeric codes to prevent any inconsistency created by typing errors. Prestructured clinical templates can be a vehicle to help users pick and choose from a predefined value set and encode accurately selected values. Retrieving these coded data is much easier than free-text data that are documented using natural language that contains numerous variations in expressions for the same concept or meaning.

While coded data can be easily retrieved and transferred to other facilities using messaging standards (such as HL7), exchanging free-text data requires multiple steps for processing.[102] For instance, assume that no structured form exists to document a skin and wound assessment but only narrative text. To identify a patient who developed a pressure ulcer during hospitalization in the narrative statements, natural language processing of clinical notes would be required. This requires computing resources and human verification of the machine-aided findings (i.e., patients with a pressure ulcer). Many natural language processing tools used in the healthcare domain adopt standardized terminologies to map terms extracted from clinical notes or scientific articles. For example, MetaMap, developed and distributed by the NLM, uses UMLS to extract certain expressions in a standardized way.[103] This exemplifies additional utility of standardized terminologies.

Monitoring the Quality of Care

Clinical databases hold massive amounts of structured and unstructured data along with date and time stamps. Once clinical data are coded in a standardized way, it is possible to monitor the quality of care by joining multiple data sources, including administrative databases. Clinicians and administrators can examine gaps between current practice and best practice, as well as trends in patient outcomes associated with changes in the organization's policy, practice pattern, and nurse staffing ratio. This kind of investigation can be summarized and shared for ongoing quality monitoring and benchmarking.[104] Example quality monitoring activities include identification of the following:

- Medication errors associated with reconciliation, prescription, and administration
- Degree of clinicians' adherence to best practice evidence and guidelines supported through reminders and alerts
- Healthcare resource use (e.g., length of stay, 30-day readmission rate of select population)

The National Database of Nursing Quality Indicators (NDNQI), established by ANA, is an exemplar of monitoring nurse-sensitive quality indicators across hospitals in the United States.[105]

Using a standardized terminology can also help to aggregate patient care data based on predefined conceptual and semantic relationships of the coded data. An administrator may want an overview of staffing to support various types of patient populations. The highest-level construct of each terminology (e.g., functional, physiologic, and psychosocial) could be used to aggregate diagnoses and interventions implemented by unit.[42] Next, the administrator could examine the types of patient problems most prevalent in each unit by sorting according to the next level of hierarchical structure of the given terminology. Practitioners can also benefit from data summarization and presentation produced at both high and granular levels to understand their level of individualized care for accreditation processes or to guide local clinical education to address the major problems, risks, and needs for health promotion for the patient population.

To ensure patient safety and reduce healthcare costs, CMS has developed various initiatives to collect quality measures such as smoking cessation and hospital-acquired pressure ulcer development.[5] CMS is collaborating with public agencies and private organizations to support the use of such quality measures, including, for example, the National Quality Forum, The Joint Commission on Accreditation of Healthcare Organizations, the National Committee for Quality Assurance, the Agency for Healthcare Research and Quality, and the AMA.[106] Reporting these quality measures requires the adoption of standardized terminology.

Discovering Knowledge through Research

Clinical researchers can benefit from EHRs with the functionality and capacity to access complete coded data across the care continuum. Current barriers, including the fact that data are currently coded with multiple terminologies, will be removed as more standardized terminologies are harmonized to support data exchange and reuse. Ideally healthcare terminologies can complement each other to enhance the coverage of domain knowledge of interest and thus promote Meaningful Use of clinical data. Coded data enable comparative effectiveness research using standardized data retrieved from multiple EHRs.

The vast volumes of clinical and administrative data residing in a large repository provide additional opportunity for clinical research. When paper-based records are used for clinical research, the number of reviewed charts is restricted because of the major resource requirements and the time-intensive chart abstraction process. In contrast, clinical research using current EHRs could involve hundreds of patient records, offering the potential to identify new relationships among clinical data. Standardized terminologies in EHRs can facilitate this kind of research. Even so, using current EHRs for research creates additional challenges and costs for data queries, processing, and analysis to handle the many inconsistent descriptions of patient care and large volumes of missing data.

CONCLUSION AND FUTURE DIRECTIONS

Since the release of the IOM report on the U.S. quality chasm, health IT has been seen as a promising solution for improving patient safety, delivering patient-centered care, and reducing healthcare costs.[1] However, a fundamental requirement for health IT is information exchange across systems. The use of standardized terminologies such as SNOMED CT and LOINC facilitates this information exchange and is one of the requirements of recent regulations for Meaningful Use criteria of EHRs.

Health practitioners have recognized the benefits of using standardized terminologies and have actively participated in the development of not only discipline-specific terminologies, but also multidisciplinary terminologies. As personal health records become popular in the twenty-first century, the health practitioner also needs to be involved in the development of consumer health vocabulary. With standardized clinical terminology, patient data will be available across the full spectrum of healthcare settings. Also, these data are and will be shared with individual patients, requiring additional efforts to translate professional vocabulary to consumer vocabulary. Personal health records maintained jointly by consumer and health professionals will provide opportunities to enhance public health surveillance by enabling a clinician's ability to track a patient's health maintenance, follow-up activity, engagement, and progress. The health professions should continue to participate in current and future endeavors to ensure that the domain concepts are represented in the approved manner within health IT.

Data standardization and exchange efforts were reviewed at various levels. Historically, coding requirements were most often associated with billing and reimbursement. With the advancement of health IT and health sciences, however, data standardization and exchange are key elements for improving the nation's healthcare. Many benefits of using data standards have yet to be realized but progress is evident. While terminology developers will continue to put their efforts into further enhancements, terminology users also need to evaluate the quality of terminologies and provide feedback to terminology developers.

REFERENCES

1. Institute of Medicine. *Crossing the Quality Chasm: A New Health System for the 21st Century*. Washington, DC: National Academies Press; 2001.
2. Agency for Healthcare Research and Quality (AHRQ). Health IT at AHRQ. AHRQ. http://healthit.ahrq.gov/portal/server.pt/community/about/562. 2010.
3. Institute of Medicine. *Health IT and Patient Safety: Building Safer Systems for Better Care*. Washington, DC: National Academies Press; 2012.
4. Blumenthal D, Tavenner M. The "Meaningful Use" regulation for electronic health records. *N Engl J Med*. 2010;363(6):501-504.
5. Centers for Medicare & Medicaid Services (CMS). EHR incentive programs. CMS. http://www.cms.gov/Regulations-and-Guidance/Legislation/EHRIncentivePrograms. 2010.
6. de Keizer NF, Abu-Hanna A, Zwetslook-Schonk JHM. Understanding terminological systems I: terminology and typology. *Methods Inf Med*. 2000;39:16-21.
7. Merriam-Webster. http://www.merriam-webster.com/dictionary. 2012.
8. Rosenbloom ST, Miller RA, Johnson KB, Elkin PL, Brown SH. Interface terminologies: facilitating direct entry of clinical data into electronic health record systems. *J Am Med Inform Assoc*. 2006;13(3):277-288.
9. Gruber T. Toward principles for the design of ontologies used for knowledge sharing. *Int J Hum Comput Syst*. 1995;43(5-6):907-928.
10. Tsarkov D, Horrocks I. FaCT++ description logic reasoner: system description. *Lecture Notes Comput Sci*. 2006;4130:292-297.
11. The National Center for Biomedical Ontology. BioPortal. http://bioportal.bioontology.org/. 2012.
12. Wilder V. UMLS 2012AB release available. *NLM Technical Bulletin*. 2012;389:e2. http://www.nlm.nih.gov/pubs/techbull/nd12/nd12_umls_2012ab_release.html.
13. McCray AT, Nelson SJ. The representation of meaning in the UMLS. *Methods Inf Med*. 1995;34(1-2):193-201.
14. Rogers JE. Quality assurance of medical ontologies. *Methods Inf Med*. 2006;45(3):267-274.
15. Bakhshi-Raiez F, Cornet R, de Keizer NF. Development and application of a framework for maintenance of medical terminological systems. *J Am Med Inform Assoc*. 2008;15(5):687-700.
16. de Coronado S, Wright LW, Fragoso G, et al. The NCI thesaurus quality assurance life cycle. *J Biomed Inform*. 2009;42(3):530-539.
17. Kim TY, Coenen A, Hardiker N. A quality improvement model for healthcare terminologies. *J Biomed Inform*. 2010;43(6):1036-1043.
18. International Health Terminology Standards Development Organisation (IHTSDO). Release of SNOMED CT: development, quality assurance and release. IHTSDO. http://www.ihtsdo.org/snomed-ct/release-of-snomed-ct/. 2009.
19. International Council of Nurses. *ICNP® Version 2*. Geneva, Switzerland: ICN; 2009.
20. NANDA International. Defining the knowledge of nursing. NANDA International. http://www.nanda.org/DiagnosisDevelopment.aspx. 2012.
21. Cimino JJ, Clayton PD, Hripcsak G, Johnson SB. Knowledge-based approaches to the maintenance of a large controlled medical terminology. *J Am Med Inform Assoc*. 1994;1(1):35-50.
22. Tuttle MS, Olson NE, Campbell KE, Sherertz DD, Nelson SJ, Cole WG. Formal properties of the metathesaurus. *Proc Annu Symp Comput Appl Med Care*. 1994:145-149.
23. Campbell JR, Carpenter P, Sneiderman C, Cohn S, Chute CG, Warren J. Phase II evaluation of clinical coding schemes: completeness, taxonomy, mapping, definitions, and clarity. CPRI Work Group on Codes and Structures. *J Am Med Inform Assoc*. 1997;4(3):238-251.
24. Chute CG, Cohn SP, Campbell JR. A framework for comprehensive health terminology systems in the United States: development guidelines, criteria for selection, and public policy implications. ANSI Healthcare Informatics Standards Board Vocabulary Working Group and the Computer-Based Patient Records Institute Working Group on Codes and Structures. *J Am Med Inform Assoc*. 1998;5(6):503-510.
25. Cimino JJ. Desiderata for controlled medical vocabularies in the twenty-first century. *Methods Inf Med*. 1998;37(4-5):394-403.
26. Oliver DE, Shahar Y. Change management of shared and local versions of health-care terminologies. *Methods Inf Med*. 2000;39(4-5):278-290.
27. Elkin PL, Brown SH, Carter J, et al. Guideline and quality indicators for development, purchase and use of controlled health vocabularies. *Int J Med Inform*. 2002;68(1-3):175-186.
28. International Organization for Standardization. *Health Informatics—Controlled Health Terminology—Structure and High-Level Indicators (ISO/TX17117:2002)*. Geneva, Switzerland: ISO; 2002.
29. International Organization for Standardization. *Health Informatics—Integration of a Reference Terminology Model for Nursing (ISO/TX 18104:2003)*. Geneva, Switzerland: ISO; 2003.
30. Goossen W. Cross-mapping between three terminologies with the international standard nursing reference terminology model. *Int J Nurs Terminol Classif*. 2006;17(4):153-164.
31. Warren JJ, Bakken S. Update on standardized nursing data sets and terminologies. *J AHIMA*. 2002;73(7):78-83; quiz 85-86.
32. American Nurses Association. ANA recognized terminologies that support nursing practice. *Nursing World*. http://www.nursingworld.org/npii/terminologies.htm. 2012.
33. Ryan P, Delaney C. Nursing minimum data set. In: Fitzpatrick JJ, Stevenson JS, eds. *Annual Review of Nursing Research*. Vol 13. New York: Springer Publishing Company; 1995:169-194.
34. Huber D, Schumacher L, Delaney C. Nursing Management Minimum Data Set (NMMDS). *J Nurs Adm*. 1997;27(4):42-48.

35. Westra BL, Subramanian A, Hart CM, et al. Achieving "Meaningful Use" of electronic health records through the integration of the Nursing Management Minimum Data Set. *J Nurs Adm.* 2010;40(7-8):336-343.

36. Kunkel DE, Westra BL, Hart CM, Subramanian A, Kenny S, Delaney CW. Updating and normalization of the Nursing Management Minimum Data Set element 6: patient/client accessibility. *Comput Inform Nurs.* 2010;30(3):134-141.

37. Vreeman DJ. Logical Observation Identifiers Names and Codes. Regenstrief Institute, Inc. http://loinc.org/. 2010.

38. McDonald C, Huff S, Mercer K, Hernandez J, Vreeman DJ, eds. Logical Observation Identifiers Names and Codes (LOINC®) users' guide. Regenstrief Institute, Inc. http://loinc.org/downloads/files/LOINCManual.pdf. 2012.

39. Scichilone RA. The benefits of using SNOMED CT and LOINC in assessment instruments. *J AHIMA.* 2008;79(7):56-57.

40. Hyun S, Shapiro JS, Melton G, et al. Iterative evaluation of the Health Level 7—Logical Observation Identifiers Names and Codes clinical document ontology for representing clinical document names: a case report. *J Am Med Inform Assoc.* 2009;16(3):395-399.

41. Matney S, Bakken S, Huff SM. Representing nursing assessments in clinical information systems using the logical observation identifiers, names, and codes database. *J Biomed Inform.* 2003;36(4-5):287-293.

42. Cornet R, de Keizer N. Forty years of SNOMED: a literature review. *BMC Med Inform Decis Mak.* 2008;8(suppl 1):S2.

43. International Health Terminology Standard Development Organisation (IHTSDO). History of SNOMED CT. IHTSDO. http://www.ihtsdo.org/snomed-ct/history0/. 2012.

44. International Health Terminology Standard Development Organisation (IHTSDO). SNOMED CT user guide. IHTSDO. http://ihtsdo.org/fileadmin/user_upload/doc/download/doc_UserGuide_Current-en-US_INT_20120131.pdf. 2012.

45. World Health Organization (WHO). International Classification of Diseases (ICD). WHO. http://www.who.int/classifications/icd/en/. 2012.

46. Centers for Disease Control and Prevention (CDC). International Classification of Diseases, ninth revision, clinical modification (ICD-9-CM). CDC. http://www.cdc.gov/nchs/icd/icd9cm.htm. 2011.

47. Centers for Medicare & Medicaid Services (CMS). ICD-10. CMS. http://www.cms.gov/Medicare/Coding/ICD10/index.html?redirect=/ICD10/. 2012.

48. American Medical Association (AMA). CPT—Current procedural terminology. AMA. http://www.ama-assn.org/ama/pub/physician-resources/solutions-managing-your-practice/coding-billing-insurance/cpt.page. 2012.

49. Centers for Medicare & Medicaid Services (CMS). Acute inpatient PPS. CMS. http://www.cms.gov/Medicare/Medicare-Fee-for-Service-Payment/AcuteInpatientPPS/index.html. 2012.

50. American Psychiatric Association (APA). DSM-ICD coding crosswalk. APA. http://www.psych.org/practice/dsm/dsm-icd-coding-crosswalk. 2012.

51. ABC Coding Solutions. ABC code structure. ABC Coding Solutions. http://www.abccodes.com. 2009.

52. National Library of Medicine (NLM). RxNorm overview. NLM. http://www.nlm.nih.gov/research/umls/rxnorm/overview.html. 2012.

53. Nelson SJ, Zeng K, Kilbourne J, Powell T, Moore R. Normalized names for clinical drugs: RxNorm at 6 years. *J Am Med Inform Assoc.* 2011;18(4):441-448.

54. Madden R, Skyes C, Ustrun TB. World Health Organization family of international classifications: definition, scope, and purpose. World Health Organization. http://www.who.int/classifications/en/FamilyDocument2007.pdf. 2007.

55. World Health Organization (WHO). *International Classification of Functioning, Disability and Health.* Geneva, Switzerland: WHO; 2001.

56. Heerkens Y, van der Brug Y, Napel HT, van Ravensberg D. Past and future use of the ICF (former ICIDH) by nursing and allied health professionals. *Disabil Rehabil.* 2003;25(11-12):620-627.

57. Heinen MM, van Achterberg T, Roodbol G, Frederiks CM. Applying ICF in nursing practice: classifying elements of nursing diagnoses. *Int Nurs Rev.* 2005;52(4):304-312.

58. Van Achterberg T, Holleman G, Heijnen-Kaales Y, et al. Using a multidisciplinary classification in nursing: the International Classification of Functioning Disability and Health. *J Adv Nurs.* 2005;49(4):432-441.

59. Mueller M, Boldt C, Grill E, Strobl R, Stucki G. Identification of ICF categories relevant for nursing in the situation of acute and early post-acute rehabilitation. *BMC Nurs.* 2008;7:3.

60. World Health Organization (WHO). Derived and related classifications in the WHO-FIC. WHO. http://www.who.int/classifications/related/en/index.html. 2012.

61. Coenen A, McNeil B, Bakken S, Bickford C, Warren JJ. Toward comparable nursing data: American Nurses Association criteria for data sets, classification systems, and nomenclatures. *Comput Nurs.* 2001;19(6):240-246, quiz 246-248.

62. Saba V. Nursing classifications: home health care classification system (HHCC): an overview. *OJIN.* 2002;7(3). http://www.nursingworld.org/MainMenuCategories/ANAMarketplace/ANAPeriodicals/OJIN/TableofContents/Volume72002/No3Sept2002/ArticlesPreviousTopic/HHCCAnOverview.aspx.

63. Saba V. *Clinical Care Classification (CCC) System Manual: A Guide to Nursing Documentation.* New York, NY: Springer Publishing Company; 2007.

64. Saba V. *Clinical Care Classification (CCC) System Version 2.5 User's Guide*, 2nd ed. New York, NY: Springer Publishing Company; 2012.

65. International Council of Nurses (ICN). ICN eHealth Programme. ICN. http://www.icn.ch/pillarsprograms/ehealth/. 2010.

66. Hardiker NR, Coenen A. Interpretation of an international terminology standard in the development of a logic-based compositional terminology. *Int J Med Inform.* 2007;76(suppl 2):S274–S280.

67. Coenen A, Kim TY. Development of terminology subsets using ICNP. *Int J Med Inform.* 2010;79(7):530-538.

68. International Council of Nurses (ICN). *Partnering with Patients and Families to Promote Adherence to Treatment.* Geneva, Switzerland: ICN; 2008.

69. International Council of Nurses (ICN). *Palliative Care for Dignified Dying.* Geneva, Switzerland: ICN; 2009.

70. International Council of Nurses (ICN). *Nursing Outcome Indicators.* Geneva, Switzerland: ICN; 2011.

71. International Council of Nurses (ICN). *Scottish Government, National Health Service Scotland, Community Nursing.* Geneva, Switzerland: ICN; 2012.

72. Gordon M. *Nursing Diagnosis: Process and Application*, 3rd ed. St. Louis, MO: Mosby; 1994.

73. Herdman TH, ed. *North American Nursing Diagnosis Association International (NANDA-I) Nursing Diagnoses 2012–2014:*

Definitions and Classification. Oxford, England: Wiley-Blackwell; 2012.

74. Bulechek GM, Butcher HK, Dochterman JM, eds. *Nursing Interventions Classification*, 5th ed. St. Louis, MO: Mosby Inc; 2008.

75. Moorhead S, Johnson MM, Maas M, Swanson E, eds. *Nursing Outcomes Classification*, 4th ed. St. Louis, MO: Mosby Inc; 2008.

76. Martin KS. *The Omaha System: A Key to Practice, Documentation, and Information Management*, 2nd ed. Omaha, NE: Health Connections Press; 2005.

77. Association of Operating Room Nurses. *Perioperative Nursing Data Set*, 3rd ed. Denver, CO: AORN Inc; 2011.

78. Petersen C, Kleiner C. Evolution and revision of the Perioperative Nursing Data Set. *AORN J.* 2011;93(1):127-132.

79. Health Level Seven International (HL7). Introduction to HL7 standards. HL7. http://www.hl7.org/implement/standards/index.cfm?ref=nav. 2012.

80. Dolin RH, Alschuler L, Boyer S, et al. HL7 clinical document architecture, release 2. *J Am Med Inform Assoc.* 2006;13(1):30-39.

81. D'Amore JD, Sittig DF, Wright A, Iyengar MS, Ness RB. The promise of the CCD: challenges and opportunity for quality improvement and population health. *AMIA Annu Symp Proc.* 2011;285-294.

82. Healthcare Information and Management Systems Society (HIMSS). Interoperability definition and background. HIMSS. http://www.himss.org/content/files/interoperability_definition_background_060905.pdf. 2005.

83. U.S. Department of Health & Human Services. Electronic health records and Meaningful Use. HealthIT.gov. http://healthit.hhs.gov/portal/server.pt?open=512&objID=2996&mode=2. 2011.

84. Healthcare Information Technology Standards Panel. http://www.hitsp.org/default.aspx. 2009.

85. National Library of Medicine (NLM). LOINC to CPT mapping. NLM. http://www.nlm.nih.gov/research/umls/mapping_projects/loinc_to_cpt_map.html. 2006.

86. Lu DF, Park HT, Ucharattana P, Konicek D, Delaney C. Nursing outcomes classification in the systematized nomenclature of medicine clinical terms: a cross-mapping validation. *Comput Inform Nurs.* 2007;25(3):159-170.

87. College of American Pathologists (CAP). SNOMED CT® mappings to NANDA, NIC, and NOC now licensed for free access through National Library of Medicine. CAP. http://www.cap.org. 2005.

88. International Health Terminology Standards Development Organisation (IHTSDO). ICN and IHTSDO team-up to ensure a common health terminology. IHTSDO. http://www.ihtsdo.org/fileadmin/user_upload/Docs_01/Press_Releases/ICN_and_IHTSDO_Announcement_March_2010.pdf. 2010.

89. Canadian Nurses Association (CNA). Mapping Canadian clinical outcomes in ICNP. CNA. http://www2.cna-aiic.ca/c-hobic/documents/pdf/ICNP_Mapping_2008_e.pdf. 2008.

90. Matney SA, DaDamio R, Couderc C, et al. Translation and integration of CCC nursing diagnoses into ICNP. *J Am Med Inform Assoc.* 2008;15(6):791-793.

91. Dykes PC, Kim HE, Goldsmith DM, Choi J, Esumi K, Goldberg HS. The adequacy of ICNP version 1.0 as a representational model for electronic nursing assessment documentation. *J Am Med Inform Assoc.* 2009;16(2):238-246.

92. Hannah KJ, White PA, Nagle LM, Pringle DM. Standardizing nursing information in Canada for inclusion in electronic health records: C-HOBIC. *J Am Med Inform Assoc.* 2009;16(4):524-530.

93. Kim TY, Coenen A. Toward harmonising WHO International Classifications: a nursing perspective. *Inform Health Soc Care.* 2011;36(1):35-49.

94. Andison M, Moss J. What nurses do: use of the ISO Reference Terminology Model for Nursing Action as a framework for analyzing MICU nursing practice patterns. *AMIA Annu Symp Proc.* 2007:21-25.

95. Badalucco S, Reed KK. Supporting quality and patient safety in cancer clinical trials. *Clin J Oncol Nurs.* 2011;15(3):263-265.

96. Bernhart-Just A, Lassen B, Schwendimann R. Representing the nursing process with nursing terminologies in electronic medical record systems: a Swiss approach. *Comput Inform Nurs.* 2010;28(6):345-352.

97. Bouhaddou O, Warnekar P, Parrish F, et al. Exchange of computable patient data between the Department of Veterans Affairs (VA) and the Department of Defense (DOD): terminology mediation strategy. *J Am Med Inform Assoc.* 2008;15(2):174-183.

98. Cho I, Park HA, Chung E. Exploring practice variation in preventive pressure-ulcer care using data from a clinical data repository. *Int J Med Inform.* 2011;80(1):47-55.

99. Leung GY, Zhang J, Lin WC, Clark RE. Behavioral health disorders and adherence to measures of diabetes care quality. *Am J Manag Care.* 2011;17(2):144-150.

100. Monsen KA, Newsom ET. Feasibility of using the Omaha System to represent public health nurse manager interventions. *Public Health Nurs.* 2011;28(5):421-428.

101. Watkins TJ, Haskell RE, Lundberg CB, Brokel JM, Wilson ML, Hardiker N. Terminology use in electronic health records: basic principles. *Urol Nurs.* 2009;29(5):321-326, quiz 327.

102. Friedman C, Shagina L, Lussier Y, Hripcsak G. Automated encoding of clinical documents based on natural language processing. *J Am Med Inform Assoc.* 2004;11(5):392-402.

103. Aronson AR, Lang FM. An overview of MetaMap: historical perspective and recent advances. *J Am Med Inform Assoc.* 2010;17(3):229-236.

104. Dunton N, Montalvo I, eds. *Transforming Nursing Data into Quality Care: Profiles of Quality Improvement in U.S. Healthcare Facilities.* Silver Spring, MD: American Nurses Association Inc; 2007.

105. American Nurses Association. National database of Nursing Quality Indicators. https://www.nursingquality.org/. 2012.

106. Centers for Medicare & Medicaid Services (CMS). Quality measures. CMS. http://www.cms.gov/Medicare/Quality-Initiatives-Patient-Assessment-Instruments/QualityMeasures/index.html?redirect=/QualityMeasures/. 2012.

DISCUSSION QUESTIONS

1. You are the only informatics nurse at your small community hospital and have been asked to use terminologies within your EHR for care planning. What terminologies would you use and why?
2. Discuss the benefits of using standardized terminologies within your EHR.
3. Discuss the major local, national, and international obstacles to implementing standardized terminologies within EHRs.
4. As a researcher you have been assigned to obtain data from two different facilities. Both facilities have mapped their data to standardized terminologies within their data warehouses. Discuss how this will benefit your research. Alternatively, what if the data in both facilities were not coded using standards? What obstacles would need to be overcome?

CASE STUDY

A small community hospital in the Midwest has used a home-grown information system for years. The system began in the early 1970s with a financial module. Over time additional modules were added. A limited number of departments selected a commercial system and interfaces were used to integrate these into the overall functionality of the hospital information system. Except for physicians, most in-house clinical or care-related documentation is online. However, about 15% to 20% of this documentation is done by free text and is not effectively searchable. In addition, the screens, including the drop-down and default values, were built using terms selected by the in-house development team in consultation with clinical staff; thus there is no data dictionary or specific standard language. In the last few years the hospital has purchased two outpatient clinics (obstetrics and mental health) and a number of local doctor practices. The clinics and doctors' offices are now being converted to the hospital administrative systems as described in Chapter 7. A few of the clinical applications that are tied directly to the administrative systems such as order entry and results reporting are also being installed.

A major change is being planned. A new chief information officer (CIO) was hired last year and she has appointed a chief medical information officer (CMIO) and a chief nursing information officer (CNIO). No other significant staff changes were made. With her team in place, one of the CIO's first activities was to complete an inventory of all applications. As part of this process each application and the system as a whole was assessed for the ability to meet Meaningful Use criteria. Based on this analysis, Stage 1 criteria are currently being met. Additional programming and upgrades are needed to meet Stage 2 criteria. Meeting anticipated Stages 3 and 4 criteria will require a significant investment in hardware, software, and additional staff. Rather than continue to build, a decision has been made to switch to a commercial vendor. The hospital is now in the process of selecting a commercial system. Because of your background as a member of the clinical staff with informatics education, you have been appointed to the selection committee. It is also anticipated that you will serve on the implementation committee.

Discussion Questions

1. What role, if any, should standard language play in the selection process?
2. What key standard languages and coding systems should be incorporated in the new system?
3. Can the work done in building the screens and developing the terms that are used for documentation of care in the old system be used in the new system or will this delay customizing the new system applications?
4. It is expected that clinical staff will participate in site visits and vendor displays. What, if any, preparation related to standard languages should be given before these activities?
5. How should clinical staff who will be using the new system be prepared for the introduction of new or different terms in the clinical documentation system?

UNIT 6

Governance and Organizational Structures for Informatics

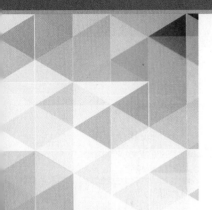

Health Information Technology Governance

Jim Turnbull and Kensaku Kawamoto

Given the rapidly changing healthcare environment, it is critical that healthcare organizations develop a health information technology (health IT) governance structure that allows priorities and direction to be promptly adapted to these changes.

OBJECTIVES

At the completion of this chapter the reader will be prepared to:
1. Describe why health information technology (health IT) governance is needed
2. Assess a health IT governance structure
3. Discuss challenges to establishing effective health IT governance

4. Describe key considerations for the establishment of health IT governance
5. Evaluate the effectiveness of health IT governance approaches

KEY TERM

Health IT governance, 371

ABSTRACT

Health information technology (health IT) represents a critical enabler for healthcare organizations to achieve strategic objectives and operational excellence. To optimize the value of health IT resources, a healthcare organization must have in place effective governance to ensure alignment with institutional strategic objectives and the effective prioritization of limited resources. This chapter provides direction and insight into the various issues that must be considered in establishing that governance structure. In addition, recommendations are provided for establishing an effective health informatics governance structure that is aligned with institutional strategic objectives, effectively prioritizes competing health IT needs, and is tailored to the unique culture and characteristics of the organization.

INTRODUCTION

As an emerging element of our healthcare delivery system, the concept of health IT governance is far from mature in all but the most advanced healthcare facilities. There is some existing literature on health IT governance, such as a book by Kropf and Scalzi published by the Healthcare Information and Management Systems Society.[1] However, a search of MEDLINE and the general Web reveals relatively little literature on this topic, and much of the existing literature focuses on the tactical implementation of transactional (operational) IT systems rather than on the growing need to optimize information management broadly within and across organizations by leveraging health IT. Consequently, the authors of this chapter offer a perspective based primarily on their extensive experience in providing administrative leadership in organizations ranging from large multihospital systems to academic medical centers (AMCs). These organizations demonstrate varying degrees of sophistication with regard to electronic health record (EHR) systems and associated health IT capabilities.

HEALTH IT GOVERNANCE: NEED AND CORE COMPONENTS

Given that healthcare is an information-intensive endeavor, health IT represents a core pillar that enables and supports a modern healthcare organization's ability to achieve its strategic and operational objectives. Healthcare organizations must ensure that their health IT efforts are aligned with the organization's key objectives. Moreover, a healthcare organization's strategic and operational initiatives often require health IT resources to be optimally effective. Whether it is care pathway implementation, population health management, or medication safety, it is rare for a key healthcare initiative to *not* require health IT support. Thus the need for health IT resources will often significantly exceed the available capacity. The critical nature of effective health IT governance then arises from the following fundamental interrelated needs:

1. The need to ensure alignment of health IT resources with institutional priorities
2. The need to effectively prioritize the use of health IT resources in the face of numerous competing demands for these limited resources

Healthcare enterprises are often recognized as being one of the most complex of all organizational structures. Consequently, when one speaks of "institutional priorities" the list is often long and is generated from multiple sources. Historically, beyond priorities established by senior leadership, requests for health IT resources are received from researchers, the finance and quality departments, specialists who are refining clinical processes or investigating clinical variances, and so forth. More recently there have been emerging requests from internal groups working on health reform, personalized medicine, and more sophisticated costing methodologies. In summary, the demand for health IT resources and expertise is growing rapidly, the requests are coming from a broader group of constituencies, and the institutional priorities are becoming much less clear.

The role of health IT governance is to help to clarify priorities, allocate resources, and, if necessary, approve the funding to support the expansion of available health IT resources. Health IT governance should also be accountable to track and monitor the benefits of these investments.

To meet these needs, effective health IT governance must include the following components:

- Organizational structures responsible for clearly defining institutional priorities. Typically this function is primarily the responsibility of the board of directors and senior leadership of a healthcare organization.
- Organizational structures responsible for ensuring that health IT efforts are aligned with institutional priorities and used optimally.
- Accompanying processes to operationalize the governance. For example, health IT governance typically incorporates formal processes for proposing new projects requiring health IT resources, evaluating and prioritizing potential projects, approving funding, and monitoring return on investment. Establishing such operational processes is much more straightforward compared to establishing a governance structure that appropriately owns and uses these processes; therefore the remainder of the chapter will focus on health IT governance structure rather than on the processes used to operationalize the governance.

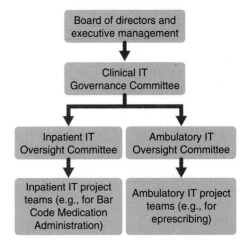

FIG 23-1 Sample health IT governance structure.

A sample health IT governance structure, adapted from recommendations by Hoehn, is as follows:

- Board of directors and executive management: responsible for setting the overall health IT strategy and clear expectations within the context of institutional priorities
- Clinical IT Governance Committee, including chief medical officer, chief nursing officer, chief medical informatics officer, chief nursing informatics officer, chief information officer, chief operating officer, and appropriate clinical and administrative department chairs: responsible for establishing and overseeing the implementation of the health IT strategic plan
- Various committees reporting to clinical IT governance committee: responsible for overseeing operational execution of clinical IT initiatives consistent with institutional priorities and the health IT strategic plan[2]

Figure 23-1 shows an example of an organizational chart demonstrating this kind of health IT governance structure. The figure shows one of many potential approaches an institution may take. Each institution may need to adapt this governance structure to incorporate other committees with overlapping responsibilities. The next section discusses this and other relevant issues that should be considered in establishing any health IT governance.

KEY INSIGHTS

Respect Current Decision-Making Structures

In establishing a health IT governance, strong consideration and respect should be given to the governance structures and decision-making processes that are already in place within the organization. It is important that strong alignment be demonstrated between the initiatives of the broader organization and the focus of the health IT program. If a health IT governance model does not demonstrate this alignment, barriers to effective communication could be erected needlessly.

Time invested in determining who "owns" health IT governance is time well spent. In some fortunate cases an existing committee can be modified to embrace the requirements for health IT governance. A much more likely scenario is that the topic has not been addressed. In those situations the health IT team typically responds to "he who yells the loudest is best heard." Clearly the governance structure needs to be tightly aligned with the position within the organization that is perceived to be "highest in the food chain" when it comes to health IT priorities and resource allocation.

Shift in Organizational Mindset

For several decades healthcare organizations have been focusing on developing IT infrastructure and implementing a plethora of applications. The latter have consisted primarily of transaction-based applications that support the revenue cycle, back-office functions such as payroll, and the delivery of clinical care. More recently data warehouses with an array of decision support and reporting tools developed by both vendors and in-house resources have emerged. The increasing sophistication of the IT environment has enabled both clinical and administrative leaders to leverage data in support of their programs and services.

Almost in lockstep, the emergence of the Internet in the early 1990s led to customer expectations that information about all topics should be at the fingertips of both clinicians and customers (often with little consideration being given as to whether the information is accurate or can be trusted). As a result, patients and families have new expectations in terms of both access to and transparency of data from their caregivers, with the expectations of patients, families, and other healthcare consumers often exceeding that of healthcare providers and institutions.

More recently, the era of Meaningful Use and health reform has brought regulatory mandates and incentives, as well as new market pressures, to the forefront. To effectively respond to these changes organizations have had to commit significant capital to health IT while requiring ever more sophisticated data analysis to refine clinical care delivery processes and improve outcomes.

These internal and external forces are causing organizations to rethink their priorities and how both capital and operational and human resources are focused. This requires a change in health IT governance for which many organizational leaders are not prepared. Information has become a strategic asset that is essential to survival within the current healthcare context and the demands on those with health IT expertise are expanding quickly. As the demands rapidly outstrip the internal capacity to meet the need, prioritization of projects becomes imperative. This is the role of governance.

The Continual Increase in Demand for Health IT

Due in large part to the successful implementation of core enabling technologies such as EHR systems and computerized provider order entry (CPOE) systems, there exists a continual increase in the demand for health IT resources. Indeed, the implementation of core clinical information systems is just the beginning of an institution's health IT road map, as the availability of these core infrastructure components opens up the possibility of ever more advanced uses of health IT, whether it be data mining, point-of-care decision support, or population health management. Moreover, especially within AMCs, a growing demand exists for health IT resources to support research missions, such as health services research, outcomes research, and personalized healthcare research. Again, this continual increase in the demands for health IT resources and the need to prioritize and manage these demands is a core role of health IT governance.

Governance Does Not Depend on Specific Technology Choices

The selection of specific health IT solutions, such as an EHR system, is certainly a critical health IT decision for an institution. However, the health IT governance should be independent of any particular technology choices made. Instead, the health IT governance should guide those types of technologies and technology choices. For example, the selection of an EHR system, population health management tool, or business intelligence platform should be within the scope of the expected responsibility of a health IT governance structure. In particular, it is imperative that the governance structure has mechanisms in place to obtain the perspectives of all relevant stakeholders and make decisions in a manner that fosters stakeholder buy-in and sustained support for these oftentimes long-term health IT investment decisions.

Coordination and Collaboration with Diverse Stakeholders

Because of their very nature, health IT initiatives often require the close coordination and collaboration of various institutional stakeholders. For example, an EHR system implementation will affect virtually every area of a healthcare organization. Thus a traditional governance structure that is informatics centered by nature may present a barrier to the kind of integrated, cross-stakeholder coordination and collaboration required. A medication safety initiative, for example, may need the close engagement of the Pharmacy and Therapeutics Committee and other relevant stakeholders from groups such as pharmacy and nursing, perhaps more so than a Health IT Governance Committee. As discussed earlier, then, substantial consideration must be given to how the health IT governance takes into account and coordinates with existing governance structures outside health IT.

RECOMMENDATIONS

One of the biggest challenges for organizations addressing health IT governance is deciding where to begin. As mentioned, there is very little literature to provide guidance on the effective governance of health IT. The following recommendations are provided with the understanding that this is an evolving area of focus in the industry. Organizations may well need to make course corrections or experiment with different approaches until a more permanent solution emerges.

Conduct a Health IT Capability Maturity Assessment

A good starting point in developing a health IT governance model is obtaining an understanding of the current health IT structure and culture. A well-defined resource that can be used for conducting such an assessment is the Informatics Capability Maturity Model developed by the United Kingdom's National Health Service.[3] This qualitative model (Table 23-1) assesses an organization's capabilities with respect to five dimensions, measured on a scale of 1 (basic) to 5 (innovative).

Of note, the effectiveness of health IT governance is measured both directly and indirectly across each of these dimensions. For example, the following are governance-related characteristics across the five dimensions that scored 5 in each category for an organization with an innovative health IT capability (level 5):

- Managing information: senior management sees information as being core to business success and exploits it to improve service quality, efficiency, and productivity
- Using business intelligence: executives and managers embrace business intelligence and use it to set and manage business strategy
- Using information technology: IT is a key focus of the business strategy encompassing all aspects and elements of its business provision
- Aligning business and informatics: governance processes support and sustain the integration of strategic business planning and health IT planning
- Managing change: governance arrangements are a core aspect of organizational control, with demonstrable reporting lines to the executive board level and with clear ownership and control responsibilities embedded within the organization

The Informatics Capability Maturity Model includes a self-assessment tool[4] that can be completed in approximately 2 hours in a forum that allows sufficient time for discussion and debate. To understand an organization's baseline state with regard to its health IT capabilities generally and its health IT governance specifically, an organization looking to enhance its health IT governance should first complete this self-assessment in a process led by its senior leadership. As part of this self-assessment an organization should explicitly identify the current health IT governance structure and processes, including in particular the various channels through which committees and institutional stakeholders currently request informatics resources and how those institutional needs are prioritized.

Upon completing this baseline assessment an organization should be able to identify the current maturity of its health IT governance and how improvements in that governance could advance the organization's ability to achieve its strategic objectives. If, for instance, the assessment reveals a low score across all five dimensions, the establishment of a health IT governance structure is probably urgently needed, albeit with a somewhat less mature model than one might find at a more advanced institution. The next step would be to identify potential health IT governance models that could be appropriate for the organization given its current health IT maturity level.

Investigate Peer Informatics Governance Models

There is unfortunately no single model for health IT governance, just as there is no single model for other areas of organizational governance. Rather than offering a prescriptive solution, the organization needs to investigate health IT governance models that are already in place at organizations of similar size and complexity. Key questions to consider when investigating other organizations' health IT governance include the following:

- How mature is the health IT capability at the organization? What are the potential implications to governance if an organization has a significantly different health IT capability?
- What is the official governance structure and process?
- Are there ad hoc governance processes in place, for example, in terms of individual institutional leaders requesting health IT governance support and prioritizing informatics activities?
- What works well with the governance? What could be improved?
- Are there aspects of the governance that are dependent on unique characteristics of the organization, such as its culture or specific individuals?

TABLE 23-1	INFORMATICS CAPABILITY MATURITY MODEL DIMENSIONS
DIMENSION	**DEFINITION**
Managing information	The degree to which users have access to the right information at the right time
Using business intelligence	The degree to which business data are effectively analyzed and presented to inform business and clinical decision making
Using information technology	The degree to which IT is innovatively leveraged to enable leaner processes and seamless information flows
Aligning business and informatics	The degree to which an organization values health IT as a strategic asset and has the capability to ensure that it can be exploited to deliver against its business objectives
Managing change	The degree to which an organization has a structured and effective approach to realizing the full benefits of health IT to enable business change

IT, Information technology.

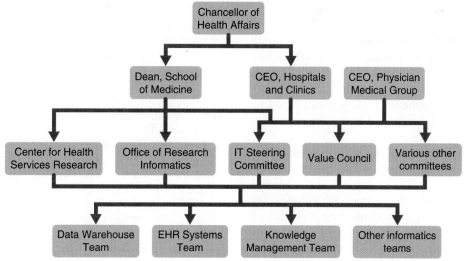

FIG 23-2 Sample informatics governance structure for an academic health system.

Figure 23-2 provides a sample health IT governance structure that may be appropriate for a large academic health system. Note that this structure is significantly more complicated than the one in Figure 23-1, which may be more feasible and appropriate for a smaller healthcare system or a healthcare system with fewer competing needs related to research and education. In this sample governance structure there are three main sources of authority: the dean of the School of Medicine, the chief executive officer (CEO) of the hospitals and clinics, and the CEO of the physician medical group, which in this case is independent of the university. In this organizational structure the primary health IT governance is intended to be the IT Steering Committee, which oversees the creation and implementation of the health IT governance strategic plan. However, other committees and organizational subunits also make significant demands on health IT resources, including a Center for Health Services Research, an Office of Research Informatics, a Value Council with oversight of initiatives to improve care value, and various other committees such as for finance and population health management. The key to enabling effective prioritization in this environment is global prioritization of the various competing initiatives by the senior leadership and, perhaps more importantly, determination of what will need to wait until the priority initiatives are completed. Also critical to enabling this sample health IT governance structure to work effectively is empowering the IT Steering Committee to adjudicate competing demands in terms of large-scale initiatives that require significant capital funding and operational resources.

Design, Implement, and Iteratively Enhance Informatics Governance

Following the baseline assessment of current health IT governance and the evaluation of the benefits and limitations of the governance models in place at peer institutions, the findings should be synthesized and a small number of candidate governance approaches should be generated for consideration by senior leaders and other key informatics stakeholders. In developing these candidate approaches, the following principles should be considered:

- Balance the sophistication of the health IT governance model with the organization's informatics capability maturity assessment.
- Develop a health IT governance structure that is reflective of the high level of organizational collaboration required for an effective health IT governance program.
- Propose a health IT governance structure that reports to the highest strategic body within the organization, whether that is an executive-level committee or a senior-level executive position.
- Consider and align with the unique characteristics and culture of the institution. For example, take into account the viewpoints and preferences of key senior leaders and whether the organization has a centralized culture with top-down decision making or a decentralized culture with consensus-driven decision making.

Following an open discussion of the candidate health IT governance model by senior leaders and other key stakeholders, the candidate approach deemed to be most suitable for the organization should be refined with operational details. Moreover, to the extent possible, consensus around the candidate approach should be developed across all stakeholder groups, in particular with groups and individuals that have traditionally had a central role in the use and prioritization of health IT governance resources.

When sufficient institutional consensus has been attained the new health IT governance model should be implemented. The impact of the new model, including unintended consequences, should be actively evaluated. The health IT governance should then be iteratively assessed and refined as needed, with the ultimate goal of ensuring that health IT is fully aligned with the strategic direction of the institution and that limited health IT resources are used optimally.

CONCLUSION AND FUTURE DIRECTIONS

Looking forward, healthcare organizations are likely to face ever more opportunities and challenges that require the effective leveraging of health IT. Given the rapidly changing healthcare environment, it will be critical for healthcare organizations to develop a health IT governance structure that allows priorities and direction to be rapidly adapted to these changes. Moreover, given the increasingly vital role of health IT in almost all aspects of a healthcare organization, it is important for health IT governance to incorporate the viewpoints of relevant stakeholders from across the enterprise in an approach that is balanced and collaborative yet still capable of focusing on strategic priorities without being pulled in a thousand directions by various competing demands. In looking toward the numerous opportunities and challenges ahead for healthcare organizations, a key factor in an organization's ability to survive and thrive will be its ability to implement effective health IT governance.

REFERENCES

1. Kropf R, Scalzi G. *IT Governance in Hospitals and Health Systems*. Chicago, IL: Healthcare Information and Management Systems Society; 2012.
2. Hoehn BJ. Clinical information technology governance. *J Healthc Inf Manag*. 2010;24(2):13-14.
3. National Health Service (NHS). Informatics Capability Maturity Model. NHS. http://www.connectingforhealth.nhs.uk/systemsandservices/icd/assessment/icmm. 2012.
4. National Health Service (NHS). Informatics Capability Maturity Model tool. NHS. http://www.connectingforhealth.nhs.uk/systemsandservices/icd/assessment/icmm/tool. 2012.

DISCUSSION QUESTIONS

1. What unique characteristics within the organizational culture at your institution are relevant in terms of their impact on health IT governance?
2. Using the Informatics Capability Maturity Model as a guide, describe the current state of health IT governance at your organization.
3. In what ways has health IT governance at your organization been affected by the Health Information Technology for Economic and Clinical Health (HITECH) Act?
4. How does the current health IT structure at your institution support or hinder the effectiveness of informatics specialists in nursing, medicine, and other disciplines?
5. What opportunities do you see for health IT governance to facilitate the achievement of strategic priorities at your institution?

CASE STUDY

Imagine that you have been hired as the chief information officer (CIO) of an academic healthcare system. The healthcare system consists of several large hospitals and several dozen outpatient clinics, all using the same EHR system. There is an affiliated but independent physician practice group as well as a School of Medicine with a strong research focus. The current health IT governance structure is as described in Figure 23-2, except that the current committees function independently of one another and, as a result, health IT resources are being overwhelmed by requests coming from a variety of sources, each with its own priority list. As one of your first tasks on the job, you have been asked to lead the formulation and implementation of a new health IT governance structure. The effectiveness of the new governance structure will be critical to your success and the success of your team and the institution as a whole.

Discussion Questions

1. How would you go about assessing the current state of health IT governance and your organization's health IT governance capabilities?
2. What issues would you need to consider in recommending improved health IT governance at your institution?
3. How could the informatics governance at your institution be more centralized, so as to allow for an enterprise-wide approach to prioritizing informatics efforts?

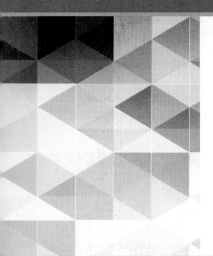

Legal Issues, Federal Regulations, and Accreditation

Michele Person Madison

As programs continue to develop and facilitate change in how healthcare is provided and how payment is received, the continued use of information technology will facilitate enhanced and creative models for new healthcare delivery designs.

OBJECTIVES

At the completion of this chapter the reader will be prepared to:

1. Discuss the federal policy initiatives related to the adoption of health information technology
2. Describe the Centers for Medicare & Medicaid Services financial incentive program to encourage the adoption of electronic health records
3. Outline the enhanced and expanded security requirements to protect patient privacy and security rights
4. Analyze the legally permissible methods for physicians and individuals to receive financial

assistance to adopt and implement an electronic health records system
5. Discuss the federal administrative, physical, and technical safeguards that apply to prevent unauthorized access, use, or disclosure of electronically transmitted patient information
6. Discuss the Centers for Medicare & Medicaid Services and the demonstration programs related to the federal healthcare reform act initiatives
7. Outline accreditation measures and agencies in the United States

KEY TERMS

Administrative safeguards, 386
Physical safeguards, 389

Technical safeguards, 389

ABSTRACT

Health information technology (health IT) is a suite of tools that the federal government intends to use to improve patient outcomes while reducing the costs of the Medicare and Medicaid programs. To achieve the improved efficiencies the federal government promulgated laws to encourage the widespread adoption of electronic health records (EHRs) while setting standards for privacy and security. Financial incentives for healthcare providers who use EHRs are subject to specific regulatory standards. The Meaningful Use (MU) standards also merge into the changes driven by the healthcare reform legislation. Throughout the funding and reform laws, the federal government's policies for improving care coordination by reducing costs and engaging patients and families remain constant elements. This chapter outlines MU

Stage 1 regulations in detail as well as introducing Stage 2 and beyond.

INTRODUCTION

This chapter provides an overview of selected federal legislation that directly affects health IT and in turn health informatics. In selecting the federal legislation to be viewed the emphasis is on the Health Information Technology for Economic and Clinical Health (HITECH) Act and the impact of this legislation on the Health Insurance Portability and Accountability Act (HIPAA) as well as the Centers for Medicare & Medicaid Services (CMS). CMS has designated The Joint Commission as an agency to accredit hospitals for participation in Medicare and Medicaid programs and the influence of this agency is discussed. The chapter concludes with a discussion of accountable care organizations (ACOs) and their implications for future directions in federal legislation.

FEDERAL INITIATIVES TO DRIVE HEALTH IT

The challenge to the healthcare system in the United States is improving the quality of care for patients while reducing the costs of delivering such care. Implementing health IT has been lauded as a critical element to address this challenge. Promoting the adoption and implementation of health IT is a bipartisan initiative that has been endorsed by both Republican and Democratic presidents beginning with President George W. Bush in 2004.

Executive Order 13335

On April 27, 2004, President George W. Bush signed Executive Order 13335 that outlined the federal initiative of granting federal dollars to incentivize healthcare providers to implement and use health IT. The Executive Order created the position of Office of the National Coordinator for Health Information Technology (ONC) with the goal of facilitating the widespread adoption and implementation of EHRs across the United States. Ultimately the goals were to develop a Nationwide Health Information Network (NwHIN) and to ensure that all residents of the United States have access to a clinical health record by 2014.

The federal initiative was built on six key components that have continued to serve as the foundation of the revolutionary changes to the healthcare delivery system in the United States. In 2004 the fundamental policies set forth by President Bush were as follows:

1. To ensure that appropriate information to guide medical decisions is available at the time and place of care
2. To improve healthcare quality, reduce medical errors, and advance the delivery of appropriate, evidence-based medical care
3. To reduce healthcare costs resulting from inefficiency, medical errors, inappropriate care, and incomplete information
4. To promote a more effective marketplace, greater competition, and increased choice through the wider availability of accurate information on healthcare costs, quality, and outcomes
5. To improve the coordination of care and information among hospitals, laboratories, physician offices, and other ambulatory care providers through an effective infrastructure for the secure and authorized exchange of health information
6. To ensure that patients' individually identifiable health information is secure and protected[1]

The American Recovery and Reinvestment Act of 2009

As mentioned above, Executive Order 13335 created the ONC. This office was charged with implementing an interoperable health IT system in both the public and the private

healthcare sectors to reduce medical errors, improve quality, and produce greater value for healthcare expenditures. While the initial framework was established in 2004 it was not until 2009, when the federal government passed the American Recovery and Reinvestment Act of 2009 (Stimulus Act), that the initiative was actually funded.[2] The Stimulus Act took the federal policy for an NwHIN to a new and elevated level. This Act included the HITECH Act, which among other initiatives dedicated $27 billion to incentivize healthcare providers to adopt and use EHRs by providing the needed funding (Box 24-1).

BOX 24-1   SECTIONS OF THE HITECH ACT

Title XXX—Health Information Technology and Quality
Sec. 3000. Definitions.

Subtitle A—Promotion of Health Information Technology
Sec. 3001. Office of the National Coordinator for Health Information Technology.
Sec. 3002. HIT Policy Committee.
Sec. 3003. HIT Standards Committee.
Sec. 3004. Process for Adoption of Endorsed Recommendations; Adoption of Initial Set of Standards, Implementation Specifications, and Certification Criteria.
Sec. 3005. Application and Use of Adopted Standards and Implementation Specifications by Federal Agencies.
Sec. 3006. Voluntary Application and Use of Adopted Standards and Implementation Specifications by Private Entities.
Sec. 3007. Federal Health Information Technology.
Sec. 3008. Transitions.
Sec. 3009. Miscellaneous Provisions.

From The American Recovery and Reinvestment Act of 2009. http://www.gpo.gov/fdsys/pkg/BILLS-111hr1enr/pdf/BILLS-111hr1enr.pdf. 2009. Accessed November 8, 2012.
HIT, Health information technology; *HITECH*, Health Information Technology for Economic and Clinical Health.

Office of the National Coordinator for Health Information Technology

Section 3001 of the HITECH Act established the ONC as a funded position with powers and authority granted by statutory support. Establishing the ONC through federal statutes instead of an Executive Order emphasized the fact that this position and its operations were approved and endorsed by both parties in Congress and represented a critical component of the federally mandated strategic plan. Section 3001 lists the duties of the ONC and groups these duties into eight areas (Box 24-2). Section 3001 of the HITECH Act directs the ONC to create a strategic plan to address the following federal initiatives:

1. The electronic exchange and use of health information and the enterprise integration of such information
2. The use of an EHR for each person in the United States by 2014
3. The incorporation of privacy and security protections for the electronic exchange of individually identifiable health information
4. Security methods to ensure appropriate authorization and electronic authentication of health information and specifying technologies or methodologies for rendering health information unusable, unreadable, or indecipherable
5. A framework for coordination and flow of recommendations and policies under the HITECH Act among the Secretary, the ONC, the Health IT Policy Committee, the Health IT Standards Committee, and other health information exchanges and other relevant entities
6. Methods to foster the public understanding of health IT
7. Strategies to enhance the use of health IT in improving the quality of care, reducing medical errors, reducing health disparities, improving public health, increasing prevention and coordination with community resources, and improving the continuity of care among healthcare settings
8. Specific plans to ensure that populations with unique needs, such as children, are appropriately addressed in the technology design, which may include technology that automates enrollment and retention for eligible individuals[2]

Health IT Policy Committee and Health IT Standards Committee

To establish national uniform standards for the electronic exchange of health information and facilitate the strategic plan, the HITECH Act included in the duties of the ONC responsibility for creating two committees that report to the ONC. The first is the Health IT Policy Committee, which was charged with making policy recommendations to the ONC relating to the implementation of a nationwide health IT infrastructure, including implementation of the eight components of the strategic plan. The Health IT Policy Committee is composed of individual stakeholders representing the full spectrum of the healthcare delivery system. These stakeholders include individual healthcare providers, patients, healthcare payer plans, legislative representatives, technology vendors, privacy and security experts, and other interested parties. Each stakeholder brings unique expertise and ultimately creates the policies defining Meaningful Use of certified EHR systems.

The second committee, the Health IT Standards Committee, was charged with recommending standards, implementation specifications, and certification criteria for EHRs, electronic exchange, and use of health information. Specific standards for the electronic exchange of health information enable each healthcare provider, regardless of location, to transmit healthcare information and allow the receiving party to receive the data directly in its EHR system. However, to ensure that healthcare providers implement EHRs that are based on the uniform national standards to permit meaningful exchange of data, each provider must use an EHR that has been certified by an ONC certification entity. The NwHIN is dependent on the adoption of uniform standards and requires that all healthcare providers use certified technology that satisfies the policies and standards set forth by the Health IT Policy Committee and the Health IT Standards Committee.

The Health IT Standards Committee also is a multistakeholder committee that includes healthcare providers, insurance companies, health IT companies that translate billing claims in nonstandard forms to a format that complies with specific electronic transaction standards (clearinghouses), academic institutions, and individuals who have specific health IT expertise and knowledge. In coordination with the Health IT Policy Committee, the Health IT Standards Committee established the standards and uniform requirements for technology to exchange data and to be deemed "certified" by the federal government. Both of these committees engaged in research and workgroups and facilitated the development of specific policies and standards to develop the foundational components of the NwHIN.

FEDERAL FINANCIAL INCENTIVES

The ultimate goal of the NwHIN is to support significant and measurable improvements in population health by an improved healthcare system. The vision includes engaging patients in their healthcare and ensuring that providers have immediate access to health information and tools to improve the quality and safety of care delivery. NwHIN also includes provisions for improved access and decreased healthcare disparities. To achieve this vision healthcare providers must adopt and implement certified EHRs. Due to the cost of an EHR many healthcare providers were reluctant to purchase a system. The HITECH Act amended the Social Security Act (42 U.S.C. 1395w-4) to provide financial incentives directly to healthcare providers that adopt, implement, and engage in Meaningful Use of certified EHR technology. If an eligible professional or entity achieves and demonstrates, to the satisfaction of the Secretary of the Department of Health & Human Services (HHS), that it adopted, implemented,

---

BOX 24-2 DUTIES OF THE NATIONAL COORDINATOR

1. Standards
2. HIT policy coordination
3. Strategic plan
4. Website
5. Certification
6. Reports and publications
7. Assistance
8. Governance for Nationwide Health Information Network

Data from the Health Information Technology for Economic and Clinical Health Act. 42 U.S.C. § 300jj-11. 2009. Retrieved from http://www.hhs.gov/ocr/privacy/hipaa/understanding/coveredentities/hitechact.pdf.
HIT, Health information technology.

upgraded, and used a certified EHR technology in a meaningful manner, the eligible professional or entity can receive financial incentives.

Eligible Entities and Eligible Professionals

Some healthcare providers are eligible to participate in both the Medicare and the Medicaid programs while others are limited to only one potential program. Eligible entities for the Medicare program include the following:

1. All licensed hospitals that are reimbursed based on the prospective payment system
2. Critical Access Hospitals

An eligible professional in the Medicare program is a doctor of medicine or osteopathy legally authorized to practice medicine and surgery, a doctor of dental surgery, a doctor of podiatric medicine, a doctor of optometry, or a chiropractor (see HITECH Act, Section 4101). All physicians participating in the Medicare program are eligible to participate in the financial incentive program regardless of the total percentage of Medicare patients treated by each physician.

To be eligible to participate in the Medicaid program, an individual physician must have a 30% Medicaid patient population. Pediatricians with a 20% Medicaid patient population are also eligible; however, these pediatricians will be eligible only for two thirds of the financial incentives (see HITECH Act, Section 4201). The Medicaid program's eligible provider category also extends to certified nurse midwives and nurse practitioners. Physician assistants practicing in rural health clinics and federally qualified health centers are eligible to participate.

Children's hospitals are eligible to participate in the Medicaid program and do not require a specific volume of Medicaid patients; other hospitals must have at least a 10% Medicaid patient volume to be eligible to participate in the Medicaid incentive program. Hospitals that satisfy the eligibility requirements may participate in both the Medicare and the Medicaid programs. However, individual physicians may participate in only one financial incentive program. Physicians are allowed to change from one program to the other but this change is permitted only one time during the program.

Medicare and Medicaid Payments

Medicare payments are based on 75% of an individual physician's allowable Medicare charges for the payment year to a maximum cap per year. To encourage healthcare providers to adopt and implement EHRs early, physicians are eligible for Medicare incentives up to $18,000 in the first two payment years and then the amounts decline each year thereafter, with a total capped amount of $44,000 during the entire program. If a physician is providing services in a Health Professional Shortage Area (HPSA), the physician is eligible for a 10% increase in payments.

Medicaid payments for eligible professionals are based on 85% of the costs attributed to the purchase of a certified EHR. In the first year the total payment to a physician by the state Medicaid program is capped at $25,000 and then is $10,000 for each subsequent year, with a total capped amount of $63,750.

For hospitals that participate in the Medicare program, the payment amount is based on a calculation that will result in a different amount for each hospital. Each hospital must calculate its payment based on the mathematical formula created by the CMS, as described in Table 24-1. For the Medicaid program, the calculation for hospitals is based on a different formula than the one described in Table 24-1 and depends on how many Medicaid patients receive care at the hospital.

The financial incentives provided through the Stimulus Act are carrots to encourage healthcare providers to adopt and implement EHRs in an expedited manner. The downside following the financial incentives period is that if healthcare providers fail to adopt and implement EHR systems by 2016, their Medicare reimbursement will decrease. Specifically, if a physician or chiropractor fails to adopt and implement an EHR by 2016, his or her Medicare reimbursement will decrease by 1% for each year up to a maximum 5% reduction. Hospitals and healthcare providers will not receive any Medicare financial incentives after 2016.

Meaningful Use

Notwithstanding the monetary incentive plans, to ensure that healthcare providers would electronically enter and exchange patient information to improve patient outcomes, the federal government determined that healthcare providers' behavior

TABLE 24-1 HOSPITAL MEDICARE PAYMENT CALCULATION		
	HOSPITALS WITH 1,149 OR FEWER DISCHARGES DURING THE PAYMENT YEAR	**HOSPITALS WITH AT LEAST 1,150 BUT NO MORE THAN 23,000 DISCHARGES DURING THE PAYMENT YEAR**	**HOSPITALS WITH 23,001 OR MORE DISCHARGES DURING THE PAYMENT YEAR**
Base amount	$2,000,000	$2,000,000	$2,000,000
Discharge-related amount	$0	$200 × (n − 1,149) (n is the number of discharges during the payment year)	$200 × (23,001 − 1,149)
Total initial amount	$2,000,000	Between $2M and $6,370,400 depending on the number of discharges	Limited by law to $6,370,400

From Centers for Medicare & Medicaid Services (CMS). EHR incentive program for Medicare hospitals. CMS. http://www.cms.gov/Outreach-and-Education/Medicare-Learning-Network-MLN/MLNProducts/downloads/EHR_TipSheet_Medicare_Hosp.pdf. Accessed November 8, 2012.

must change. Therefore to obtain Medicare payments the eligible professional or entity must use certified EHRs "meaningfully." Section 4101 of the HITECH Act defines Meaningful Use as eprescribing, engaging in health information exchange, and submitting information on clinical quality measures and other measures specified by the Secretary of HHS. Therefore by requiring healthcare providers to adopt certified health record systems and perform and report on specific measures, the end goal is to change provider behavior and increase the electronic exchange of patient information.

As described above, the Health IT Policy Committee and the Health IT Standards Committee focused on establishing the underlying policies and standards to establish the NwHIN. The ultimate goal identified by the Health IT Policy Committee is to enable significant and measurable improvements in population health through a transformed healthcare delivery system. The goal of the financial incentive program is to encourage eligible healthcare providers to change their behavior to achieve the strategic goals of electronically exchanging health information to improve patient care while supporting the NwHIN. However, adoption of certified EHRs without using the EHRs in a meaningful manner was insufficient to facilitate the NwHIN. Therefore the financial incentives were only remitted to healthcare providers that became meaningful EHR users.

The Health IT Policy Committee identified the following five main policy initiatives to define and model MU:

1. Improve quality, safety, and efficiencies and reduce health disparities
2. Engage patients and families
3. Improve care coordination
4. Improve population and public health
5. Ensure adequate privacy and security protections for personal health information[3]

Generally, each policy conforms to the initiatives from both the 2004 and the 2009 legislation designed to reduce medical errors, improve communication, and facilitate secure electronic transmission of patient information. The Health IT Policy Committee and the Health IT Standards Committee developed specific measures for each healthcare provider to perform and report on to successfully be deemed a meaningful EHR user. Each measure is directly related to driving the use of IT in the clinical care setting. Because individual healthcare providers have different types of practices, the Health IT Policy Committee and the Health IT Standards Committee divided the MU metrics into "core" required elements and "menu" elements. Permitting healthcare providers an opportunity to report on required core elements and then choose to report on a select few "menu" elements addresses the unique aspects of each provider's practice or facility and adds flexibility to the financial incentives program. Table 24-2 provides a detailed description of the core and menu elements.

Although each year the Medicare program requires attesting to the MU metrics, the Medicaid program is much more flexible. In the first year healthcare providers do not have to satisfy the MU metrics. Instead, if a provider adopts, implements, or upgrades an EHR system during the first payment year, the individual physician will be eligible to receive payments to a maximum of approximately $21,000 to $25,000 during that first year. Because Medicaid is a state program, each state may require different forms of verification that the

Text continued on page 386

TABLE 24-2	MEANINGFUL USE		
CORE SET			
HEALTH OUTCOMES POLICY PRIORITY	**STAGE 1 OBJECTIVES**		
	ELIGIBLE PROFESSIONALS	ELIGIBLE HOSPITALS AND CAHs	STAGE 1 MEASURES
Improving quality, safety, efficiency, and reducing health disparities	Use CPOE for medication orders directly entered by any licensed healthcare professional who can enter orders into the medical record per state, local, and professional guidelines	Use CPOE for medication orders directly entered by any licensed healthcare professional who can enter orders into the medical record per state, local, and professional guidelines	More than 30% of unique patients with at least one medication in their medication list seen by the EP or admitted to the eligible hospital's or CAH's inpatient or emergency department (POS 21 or 23) have at least one medication order entered using CPOE
	Implement drug–drug and drug–allergy interaction checks	Implement drug–drug and drug–allergy interaction checks	The EP/eligible hospital/CAH has enabled this functionality for the entire EHR reporting period
	Generate and transmit permissible prescriptions electronically (eRx)		More than 40% of all permissible prescriptions written by the EP are transmitted electronically using certified EHR technology

Continued

TABLE 24-2   MEANINGFUL USE—cont'd

CORE SET

HEALTH OUTCOMES POLICY PRIORITY	STAGE 1 OBJECTIVES		STAGE 1 MEASURES
	ELIGIBLE PROFESSIONALS	ELIGIBLE HOSPITALS AND CAHs	
	Record demographics • Preferred language • Gender • Race • Ethnicity • Date of birth	Record demographics • Preferred language • Gender • Race • Ethnicity • Date of birth • Date and preliminary cause of death in the event of mortality in the eligible hospital or CAH	More than 50% of all unique patients seen by the EP or admitted to the eligible hospital's or CAH's inpatient or emergency department (POS 21 or 23) have demographics recorded as structured data
	Maintain an up-to-date problem list of current and active diagnoses	Maintain an up-to-date problem list of current and active diagnoses	More than 80% of all unique patients seen by the EP or admitted to the eligible hospital's or CAH's inpatient or emergency department (POS 21 or 23) have demographics recorded as structured data
	Maintain active medication list	Maintain active medication list	More than 80% of all unique patients seen by the EP or admitted to the eligible hospital's or CAH's inpatient or emergency department (POS 21 or 23) have at least one entry (or an indication that the patient is not currently prescribed any medication) recorded as structured data
	Maintain active medication allergy list	Maintain active medication allergy list	More than 80% of all unique patients seen by the EP or admitted to the eligible hospital's or CAH's inpatient or emergency department (POS 21 or 23) have at least one entry (or an indication that the patient is not currently prescribed any medication) recorded as structured data
	Record and chart changes in vital signs: • Height • Weight • Blood pressure • Calculate and display BMI • Plot and display growth charts for children 2-20 years, including BMI	Record and chart changes in vital signs: • Height • Weight • Blood pressure • Calculate and display BMI • Plot and display growth charts for children 2-20 years, including BMI	For more than 50% of all unique patients aged 2 years and over seen by the EP or admitted to eligible hospital's or CAH's inpatient or emergency department (POS 21 or 23), height, weight and blood pressure are recorded as structured data
	Record smoking status for patients aged 13 years or older	Record smoking status for patients aged 13 years or older	More than 50% of all unique patients aged 13 years or older seen by the EP or admitted to the eligible hospital's or CAH's inpatient or emergency department (POS 21 or 23) have smoking status recorded as structured data

TABLE 24-2   MEANINGFUL USE—cont'd

	CORE SET		
HEALTH OUTCOMES POLICY PRIORITY	**STAGE 1 OBJECTIVES**		
	ELIGIBLE PROFESSIONALS	**ELIGIBLE HOSPITALS AND CAHs**	**STAGE 1 MEASURES**
	Implement one clinical decision support rule relevant to specialty or high clinical priority along with the ability to track compliance with that rule	Implement one clinical decision support rule relevant to specialty or high clinical priority along with the ability to track compliance with that rule	Implement one clinical decision support rule
	Report ambulatory clinical quality measures to CMS or the States	Report hospital clinical quality measures to CMS or the States	For 2011, provide aggregate numerator, denominator, and exclusions through attestation as discussed in section II(A)(3) of this final rule
			For 2012, electronically submit the clinical quality measures as discussed in section II(A)(3) of this final rule
Engage patients and families in their health care	Provide patients with an electronic copy of their health information (including diagnostic test results, problem list, medication lists, medication allergies), upon request	Provide patients with an electronic copy of their health information (including diagnostic test results, problem list, medication lists, medication allergies, discharge summary, procedures), upon request	More than 50% of all patients of the EP or the inpatient or emergency departments of the eligible hospital or CAH (POS 21 or 23) who request an electronic copy of their health information are provided it within 3 business days
		Provide patients with an electronic copy of their discharge instructions at time of discharge, upon request	More than 50% of all patients who are discharged from an eligible hospital's or CAH's inpatient department or emergency department (POS 21 or 23) and who request an electronic copy of their discharge instructions are provided it
	Provide clinical summaries for patients for each office visit		Clinical summaries provided to patients for more than 50% of all office visits within 3 business days
Improve care coordination	Capability to exchange key clinical information (for example, problem list, medication lists, medication allergies, diagnostic test results), among providers of care and patient authorized entities electronically	Capability to exchange key clinical information (for example, discharge summary, procedures, problem list, medication lists, medication allergies, diagnostic test results), among providers of care and patient authorized entities electronically	Performed at least one test of certified EHR technology's capacity to electronically exchange key information
Ensure adequate privacy and security protections for personal health information	Protect electronic health information created or maintained by the certified EHR technology through the implementation of appropriate technical capabilities	Protect electronic health information created or maintained by the certified EHR technology through the implementation of appropriate technical capabilities	Conduct or review a security risk analysis per 45 CFR 164.308 (a)(1) and implement security updates as necessary and correct identified security deficiencies as part of its risk management process

Continued

TABLE 24-2   MEANINGFUL USE—cont'd

MENU SET

HEALTH OUTCOMES POLICY PRIORITY	STAGE 1 OBJECTIVES		STAGE 1 MEASURES
	ELIGIBLE PROFESSIONALS	ELIGIBLE HOSPITALS AND CAHs	
Improving quality, safety, efficiency, and reducing health disparities	Implement drug-formulary checks	Implement drug-formulary checks	The EP/eligible hospital/CAH has enabled this functionality and has access to at least one internal or external drug formulary for the entire EHR reporting period
		Record advance directives for patients aged 65 years or older	More than 50% of all unique patients aged 65 years or older admitted to the eligible hospital's or CAH's inpatient department (POS 21) have an indication of an advance directive status recorded
	Incorporate clinical lab test results into certified EHR technology as structured data	Incorporate clinical lab test results into certified EHR technology as structured data	More than 40% of all clinical lab test results ordered by the EP or by an authorized provider of the eligible hospital or CAH for patients admitted to its inpatient or emergency department (POS 21 or 23) during the EHR reporting period whose results are either in a positive/negative or numerical format are incorporated in certified EHR technology as structured data
	Generate lists of patients by specific conditions to use for quality improvement, reduction of disparities, research or outreach	Generate lists of patients by specific conditions to use for quality improvement, reduction of disparities, research or outreach	Generate at least one report listing patients of the EP, eligible hospital or CAH with a specific condition
	Send reminders to patients per patient preference for preventative/follow-up care		More than 20% of all unique patients aged 65 years or older or 5 years or younger were sent an appropriate reminder during the EHR reporting period
Engage patients and families in their health care	Provide patients with timely electronic access to their health information (including lab results, problem list, medication lists, medication allergies) within four business days of the information being available to the EP		More than 10% of all unique patients seen by the EP are provided timely (available to the patient within four business days of being updated in the certified EHR technology) electronic access to their health information subject to the EP's discretion to withhold certain information
	Use certified EHR technology to identify patient-specific education resources and provide those resources to the patient if appropriate	Use certified EHR technology to identify patient-specific education resources and provide those resources to the patient if appropriate	More than 10% of all unique patients seen by the EP or admitted to the eligible hospital's or CAH's inpatient or emergency department (POS 21 or 23) are provided patient-specific education resources

TABLE 24-2	MEANINGFUL USE—cont'd		
	MENU SET		
HEALTH OUTCOMES POLICY PRIORITY	**STAGE 1 OBJECTIVES**		
	ELIGIBLE PROFESSIONALS	**ELIGIBLE HOSPITALS AND CAHs**	**STAGE 1 MEASURES**
Improve care coordination	The EP, eligible hospital, or CAH who receives a patient from another setting of care or provider of care or believes an encounter is relevant should perform medication reconciliation	The EP, eligible hospital, or CAH who receives a patient from another setting of care or provider of care or believes an encounter is relevant should perform medication reconciliation	The EP, eligible hospital, or CAH performs medication reconciliation for more than 50% of transitions of care in which the patient is transitioned into the care of the EP or admitted to the eligible hospital's or CAH's inpatient or emergency department (POS 21 or 23)
	The EP, eligible hospital, or CAH who transitions their patient to another setting of care or provider of care or refers their patient to another provider of care should provide a summary of care record for each transition of care or referral	The EP, eligible hospital, or CAH who transitions their patient to another setting of care or provider of care or refers their patient to another provider of care should provide a summary of care record for each transition of care or referral	The EP, eligible hospital, or CAH who transitions or refers their patient to another setting of care or provider of care provides a summary of care record for more than 50% of transitions of care and referrals
Improve population and public health*	Capability to submit electronic data to immunization registries or Immunization Information Systems and actual submission in accordance with applicable law and practice	Capability to submit electronic data to immunization registries or Immunization Information Systems and actual submission in accordance with applicable law and practice	Performed at least one test of certified EHR technology's capacity to submit electronic data to immunization registries and followed up submission to determine if the test was successful (unless none of the immunization registries to which the EP, eligible hospital, or CAH submits such information have the capacity to receive the information electronically)
		Capability to submit electronic data on reportable (as required by state or local law) lab results to public health agencies and actual submission in accordance with applicable law and practice	Performed at least one test of certified EHR technology's capacity to provide electronic submission of reportable lab results to public health agencies and followed up submission to determine if the test was successful (unless none of the public health agencies to which eligible hospital or CAH submits such information have the capacity to receive the information electronically)
	Capability to submit electronic syndromic surveillance data to public health agencies and actual submission in accordance with applicable law and practice	Capability to submit electronic syndromic surveillance data to public health agencies and actual submission in accordance with applicable law and practice	Performed at least one test of certified EHR technology's capacity to provide electronic syndromic surveillance data to public health agencies and followed up submission to determine if the test was successful (unless none of the public health agencies to which eligible hospital or CAH submits such information have the capacity to receive the information electronically)

From Centers for Medicare & Medicaid Services. Department of Health and Human Services: Medicare and Medicaid programs; Electronic Health Record Incentive Program; Final rule. *Federal Register.* 2010;75(144).
BMI, Body mass index; *CAH,* Critical Access Hospital; *CMS,* Centers for Medicare & Medicaid Services; *CPOE,* computerized provider order entry; *EHR,* electronic health record; *EP,* eligible professional; *eRx,* eprescribing; *POS,* place of service.
*Unless an EP, eligible hospital, or CAH has an exception for all of these objectives and measures, they must complete at least one part of their demonstration of the menu set in order to be a meaningful EHR user.

healthcare provider adopted, implemented, or upgraded an EHR system. For each subsequent year providers must attest to achieving the MU metrics to obtain Medicaid incentives. The Medicaid program also extends payments for 5 years as long as the healthcare provider begins by 2016. Thus Medicare financial incentives cease as of 2015 but Medicaid funding may continue until 2021.

Further, to effectively change healthcare provider behavior, the reporting obligations have been divided into three stages. The first stage, which commenced in 2011 with an end date of 2014, required reporting on specific measurements to achieve MU. The intention of Stage 1 is to enable the collection of meaningful data in a coded format to permit tracking of key clinical conditions and communication of that information for care coordination purposes.[4] Stage 1 metrics also require the implementation of clinical decision support tools to facilitate disease and medication management, reporting clinical quality measures, and public health information. Stage 1 established a foundation of adopting technology with uniform functions that enable healthcare providers to change their behavior. Stage 2 metrics, which have been delayed until 2014, are designed to encourage continuous quality improvement and the exchange of information. Stage 2 focuses on the structured formats created to electronically transmit patient data between healthcare providers.[4] Stage 2 takes the Stage 1 objectives that were optional and incorporates these measures into the required core elements. The final rules for Stage 2 were announced in August 2012 and make it clear that no healthcare providers will be required to follow the Stage 2 requirements before 2014. Table 24-2 provides a comparison of the core and menu MU requirements.

The CMS final rule also provides a flexible reporting period for 2014 to give healthcare providers sufficient time to adopt or upgrade to the latest EHR technology certified for 2014. A fact sheet on CMS's final rule is available at www.cms.gov/apps/media/fact_sheets.asp. A fact sheet on ONC's standards and certification criteria final rule is available at http://healthit.hhs.gov/standardsandcertification.

Currently scheduled to begin in 2015, Stage 3 will require higher standards for healthcare providers to be deemed meaningful users of certified EHRs. The optional standards under Stage 2 will be mandatory measures in Stage 3. Stage 3 promotes improvements in quality, safety, and efficiency. Stage 3 goes beyond merely exchanging data electronically and focuses on improving the general population health. Instead of healthcare providers changing their behavior in the practice setting, Stage 3 intends to use technology to engage in decision support analysis for studying chronic disease and best practices. Stage 3 is the final phase for the MU incentive program but likely will not be the final phase of expanding and enhancing the health IT infrastructure necessary to facilitate an effective NwHIN.

HIPAA SECURITY RULE AND PRIVACY RULES

Responding to concerns about the security and privacy of protected health information (PHI), the HITECH Act enhanced the privacy and security measures that are required for all healthcare providers. In 1998 the federal government initially proposed a Security Rule to address the security of electronic PHI, thereby enhancing the HIPAA Privacy Rule, which addressed the use and disclosure of PHI. On April 21, 2003, the HIPAA Security Rule became effective and serves as the minimum level of security safeguards required by federal law. The Security Rule applies to all "covered entities," which includes health plans, healthcare clearinghouses, and healthcare providers that electronically transmit PHI. After the passage of the HITECH Act, the Security Rule also applied directly to business associates. The Security Rule requires each applicable organization to implement specific administrative, physical, and technical safeguards to protect the security, integrity, and confidentiality of electronic PHI (Table 24-3).

Administrative Safeguards

The first and most critical component of the Security Rule is the security management process, which requires each covered entity and business associate to perform administrative safeguards, or a risk analysis of its organization, and to evaluate how it uses, discloses, and accesses electronic PHI. The risk analysis should include evaluating and addressing each administrative, physical, and technical safeguard set forth by the Security Rule. In response to the risk analysis, the risk management process should include implementing corrective work plans to mitigate potential issues or vulnerabilities that may result in a breach of electronic PHI. The security management process also includes an information system activity review, which requires the organization to map how PHI is used, disclosed, accessed, and stored as part of the organization's operations. By engaging in the information system activity review, the organization may identify vulnerabilities that should be addressed through the risk management process.

An example of an information system activity review is evaluating where and how nurses use an EHR. If a home health nurse treats patients in a home setting and documents the clinical findings in the EHR through a mobile device, analyzing how the clinical information is documented and the location and the means of transmission should be considered part of the information system activity review. The technology, including the software, used on the mobile device should be evaluated to ensure that it is secure. Further, the device should be evaluated to determine whether the EHR is accessed through a secure portal or the information is documented directly on the mobile device. Finally, the technology protection used in transmitting the data should be evaluated to ensure that it is secure and not susceptible to hackers or a security incident. This review should be documented and any and all remedial actions should be implemented in a timely manner.

In addition to the information security analysis, organizations are required to assign an individual to be responsible for the security of electronic PHI. This individual serves in a similar capacity as a privacy officer under the HIPAA Privacy

TABLE 24-3 SECURITY SAFEGUARDS

ADMINISTRATIVE SAFEGUARDS

STANDARDS	SECTIONS	IMPLEMENTATION SPECIFICATIONS (R) = REQUIRED; (A) = ADDRESSABLE	
Security Management Process	§ 164.308(a)(1)	Risk Analysis	(R)
		Risk Management	(R)
		Sanction Policy	(R)
		Information System Activity Review	(R)
Assigned Security Responsibility	§ 164.308(a)(2)		
Workforce Security	§ 164.308(a)(3)	Authorization and/or Supervision	(A)
		Workforce Clearance Procedure	(A)
		Termination Procedures	(A)
Information Access Management	§ 164.308(a)(4)	Isolating Health Care Clearinghouse Functions	(R)
		Access Authorization	(A)
		Access Establishment and Modification	(A)
Security Awareness and Training	§ 164.308(a)(5)	Security Reminders	(A)
		Protection from Malicious Software	(A)
		Log-in Monitoring	(A)
		Password Management	(A)
Security Incident Procedures	§ 164.308(a)(6)	Response and Reporting	(R)
Contingency Plan	§ 164.308(a)(7)	Data Backup Plan	(R)
		Disaster Recovery Plan	(R)
		Emergency Mode Operation Plan	(R)
		Testing and Revision Procedures	(A)
		Applications and Data Criticality Analysis	(A)
Evaluation	§ 164.308(a)(8)		
Business Associate Contracts and Other Arrangements	§ 164.308(b)(1)	Written Contract or Other Arrangement	(R)

PHYSICAL SAFEGUARDS

STANDARDS	SECTIONS	IMPLEMENTATION SPECIFICATIONS (R) = REQUIRED; (A) = ADDRESSABLE	
Facility Access Controls	§ 164.310(a)(1)	Contingency Operations	(A)
		Facility Security Plan	(A)
		Access Control and Validation Procedures	(A)
		Maintenance Records	(A)
Workstation Use	§ 164.310(b)		
Workstation Security	§ 164.310(c)		
Device and Media Controls	§ 164.310(d)(1)	Disposal	(R)
		Media Re-use	(R)
		Accountability	(A)
		Data Backup and Storage	(A)

TECHNICAL SAFEGUARDS

STANDARDS	SECTIONS	IMPLEMENTATION SPECIFICATIONS (R) = REQUIRED; (A) = ADDRESSABLE	
Access Control	§ 164.312(a)(1)	Unique User Identification	(R)
		Emergency Access Procedure	(R)
		Automatic Logoff	(A)
		Encryption and Decryption	(A)
Auto Controls	§ 164.312(b)		
Integrity	§ 164.312(c)(1)	Mechanism to Authenticate Electronic Protected Health Information	(A)
Person or Entity Authentication	§ 164.312(d)		
Transmission Security	§ 164.312(e)(1)	Integrity Controls	(A)
		Encryption	(A)

From Centers for Medicare & Medicaid Services. *HIPAA Security Series*. Volume 2, paper 1. 2007.

Rule. One of the security officer's responsibilities is to address the workforce security measures to ensure that the organization has safeguards in place to limit access to PHI to authorized individuals only. Each organization must have a method to perform workforce clearance procedures and educate employees about their obligation to maintain the privacy and security protections before they are granted access to the IT systems. For example, when an individual is hired the organization should provide training on HIPAA and its requirements. Each employee should be trained on the IT systems and the security measures. Prior to granting an employee a unique password to access the IT systems, he or she should be required to pass a test and provide evidence of competency on the proper privacy and security safeguards to comply with the applicable laws. Unless an employee can demonstrate competency, he or she should not be "cleared" to use, access, or disclose patient information.

As part of the organization's security management process, the organization must maintain a sanction policy to either discipline or terminate employees who violate the protections afforded to patient PHI. If an employee improperly accesses medical records, the organization must have a method to discipline the individual, depending on the circumstances of the breach. A sanction policy should provide for discipline ranging from verbal counseling to termination. An example of a proper termination occurred in 2006 at Northeast Arkansas Clinic. A licensed practical nurse improperly accessed a patient's records and provided the information to her husband. The husband threatened the patient about using the information in an ongoing legal proceeding. Because of this intentional and improper taking of patient information, the nurse was terminated from her employment. The termination was proper and in accordance with the HIPAA sanction policy requirements.

Likewise, organizations must ensure that when an individual is terminated, his or her access to the EHR and PHI is terminated in a timely manner. If an employee leaves his or her employment but can still access the IT systems remotely, this will be deemed a breach and a security violation of the organization. Furthermore, organizations are required to evaluate how they permit access to information systems. Specifically, organizations must establish access to the minimum necessary information for an individual to perform his or her job function.

Access to information must be strictly controlled. First, the covered entity must isolate any of its operations that involve healthcare clearinghouse functions from its other business operations. HIPAA defines clearinghouse functions as follows:
1. Processing or facilitating processing of health information in a nonstandard format into standard data elements or a standard transaction, or
2. Receiving a standard transaction and processing or facilitating the processing of health information into a nonstandard format for the original sender

Many healthcare providers perform billing and collection activities for multiple third parties by taking data and modifying the PHI into a standard format as required by the HIPAA Transaction and Code Set Standards. Converting data from nonstandard to standard billing formats differs from the day-to-day healthcare operations for providers of healthcare services. Therefore the healthcare provider must isolate the clearinghouse functions to prevent comingling of data and to maintain the integrity of the clearinghouse function.

Further, in an effort to ensure that access to PHI is limited to only the individuals who require it, access must be established based on job function or role in the organization. Access to PHI should be managed through a uniform process. Access for some members of the workforce will be limited to specific modules or software programs. In addition, the organization should have a process to modify an individual's access in the event that the individual's job changes. For example, if a billing clerk is transferred to the registration department, the organization must maintain a process to modify the modules, databases, and software programs that the employee's password can access. Thus access to the modules and databases affiliated with billing should be terminated and the registration modules should be added to this employee's access rights.

Once access has been established, the organization must also engage in security awareness training. Security awareness training requires educating employees about security reminders, avoiding leaving workstations unattended, protecting from malicious software, and learning how to take preventive and proactive actions to prevent unauthorized access or disclosure of PHI. For example, on a regular basis employees should be informed that emails from unknown senders should not be opened and should be deleted. Furthermore, emails with attachments that contain non–work-related matters should not be opened as the attachments may contain malicious viruses, Trojans, or malware. Security awareness training requires providing a password to an individual that is unique and can be monitored through log-in monitoring of the information access management process within the organization. Each individual employee or workforce member should be cautioned not to share passwords to avoid any unauthorized access to the electronic PHI.

Each organization must also address how it responds and reports security incidents. The HIPAA Privacy Rule defines a security incident as "the attempted or successful unauthorized access, use, disclosure, modification, or destruction of information or interference with system operations in an information system."[5] Each organization is required to ensure that any attempted or successful security incident is addressed and reported. Therefore any ping to the network or attempt by a third party to access a network or database must be identified and tracked to ensure that the information can be reported even if the actual PHI is not accessed. For many organizations this is an impracticable task due to the extensive number of pings and unsuccessful attempts that occur on a daily basis to the network. This portion of HIPAA may be refined as time goes by. In addition, when the HITECH Act was passed, security incidents and the reporting requirements regarding breaches of unsecured PHI enhanced the obligations of all organizations. This is explored later in this chapter.

Organizations must also have backup plans, disaster recovery plans, and an emergency mode of operation to test and revise procedures in the event of an emergency. Additional information about these types of plans is included in Chapter 18. Contingency plans must be implemented by each organization to ensure that electronic PHI is accessible for healthcare providers in the event of an emergency. For example, if hospitals utilized EHR systems when Hurricane Katrina hit New Orleans, the individual hospitals with EHR systems would have been required to implement a contingency plan so that the EHRs could be accessed either internally or remotely, notwithstanding the loss of power and flooding occurring within the city. If the hospitals had EHR systems, these hospitals would have initiated the emergency mode of operation. Prior to commencing the contingency plan the hospital would have identified which databases and types of information were critical to the delivery of care during an emergency. The contingency plan would require that the most critical data sources and types of data be retrieved first during the emergency situation. All of these efforts and planning are intended to ensure proper access to the critical data and security of the information. To ensure that the security of patient information can be maintained, the contingency plan and the emergency mode of operation must be evaluated on a regular basis. Covered entities must be proactive to prevent improper access and maintain security regardless of the circumstances.

Physical Safeguards

Each organization must evaluate its physical safeguards, or the physical building and the areas where the records and databases are maintained. For example, there should be a facility security plan that identifies the potential portals to the physical buildings. Each door and access point should have some form of security precaution, such as a biometric recognition lock, password lock, or key lock with limited key access. Only the individuals who require access to the databases should be provided with security keys, including passwords and biometric programming to access the database centers. If access is granted, the organization must have processes to validate that the individual requesting access is authorized via a contract or job description to access the PHI. Validating that access for the proper individual is a critical component of any facility security plan. Likewise, there should be records of maintenance of the physical facility, such as changing of locks, changing of cameras, and repair of facility doors to prevent improper alteration or tampering with the facility's security safeguards.

Organizations also must ensure that the workstations where individuals provide services and electronically exchange PHI are secure. A workstation should be used only for the purposes of the job that the individual is hired to perform. Workstations should not be used for personal use. For example, individuals who use email systems and download inappropriate pictures, jokes, or links may inadvertently download malicious software, which could cripple an organization's network or databases. Accordingly, use of the workstation and its software applications should be identified in the organization's policies and each employee should be trained on policies. The workstation should also be maintained in a secure location so that inappropriate individuals cannot access patient information. For example, a workstation should be in locked offices or in cubicles where the devices are not open to the general public. Healthcare providers using bedside terminals or laptops to document at the patient's bedside should ensure that the terminal or laptop is not left logged in and unattended.

In addition to workstation use and security, organizations must evaluate the device and media controls. Specifically, many individuals use portable devices. Portable devices can retain patient PHI on the portable database and can link to remote databases for storage. Because portable media devices are relatively small and mobile, the risk of loss or theft is higher than with a stationary database server in a database center. Therefore extra security precautions are needed to prevent breaches of patient information. Each organization should evaluate how mobile devices are used and whether the devices are programmed to prevent storing patient information on them. The level of security installed on a mobile device will differ based on the unique circumstances that apply to each organization.

Each organization must ensure that when media, such as optical disks, are disposed of or reused, the information previously on the media has been completely cleaned and that there is no potential vulnerability of inappropriate access upon subsequent use of the media. Likewise, each employee should be accountable for maintaining any and all devices and the media controls process should be documented for each employee to be aware of and responsible for as a part of his or her job functions. Furthermore, the device and media controls should be backed up so that the organization can retrieve the information in the event that a device is manipulated or damaged.

Technical Safeguards

In addition to the administrative and physical safeguards, technical safeguards must be addressed by each organization. The technical safeguards are similar to the administrative and physical safeguards in that the specifications must protect the access to the organization's IT systems. As mentioned above, each organization must ensure that each individual user has a unique identifying password to access information. There must also be an emergency access procedure in the event that an emergency occurs. For example, if an unexpected weather event causes the hospital to lose power, the hospital must have a process to access the necessary information to continue to provide care to patients. This emergency access to health records should continue to protect patients' rights to privacy and security. Therefore in the event of a loss of power, the hospital should have a generator to provide limited power to some of the IT systems, preferably the most critical systems. The IT systems that are provided backup power resources should include the databases that contain the critical information to continue the delivery of patient care. Some examples of critical data applications include the medication or pharmacy module, the patient's recent vital signs, the patient's current medication and allergy lists, and the current treatment plan. Healthcare providers should access the database with a password and print the minimum information necessary to provide care. This process minimizes the number of systems that must be used in an emergency while still limiting access to only those individuals who need access to perform their job functions. This process also continues to protect patient privacy. Likewise, if the hospital's IT system crashes and is inaccessible, the hospital should maintain a redundant backup site with access to patient records in real time to continue the delivery of quality care.

There should also be an automatic log-off from the computer system in the event that an individual leaves a workstation or device unattended. An automatic log-off that terminates a user's session helps to mitigate the possibility that an unauthorized person could access a workstation when an employee walks away from it. Workstations in hallways that are readily available for healthcare providers to document clinical information should be programmed to have an automatic log-off in the event that a provider leaves the workstation for more than a few minutes. This automatic log-off will prevent patients and visitors from using the workstations and improperly accessing patient information. Furthermore, each organization is required to evaluate encryption protections. Encryption is not a mandatory safeguard under HIPAA. However, use of encrypted information became more important when the HITECH Act was passed.

Organizations are also required to use automatic controls for their databases and electronic access of information to mitigate the risk of improper access. As the organizations transmit information electronically, they should also ensure that there is integrity of the information and its values from one transmission site to another. For example, if a physician enters an order for 1 mg of Versed as an injection for a patient, the electronic transmission of that information received in the pharmacy must have the reliability and integrity to reflect 1 mg of Versed instead of 10 mg. Ensuring the integrity of the information in a healthcare setting is imperative to ensure that proper treatment is rendered to patients and that protocols are carried out to improve patient outcomes and reduce the cost of healthcare.

Depending on their operations and scope, organizations are also required to address their unique technical safeguards based on how PHI is used and disclosed. First, each organization should ensure that the individuals who are accessing the records can be authenticated as the proper users. Second, the covered entity must address whether encryption is appropriate to protect the patient's information during transmission or if the organization requires other integrity policies and procedures. Often costs associated with implementing encryption and the potential impact to the timely response of the electronic systems will deter organizations from implementing encryption on their networks. Therefore, in many instances, organizations will use unique passwords, strict policies, and manual controls to protect the integrity and security of PHI. However, after the HITECH Act enhanced reporting obligations and increased penalties, more organizations are implementing encryption to protect their PHI.

In 2009 when the Stimulus Act became effective and the federal government financially rewarded healthcare providers that exchanged information electronically, the federal government received a great deal of feedback about ensuring that the information that was transmitted electronically be protected. Accordingly, the HITECH Act provisions emphasized and enhanced the security measures that were originally created with the HIPAA Security Rule in 2005. In fact, Subtitle D—Privacy of the HITECH Act is dedicated to improving privacy and security provisions related to patient information.

Business Associates

Previously, a business associate was defined under the HIPAA Privacy 45 C.F.R. § 160.103 of 1996 as a person who, on behalf of a covered entity or an organized healthcare arrangement and other than a workforce member of such an entity, performs or assists in the performance of a function or activity involving the use or disclosure of individually identifiable health information. This definition included, among other service providers, accountants, billing companies, data analytic companies, management companies, and attorneys. Under Section 13408 of the HITECH Act, the types of entities that are considered business associates expanded. Specifically, in light of the development of health information exchanges and regional health information organizations, the HITECH Act expanded the definition of a business associate to include "an entity that provides data transmission of PHI to a covered entity or its business associate and that requires access on a routine basis to such PHI, such as a health information exchange, a regional health information organization, an e-prescribing gateway or a vendor that contracts with a covered entity to allow the covered entity to offer a personal health record as part of its EHR system."[2]

After expanding the definition of business associates, the HITECH Act made the HIPAA privacy and security requirements apply directly to all business associates. This direct application of the administrative, physical, and technical safeguards to business associates has caused many IT vendors and service providers to change their operations. Specifically, prior to the HITECH Act, business associates were not directly responsible for ensuring that each Security Rule safeguard was addressed and implemented. Following the HITECH Act, business associates were required to document their policies and procedures and invest in both physical and technical safeguards. Moreover, the Office for Civil Rights and HHS were granted authority to directly enforce HIPAA and HITECH Act obligations on business associates. For more information on the expanded application and enhanced obligations of business associates, refer to Sections 13400, 13401, 13402, 13404, and 13408 of the HITECH Act at www.hhs.gov/ocr/privacy/hipaa/understanding/coveredentities/hitechact.pdf.

Breach and Notification

The HITECH Act ensures that in the event of a breach of unsecured PHI, the individual patient must be notified of the breach. If a patient's information is readable or decipherable and it is improperly accessed, the patient should receive written notification from the covered entity within 60 days after discovery of the breach. Discovery of the breach occurs when the covered entity or a business associate or any individual, including a workforce member other than someone committing the breach, has knowledge of or reasonably should have known about the breach. The individual notice should be provided to the patient via first-class mail or in the event that the patient requested electronic mail, such notice can be provided electronically. The HITECH Act, Section 13402 requires that the notice include the following components:

1. A brief description of what happened, including the date of the breach and the date of the discovery of the breach, if known
2. A description of the types of unsecured PHI involved in the breach
3. The steps the individual should take to protect himself or herself from potential harm resulting from the breach
4. A brief description of what the covered entity involved is doing to investigate the breach to mitigate losses and to protect against any further breaches
5. Contact procedures for the individual to ask questions and to learn additional information, which should include a toll-free telephone number, an email address, a website, and/or a postal address[2]

This notification of individual patients may be delayed if there is a criminal investigation and such notification would impede that investigation.

In the event that there is a breach involving 500 or more unsecure records, notification must be provided to prominent media outlets serving the regions where these individual patients reside. The notice must also be submitted to HHS, which will investigate and assess monetary penalties. Note that these breach notification requirements apply only to unsecure PHI. Accordingly, in the event that the information is completely deidentified or is encrypted by a minimum of 128-bit encryption that conforms with the guidance provided by HHS in June 2010, these notification requirements do not apply.

Patient Rights

In addition to the new notification requirements, the individual patient's rights and the obligation of the covered entity to protect patient rights were enhanced by the HITECH Act. Specifically, individual patients are now provided the ability to pay for a healthcare service in cash and the ability of the healthcare provider to submit the claim to an insurance company is restricted. Accordingly, when the patient has paid out-of-pocket in full, the PHI can be restricted and should not be submitted to any other party for payment. This was specifically enacted to ensure that individual patients would not be deterred from receiving genetic counseling or other sensitive testing or treatment. Instead, the patient may pay out-of-pocket in full without the insurance company receiving notification of the testing or treatment provided.

Likewise, the HITECH Act clarifies the fact that covered entities cannot sell EHRs or PHI. Providing information to patients pursuant to an authorization and providing information for research or public health purposes or for treatment purposes are not considered the sale of PHI. In addition, the HITECH Act provides that individual patients can now receive a copy of their medical records in electronic format. The charges for the electronic production of the medical record were modified to include only the labor cost associated with producing those records. This charge for records differed from the initial Privacy Rule, which permitted covered entities to charge for copies of medical records based on the reasonable costs for copying them. Following the HITECH Act, individual patients can now receive a copy of their EHRs in electronic form and pay only the labor cost associated with preparing the records in that form.

Further, according to the HIPAA Privacy Rule individual patients can receive an accounting of who has accessed or used their records during the previous 6 years commencing on April 21, 2003. However, pursuant to 45 C.F.R. § 164.528 of 2011, the initial HIPAA Privacy Rule regulation governing a patient's right to an accounting, individual access to patients' records for treatment, payment, and healthcare operations was not included in the accounting. Under the HITECH Act, the rules and regulations are modified to allow individual patient requests for a list of anyone who accessed the patient record for treatment, payment, and healthcare operations. In the HITECH Act this requirement to include any and all access for treatment, payment, and healthcare operations would be effective after the rules and regulations were enacted and depending on whether the healthcare provider was an early or late adopter of EHRs. In the case of a covered entity who adopted an EHR as of January 1, 2009, the covered entity is not required to provide for this type of accounting until 2016 as an inducement to encourage healthcare providers to adopt EHRs early. Covered entities that failed to obtain an EHR before January 1, 2009, are required to be in compliance with this provision as of January 1, 2011, or the date when they obtain an EHR. However, subsequent to the HITECH Act, the proposed rules and regulations that clarified how this process would work for patients were not finalized. Multiple healthcare providers and technology companies resisted this concept of providing an accounting of all treatment, payment, and healthcare operations. Accordingly, due to this resistance, the federal government is evaluating the comments and as of this writing the final rule on how to provide an accounting of records to patients has not been finalized.

The government also promulgated regulations under the HITECH Act to clarify that communication by a covered entity or business associate about a product or service encouraging a patient to purchase a product or service is not a healthcare operation. Instead, it is considered marketing and requires a patient's authorization.

TABLE 24-4	CIVIL MONETARY PENALTIES
STANDARD	**PENALTY AMOUNT**
Did not know and would not have known	$100 to $25,000 per violation per calendar year
Violation was due to reasonable cause	$1,000 to $100,000 per violation per calendar year
Willful neglect	$10,000 to $250,000 per violation per calendar year
Willful neglect and not corrected	$50,000 to $1,500,000 per violation per calendar year

ENHANCED PENALTIES

Even more significant than the enhanced patient protections is the fact that the HITECH Act dramatically increased the civil monetary penalties associated with HIPAA violations (Table 24-4). Specifically, under the HITECH Act a new standard for willful neglect was created. In the event that an organization engages in a violation (i.e., where the entity acted in reckless disregard and failed to cure the potential violation) the organization can be held responsible for fines and penalties up to $1.5 million. Moreover, to enforce the fines and penalties associated with HIPAA and the HITECH Act, state attorneys general are provided expanded authorization to enforce HIPAA laws and regulations. The state action is capped at a penalty of $25,000 plus attorney's fees. However, this expands the agencies that have the capacity and authority to enforce HIPAA and HITECH Act violations.

FEDERAL SELF-REFERRAL LAWS

Prior to the Stimulus Act, the federal government promulgated specific rules and regulations to encourage healthcare providers to work together to obtain EHR systems. The physician self-referral laws generally prohibited healthcare providers from engaging in financial relationships with other individuals or entities that may be in a position to refer business. For example, hospitals were previously prohibited from giving healthcare providers financial assistance to purchase an EHR because it was considered a prohibited kickback that may influence providers to refer business to the hospital. Unfortunately, without financial assistance it was often difficult for healthcare providers, especially those in small practices, to afford EHRs. To reduce the burden of expensive EHR systems the federal government recognized the need to permit larger institutions and entities that have financial capacity to assist physicians in purchasing EHR systems.

Anti-Kickback Statute

The Anti-Kickback Statute, as described in Section 1128B(b) of the Social Security Act, also governs financial relationships with individuals who can influence referrals or ordering of services billed to state and federal healthcare programs. The

Anti-Kickback Statute includes language making it a criminal offense to solicit or receive any monies to induce or reward referrals of items or services that are reimbursable by a federal healthcare program. If monies are paid purposefully for referrals of items or services from a federal healthcare program, the Anti-Kickback Statute has been violated. For example, if a device company gave all advanced practice registered nurses (APRNs) mobile devices for free to generate business, this may be considered a prohibited kickback. Violation of the statute is considered a felony and punishable by a maximum fine of $25,000, imprisonment up to 5 years, or both. A conviction also includes automatic exclusion from federal healthcare programs, including Medicare and Medicaid.

However, the federal government has recognized arrangements that are legitimate business arrangements in the Anti-kickback accompanying regulations of 42 CFR § 1001.952. HHS promulgated safe harbor regulations that define practices that are not subject to the Anti-Kickback Statute. Safe harbors are intended to permit practices that would be unlikely to result in fraud or abuse. Arrangements that satisfy all elements of a safe harbor are deemed "safe" from prosecution. If the arrangement does not satisfy all elements, the arrangement is not illegal per se but the federal government will evaluate the arrangement on a case by case basis to evaluate the parties' intent. It is imperative that the parties ensure that the financial relationship is not intended to induce referrals and make all efforts to comply with all elements of the safe harbor regulations so that the arrangement can be deemed safe from prosecution.[6]

One such safe harbor is the eprescribing safe harbor. If an entity provides items and services in the form of hardware, software, or IT and training services necessary and used solely to receive and transmit electronic prescription information, the assistance may be permitted. The Anti-Kickback Statute eprescribing safe harbor applies broadly to any recipient and not just to a physician recipient.

Likewise, the Anti-Kickback Statute's accompanying regulations permit physicians to receive assistance to obtain EHRs. The assistance cannot be direct monetary consideration but may include software or IT and training services necessary and used predominantly to create, maintain, transmit, or receive EHRs. If all conditions listed in Box 24-3, as defined by the Anti-Kickback safe harbor regulations of 42 CFR § 1001.952, are met, safe harbor applies.

Here, the Anti-Kickback Statute safe harbor only applies to assistance provided to healthcare providers that participate in Medicare or Medicaid or a federal or state healthcare plan. Therefore the pool of individuals eligible to provide such assistance is limited. Likewise, the software must be certified to be eligible to be provided as a donation. The recipient must remit payment for at least 15% of the costs. Above all else, any donation of software or training cannot be related to the volume or value of referrals of business. Depending on the state in which the healthcare provider practices medicine, the state may also maintain specific prohibitions on financial relationships by and between physicians and entities that are providing financial assistance for which there may be a

BOX 24-3	FEDERAL REQUIREMENTS FOR EHR ASSISTANCE TO COMPLY WITH THE ANTI-KICKBACK STATUTE

1. The items and services are provided to an individual or entity engaged in the delivery of health care by—
   i. An individual or entity that provides services covered by a Federal health care program and submits claims or requests for payment, either directly or through reassignment, to the Federal health care program; or
   ii. A health plan.
2. The software is interoperable at the time it is provided to the recipient. For purposes of this subparagraph, software is deemed to be interoperable if a certifying body recognized by the Secretary has certified the software within no more than 12 months prior to the date it is provided to the recipient.
3. The donor entity does not take any action to limit or restrict the use, compatibility, or interoperability of the items or services with other electronic prescribing or EHR systems.
4. Neither the recipient nor the recipient's practice makes the receipt of items or services, or the amount or nature of the items or services, a condition of doing business with the donor.
5. Neither the eligibility of a recipient for the items or services, nor the amount or nature of the items or services, is determined in a manner that directly takes into account the volume or value of referrals or other business generated between the parties.
6. The arrangement is set forth in a written agreement that—
   i. Is signed by the parties;
   ii. Specifies the items and services being provided, the donor's cost of those items and services, and the amount of the recipient's contribution; and

iii. Covers all of the EHR's items and services to be provided by the donor (or any affiliate).
7. The donor does not have actual knowledge of, and does not act in reckless disregard or deliberate ignorance of, the fact that the recipient possesses or has obtained items or services equivalent to those provided by the donor.
8. For items or services that are of the type that can be used for any patient without regard to payor status, the donor does not restrict, or take any action to limit, the recipient's right or ability to use the items or services for any patient.
9. The items and services do not include staffing of the recipient's office and are not used primarily to conduct personal business or business unrelated to the recipient's clinical practice or clinical operations.
10. The EHR's software contains electronic prescribing capability, either through an electronic prescribing component or the ability to interface with the recipient's existing electronic prescribing system, that meets the applicable standards under Medicare Part D at the time the items and services are provided.
11. Before receipt of the items and services, the recipient pays 15 percent of the donor's cost for the items and services. The donor does not finance the recipient's payment or loan funds to be used by the recipient to pay for the items and services.
12. The donor does not shift the costs of the items or services to any Federal health care program.
13. The transfer of the items and services occurs, and all conditions in this safe harbor have been satisfied, on or before December 31, 2013.

From 112th Congress. *Title 42—Public Health, Exceptions.* Section 1001.952. 2011.
EHR, Electronic health record.

referral relationship. Accordingly, healthcare providers are encouraged to evaluate their state's specific laws and regulations to ensure that they are in compliance with the state-specific prohibitions in addition to the federal guidelines.

For hospitals that are nonprofit and tax-exempt organizations as recognized by the Internal Revenue Service (IRS), providing financial assistance to individual physicians who may be members of the medical staff could jeopardize the tax-exempt status. Accordingly, individual hospitals are encouraged to consider the IRS memorandum regarding the adoption and donation assistance related to EHR systems. The IRS memorandum recommends that hospitals that are tax exempt ensure that they offer the same assistance to all members of the medical staff to prevent one or more members of the staff from receiving an excess or personal benefit. Otherwise, hospitals may vary the amount of assistance provided to their physicians as long as the reason that the amount varies is based on criteria that address the needs of the community. In addition, if legally permitted, the IRS recommends that the hospital making the donation maintain access to the EHR to further support the electronic exchange of and access to healthcare information.

By permitting hospitals and larger institutions to pay for at least 85% of the cost of a certified EHR, healthcare providers should be encouraged to adopt and implement an EHR system. Unfortunately, the Patient Protection and Affordable Care Act of 2010 reduced hospital reimbursement rates beginning in 2010. In 2014 the disproportionate share payment to hospitals is scheduled to decrease significantly. Moreover, due to the high unemployment rate in the United States, hospitals' patient payer mix includes a higher number of uninsured or underinsured patients than in previous years. Therefore many hospitals are financially constrained and often do not have the resources to financially assist all members of the medical staff. Accordingly, the Anti-Kickback Statute safe harbor for EHR assistance has not been widely adopted.

ACCREDITATION STANDARDS

CMS has designated The Joint Commission (TJC) as an agency to accredit hospitals for participation in Medicare and Medicaid programs. TJC recognized well before the HITECH Act that health IT systems can be used effectively to prevent patient harm and have for years used information management standards as part of its accreditation standards. On December 11, 2008, TJC issued Sentinel Event Alert 42, which focused specifically on health information and converging technologies. This Sentinel Event Alert stressed the importance of proper due diligence and IT planning for organizations. TJC was concerned that improper purchases of technology without full consideration of how the technology would affect workflows and direct patient care may cause adverse patient outcomes and hamper proper communication between healthcare providers. Therefore TJC established specific recommendations for organizations related to IT planning.

Generally, TJC recommended that organizations engage in a full due diligence process on how IT may affect the delivery of care. The recommendations included establishing a multidisciplinary team of clinical staff members who would use and be affected by the technology. The due diligence process should include a review of all workflow processes and procedures to identify risks and inefficiencies so that they can be addressed prior to full implementation of the technology. Likewise, TJC stressed the importance of timely training and continuous evaluation of the technology during the implementation to address any critical problems that arise. TJC also recommended establishing a standard and documented set of guidelines for workflow processes. Further, establishing standardized order sets that are approved by the proper committees was also recommended.

TJC recommends using IT to improve patient outcomes and implement safety measures such as providing alerts. However, going beyond merely receiving alerts or reminders, TJC recommended that organizations study which alerts are ignored or skipped and which alerts require a hard stop to prevent medical errors. Engaging in this review ensures that a system protects healthcare providers from "undue distractions when using the technology." Likewise, to support patient safety, in 2008 the Sentinel Event Alert recommended developing a system to mitigate potential prescription errors when a prescription exceeds or contradicts the usual computerized provider order entry (CPOE) orders permitted by an EHR. An additional recommendation was to maintain oversight and approval of computerized order sets and to ensure that the abbreviations, doses, forms, and labels used for communication are proper to prevent medical errors. Each of these recommendations requires organizations to establish committees to ensure that proper and uniform standards are implemented for setting clinical decision alerts in the EHR and that the proper forms are used for proper communication between healthcare providers.

Finally, the Sentinel Event Alert also stressed the importance of continuous monitoring. TJC expects organizations to continually track and monitor potential errors, near-miss events, and failures within workflow processes or the technology. The tracking and trending of potential issues is intended to be used to improve processes and prevent adverse patient outcomes. The Sentinel Event Alert also recommended the evaluation of security and confidentiality protocols to comply with HIPAA.

In addition to the Sentinel Event Alert, TJC maintains standards that hospitals must satisfy to be deemed in compliance with the CMS Conditions of Participation. First, TJC through its leadership standards expects for the organizations' leadership to address and implement programs that support patient safety initiatives and reporting. Organizations are expected to use IT within their processes and the organizations' leadership should engage in, review, and approve the technology and workflow processes, including reporting and reviewing potential areas of improvement.

TJC also maintains an entire chapter that is dedicated to the proper use, maintenance, and disclosure of patient information and organization records. The information management standards are continually evolving and have historically tracked the HIPAA requirements. Specifically, organizations are required to ensure that patients' health information is secure and that patients' right to privacy is protected. The right to confidentiality of a patient's records is also a CMS Condition of Participation for Hospitals.[7] To receive accreditation each organization is required to plan for and implement a plan to address how it will manage its information. This is similar to the administrative risk analysis, information security review, and administrative safeguards that are required by HIPAA and discussed above. In addition, TJC standards require each organization to maintain patient information and protect it from loss, damage, or tampering. Protecting patient information in both written form and electronic form is required by the HIPAA regulations and security safeguards as well. Further, similar to the technical safeguards that require an emergency mode of operation and contingency planning, TJC requires organizations to maintain processes and procedures to ensure that critical patient information is accessible for use in the event of an emergency. Accordingly, if the technical safeguards are addressed and the organization maintains a workflow process and procedure for emergency situations and a backup contingency plan, this standard should be satisfied. Organizations should continually evaluate TJC Sentinel Event Alerts, patient safety initiatives, and modified standards to ensure that their processes to address the HIPAA administrative, physical, and technical safeguards comply with the accreditation requirements. Finally, the accreditation standards may also provide persuasive guidance to encourage an organization to modify or enhance its security safeguards beyond the minimum requirements set forth by HIPAA.

CONCLUSION AND FUTURE DIRECTIONS

With the Patient Protection and Affordable Care Act, Section 1115A the federal government created the Center for Medicare & Medicaid Innovation (CMI). CMI's purpose was to test innovative payment and service delivery models to reduce Medicare and Medicaid expenditures while preserving or enhancing the quality of the care furnished to individuals. In performing these obligations CMI focused on very specific demonstration projects and programs to spur innovation within the healthcare industry. Some of these models included facilitating the electronic exchange of information to improve healthcare services while reducing the costs. One such model is the statutory model called the Shared Savings Program, commonly known as accountable care organization (ACO) model. ACOs are legal organizations composed of physicians, hospitals, or other healthcare providers who voluntarily integrate with each other to provide high-quality coordinated care to at least 5000 Medicare beneficiaries to receive a share in the savings that this provides to the Medicare program.

The initial ACO model was promulgated via statutory code in the Patient Protection and Affordable Care Act. When the ACO-implementing rules and regulations were promulgated the federal government received numerous comments and resistance from the industry. In an effort to spawn potential ideas and drive adoption of the ACO model, CMI created and facilitated a Pioneer ACO Model. The Pioneer ACO Model granted monetary awards to 32 organizations with experience in integrating services to report on quality metrics, collect data, and implement patient-centered protocols to reduce the overall cost of care. This demonstration project began on January 1, 2012, and will continue for 3 years. It includes organizations that have hospitals and physicians as well as other healthcare providers who have integrated their systems and their operations to provide care to Medicare beneficiaries. The concept is to reduce duplicate tests, communicate information in an effective manner, and implement patient-centered protocols to ensure that patients are receiving the highest and best quality of care, which will ultimately reduce the number of visits and the cost to the Medicare system. If the ACO is successful and achieves the quality thresholds being collected by the federal government, the ACO will receive a share of the savings that is realized by the Medicare program. To integrate healthcare providers who are separate and independent entities and to collect data electronically from multiple independent entities, it is imperative to use a health IT resource. Accordingly, in evaluating the ACO models it has been recommended and encouraged that healthcare providers adopt EHR systems and integrate the technology resources to facilitate the complete and accurate collection of quality data to enable the providers to be paid and to receive a share in the savings under the Medicare program.

In addition to the ACO model, CMI also provided a program for bundled payments. Under the Bundled Payment Program individual healthcare providers will coordinate and integrate their services to provide services to Medicare beneficiaries in a hospital setting and post–acute care setting. There are four proposed models in the Bundled Payment Program. Under each of these models the individual physicians, hospitals, and long-term acute care facilities will collaborate to provide specific care for a patient based on an episode of care.

Specifically, under Model 1 the episode of care would be the inpatient stay for a general acute care hospital. Hospitals and physicians collaborate to provide care to the individual patient in the hospital. In Model 2 the episode of care would be the inpatient stay and the post–acute care stay. Accordingly, this would include the hospitals, physicians, long-term

acute care facilities, skilled nursing facilities, and rehabilitation providers. This may also include clinical laboratory providers, durable medical equipment, prosthetics, and Medicare Part D drugs. The entire episode of care would occur from the commencement of the inpatient stay until 30 days post discharge. To the extent that the providers can coordinate the care and achieve a savings by facilitating effective communication and patient-centered protocols for the delivery of healthcare services, the individual providers will share in the savings that the Medicare program would realize. This same model exists in Model 3, except that Model 3 only includes the post–acute care providers, including long-term acute care hospitals, home health agencies, and skilled nursing facilities in the episode of care for a period of 30 days. Finally, Model 4 is similar to Model 1 in that it is bundled payment for the inpatient stay. In this instance one payment is initiated to the hospital. All other healthcare providers would issue a "no pay" claim to Medicare. The hospital would then divide up the revenues received for the services delivered by all practitioners to each practitioner.

To facilitate bundled care and reconcile one payment, integration is required both clinically and financially by and between healthcare providers. Part of this clinical and financial integration has been supported by the use of integrated IT systems so that the data on the bills, charges, and claims that are submitted to Medicare and bundled in one payment can be reconciled. Likewise, pooling quality data and information about specific episodes of care is easier to perform when there is one IT system electronically exchanging the data by and between healthcare providers. Accordingly, these innovative models developed by CMI are focused on integrating providers, which requires the use of IT.

As these programs continue to develop and facilitate the change in how healthcare is provided and how payment is received, the continued use of IT will facilitate these enhanced and creative models for new healthcare delivery designs. Individuals who are engaged in these programs should focus on the quality metrics that are being collected by the government and should ensure that the technology systems have the ability to use EHR systems that can facilitate the proper and accurate integration and data analysis of the quality indicators necessary to achieve payment by the healthcare providers.

REFERENCES

1. Executive Order 13335. *Incentives for the Use of Health Information Technology & Establishing the Position of the NHI IT Coordinator.* April 27, 2004.
2. 111th Congress. *The American Recovery and Reinvestment Act of 2009.* 2009.
3. Office of the National Coordinator for Health Information Technology. HIT Policy Committee Meaningful Use Matrix. http://www.healthit.gov/policy-researchers-implementers/health-it-policy-committee-recommendations-national-coordinator-heal. Accessed November 8, 2012.
4. U.S Department of Health & Human Services. Medicare and Medicaid programs; Electronic Health Record Incentive Program—

Stage 2; Proposed rule. *Federal Register.* 2012;77(45). March 7, 2012.

5. 107th Congress. *Title 45—Public Welfare, HIPAA Privacy Rule.* Sections 160, 164. 2002. Retrieved from http://www.hhs.gov/ocr/privacy/hipaa/administrative/privacyrule/privruletxt.txt.

6. 112th Congress. *Title 42—Public Health, Exceptions.* Section 1001.952. 2011. Retrieved from http://www.gpo.gov/fdsys/pkg/CFR-2011-title42-vol5/pdf/CFR-2011-title42-vol5-part1001.pdf.

7. 112th Congress. *Title 42—Public Health, Condition of Participation: Patient's Rights.* Section 482.13. 2011. Retrieved from http://www.gpo.gov/fdsys/pkg/CFR-2011-title42-vol5/pdf/CFR-2011-title42-vol5-part482.pdf.

■ DISCUSSION QUESTIONS

1. Describe how the Nationwide Health Information Network reflected national policy.

2. List and describe the federal agencies that are responsible for facilitating electronic exchange of health information in the United States.

3. Identify and describe the three main sections of the HITECH Act that have affected patients' privacy and security?

4. Accessing the latest material on the websites listed in this chapter, what are the current time periods for the Meaningful Use program under Medicare and Medicaid, respectively?

5. What are the critical steps that all eligible health professionals and business associates must take to comply with the HIPAA Security Rule?

■ CASE STUDY

A hospital and an independent physician association (IPA) comprising 600 physicians have elected to apply to participate in the accountable care organization (ACO) program sponsored by the Centers for Medicare & Medicaid Services. The hospital and IPA will agree to provide healthcare to a minimum of 5000 Medicare beneficiaries. Because the individual entities are required to report to Medicare as one entity on 33 quality metrics, including seven patient encounter caregiver experience elements, the ACO is interested in facilitating the widespread adoption of electronic medical records within the ACO. Accordingly, the hospital intends to provide assistance to the individual physicians to obtain electronic health records. In addition, the individual physicians will be required to achieve Meaningful Use and comply with policies and procedures of the ACO. Regardless of the electronic health record they would like to purchase, the individual physicians will be required to exchange health information electronically to improve effective communication between healthcare providers, reduce duplicate visits, and lower the overall cost of delivering care to the Medicare beneficiaries.

Discussion Questions

1. Explain how the arrangement should be established to permit the hospital to assist the healthcare providers in obtaining electronic health records.

2. Describe the timeline and the potential financial impact to the individual healthcare providers who are involved in Meaningful Use of the program.

3. Discuss the benefits of using health IT within the ACO program.

4. Discuss the implementation specifications that each individual healthcare provider as a member of the ACO must implement within his or her own facility and as part of a larger ACO to protect the security, confidentiality, privacy, and integrity of patient information.

Health Policy and Informatics

Joyce Sensmeier and Judy Murphy

By understanding current informatics-related health policy issues, the role of the professional organizations, the current federal infrastructure support for health informatics, and specific approaches for participating in the advocacy process, health informatics leaders can positively affect healthcare policy.

OBJECTIVES

At the completion of this chapter the reader will be prepared to:
1. Describe key health policy issues for informatics
2. Differentiate the Institute of Medicine recommendations in the *HIT and Patient Safety* and *The Future of Nursing* reports

3. Define the process for developing and implementing informatics concepts in health policy
4. Describe the impact of informatics on health policy

KEY TERMS

EHR adoption, 405
Health information technology (health IT), 397

Health policy, 398
Unintended consequences, 401

ABSTRACT

All health practitioners should have an understanding of current health policy initiatives and advocate for efforts that leverage informatics and technology to improve patient safety and health outcomes. Health practitioners provide care in every setting and should be involved in shaping the effective use of information technology and related policies wherever they practice. This chapter describes how health practitioners can take on leadership roles and influence health policy to improve safety and efficiency, thereby bringing practice standards and evidence for decision making to the point of care and empowering patients and healthcare consumers as partners.

INTRODUCTION

Healthcare leaders are being affected on multiple fronts by a changing healthcare landscape. Healthcare reform and economic stimulus legislation is rapidly advancing regulations that incentivize the adoption and Meaningful Use of electronic health records (EHRs) to improve the health of Americans. Health practitioners understand that Meaningful Use of health information technology (health IT), when combined with best practice and evidence-based care, can improve health and healthcare for all Americans. Informatics leaders should be knowledgeable about and current in public policy initiatives in order to translate their impact into practice and care delivery.[1]

Health practitioners should have a voice in the selection, planning, implementation, and evaluation of EHR systems and health information exchange to achieve quality outcomes. Informatics leaders should be able to articulate their organization's vision and strategy for clinical transformation as well as actively engage in managing change and measuring success through established metrics. While informatics is highly specialized, there are foundational competencies that all practitioners and students should possess to meet the standards of providing safe, quality, and competent care.[2] Among these competencies is the ability to understand current health policy initiatives and advocate for changes that leverage informatics and technology to improve patient safety and health outcomes.

KEY HEALTH POLICY ISSUES FOR INFORMATICS

EHR Adoption

A new era for EHRs began in 2004 when President George W. Bush addressed the topic in his State of the Union address: ". . . an electronic health record for every American by the year 2014 . . . by computerizing health records, we can avoid dangerous medical mistakes, reduce costs and improve care."[3] President Bush then established the Office of the National Coordinator for Health Information Technology (ONC) and appointed the first National Coordinator for Health Information Technology. The focus on EHRs grew when just after his inauguration in 2009 President Obama proclaimed that he wanted the federal government to invest in EHRs so that all health records would become digitized within 5 years. He vowed to continue to push for the 2014 deadline established by President Bush: "To lower health care cost, cut medical errors, and improve care, we'll computerize the nation's health records in five years, saving billions of dollars in health care costs and countless lives."[4]

Support for EHRs continued with the passage into law of the American Recovery and Reinvestment Act (ARRA) and its key Health Information Technology for Economic and Clinical Health (HITECH) Act provisions in the early weeks of President Obama's administration. Backed by an allocation of $19 billion, this legislation authorized the federal government to provide reimbursement incentives for hospitals and eligible providers who take steps to become "meaningful users" of certified EHR technology to improve care quality and better manage costs.

The incentivized adoption of EHRs is at the core of reform initiatives and can help to improve care quality and better manage care costs, meeting clinical and business needs by capturing, storing, and displaying clinical information when and where it is needed to improve individual patient care and provide aggregated, cross-patient data analysis. EHRs manage healthcare data and information in ways that are patient centered and information rich. Improved information access and availability enable both the healthcare provider and the patient to better manage the patient's health by using capabilities provided by enhanced clinical decision support and customized education materials.

Today, as the United States undergoes dramatic change during healthcare delivery and payment reform, technology plays a huge role in shaping the country's future healthcare system. The terms *EHR* and *Meaningful Use* are becoming commonplace in the national lexicon and with the advent of new technological innovations, informatics leaders are in positions of great influence within their organizations. The following background information describes these changes and how informatics leaders can play an influential role.

Meaningful Use and Incentives

The majority of the HITECH Act funding is being used to incentivize and reward hospitals and eligible providers for Meaningful Use of certified EHRs with increased Medicare and Medicaid payments. The hospital program started in fiscal year 2011 (running from October 1, 2010, to September 30, 2011) and the eligible provider program started in calendar year 2011 (running from January 1, 2011, to December 31, 2011). The criteria for meeting Meaningful Use are divided into the following five initiatives adapted from the work of the National Priorities Partnership (NPP):

1. Improve quality, safety, and efficiency and reduce health disparities
2. Engage patients and families
3. Improve care coordination
4. Improve population and public health
5. Ensure adequate privacy and security protections for personal health information[5]

Specific objectives were defined to demonstrate that EHR use has a "meaningful" impact on one of the five initiatives. For Stage 1, hospitals must complete 14 core objectives and choose 5 of 10 objectives from the menu set of objectives. Eligible providers must complete 15 core objectives and choose 5 of 10 objectives from the menu set of objectives. Some of the objectives are the same or overlap between hospitals and eligible providers. Each objective includes corresponding measurement criteria and applicable standards. If the objectives are met during the specified year and the hospital or healthcare provider submits the appropriate measurements, the hospital or healthcare provider will receive the incentive payment. The hospital incentive amount is based on Medicare and Medicaid patient volumes; the healthcare provider incentives are fixed per provider. The incentives are paid over 5 years and the hospital or healthcare provider will need to continue to submit measurement results annually for each of the 5 years to continue to qualify for payment. The objectives mature every few years, with new Stage 2 criteria and standards published in 2014.

One Meaningful Use criterion for both hospitals and healthcare providers is to report quality measures to the Centers for Medicare & Medicaid Services (CMS) (for Medicare) or to the state (for Medicaid). Hospitals must report 15 clinical quality measures and eligible providers must report 6 clinical quality measures (3 core or alternate core measures and 3 of 38 measures from an alternate set). Quality measurement is considered one of the most important components of the incentive program under the HITECH Act since the purpose of the health IT incentives is to promote reform in the delivery, cost, and quality of healthcare in the United States. Dr. David Blumenthal, former national coordinator for health IT, emphasized this point when he said that healthcare IT is the means, but not the end. Getting healthcare IT up and running in doctors' offices is not the main objective behind the incentives provided by the federal government under the American Recovery and Reinvestment Act, according to Dr. Blumenthal—improving health is.[6]

Health IT Policy Committee. The HITECH Act reenergized the ONC in 2009 with specific accountabilities and significant funding and created two new federal advisory committees under its control: the Health IT Policy Committee and the Health IT Standards Committee. These two federal advisory committees comprise individual public and private stakeholders (including physicians and nurses) tasked to provide recommendations on the health IT policy framework, standards, implementation specifications, and certification criteria for electronic exchange and use of health information. The focus here is on the Health IT Policy Committee. Additional information on the Health IT Standards Committee is provided below.

The Health IT Policy Committee is charged with making recommendations to the ONC on a policy framework for the development and adoption of a Nationwide Health Information Network (NwHIN), including standards for the exchange of patient medical information. The Committee worked closely with the ONC and CMS to develop and refine the Meaningful Use criteria used for the EHR incentive program payments. Committee workgroups address and make recommendations to the full Committee on key reform issues such as Meaningful Use of EHRs, certification and adoption of EHRs, information exchange, the strategic plan framework, privacy and security policy, and enrollment in federal and state health and human services programs.

Regional Extension Centers. The HITECH Act–funded Health IT Extension Program consists of Regional Extension Centers (RECs) and a national Health Information Technology Research Center (HITRC). This program supports the training and consulting needs of the many healthcare providers seeking to adopt EHRs and achieve Meaningful Use by offering education, outreach, and technical assistance. RECs help healthcare providers in their geographic service areas to select, successfully implement, and meaningfully use certified EHR technology to improve the quality and value of healthcare.

There are 62 RECs located in virtually every geographic region of the United States to ensure adequate support to healthcare providers in communities across the country. The HITRC promotes communication and learning among the RECs and collaborates with them by offering technical assistance, guidance, and information on best practices to support and accelerate healthcare providers' efforts to become meaningful users of EHRs. This support is especially helpful to small healthcare provider practices with limited resources for the selection, implementation, and evaluation of EHRs.

Health Policy and Standards

With the recognition that local and regional electronic exchange of health information is essential to the successful implementation of a nationwide exchange and to the success of national healthcare reform in general, the HITECH Act authorized and funded a State Health Information Exchange Cooperative Agreement Program. This state-based grant program offers much-needed local and regional assistance and technical support to healthcare providers while enabling coordination and alignment within and among states. Ultimately this will allow information to follow patients anywhere they go within the United States healthcare system.

The Health IT Standards Committee, along with the ONC, is responsible for recommending standards to the state health information exchanges (HIEs) and for providing the standards infrastructure necessary for this transformation to occur. Rather than using rule making through a top-down process for vetting and selecting the data transport, content exchange, and vocabulary standards, they chose a consensus-based bottom-up approach through the Standards and Interoperability (S&I) Framework Initiatives.

Health IT Standards Committee. The Health IT Standards Committee is charged with making recommendations to the ONC on standards, implementation specifications, and certification criteria for the electronic exchange and use of health information. In harmonizing or recognizing standards and implementation specifications, the Health IT Standards Committee is also tasked with providing for all associated EHR certification testing by the National Institute of Standards and Technology (NIST). Serving the Committee are workgroups addressing clinical operations, clinical quality, data exchange, privacy and security requirements, and implementation strategies that accelerate the adoption of the proposed standards.

The Health IT Standards Committee has made considerable progress in addressing concerns over interoperability implementation through their support of the standards development work being done by the S&I Framework. One of the S&I Initiatives, the Direct Project, was launched to develop the standards and services required to enable secure health information exchange at a more local and less complex level, such as a primary care provider electronically sending a referral or care summary to a local specialist. The state HIEs have embraced this simpler standard and have added it to their implementation plans, providing options for the data exchange offered in each state. The Health IT Standards Committee has been supportive of optionality when addressing different use cases for interoperability.

ONC Standards and Interoperability Framework. Today there is very little controversy over the importance of interoperability and the electronic exchange of standardized patient data between clinical and administrative stakeholders in healthcare. Although healthcare has a long-standing clinician- or hospital-centric view of data and has embraced hospital-centric patient records that were nontransportable to other care venues, today our healthcare model includes a continuum of care view with increased emphasis on ambulatory and home care and with the patient at the center of that care.[7] In that model the need for data to move with the patient across venues of care has become clear.

Interoperability is the ability of health information systems to work together within and across organizational boundaries to advance the effective delivery of healthcare for individuals and communities by sharing data between EHRs. To achieve interoperability, standards for data transport, content exchange, and vocabulary management are needed. These standards are explained in more detail in Chapter 22. This is why standards development is so important; it enables the interoperability needed for regional and nationwide health data exchange and is essential to the development of patient-centric records.

Launched in January 2011, the ONC-sponsored S&I Framework is an investment by the country in a set of harmonized interoperability specifications to support national health outcomes and healthcare priorities, including Meaningful Use and the ongoing mission to create better care, better population health, and cost reduction through delivery improvements. The S&I Framework creates a forum in which healthcare stakeholders can focus on solving real-world interoperability challenges. Each S&I Initiative focuses on a single interoperability challenge with a set of value-creating goals and outcomes that will enhance efficiency, quality, and effectiveness of the delivery of healthcare through the development or modification of standards for data transport, content exchange, and vocabulary management.

The S&I Framework started with three initiatives but now is managing 10 initiatives, such as transitions of care, lab results, and healthcare provider directories. Each S&I Initiative has a rigorous process that includes the following:

- Development of clinically oriented user stories and robust use cases
- Harmonization of interoperability specifications and implementation guidance, including synchronization among the initiatives
- Provision of real-world experience and implementer support through new initiatives, workgroups, and pilot projects
- Mechanisms for feedback and testing of implementations, often in conjunction with ONC partners such as NIST

The work is done online through a moderated wiki with more than 1300 volunteer participants.[8] The focus of the S&I Framework is on delivering guidance to the health IT community through the development of standards content and technical specifications, the development of reusable tools and services, and the effort to unite stakeholders on common healthcare challenges. This work is necessary to move forward on EHR data exchange between venues of care and to take our country to the next level in creating a patient-centric rather than facility-centric healthcare record.

Patient Safety

In 1999 the Institute of Medicine (IOM) report *To Err Is Human* estimated that 44,000 to 98,000 lives are lost every year due to medical errors in hospitals, which led to the widespread recognition that healthcare is not safe enough and catalyzed a revolution to improve the quality of care.[9] Despite considerable effort, patient safety has not yet improved to the degree hoped for in the follow-up IOM report, *Crossing the Quality Chasm*.[10] One strategy the nation has turned to for safer, more effective care is the widespread use of health IT. As described earlier, the federal government

is investing billions of dollars toward Meaningful Use of EHRs so that all Americans can benefit.

When designed and implemented appropriately, health IT can improve healthcare providers' performance, support better communication between patients and healthcare providers, and enhance patient safety, all of which ultimately leads to better care. For example, the number of patients who receive the correct medication in hospitals increases significantly when hospitals implement computerized prescribing and use bar-coded medication administration. However, there is a concern that poorly designed and implemented health IT can actually create new hazards in the already complex delivery of healthcare. To protect patients, health IT must be designed and used in ways that maximize patient safety while minimizing harm. Information technology can better help patients if it becomes more usable, more interoperable, and easier to implement and maintain.

IOM Report on Health IT and Patient Safety

In the wake of more widespread use of health IT and to mitigate the risks posed by these safety concerns the U.S. Department of Health & Human Services (HHS) asked the IOM to evaluate health IT safety concerns and to recommend ways in which both the government and the private sector can make patient care safer using health IT. The resulting IOM report, *HIT and Patient Safety*, states that safe use of health IT relies on several factors, including clinicians and patients.[11] Safety analyses should not look for a single cause of problems but should consider the system as a whole and consider the interplay of people, process, and technology when looking for ways to make it safer. Vendors, users, government, and the private sector all have roles to play. The IOM's recommendations include improving transparency in the reporting of health IT safety incidents and enhancing monitoring of health IT products. A summary of these recommendations follows:

- HHS should ensure that vendors support users in freely exchanging information about health IT experiences and issues, including safety
- ONC should work with the private sector to make comparative user experiences publicly available
- HHS should fund a new Health IT Safety Council within an existing standards organization to evaluate criteria for judging the safety of health IT
- HHS should establish a mechanism for vendors and users to report health IT–related deaths, serious injuries, or unsafe conditions
- HHS should recommend that Congress establish an independent federal entity, similar to the National Transportation Safety Board, to perform investigations in a transparent, nonpunitive manner.

According to the report these would be the first stages for action, to advance current understanding of the threats to patient safety. While some organizations have very good tracking databases to prioritize technical issues and human factors issues related to technology, others do little to track health IT problems and resolutions. Because of this lack of self-monitoring the IOM recommended that HHS get involved to monitor and report on health IT safety beginning in 2012. HHS could decide to direct the Food and Drug Administration to exercise authority to regulate health IT but that was not the first approach explored in the safety plan developed by the ONC in 2012.

The IOM report also examines a broad range of health information technologies, including EHRs, secure patient portals, and HIEs. It asks the Secretary of HHS to publish a plan within 12 months to minimize patient safety risks associated with health IT and report annually on the progress being made. The plan was published for public comment in late 2012 and finalized in 2013.

Unintended Consequences of Health IT Implementation

The unprecedented funding provided by the HITECH Act has spawned a flurry of EHRs and other health IT implementations. While expectations are high for achieving all of the quality, safety, and cost benefits from these implementations, experience and research shows that unplanned and unexpected consequences have resulted from major policy and technological changes.[12,13] Health IT is not immune from this phenomenon. Thus it is important to consider the potential unintended consequences that may be engendered by adoption of health IT, particularly when it is accelerated.[14]

More research in this area of health IT began in 2004 with Agency for Healthcare Research and Quality (AHRQ) grants for planning, implementing, and testing the value of both EHRs and HIEs yet there is still much that has not been explored or proven. However, there are some things to consider during implementation. Monitoring for and tracking of the unplanned or unexpected consequence, especially when it has an undesirable outcome, is important. Enhanced communication among multiple stakeholders in different venues and disciplines will strengthen the collective ability to identify and address unintended consequences of health IT. Federal and organizational leadership can facilitate the sharing of information about technical and organizational safeguards that address unintended consequences. Further, mechanisms are needed to share findings of health IT system implementers so that data captured by individual organizations can have a broader impact.

IMPACT OF INFORMATICS ON HEALTH POLICY

Meaningful "Meaningful Use"

So what is Meaningful Use? Simply put, it is determining how you want to leverage the EHR implementation to accomplish other strategic and clinical goals in your organization beyond just meeting the Meaningful Use criteria. It is not just doing the minimum and checking off the Meaningful Use criteria in order to attest and get the incentive payments but rather using the implementation process to create the health, healthcare, and payment changes needed to advance healthcare reform.

With regard to the implementations of health IT systems for health practitioners, the importance of planning and executing the project as a *practice* change that is being *facilitated* by technology cannot be overemphasized. The technology change should take a supportive role to the people, processes, and practice changes being enabled by the technology. Thus it is important to ensure that EHR implementation is seen as the *means to an end* and not as an *end unto itself*. It is not about the EHR implementation alone but about the way in which the clinician's practice evolves through the use of the supportive technology. Implementing in this way ensures that there is clarity around the purpose of the EHR, as demonstrated by the Meaningful Use objectives, quality outcome measures, and evidence-based practices.

Another way of looking at this is to consider how users are going to leverage the EHR to create the practice and payment changes needed for the future transformation of healthcare. Whether it is the implementation of a patient-centered medical home, value-based purchasing, bundled payments, or accountable care organizational changes, health IT is not only needed but also essential to creating the data, information, knowledge, and wisdom infrastructure necessary for these healthcare practices.

Quality Initiatives
National Priorities Partnership

As mentioned earlier in this chapter, the Stage 1 Meaningful Use objectives were organized around five quality initiatives adapted from the work of the NPP. The NPP is a collaborative effort of 51 major national organizations that brings together public and private sector stakeholder groups as partners in a forum that balances the interests of consumers, purchasers, health plans, clinicians, providers, communities, states, and suppliers in achieving the aims of better care, affordable care, and healthy people and communities.

Under contract to provide input to the Secretary of HHS on the 2012 National Quality Strategy, NPP published its report on national priorities on September 1, 2011. To provide more meaningful input on each priority the structure for this work allowed the full NPP to serve as an overarching committee, while its partners divided into three subcommittees responsible for advising on goals, measures, and strategic opportunities specific to three domains of the National Quality Strategy: healthy people and healthy communities, better care, and affordable care. This important work evolved from NPP's previous input to HHS on national priorities and goals, including a report submitted in 2010 as well as its 2008 report, Aligning Our Efforts to Transform America's Healthcare.

National Quality Strategy

In March 2011 HHS released the National Quality Strategy for health improvement, the first effort to create a national framework to help guide local, state, and national efforts to improve the quality of care in the United States.[15] The National Quality Strategy recognizes health IT as critical to improving the quality of care, improving health outcomes, and ultimately reducing costs. Putting the National Quality Strategy into action, HHS subsequently launched the following two key initiatives that set specific national targets:

- Partnership for Patients, which is working with a wide variety of private and public stakeholders to make hospital care safer by reducing hospital-acquired conditions by 40% and improving care transitions upon release from the hospital so that readmissions are reduced by 20%
- Million Hearts campaign, which is a public–private initiative to prevent 1 million heart attacks and strokes between 2012 and 2016 by improving access to care and increasing adherence to basic preventive medicine

The evidence shows that health IT, along with delivery system improvements, will be a key ingredient in the success of these campaigns and other efforts around the country to improve health outcomes. One study published in *The New England Journal of Medicine* looked at diabetes care in Cleveland and found the following:

- 51% of patients being treated by physician practices using an EHR received care that met all endorsed standards of diabetes care compared to 7% of patients treated by practices not using an EHR
- 44% of patients treated by practices using an EHR met at least four of five outcome standards for diabetes compared to 16% of patients treated by paper-based practices with similar outcomes[16]

This study speaks volumes about the positive impact that well-implemented health IT can have on the quality of clinical practice when it supports clinician decisions. With decision support, health IT can facilitate the consistent execution of evidence-based best practices by healthcare providers, including both nursing and medicine.

PROCESS OF DEVELOPING AND IMPLEMENTING INFORMATICS POLICY

Ensuring That Health Practitioners Are Positioned on Key Committees and Boards

Over the past decade the informatics community, especially nursing informatics, has become more actively engaged with health policy efforts. Informatics nurses are claiming a seat at the policy table and are being sought after for key national appointments and hired for executive positions. Through this effort there has been an awakening to the importance of recognizing opportunities to communicate and collaborate with others to produce favorable outcomes.[17]

Another notable change is that nurses today proactively reach out to other leaders in positions of influence, including government agencies, national organizations, and committees, to share knowledge and offer expertise, and they have learned a great deal from these discussions. One key takeaway is that national leaders and groups respond positively to nursing's large population. For example, the Alliance for Nursing Informatics (ANI) and the American Nurses Association (ANA) are working closely to articulate a unified voice that more broadly represents the profession, which consists of more than 3 million nurses. Increasingly, representatives from these two groups are being invited to participate in national efforts that advance policies focused on improving patient safety and outcomes.

As one example, on September 12, 2011, ONC launched a consumer campaign to empower and educate patients, caregivers, and individuals in managing their day-to-day health and acting as partners in their health through the use of health IT.[18] ANI and ANA jointly pledged to coordinate a campaign with other national nursing organizations to promote use of personal health records (PHRs) and patient portals. The ultimate goal of the ANI Pledge to Support the Consumer eHealth Program[19] is to help clinicians offer a wider range of considerations and options for patients while also providing patients with resources that encourage proactive behavior, thus empowering them to be active partners in their health plan.

Providing Expert Testimony

Opportunities may also arise to offer testimony or serve as an expert witness in a public forum on a current policy topic such as evaluating the impact of an EHR on patient safety or how to standardize documentation of quality measures. For example, testimony may be requested by a national organization such as the National Quality Forum, a national committee such as the Committee on the Robert Wood Johnson Foundation Initiative on the Future of Nursing, or a forum hosted by a professional society such as the ANA. Health practitioners should seek and embrace these opportunities since their clinical background and experience make them credible witnesses. To be successful it is important to plan ahead carefully to ensure that comments are grounded in evidence and closely aligned with any relevant organizational policy statements.

Preparation should begin by gathering background materials and reviewing current literature, white papers, articles, research and policy statements, or key legislation on the topic. The hosting organization may request that certain documents be submitted in advance, including a draft copy of the testimony, the expert's curriculum vitae and biography, and a financial disclosure statement. It is ideal to work with a knowledgeable "prep" team when developing the testimony to ensure that all predetermined questions or topics are fully and clearly addressed.

During the preparation, previous relevant testimony, position statements, and background materials from the expert's sponsoring organization should be reviewed. It is also helpful to seek out and interview individuals who are knowledgeable in the topic area, including board members and industry, organizational, and volunteer leaders. Multiple rounds of editorial and content review should take place prior to calling the testimony "final" and ready for submission. Keep in mind that the comments likely will be documented in a public record, so the testimony should be clearly stated and credible.

Next, oral comments should be prepared, keeping in mind that they likely will need to be delivered in a maximum time frame of minutes rather than hours. It is helpful to summarize the testimony into its most important points so that it can be delivered within the allotted time, after repeated practice sessions. Be mindful that a timing device such as a stop light may be used to track and enforce the time limit. Another helpful strategy is to have a team of subject matter experts drill the testifier on potential questions that might be posed. This practice session will reinforce the ability of the nurse expert to answer succinctly while still emphasizing the key points. Gather and review background materials on the hosting entity, including its leaders and committee members; their pictures, congressional districts, and political parties; and any relevant legislation they may have recently introduced or supported. Keeping these key strategies in mind will go a long way toward ensuring success and may also lead to future opportunities to advance the cause.

Responding to Requests for Comments

With the advent of the HITECH Act there are an increasing number of opportunities for organizations and individuals to submit comments on the ensuing regulations and other related federal guidance documents. Laws passed by Congress rarely contain enough specific language to fully guide their implementation.[20] Regulations and the rule making process are used to clarify definitions, authority, eligibility, benefits, and standards. Their development is shaped by the monitoring, involvement, and input of professional societies, healthcare providers, third party payers, consumers, and other special interest groups.

Each organization's internal policies may offer direction as to if or when a formal written response to federal policymakers is warranted. As an example, ANI has developed a policy that describes its process for member organizations to achieve consensus on policy issues affecting nursing informatics.[19] This policy states:

> ANI, as a collaboration that represents multiple nursing informatics organizations, responds as one voice to federal health policy initiatives by sharing nursing informatics perspectives for shaping health policy. Due to limited timing to respond, it is not always possible to have a full review by all members within each of the ANI member organizations. ANI will make every effort to provide notification about its intent to respond to a call for comments for healthcare reform initiatives, requirements and rulings from ONC or other government agencies and organizations, as soon as ANI decides to pursue a specific call. The length of time available to respond will determine the steps in the procedure for obtaining comments.[19]

To enhance the credibility of submitted comments, address any questions in the notice and take the time to offer positive feedback on points of agreement with the proposed regulation. If a template is provided, use it for the response submissions. Finally, be sure to publicize the response and use it as an opportunity to increase awareness and provide education about the public policy effort and related publications or activities.

The ANA has offered the following guidance on how individual nurses can affect federal rules and regulations:

- Learn about the federal rule-making process and how to make your voice heard.
- Become informed about the public policy and health policy issues currently under consideration at the federal level of government.
- Check out the *Federal Register*. It is the very best source of information about proposed rules and changes to existing rules for federal programs. It is posted every day and contains complete directions on where to send comments and deadlines for the public comment period.
- Work with your state nurses association by offering your expertise to assist in developing new regulations, modifying existing regulation, or preparing comments on proposed regulations.[20]

Developing Position Statements

Another mechanism for advancing health policy is through the development and publication of position statements. A position statement is an explanation or a recommendation for a course of action that reflects an organization's stance on an issue of concern. Position statements are typically developed after an internal discussion with content experts, then advanced to the broader membership for review and input, and finally submitted to the oversight governance group or board for approval. This review and approval process allows interested parties to voice their concerns and opinions on the issue at hand and enables the group to reach consensus. A recent example is the Healthcare Information and Management Systems Society (HIMSS) Nursing Informatics Position Statement titled *Transforming Nursing Practice through Technology & Informatics*. This HIMSS Position Statement was developed by the HIMSS Nursing Informatics Community and subsequently reviewed and approved by its board of directors. Position statements may also be created in collaboration with other groups and issued as joint statements.

LEADING POLICY ACTIVITIES THROUGH ORGANIZATIONAL WORK AND LEADERSHIP

Organizations that actively influence health informatics policy through organizational work and leadership include the American Academy of Nursing (AAN), American Health Information Management Association (AHIMA), American Medical Informatics Association (AMIA), HIMSS, and others. A brief summary of the public policy focus of selected organizations is provided in Table 25-1.

Strategies

Health practitioners require certain skills to be able to communicate effectively with policy-makers and take advantage of relevant advocacy opportunities. According to Walker, in order to advocate, informaticists must be strategists, leaders, great communicators, and they must engage stakeholders across multiple spectrums to ensure that the needs of patients and nurses are met.[17] Health informaticists have a deep

TABLE 25-1	PUBLIC POLICY FOCUS OF SELECTED ORGANIZATIONS
ORGANIZATION	PUBLIC POLICY FOCUS
Alliance for Nursing Informatics (ANI)	ANI aims to foster further development of a united voice for nursing informatics and provide a forum for its expression. Further, ANI provides a forum to respond to opportunities that support and encourage nursing informatics participation in activities such as: developing resources, guidelines, and standards for nursing informatics practice, education, scope of practice, research, certification, public policy, and workforce development. www.allianceni.org/statements.asp
American Academy of Nursing (AAN)	The Academy serves the public and the nursing profession by advancing health policy and practice through the generation, synthesis, and dissemination of nursing knowledge. www.aannet.org/about-the-academy
American Health Information Management Association (AHIMA)	AHIMA's advocacy and public policy team monitors, responds, and participates in national policy and industry initiatives that are important to the health information management profession. www.ahima.org/advocacy/default.aspx
American Medical Informatics Association (AMIA)	AMIA . . . works to shape public policy regarding ongoing health and health policy concerns such as ensuring access to care and protecting funding for core health IT and informatics-related training programs and services. In addition, AMIA works to respond to ongoing and emerging issues such as bio-surveillance and emergency preparedness, access to care, public health infrastructure, disease control and prevention, health disparities, and global health. www.amia.org/public-policy/policy-priorities
American Nurses Association (ANA)	Practicing nurses have first-hand experience regarding the effects of healthcare laws and regulations in providing quality care. This gives the nursing community a unique perspective on healthcare policy. ANA is in part an advocacy organization, charged with using these insights to set policy and influence healthcare legislation. www.nursingworld.org/MainMenuCategories/Policy-Advocacy
Healthcare Information and Management Systems Society (HIMSS)	HIMSS frames and leads healthcare practices and public policy through its content expertise, professional development, research initiatives, and media vehicles designed to promote information and management systems' contributions to improving the quality, safety, access, and cost-effectiveness of patient care. www.himss.org/ASP/aboutHimssHome.asp Each year, HIMSS creates policy principles for all stakeholders to consider for inclusion as provisions in legislation proposed by the U.S. Congress or state legislatures, or for inclusion in federal and state regulations, to foster enhanced healthcare using IT. www.himss.org/ASP/ContentRedirector.asp?ContentId=76351&type=HIMSSNewsItem
Joint Public Health Informatics Taskforce (JPHIT)	The Joint Public Health Informatics Taskforce (JPHIT) is a consortium of nine public health associations committed to improving population health through coordinated informatics policy and action. www.phii.org/what-we-do/joint-public-health-informatics-taskforce-jphit/111

understanding of clinical processes, technology, and health IT systems in addition to experience as advocates for patients, groups, communities, and overall populations.

It seems clear from these discussions that nurses must advocate as leaders to advance an improved health system. Changes in health policy are one part of the necessary reform[21] but how do nurses prepare to engage in public policy efforts? The beginner must acquire a basic knowledge of health policy and funding. An understanding of health policy principles can be gained through formal coursework, continuing education, or even self-study of the myriad resources available virtually on the Internet. Volunteering to participate in state-level advocacy activities that also prepare participants to meet with legislators offers another opportunity to learn how to influence policy.

Beyond acquiring knowledge of basic policy principles, demonstrating leadership skills and leveraging a professional network are necessary to achieve success. Professional colleagues may be willing to act as coaches to offer advice,

criticism, information, encouragement, and support. Communication skills are essential to be able to craft and articulate key points that will "make the case" as well as to capture and engage the target audience. Exemplary leadership activity will move the cause forward in an actionable way toward policy improvement.[21] Demonstrating such leadership requires more than showing passion for an issue. It also involves being able to connect evidence to the policy agenda and framing it in a logical context. HIMSS believes that nurses must lead and be visible, vocal, and present at the table for all significant healthcare reform initiatives.[22] Collaboration and unified messaging among all stakeholders are keys to success. Getting involved with the policy efforts within one's own organization is a simple way to get started.

DISCIPLINE-SPECIFIC POLICIES: NURSING

This section provides an example of current influences within the specific discipline of nursing. All health disciplines are encouraged to research current policies specific to their areas. Readers in other health disciplines are encouraged to note the outline and content provided here as a model.

Use of Health IT to Advance the Future of Nursing

An important report titled *The Future of Nursing: Leading Change, Advancing Health* was published as the result of a partnership launched in 2008 between the Robert Wood Johnson Foundation and the IOM.[23] The purpose of the report was to determine recommendations to transform the nursing profession, leading to advanced roles and leadership positions for nurses in the redesign of the healthcare system.

The Future of Nursing Report Recommendations

Many leading nursing organizations, including ANI, provided testimony to the Committee on the Robert Wood Johnson Foundation Initiative on the Future of Nursing. The vision of ANI—to improve health and healthcare through nursing informatics and innovation—is closely aligned with the recommendations of the report as it envisions the future of the profession. ANI testimony emphasized that nurses are key leaders in the effective use of IT to positively affect the quality and efficiency of healthcare services. These contributions, along with others from national nursing leaders, were used by the Committee in the development of the report, which has been described by some as the "tipping point in nursing care," calling for the nursing profession to be reengineered with a more educated workforce capacity.

The Future of Nursing report outlines several opportunities to transform nursing practice through informatics and technology. As EHRs become more refined and integrated, nurses will have the opportunity to help define additional Meaningful Use objectives. Nurses need to be in the right leadership positions in order to influence policy.

Implications for Time and Place of Care. Care supported by interoperable digital networks will shift in the importance of time and place. It is likely that a significant subset of care delivery might be independent of physical location when health IT is fully implemented. Nurses provide care in every setting, particularly in the community; therefore nurses should be involved in shaping the effective use of health IT and related policies wherever they practice. Nurses have identified that lack of an integrated EHR is a barrier to success.[22] As described earlier in this chapter, national initiatives to address EHR adoption and integration challenges are being advanced. Nurses should become increasingly more engaged in national, regional, and local policy efforts in order to drive this agenda of patient-centric, location-independent healthcare information.

In the 2011 HIMSS Nursing Informatics Workforce Survey, and for the first time in this triennial survey, almost one third of respondents mentioned lack of integration and interoperability as the top barrier to their success, followed by lack of financial resources (26%) and lack of administrative support (23%).[1] The majority of the 660 nurse informaticists who participated in this research work in a hospital setting where they frequently experience the negative impact of disconnected systems on transitions of care, medication reconciliation, and their ability to achieve optimal patient outcomes. The IOM recommendations in *The Future of Nursing*, once implemented, will go far toward addressing these integration barriers.

Expand Opportunities for Nurses to Lead and Diffuse Collaborative Efforts. Interoperable EHRs linked with PHRs or patient portals will influence how collaborative care teams are able to work and share clinical information. Care teams are no longer bound by physical space but rather can engage in virtual learning environments to support the care delivery of the future. The increasing use of communication tools, the proliferation of mobile devices, and the increasing availability of online health tools will multiply opportunities for healthcare providers to collaborate with each other and to engage with patients.[24] Personal health information is a valuable resource to individuals, their families, and the healthcare professionals who provide treatment and deliver care in residential and community settings. Examples of personal health information management systems and tools that can be leveraged include PHRs and web-based portals linked to EHRs or clinical information systems. Well-defined policies are necessary to ensure that the security and confidentiality of protected health information is safeguarded in this rapidly evolving virtual healthcare environment. Nurses should seek opportunities to participate in efforts to define policies that affect patient care, including volunteering for policy development committees within their own organizations.

While health IT will have its greatest influence on how nurses plan and document their care, all facets of care are becoming increasingly digital. From the expanded use of remote devices and smart beds, data capture is being automated and nurses are more able to focus on complex cognitive decisions using knowledge management and decision support. Policy-makers should and do work with nurse leaders to leverage these opportunities to transform nursing practice through the use of new and existing technologies intended to support decision making and care delivery. For example, nurses can provide input as to how the proposed use of health IT may affect their workflow or offer guidance on the optimal use of these technologies to improve care delivery.

Prepare and Enable Nurses to Lead Change to Advance Health. Other key recommendations in *The Future of Nursing* report emphasize the importance of preparing and enabling nurses to lead change to advance health. Public, private, and governmental healthcare decision makers should include nurses at every level. Nurses consistently rank at the top of the Annual Gallup Poll on Honesty/Ethics in Professions, doing so each year since they were first included in the poll in 1999, except in 2001 when firefighters were included on a one-time basis to recognize their heroic actions on September 11.[25] Nurses are the most trusted professionals, outranking medical doctors by 15 percentage points, but frequently they do not recognize that power or leverage opportunities to influence policy or strategic direction.

The TIGER Initiative's goal of engaging more nurses in leading both the development of a national health IT infrastructure and healthcare reform is referenced in *The Future of Nursing*, as is its goal to accelerate adoption of smart, standards-based, interoperable technology that will make healthcare delivery safer, more efficient, timely, accessible, and patient centered while also reducing the burden on nurses.[26] Through efforts such as TIGER, nurses are cultivating informatics competencies to better influence policy efforts in today's rapid EHR adoption.

The promotion of data standardization to enable knowledge sharing has played a critical role in the establishment of healthcare policy. The TIGER Standards and Interoperability Collaborative and its associated workgroups have addressed important aspects of the TIGER action plan to support nursing engagement and to enable the nursing voice to be heard throughout standards adoption processes and national health IT activities.[2]

The TIGER Standards and Interoperability Collaborative has published a Call to Action, which states the following:

- To ensure safe, efficient, and quality care, nurses must be advocates for patient-consented, secure, and reliable exchange of health information
- Collaboration across professional disciplines, healthcare organizations, and society is necessary to achieve our collective goal of improving care delivery through use of interoperable EHRs
- For the betterment of clinical practice and the profession, nurses must embrace collaboration and build a consensus agreement regarding standardization of nursing language
- Nurses have a professional responsibility to be engaged in standards development, harmonization and synchronization, and implementation activities, including encouraging adoption of and patient engagement in PHRs and EHRs
- Nurses should encourage collaboration to achieve interoperable health information exchange for clinical, research, and education
- Nurses should perform environmental scanning for lessons learned from use of emerging technologies in other industries such as communications, banking, and retail
- Nurses must ensure ongoing collaboration across all nursing specialties regarding adoption of standards for health information exchange[2]

The Future of Nursing report emphasizes that the United States has the opportunity to transform its healthcare system, and nurses can and should play a fundamental role in this transformation. However, this transformation will require that nurses embrace technology as a necessary tool to innovate the delivery of nursing care.

Center to Champion Nursing in America

Future of Nursing: Campaign for Action is an initiative to advance comprehensive healthcare change. It envisions a healthcare system in which all Americans have access to high-quality care, with nurses contributing to the full extent of their capabilities.[27] The campaign is coordinated through the Center to Champion Nursing in America (CCNA), an initiative of AARP, the AARP Foundation, and the Robert Wood Johnson Foundation, and includes 48 state action coalitions and a wide range of healthcare providers, consumer advocates, policymakers, and business, academic, and philanthropic leaders.

The Campaign for Action is moving forward simultaneously on national, state, and local levels through efforts to accomplish the following:

- Strengthen nurse education and training
- Enable nurses to practice to the full extent of their education and training
- Advance interprofessional collaboration among healthcare professionals to ensure coordinated and improved patient care
- Expand leadership ranks to ensure that nurses have a voice on management teams, in boardrooms, and during policy debates
- Improve healthcare workforce data collection to better assess and project workforce requirements[27]

State-level action coalitions are also working to advance the campaign's efforts at the local, regional, and state level. These action coalitions will capture best practices, determine research needs, track lessons learned, and identify replicable models that can be embedded in national policy efforts.

HIMSS Nursing Informatics Position Statement

To further advance recommendations in *The Future of Nursing* report, HIMSS published a position statement titled *Transforming Nursing Practice through Technology & Informatics*. This statement asserts that:

> Nurses are key leaders in developing the infrastructure for effective and efficient HIT [health IT] that transforms the delivery of care. Nurse informaticists play a crucial role in advocating both for patients and fellow nurses who are often the key stakeholders and recipients of these evolving solutions. Nursing informatics professionals are the liaisons to successful interactions with technology in healthcare. As clinicians who focus on transforming information into knowledge, nurse informaticists cultivate a new time and place of care through their facilitation efforts to integrate technology with patient care. Technology will continue to be a fundamental enabler of future care delivery models and nursing informatics leaders will be essential to transforming nursing practice through technology.[1]

To achieve the goals of this position statement nurse leaders should be engaged at all levels in health IT policy and strategy-setting committees and initiatives. As well, they must be knowledgeable and well versed in current public policy initiatives and seek opportunities to participate in advocacy and educational efforts directed toward policy-makers.

CONCLUSION AND FUTURE DIRECTIONS

By understanding current informatics-related health policies issues, the role of the professional organizations, the current federal infrastructure support for health informatics, and specific approaches for participating in the advocacy process, health informatics leaders can positively affect healthcare policy. As demonstrated by a variety of nursing initiatives, leadership makes a difference. Health practitioners can and must take on leadership roles and influence policy to improve safety and efficiency, thereby bringing evidence for decision making to the point of care and empowering patients and consumers as partners. Collectively, health practitioners must respond to the policy challenges outlined in this chapter to advance nursing's role in leading change and advancing health. Whatever their role, nurses must be confident that they can influence health policy at the local and organizational, regional, state, and national level.

Where are we now, more than 25 years after starting the implementation of health IT in healthcare and about 2 years into the EHR incentive program? Winston Churchill put it best when he said, "Now this is not the end. It is not even the beginning of the end. But it is, perhaps, the end of the beginning."[28(p264)] We have much more hard work to do. Through strong leadership and active participation we will be able to organize and complete the hard work necessary to create the policy changes that will transform healthcare.

REFERENCES

1. Healthcare Information and Management Systems Society (HIMSS). 2011 HIMSS nursing informatics workforce survey. HIMSS. http://www.himss.org/content/files/2011HIMSSNursing InformaticsWorkforceSurvey.pdf. 2011.
2. TIGER Initiative. Nursing standards and interoperability: a TIGER collaborative report. TIGER Initiative. http://www.theti gerinitiative.org/docs/TigerReport_StandardsAndInteroper ability_001.pdf. 2008.
3. Bush GW. The 2004 State of the Union address. http://www. washingtonpost.com/wp-srv/politics/transcripts/bushtext_ 012004.html. 2004.
4. Obama B. Remarks of President Barack Obama: weekly address. WhiteHouse.gov.http://www.whitehouse.gov/president-obama-delivers-your-weekly-address. January 24, 2009.
5. National Priorities Partnership. *National Priorities and Goals: Aligning Our Efforts to Transform America's Healthcare*. Washington, DC: National Quality Forum; 2008.
6. Blumenthal D. National HIPAA Summit in Washington, D.C. 2009.http://www.healthcareitnews.com/news/healthcare-it-means-not-end-says-blumenthal.
7. Murphy J. The center of the universe: a closer look at a patient-centric care model. *J Healthc Inf Manag*. 2008;22(2):6-7.
8. Standards & Interoperability Framework. Wiki. http://wiki. siframework.org/. 2012.
9. Institute of Medicine. *To Err Is Human: Building a Safer Health System*. Washington, DC: National Academy Press; 1999.
10. Institute of Medicine. *Crossing the Quality Chasm: A New Health System for the 21st Century*. Washington, DC: National Academy Press; 2001.
11. Institute of Medicine. *HIT and Patient Safety: Building Safer Systems for Better Care*. Washington, DC: The National Academies Press; 2011.
12. Ash JS, Berg M, Coiera E. Some unintended consequences of information technology in health care: the nature of patient care information system-related errors. *J Am Med Inform Assoc*. 2004;11(2):104-112.
13. Koppel R, Metlay JP, Cohen A, et al. Role of computerized physician order entry systems in facilitating medication errors. *J Amer Med Assoc*. 2005;293(10):1197-1203.
14. Bloomrosen M, Starren J, Lorenzi NM, Ash JS, Patel VL, Short-liffe EH. Anticipating and addressing the unintended consequences of health IT and policy: a report from the AMIA 2009 Health Policy Meeting. *J Am Med Inform Assoc*. 2011;18(1): 82-90.
15. National Quality Strategy. http://www.ahrq.gov/workingfor quality/nqs/. 2011.
16. Cebul R, Love TE, Jain AK, Hebert CJ. Electronic health records and quality of diabetes care. *N Engl J Med*. 2011;365(9): 825-833.
17. Walker A. Shaping nursing informatics through the public policy process. In: Saba V, McCormick KA, eds. *Essentials of Nursing Informatics*. 5th ed. New York, NY: McGraw-Hill; 2011:279-287.
18. Office of the National Coordinator for Health Information Technology. National health IT week. HealthIT.gov. http:// www.healthit.gov/healthitweek/. 2011.
19. Alliance for Nursing Informatics (ANI). Alliance for Nursing Informatics pledge to support the Consumer eHealth Program. ANI. http://www.allianceni.org/documents/ANIPledgetoSupport ONCConsumereHealthProgram_000.pdf. September 12, 2011.
20. American Nurses Association. Agencies & regulations. Nursing World. http://www.nursingworld.org/Agencies-RegulatoryAffairs. aspx. 2012.
21. Gillis CL. Developing policy leadership in nursing: three wishes. *Nurs Outlook*. 2011;59(4):179-181.
22. Healthcare Information and Management Systems Society (HIMSS). *Position Statement on Transforming Nursing Practice through Technology and Informatics*. Chicago, IL: HIMSS; 2011.
23. Institute of Medicine. *The Future of Nursing: Leading Change, Advancing Health*. Washington, DC: The National Academies Press; 2011.
24. California HealthCare Foundation (CHCF). What's ahead for EHRs: Experts weigh in. CHCF. http://www.chcf.org/~/media/ MEDIA%20LIBRARY%20Files/PDF/W/PDF%20WhatsAhead-EHRsExpertsWeighIn.pdf. 2012.
25. Gallup Poll. http://www.gallup.com/poll/1654/honesty-ethics-professions.aspx. November, 2012.
26. TIGER Initiative. The TIGER Initiative: collaborating to integrate evidence and informatics into nursing practice and education: an executive summary. TIGER Initiative. http://www.theti gerinitiative.org/docs/TIGERCollaborativeExecSummary_ 20090405_000.pdf. 2008.
27. Center to Champion Nursing in America. http://champion nursing.org/about-FON-CFA. 2012.
28. Churchill WS. *The End of the Beginning*. London, England: Cassel; 1943. http://www.winstonchurchill.org/component/ content/article/3-speeches/987-the-end-of-the-beginning.

DISCUSSION QUESTIONS

1. Outline the basic health policy competencies for health informatics leaders.
2. Discuss three key policy issues that affect EHR adoption.
3. Describe the policy concerns regarding the use of health IT and patient safety.
4. Discuss the implications of *The Future of Nursing* report on the use of health IT by nursing and other health-related disciplines.
5. Outline the process for developing and implementing informatics policy.
6. Describe four strategies for leading policy activities through organizational work and leadership.

CASE STUDY

Mr. Smith Goes to Washington is a 1939 American film starring James Stewart and Jean Arthur about one man's effect on American politics. Today, health practitioners make their own trips to our nation's capital and while the focus may be somewhat different, the experience is no less exciting. Here is a case study outlining one possible scenario.

It all started with a phone call requesting that a nurse testify at a congressional hearing on Standards for Health IT: Meaningful Use and Beyond, hosted by the House Subcommittee on Technology and Innovation. The testimony would include both written and oral comments. The call launched a flurry of activity aimed at ensuring that the testimony would be successful and Johnson was selected to testify. Multiple documents were prepared in advance, including a draft of the testimony and Johnson's curriculum vitae, biography, and financial disclosure form. The team worked to create testimony that addressed the House Subcommittee's two questions:

1. What progress has ONC made since the HITECH Act was passed in meeting the need for interoperability and information security standards for EHRs and health IT systems?
2. What are the strengths and weaknesses of the current health IT standards identification and development process and what should the top standards-related priorities be for future health IT activities?

During preparation of the written comments, previous testimony, position statements, and background materials were leveraged. Several board members, leaders in privacy and security efforts, leaders in standards and standards harmonization efforts, and volunteer leaders from the HIMSS Electronic Health Record Association were interviewed. Multiple rounds of editorial and content review took place prior to calling the testimony "final" and ready for submission.

Next, oral comments were prepared, keeping them to a maximum of 5 minutes. The testimony was boiled down to the key points that could be delivered in that brief time frame yet still make sense. Repeated practice sessions drove home the realization that 5 minutes is very little time!

Then came the "murder squad," a dry run facing a team of experts who drilled Johnson with questions that she might be asked by House Subcommittee members. She said later that it may have been more nerve-racking to face peers than to face the House Subcommittee itself! In this practice session the key lessons learned were to get to the point quickly and use the responses to panel members' questions as an opportunity to reemphasize key points from the testimony. Other homework included reviewing the list of House Subcommittee members to recognize their faces and learn their districts, political parties, recent activities, and any relevant legislation they had recently introduced or supported.

On the day of the testimony a meeting was held with the team in the House of Commons cafeteria to share last-minute updates and further refine the strategy. Johnson then proceeded to the office of the House Subcommittee chairman, where the panelists were introduced to each other. The chairman joined the panelists at the prehearing session, facilitating the dialog in a casual setting to put the panelists more at ease. During this session the panelists learned that the hearing had been at risk of cancellation since the House had adjourned the night before and that many of the House Subcommittee members had left Washington for their home states. However, the chairman's staff commented that the chairman is very committed to the advancement of health IT as well as to the House Subcommittee's HITECH Act oversight role and therefore he did not cancel the hearing.

At the scheduled time the panelists entered the hearing room and took their seats at a row of tables on the main floor. The House Subcommittee chairman, members, and staff were seated at the front of the room, one level above the main floor, and the public audience was seated at the back of the room. In front of each panelist was a microphone, timer, and stop light that tracked each speaker's time limit. During the testimony the stop light changed from green to yellow and then to red when each speaker's 5-minute time limit was reached.

Throughout the hearing the chairman was very gracious, noting his appreciation of the panelists' contributions. In part because of her thorough preparation, Johnson gave her prepared oral testimony flawlessly. Although not asked any direct questions, she chimed in to help answer several other questions that were asked of other panelists in order to offer key points germane to the discussion. The hearing was broadcast live on the Internet, a transcript of the testimony is available in the public record of the hearing, and a video clip of the testimony can be found on YouTube.

While *Mr. Smith Goes to Washington* made James Stewart a major movie star, Johnson's aspirations were quite simple: that the recommendations on how to improve patient care and reduce costs would be heard and that steps toward implementation would be taken.

Discussion Questions

1. How can nurses best leverage their clinical background when providing testimony as expert witnesses?

2. When preparing testimony, should a nurse expert witness focus primarily on developing nursing-specific content or should his or her nursing background be used more as a context for the discussion? What are the advantages and disadvantages of each approach?

Education and Informatics

Informatics in the Curriculum for Healthcare Professionals

Helen B. Connors, Judith J. Warren, and E. LaVerne Manos

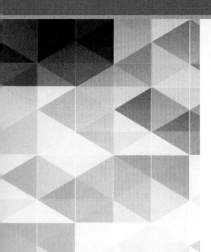

Informatics competencies and new workforce roles will continue to evolve as the continuous learning loop and new technology change the way in which healthcare and education are delivered.

OBJECTIVES

At the completion of this chapter the reader will be prepared to:

1. Summarize the forces driving the integration of informatics in the curriculum for health professionals
2. Recommend appropriate pedagogic approaches for the incorporation of informatics competencies for generalist to specialist
3. Articulate the importance of continued professional development
4. Analyze the challenges of informatics education
5. Operationalize the interprofessional team approach to informatics education and practice

KEY TERMS

Health information exchange (HIE), 412
Interprofessional education (IPE), 416

Learning health system (LHS), 411
Nationwide Health Information Network (NwHIN), 412

ABSTRACT

Health and healthcare in this country and around the world are being transformed by information and communication technology (ICT). Increasingly these industries are turning to digital information and the use of electronic communication to fundamentally change the services they provide. The Health Information Technology for Economic and Clinical Health (HITECH) Act of 2009 laid the foundation to operationalize the infrastructure for a digital healthcare system. This unprecedented change has major implications for the workforce and workforce development. The widespread adoption of electronic health records (EHRs), digital communications between patients and healthcare providers, accessible web-based health information, remote diagnosis and treatment, and the availability of large health data repositories necessitate widespread training and upgrading of skills for health practitioners and support for workers who will interface with patients and these technological advances. Health professional education engagement should be a vital
component of the learning health system (LHS).[1] This chapter will focus on the interface between the LHS and a health professional curriculum that will help to drive that system.

INTRODUCTION AND BACKGROUND

Overview of Informatics and Health Information Technology

To understand the discipline of informatics and the various roles within informatics, it is important to understand the national, regional, and local contexts of the use of health information and the political agenda for the use of health information technology (health IT). Health information and health IT have received significant federal strategic attention for more than a decade. The various Institute of Medicine (IOM) reports each have linked health IT to the improvement of healthcare. In the first IOM report, *To Err Is Human*, one of the main conclusions is that the majority of medical errors are caused by faulty systems, processes, and conditions that lead people to make mistakes or fail to prevent mistakes.[2] The report emphasized the importance of IT in implementing safe systems to ensure safe practices at the delivery level. The next IOM report, *Crossing the Quality Chasm*, not only addressed the importance of health IT, but also noted how crucial it is to all aspects of clinical decision making, the delivery of population-based care, consumer education, professional development, and research.[3] In 2003 the IOM issued a third report, *Health Professional Education: A Bridge to Quality*.[4] This report called for including informatics as a core competency in the educational programs of all health professionals and launched a movement in this country referred to as the Decade of Health Information Technology.

After slow but steady progress over a decade in converting paper-based health records to electronic delivery, President Obama signed into law the American Recovery and Reinvestment Act (ARRA) on February 17, 2009. The widespread use of EHRs and health information exchanges (HIEs) encouraged by this act are projected to expand greatly in the next several years. The HITECH Act and its funding have positioned informatics and health IT in the forefront of all healthcare sectors, including health professional education. The major foundational trends to watch are Meaningful Use (MU) and the Nationwide Health Information Network (NwHIN), both of which can be expected to have a major impact on the informatics-related education of all health professionals. As the NwHIN matures the Office of the National Coordinator for Health Information Technology (ONC) envisions it evolving into an LHS. The LHS aligns science, informatics, incentives, and culture for continuous improvement and innovation, with best practices seamlessly embedded in the delivery process and new knowledge captured as a by-product of care delivery. The concept of the LHS is the outcome of the IOM's Roundtable on Value & Science-Driven Health Care. Roundtable members worked to identify key challenges and opportunities for achieving better outcomes and greater value in healthcare. The reports of the Roundtable are conveyed in 11 volumes of the IOM Learning Health System Series, published by the National Academies Press. A graphic of the LHS as visualized by the ONC is shown in Figure 26-1.

Education Reform Initiatives

For the past decade the above-mentioned driving forces have spurred health professional organizations and special interest groups to call for transformation in education and the inclusion of health informatics and health IT competencies in the curriculum for all health professionals. If the United States is serious about transforming its healthcare system to be safe, efficient, patient centered, timely, equitable, and effective, it needs to invest in the education and training of individuals to ensure that the workforce is poised to meet the challenge.

Nursing, in particular, has led the way in this transformation. In 1992 the American Nurses Association (ANA) recognized nursing informatics as a nursing specialty that integrates nursing science, computer science, and information science to manage and communicate data, information, and knowledge in nursing practice. The definition was further articulated and roles and responsibilities were defined in the first editions of *The Scope of Practice for Nursing Informatics*[5] and *The Standards of Practice for Nursing Informatics*.[6] As technology and informatics developed over time these documents were combined into the ANA's *Scope and Standards of Nursing Informatics Practice*[7] and expanded in 2008 as *Nursing Informatics: Scope and Standards of Practice*[8] to reflect the growing changes in nursing informatics roles and responsibilities brought about by the dramatic bolstering of the nation's health IT agenda.

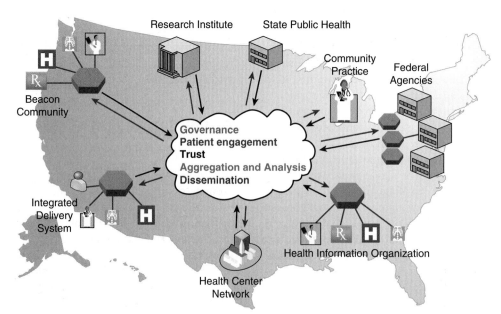

FIG 26-1 A learning health system for the U.S. (Copyright the Office of the National Coordinator of Health Information Technology.)

In 1997 the Health Resources and Services Administration's (HRSA's) Division of Nursing, the agency responsible for setting national policy to guide the nursing workforce, convened the National Nursing Informatics Work Group (NNIWG) to make recommendations to the National Advisory Council on Nurse Education and Practice (NACNEP) regarding the nation's nursing informatics agenda for education and practice. As a result of NACNEP's recommendations to the Secretary of Health & Human Services, legislation in 1998 specifically named informatics as one of seven priority areas for strengthening capacity and endorsed the inclusion of core informatics knowledge and skill in all undergraduate, graduate, and continuing education programs.

Despite these efforts to bring nursing informatics to the forefront and increase informatics knowledge and competencies in the curriculum, a number of studies demonstrated slow progress on integrating these competencies in the curriculum.[9-13] Faculty have been cited as the largest barrier to greater IT integration in education because they lack the knowledge and skills regarding new technologies and their potential.[14] However, recent federal initiatives to coordinate efforts for the implementation and use of advanced health IT have included support for nursing faculty development in the use and integration of information and other technologies in nursing education. In addition, private funders and professional organizations have developed initiatives to enhance informatics in the curriculum. Table 26-1 outlines some of the initiatives that have helped to develop faculty and support workforce competencies for informatics practice.

TABLE 26-1	EXAMPLES OF FACULTY AND WORKFORCE DEVELOPMENT PROGRAMS FOR INFORMATICS COMPETENCIES
PROGRAM	**PURPOSE**
Health Resources and Services Administration (HRSA), Bureau of Health Professions (BHPR) Faculty Development: Integrated Technology into Nursing Education and Practice (ITNEP), 1996 http://bhpr.hrsa.gov/nursing/grants/itnep.html	This initiative was to provide support to nursing collaboratives for faculty development in the use of information and other technologies in order to expand the capacity of collegiate schools of nursing to educate students for 21st century healthcare practice. Nursing collaboratives will use healthcare information systems to enhance nursing education and practice, optimize patient safety, and drive improvements in healthcare quality. Nine faculty development collaboratives were funded.
Robert Woods Johnson Foundation (RWJF) Quality and Safety Education for Nurses (QSEN) Project http://qsen.org/	The overall goal of the QSEN Project is to meet the challenge of preparing future nurses who will have the knowledge, skills, and attitudes necessary to continuously improve the quality and safety of the healthcare systems within which they work. QSEN has developed informatics competencies for prelicensure and advanced nursing practice, working on competencies for specialty informatics practice and collaborating with other professional associations, such as the American Association of Medical Colleges, to integrate these competencies across health professional programs.
Technology Informatics Guiding Educational Reform (TIGER), 2009 http://www.tigersummit.com/About_Us.html	This initiative aims to enable practicing nurses and nursing students to fully engage in the unfolding digital electronic era in healthcare. The purpose of the initiative is to identify information and knowledge management best practices and effective technology capabilities for nurses. TIGER's goal is to create and disseminate action plans that can be duplicated within nursing and other multidisciplinary healthcare training and workplace settings.
American Medical Informatics Association (AMIA) 10 × 10 Program http://www.amia.org/education/10x10-courses	AMIA conducts training in a wide range of settings across the U.S. in collaboration with key academic partners in the biomedical and health informatics education community. AMIA is committed to the education and training of a new generation of clinical, public health, research, and translational bioinformatics informaticists to lead the transformation of the American healthcare system through the deployment and use of advanced clinical computing systems. Informatics topics covered include clinical or health informatics, clinical research informatics, translational bioinformatics, nursing informatics, and public health informatics.
Office of the National Coordinator for Health Information Technology (ONC), 2009-2013 Health IT Workforce Development Program	To help address the growing demand for a highly skilled workforce to support the adoption and Meaningful Use of electronic health records (EHRs), the ONC invested $116 million in the Health IT Workforce Development Program. The goal of this program is to train a new workforce of health IT professionals who will be ready to help healthcare providers implement EHRs and health information exchanges. The program is now graduating health IT professionals interested in supporting the growing and evolving health IT industry. Graduates of the program are for the most part mid-career healthcare or IT professionals who have received specialized training in one of the 12 ONC-defined workforce roles.

Challenges of Technology-Enhanced Education

Health IT applications are no longer a luxury but a necessity. This trend has made health professional educators keenly aware of the need to integrate health IT into the curriculum in a meaningful way and to prepare informatics specialists to serve as experts in the evolving LHS. At the same time several challenges must be overcome to teach with health IT tools and assist students to develop appropriate competencies. The paucity of faculty prepared to teach to informatics competencies is well documented.[14] Although advanced informatics nursing education programs are accelerating, finding qualified faculty to teach in these programs is extremely difficult. Teaching informatics requires both knowledge of the content and experience in the use of informatics skills in clinical practice.

In addition to experienced faculty, most academic institutions do not have the infrastructure to support the integration of health IT tools essential for informatics competencies in the curriculum. To be competent, students need to use the same tools that they will use in clinical practice. In many instances the cost of these tools is prohibitive in academic arenas or, if the tools are available, many faculty lack the knowledge and expertise needed to strategically incorporate the tools in their teaching. Successful implementation requires integration in the curriculum and a change in workflow. Teaching students to be competent with health IT tools and practices is not an add-on to an already overcrowded curriculum. Faculty need to critically examine what content is taught and how it contributes to a workforce that supports the LHS. For example, if one of the goals of the LHS is to achieve the best outcome for every patient, we need better evidence on which to base healthcare decisions and more effective application of the knowledge we have. However, with the current pace of change, the problem is the health professional's ability to acquire the needed evidence in a timely manner.[15] Most institutions find considerable variance in the level of integration of evidence into education across health professions. While knowledge of the importance of evidence-based practice is evident in faculty publications, it has not yet found its way extensively into the curriculum framework of most health professional programs. As evidence-based healthcare practice evolves, educators need to be ready to transform curriculum to ensure that graduates have a new skill set that is recognized and used in the healthcare setting.[15] However, for the most part curriculum is not readily adaptable to change thus creating a gap between education and practice that needs to be resolved in this rapidly changing healthcare environment.

TEACHING AND LEARNING IN AN EVOLVING HEALTHCARE AND TECHNOLOGY ENVIRONMENT

Since its inception the World Wide Web has transformed and will continue to transform the way in which we deliver healthcare and the way in which we learn. Several reports and white papers published in the past decade suggest paradigm shifts in health professional education. As the technology-driven healthcare system evolves it is only right that we overhaul the educational platforms that prepare graduates who are the core of the healthcare environment.[16] Health professionals, in all domains of practice and at all levels, must be "technology competent" to be able to participate in decision making and evaluation of health IT systems and their Meaningful Use. These systems should be patient centered and should support healthcare providers in information management, knowledge development, and evaluation of evidence-based innovative practice strategies.

The Role of Informatics in the Curriculum

Health IT goes beyond the role of keeping records and confirming payments. Today, technology allows health records to be shared among healthcare providers and patients as well as across healthcare settings. As health records become digitized and amass huge amounts of data, "big data" or large datasets are available to analyze health records and discover trends helpful for evidence-based practice and population-based health. Health IT has transformed the provision of healthcare in ways that were not imagined even a few decades ago, and the future is sure to hold many more changes.

The term *informatics* as it relates to healthcare is ubiquitous and ambiguous, largely because of the various health professionals and related disciplines that use health IT and health data.[17] The American Medical Informatics Association (AMIA) and its classification of informatics domains—clinical informatics, public health and population health informatics, and translational informatics—provides a sense of structure to the overall categories of health informatics. Through its Academic Forum, AMIA has appointed a special task force to develop a formal definition to specify the core competencies that should drive curriculum and course design for graduate training in the advanced informatics field.

In keeping with key federal initiatives that encourage the widespread adoption of EHRs and support the goal of a well-trained informatics workforce, informatics roles as well as ancillary or support roles have escalated. The ONC has defined 12 job roles for the health IT workforce. Six roles were initially funded through the Community College Consortium and the remaining six were funded through the university-based training initiatives.

As new health IT and informatics roles evolve, informatics competencies need to be addressed at all levels of health professional curricula. Informatics competencies need to be placed along a continuum from basic to advanced. All health professionals will need some level of basic informatics knowledge and skills and certain clinicians and informaticists will need advanced specialty education.

Several disciplines have completed foundational work on needed competencies: nursing, public health, and clinical informatics (for physicians). Within nursing in the United States, the Delphi work in 2002 by Staggers and colleagues spurred additional work on informatics competencies (e.g., for nurse practitioners and BSN students).[13] The initial list of competencies was updated in 2011 and a review of informatics competencies was completed in 2012.[18,19] Unfortunately no consensus exists as yet about informatics competencies for nurses despite the large amount of work in the area.

Public health experts completed a consensus list of informatics competencies in the mid-2000s and their most current work from 2009 is available online at www.cdc.gov/informaticscompetencies. More recently, in 2012 AMIA released a list of informatics competencies for physicians to be certified in clinical informatics. Information is available on the AMIA's general website and at www.amia.org/issues/subspecialty-certification-clinical-informatics. Clearly more work is needed to harmonize informatics competencies across disciplines and reach consensus about required core competencies.

The Science of Informatics and Curriculum Design

The science of informatics is inherently interdisciplinary, drawing on (and contributing to) a large number of other component fields, including computer science, decision science, information science, management science, cognitive science, and organizational theory. Discipline-specific sciences and practices, such as nursing, medicine, dentistry, and pharmacology, are what differentiate how informatics is applied. Knowledge of the interdisciplinary approach to informatics; the science that underpins informatics; the relationship among the elements of data, information, knowledge, and wisdom; and the corresponding automated support systems drive the framework for curriculum development across nursing and other health professional curricula.[8] Working in teams across disciplines will provide a better understanding of the various roles and functions of the informatics team and assist in placing the right competencies with the right role and educational level. In addition, providing informatics education in an interprofessional environment will assist in ensuring that health professionals in different disciplines understand and appreciate the different levels and types of competencies across disciplines.

FRAMEWORK FOR INFORMATICS CURRICULUM

If the U.S. is truly envisioning an LHS, this is an opportunity for health professional education to be guided by this model. In a system that increasingly learns from data collected at the point of care and applies the lessons learned to improve patient care, healthcare professionals will be the cornerstone for assessing needs, directing approaches, ensuring integrity of the tracking and quality of the outcomes, and leading innovation.[15] However, practitioners and health professional educators need to know that how and what they learn will dramatically change as technology, evidence-based practices, and innovations evolve over time. Orienting the education system to meet the needs of an evolving evidence-based

healthcare system requires new ways of thinking about how we can create and sustain a healthcare workforce that recognizes the by-products of an LHS and uses these by-products to adjust curriculum and address lifelong learning needs. What is needed is a nimble curriculum that can readily adapt to change. Figure 26-1 provides a model of such an LHS.

In February 2012 the Technology Informatics Guiding Educational Reform (TIGER) board of directors approved a new vision statement:

> To enable nurses and interprofessional colleagues to use informatics and emerging technologies to make healthcare safer, more effective, efficient, patient-centered, timely and equitable by interweaving evidence and technology seamlessly into practice, education and research fostering a learning health system. A primary goal of TIGER is to create collaborative learning communities that maximize the potential of technology through knowledge development and dissemination, driving rapid deployment and implementation of best practices.[20]

This revised vision and goal coincides with the vision and goals of a national LHS and should be the hallmark for health professional curriculum reform. Today, most health professional accrediting bodies have adopted accreditation standards, guidelines, and scopes of practice that reflect the IOM's core competencies as further refined and delineated in the LHS reports.[1,4,15] Nursing and other health professional education must recognize that the healthcare paradigm has shifted from practice focused to outcomes focused and that health IT and informatics are critical to that shift.

Pedagogy

Today's information age students are calling for learner-driven education environments that provide access to powerful learning tools, information and knowledge bases, and scholarly exchange networks for the delivery of learning. Teaching with technology and teaching about technology require a change in teaching workflow and practices.

Pedagogy is a broad term that includes multiple theories of behavior based on the learning process. The three major categories of theory that drive education are behaviorist, cognitive, and constructivism. Behaviorists believe that learning is a change in behavior caused by external stimuli—the "know what." Early computer programs were based on behaviorist theory. It is useful in learning what basic content and concepts are important. Cognitive psychology claims that learning involves memory, motivation, thinking, reflection, and abstraction. It is concerned with how to apply content, access and synthesize information, think critically, and make decisions—the "know how." Constructivism asserts that learners interpret information and the world according to their personal reality and that they learn by observing, processing and interpreting information, and then customizing the information into personal knowledge for immediate application. Learners use previous knowledge to create new knowledge and act on it—the "know why." Cognitive psychology and constructivism allow faculty to create higher-order learning activities that can be enhanced with the use of

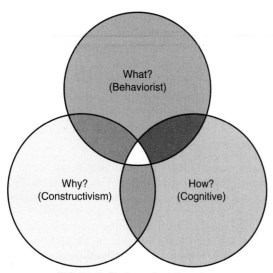

FIG 26-2 Pedagogical theories.

technology. These learning theories and their derivatives support sound teaching and learning strategies (Fig. 26-2).

Teaching Tools and Learning Strategies

The rapid growth in knowledge, research, and technology does not mean adding more layers to an already overcrowded curriculum. Just as curriculum must change, so too should teaching and learning strategies change to become more efficient and effective. The rapid advancement of knowledge and decision support technology is changing the way in which students and health professionals access, process, and use information. New tools and new approaches must be incorporated to teach fundamental concepts and methods that can be applied in different situations. For example, integrating the EHR in the curriculum as a teaching tool is a key mechanism for teaching students to use data to think critically and lays the foundation for teaching evidence-based care. The EHR also can be used to support learning of decision support tools, safety alerts, clinical workflow, population management, quality improvement, and interprofessional learning. Education programs can emphasize the importance of the EHR in healthcare but unless there is an opportunity for students to use the EHR as they learn clinical skills, they will not develop the competencies required for practice in a computerized healthcare environment.[21] The EHR alone is not sufficient for health professional students to learn the capabilities of the system. Nursing and other health professional students need to completely understand the full potential of the EHR and HIE and how both technologies can empower providers to be meaningful users of these systems.

The EHR provides a technology teaching platform that supports evidence-based teaching strategies such as active learning, time on task, rapid feedback, collaboration, and interprofessional education (IPE) when it is integrated across the curriculum.

Other examples of teaching and learning strategies that can be incorporated in the curriculum are collaborative practice, knowledge management, simulation, and Web 2.0 tools. An example of a *collaborative practice tool* is Team-STEPPS (http://teamstepps.ahrq.gov/), an evidence-based teamwork system that improves communication and teamwork skills among health professionals. TeamSTEPPS is an established system for improving patient safety as well as the efficiency and effectiveness of the healthcare team. Because graduates are expected to work in interprofessional teams, this skill needs to be part of all health professional curricula.

Similarly, *knowledge management tools* build individual and organizational intelligence by enabling people to improve the way in which they capture, share, and use knowledge. Knowledge management involves not only building your own knowledge repository (personal knowledge management), but also using the knowledge, ideas, and experience of others to improve the organization's performance. An LHS incorporates knowledge management tools to build on what works well and discover which evidence leads to better practice, strategy, and policy.

Simulation is a tool used to assist in resolving the patient safety issue while enhancing student learning. During the past decade simulation in health professional programs has increased exponentially. Simulation is an educational process that replicates the clinical work environment and requires students to demonstrate an identified skill set. Simulation-based IPE is a new phenomenon with increasing evidence to support outcomes. Qualitative feedback regarding IPE indicates that participants report feeling comfortable learning with students from other professions and find value in the interprofessional simulation sessions.

Web 2.0 tools are on the rise in all aspects of our lives, including healthcare and education. The emergence of new classes of web-based applications has introduced new possibilities for healthcare delivery as well as new environments for teaching and learning. A variety of Web 2.0 tools is available and the menu continues to grow. Some of these tools are blogs, podcasts, social media networks (e.g., Facebook, Twitter, YouTube), and virtual worlds (e.g., Second Life).

These technologies are changing the way in which consumers and healthcare providers access information and learn. Seamlessly integrating these technologies in the curriculum is an efficient and effective mechanism for bringing health professional education into the digital age and assisting students to gain the competencies they need in practice.

IT TAKES A VILLAGE: ROLES AND COMPETENCIES

In 2008 the ANA developed a competency matrix categorizing three major areas (computer literacy, information literacy, and professional development and leadership) with four educational levels (undergraduate, graduate, informatics specialist, and informatics innovator) and functional roles identified through a job market analysis.[8] Although a standard list of informatics competencies does not exist, the ANA and other organizations (Healthcare Information and Management

Systems Society [HIMSS], AMIA, TIGER, American Association of Colleges of Nursing [AACN], Quality and Safety Education for Nurses [QSEN], National League for Nursing [NLN] and ONC) continue to refine these competencies as health IT and informatics evolve and move to the forefront of the LHS.

What is clear is that all undergraduate, graduate, and practicing nurses need to have a certain level of knowledge about and competency in informatics and its impact on evidence-based practice, quality care, and safety. In addition, informatics specialists are needed to work in interprofessional teams to provide vision, leadership, and management and to advance the science of health informatics through wisdom, research, and innovation. Informatics specialists, educated in informatics specialty programs at the master's or doctoral level (DNP, PhD), will continue to be in high demand. Currently there are not enough health professionals in this specialty area of practice.

Over the past few years the HITECH Act programs have had a significant impact on health IT roles and competencies. In 2010 the U.S. Department of Health & Human Services (HHS) estimated a shortfall of approximately 51,000 qualified health IT workers over the next 5 years based on data from the Bureau of Labor Statistics, the Department of Education, and independent studies. In an attempt to address this shortfall the ONC awarded grants totaling $84 million to 16 universities and junior colleges to help support the training and development of more than 50,000 new health IT professionals. A total of 12 key health IT workforce roles were identified. Each role has specific required educational preparation and outcomes. Six roles require 1-year university-based training and the remaining six roles require 6 months of intense training in a community college or distance-learning organization. Upon completion of these programs it is anticipated that trainees will be able to support nationwide deployment of certified EHR technology and ensure the trusted exchange of health information.

Specific health IT roles requiring university-based education and training include the following:

- *Clinician and public health leader.* Individuals in this role are expected to lead the successful deployment and use of health IT to achieve transformational improvement in the quality, safety, outcomes, and value of health services. Training appropriate to this role will require at least 1 year of study leading to a university-issued certificate or master's degree in health informatics or health IT as a complement to the individual's prior clinical or public health academic training. The individual entering this program may already hold a master's or doctoral degree or the program may be part of his or her existing program of study leading to an advanced clinical practice or public health professional degree. Career opportunities include chief information officer and chief informatics officer.
- *Health information management and exchange specialist.* Individuals in this role support the collection, management, retrieval, exchange, and analysis of electronic information in healthcare and public health organizations.

These individuals would not enter into leadership or management roles unless they had postbaccalaureate or master's education in health information management (HIM) or health informatics.

- *Health information privacy and security specialist.* Individuals in this role are charged with maintaining trust by ensuring the privacy and security of health information as an essential component of any successful health IT deployment in healthcare and public health organizations. Education for this role requires specialization within baccalaureate-level programs or a certificate of advanced studies or postbaccalaureate training in HIM or health informatics. Individuals in this role would be qualified to serve as institutional and organizational information privacy or security officers.
- *Research and development specialist.* Individuals in this role support efforts to create innovative models and solutions that advance the capabilities of health IT and conduct studies on the effectiveness of health IT and its impact on healthcare quality. Education required for this role is a doctoral degree. Career opportunities include faculty roles as well as enterprise analytics and research and development positions.
- *Program and software engineer.* Individuals in this role will be the architects and developers of advanced health IT solutions. They need to have knowledge and understanding of health domains to complement their computer and information science expertise in order to work with the healthcare team (including the patient) to develop solutions that address the specific concerns. Training appropriate to this role is specialization within a baccalaureate program or a certificate of advanced studies or postbaccalaureate education in health informatics. A certificate of advanced study or a master's in health informatics may be very appropriate for individuals with IT backgrounds.
- *Health IT subspecialist.* A small subset of specialized individuals with generalist knowledge of healthcare or public health and in-depth knowledge and expertise in disciplines that inform health IT policy or technology is critical to the success of the health IT initiative. Such disciplines might include ethics, economics, business, policy and planning, cognitive psychology, and industrial and systems engineering. These individuals might expect to find employment in research and development organizations and teaching. These positions would require at least a master's degree but more likely a doctoral degree.

Specific roles designed for community college training include the following:

- *Practice workflow and information management redesign specialist.* Individuals in this role assist in reorganizing the work of a healthcare provider to take full advantage of meeting the Meaningful Use criteria. These individuals may have backgrounds in healthcare or IT but they are not licensed clinical professionals.
- *Clinician or practitioner consultant.* This role is similar to the redesign specialist discussed above; however, these

individuals have backgrounds and experience as licensed clinical or public health professionals. In addition to the responsibilities discussed above they address workflow and data collection issues, including quality outcomes and improvement, from a clinical perspective. They serve as a liaison between users, IT staff, and vendors.

- *Implementation and support specialist.* Individuals in this role provide support before and during implementation of health IT systems in clinical and public health settings. They execute implementation plans by installing hardware and software, incorporating usability principles, testing software against performance specifications, and interacting with vendors to resolve issues during deployment. Backgrounds for these individuals include IT and information management.
- *Implementation managers.* Individuals in this role provide on-site management of mobile adoption support teams before and during implementation of health IT systems. Backgrounds for this role include experience in health and/or IT environments as well as administrative and management experience. These individuals apply project management and change management skills to create implementation plans to achieve project goals, lead implementation support teams, and manage vendor relations.
- *Technical and software support staff.* Individuals in this role maintain health IT systems in clinical and public health settings. Previous backgrounds include IT and information management. Workers interact with end-users to diagnose and document IT problems as well as implement solutions and evaluate their effectiveness.
- *Trainer.* Individuals in this role design and deliver training to employees in clinical and public health settings. Backgrounds for these workers include experience as a health professional or health information specialist. Experience as an educator or trainer is also valued.

The educational training materials developed for the community college training program were supported by the ONC Curriculum Development Centers Program's grants to five universities (Oregon Health & Science University, University of Alabama at Birmingham, Johns Hopkins University, Columbia University, and Duke University). The entire set of teaching materials for the curriculum components is available from the National Training and Dissemination Center at www.onc-ntdc.org/. This is a great resource and foundation for a strong, short-term training program that is currently needed, but it should not replace the integration of the content and competencies across health professional curriculum or the need for advanced education in health informatics. Since the ONC workforce development plan is designed to rapidly increase the number of healthcare IT professionals who will be able to assist healthcare providers in reaching Meaningful Use, these competencies need to be cross-mapped in higher education programs to reach the goal of an LHS. As academic institutions, healthcare organizations, and accrediting agencies establish competencies for health IT and health professionals, they need to look to these nationally defined workforce roles and competencies for guidance. For

a health informatics curriculum to be relevant it must encompass both current and future roles of health IT professionals in all types of health organizations. As the LHS continues to evolve, these roles and competencies will adjust to better align with the market demands of students, communities, and employers. The problem is that healthcare organizations are looking for seasoned health IT professionals and those individuals are rare at this time.

Box 26-1 organizes the competencies derived from the ANA's *Nursing Informatics: Scope and Standards of Practice*, the AACN Essentials documents, and the ONC work role descriptions and categorizes the competencies across curriculum levels. It also includes health IT support professionals, recognizing that these individuals work closely with informatics specialists, researchers, and innovators. In some organizations these support roles may be subsumed by informatics nurses or informatics specialists.

Educating the Generalist

All health professionals need to have a basic level of competency in informatics. The ANA suggests that nurses need computer and information literacy competence.[8] All health professionals at the generalist level need knowledge, skills, and abilities related to data, information, and basic knowledge. According to QSEN, nurses at the prelicensure level should be able to use information and technology to communicate, manage knowledge, mitigate error, and support decision making in a caring and secure environment. QSEN outlines a series of knowledge, skills, and attitudes essential to meeting this overall competence.[22] These competencies, as well as some of the ONC health IT role competencies, are further delineated in the AACN's *The Essentials of Baccalaureate Education for Professional Nursing Practice* and the NLN position statement titled *Preparing the Next Generation of Nurses to Practice in a Technology-Rich Environment: An Informatics Agenda*.[23,24] Upon examination of these competencies it is obvious that integrating an EHR into the academic environment is essential to fully prepare healthcare workers to use EHRs in clinical practice. Several schools use academic versions of EHRs in the classroom and simulated case scenarios to create powerful high-fidelity learning environments.[16,21,25-28] The online activity that is posted on the Evolve site for this chapter exemplifies one school's approach to simulation-based interprofessional education. Just as pilots are trained in simulators to fly airplanes, simulation, including the use of an EHR, can be used to teach health professionals IPE and informatics skills.

Educating Healthcare Specialists at the Graduate Level

While there is variation across the healthcare disciplines, the overall pattern is that increased levels of education correlate with increased specialization. These higher levels of education also prepare specialists for their leadership role. As the use of technology expands, all master's- or doctorate-prepared health practitioners, regardless of specialty, must have the knowledge and skills to meaningfully use current

BOX 26-1 **COMPETENCIES MATRIX OF HEALTH INFORMATION TECHNOLOGY (HEALTH IT) AND INFORMATICS SKILLS**

GENERALIST	ADVANCED PRACTICE	HEALTH IT SUPPORT	SPECIALIST	RESEARCHER AND INNOVATOR
• Demonstrate skills in using patient care technologies, information systems, and communication devices that support safe nursing practice. • Use telecommunication technologies to assist in effective communication in a variety of healthcare settings. • Apply safeguards and decision making support tools embedded in patient care technologies and information systems to support a safe practice environment for both patients and healthcare workers. • Understand the use of CIS to document interventions related to achieving nurse-sensitive outcomes. • Use standardized terminology in a care environment that reflects nursing's unique contribution to patient outcomes. • Evaluate data from all relevant sources, including technology, to inform the delivery of care. • Recognize the role of IT in improving patient care outcomes and creating a safe care environment. • Uphold ethical standards related to data security, regulatory requirements, confidentiality, and clients' right to privacy. • Apply patient care technologies to address the needs of a diverse patient population. • Advocate for the use of new patient care technologies for safe, quality care.	**Master's** • Analyze current and emerging technologies to support safe practice environments and optimize patient safety, cost effectiveness, and health outcomes. • Evaluate outcome data using current communication technologies, information systems, and statistical principles to develop strategies to reduce risks and improve health outcomes. • Promote policies that incorporate ethical principles and standards for the use of health and information technologies. • Provide oversight, guidance, and leadership in the integration of technologies to document patient care and improve patient outcomes. • Use information and communication technologies, resources, and principles of learning to teach patients and others. • Use current and emerging technologies in the care environment to support lifelong learning for self and others. **DNP** • Design, select, use, and evaluate health IT programs, including consumer use of healthcare information systems. • Analyze and communicate critical elements necessary to the selection, use, and evaluation of healthcare informatics systems and patient care technology.	**Workflow and Information Management (IM) Specialist** • Document workflow and IM models of practice. • Conduct user requirements analysis. • Develop revised workflow and IM models based on Meaningful Use of a certified EHR product. • Develop a set of plans to keep the practice running if the EHR system fails. • Work directly with practice personnel to implement the revised workflow and IM model • Evaluate the new processes, identify problems and solutions, and implement changes. • Design processes and information flows that accommodate quality improvement and reporting. **Implementation Support Specialist** • Install hardware and software to meet practice needs. • Incorporate usability principles in software configuration and implementation. • Test the software against performance specifications. • Interact with the vendors to rectify technical problems that occur during the deployment process. • Proactively identify software or hardware incompatibilities. • Assist the practice in identifying a data backup and recovery solution. • Ensure that the mechanism for hardware and software recovery and related capabilities is appropriately implemented to minimize system downtime. • Ensure that privacy and security functions are appropriately configured and activated. • Document IT problems and evaluate the effectiveness of problem resolution. • Assist end-users with audits.	**Clinician and Practitioner Consultant** • Analyze and recommend solutions for health IT implementation problems in clinical and public health settings. • Advise and assist clinicians in taking full advantage of technology, enabling them to make best use of data to drive improvement in quality, safety, and efficiency. • Assist in selection of vendors and software by helping practice personnel to ask the right questions and evaluate answers. • Advocate for users' needs, acting as a liaison between users, IT staff, and vendors. • Ensure that the patient and consumer perspective is incorporated into the EHR, including privacy and security issues. • Train practitioners in best use of the EHR system, conforming to the redesigned workflow. • Provide leadership, ensuring that implementation teams function cohesively. **Implementation Manager** • Apply project management and change management principles to create implementation project plans to achieve the project goals. • Interact with diverse personnel to ensure open communication across end-users and with the support team. • Lead implementation teams consisting of workers in the roles described above. • Manage vendor relations, providing schedule, deliverable, and business information to health IT vendors for product improvement. • Coordinate implementation-related efforts across the implementation site and with the health information exchange partners, troubleshooting problems as they arise.	• Conduct research on design, development, implementation, and impact of informatics solutions. • Conduct research on mobile health and telehealth technologies and the impact on informatics. • Conduct research on emerging patterns of care and outcomes. • Analyze outcomes leading to new evidence-based guidelines. • Develop new methods of organizing data to enhance research capacities. • Design and develop informatics solutions. • Develop new ways to interact with computer systems and access data. • Assist in setting the future agenda for health informatics. • Disseminate process and outcomes of research and product development.

Continued

BOX 26-1	COMPETENCIES MATRIX OF HEALTH INFORMATION TECHNOLOGY (HEALTH IT) AND INFORMATICS SKILLS—cont'd

GENERALIST	ADVANCED PRACTICE	HEALTH IT SUPPORT	SPECIALIST	RESEARCHER AND INNOVATOR
• Recognize that redesign of workflow and care processes should precede implementation of care technology to facilitate nursing practice. • Participate in evaluation of information systems in practice settings through policy and procedure development.	• Demonstrate the conceptual ability and technical skills to develop and execute an evaluation plan involving data extraction from practice information systems and databases. • Provide leadership in the evaluation and resolution of ethical and legal issues within healthcare systems relating to the use of information, IT, communication networks, and patient care technology. • Evaluate consumer health information sources for accuracy, timeliness, and appropriateness.	**Technical and Software Support Staff** • Interact with end-users to diagnose IT problems and implement solutions. • Document IT problems and evaluate the effectiveness of solutions. • Support systems security and standards. • Assist end-users with the execution of audits and related privacy and security functions. • Incorporate usability principles into ongoing software configuration and implementation. • Ensure that the hardware and software "fail-over" and related capabilities are appropriately implemented to minimize system downtime. • Ensure that privacy and security functions are appropriately configured and activated in hardware and software. • Interact with the vendors as needed to rectify technical problems that occur during the deployment process. • Work with the vendor and other sources of information to find the solution to a user's question or problem as needed.	• Apply an understanding of health IT, Meaningful Use, and the challenges practice settings will encounter in achieving Meaningful Use. **Trainer** • Be able to use a range of health IT applications, preferably at an expert level. • Communicate clearly both health and IT concepts as appropriate, in language the learner or user can understand. • Apply a user-oriented approach to training, reflecting the need to empathize with the learner or user. • Assess training needs and competencies of learners. • Accurately assess employees' understanding of training, particularly through observation of use both in and out of the classroom. • Design lesson plans, structuring active learning experiences for users and creating use cases that effectively train employees through an approach that closely mirrors actual use of the health IT in the patient care setting. • Maintain accurate training records of the users and develop learning plans for further instruction.	

CIS, Clinical Information System; *DNP,* doctor of nursing practice; *EHR,* electronic health record.

technologies to deliver and coordinate care across multiple settings, analyze point-of-care outcomes, and communicate with individuals and groups, including the media, policymakers, other health professionals, and the public, regarding health IT and the secure and trusted use of HIEs. Integral to these skills is an attitude of openness to innovation and continual learning since information systems and care technologies are constantly changing.[29] For example, all nurses educated at the master's level should be prepared to use information and technology to communicate, manage knowledge, mitigate error, and support decision making.[30] The IOM and QSEN advanced practice competencies build on the prelicensure competencies and are embedded in the AACN's revised *The Essentials of Master's Education for Professional Nursing*[29]

and *The Essentials of Doctoral Education for Advanced Nursing Practice.*[31] The need for an informatics skill set across all levels of the curriculum further points out the importance of integrating informatics tools in the curriculum and a shift in teaching approaches to include collaboration and teamwork. At this level students use EHR data to monitor open loop processes, generate research questions, look for links to evidence-based decision making, detect unanticipated events, and support clinical workflow and population management. Clinicians at this level use a variety of digital technologies to advance their skills as an integrator, aggregating information from patients and their health records, recognizing patterns, making decisions, and translating those decisions into action.

Educating the Informatics Specialist

Informatics specialists are formally prepared at the graduate level (master's or doctorate) in their discipline (i.e., nursing informatics), health informatics, or biomedical informatics programs. Informatics specialists design, manage, and apply discipline-specific data and information to improve decision making by consumers, patients, nurses, and other healthcare providers.[8] They must have strong verbal and communication skills and analytical skills as well as clinical knowledge and technical proficiency. Most health informatics specialists work in a hospital or healthcare setting in management or administrative positions; however, a significant percentage hold positions with health-related vendors, suppliers, insurance companies, and consulting firms. As EHRs and other information and communication technologies become increasingly important, informatics specialists will become even more vital in bridging the gap between clinical care skills and technology. These specialists are expected to practice in interprofessional team environments, interact with health IT support professionals, and lead change. They need to be knowledgeable about clinical information systems and how they support the work of clinicians.

The healthcare industry is looking for informatics specialists to correctly design, build, test, implement, and maintain health IT systems to meet Meaningful Use criteria. The specific job description and activities of an informatics specialist in any setting will, of course, be determined by the employing organization but these activities can be expected to include responsibilities such as analysis, project management, software tailoring and development, designing and implementing educational programs, administration, management and leadership, consulting, and program evaluation and research.

Educating the Informatics Researcher and Innovator

The role of the informatics researcher is prominent in the emergence of an LHS that focuses on best care practices and the generation and application of new knowledge. Constant innovation is needed to keep pace with evolving technologies and ever-changing regulatory mandates. As new health technologies emerge, new innovations will grow, and research and development will be essential to support commercialization. Preparation for the researcher and innovator role is at the graduate level, usually in a PhD or DNP informatics program depending on the primary focus of research or innovation. Education at the PhD level focuses on developing and analyzing evidence; at the clinical level (DNP) the focus is on implementing evidence.

The role of an informatics researcher includes knowledge of research designs and application to develop better and more efficient ways of entering, retrieving, and using health informatics to improve health outcomes and engage consumers. An informatics researcher has a key role in developing new data collection methods and assisting with finding the appropriate data to collect for various projects and research grants. This research ranges from experimental research to process improvement and from informal evaluation to evidence-based practice.[8] Informatics researchers must be effective written and oral communicators, as dissemination of their work through consultation, publication, and presentation is an important part of their role. They should have a clear understanding of research design and how to develop accurate and correct questions for surveys and research projects. The ability to work in a team environment with those both familiar and not as familiar with research is essential. Excellent computer skills and knowledge of databases and software programs available for research are important. A healthcare background and experience working with patients and consumers in some capacity are helpful. Knowledge of healthcare organizations, state and federal regulations and policies regarding healthcare practices, data collection, data stewardship, and confidentiality is critical. In addition, a spirit of entrepreneurship along with knowledge of commercialization and technology transfer are important to the innovator role.

Continuing Professional Development

Lifelong learning is a key component of an LHS. This new movement to accelerate the national efforts to increase adoption of health IT across all healthcare arenas (including consumer engagement, public health surveillance, and research) affects practicing nurses and other health professionals. As practice changes and new technology evolves, continuous learning is necessary to have competent, up-to-date, skilled professionals who are able to respond quickly to the needs of the system. Nurses who are interested in expanding their education to include informatics have many opportunities for learning through formal academic education as well as continuing education programs. The HITECH Act, federal and private initiatives, professional organizations, the health IT industry, and universities have increased opportunities for health IT and informatics continuing education. A web search for health IT or informatics seminars and webinars or conferences will provide a variety of opportunities to help meet the learner's specific needs. Opportunities for continuing professional development are included in Table 26-1.

CONCLUSION AND FUTURE DIRECTIONS

Health, healthcare, and education in this country are going digital, setting the stage for an LHS dependent on continuous learning and facilitated by information and communication technologies. This developing potential presents opportunities and challenges for health professional education. It is forcing educators to redefine and rethink how they educate health professionals.

Nursing and health informatics specialty programs will continue to expand and core informatics competencies will be taught across all levels of the curriculum for health professionals. The LHS will require a new skill set that will necessitate a major redesign of educational programs for health professionals, including a focus on interprofessional collaborative education and practice. Informatics competencies and new workforce roles will continue to evolve as the continuous learning loop and new technologies change the way in which healthcare and education are delivered. Continuous learning through formal academic programs, short-term courses, conferences, workshops, and seminars is core to ensuring that clinical practice reflects the current best evidence. In the future one can expect to see continued learning and just-in-time learning incorporated directly into the information systems used to provide care. For example, as standards of care change, healthcare providers may not attend a workshop to learn about these new standards but rather will be brought up to date on these new standards through the decision support systems incorporated in the EHR.

REFERENCES

1. Grossman C, Powers B, McGinnis M, eds. *Digital Infrastructure for the Learning Health System: The Foundation for Continuous Improvement in Health and Health Care: Workshop Series Summary*. Washington, DC: The National Academies Press; 2011.

2. Kohn LT, Corrigan JM, Donaldson MS, eds. *To Err Is Human: Building a Safer Health System*. Washington, DC: The National Academies Press; 2000.

3. Committee on Quality of Health Care in America, Institute of Medicine. *Crossing the Quality Chasm: A New Health System for the 21st Century*. Washington DC: The National Academies Press; 2001.

4. Greiner AC, Knebel E, eds. *Health Professions Education: A Bridge to Quality*. Washington DC: The National Academies Press; 2003.

5. American Nurses Association. *The Standards of Practice for Nursing Informatics*. Washington, DC: American Nurses Publishing; 1995.

6. American Nurses Association. *The Scope of Practice for Nursing Informatics*. Washington, DC: American Nurses Publishing; 1994.

7. American Nurses Association. *Scope and Standards of Nursing Informatics Practice*. Washington, DC: American Nurses Publishing; 2001.

8. American Nurses Association. *Nursing Informatics: Scope and Standards of Practice*. Washington, DC: American Nurses Publishing; 2008.

9. Booth RG. Educating the future ehealth professional nurse. *Int J Nurs Educ Scholarsh*. 2006;3(1).

10. Healthcare Information and Management Systems Society (HIMSS). *Informatics nurse impact survey final report*. HIMSS. http://www.himss.org/asp/ContentRedirector.asp?ContentId=76364. 2011.

11. Healthcare Information and Management Systems Society (HIMSS). *Informatics nurse impact survey final report*. HIMSS. http://www.himss.org/asp/ContentRedirector.asp?ContentID=69103. 2009.

12. Skiba D, Rizzolo MA. Education and faculty development. In: Hannah KJ, Ball MJ, eds. *Nursing Informatics: Where Technology and Caring Meet*. 4th ed. New York, NY: Springer; 2011:65-80.

13. Staggers N, Gassert CA, Curran C. A Delphi study to determine informatics competencies for nurses at four levels of practice. *Nurs Res*. 2002;51(6):383-390.

14. Committee on the Robert Wood Johnson Foundation Initiative on the Future of Nursing, Institute of Medicine. *The Future of Nursing: Leading Change, Advancing Health*. Washington, DC: The National Academies Press; 2010.

15. Institute of Medicine. *Learning What Works: Infrastructure Required for Comparative Effectiveness Research*. Washington DC: The National Academies Press; 2007.

16. Connors HR. Transforming the nursing curriculum: going paperless. In: Weaver CA, Delaney CW, Weber P, Carr RL, eds. *Nursing and Informatics for the 21st Century: An International Look at Practice, Trends and the Future*. Chicago, IL: HIMSS Press; 2006:183-194.

17. Connors H, Warren J, Popkess-Vawter S. Technology and informatics. In: Giddens JF, ed. *Concepts for Nursing Practice*. St. Louis, MO: Elsevier; 2012:443-452.

18. Chang, J, Poynton MR, Gassert CA, Staggers N. Nursing informatics competencies required of nurses in Taiwan. *Int J Med Inform*. 2011;80(5):332-340. doi:10.1016/j.ijmedinf.2011.01.011.

19. Goncalves L, Wolf LG, Staggers N. Nursing informatics competencies: analysis of the latest research. Paper presented at: NI 2012: Advancing Global Health through Informatics. June, 2012; Montreal, Canada.

20. Technology Informatics Guiding Educational Reform (TIGER). *About TIGER*. TIGER. http://www.tigersummit.com/About_Us.html. 2012.

21. Warren JJ, Meyer MJ, Thompson TL, Roche AJ. Transforming nursing education: integrating informatics and simulations. In: Weaver CA, Delaney CW, Weber P, Carr RL, eds. *Nursing and Informatics for the 21st Century: An International Look at Practice, Trends and the Future*, 2nd ed. Chicago, IL: HIMSS Press; 2010:145-161.

22. QSEN Institute. Pre-Licensure KSAS. http://qsen.org/competencies/pre-licensure-ksas/. 2012.

23. American Association of Colleges of Nursing (AACN). *The essentials of baccalaureate education for professional nursing practice*. AACN. http://www.aacn.nche.edu/education/pdf/baccessentials08.pdf. 2008.

24. National League for Nursing (NLN) Board of Governors. *Preparing the next generation of nurses to practice in a technology-rich environment*. NLN. http://www.nln.org/aboutnln/PositionStatements/informatics_052808.pdf. 2008.

25. Connors HR, Weaver C, Warren JJ, Miller KL. An academic-business partnership for advancing clinical informatics. *Nurs Educ Perspect*. 2002;23(5):228-233.

26. Fauchald SK. An academic-industry partnership for advancing technology in health science education. *Comput Inform Nurs*. 2008:26(10):4-8.

27. Jeffries PR, Hudson K, Taylor LA, Klapper SA. Bridging technology: academe and industry. In: Hannah KJ, Ball MJ, eds. *Nursing Informatics: Where Technology and Caring Meet*. 4th ed. New York, NY: Springer; 2011:167-188.

28. Warren JJ, Connors HR. Health information technology can and will transform nursing education. *Nurs Outlook*. 2007;55(1):59-60.

29. American Association of Colleges of Nursing (AACN). *The essentials of master's education for professional nursing*. AACN. http://www.aacn.nche.edu/education-resources/MastersEssentials11.pdf. 2011.

30. Cronenwett L, Sherwood G, Pohl J, et al. Quality and safety education for advanced nursing practice. *Nurs Outlook*. 2009;37(6):338-348.

31. American Association of Colleges of Nursing (AACN). The essentials of doctoral education for advanced practice nurses. AACN. http://www.aacn.nche.edu/publications/position/DNPEssentials.pdf. 2010.

DISCUSSION QUESTIONS

1. Why are informatics competencies necessary when responding to the ONC's initiatives and to proposed healthcare reform regulations?
2. Discuss the learning health system in relation to developing a curriculum and assignments to teach students about participating in this system.
3. Compare and contrast the competencies outlined in Box 26-1: generalist, advanced practice, health IT support, specialist, and researcher and innovator.
4. Describe how health informatics can be used to transform interprofessional education (IPE).
5. What main resources would you need to integrate an academic electronic health record in healthcare simulations (with and without human patient simulators)? Include staff in the discussion.
6. Develop an action plan to improve informatics competencies for faculty and for students.
7. Differentiate, in terms of informatics roles and education, the nurse generalist, the advanced practice nurse, and the informatics nurse specialist.
8. Develop a plan of study for a nurse researcher to be able to engage in big data analytics.
9. Develop a plan of study for an innovator. Include in the plan informatics skills, change management, quality improvement, business management, intellectual property knowledge, financial planning, and so forth.
10. Compare and contrast informatics knowledge and competencies, information literacy, and computer literacy.

CASE STUDY

Best Hospital is a 325-bed suburban community hospital that has just merged with a local major academic medical center, the University of Excellence Medical Center (UEMC). There are 15 hospitals in the UEMC system, ranging from small rural hospitals with 50 or fewer beds to large multiple-specialty tertiary referral hospitals. Two hospitals in the system have achieved magnet status and several hospitals are working to achieve this status. Within the UEMC system a high value is placed on collaboration with the schools of the health professions at the University of Excellence (UE).

Best Hospital has a long history of association with local universities, functioning mainly as a site for student clinical experiences. For example, undergraduate students enrolled at the UE College of Health Professions often complete a portion of their clinical work at the hospital. Each year the hospital hires a number of graduates from this program. Several nurses in first-level management positions at the hospital are enrolled in the master's program.

The vice-president for clinical practice at Best Hospital is a PhD-prepared nurse who has been appointed to the faculty at the UE School of Nursing. Your current position is director of staff development at Best Hospital. You are responsible for the educational programming of all clinical staff. Over the past 2 years Best Hospital has been fully involved in meeting Meaningful Use criteria. As director of staff development you have played the major leadership role in developing and implementing all related educational programs.

The health professional schools at UE are working together to revise their curricula to integrate informatics throughout.

The goal is to develop an interprofessional approach that incorporates informatics across and throughout the different educational programs within these schools. The schools have requested a meeting with clinical leaders from the hospital to gain a practice perspective on what information should be included in the curriculums. The vice-president for clinical practice has included you on the list of leaders to attend the meeting. She has also asked that each person attending the meeting prepare (1) a list of key references related to this topic and (2) a list of competencies, concepts, and skills that should be included in the educational preparation of graduates of the healthcare educational programs at both the graduate and the undergraduate levels.

Discussion Questions

1. Discuss what you think should be included on either or both of these lists.
2. Describe how informatics competencies could or should be incorporated into the clinical experiences of students. Be specific. For example, how should student access to the clinical information systems be developed? Who should provide the needed instruction time and cover the cost of orienting each group of students?
3. Realizing that both Best Hospital and UE include in their mission statements service, scholarship, and education, what other innovative collaborative programs might be developed by these institutions?

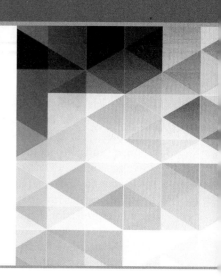

Distance Education: Applications, Techniques, and Issues

Irene Joos

Web 2.0 tools are opening up educational opportunities for lifelong learning to a diverse global community.

OBJECTIVES

At the completion of this chapter the reader will be prepared to:

1. Discuss historical developments and their impact on today's distance education scene, including developments in nursing and other healthcare professional fields

2. Evaluate course management systems (CMSs) using appropriate criteria

3. Examine issues related to development and implementation of distance education options in a college or university

KEY TERMS

Course management system (CMS), 426
Distance education, 426
Distance learning, 426
Distributive (distributed) education, 426

Distributive learning, 426
eLearning, 427
Learning management system (LMS), 428
Online education, 427

ABSTRACT

The changes in our educational environment are reflective of shifts in our demographics, economic conditions, and technological developments. Web 2.0 tools are opening up educational opportunities for lifelong learning to a diverse global community. This chapter presents a brief history of distance education, defines emerging terms, and discusses course management and learning management systems, including some of the trends and issues related to selection. It concludes with a discussion of four issues related to the development and implementation of distance education: legal, disability, quality, and readiness.

INTRODUCTION

Technology developments and the Internet are causing an unprecedented upheaval in how institutions of higher learning deliver instruction. Since the late 1990s and early 2000s distance education has become a major issue. It is one of the "most complex issues facing higher education institutions today."[1(pv)] While this statement was written years ago, it holds true today. Most colleges and universities are now beyond asking whether they should offer distributive or distance learning options and instead are addressing the issue of how to handle these offerings.

Given the current work environment and the economic times, growing numbers of health-related programs are offering part or all of their program content online. Increasingly students come to school with work and family obligations or live in areas distant from educational opportunities. Distance education is a viable option for this demographic of health professions students.[2] This type of education provides increased flexibility in meeting the educational needs of the changing student population and is influencing how authors write to facilitate all learning styles and how textbooks are delivered (etexts with multiple interactive activities, videos or podcasts, etc).

Technology developments have an impact on the institutions themselves and student expectations, and also on how students learn. Several recent books have addressed what constant technology-facilitated connections might be doing to our brains; what constant connections are doing to relationships between family members, friends, and colleagues; how we understand privacy, community, intimacy, and solitude; and how the digital revolution changes people and who they can become.[3-5] Frand identified the following 10 attributes of the information age mindset:

- Computers are not technology
- The Internet is better than TV
- Reality is no longer real
- Doing is more important than knowing
- Trial and error and experimentation are preferable to logic
- Multitasking is a way of life
- Typing is preferable to handwriting
- Staying connected is essential
- There is zero tolerance for delays
- There is a blurring of the lines between consumer and creator[6]

Think about the impact those mindsets are having on the educational system and traditional methods of teaching.

This chapter presents a brief history of distance education, defines evolving terms, examines course management and learning management systems for delivering distance education, and presents issues related to development and implementation of distance education in colleges, universities, and organizations.

HISTORICAL DEVELOPMENT

Four phases divide the historical development of distance education and its changing nature. Correspondence education characterized the first phase, encompassing the mid to late 1800s. Correspondence education involved receiving printed materials, reading those materials, and sending back any required assignments. The founding of the Society to Encourage Studies at Home in 1873 by Anna Ticknor[7] and the founding of the Chautauqua College of Liberal Arts in 1883[8] were two instrumental events that moved correspondence education forward, as both of these programs offered correspondence opportunities. They responded to the need for a more educated workforce and to the interest of women and the common man for an education. An inexpensive postal service facilitated this development. While the number of offered courses grew along with enrollment, so too did the concerns about quality education and the effectiveness of this means of delivery—a theme that continues today. While audiovisual developments occurred in the early 1900s, there was little evidence of their use for distance education until the early 1960s.

Phase 2, encompassing the 1960s, the 1970s, and the early 1980s, enhanced the delivery method for distance education by involving broadcast media: cable and satellite television.[9] The terms changed from *correspondence* to *telecourses* and from *correspondence education* to *distance education* during this time. While students were ready to embrace this method of delivery because of family responsibilities, work responsibilities, geographic challenges in accessing academic institutions, and disability issues, the academic institutions

continued to question the effectiveness of this new delivery method and the changes required in teaching methods. While educational television programs could be "shared" across academic institutions, this method of delivering content did not become popular even with the development and use of videotapes, the telephone, and other technologies. As late as the 1970s learners were taking "external studies" courses in which learners purchased printed course packages, some of which included audiotapes and most of which had no television component.

Phase 3, which took place in the 1980s and 1990s, found many colleges and universities laying fiber optic cables on campus. This high-speed connection made possible live two-way video communication between local distance education classrooms and remote classrooms. The main issues with this technology were the expense of the classrooms, the support necessary to run the equipment during scheduled class times, and the restrictions on faculty as to movement out of camera and microphone range. Students and faculty at both sites could see and hear each other, although sometimes with a slight transmission delay. This was education at a distance but in real time (synchronous). In addition, developing technology made it possible for more people to purchase home personal computers with dial-up Internet access, enabling students to access course materials from a distance and to interact with faculty and other students through email, telephone, or other communication systems.

Phase 4, which began in the late 1990s and continues to the present, saw advances in the Internet and the development of Web 2.0 tools. This moved the focus from information retrieval to user-generated content and interaction, to users and communities. This phase saw a spurt in development of distance education courses and programs to meet the needs of a mobile society that was and is concerned about costs, currency, and lifelong learning, as well as a need to stay competitive in the job market. Also of concern here is the integration of technologies into traditional classrooms and a hybrid approach to delivering courses and facilitating learning for a wide range of learners.

In health education, faculty have been providing distance education courses and programs for more than 35 years.[10,11] Early programs relied on mostly print materials and some audiotapes, with a few on-campus meetings during the semester. Students purchased the packet of materials, completed the assigned work, and in most cases attended two or three on-campus sessions. Some courses set up testing centers located off-campus for the taking of proctored tests. With changing technology developments, delivery system formats changed from mostly printed materials to broadcast courses (e.g., distance learning classrooms that broadcast live classes to remote sites). Computer-aided instructional programs and interactive videodiscs ran on free-standing computers.[12] The Fuld Foundation provided competitive grants for the equipment and videodisc programs such as *Managing the Experience of Labor and Delivery* and *The Suicidal Adolescent*.

The current generation of course delivery methods increasingly incorporates mobile devices; Web 2.0 tools such as podcasts, wikis, blogs, and video conferencing; and integrated campus course management systems (CMSs). These CMSs integrate student functions such as registration, billing, courses, library, tutoring, and other related student services. What will the next generation of CMSs look like? What tools are in development that will facilitate delivery of courses and improved learner outcomes? The answers to these questions will become apparent as we move toward Web 3.0 tools and applications and ever-changing technological developments. One example of changes relates to the terms that describe the evolving educational delivery methods.

EVOLVING TERMS

Although the phrases *distributive (distributed) education, distance education, distributive (distributed) learning,* and *distance learning* are used interchangeably, there is a growing consensus that distributive education and learning have broader meanings. This section examines the various definitions and how they differ.

Distance education is instruction and learning that takes place when the teacher and the learner are in two different settings and possibly teaching and learning at two different times.[2] Other authors remove the time element, defining distance education as teaching and learning where the teacher and learner are geographically separated and rely on technology for instructional delivery.[13] Time is not a critical element in this definition; distance is the critical element. Knebel's 2001 definition fits with the distance learning *classrooms* that educational institutions use to provide instruction to remote locations through satellite connections and equipment that permits the teacher and learner to interact with and see one another in real time. The teacher and learner are separated by distance but not by time. Note that time here refers to when students attend to their learning, not the time frame surrounding start and end of semesters, due dates for completion of assignments, etc. Some people believe that if the student and teacher are in the same space and time, it is *not* distance education; others believe that if they are in different locations, it is distance education. Also critical in distinguishing distance education from independent learning or programmed computer instruction is that distance education is planned, mediated instruction; this means that the teacher provides direction, comments on coursework, and issues a grade on completion of the course and that course organization and designed learning experiences guide the student's learning. As an example, the National Council of State Boards of Nursing (NCSBN) adopted the American Association of Colleges of Nursing's (AACN's) definition of distance education: "a set of teaching/learning strategies to meet the learning needs of students that are separate from the traditional classroom setting and the traditional role of faculty. In distance education the students and faculty are separate from each other."[11(para3)] Note the focus on learning. This definition aligns with that of Knebel's in that time is not the issue; distance is the issue. Again, time here refers to when students attend to their learning and not to the parameters related to start and end dates for courses, assignments, etc.

Distance learning focuses on students who may be separated in time and space from their peers and professor and what they learn when taking distance education classes.[1] The focus is the student's learning or outcome, not the institutional processes and policies surrounding distance education. Learning experiences can include using email to interact with others; discussion forums to discuss questions and express ideas; video conferences, chats, and blogs to interact with classmates and the professor; and other creative experiences the faculty may develop. Many people use the terms *distance education* and *distance learning* interchangeably.

Distributive (distributed) education is a change in pedagogy where the course developer customizes the learning environment to the learning styles of the learners using technology; the learners may be taking distance, hybrid (combination of online and face to face), or on-site courses. This method includes interactive activities using available technologies. The pedagogy supports a hands-on learning-by-doing approach in which the learners interact and collaborate during the course of study using appropriate technology. For example, one might have the learners review a lesson and video on patient teaching, discuss critical elements of a good patient teaching guide on a discussion forum, and then work on a wiki to produce a project such as a patient teaching guide on some aspect of nursing care where there is a written lesson, podcast, and demonstration video.

Distributive learning is learning through the use of technologies (such as video and Web 2.0 tools) and interactive activities and it may include augmented classrooms, hybrid courses, or distance education courses. The NCSBN uses the definition "a student-centered approach to learning that incorporates the use of technology in the learning process"[14(para20)] and also uses Dede's characteristics of distributive education:

- Supports different learning styles by using mixed media
- Builds on the learner's perspective though interactive experiences
- Builds learning and social skills through collaboration
- Integrates learning into daily lives[15]

Although the terms *distributed learning* and *distance education* are used interchangeably, distance education has a narrower definition. Since the primary characteristic of distance education is that learners and teachers are separated by time and distance, learners learn the material on their own time and in their own place. Distance education may or may not include the use of emerging technologies. The primary goal of distributed learning is the customization of the learning environment to better meet the learner's needs through the use of technologies and an interactive collaborative environment that can take place on or off campus—that is, through course enhancements embedded in traditional classroom settings, hybrid (combination of face-to-face and distance learning), or distance courses. Distributed learning is more inclusive in its delivery methods. See the Office of the Undersecretary of Defense for Personnel and Readiness's Advanced

Distributed Learning Network at www.adlnet.gov/ for information on the Next Generation of Learners, Learning Environment, and Personal Learning Assistant initiatives.

Two other useful terms one might encounter are *online education* and *elearning*. Online education requires the use of the Internet or an intranet to deliver educational materials. eLearning is "interactive learning in which the learning content is available online and provides automatic feedback to the student's learning activities."[16(p25)] Others, like Saffarzadeh, define elearning as "a change in the learner's knowledge that is attributable to an experience with an electronic device."[17(para1)] This means that elearning requires a computer or other electronic device such as a smartphone or tablet. eLearning involves a greater variety of equipment than online resources or the Internet in that any electronic device may be used: DVDs, CD-ROMs, etc. One can use these devices in distance education courses or on campus in computer or simulated labs.

With such variations and overlap in these definitions, schools that offer distance or distributive education and elearning must consistently define these terms and the related technology required to implement the program or course. This process should answer the question, will these terms be used interchangeably or not? If not, what are the distinctions being made by faculty and why is that important? Faculty should discuss and define these terms during their strategic planning process when developing distance or distributive education courses and programs. Box 27-1 provides a sample outline for a strategic plan and Box 27-2 provides an outline for a progress report. Questions to ask and answer during strategic planning include the following:

- What terms are faculty and the school using to describe the distance learning initiative? What terms do the accreditation agencies use? How are colleagues in other schools defining the terms? How will these definitions be conveyed to the student?
- What technology will the institution use to deliver these courses? How will the school notify students about the required technology—for example, a webcam and broadband connection?
- Does enrollment in online and distance education courses mean that students will never be required to come to campus? Are faculty using some hybrid approach that may require some attendance on campus?
- What course or learning management system will the school use? Who will make that decision? What input do faculty have?

Once the school decides to provide options for students regarding course delivery methods to complete their degrees, the selection of the course or learning management system

---

BOX 27-1   OUTLINE FOR A STRATEGIC PLAN FOR DISTRIBUTIVE EDUCATION

Issues

This section sets the background for the plan and generally includes the following subsections:

Introduction. This subsection sets the stage for why faculty and the school are doing this. It addresses what is happening in the broader world, then locally, and then within the institution. It should answer the following questions: Why is the institution and faculty doing this? What are the goals? How will faculty and the institution define related terms? Some include a SWOT (strengths, weaknesses, opportunities, and threats) analysis in the introduction. Others place it within the Details section as a separate subsection called *SWOT analysis.* Others place it in an appendix to the plan.

Mission statement. What is the mission for this initiative? How does that fit with the mission of the college or university? The mission statement should include some of the language of the school's mission.

Goals. What are the goals for this initiative? This can include goals such as providing flexibility in helping students to achieve their educational goals, targeting the adult and second degree populations, and developing faculty. Areas to address in the goals are as follows:

- *Students.* Who are the target students? What are the rules as to who can take these courses or enroll in the program? How will students be oriented to these means of learning?
- *Faculty.* How will faculty be trained? What training will faculty need? How will ongoing support be provided? How will this count toward faculty teaching loads? Who will monitor quality?

- *Courses and programs.* What programs and courses will be offered in this delivery method? Who makes these decisions? How are decisions approved? How do faculty address issues such as the TEACH Act and copyright. What is the target class size? How will that decision be made?
- *Support issues.* What CMS will be used? Can it interface with the school's other systems? When will faculty have access to a shell for course development? What library changes will be needed to support remote students? How will access to other support services such as registration, paying tuition, and accessing tutoring be handled? What support services will students need?
- *Policy and procedures.* Who will develop and approve them? When?

Details

This section provides the details for each of the goals identified.

Goals. List and number each goal. For example, 1a, 1b, 2a, 2b, 2c, etc.

Recommendations. After careful review, comparison, and research, what is the recommendation for each goal? For example, after careful review, Blackboard is the recommended CMS. Recommendations should also include who will be responsible for moving each goal forward.

Budget items. Include projected costs for achieving each goal.

Time frame. Include a target date for achievement of each goal.

usually begins. This generally requires considering all available options.

COURSE MANAGEMENT SYSTEMS (CMSs): MAJOR VENDORS AND PLAYERS

CMSs, also known as learning management systems (LMSs), are software programs or applications that permit a faculty member to deliver a course without knowing any programming code. These programs provide the tools necessary to plan, implement, and assess the learning process by giving the professor the ability to create and deliver content, monitor student participation, and assess learning outcomes.[18] Most CMS and LMS software products now have interactive features like chat, blogs, wikis, conferencing, and discussion forums. There are many CMS software programs and the market is constantly changing. See Table 27-1 for CMS usage rankings based on a survey by Campus Computing in 2011 and presented by Green at the 2011 EDUCAUSE Conference.[19]

The CMS selection decision often rests with administrators, information technology (IT) personnel, and faculty, although some institutions may have student representatives on the planning committee. The process for selection should be part of the strategic plan for distance education. Considerations for selection should include the following:

- *Integration with current systems.* How important is that? Which campus systems? Does the CMS support interoperability with third party products (e.g., registrar's applications, billing, registration)?
- *Compatibility with different student systems* such as operating systems, mobile devices, and related security programs like firewalls and antivirus programs.
- *User base.* What is the installed user base (how many institutions and end-users are using the product)? What type of support does it provide? How stable is the company offering the CMS?
- *Customization.* Will the CMS require extensive custom programming? Are sufficient resources in place for that work?

- *Scalability.* How scalable is the CMS? Can it easily expand or contract based on varying needs?
- *Usability.* How user friendly is the CMS? Does it have the tool set that faculty needs to deliver the courses? Are those tools intuitive to use for both students and faculty to complete typical tasks?
- *Outcome measures.* Does the CMS support outcome measures?
- *SCORM (Sharable Content Object Reference Model) compliant.* Is the system SCORM compliant (encourages the standardization of LMSs)? Is that important?
- *Cost.* What is the cost for hosting versus housing the CMS? What are the mechanism for and frequency of upgrades? What are the costs of these upgrades?[20,21]

One way to start the selection process is to first decide on the type of system that will meet the needs of the institution and its students: campus-based portal, proprietary CMS, open source system, or partnership. Many of these systems are moving toward the campus-based portal model.

TABLE 27-1	CAMPUS COMPUTING PROFILE OF THE CMS MARKET, FALL 2011	
CMS	**MARKET SHARE***
Blackboard (including WebCT and Angel)	51%
Moodle	19%
Desire2Learn	11%
Sakai	7%
None	7%
Jenzabar	2%
Other	2%
eCollege	2%
In-house structure	1%

Data from Green K. The campus computing project. The Campus Computing Project. http://www.campuscomputing.net/sites/www.campuscomputing.net/files/Green-CampusComputing 2011_4.pdf. October 2011.
CMS, Course management system.
*Rounded up.

Campus-Based Portals

Campus-based portals are customized, personalized entries or gateways where users, including students and faculty, can access all of the content they typically need. A portal is a user-centric web page that includes access to a CMS. The portal integrates and provides a secure access point to the data, information, and applications users need in their roles as a student or faculty. Portals generally include enterprise resource systems (finance, human relations, etc.), community building communications, admissions, retention, web-based academic counseling, CMSs, and metrics to measure success, to name only some features. Two examples of portals are Ellucian and Jenzabar.

Ellucian

Ellucian (www.ellucian.com) is the new name for two educational technology providers, Datatel and SunGard Higher Education, that merged in 2012. Its focus is assisting educational institutions to grow in a changing educational climate by offering applications that integrate and interface all of the systems that faculty and students need. The solution includes a CMS. This campus portal was used by 2300 colleges, universities, foundations, and state systems in 40 countries as of 2012.[22]

Jenzabar e-Racer

Jenzabar (www.jenzabar.com) is another example of a portal system that supports a college or university across each department, including every administrative office and academic department. Jenzabar attempts to align the school's mission and goals with technology investments. Jenzabar e-Racer is Jenzabar's advanced learning management portal. This product integrates with the other Jenzabar products, such as the student information system and the business operations systems, allowing for a single sign-on to access courses, collaborate with classmates and faculty, participate in online discussions, take tests, etc. Figure 27-1 shows the Higher Education Solutions menu on the main screen and the range of offerings that Jenzabar provides. These products are similar for most portal systems.

Proprietary CMSs and LMSs

Proprietary CMSs are "software products that are purchased or licensed by one vendor."[23(pviii)] These vendors provide a license either to install the system on the customer's servers or to host the customer's license on their servers. For many years proprietary CMSs were the dominant systems on the market. Many of these original systems merged and only a handful make up the current market share of proprietary systems. For example, Blackboard acquired WebCT (which was phased out in 2012) and ANGEL Learning (which it planned to phase out in 2014 but recently that decision was reversed) and in 2012 announced its purchase of Moodlerooms and NetSpot, two open source systems.

Most CMSs provide content management, user management and enrollment, assessment of learners, communications such as email and discussion forums, and social learning tools such as wikis, blogs, journals, and mobile features. Three examples of proprietary CMSs and LMSs are Blackboard, Desire2Learn, and SharePoint LMS.

Blackboard

Blackboard (www.blackboard.com), founded in 1997 as a small educational technology company, is the market share leader in proprietary CMSs, although its percentage of the market share is dropping.[19(p16)] Blackboard provides a full range of CMS services (Fig. 27-2) with additional building

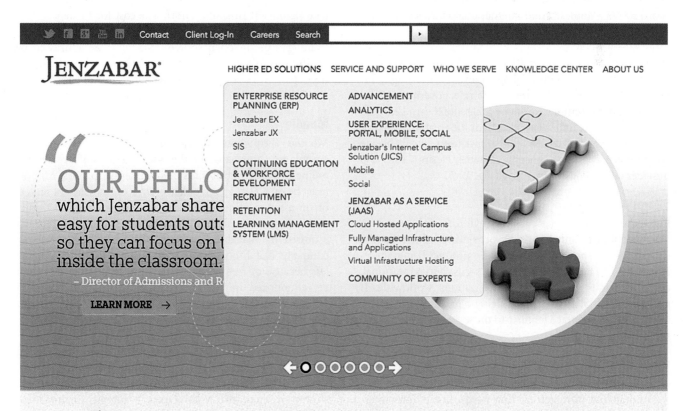

FIG 27-1 Jenzabar products menu. (Copyright 2013 Jenzabar, Inc. All rights reserved. Used with permission.)

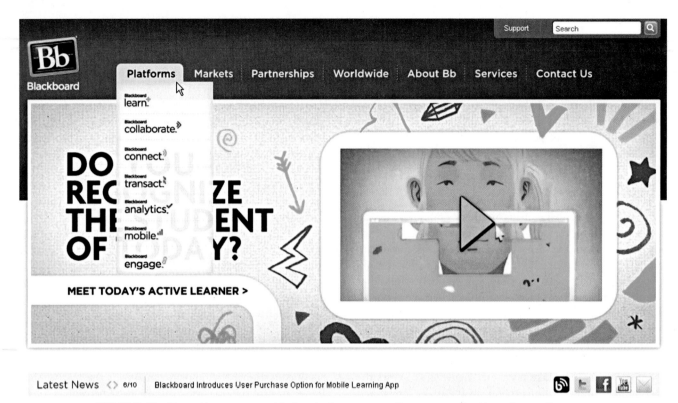

FIG 27-2 Blackboard home page with the platforms menu. From www.blackboard.com. Property of Blackboard and used with permission.

blocks to enhance the teaching and learning process. Blackboard serves a domestic and international market.

Desire2Learn

Desire2Learn Incorporated (desire2learn.com), founded in 1999, markets itself as providing innovative learning solutions to K-12, higher education, corporate, government, and healthcare organizations worldwide.[24] Desire2Learn Learning Suite provides a seamless experience for the creation, delivery, and management of courses that allows users to collaborate and connect around content and activities. Desire2Learn also provides a full range of products (Fig. 27-3).

SharePoint LMS

ELEARNINGFORCE (www.elearningforce.com), based in Denmark and founded in 2003, provides products for the delivery of elearning, with its primary product being SharePoint LMS.[25] The company provides services to educational, corporate, and public sector organizations worldwide. It prides itself on SharePoint LMS being a product that is easy to use with an interface familiar to those who use the Microsoft environment.

Open Source

Open source software refers to software code that is "free" to use and altered to match existing needs. Institutions interested in cost savings may select an open source CMS. However, the development of the custom interface and long-term maintenance costs of a custom-built CMS can be high.

Additionally, updates for new requirements or security can take significant time and effort. The cost for IT department time, the skill set to manage server and network issues, and training time on open source CMS must be addressed by institutions. What is free is the code; there is no yearly license fee to pay. Two examples of open source software are Moodle and Sakai.

Moodle

Moodle (http://moodle.org/) has become very popular among educators around the world as a tool for creating online dynamic websites for their students. To work, Moodle must be on a web server, either on one of the school's servers or on a server at a web hosting company such as Moodlerooms (www.moodlerooms.com/home), which was recently acquired by Blackboard. There is a fee to use a hosting company like Moodlerooms but the overall cost may be less because of free access to the code. Blackboard has not yet announced its intentions regarding its acquisition of Moodlerooms.

Sakai

Sakai (www.sakaiproject.org) is a community aligned around a single project, the Sakai Collaboration and Learning Environment (CLE); however, it currently is expanding to include a new product, the Sakai Open Academic Environment (OAE), that reimagines the approach to scholarly collaboration.[26] This product is a community that exists to enhance teaching, learning, and research. The company defines the

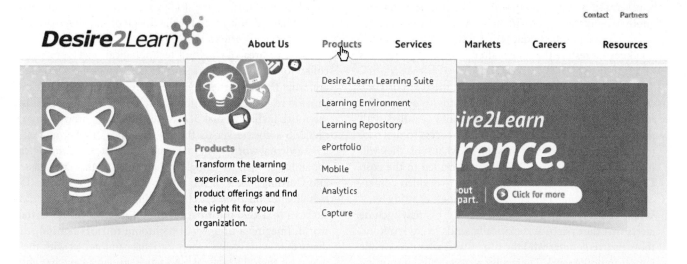

FIG 27-3 Desire2Learn product menu. (Copyright 2013 Jenzabar, Inc. All rights reserved. Used with permission.)

needs of academic users, creates software tools, and shares best practices while pooling knowledge and resources in support of this goal. Blackboard recently hired the long-time leader and one of the founders of the Sakai community to a senior role to lead Blackboard's open source learning management team.

Partnerships

Book publishers often partner with software vendors to provide a package of tools to assist with the delivery of distance education. Elsevier's Evolve LMS and Pearson's learning environments (LearningStudio) supply everything from customized, concept-to-completion LMSs to digital content. These online learning environments offer resources to both faculty and students (e.g., interactive grade book features, learning tools that simulate clinical experience and charting, cloud-based technology).

With all of these options, how do the faculty and school begin to select the system that will work within their environment and with their faculty and students? The next section discusses selection criteria and the role of the faculty.

Selection Criteria and Role of the Faculty

From a faculty perspective, the criteria for the selection of a CMS or LMS fall into several categories: ease of use, stability, tool set, and support. Other school considerations relate to compatibility or integration and to cost issues that require financial and technical support.[20] Faculty are most useful in providing input and selection criteria about what they do best: developing and teaching courses in the area in which they are experts.

- *Ease of use.* There is a learning curve to using CMS software. The interface should be intuitive to use. Does it use common educational terms to describe tools such as discussion forums or boards? Does its design support distance education or is it an adaptation of other products? Faculty should ask questions and complete typical educational tasks to assess ease of use for grading papers, projects, and tests; returning files; and setting up and using the grading centers. Also important are tools such as wikis, blogs, conferencing, and chat that are available for collaboration activities. How easy is it for students and faculty to learn to use these tools? This could include an analysis of the number of clicks it takes to upload content, what file formats are acceptable for upload, and what file size limits are enforced. Another area to analyze is the ease of content movement between courses and between semesters and the ease of archiving and exporting courses. Too many required clicks or difficulty in understanding the screen discourages faculty from using tools. Does the set-up reduce time and effort or demand more time and effort in delivering the course? More information about usability is in Chapter 21.
- *Stability.* How stable is the company offering the CMS? Will it be in business next year or will the school have to

select another system next year if the company fails or another company acquires it? Stability also includes system reliability such as the frequency of system crashes and the quickness to restore the system after such a crash. Students and faculty expect 24/7 access.

- *Tool set.* What are the bundled tools in the CMS or LMS and which ones require additional funds to access? For example, is Blackboard's Collaborate tool bundled with the basic version of Blackboard or does access to that tool increase the price? Faculty must know what tools they will need so that the correct "bundle" is included in the cost. Do faculty want collaborative tools such as video conferencing, podcasting, blogging, wiki abilities, chatting, etc.? What "smart" features do faculty need? This may include alerts that the system automatically sends to students and tools that remember who the user is and where he or she left off in doing work. Do faculty want mobile computing as part of the tool set? Do they want textbook cartridge capabilities or online testing tools? These are files that a textbook publisher provides faculty who select its textbook. Once uploaded the cartridge sets up the course in the CMS. These cartridges contain lessons, PowerPoint slides, discussion forums, tests, etc. It is the role of faculty to identify what tools they need to teach a course.[27]
- *Support.* What training materials does the CMS offer? Does it have a 24/7 help system, either by phone or by chat? What support does it offer students?

After considering these factors, faculty are responsible for determining the essential criteria or features necessary to deliver a quality course using appropriate technology as well as any "nice to have" but not essential criteria or features. In many universities CMS decisions are made for the academic environment as a whole. Thus knowing school- and profession-specific requirements is critical.

CMS and LMS products are improving with new technological developments and arrangements with partners that bring new tools to the product. For example, most products now provide access to Web 2.0 tools that facilitate collaboration efforts. These include tools such as wikis, blogs, eportfolios, and journaling. Most products now offer mobile learning options.

The Future of CMS

What is the future of CMS software? Weiss predicts several trends of note and how they might affect the future of CMS software, including the following two trends:

- A demand for more mobile tablet-based learning platforms.
- A move to more user-friendly open source CMSs that do not require customization (as is required with Moodle) to achieve a user-friendly interface. While Weiss lists some of these systems, they are not yet mainstream.[28]

Institutions are or have considered adding mobile ability in the criteria for selection of CMS or LMS software. For instance, take a look at a system called iQpakk (https://itunes.apple.com/us/app/iqpakk/id443528985?mt=8) for the iPad. Does this mean that colleges and universities that make

this decision will require students to have a tablet of some sort? What will this mean for the design of learning materials and learning experiences?

Another area of growing technological developments is collaborative tools that are smarter (i.e., remember who users are, what they like, and what they were doing [Web 3.0]) and provide relevant information to each user. Users should also see more lifelike virtual 3D worlds integrated into the LMS or CMS software versus the current ones like Second Life. These virtual worlds will make use of the latest technological capabilities, such as Google's augmented reality 3D glasses and Corning's view of the future (see the web resources for this chapter on Evolve). The Corning vision integrates glass surfaces to access information and to interact in the virtual world. Imagine a time when bathroom mirrors remind students that work is due, when students can interact with their world on their TV screens, and when students can chat with classmates and the professor through their kitchen counter. What will this mean for the design and teaching of distance education and the new wave of distributive courses?

INSTRUCTIONAL DESIGN FOR DISTANCE EDUCATION AND LEARNING

While most of the principles of instructional design hold true for distance education, the principal teaching change in a learning environment is the use of technology to engage and empower the learner.

This section is not meant to be an entire discourse about instructional design but rather about what distance education and distributive learning might mean in the design of each course. Several issues are of concern and are discussed below.

Learners and How They Learn

The key is to know the learners and their skill sets. Are these undergraduate or graduate students? Are these older adults returning to the educational world? Are these working adults pursuing updated skills? What technology skills do they bring to the course? What comfort level do they have with new methods of course delivery and learning? Have they taken distance education or online courses before? Are they ready to take responsibility for their learning? Do they understand that they must be an active and not passive learner in this environment?

As the introduction to this chapter pointed out, there can be a different mindset among digital natives (learners who grew up with technology) and students who were schooled using more traditional methods. How do faculty design for those differences? Oblinger et al. identify the following implications for learning and the design of these courses:

- Using the web as an exploratory tool to access the wealth of information available
- Offering learners a comprehensive learning experience
- Engaging learners
- Empowering learners to take charge of their own learning[1]

Faculty will usually see a range of students with a range of abilities. Knowing this, faculty must provide a range of learning activities to meet the needs of all students. For example, a faculty member may provide a written lesson about some concept, a podcast with the same content, discussion questions to engage students in the content, and an exploratory activity that requires students to explore the web for a quality resource that covers this content. The faculty may develop webquest learning experiences. See Google's Teaching with Technology website (https://sites.google.com/site/learnteachtech/webquest-projects) for many examples and zunal.com for an example of a nursing webquest (http://zunal.com/index-search.php?t=5&key=nursing&sGradeLevel=105&sCurriculum=100&Search=Search).

Goals and Objectives (Outcomes)

In distance education, writing clear, measurable goals and objectives or outcomes is critical to ensure that students know the course expectations, where they are going, and how faculty will assess their learning. Each lesson or activity should identify the purpose, identify the goals and objectives, provide clear directions for what students are to do, and provide a scoring rubric for evaluation of students' achievement of the objectives or outcomes. These should also include due dates and time periods.

Instructional and Learner Activities

Instructional and learner activities should provide learners with the skills, knowledge, and experience necessary to meet the course objectives. These activities or experiences should consider the learners' need for engagement, activity, and relevance to the content, objectives, and work world. This means that the professor will need to take advantage of the tool set available through the CMS software as well as tool sets available from outside sources. It may also mean that the professor must step outside his or her comfort zone in learning new ways to deliver the course and develop relevant learning experiences. Faculty should include a wide variety of collaborative tools that encourage interaction with the content and with others. These tools include wikis, blogs, discussion forums, and webquests. Other student activities could include developing podcasts, videos, and group projects. When designing course activities, keep in mind that active participation facilitates learning better than passive participation.

Evaluation

Regular and timely feedback to students on their progress is important to student success and engagement in the course. Faculty members who design the learning activities should develop a grading rubric for each activity and place it with the directions for that learning activity. Convey to students how soon they will receive comments and grades on submitted work. Faculty will also need to enter scores in the grading center that most CMS or LMS software includes.

In addition to the evaluation of student learning, faculty should give consideration to evaluation of the course and related learning activities. Does the school have course evaluation or best practices guidelines? Are these guidelines appropriate for distance education courses? Many of these course evaluation points are tied to faculty contracts and will not necessarily help to improve the course. Does the faculty member use something like Quality Matters, which is a peer review process to certify the quality of online and blended courses?[29] There is no one best practice guide for distance education but all guides consider these points as being critical to quality: institutional commitment and resources, curriculum and instructional rigor with interactivity and regular communication between faculty and learners, faculty support services, student support services, and evaluation of the course and programs.

On a course-by-course basis, faculty may develop some activities that provide learner feedback to the professor. A student statement illuminating what the student learned from completion of the activity provides feedback as to what is working and what is not. For example, at the end of each blog entry, have the student identify one to three things that he or she has learned and why he or she found them to be important. As a final example, require the students to rate themselves on a scale of 1 to 5 on how well they achieved each course objective and to support that rating with some data (an activity or resource that helped them learn, a product they produced, etc.).

Equally important to a well-designed and well-delivered course are the support services available to students.

STUDENT (LEARNER) SUPPORT SERVICES

Student support services are important to the achievement of learner outcomes, learner satisfaction, and learner retention. In planning for learner support services the faculty may need to assess what support services online learners expect. Nelson states: "putting all student services online will not eliminate the need for support services specifically designed for distance education students."[30(p186)] All learners, both on and off campus, must have access to the same resources.

Library

While most schools have online access to full text databases, interlibrary loans, and book borrowing, there is a wealth of other library resources of which the learner should be made aware. The following are two examples.

- Top Sites Blog contains a list of the top 10 free online libraries (http://topsitesblog.com/free-online-libraries). These online libraries contain mostly historical information but can assist students with their general education requirements as well as provide historical information about healthcare.
- The 100 Useful Online Libraries for Nurses and Nursing Students (www.nursingschools.net/blog/2009/08/100-useful-online-libraries-for-nurses-and-nursing-students/) includes nursing, chemistry, biology, general medical, anatomy, medical and nursing video, and general online libraries. Consider placing these links on the course site, the library website, or the school's online learning website.

The Association of College and Research Libraries (ACRL) publishes a set of standards for libraries servicing the distance education population.[31] During the planning phase the school should compare its services to those standards and develop a plan to acquire the services and materials that do not currently meet those standards. In addition, faculty must discuss what additional services online students may need that on-campus students do not. This can vary from institution to institution based on how the course is delivered. For example, do learners need a different user ID and password to access the school's online full text databases or do they have one user ID and password to access all resources whether on or off campus?

Tutoring Services

All learners studying at a distance should have the same access to tutoring services as on-campus learners. There are several online tutoring services that students may use for a fee or that the school may provide. Some examples include Tutor.com (www.tutor.com), Smarthinking, Inc. (www.smarthinking.com), Student of Fortune (www.studentoffortune.com), and Tutor.com (http://www.tutor.com/higher-education). The tutoring service must be similar to those that the school offers on campus and must have the same pricing structure. Faculty should ask questions about these services regarding the fees, live real-time help, hours of operation, and qualifications of the tutors. For example, does the service have nursing tutors who can address nursing content issues or help students to learn drug calculations?

If there are peer tutoring services for on-campus students, how will those same services be available to the distance education learner? What technology will be in place to provide for these services? For example, the school could provide a video conference solution where the writing center peer tutor can see the student and paper while talking about needed improvements. If a video conference system is not available, the learner could email the paper to the tutor and arrange a phone conversation to discuss it.

Online Textbook Distributors

The cost and acquisition of required textbooks in a timely fashion merits attention. How is the campus bookstore responding to the growing student population that may not reside on campus nor live nearby? Does it provide online ordering and shipping to the student's residence? What does that do to the costs? Does it provide etext options? Can learners rent their textbooks through the bookstore? Other options that learners may use are the growing number of online textbook distributors such as Chegg and CourseSmart. Of course, the student has the option to order from websites like Amazon and Barnes & Noble College as well as from traditional booksellers. The following are a few examples of distributors in the higher education market.

- *Follett* (www.follettbooks.com). Follett is the leading operator of college bookstores and a major distributor of textbooks. It operates a service called CafeScribe, which is a digital textbook platform; this is different from ebooks,

which are digital editions of traditional textbooks that students or faculty read on a computer, tablet, or smartphone. CafeScribe provides the ability for faculty and students to share notes and insights in line with the text, search the text for specific information, take notes directly in the text, bookmark places in the text, and highlight information.[32]
- *Chegg* (www.chegg.com). Chegg provides students with the ability to rent textbooks as well as buy new and used textbooks at a reduced cost. Students can also sell their books back to Chegg. It also offers homework help for many courses, scholarships, and course selection help. Chegg acquired several companies in 2010 and 2011: CourseRank, Cramster, Notehall, Student of Fortune, and Zinch.[33]
- *CourseSmart* (www.coursesmart.com). CourseSmart, founded in 2007, provides etextbook and digital learning tools. It provides both online and off-line access. It has a partnership arrangement with Pearson, Cengage Learning, McGraw-Hill, and John Wiley & Sons along with distribution partnerships with Jones & Bartlett Learning, Elsevier Science, Wolters Kluwer Health (Lippincott Williams & Wilkins), F.A. Davis, Sinauer Associates, Sage Publications, Taylor & Francis, and Princeton University Press.[34]

What guidance should the school provide to learners in distance education courses with regard to acquisition of textbooks? For example, are these books that the student will need throughout their time in college? Depending on the answer, the students then must ensure that they are renting or using digital forms of the textbook that are available to them for the duration of their time in college. The Higher Education Opportunity Act, discussed later in this chapter, mandates that students be provided with information about the required textbooks when they register for a course. What should they know about older editions? Are they acceptable or not? When will students actually need access to the textbooks? They may need certain textbooks immediately but may not need others until later in the course. Knowing this may help students to balance the cost of textbooks. Will students need a code to access the textbook website? If so, does a used textbook come with the code or will the student need to buy that separately? Buying codes separately is generally more expensive and may not save students money when the used book costs and new code costs are combined. What is the return policy of these online distributors?

Help Desk

Given the nature of technology and that technical issues will arise during the course of the semester, the school will need to address technical assistance for off-campus learners. These students cannot walk to the help desk for assistance. The school must make an early decision as to the location of the help desk. Should it provide for an internal help desk, an outsourced help desk, or some combination? This is not an easy decision. It requires a cost analysis to assess staffing a help desk with staff and students versus outsourced staffing. Software will be necessary to run the help desk and a budget needs to be allocated to train the staff. The school will need to make decisions about help desk staff's ability to reset passwords and access the CMS, with designated privileges for functions they can perform such as configuring a student's browser and firewall and running virus checks. What is the range of help that a student working at the help desk can provide? Should there be a student nurse with specific training to help with nursing-specific issues?

Since distributive learning occurs at any time (24/7) and any place (may or may not be on campus), many schools are opting for outsourcing. If outsourcing is the solution, then the college must ensure that it outsources the correct work and tasks. For example, will the help desk be able to reset passwords? Will it have remote access to see what the student is doing or to control the student's desktop? What should it know about the CMS or LMS? Will it have privileges to enter the CMS? What legal implications does CMS access have? The school will also need to monitor the effectiveness of its contract and related services.

A key question to ask in the CMS selection process is whether a CMS provides a help desk service. If so, what is the fee and what is the advantage of using that service for the distance education program? If this is a campuswide CMS, might using the CMS's help desk be a better approach? Another approach is to use a general help desk provider. The following are a few examples.

- *Perceptis* (http://perceptis.com). Perceptis provides help desk support for students, faculty, and staff. It can help with questions about email, admissions, how to connect to the network, benefits, payroll, financial aid, and more. Its market focus is educational institutions.
- *Ellucian* (www.sungardhe.com/). This portal solution (see Campus-Based Portals earlier in the chapters) also offers help desk services. It offers assistance 365 days per year to faculty, staff, and students. Since it knows the portal software, it may be in a better position to assist students than a free-standing help desk service.
- *Blackboard* (www.blackboard.com/Services/Student-Services/Services/IT-Help-Desk.aspx). Blackboard offers a student help desk support service. Faculty may want to confirm that the school's CMS provider can bundle a help desk product with its CMS product; many CMSs are moving in this direction (to a portal or bundled product).

In summary, learners will need access to the help desk 24/7 or nearly so and this will necessitate a variety of communication channels: phone, chat, video conference, self-help website, etc. The efficiency and effectiveness of the help desk support must be subject to evaluation to validate that it is meeting the needs of this student population.

Administrative Services, Academic Support, and Community Building

The retention rate for students who learn in their own space and time has been a problem. How should the school adjust certain traditional student services to provide for a feeling of connectedness and belonging for distance education students? Will this aid in retention and better student outcomes?

- *Administrative services.* These services include registration, financial aid, adds and drops, and admissions. Since most schools provide these services online, the procedures for accessing them should be the same as those used by on-campus students. The key institutional issue here is whether this should be a portal solution with one interface or each system should stand on its own. The key issue from a learner and faculty perspective is ease of access; there should be one user ID and password for all of the services that one needs to access.
- *Academic support.* This includes advising and career services. Many of these services are already extended to students through web portals or department websites and through social media tools such as Facebook and Twitter. The school may need to develop additional options for use of social media tools to extend the services in both time and space. For example, use of video conferencing or chat rooms for advising sessions with extended hours may be appropriate. It may also be important to put in place an alert and "job well done" system (such as Starfish, www.starfishsolutions.com) to keep students on track and motivate them to finish. Some schools also have as a part of the student information system an online audit for ease of scheduling courses, reminders for requirements they met, and links to appropriate content.
- *Community building.* This is an area that schools may neglect more than the other learner support services. How does the institution build a sense of belonging and identification with the program or school? Faculty and the school should consider services such as a cybercafe either in or outside the CMS program (some CMSs have a community tab or feature separate from a course) or a blog that students can use to interact outside of the course. Faculty might also consider a regular newsletter or podcast that highlights an event, student, or opportunity. What about a webinar on an issue of concern to healthcare or nursing that is open to students in the program? What about an online student government community? There are other community building options but these must engage the students and help them to identify with their online learning community.

ISSUES

This section of the chapter addresses additional issues that relate to distance education.

Legal

Digital Millennium Copyright Act of 1998

The Digital Millennium Copyright Act (DMCA) addresses the demands of the digital and Internet age and conformance to the requirements of the World Intellectual Property Organization.[35] This is a complex Act that is generally outside the scope of this chapter. This chapter highlights those areas of the law that might affect a distributive learning program. DMCA protects any copyrightable work. Copyrightable work includes written text or literary works, visual works, graphic works, musical works, and codes that pass between computers.[36] Key sections that affect distributive learning include the following:

- Prohibiting the circumvention of protection technologies, including encryption or password-breaking programs, and the manufacturing of devices that defeat such protection measures
- Limiting liability of online service providers because of the content that users transmit over their services
- Expanding existing exemptions for making copies of computer programs under certain conditions
- Updating rules and procedures for archival preservations
- Mandating studies to examine distance education in a networked world[35]

DMCA also established the Takedown Notice, through which copyright holders can demand removal of infringing content. This requires the copyright holder to follow the appropriate process and procedures.

Since this is a complex law, students should check with the school's legal counsel if they are in doubt about violating DMCA while preparing and posting educational materials for a distance course. Many schools also have a checklist that can be used as a guide to maintain compliance with this law. This checklist is often posted on the library website.

Technology, Education, and Copyright Harmonization (TEACH) Act

The TEACH Act, passed in 2002 and signed into law by President George W. Bush, addresses some of the issues that require attention when planning and delivering distance education. The purpose of this Act was to clarify acceptable use of copyrighted materials as it relates to distance education. Many of the responsibilities for compliance with this Act are placed on the institution and its IT staff. The TEACH Act permits the performance and display of copyrighted materials for distance education under the following conditions:

- The institution is an accredited, nonprofit educational institution
- Only students who have enrolled in the course can have access to these materials
- The use must be for either "live" or asynchronous sessions (permits storage of the materials on a server)
- The institution must provide information to faculty and students stating that course materials may be copyrighted and provide access policies regarding copyright
- The institution must limit access to the materials for the period of time necessary to complete the session or course
- The institution must prevent further copying or redistribution of copyrighted materials
- No part of the use may interfere with copy protection mechanisms[37-39]

For the professor, the law includes the following:

- The materials must be part of mediated (systematic) instructional activities (i.e., relevant to the course)
- The use must not include the transmission of textbook materials or other materials generally purchased or works developed specifically for online uses

- Faculty can use only reasonable and limited portions of such materials as they would typically use in a live classroom
- The materials must be available *only* to registered students and not to guests or observers
- Faculty must post a notice or message in the CMS that identifies the copyrighted materials and therefore precludes the student from copying or distributing these materials to others, as that would be a breach of copyright law
- Faculty must pay attention to "portion" limitations (how much one can use)[37-39]

Consult the school's policy and legal and library authorities when in doubt about materials necessary for the course. The American Library Association has an excellent website that further explains the roles of the institution (administrators or policy-makers and IT staff), faculty, and librarians.

Higher Education Opportunity Act (HEOA)

The Higher Education Opportunity Act of 2008 is a reauthorization of the Higher Education Act of 1965. It requires postsecondary institutions to be more transparent about costs and requires that a net price calculator as well as security and copyright policies be posted on its website.[40] While many of the provisions in this Act do not directly affect faculty (since they relate to administrative offices that deal with fees, growth, public relations, credits, etc.), the following do affect faculty: the textbook information provision, the definition of distance education, and the requirement to establish that students are indeed who they say they are.[41,42]

HEOA compliance entails the following:

- Faculty must select and submit textbook requirements to the campus bookstore *before* posting the next semester's schedule and registration. Each institution establishes the process for this. Under certain circumstances the institution may post a "to be determined" notice if it was not practical for the textbook to be selected before the school posts the next semester's schedule.
- Schools must pay attention to the change in terminology from distance learning to distance education. Education describes the process from the institution's perspective; it includes the use of one or more technologies to deliver instruction to students who are in a separate location and to support regular and substantive interaction between faculty and students. Learning describes the process from the students' perspective; it focuses on how the student interacts with the course content, classmates, and instructor in mastering the course content.
- Institutions must have a process in place to verify that the enrolled student is actually the person completing the course. Faculty may assist in determining how this process will work and with the development of a policy to cover this provision.

Intellectual Property

The issue of intellectual property is coming to the forefront as a major concern in the digital age. Faculty are increasingly concerned about the ownership of distributive courses materials and the use of those materials. Many faculty assume that these course materials are their creative property, meaning that a requirement exists for others to obtain permission to use them. Since these materials exist in digital form on a school's accessible server, others may have access to these materials with or without faculty consent. In today's world, some of these materials may have commercial value not before seen and institutions are increasingly taking ownership of these materials. A clear institutional policy will convey to all persons involved who owns what and what constitutes allowable use of the materials.

Some questions to consider in developing an intellectual property policy are as follows:

- What works are included under the policy (e.g., artworks, writings, software, course learning objects, PowerPoint slides, podcasts)?
- To whom does the policy apply (e.g., all employees, professors, researchers, postdoctoral fellows, administrators)?
- Under what circumstances does the school own the materials? Under what circumstances does the faculty member own the materials? Can there be joint ownership? Is this a work for hire or within the scope of the faculty member's employment?
- What institutional resources did the faculty member use to create the materials?
- What key words should the policy clearly define?
- Is there a clear, definitive written agreement between the faculty member and the institution as to ownership and rights?
- Who is responsible for obtaining copyrights, trademarks, etc.?[21,43,44]

Family Educational Rights and Privacy Act (FERPA)

The Family Educational Rights and Privacy Act (FERPA) is a federal law that requires colleges and universities to give students access to their educational records. Colleges and universities must maintain the confidentiality of personally identifiable educational records. See www.ed.gov/policy/gen/guid/fpco/ferpa/index.html for the U.S. Department of Education's summary of FERPA. While distance education courses were not a direct concern to those who wrote the FERPA rules, any time a faculty member or a university generates student information electronically, precautions must be taken.

Consider the following guidelines for distributive education and student records:

- Only enrolled students and the faculty teaching the course should have access to the course. However, the CMS administrator also has access to the course to manage and troubleshoot problems in using the CMS. The school must make the administrator aware of FERPA policies.
- If a college uses a hosting client (someone off campus that maintains the CMS), this arrangement makes the hosting client a third party vendor. While the client should not have access to information that links a student to a grade, the client's systems administrator does have access to the servers and ultimately to everything on them.

- Students should be able to view only their own grades in the online grade book. They should not be able to see other students' grades.
- Some issues may arise regarding discussion forums, depending on how the faculty use them. Faculty should *not* post evaluative comments or grades for students' comments in the discussion forum. Faculty should also state in the course requirements that students are required to post to the discussion forum, share their papers, etc.
- If faculty use Excel to keep a record of student grades, they should remove the students' ID numbers from the spreadsheet, leave no storage devices where others may access them, password protect the spreadsheet (but faculty *must* remember the password), and use an encryption program that comes with some external drives. This will protect the confidentiality of student data.
- If faculty lose a portable device such as a thumb drive that contains student grade sheets where the student names and grades are identifiable, they must notify the proper college or university authorities to determine whether anything further needs to be done.
- If faculty require students to send or post information to sites outside the college (blogs; social networking sites such as LinkedIn, Facebook, and YouTube; etc.), they must make it clear that the student and the college should not be identifiable. This type of assignment can be ripe for FERPA violations.

Disability Issues

Distance learning opportunities can open doors for millions of Americans with disabilities. When planning for the delivery of distance education courses, faculty must not create access barriers for the disabled. Laws such as the Americans with Disabilities Act (ADA) prohibit discrimination due to disability and sections 504 and 508 of the Rehabilitation Act provide protections to students with disabilities.[45]

What constitutes a reasonable accommodation for a particular student will depend on the situation and the type of program. The accommodation, however, may not be unduly costly or disruptive for the school or be for the student's personal use only. In colleges and universities the student has the primary responsibility to identify and document the disability and to request specific supports, services, and other accommodations. Most schools have a person responsible for assessing students with disabilities and providing an accommodation letter to faculty. Each accommodation letter details modifications for each student with a disability. The modifications may include the following items:

- Providing the student with extended time to turn in assigned work
- Providing extra time for timed exams
- Administering an exam in an alternative format, such as a paper exam when others will take the exam on a computer through the CMS
- Allowing spelling errors on papers or exams without deduction of points

Given the disability of the student and the nature of distance education, the student may need computer assistive devices. Students with disabilities may need adapted keyboards, magnification software, screen reader programs such as JAWS (www.freedomscientific.com/products/fs/jaws-product-page.asp) or Dolphin's SUPERNOVA (www.yourdolphin.com/products.asp) that convert the text and images to speech, voice recognition, and alternative communication programs. Most operating systems support persons with disabilities by incorporating accessibility utilities into the system.

For faculty this may mean providing alternative experiences for a student with a disability (e.g., use of a captioned video for the hearing impaired student). Faculty that teach distance education courses should review the tutorial titled Ten Simple Steps toward Universal Design of Online Courses (see the web resources for this chapter on Evolve) that addresses these issues. It lists 10 steps and provides examples and details for each one.

Quality

The traditional model of quality evaluation is site based but distance education and distributive learning are not site based.[46] Distance education is changing the thinking about quality assessment methods. Pond suggests that this new paradigm creates opportunities and challenges for quality assurance and accreditation.[47] Pond further suggests that the traditional items of quality assurance, such as physical attendance, contact hours, proctored testing, and library holdings, are impractical or simply not rational in a distributive course. Pond makes the following three suggestions:

- Use a consumer-based means of judging quality much like Amazon or eBay
- Accredit the learner by having the learner demonstrate competencies rather than earn credits or certify the teacher's competencies
- Move quality assurance toward an outcomes- or product-based model

This new model will look at quality indicators such as continuity between "advertising" and reality, personal and professional growth of the learner, relevance, and multidirectional interactions.

Eaton states that accreditation institutions or agencies need to do the following:

- Identify the distinctive features of distance learning delivery
- Modify accreditation guidelines, policies, or standards to meet the needs of this distinctive environment
- Pay attention to student achievement and learning outcomes[48(p6)]

In the Eaton article, Appendix A features guidelines for quality assurance in distance education and Appendix B includes 12 important questions about external quality review that are worth examining.

Faculty must answer these questions: How will quality be evaluated in the distance education environment? How will the approach be the same as or different from that used for on-campus courses or programs? What are the current criteria that educational accrediting agencies will use to accredit or review the program? How do faculty address these criteria? What issues arise when states serve as the primary arbiters of policy and governance issues in U.S. education but the student population resides in one state and does not physically go to the campus in another state where the student is taking distance education courses?[49]

Readiness

This section examines both the institution's readiness and the learner's readiness for teaching and learning in a distance education model.

Institution

Some institutions may enter the distance education market to maintain competitiveness; others may do so because their recruitment staff has identified a market need. Some see this movement as a means to increase revenues in these difficult financial times without the need for brick and mortar facilities. Regardless of the reason, the critical issues for readiness are as follows:

- Does the movement to distance education fit with the institution's missions and goals?
- Is the institution ready to invest in the technologies necessary to produce a quality program?
- Does the institution have the resources—people, money, and time—to develop and implement the program?
- Does the institution have faculty buy-in? Does it have administrative commitment? Does it have staff buy-in?
- Are faculty ready and prepared? Some institutions, such as Pennsylvania State University (PSU), have developed a faculty readiness assessment; the PSU document is available at http://weblearning.psu.edu/news/faculty-self-assessment. Does the institution have such an assessment or survey?

Without this readiness and commitment, distance education will not work or at best will result in a program of marginal quality. Just as the institution needs to be ready, it also needs to assess the students and potential student population for their readiness. That being said, the move to this method is moot for many institutions because competition is forcing distance education solutions and most universities have already made this transition.

Students (Learners)

Many students (learners) today work and may learn differently than other digital nonnatives. Many of today's students enter distributive education courses without the mindset for success. Some have inappropriate expectations about requirements for succeeding in these types of courses. This presents several issues, as follows:

- What information does the institution provide to these learners to assess their readiness to learn in distance courses?
- Does the institution provide learners with a self-assessment tool such as Kizlik's readiness assessment (www.adprima.com/dears.htm) or PSU's readiness assessment (http://

ets.tlt.psu.edu/learningdesign/assessment/onlinecontent/online_readiness)?

- How will the institution make learners aware of the requirements for learning in this manner? For example, do learners know that distance courses require discipline and organization in setting aside time to complete the learning, as well as reading and comprehension skills to understand the concepts and develop the skills necessary for this program or course? Do students have the ability to follow directions and ask questions and the ability to work on their own under the guidance of a faculty member?

- How does the institution make elearners aware of their responsibilities? For example, students will have to meet course deadlines, check in to the course regularly, interact with faculty and classmates, ask questions as necessary, and conduct themselves in a professional manner in all interactions.

The institution should list or outline learner requirements in a policy and procedures document and make this document available to students to ensure that they understand their responsibilities.

CONCLUSION AND FUTURE DIRECTIONS

The changes in our educational environment are reflective of shifts in our demographics, economic conditions, and technological developments. Web 2.0 tools are opening up educational opportunities for lifelong learning to a diverse global community. Emerging terms, course management and learning management systems, and issues related to the development and implementation of distance education and distributive learning are all elements resulting from these budding educational opportunities.

The next generation of CMSs and LMSs will be integrated portals that are smarter, track more information, and analyze student data across functions such as email, wikis, chats, forums, and so forth. They will include immersive, 3D learning worlds with better communication channels and collaboration for any time and any place learning with tablets and mobile devices.[50] This will result in just-in-time, customized learning environments where the focus is on outcomes rather than traditional credit hours. This environment will not be about course management or learning management systems but about the learners and the learners' needs.

REFERENCES

1. Oblinger D, Barone C, Hawkins B. *Distributed education and its challenges: an overview.* American Council on Education, Center for Policy Analysis. http://www.acenet.edu/bookstore/pdf/distributed-learning/distributed-learning-01.pdf. 2001.

2. Holly C. The case for distance education in nursing. *MERLOT Journal of Online Learning and Teaching.* 2009;5(3). http://jolt.merlot.org/vol5no3/holly_0909.htm.

3. Carr N. *The Shallows: What the Internet Is Doing to Our Brains.* New York, NY: W.W. Norton & Company; 2011.

4. Turkle S. *Alone Together: Why We Expect More from Technology and Less from Each Other.* New York, NY: Basic Books; 2011.

5. Lanier J. *You Are Not a Gadget: A Manifesto.* New York, NY: Vintage Books; 2011.

6. Frand J. The information-age mindset: changes in students and implications for higher education. *EDUCAUSE Review.* 2000; September/October:14-18, 22, 24. http://net.educause.edu/ir/library/pdf/ERM0051.pdf.

7. Eliot S, Agassiz E. *Society to Encourage Studies at Home.* Cambridge, MA: Riverside Press; 1897.

8. Moore M. *From Chautauqua to the Virtual University: A Century of Distance Education in the United States.* Columbus, OH: Center on Education and Training for Employment, Ohio State University; 2003. http://www.calpro-online.org/eric/docs/distance.pdf.

9. Jeffries M. *Research in distance education.* Digitalschool.net. http://www.digitalschool.net/edu/DL_history_mJeffries.html. n.d.

10. Billings D. Optimizing distance education in nursing. *J Nurs Educ.* 2007;46(6):247-248.

11. American Association of Colleges of Nursing (AACN). *Distance technology in nursing education white paper.* AACN. http://apps.aacn.nche.edu/Publications/WhitePapers/whitepaper.htm. 1999.

12. Billings D. Distance education in nursing: 25 years and going strong. *Comput Inform Nurs.* 2007;25(3):121-123.

13. Knebel E. *The Use and Effect of Distance Education in Healthcare: What Do We Know?* Bethesda, MD: U.S. Agency for International Development, Quality Assurance Project; 2001. http://www.hciproject.org/sites/default/files/Distance%20Education.pdf.

14. National Council of State Boards of Nursing (NCSBN). Distance learning/web definitions: a resource for the model education rules. NCSBN. https://www.ncsbn.org/836.htm.

15. Dede C. *Emerging technologies and distributed learning.* Project ScienceSpace. http://www.virtual.gmu.edu/ss_pdf/ajde.pdf. 1996.

16. Paulson M. *Online education and learning management systems: global e-learning in a Scandinavian perspective. George Mason American Journal of Distance Education.* Oslo, Norway: NKI Forlaget; 2003. Retrieved from http://www.virtual.gmu.edu/ss_pdf/ajde.pdf.

17. Saffarzadeh A. A new definition of e-learning. AeroMD.com http://areomd.com/2012/04/30/a-new-definition-for-e-learning/. April 30, 2012.

18. Learning management system (LMS). *TechTarget.* http://searchcio.techtarget.com/definition/learning-management-system. 2005.

19. Green K. *The campus computing project.* The Campus Computing Project. http://www.campuscomputing.net/sites/www.campuscomputing.net/files/Green-CampusComputing2011_4.pdf. October 2011.

20. Jafari A, McGee P, Carmean C. *Managing courses, defining learning: what faculty, students, and administrators want.* EDUCAUSE. http://www.educause.edu/ero/article/managing-courses-defining-learning-what-faculty-students-and-administrators-want. 2006.

21. Simonson M, Smaldino S, Albright M, Zvacek S. *Teaching and Learning at a Distance: Foundations of Distance Education.* 5th ed. Upper Saddle River, NJ: Pearson Education; 2012.

22. Ellucian. *Ellucian: New company name announced for Datatel and SunGard higher education combination.* Ellucian. http://www.ellucian.com/News/Ellucian-New-Company-Name-Announced-for-Datatel-and-SunGard-Higher-Education-Combination/. 2012.

23. Simonson M. Course management systems. *The Quarterly Review of Distance Education.* 2007;8(10):vii-ix. http://web2integration.pbworks.com/f/COURSE%2BMANAGEMENT%2BSYSTEMS.pdf.

24. Desire2Learn. *Discover Desire2Learn.* Desire2Learn. http://desire2learn.com/about/discover/. 2012.

25. ELEARNINGFORCE. *About ELEARNINGFORCE.* ELEARNINGFORCE. http://www.elearningforce.com/company/Pages/default.aspx. 2012.

26. Sakai. *About Sakai.* Sakai. http://www.sakaiproject.org/about-sakai. 2012.

27. Daswon C. LMS? SIS? SIF? LTI? Alphabet soup and blended learning. ZDNet. http://www.zdnet.com/lms-sis-sif-lti-alphabet-soup-and-blended-learning-7000000420/. July 8, 2012.

28. Weiss C. *Latest e-learning insight and news.* E-Learning 24/7 Blog. http://elearninfo247.com/2011/10/24/latest-e-learning-insight-and-news/. October 24, 2011.

29. Quality Matters Program. MarylandOnline. http://www.qmprogram.org. 2010.

30. Nelson R. Student Support Services for Distance Education Students in Nursing Programs. In: Oermann M, Hernrich K, eds. Annual Review of Nursing Education. Vol 5. New York, NY: Springer Publishing Company; 2007:183-206.

31. Association of College & Research Libraries (ACRL). *Standards for distance learning library services.* ACRL. http://www.ala.org/acrl/standards/guidelinesdistancelearning. 2008.

32. Digital textbooks from CafeScribe. follettbooks.com. http://www.follettbooks.com/fb3/ebooksMain.jsp. 2012.

33. Chegg. *Fact Sheet: About Chegg.* Chegg. http://www.chegg.com/factsheet. 2012.

34. CourseSmart. *About CourseSmart.* CourseSmart. http://www.coursesmart.com/overview. 2012.

35. American Library Association (ALA). *DMCA: The Digital Millennium Copyright Act.* ALA. http://www.ala.org/ala/issues advocacy/copyright/dmca/index.cfm. 2011.

36. The Digital Millennium Copyright Act of 1998: U.S. Copyright Office Summary. United States Copyright Office. http://www.copyright.gov/legislation/dmca.pdf. 1998.

37. Copyright Clearance Center. *The TEACH Act: new roles, rules and responsibilities for academic institutions.* Copyright Clearance Center. http://www.copyright.com/media/pdfs/CR-Teach-Act.pdf. 2005.

38. American Library Association (ALA). *TEACH Act best practices using Blackboard™.* ALA. http://www.ala.org/advocacy/copyright/teachact/teachactbest. 2012.

39. Gassaway L. *Balancing copyright concerns: the TEACH Act of 2001.* EDUCAUSE. http://net.educause.edu/ir/library/pdf/ERM01610.pdf. November/December 2001.

40. EDUCAUSE. *Implementing the Higher Education Opportunity Act: A checklist for business officers.* EDUCAUSE. http://www.educause.edu/Resources/ImplementingtheHigherEducation/192839. 2009.

41. Middle States Commission on Higher Education. Distance education and the HEOA. *Middle States Commission on Higher Education Newsletter.* http://www.msche.org/news_newsletter.asp. January 2010.

42. Middle States Commission on Higher Education. New HEOA regulations impact distance education programs, substantive change & monitoring growth, transfer of credit. *Middle States Commission on Higher Education Newsletter.* http://www.msche.org/news_newsletter.asp. Fall 2009.

43. Diaz V. *Distributed learning meets intellectual property policy: who owns what?* Campus Technology. http://campustechnology.com/articles/2005/08/distributed-learning-meets-intellectual-property-policy-who-owns-what.aspx. 2005.

44. Ulius S. *Intellectual property ownership in distributed learning.* EDUCAUSE. http://net.educause.edu/ir/library/pdf/erm0346.pdf. 2003.

45. U.S. Department of Justice. *A guide to disability rights laws.* U.S. Department of Justice. http://www.ada.gov/cguide.htm. July 2009.

46. Baer MA. Forward. In: Eaton JS, ed. *Maintaining the Delicate Balance: Distance Learning, Higher Education Accreditation, and the Politics of Self-Regulation.* Louisville, CO: EDUCAUSE Publications; 2002:v. http://www.acenet.edu/news-room/Documents/Maintaining-the-Delicate-Balance-Distance-Learning-Higher-Education-Accreditation-and-the-Politics-of-Self-Regulation-2002.pdf.

47. Pond W. *Distributed education in the 21st century: implications for quality assurance.* University of West Georgia. http://www.westga.edu/~distance/ojdla/summer52/pond52.html. 2002.

48. Eaton J. *Maintaining the delicate balance: distance learning, higher education accreditation, and the politics of self-regulation.* American Council on Education, Center for Policy Analysis. http://www.acenet.edu/bookstore/pdf/distributed-learning/distributed-learning-02.pdf. 2002.

49. Levine A, Sun J. *Barriers to distance education.* American Council on Education, Center for Policy Analysis. http://www.acenet.edu/bookstore/pdf/distributed-learning/distributed-learning-06.pdf. 2002.

50. Moore E, Utschig T, Haas K, et al. Tablet PC technology for the enhancement of synchronous distributed education. *IEEE Transactions on Learning Technologies.* 2008;2(1):105-116.

DISCUSSION QUESTIONS

1. How does your institution define distance education, distance learning, distributive education, and distributive learning? What standards, if any, did it use in creating those definitions? How do those definitions affect you as a student? (Alternatively, examine surrounding programs in your geographic area—that is, your institution's competition.)

2. Interview five interdisciplinary faculty members to obtain information about the features in a CMS or LMS that are critical to the delivery of their courses. Using that information, determine what criteria should be used to compare and evaluate two CMS or LMS programs. Discuss what you learned in developing these criteria and in comparing two products against them. Include answers to the following question: How useful were these criteria, what was missing, and how would you revise the criteria next time?

3. Research how your institution implements either the HEOA or the TEACH Act. How are faculty notified of these laws and your institution's policy regarding them? Where can you find this information? Who do you go to for assistance if you need clarification? How are students

informed of copyright issues? How were you informed of these?

4. Research the intellectual property policy for your institution as it relates to distributive education. Where is the policy located? Who developed the policy? When? What is covered in the intellectual policy as it relates to digital course materials or distributive education?

CASE STUDY

You are a faculty member serving on the online learning committee. The university requires an assessment of which learning strategies are working and which are not and an examination of the current standards, emerging trends, and how the school should plan for the distributive education and learning movement. The committee is charged with setting the course for this initiative for the next 2 years. There are many subcommittees, each with a specific charge. You are serving on the subcommittee charged with developing the stakeholder matrix, a document identifying all "stakeholders"—those who have an interest in this initiative, how they fit in the organizational structure, what influence they exert, and so forth. These are the people from whom you will collect data and involve in the process and many times in the decision making.

Using either a word processer such as Microsoft Word or a spreadsheet application such as Microsoft Excel, create a 5-column table with the following headings for the columns: Stakeholder Name and Organization; Organizational Role; Influence and Power; Unique Information about

This Person/Organization; and Strategies for Communicating and Working with This Person. Each stakeholder will be entered as a new row in the matrix.

Once you have designed the stakeholder matrix, analyze its importance and how it will be used. Using what you have learned in this chapter, create a strategy for each column. For example, determine how you would systematically identify each stakeholder. Develop one to three questions to guide your collection of the data for each column. Then complete this matrix for your college.

Discussion Questions

1. Discuss the pertinent laws that should be considered for this initiative.
2. Describe next steps in the process that would help assure the success of the initiative.
3. Using what you learned in this chapter and by searching the web for distributive learning materials, list two likely future directions.

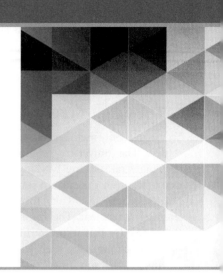

Informatics Tools for Educating Health Professionals

W. Scott Erdley and Kay M. Sackett

In education the final record of a student's learning is the limited information included on the transcript. In the manual world of education, for the most part, all other data collected by individual faculty and academic departments are maintained, if at all, in file cabinets or individual faculty files. This can be called the ultimate system for creating an island of lost data and information.

OBJECTIVES

At the completion of this chapter the reader will be prepared to:

1. Discuss the effectiveness of computerized teaching tools that can be used to deliver education within the traditional classroom environment
2. Explore computerized applications that can be used to manage educational information and support the work of health-related faculty
3. Examine the increasing impact of automation, including comprehensive education information systems on the academic policies and procedures of the academy
4. Outline the impact of computerization on the role and career development of healthcare faculty with the academy
5. Analyze how technical tools and education information systems can be used to increase the effectiveness and efficiency of faculty

KEY TERMS

Academy, 443
Avatar, 449
Big data, 442
Clicker, 446

Comprehensive education information system (CEIS), 443
eBooks, 444
ePortfolio, 448
Interactive whiteboard, 444

ABSTRACT

The educational preparation of healthcare providers is the foundation of a safe, effective, and efficient healthcare delivery system. This chapter addresses the use of education information systems and technical tools that support the work of healthcare faculty charged with the preparation of competent healthcare providers. The impact of the computerization of higher education is described, computerized teaching tools are presented, the impact of computerization on the faculty role is discussed, and the implications for health-related faculty are explored. While all levels of education are being affected by computerization and are employing technology tools (e.g., course management systems, the Internet, computer-based instructional games), it is at the collegiate level that the impact of technology is being felt most keenly. Of particular interest are tools available for use by faculty directly engaged in the process of educating healthcare providers.

The increased computerization in institutions of higher education is now creating sets of big data (large datasets). The implications of these data and the potential for predicative analytics is explored, with a focus on future directions.

INTRODUCTION

Over the last several decades the implementation of healthcare computer-based information systems has transformed the healthcare delivery system. That impact is now being experienced in the educational process of healthcare providers. A primary mission of higher education is the education of students to ultimately create an improved healthcare

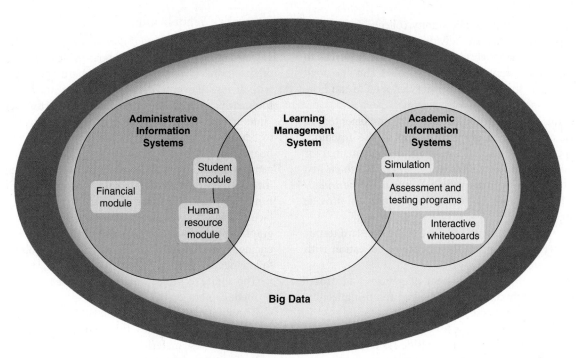

FIG 28-1 Comprehensive education information system.

system. These may be students in current degree programs or continuing education. No matter the program, the educational process is supported by a complex administrative infrastructure. The computerization of the academy can be considered from both an academic perspective and an administrative perspective. The academic perspective focuses on the assessment of students and the delivery of learning. The administrative perspective focuses on the development of systems and processes that support the day-to-day operation of the institution. This includes student information systems, financial information systems, and human resources and payroll systems.[1] Both the education of students and the surrounding administrative infrastructure have benefited from the opportunities provided by technology integration. In addition, as new systems in both areas have evolved their functions have increasingly overlapped, moving toward a comprehensive education information system. Such a system creates the opportunity for increased effectiveness of the learning process and efficiency of the academy. For example, predictive analysis of big data can result in innovative curricula that may prevent academic problems for future students. In this chapter the computerization of the academy is described, computerized teaching tools are presented, the impact of computerization on the faculty role is discussed, and the implications for health-related faculty are explored.

COMPREHENSIVE EDUCATION INFORMATION SYSTEM (CEIS)

Comprehensive education information systems (CEISs) include the hardware, applications, overlapping and integrated functionality, and data produced by all information systems within an academic setting. This is depicted in Figure 28-1, which divides the CEIS into three overlapping areas. These are the administrative information systems, the learning management system (LMS), and the academic information tools used in teaching. Overlap of functionality and data flow occurs across the system. For example, a group of students preregisters for an online three-credit theory course and a five-credit related clinical course. As each student registers, the course shell roster for the online course is populated with the student's name. The faculty member then assigns the students to their clinical sections and these data are sent back to the registration system for transcript and tuition purposes.

Increasingly, a common database depicted on the model as big data allows data integration across the institution. The model demonstrates the concept of a CEIS as it applies to an academic institution; however, the concept can be applied to several educational institutions within a larger system. For example, in Ohio the Higher Education Information (HEI) system (www.ohiohighered.org/hei) includes a comprehensive database with student enrollment, courses, financial aid, personnel, facilities, and finance data submitted by Ohio's colleges and universities. Data are used for a variety of purposes, including reporting on higher education outcomes, funding formula and financial aid, policy analysis, and strategic planning.

One module within the HEI system is the Course Inventory Expert System, which includes decision rules for classifying undergraduate courses with the goal of achieving consistent treatment of undergraduate courses across the system (http://regents.ohio.gov/hei/ci/documentation/ciexpertsystemhome.php). This makes it possible to implement a comprehensive credit transfer system across Ohio's entire public higher education system of 14 universities, 24 regional campuses, and 23 community colleges. In contrast to traditional approaches, an individual faculty member does not need to review a syllabus and other course materials to decide whether a student can transfer a course. This one small example suggests the potential impact that a CEIS can have on the role of faculty within the academy.

To ensure that information systems implemented in health-related education programs support the teaching-learning process and take full advantage of the potential for innovative opportunities offered by CEIS, health-related faculty must assume a proactive role. Nelson and others identified the following four key areas where faculty can provide leadership:

- Identifying data elements and developing standard terminology needed to capture the essence of education with the healthcare professions
- Participating in the development of policies and procedures for securely collecting, accessing, and using faculty, staff, administrative, and student data
- Contributing to the process for selecting, implementing, and integrating education information systems
- Designing educational opportunities to ensure that faculty clearly understand the potential of automated academic systems and the importance of participating in these activities[1]

Participating in these activities obviously requires time and effort but these activities may not contribute to achieving tenure and promotions. Given this reality, faculty teaching in the health disciplines must decide whether they will play a leadership role or step back and have the transformation of higher education managed by others. Just as the design of effective healthcare information systems requires input from healthcare providers and health informatics experts, the design of effective systems that support the teaching-learning process requires the advice of educators and informatics experts within healthcare.[1] Often the best way to begin moving into an education leadership role involves working with the implementation of computerized teaching tools.

COMPUTERIZED TEACHING TOOLS

Computerized teaching tools are hardware and software that are used in the design, implementation, and evaluation of student learning. These tools make it possible to develop creative and innovative learning experiences as well as to assess and track student learning.

Hardware

Hardware refers to tangible, physical items used in the educational process. These devices are used by students and faculty to engage with each other and the educational content with the goal of increased learning. Hardware includes computer-related tools used in all areas of society, such as laptop computers, tablets, cellphones, and tools designed specifically for education such as interactive whiteboards and clickers.

Interactive Whiteboards

Historically, conventional classrooms within a college or university setting included a chalkboard at least across the front of the room. Over time the chalkboard was supplemented with the use of overheads. The computerization of these basic tools early in the 1990s resulted in the "smart whiteboard" or "interactive whiteboard," which offered innovative approaches to education and the related administrative functions.[2] The boards come in a wide variety of sizes to complement or meet general unique users and environment requirements. These interactive whiteboards are sold with a variety of possible functions that allow for real-time consultation between faculty and students, real-time editing of documents by geographically distinct persons, and the ability for video conferencing. Typical features of these interactive tools include the following:

- The ability to project materials from a computer, a document camera, or the Internet.
- The ability to write directly on the board, creating figures, documents, and notes that can be edited as they are created. These materials can be saved or printed for distribution to students.
- A touch interface making it possible for a user to interact with the board by using a finger. A single digit is used for the most part; multifinger use is not common at this time.

See Box 28-1 for additional features.

BOX 28-1	COMMON FEATURES OF AN INTERACTIVE WHITEBOARD

Wireless (Wi-Fi connectivity, interface with users)
Touch, keyboard, and mouse capable
Conferencing capable with multiple concurrent users
Document editing with two or more concurrent users
Short projection distance to eliminate walking in front of projection
Multiple USB ports with easy access

The features offered on interactive whiteboards have been evolving over time and now often include collaborative functionality such as conferencing between users anywhere a connection is available. Faculty can use these boards for video conferencing between classes held on different university campuses or with colleagues located in different areas of the world. However, not all universities provide an interactive whiteboard with a video camera available at both sites. As a result, video conferencing may be one-sided. Other uses include note creation thus allowing the instructor to insert notes into a document projected to both sites and create a collaborative distributed classroom. Because of the interactive capabilities, participants at the distance classroom are able to respond by entering their own viewable notes. On the downside, these tools can be expensive, ranging from $3000 for low-end models to $15,000 or more for models with all possible features.

eReaders and Digital Books

Referred to as ebooks, these devices are an emerging technology for educational users. Initially designed for reading books, ebook readers are now branching out to challenge tablet computers. eBook readers have electronic "ink" or electronic paper to render a "page" that is similar to a printed page found in a book. Only a few technology companies have created digital ink and many reading devices license the technology from these companies (e.g., Adobe and E Ink). Sony (Reader), Amazon (Kindle) and Barnes & Noble (Nook) are examples of suppliers of these digital reading devices. The advantages of using these media include portability, the ability to adjust font sizes for easier viewing, and the large storage capabilities. Some disadvantages are limited backlighting of the page, a need to maintain adequate battery charge, and limited ability for text markup. In the past these devices were single function, although this is changing. The September 2012 release of four new models of the Kindle by Amazon is evidence of the shift toward a multifunctional ereader device. Newer versions of the Kindle (Fire) and Nook (Touch) provide the ability to browse the Internet, check email, connect via cellular plan and Wi-Fi, and watch movies on the device. Some of the new models also support text markup or highlighting.

Additional applications (or apps) are available that allow ereader functions on non-ereader devices (e.g., for iPads and Google devices). However, these apps have limited functionality compared to the ereader devices. Despite this limitation users are able to connect using the app and access and read current materials without having to have a dedicated ereader. This allows mobile devices such as laptops, smartphones, and tablets to become, in essence, ebook readers, making the purchase of a separate ereader unnecessary.

In the education arena textbook suppliers are beginning to offer electronic texts for students at all levels. Vendors offering electronic textbooks, often including web-based resources, include Lippincott Williams & Wilkins, McGraw-Hill, Pearson, and Elsevier. Textbooks are available in ereader (Kindle and Nook) and browser-based (usually requires a "plug-in" and has to function within a learning management system software such as Blackboard) formats. The ability to link to web-based resources has appeal for students. Faculty resources are available in a similar fashion, in particular allowing faculty to quiz students via etextbook-created tests and quizzes.

The limitations of these offerings include cost (which can approximate hard copy costs), limited available formats (some are available only in a proprietary publisher ebook format, others in just Adobe Reader file format), limited selections in print, and limited ability to mark up or highlight the text. An early study reported student reluctance to pay for the use of ebooks as well as frustration with the search function within ebooks.[3] In addition, depending on the size of the screen, viewing charts, figures, and other nontext content can be difficult.

The obvious advantages are user mobility and content portability. The ability to integrate graphics, multimedia, and text material is becoming more prominent. eReaders are now able to download files so the need to maintain online access while reading a text is not required. The prevalence of

students interacting with ebooks is increasing and students are now able to connect to additional resources cited in a text via a URL. Text highlighting is becoming more available. Students may also copy and save, in some cases, text information for later use and/or sharing with others. In the clinical realm, texts, compendiums, and reference materials are now more available to students and other users of this information for patient care at the point of care. However, how these tools can be effectively integrated into the educational process at the point of care is in many ways an unanswered question both from a technical and an academic perspective. For example, if a student is reading a patient's EHR and needs to check a reference for additional information about a drug, lab test, or diagnosis, should the student reference materials be on a separate device, or integrated with the decision support content in the EHR?

A search of the literature using the terms "electronic books" and "nursing education" demonstrates limited information on how these tools are being used. However, some research is beginning to be reported. In one study undergraduate nursing students were very pleased to use ebooks and personal digital assistant (PDA) devices as tools during their clinical rotation.[4]

Smartphones

A smartphone upgrades a cellular phone with a host of additional functionality beyond the functions of calling and texting between callers. Smartphones have become handheld computers. Some are better at handling graphics (such as movies, pictures, and games) while others offer improved functionality regarding Internet browsing and social media use. Many smartphones are able to take advantage of wireless networks for data transmissions. At this point in time, smartphones with the largest market share operate using either Google's Android or Apple's iOS platform. There are advantages and disadvantages with each operating system and device. Android-based smartphones tend to employ a larger screen size and more powerful chipsets or computer processing units (CPUs) and are able to use additional storage via mini storage disk (SD) cards. iPhones have a smaller screen size, are not able to take advantage of additional storage, and do not interact well with Adobe Flash–based web applications. iPhones, though, have access to the largest app store, iTunes. Many current smartphones are powered by dual-core low power CPUs. This power, coupled with the size, allows for a large amount of computational horsepower in a small portable device.

Due to their computational power and increasing popularity, the integration of smartphones into both healthcare delivery and education is of growing importance. At least a quarter of the world's cellphones, more than 1 billion, are defined as smartphones.[5] In the U.S. almost 40% of consumers over the age of 18 own a smartphone as of 2011.[6]

Regardless of the operating system, many smartphones are able to interact with a variety of mainstream educational learning management systems such as Blackboard. Software for these devices that allows users to interact with their

Blackboard courses through their mobile devices is available. Smartphones can even be "substituted" for handheld classroom interactive devices using software (e.g., web>clicker, www.iclicker.com/products/webclicker).

A variety of applications are available for smartphones for health students and practitioners. The more common types are drug reference software such as Davis's Drug Guide and Epocrates. iTunes and Android app stores offer an increasing variety of healthcare applications beyond drug references, including formula calculators, physical assessment guides, protocols such as ACLS and PALS, and audio assist applications for lung and heart sounds. Many of these apps are free while others are available for a nominal fee. The free version of an app may not have the full features of the same app with an associated cost. Textbooks and other typically hard copy–only reference manuals are becoming increasingly available for smartphone platforms.

Due to their increasing popularity among students, healthcare providers, and patients, smartphones are increasingly included as requisite tools for education and healthcare practice. Smartphones can interact not only with educational management systems (e.g., Blackboard, Moodle, Joomla) but also with different electronic health record systems. While a wide variety of apps are available, some caution is warranted. Some institutional policies may preclude smartphone use because of potential patient privacy and information security breaches. Every organization has a policy and protocol detailing Health Insurance Portability and Accountability Act (HIPAA) requirements and the use of mobile devices. (See Chapter 24 for more information on this subject.)

Tablets

Tablet computers are another tool available to faculty and students. Tablets are increasing in popularity and use in higher education. Early tablets were bulky and heavy but the iPad, first available in early 2010, revolutionized widespread tablet use. Lightweight and novel in design, the iPad is a device with strong support from a wide range of software companies. The iPad employs a touch screen user interface that allows users' fingers to maneuver through the Internet and documents. A virtual keyboard, with an optional Bluetooth keyboard, provides standard data entry capability. Using almost the same iOS platform as the iPhone, the iPad is rapidly becoming a dominant tablet on the market, if not already *the* dominant tablet. However, Windows 8.0 which makes it possible to convert a laptop into a tablet computer may reconfigure this market once again.

Tablets, such as the iPad, are becoming increasingly popular with educators, students, and healthcare providers. With the availability of applications similar to the Microsoft Office suite these devices are becoming increasingly functional for a wide variety of activities. Some current examples include Smart Office 2 and Documents To Go – Office Suite. The price for these applications can range from free to $50 or more and they are available only at the App Store run by Apple. Equivalent applications are available for the Android-platform tablets via the Android App store.

One concern with using these sorts of applications is storage. iPads do not have USB ports for accessing flash storage. Instead, users must access online or cloud environments to store and retrieve material. An example of cloud storage is Dropbox (www.dropbox.com), a free service that works on a wide variety of devices and operating systems. The free account for this service includes 2.5 GB of space, which is a fair amount of space for access and storage of a wide variety of documents for educational use.

Despite the positives, some issues remain. As with any mobile device, battery life varies depending on how the device is used. Simple browsing and word processing will drain the battery at a slower rate than using multiple applications simultaneously. The iPad has a sealed battery, which means that the entire device must be returned to Apple Service for any battery service. Another limitation relates to use. Tablets, for the most part, are not replacements for office computers but rather adjuncts to them. The built-in virtual keyboard is not conducive to long periods of use.

Tablets, including the iPad, are more suited to an educational environment than smartphones. Because common ereader devices have applications available for tablets, reading textbooks and accessing course management applications is feasible. Many tablets include a built-in webcam, providing users with the ability to video conference on many courses and seminars. The physical footprint of these devices makes them more appealing to some users than a laptop. However, Windows 8.0 makes it possible to convert a laptop to a tablet computer providing both the functionality of a laptop and a tablet.

Laptops and Desktop Computers

Historically, the desktop computer was the mainstay of academic computing; however, desktop computers are declining in popularity. Laptops are now more popular computing devices for educational use. A fairly robust laptop can be purchased for around $500, about the same cost as a comparably equipped and more powerful desktop. The portability of laptops or tablets is often the deciding factor for students and faculty. The increasing availability of broadband access is an additional strong influence for users. Students and faculty are able to access courses and content from anywhere with Internet access. Many online courses promote this aspect of their respective programs. For in-person classes students often bring a computing device into the classroom to take notes, research a topic, and link the items for reference at a later time. A subcategory of the laptop category, called ultrabook, is a smaller and lighter device that sacrifices a device drive (typically a DVD) and a spinning hard drive for a solid-state drive (SSD). Examples are the MacBook Air and the Samsung Series 5 laptop computers.

Clickers

A clicker is a device used with an audience response system; however, the term *clicker* is often used to refer to the complete system. These systems are used to provide faculty with real-time feedback from students during a presentation. The device itself is about the size of a deck of cards or smaller and is wirelessly linked via sensors in the room to a computer that records the responses. Software is available for those who want to use their smartphones as the feedback device. Instructors phrase questions as if administering a poll and ask students to respond using the clickers. Questions can be basic ("Do you understand the concept? – yes or no") or more complex ("What are the best options to solve a stated problem?"). Many users employ a multiple-choice approach and feedback questions can be embedded in a Microsoft PowerPoint presentation. Real-time feedback can be depicted in graphic format to help the instructor and audience understand the results of the poll. Examples of companies offering this technology include eInstruction (www.einstruction.com), i>clicker (www.iclicker.com), and Turning Technologies (www.turningtechnologies.com).

Audience response systems are also available for conference settings and have been integrated into webinar delivery type products. Uses include determining the winner of a competition, helping the audience to understand a concept or information by helping the presenter to shape the presentation to meet the audience's needs, and facilitating interactivity. The positives of this technology are several. No matter the device, responses are typically anonymous, although the system can be set up to tie the response to the user, for example, and to take classroom attendance. The anonymity may provide more honest responses. Audience response technology provides course instructors or conference presenters with immediate feedback. The immediacy of the response allows presenters to customize content to clarify audience concerns, meet audience needs, and facilitate user interaction and involvement with the educational content.

Barriers to this technology include instructor resistance to changing a class format; the time commitment to reformat a course; the cost of the devices, sensors, setup time, and software; system maintenance; and possible student resistance to the cost of the technology (i.e., another fee) and the need to learn and use more technology. For some instructors the device is a novelty, good for occasional use rather than a mainstream method of learning.

Educational Software

Many choices exist for faculty and students but there are some general considerations when selecting educational software. This type of software can be proprietary, such as Microsoft Word, or open source such as OpenOffice. Even though downloading and installing open source software is free, there are costs associated with obtaining support and maintenance for the software. Support and maintenance can also be an additional cost with proprietary software and should be negotiated before signing a contract. In addition, many educational software products have hardware limitations that should be carefully evaluated during the selection process. A number of products are discussed in this section, including learning and content management systems, mind maps, gaming, and eportfolios.

Learning and Content Management Systems

A learning management system (LMS) is generally defined as software used to address educational functions ranging from class administration and document and grade tracking to report generation and delivery of online courses.[6] These systems are mainly used as course management systems delivering hybrid or online courses as discussed in Chapter 27. However, they can also be used for other group activities such as setting up access to online advising and other university services for enrolled students. LMSs can provide content management functionality. For example, the LMS can be used to determine when and how content is displayed. However, a separate content management system or application can also be used with LMSs. A content management system is software that uses a central repository and focuses on the actual content for electronic delivery. A content management system encompasses the process of content development (create, edit, store, and deliver) and storage of learning materials such as PowerPoint slides, videos, etc. that can be used in different courses for different purposes. Depending on the vendor a content management system may be a component of an LMS or can function in a solo capacity with an interface to an LMS.[7] It should be noted that when used in higher education literature the acronym *CMS* usually refers to a course management system as denoted in Chapter 27 but can also refer to a content management system as described here.

LMSs are increasingly used by higher education institutions for distance education and as a supplement to traditional classroom education. LMSs allow for asynchronous access, online meetings, and remote testing and grading. Student assessment is a large component of an LMS. Blackboard, for instance, includes a dashboard for faculty to monitor student progress. Barriers to use of an LMS include the need for a broadband connection by students and the use of certain operating systems, although these barriers are fading over time. The largest barrier is the cost to purchase and maintain an LMS, especially a proprietary system. A detailed discussion of distance education, and the use of LMSs, is provided in Chapter 27.

Mind Maps

Mind maps are graphic or visual representations connecting words, ideas, tasks, or other items to a central core word or idea.[8] This type of activity may also be called a concept map. The visualization provides students with a tool to see how various components are related to a particular core idea or item (e.g., categories of medications and pain management, specific drug side effects related to a specific disease process). An example of a mind map is shown in Figure 28-2.

While mind map software can be used by individual students, it can also be used by students collaborating in face-to-face or online groups to create mind maps using an assortment of point devices (from fingers to color-coded digital markers). Maps can be saved and referenced for later review or incorporated into a student's eportfolio (discussed below) as an example of his or her work. The interactive

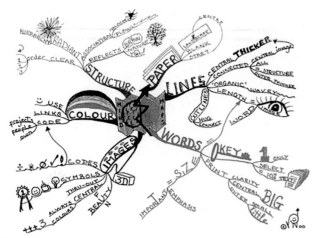

FIG 28-2 An example of a mind map. (From Litemind. What is mind mapping? [and how to get started immediately]. Litemind.com. http://litemind.com/what-is-mind-mapping/. 2012.)

creation of mind maps or concept maps can also be a tool for educators in healthcare. Studies indicate that concept maps facilitate critical thinking as well as student engagement.[9,10] Mind maps are also visually appealing for students. However, software costs may be a barrier, although other hardware platforms such as interactive whiteboards or LMSs can reduce overall costs.

Digital Portfolios

The electronic portfolio, or eportfolio, reflects a shift from the pen-and-paper portfolio model to a digital environment. The components of an eportfolio are basically the same as a traditional portfolio but are stored and presented in a digital format. The general structure, with some variation depending on the profession or department, includes a curriculum vita, a personal statement of some sort, a description of personal skills, and examples of the individual's work. The work example category, using the digital format, allows for digitization of pictures, movies, and other similar interactive presentations of personal work. The eportfolio provides an improved process for an individual to present a detailed picture of his or her work. Software supporting this concept includes ePortfolio (www.eportfolio.org) for students and Desire2Learn ePortfolio (www.desire2learn.com/products/eportfolio) geared more toward faculty. Many higher education institutions offer homegrown as well as proprietary products for users to use.

Many educational institutions required eportfolios as a component of student learning and evaluation. However, the requirement that students complete an eportfolio and the procedures for using portfolios and eportfolios vary greatly from one institution to another. For example, requiring that a student complete an eportfolio could ensure that students would be able to show future employers examples of their work. However, many institutions do not provide students with access to their eportfolios after graduation.

A significant advantage of using eportfolios is that faculty can use them to provide individualized feedback and advice to students. Drawbacks include a lack of quality assurance and the amount of time that eportfolios consume for both student and faculty.[11] Research on using portfolios (and eportfolios) in educational applications is limited. Nonetheless, this application facilitates student self-evaluation and continues to be a useful tool in education.

Web-Based Student Testing

Other educational tools include applications that facilitate online, or web-based, student testing. Web-based testing is usually independent of an operating system and the testing software is accessed using a web browser. Most LMSs (e.g., Blackboard, Moodle) support web-based testing options. Within an application, tests can be customized to question type (e.g., multiple choice, multiple answer, write-in, matching, essay). Common features of online testing solutions include the ability to control student access, length of tests, time available to take the test, feedback customization, and score analyses. Instructors can randomize the order of questions for each person taking the test. Obviously randomization helps to discourage screen sharing and easy answer sharing between students. Testing within an LMS is advantageous because the test score is automatically integrated into the LMS grading module and students receive immediate feedback on their performance. In nursing, web-based NCLEX review content is available. Companies providing this testing include ATI (www.atitesting.com/Home.aspx) and Kaplan (www.kaptest.com/NCLEX/Home/index.html). Both companies provide materials and tests for faculty to use and integrate in their programs.

Online testing tools usually can be configured to administer surveys to students. Other free-standing survey-specific tools are available for limited, if any, cost (e.g., SurveyMonkey, www.surveymonkey.com). More powerful and costly tools are also available. Proprietary applications often include a free version with limitations but these are useful for trying out the software. A well-known example is Qualtrics (www.qualtrics.com).

The advantages of web-based testing include faculty control and customization, the ability to incorporate feedback on a question-by-question basis, and immediate scoring available to the student. Faculty may incorporate these tests into mastery learning where students who have not done well on the test can relearn and retest before moving on to new content.

Security issues can present a major disadvantage for online testing. Students may be able to share tests either visually (sitting next to each other), by interacting remotely, or by using a browser with less security (allowing screenshots to be saved and shared). Because these tests are digital the potential for electrical or equipment failure can also be a disadvantage. Students can take advantage of this by accessing and reviewing a test and then turning the power off, reporting this as power failure and using the intervening time to look up answers to the test.

Student Journaling Software

Journaling is a methodology used to engage students in reflective learning. Reflective journaling is often used to evaluate students' clinical or practicum progress; at the same time, it improves critical thinking by providing students with insight into their own experiences and performance. Paper journals with handwritten faculty comments and questions were cumbersome and have been replaced by digital applications that provide easy access for faculty and more timely responses for students. These applications can be as simple as using blog applications to create an online diary. Free services are available, such as Blogger (www.blogger.com) or Google Drive (www.google.com/drive). In both of these examples the preference section includes the option of adjusting privacy settings to protect the students' work from the general public. Before using these types of free services for class assignments faculty should review the site's Terms and Conditions as well as the Privacy Statement that students must accept before using these free applications. These documents are legal contracts and using the site is the same as signing a printed contract. A number of LMSs also include this option but usually do not raise the same legal issues.

Gaming

Learning games are a means of engaging students within a classroom environment. They may be used to vary course content delivery and to allow students an active learning environment. As such, they are useful teaching strategies in healthcare.[12] Gaming commonly involves competition (a winner and a loser). This element helps to compel students to engage in the content, thereby improving learning. A number of topics can be used for gaming, from learning metabolic pathways to critical care for surgical patients.[12]

Gaming software typically involves the use of a game format, such as Jeopardy, Wheel of Fortune, a board game, or a card game, to engage students. PowerPoint templates of some television games are even available for faculty. Gaming does not always require information technology; it can be very low tech and still work well. Simple gaming formats can be relatively easy and inexpensive to use. In addition, a number of higher complexity computer games have been developed to provide interactive learning for students. For instance, Sim Hospital, a computer simulation game, provides healthcare students with the experience of administering a hospital.

Other applications use a computer gaming interface without being a game. For instance, one vendor, Anesoft (www.anesoft.com), produces a wide variety of browser-based software targeting for clinical specialties such as critical care and anesthesia. The two-dimensional application simulates patient care by providing the student with a picture of the patient along with vital signs and laboratory results. The student is able to evaluate patient data, make decisions, and view the results of those decisions. These materials can be especially useful in teaching groups of interprofessional students to work together in teams. Regardless of the format, gaming provides active learning and student engagement in an approach that is usually well received by students.

Virtual Worlds

Virtual worlds are computerized settings that simulate a world without traditional boundaries. A virtual world is limited by only two major constrictions: creativity and coded software. Typically the virtual world is viewed as three dimensional. Avatars (computer-generated objects that may or may not be humanlike) are characters that users adopt and portray as their own personalities in the virtual world. Avatars then interact with each other.

One of the earliest well-developed virtual worlds was Second Life (http://secondlife.com), a browser-based experience requiring the user to install a viewer on his or her computer. Access to Second Life is available to the viewer without charge. However, there are costs associated with developing student learning environments within Second Life. Users create their own avatar or virtual person and experience the environment of Second Life. Another example of a virtual world software application is OpenSimulator (http://opensimulator.org/wiki/Main_Page). OpenSimulator is an open source application used to simulate virtual environments similar to Second Life with much of the same functionality. Creating student environments in either of these applications can involve a significant learning curve. As a result, faculty often find it helpful to select one of these applications and work together in developing learning environments.

Originally these virtual worlds were designed for fantasy experiences but they have evolved to support other groups of people, such as those with compromised health. For example, in a virtual world physically handicapped persons are without limitations and can enjoy activities such as dancing, swimming, and walking. Healthcare sites, created by health professionals, within Second Life represent hospitals, clinics, and recreational areas, providing a means of support for patients. Healthcare learning environments can be specific for a particular topic such as midwifery or emergency healthcare and health-related schools have created virtual worlds for learning many different topics ranging from psychiatric care to community health nursing to emergency crises.

Second Life is currently the most common application used by health educators to create environments for students. For example, Tacoma Community College uses Second Life to provide simulated emergency experiences for nursing students with guidance from faculty (http://bit.ly/EvergreenOrientation). This experience includes a virtual patient, the ability to view an electrocardiogram and other vital signs on a monitor, and the ability to talk and interact with the patient and other persons in the location. Participants, if allowed, can even draw up and administer virtual medications. Limitations of this environment include cost and the resources necessary to build and maintain it.

The virtual environment provides a different experience for health education students. It allows students to experience different roles via their avatars. They can practice different aspects of care ranging from communication (since avatars can speak) to clinical skills. This makes the use of virtual worlds an excellent tool for simulation-type learning with groups of students from a variety of disciplines. However, there are limitations to this simulated environment. For example, there are no sensory experiences such as odors or touch, which can be a barrier for some experiences.

IMPACT ON THE TEACHING AND LEARNING PROCESS

Today, technology drives a teaching-learning process that is increasingly student centered, faculty facilitated, collaborative, open sourced, and globally focused, using a blend of synchronous and asynchronous modalities and focused on contextual learning, to enhance the acquisition of new knowledge for both students and faculty. The ripple effects of the paradigm change are evident, with intergenerational differences in teaching and learning styles, the time requirements of teaching, faculty evaluations, and impact on tenure.

The use of technology in education is changing both educators' and students' roles and responsibilities. For example, educational theorists have acknowledged that individuals learn in different ways. Perhaps one of the most adopted theoretical approaches used in education to explain these individual differences is Gardner's multiple intelligences. Gardner determined that people learn through nine different intelligences: linguistic, logical-mathematical, spatial, bodily-kinesthetic, musical, interpersonal, intrapersonal, naturalistic, and existentialist. Gardner determined that while everyone uses all nine intelligences with some degree of competence, one or two of the intelligences are more dominant in each individual (Box 28-2).[13]

BOX 28-2   EXAMPLES USING GARDNER'S NINE MULTIPLE INTELLIGENCES

- Develop podcasts, wikis, or blogs for the expressive linguistic learner
- Play online strategy games, search databases for information, or use graphics packages for the logical-mathematical learner
- Create a digital story, develop a digital art project, or create a concept map for the visual creative spatial learner
- Interact with software programs to write and create music or to create a music video or podcast for the auditory musical learner
- Create experiences with simulation, virtual field trips, or virtual role-playing games for the bodily-kinesthetic learner
- Expound on discussion boards or develop imbedded audio and video PowerPoint presentations for online class introductions for the interpersonal learner
- Write a blog, develop online survey tools, and encourage independent exploration of any of the aforementioned activities for the intrapersonal learner
- Develop photo journals or use mapping and graphic organizing software for the naturalistic learner
- Use web research, presentation applications, email, and chat to encourage big-picture thinking (questioning, analyzing, and figuring out why things work) for the existentialist learner

---

For several decades educators have attempted to individualize the process of educating students by creating instructional materials and experiences that address individual students' intelligences or learning styles. Today's technology can make that goal a reality.

Matching students' nine intelligences or learning styles through the use of technology allows for more meaningful educational experiences.[14,15] Essentially, faculty and students are engaged in subtle and not-so-subtle shifts in technology-driven changes that will continue to transform the process of teaching and learning.

National and International Perspectives on Education

Creating and delivering learning that is relevant to students is a challenge for educators and education systems worldwide. For global education, the following suggestions are offered:

- Consider using more cellphones and mobile applications since not everyone has computer access
- End the traditional lecture and replace it with easily accessible, open source, short educational videos
- Use free web tools for course discussions and projects to better prepare students for jobs after college
- Encourage scholarly associations to set up bloglike online forums to allow scholars to share ideas and openly conduct peer review

There is a need to evaluate the changes in education and redefine both student and faculty self-expectations for learning.[16-18] Proponents of interprofessional learning nationally and internationally suggest that students and faculty need to learn with, from, and about each other. The emphasis on teacher-centered, didactic instruction changes to a student-centered, interdisciplinary, faculty-facilitated, and collaborative approach to learning. Shared experiences and collaborative learning could translate to improved quality of care and help to break down the traditional professional silos. The use of information systems and technology strategies, such as online course delivery, could help to facilitate shared interprofessional knowledge building and knowledge mobilization and transfer this collaboratively generated new knowledge into practice.[18-20]

IMPACT ON THE FACULTY ROLE

Faculty are now being asked to be proactive in the adoption and integration of technology while maintaining traditional research, practice, and service requirements. The impact of this demand on faculty satisfaction, time related to teaching, student evaluations, and tenure can be dramatic. While many faculty have enthusiastically embraced the use of technology in the classroom, faculty have also expressed concerns about being undervalued, the changing focus of pedagogy, compensation and workload issues (especially the amount of time necessary to create and maintain technology-enhanced courses), the lack of institutional support for these new teaching methods, and the need to continually update their own technology skills without compensation or institutional support.[21,22]

Nelson et al.[1] and Moseley[23] remind us that the cultures of technology and academia differ, as demonstrated by a quote from Nelson: "The cultures of information technology and academia are characterized by competing traits. Words like *ubiquitous, youthful, volatile, instantaneous,* and *profitable* are used to define information technology. Conversely, words such as *steadfast, autonomous, venerable, persistence, resistant, patient,* and *non-lucrative* are words we associate with academia."[1(p194)] Faculty are now being asked to reach across this divide. Institutions of higher education must help by investing in high levels of support and training for faculty and students who use technology.

While faculty are working to maximize the benefits of technology in the classroom the inclusion of technology can have a significant impact on student course evaluations. Student evaluations for faculty teaching online have been mixed, from lower scores for faculty teaching online versus face to face to no difference in scores.[24,25] This can be especially troublesome in settings where student evaluations of faculty play a significant role in determining faculty promotion and tenure decisions.

Other related barriers to the tenure process that can be affected by the implementation of technology include the following:

- Outdated policies and explicit expectations for performance
- Escalating expectations for the quantity and quality of publications, practice, service, and especially funded research
- Lack of or infrequent feedback or formal mentoring by seasoned faculty
- Marrying online education information systems and technology tools with a changing teaching-learning process
- The need for work–life balance[26]

New models may be in order for technology and tenure. The following two examples exemplify technology-driven scholarly activities that may be considered during the tenure process for health professions faculty:

- A collaborative, international, digitally developed, implemented, and evaluated project rather than a written dissertation by one person
- Rewriting scholarly activity guidelines for tenure to include the creation and use of open source resources and publication opportunities available globally and free of charge[27-29]

Teaching, learning, and the tenure process are in a state of flux for both faculty and students. How university administrators will factor the impact of technology into faculty promotion and tenure decisions remains a focus for discussion far into the future.

CONCLUSION AND FUTURE DIRECTIONS

Bartholomew wondered whether higher education is really ready for the information revolution.[30] Despite recommendations from a multitude of organizations, government, and the business sector, some institutions of higher education have been slow to adopt and use information management and technology tools and to view online learning as a strategic asset.[31] A myriad of reasons are described, including the cost of purchasing technologies; administrative, staff, faculty, and student dislike or fear of change; a parochial view of traditional education; and the need to generate a new model for education other than student credit hours.[29,31,32]

In the United States there are an estimated 4400 institutions of postsecondary education. Three vendors provide approximately 3000 administrative systems, such as student information systems for managing student records. In addition, many larger research universities have built their own solutions and others are using a best of breed approach to create their administrative information systems.[33] As a result, "colleges and universities are swimming in an ever widening sea of data" and creating pools of big data.[34(p11)] In the future the analysis of these data with data mining tools will create a better picture of what does and does not work in education. For example, a number of the health professions require that students complete courses from the physical sciences, such as chemistry, anatomy, or physiology, before they are introduced to the health-related sciences, such as pathophysiology. From an intuitive prospective this makes sense but is it possible that students may comprehend chemistry better if it followed a course such as pathophysiology? In actual practice this progression rarely happens but in big data repositories there may be the numbers to answer this question and other questions that one currently would not think to ask.

While many universities are now using administrative systems and the technology used to deliver distance education has become increasingly robust, much of the teaching-learning process is still managed manually. A number of computerized teaching tools have been discussed in this chapter. Currently these tools are being used to provide innovative approaches to delivering content and to engage students in learning that content, but they do not track data related to a student's individual learning process. For example, in most cases clickers record a student's response and discard that response with the introduction of the next question. A few of these applications, especially in the area of LMS, are beginning to track each student's progress with the assessment tools used in an individual course. For example, LMSs are designed to track a student's amount of participation in various discussion groups.

However, in most university settings, very little data (other than the course grade) about the individual student's learning across educational programs are recorded and maintained. The current system could be compared to a paper patient chart with additional limitations. In the healthcare system, health-related data are maintained in one chart for each patient. In education the final record of a student's learning is the limited information included on the transcript. In the manual world of education, for the most part, all other data collected by individual faculty or academic departments are maintained, if at all, in file cabinets or individual faculty files. This can be called the ultimate system for creating an island of lost data and information. In the future, with the computerization of the academy, the student record will become rich with data related to individual learning, thereby creating new options for academic success.

Over the next several years education information systems and technical tools will continue to increase in number and complexity. User interfaces will become more intuitive and learning curves less steep. Increased technical presence will drive increased use. Interactions with applications may become more "natural," using voice and motion recognition. Greater functionality for education is likely for smartphones and tablets. As hardware increases in capacity and shrinks in size, mobile learning (mlearning) will likely become easier and easier. Questions for the future are: How much and what data should be collected about individual administrators, faculty, staff, and students, and why? Do faculty and students want 24/7 learning? Can learning truly become ubiquitous? Should the learning process truly become lifelong?

Acknowledgement: We would like to acknowledge the assistance of Dr. Ernesto Perez, Dr. Mary Smith, Dr. Vincent Sperandeo, and Dr. Dara Warren from the DNP graduating class of 2011, Capstone College of Nursing, The University of Alabama. We appreciate their thoughtful comments and suggestions for this chapter.

REFERENCES

1. Nelson R, Meyers L, Rizzolo MA, Rutar P, Proto MB, Newbold S. The evolution of education information systems and nurse faculty roles. *Nurs Educ Perspect.* 2006;27(5):189-195.
2. Criswell C. What is a SmartBoard? Suite101. http://suite101.com/article/what-is-a-smartboard-a71150. September 30, 2008.
3. Appleton L. The use of electronic books in midwifery education: the student perspective. *Health Info Libr J.* 2004;21:245-252.
4. Williams MG, Dittmer A. Textbooks on tap: using electronic books housed in handheld devices in nursing clinical courses. *Nurs Educ Perspect.* 2009;30(4):220-225.
5. Hepburn A. Infographic: Mobile Statistics, Stats & Facts 2011. Retrieved from http://www.digitalbuzzblog.com/2011-mobile-statistics-stats-facts-marketing-infographic/. April 4, 2011.
6. Spong A. Mobile health adoption doubles between 2010 & 2011. Twitpic. http://twitpic.com/7hayut. 2012.
7. Ellis RK. A field guide to learning management systems. *ASTD Learning Circuits,* Retrieved from http://cgit.nutn.edu.tw:8080/cgit/PaperDL/hclin_091027163029.PDF. 2009.
8. Passuello L. What is mind mapping? (and how to get started immediately) [Web log post]. Retrieved from http://litemind.com/what-is-mind-mapping). 2007.
9. Atay S, Karabacak U. Care plans using concept maps and their effects on the critical thinking dispositions of nursing students. *Int J Nurs Pract.* 2012;18:233-239.
10. Revell SMH. Concept maps and nursing theory: a pedagogical approach. *Nurs Educ.* 2012;37(3):131-135.
11. Buckley S, Coleman J, Davison I, et al. The educational effects of portfolios on undergraduate student learning: a Best Evidence Medical Education (BEME) systematic review: BEME Guide No. 11. *Med Teach.* 2009;31:340-355.
12. Akl EA, Pretorius RW, Sackett K, et al. The effect of educational games on medical students' learning outcomes: a systematic review: BEME Guide No 14. *Med Teach.* 2010;32:16-27.
13. Gardner H. *Frames of Mind: The Theory of Multiple Intelligences.* New York, NY: Basic Books; 1983.
14. Smith MK. Howard Gardner and multiple intelligences. *The encyclopedia of informal education.* http://www.infed.org/thinkers/gardner.htm. 2002, 2008.
15. Johnson L, Lamb A. Technology and multiple intelligences. Teacher Tap: Professional Development Resources for Educators & Librarians. http://eduscapes.com/tap/topic68.htm. 2007.
16. The Lancet. International Collaboration for Health Professions Education's Commission on Education for Health Professions for the 21st Century. The Lancet. http://www.thelancet.com/journals/lancet/issue/vol376no9756/PIIS0140-6736(10)X6159-1. 2010.
17. Nicholas P, White T. e-Learning, e-books and virtual reference service: the nexus between the library and education. *Journal of Library & Information Services in Distance Learning.* 2012;6(1):3-18.
18. Hsieh PH. Globally-perceived experiences of online instructor: a preliminary exploration. *Computers and Education.* 2010;54:27-36.
19. Centre for the Advancement of Interprofessional Education (CAIPE). Interprofessional education: a definition. CAIPE. http://www.caipe.org.uk/about-us/the-definition-and-principles-of-interprofessional-education/. 2002.
20. Lewis K, Baker R. Expanding the scope of faculty educator development for health care professionals. *The Journal of Educators Online.* 2009;6(1):1-17.
21. Schell G. Universities marginalize online courses: why should faculty members develop online courses if the effort is detrimental to their promotion or tenure? *Commun ACM.* 2004;47(7):53-56.
22. Neely P, Tucker J. Unbundling faculty roles in online distance education programs. *International Review of Research in Open and Distance Learning.* 2010;11(2).
23. Moseley WL. Student and faculty perceptions of technology's usefulness in community college general education courses. *Open Access Theses and Dissertations from the College of Education and Human Sciences.* Paper 74. 2010.
24. Regan K, Evmenova A, Baker P, et al. Experiences of instructors in online environments: identifying and regulating emotions. *Internet High Educ.* 2012 [in press]. doi:10.1016/j.iheduc.2011.12.001.
25. Topper A. Are they the same? comparing the instructional quality of online and face-to-face graduate education courses. *Assessment & Evaluation in Higher Education.* 2007;32(6):681-691.
26. American Association of University Professors (AAUP). Documents related to academic freedom and tenure. AAUP. http://www.aaup.org; http://www.aaup.org/AAUP/pubsres/policydocs/contents/RIR.htm. 2002, 2005, 2007, 2008, 2010.
27. Sorcinelli M. New conceptions of scholarship for a new generation of faculty members. *New Directions for Teaching and Learning.* 2002;90:41-48.
28. Pannapacker W. Invisible gorillas are everywhere. *The Chronicle of Higher Education.* 2012;24.
29. Pepicello W. University of Phoenix. In: Oblinger DG, ed. Game changers education and information technologies. EDUCAUSE 2012; 2012. Retrieved from http://www.educause.edu/library/resources/chapter-10-university-phoenix.
30. Bartholomew N. Is higher education ready for the information revolution? *International Journal of Therapy and Rehabilitation.* 2011;18(10):558-565.

31. Association of Public and Land-Grant Universities, A*P*L*U-Sloan National Commission on Online Learning. *Online Learning as a Strategic Asset: Volume 1: A Resource for Campus Leaders; Volume 2: The Paradox of Faculty Voices: Reviews and Experiences with Online Learning.* 2009.

32. Oblinger DG. IT as a game changer. In: Oblinger DG, ed. *Game Changers: Education and Information Technologies.* Louisville, CO: EDUCAUSE; 2012:37-51.

33. Bonig R. Latest trends in student information systems: driven by competition. *Educause Review.* May 9, 2012. Retrieved from http://www.educause.edu/ero/article/latest-trends-student-information-systems-driven-competition.

34. Walters J. Big data. *Campus Technology.* 2012;26(2):11-16.

DISCUSSION QUESTIONS

1. How might comprehensive academic information systems affect the work of faculty within an academic setting?
2. What role should faculty play in the selection, implementation, and evaluation of information systems and computerized teaching tools?
3. What are some advantages and disadvantages of the current computerized education tools?
4. How are interprofessional education, the tenure process, and information technology educational tools connected?
5. Describe how computerized teaching tools might be employed in an interdisciplinary environment.
6. What do you think are the key questions one might consider when using big data in health education programs?
7. The future has many pathways. What do you see in the future regarding information systems and technology tools in healthcare education?

CASE STUDY

You are a baccalaureate-prepared health practitioner in the school system and are also certified to teach kindergarten to twelfth grade. You are intrigued by the teaching-learning process and decide that you are now interested in teaching new health professionals in an institution of higher education about the importance of school health. You begin your education to obtain the necessary degrees and experience. You select a program with an emphasis on education, teaching, and learning. Through your coursework you acquire knowledge about education's history and learn how cognition processes transform knowledge gained from social, biological, cultural, and historical contexts. You are also introduced to a number of new computer-based technologies designed for educational use. Informatics and its application to education and the process of teaching and learning fascinate you. You eagerly begin to incorporate student-centered learning, technology-related activities in your classes and frequently work collaboratively with interdisciplinary faculty peers and staff in planning, assessing, implementing, and evaluating the addition and adoption of new student-centered learning activities. You and the students learn both individually and collaboratively during, for example, the adoption of online testing, eportfolio development, the use of video conferencing, online courses, and other similar activities, including online class chats and discussions with international nursing faculty and their students.

You begin to do research and publish your findings in online journals as well as on a blog that focuses on the use of technology in health education programs. However, in your annual review you are advised that you now need to take a more traditional approach to teaching, research, and publications. Using technology to create the innovative classes you are teaching is taking up too much of your time and this is time that would be better spent in developing grants from traditional sources.

Discussion Questions

1. Resistance to change is a formidable foe to progress. What are some possible options to facilitate change in education and the introduction of technology?
2. Suppose that the educational setting in this case study decides to become interdisciplinary. Describe educational technologies and methods that would facilitate the process.
3. If you could collect and track learning data related to individual students across their educational program, what data elements would you consider a priority? For example, would you want to track learning preferences; writing ability, including specific strengths and weaknesses; or clinical strengths and weaknesses?

Simulation in Healthcare Education

Valerie Howard, Kim Leighton, and Teresa Gore

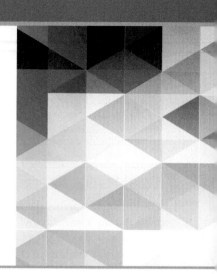

The emergence of technology for educational purposes creates a need for faculty and health science educators to understand how to not only operate the technology but also implement it within the academic and service settings while still using sound academic principles.

OBJECTIVES

At the completion of this chapter the reader will be prepared to:
1. Define the different types of simulation modalities available
2. Describe the challenges and opportunities inherent to simulation
3. Apply the Standards of Best Practice: Simulation to the simulation lab

4. Discuss the use of simulation-based education in interprofessional experiences
5. Analyze the similarities and differences related to the available simulation resources
6. Develop evidence-based simulation activities for graduate-level education

KEY TERMS

Clinical scenario, 459
Debriefing, 461
Fidelity, 455
Learning environment, 457

Simulation, 454
Simulation experience, 457
Standards of Best Practice: Simulation, 460

ABSTRACT

The use of simulated learning experiences has rapidly emerged in healthcare education as a method of training healthcare providers in a safe environment without subjecting patients to harm. Multiple definitions of simulation-related terms exist, so the importance of the use of standardized terminology is stressed. Best practice standards for implementing simulated learning experiences are discussed in this chapter. These should be provided in a standardized manner while adhering to guidelines to maximize learning. Simulated learning experiences directly correlate with the *Core Competencies for Interprofessional Collaborative Practice*. Finally, issues, challenges, and opportunities for the future of healthcare education and the use of simulation are outlined.

INTRODUCTION

Simulation is a time-honored method of teaching that has been used in health education for decades. It is defined as the use of "one or more typologies to promote, improve, and/or validate a participant's progression from novice to expert,"[1(pS6)] where the novice to expert continuum is consistent with that promoted by Benner.[2] Experiential learning theory is used in health professions education to emphasize the importance of clinical practice in the educational process.[3] Simulation is one method of experiential, hands-on application learning and can range from a simple activity used to mimic reality (e.g., the process of injecting an orange to create the feel of puncturing skin) to the use of high-fidelity simulation to create the comprehensive experience of interacting with a healthcare team during a clinical emergency. In each case the simulated clinical experience "includes pre-briefing, the clinical scenario, and debriefing; it is the engagement part of a clinical scenario."[1(pS6)]

Types of Simulations

Several types of simulation are used in healthcare education, including written case studies, computer models such as Second Life, standardized patients, partial task trainers, and medium- to high-fidelity patient simulators. Simulators are used to help students to improve critical thinking, clinical judgment, communication, and teamwork skills while assisting learners to meet psychomotor, cognitive, and affective learning objectives. Most of the growth in simulation is with standardized patients, task trainers, and simulators.

Standardized patients consistently portray a patient or other individual in a scripted scenario for the purposes of instruction, practice, or evaluation.[4] Standardized patients may be actors who require little training. Others may be people who respond to requests for assistance with healthcare training and require significant resources for training. Still others may actually have the disease, illness, symptom, or injury under study. In most cases standardized patients are paid for their assistance to the educational process.

Partial task trainers typically represent anatomic parts of the human body and are used to practice skill acquisition.[5] This type of simulator assists learners to meet psychomotor objectives, those accomplished when a student demonstrates the ability to perform a task such as inserting a urinary catheter, giving an injection, or attaching a heart monitor. Partial task trainers can range from low to high levels of realism. Examples of low-realism partial task trainers are when learners practice giving intradermal injections using a silicone pad that is flexible enough to allow a bleb to form when fluid is injected or using a hot dog with skin for the same purpose. An example of a more realistic partial task trainer is a model that promotes practice of intravenous needle insertion through a virtual model that includes haptic technology. Haptics is a feature allowing tactile sensation, for example, when the needle enters a vein.

Simulators include full-body mannequins and can range from static mannequins that do not respond to any intervention to high-fidelity computerized simulators designed to realistically respond to learner interventions. High-fidelity mannequins can have blinking eyes, a chest that rises and falls with breaths, heart and lung sounds, and palpable peripheral pulses and can be capable of being intubated, having chest tubes inserted, and having other assessments and procedures performed on them. High-fidelity simulators are particularly useful for interprofessional training on cooperative activities such as codes. An example is the mannequin shown in Figure 29-1 marketed by Laerdal. These simulators are considered the most lifelike compared to human patients. The most realistic simulators in healthcare education are, of course, real persons. Obviously, numerous skills and conditions cannot be recreated for safety reasons. Instead, educators often use a hybrid simulation involving two types of simulators. A

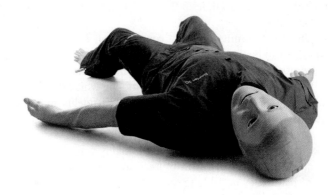

FIG 29-1 Sample high-fidelity simulator. (Photo courtesy of Laerdal Medical Corporation.)

student can explain the procedure, risks, and potential complications to the standardized patient while performing the procedure on the partial task trainer. Standardized patients can assist learners to meet objectives while enhancing communication, clinical judgment, critical thinking, and teamwork skills.

Fidelity

Fidelity is the standard term used to describe the realism involved in simulated learning activities. There are a variety of ways to create fidelity in the learning experience, which can be confusing for educators. It recently has been recognized that fidelity has very little to do with *what* equipment is used and much more to do with *how* that equipment is used. Fidelity can involve a variety of dimensions, including the following:

- Physical factors such as environment, equipment, and related tools
- Psychological factors such as the emotions, beliefs, and self-awareness of participants
- Social factors such as participant and instructor motivation and goals
- Culture of the group
- Degree of openness and trust, as well as participants' modes of thinking[1(pS5)]

On a trajectory from low fidelity to high fidelity, task trainers are considered of lower fidelity than high-fidelity simulators and finally standardized patients. However, this type of classification is not without controversy. Alinier places computer-controlled simulators above standardized patients in his continuum.[6] For example, a high-fidelity mannequin used in a cardiopulmonary arrest situation may not even be turned on, depending on the level of the learner. A low-fidelity task trainer used in a high-fidelity environment may allow the combination to rank higher than the task trainer alone. Other types of simulation (e.g., written, screen-based) fall into the trajectory, depending on how they are used. The decision about the level of fidelity needed for any simulated clinical experience should always be based on the learning objectives. Thus it is not always necessary to have high fidelity, especially when cost as well as technology needs are both considered. The example in Table 29-1 involves inserting a central line.

The most common fidelity consideration is the type of simulator to be used; however, educators have become aware of additional types of fidelity such as environment. Fidelity of the environment considers the location in which the simulated clinical experience takes place. A high-fidelity mannequin may need to be used within a psychomotor skills lab, a classroom, or even office space. An environment most similar to where real patient care takes place is highly desirable. Additionally, the equipment, furniture, and supplies should all be as realistic as possible to the traditional clinical environment. Creating methods to add patients' emotions, beliefs, spirituality, culture, and communication are also ways to make the experience more realistic. Table 29-2 outlines ideas for meeting learning needs in the developmental, spiritual, sociocultural, and psychological dimensions.

Benefits of Simulation

Simulation offers the chance for learners to practice in a safe environment without placing patients at risk. Simulation significantly increases learners' knowledge,[7,8] competence,[9] self-efficacy,[10] and confidence[11] at no added risk to patients. While the former are intermediate outcomes, a longer-term outcome of better training is higher quality of patient care. Deliberate practice, the process of practicing a skill multiple times until mastery is reached, is facilitated within the simulation environment through the use of task trainers, further reducing the risk of harm to patients.[9] Simulation also offers the opportunity to create standardized learning experiences in a controlled environment and provides exposure to low-occurrence, high-risk situations with opportunities to practice critical thinking skills, problem solving, and decision making.

An evaluation of any educational training program should align with evaluation models of training, for example, Kirkpatrick's model.[12] Kirkpatrick identified the following four different levels of outcomes of training programs:

- *Level 1: Reaction*, measures the learners' reactions to the training program. For example, were the learners satisfied with the program and how do they plan to use the information provided?
- *Level 2: Learning*, measures the amount of knowledge, attitudes, or skills that have changed and the level of the change as a result of the training.
- *Level 3: Behavior or Training Transfer*, measures the amount of "on the job" behavior change by the learner following the training sessions.
- *Level 4: Results*, measures the organizational impact of the training program, on either performance or cost savings.

Much of the research related to simulation has focused on the first two levels, measuring the learner's perspective, satisfaction, and knowledge gain related to the experience. However, ultimately simulation researchers will want to demonstrate the benefit of simulation training and its impact on patient outcomes (level 4). As an example, most recently simulation training has been correlated with lower central line infection rates,[13] decreased complications resulting from shoulder dystocia obstetrical emergencies,[14] and healthcare cost savings related to decreased malpractice claims.[15]

TABLE 29-1	FIDELITY CORRELATED WITH OBJECTIVES
OBJECTIVE: THE LEARNER WILL . . .	TYPE OF SIMULATOR
Accurately place central line catheter	Task trainer
Maintain sterile technique when placing a central line	Task trainer
Clearly communicate risks when obtaining consent from patient	Standardized patient
Use various communication techniques to calm patient's anxiety	Standardized patient
Recognize need for central line insertion during hypertensive crisis	High-fidelity simulator
Insert central line when rapid blood transfusion is required	High-fidelity simulator

TABLE 29-2	DIMENSIONS OF LEARNING AND FIDELITY	
DIMENSION	SIMULATED PATIENT	IMPROVING FIDELITY
Developmental	42-year-old male patient with myocardial infarction (MI); works as laborer	Place frame with picture of young family at bedside. Does the learner recognize that patient likely will not be able to return to work? Does he or she consider how the family will have their financial needs met?
Spiritual	Patient will be having emergent surgery	Place religious or spiritual book or icon at the bedside. Does the learner recognize the need to ask the patient about his or her beliefs and practices?
Sociocultural	Patient is being discharged with five new prescriptions	Provide discharge instruction sheet. Does the learner determine whether the patient has the resources to get new prescriptions filled?
Psychological	Postoperative knee replacement patient cannot return home to care for self	The patient reveals that there are 10 steps before entering his home. Does the learner explore how the patient feels about the loss of his or her independence?

Challenges and Opportunities

While simulation is an ideal environment for creating standardized learning opportunities and applying theoretical knowledge in the practice setting, inherent challenges exist related to the ease of implementation.

Cost

High-fidelity simulation mannequins can be expensive to purchase and maintain. Highly computerized mannequins can cost between $30,000 and $125,000 while task trainers can cost as little as $250 depending on the level of complexity and fidelity. Standardized patient experiences also have higher costs because of the need to hire and train actors. Hourly pay for actors differs depending on the region and the level of the actors' experience but can range between $12 and $40 per hour. Educators need to factor in time for preparation, training, and participation per actor. If the simulation center is recording each simulation experience for use in debriefing, as is typical, the audiovisual software systems can cost between $10,000 and $50,000 per simulation room depending on the functions needed and levels of complexity. In addition to costs related to the simulation modalities, financial resources must be committed to support the center and faculty time and training. Resource considerations can include workload release time to learn and understand how to use the simulation technology and how to implement simulations into the curriculum, funding for conference attendance, purchase of related journals and books, and membership dues for simulation organizations.

After the initial purchase costs, annual maintenance funds are required. These costs include ongoing maintenance, depreciation, and upgrades to the technology. Extended warranties can be purchased to cover the ongoing maintenance needed to ensure proper working order of the computerized mannequins. Most simulator mannequins are classified as capital purchases, so it is important to discuss the purchase, maintenance, and any insurance coverage with your institution's business office prior to making a commitment. Also, when planning for a simulation mannequin purchase, consider budgeting for costs related to replacement parts. Each piece of simulation equipment may have different suggestions related to replacement parts, including "skins," appendages, and moulage, so it is important to have conversations with simulation vendors prior to purchase so that appropriate budgetary planning and projections can begin.

Many health professional programs include student simulation lab fees. Others may seek grant funding from foundations, corporations, or private donors to support these efforts. Funding success can be maximized by developing a relationship with the potential funder, correlating the funding proposal with the mission and vision of the funding agency, and forming collaborative partnerships to demonstrate a unique and sustainable project.

Technology

The high-fidelity simulation mannequins can be difficult to operate by faculty who lack technological experience

---

BOX 29-1 JOB DESCRIPTION FOR SIMULATION TECHNICIAN

Under the direction of the Simulation Center Director, the technician will provide technical support for all simulation experiences and operations, including preparation, maintenance and repair of computerized mannequins, task trainers, simulation-related hardware and software systems, audiovisual equipment, administrative website management, and digital recording systems.

---

or knowledge. In addition, skills are required to operate the digital audiovisual equipment to record simulation experiences.

Partnering with simulation vendors may allow specific training opportunities to enhance understanding of the simulator technology and promote ease of use. Hiring a full-time or part-time simulation technician may be necessary. Generally, previous experience with computers, information technology, and even sound or recording can enhance the effectiveness of the simulation technology. Box 29-1 offers a sample job description for a simulation technician.

Informatics principles and processes can be used for simulation projects and for developing simulation centers. For example, the systems life cycle (SLC) introduced in Chapter 2 can be applied to the purchase and installation of products. To review, the phases of the SLC are as follows:

1. Analyze
2. Plan
3. Develop or purchase
4. Test
5. Implement or go-live
6. Maintain and evolve
7. Evaluate
8. Return to analyze

The SLC is tailored to the project at hand; however, the processes and activities are similar to those used for any other project.

Faculty Development

Simulation is just one example of an experiential teaching and learning strategy, but many faculty lack the understanding of educational principles related to the best methods for implementing experiential learning strategies within the curriculum. Therefore knowledge of the following educational principles will assist the simulation facilitator in developing academically sound experiences:

- Educational theory
- Application of theory to practice
- Development of clear and measurable objectives
- Instructional design
- Formative and summative learner evaluation
- Program evaluation
- Facilitation of learning
- Debriefing strategies
- Creating a safe learning environment in the simulation lab

To maintain a safe environment for learning and ensure commitment to academic principles, each simulation facilitator should have an orientation period to learn the aforementioned principles and observe experienced simulation facilitators, similar to a mentorship model. If schools do not have the appropriate experts within their organizations, resources should be committed to educate the simulation facilitator. Likewise, institutions will need to develop policies that require the simulation facilitator to have appropriate training before interacting with learners in the lab.

Several organizations, such as the International Nursing Association for Clinical Simulation and Learning (INACSL), the National League for Nursing (NLN), the American Association of Colleges of Nursing (AACN), and the Society for Simulation in Healthcare (SSH), offer annual meetings, conferences, and faculty development webinars to assist with this challenge. In addition, several higher education institutions offer graduate-level certificates with concentrations in simulation. Two scholarly journals are devoted to simulation: *Clinical Simulation in Nursing* and *Simulation in Healthcare*. Finally, other organizations offer continuing education programs with continuing education credits for their ongoing developmental programs.

Faculty or Administrative Buy-In

The use of simulation modalities to enhance learning can be considered an organizational change and resistance to change efforts has been widely reported in all disciplines, including business, organizational behavior, psychology, and healthcare. Faculty may be resistant to learning the new technology, administrators may not understand the importance of dedicating time and resources to the successful implementation of the simulation efforts, and students may be anxious about the possibility of being recorded as they practice in the simulation center.

Successful change efforts can be facilitated by having a thorough understanding of change theories and using this theoretical knowledge to guide the efforts. One change model used in healthcare was developed by John Kotter, who suggests following eight steps when leading a change effort (Table 29-3).[16] These steps can be applied to simulation efforts with health practitioners. Creating a mission and vision statement for the simulation program and developing a strategic plan can also guide future efforts related to integrating advanced practice experiences within the simulation program.[17] Evaluating the participants' satisfaction related to the simulation experiences through the use of postsimulation surveys can

TABLE 29-3	KOTTER'S PRINCIPLES APPLIED TO SIMULATION
KOTTER'S PRINCIPLE	**APPLICATION TO SIMULATION EDUCATION**
Creating a sense of urgency	• Identify the need for simulation based training within institution • Share simulation based research and evidence with stakeholders
Developing a guiding coalition	• Identify simulation champions and other like-minded individuals in your organization to form your simulation team • Choose representatives from all stakeholders (faculty, administrators, clinicians, educators, learners, students, staff, patients, families)
Developing a vision	• Develop a mission, vision, name, and strategic plan for your simulation program or center • Create a business plan • Include input from all stakeholders
Communicating that vision	• Share the plan with all stakeholders • Use a marketing or branding approach for the name of your organization • Consult with your public relations department
Empowering stakeholders to act upon that vision	• Develop an organizational structure to support each team member • Schedule regular meetings for progress updates and document the minutes from each meeting • Develop clear and concise roles and responsibilities for simulation related activities and ensure accountability • Seek resources from administration, outside funding agencies, participant fees to support the structure
Create short term wins	• Develop one or two simulation activities based upon sound educational principles and implement this according to the best simulation evidence available • Celebrate the successes of each individual in your simulation team
Consolidation of improvements	• Collect data on each simulation experience and use the data to improve quality
Institutionalizing new approaches	• Develop and implement policies and procedures related to simulation (i.e.: simulation facilitator, facilitation, simulation design, scheduling, debriefing) • Maximize use of your simulation center • Continue to share the positive simulation evaluation data, both quantitative and qualitative, with administrators, faculty, clinicians, educators, and all stakeholders

Adapted from Kotter, JP. Leading Change. Boston, MA: Harvard Business Review Press; 1996.

also provide necessary data to share with administrators in an effort to gain support. Faculty members can be given an opportunity to visit the simulation lab and experience first-hand the learners' reaction to this powerful educational tool. Finally, sharing the positive experiences of students both quantitatively and qualitatively, through reflections and stories, can also generate buy-in.

THE SIMULATION PROCESS

Learning Theories Applied to Simulation

Simulation is often accepted without any validation and based on the technology instead of a theoretical underpinning. Kneebone identified the following four areas for using theoretical underpinning:

1. Gaining technical proficiency with psychomotor skills
2. Learning theory with repetitive practice and frequent reinforcement
3. Tailoring support to the individual learner's need using situated learning
4. Addressing the affective domain of emotions with learning[18]

In addition, Kneebone identified the following four criteria for evaluating existing and new simulations:

1. Allow sustained, repetitive, and purposeful practice in a safe, controlled environment
2. Level interaction with the expert or mentor depending on the proficiency of the student
3. Simulation should mimic actual life experiences
4. The simulated environment should foster a learner-centered approach that inspires and supports students[18]

Through deliberate practice students can develop a foundation for incorporating evidence-based practice (EBP) in bedside patient care. This should result in better patient outcomes from safe, quality nurses.[19-22]

A foundation for a theoretical background for simulation can be based on experiential learning. Several experiential learning theories have been applied to the use of simulation, as follows.[23-25]

- *Knowles' adult learning theory.* This theory originally stated that adults learn differently due to andragogy (theory of adult learning).[26] Characteristics of adult learners are that they are self-directed, want to be involved in planning and evaluating their learning experience, use past experiences to build new learning, need to understand the reason for learning, want immediate application of knowledge to solve problems, and are more invested when the learning is associated with a new role. In 1984 Knowles changed his position to recognize that the assumptions about andragogy are situation specific and not unique to adults.[27] In 2010 Clapper expanded on this assumption regarding what adult learners wanted educators to know. These learners want educators to create a safe learning environment that uses active and collaborative learning experiences, encourage reflection on current and past experiences, and focus more on the assessment of improvements made instead of pure evaluation.

- *Kolb's experiential learning.* This refers to a person's ability to transfer knowledge from theory into practice, thereby leading to acquisition of knowledge.[28] Waldner and Olson combined Benner's first three stages of learning (novice, advanced beginner, and competent) and Kolb's framework using high-fidelity patient simulation in academia.[29]

- *Situated cognition.* Learning occurs as a social activity incorporating the mind, the body, the activity, and the tools in a context that is complex and interactive. This incorporates all domains of learning: psychomotor, cognitive, and affective.[27]

- *Lasater's Interactive Model of Clinical Judgment Development.* Four areas of clinical judgment are noticing, interpreting, responding, and reflecting.[30,31] This model can be applied to simulation for noticing and assessing patient situations and conditions, interpreting the assessment findings, responding by developing a plan of care and interventions, and reflecting during the debriefing process.

- *Jeffries/NLN simulation framework.* This is a conceptual framework developed for use in nursing education to design, implement, and evaluate simulation experiences.[32] This model depicts the triadic relationship of students, faculty, and educational practices and their influence on the simulation design and desired outcomes. The five possible outcomes of simulations are increased knowledge, skill performance, learner satisfaction, critical thinking abilities, and self-confidence of the participants.

- *Gaba's 11 dimensions of simulation.* These are as follows:
  1. The purpose and aims of simulation activity
  2. Unit of participation
  3. Experience level of participants
  4. Healthcare domain in which simulation is applied
  5. Healthcare disciplines of participants
  6. Type of knowledge, skills, attitudes, or behavior addressed in simulation
  7. Age of patient being simulated
  8. Applicable or required technology
  9. Site of simulation participation
  10. Extent of direct participation
  11. Feedback method accompanying simulation[33(pp13-16)]

For students to envision themselves successfully assuming a new role, practicing that role in a realistic environment will assist with role identification, mental visualization for performing in the role, and bridging the gap from didactic to practice. Through participating and acting in a specific simulation case the participants can then generalize the information in order to apply it to new situations.[23,34]

Best practices are available for many aspects of simulation practice. A clinical scenario should be developed based on the specific learning objectives of the participants. During the planning and development of a scenario it is important to construct an experience that is appropriate to the participant's level of learning as well as the participant's objective. Since many simulation experts believe that the majority of learning occurs during the debriefing process, a planned debriefing strategy should guide the facilitator in the process. The last aspect is the identification and application of a theoretical framework to plan and guide a simulation to provide the theoretical underpinning for that simulation and simulation program.[1,32,34-36] These aspects will be explored further in the next section.

Summary of Standards of Best Practice: Simulation

Standards of Best Practice: Simulation was developed by the INACSL board of directors at the request of its membership after an extensive needs analysis was conducted via member email and listserv. The purpose of the analysis was to determine the priority and ranking of the INACSL membership. Top priorities were established as standards and the lower priorities are under development as guidelines. The work of the Standards Committee is ongoing, with a current focus on developing guidelines to support the standards. Simulation standards have been developed to assist with the planning and implementation of simulation experiences.[6] Following Standards of Best Practice: Simulation will likely lead to better learning experiences and improved learning outcomes for participants.

The first seven standards were presented at the 2011 conference and published for all members in the fall of 2011 by Elsevier. These initial standards are terminology, professional integrity of the participants, participant objectives, facilitation methods, simulation facilitator, the debriefing process, and evaluation of expected outcomes.

Standards and Their Application to the Simulation Process

The simulation experience will depend on the objectives to be obtained by the participants. The objectives are the guiding principle of the entire simulation. Once the objectives have been established, the level or type of facilitation should be determined based on the level of experience of the participants and the type of evaluation of the participants. The simulation process should follow the steps outlined in Box 29-2 in designing the scenario or experience to assist the participants in achieving the objectives.

Standard I: Terminology

The main terminology used in simulation is defined based on a review of literature. To begin the simulation experiences, have standard definitions for the application and possible publication and replication of research and evidence-based

BOX 29-2	STEPS FOR THE SIMULATION PROCESS

1. Assign the presimulation or prescenario exercises to be completed by the participants
2. Prebriefing sessions immediately prior to the simulation
3. Simulation scenario with appropriate facilitation by a trained facilitator
4. Debriefing and/or guided reflection
5. Postsimulation exercises

practices.[37] Also, with more emphasis on interprofessional collaboration, standardized terminology is the key to increasing understanding between team members by not having only one discipline's terminology used.

Standard II: Professional Integrity of the Participants

Prior to beginning any simulation the participants need to be oriented to the simulation program and understand the need for professional integrity to maintain confidentiality and integrity of the simulation.[38] Professional integrity is needed in order for all participants to have the same learning experience. If participants share what occurred in the simulation with future participants prior to the simulation, then those participants do not have the same opportunity to use critical thinking and clinical judgment. This could affect their confidence level and take away learning experiences. Participants must be informed of the type of evaluation and expectations prior to any simulation.

Standard III: Participant Objectives

The simulated clinical experience should focus on course, clinical, or program objectives and be based on the participants' level of experience rather than on the fidelity of the equipment. The technology does not guide the learning but rather is a supplement to the educational experience. It is important to identify the methodology for implementing the scenario prior to the simulation to construct the best learning experience for participants. This will provide a foundation or guide for the simulation experience by identifying the appropriate scenario, the level of fidelity (mannequin, standardized patient, or a hybrid), the type of facilitating, the facilitator, and the environment.[33,34,39]

There is no evidence that suggests or dictates a specific time recommendation for each scenario. The scenario time should be based on the time required to meet the objectives; however, a time limit should be identified for each scenario. Some commercially purchased simulation products incorporate presimulation (prescenario) and postsimulation (postscenario) exercises for undergraduate education; however, this is not available for graduate-level education at this time. Presimulation or prescenario exercises are designed to prepare the student for participation in the simulation. Prescenario exercises are to be completed by the participants prior to participating in the simulation and can include, but are not limited to, reading assignments for major concepts in the simulation, pretest questions, skills review, and audiovisual material.

Standard IV: Facilitation Methods

Facilitation type should be determined by the level of the participant and the type of evaluation.[40,41] Several types of facilitation are instructor driven, partial instructor driven, or participant driven. As might be obvious from the labels, beginning participants usually require more instructor cueing or prompting (instructor driven). As the level of experience increases, less instructor prompting is required (partial instructor driven). During a summative evaluation, such as high-stakes testing, minimal to no prompting by the instructor is performed (participant driven).

Standard V: Simulation Facilitator

The facilitator is the major component that provides the link between the scenario and the participant to provide guidance for meeting the objectives of the simulation. The role of the facilitator is to adjust the scenario to respond to the actions or inactions of the participants according to the objectives of the scenario. The facilitator also leads the participants in the debriefing process in a positive manner to reflect on ways to improve the care provided for better patient outcomes.[41]

Standard VI: The Debriefing Process

The purpose of a debriefing is to promote participant reflective thinking by allowing the participants to think about and clarify actions that occurred during the simulation (Box 29-3).[42] Feedback is provided to the participants by the facilitator to ensure that concepts are understood and the

---

BOX 29-3   SAMPLE DEBRIEFING QUESTIONS FOR A PEDIATRIC PATIENT IN ISOLATION FOR PNEUMONIA WITH CYSTIC FIBROSIS

Ask at least one question from each section.

Aesthetic Questions
"I would like each of you to talk to me about the problems _____ was experiencing today."
"What was your main objective during this simulation?"
"How did patient safety and isolation issues affect the patient care you provided?" (scenario specific)

Personal Questions
"Was there any point during the scenario when you felt unsure of your decisions? If yes, how did you manage your feelings and focus on the patient's needs?"
"What made you choose the actions, interventions, and focus that you chose for _____?"

Empirical Question
"I would like each of you to talk with me about the knowledge, skills, attitudes (KSA), and previous experiences that provided you with the ability to provide evidence-based care to _____."

Ethical Question
"Talk to me about how your personal beliefs and values influenced the care provided to _____."

Reflection Questions
"Please tell me how you knew what to do for a cystic fibrosis patient with pneumonia in isolation and why."
"If we could repeat this scenario now, what would you change and why?"
"How will you use this in your professional practice?"

---

participants are given the right "take-home message" to incorporate into their professional practice. The debriefing process has been reported as the most important component of simulation because of the learning that occurs when concepts are clarified.[42-44] Literature suggests that debriefing should last at least as long as the simulation scenario but current practices range from half as long as the simulation scenario to twice as long as the scenario.[45]

Standard VII: Evaluation of Expected Outcomes

The evaluation and assessment of the participants' performance during the simulation should be based on the focus and desired outcomes of the simulation scenario. The participants should be aware of the evaluation or assessment methods being used before beginning the simulation.[35,46,47]

While there is growing interest in adoption of clinical simulation within educational programs, there is a gap in empirical research identifying valid and reliable tools to evaluate simulation effectiveness, especially in translating knowledge and skills from simulation experiences to actual clinical practice; research is needed.[36,48,49] Also, the National Council of State Boards of Nursing (NCSBN) is conducting a longitudinal national simulation study to determine the appropriate use of simulation for best student outcomes.[50]

Types of evaluations are skills checklists, formative assessment of performance, or summative evaluation. Skills checklists may be used during a skills validation, such as an indwelling catheter or chest tube insertion for students or an endotracheal intubation for respiratory therapy students.

Formative assessments measure a participant's progress toward overall or long-term program objectives. This type of assessment provides the participant with feedback that will aid in professional growth and promote self-reflection.

Summative evaluations are traditionally measured at the end of a learning experience, to correlate with the end of the course or program. This type of evaluation may have a grade assigned or use another method to determine student progression. An example of a summative evaluation is an objective structured clinical examination (OSCE). An OSCE summative evaluation can be a graduate student's evaluation at the end of the advanced assessment course to determine his or her ability to perform in a traditional clinical setting. Some medical boards require an OSCE to become certified. Regardless of the type of evaluation, the instrument used should have reported psychometric data demonstrating reliability and validity.

The evaluation tools currently used in simulation were described in a review by Kardong-Edgren and colleagues and were categorized within the cognitive, psychomotor, and affective learning domains.[51] The *cognitive domain* focuses on application with thinking such as perform, identify, maintain, communicate, prioritize, and provide. An example is that the participant will be able to identify the signs and symptoms of congestive heart failure and provide appropriate interventions for best patient outcomes. The *psychomotor domain* focuses on the precision of performing the assessment or skill, such as insertion of an intravenous catheter

---

BOX 29-4   **LEARNING DOMAINS**

Cognitive domain. Simulation evaluation tools included the Basic Knowledge Assessment Tool 6 (paper-and-pencil test); the Outcome Present State Test Model for Debriefing (worksheets that participants complete during the structured debriefing); the Lasater Clinical Judgment Rubric, based on Tanner's Clinical Judgment Model for student evaluation during simulation; and the Simulation Evaluation Instrument, developed to evaluate the American Association of Colleges of Nursing core competencies for undergraduate nursing students during simulation.

Psychomotor domain. There were no tools identified for the psychomotor domain for simulation that reported validity and reliability testing.

Affective domain. The evaluation tools identified in this section were developed to measure student satisfaction and perceived effectiveness of the simulated clinical experience. The tools identified included a satisfaction survey, the Emergency Response Performance Tool (ERPT), and the Simulation Design Scale. Other tools were reviewed for group evaluation.

---

and effective therapeutic communication using Situation-Background-Assessment-Recommendation (SBAR) communication. The *affective domain* reflects the emotion of reflective thinking by responses to and prioritization of patient care (Box 29-4).

The Leighton Clinical Learning Environment Comparison Survey (L-CLECS) was designed to compare how well undergraduate students' learning needs were met in the simulated clinical environment and the traditional clinical environment.[52] L-CLECS is one of the tools being used during the current national simulation survey by the NCSBN.[50] Validity and reliability evaluation measures have been conducted on this instrument.

The Creighton Simulation Evaluation Instrument (C-SEI) is a tool that evaluates simulation experiences by measuring assessment skills.[53] C-SEI is the second tool being used in the NCSBN's National Simulation Study and has established reliability and validity.[50] The C-SEI tool is designed to be modified to meet the specific outcomes of the simulation. The goal of this tool was to evaluate student assessment skills for improvement. As the assessment skills improve, so will clinical performance.

APPLICATION OF SIMULATION

General Application of Simulation to Education

The use of simulation in undergraduate nursing, graduate schools for advanced practice nurses (especially nurse anesthetists), medical schools, and interprofessional education has been well documented in the literature. However, literature is not available for simulation applied to doctoral education.

Multiple research studies revealed that students have higher satisfaction with higher levels of fidelity.[8,54] However, studies

have not shown that high-fidelity simulation increases students' clinical reasoning skills.[8] There is a growing body of health literature evaluating the differences in student outcomes using low- and high-fidelity simulation experiences. Multiple studies indicated no statistically significant differences in student learning outcomes using traditional pencil-and-paper testing scores compared to varying levels of fidelity teaching strategies.[55-59]

Some studies have demonstrated a statistically significant difference in students' self-perceived improvements depending on the level of fidelity used in simulation.[60-64] The participants of these studies preferred high-fidelity teaching strategies as compared to low-fidelity strategies.

Several studies recommend that educators need to compare the level of fidelity when considering cost and short- and long-term participant outcomes.[56,57] Some authors have questioned the appropriate evaluation method: an OSCE or a paper-and-pencil test.[57,65] However, there have not been consistent results with OSCEs in terms of finding differences in participants' performances to compare acquisition of knowledge and applying that knowledge to clinical practice.[55]

Application of Simulation to Interprofessional Education

Many professional medical organizations stated an increasing need for interprofessional education (IPE), as evidenced by the newly introduced Core Competencies for Interprofessional Collaborative Practice sponsored by the Interprofessional Education Collaborative (IPEC) (Table 29-4).[66] IPEC was a collaborative effort between multiple associations, including the AACN, American Association of Colleges of Osteopathic Medicine, American Association of Colleges of Pharmacy, American Dental Education Association, Association of American Medical Colleges, and Association of Schools of Public Health.

To improve patient safety, evidence-based practice, translational research, and more IPE opportunities are needed. New teaching strategies have evolved. Some of these are in response to the changing technology that has proliferated over the past 25 years. The strategies include the following:

1. Communication tools such as SBAR for more effective professional and interprofessional communication
2. Simulation scenarios to practice skills and techniques, assessment, therapeutic communication, interprofessional collaboration, reflection on actions and inactions of participants, and incorporation of evidence-based practice throughout the curriculum and applying these in simulation
3. Informatics capabilities to improve patient care with point-of-care access to information through handheld devices and electronic health records (EHRs)

If the interprofessional members of the healthcare team have access to the pertinent information about a patient, healthcare delivery can be more holistic and potentially decrease harm to the patient. Health sciences students can learn the roles and responsibilities of other healthcare team members for collaborative purposes through IPE simulations to ensure the best patient outcomes. For graduate school

TABLE 29-4	CORE COMPETENCIES FOR INTERPROFESSIONAL COLLABORATIVE PRACTICE		
CORE COMPETENCY	**FOCUS**	**APPLICATION WITH SIMULATION**	**OPPORTUNITY FOR IPE**
Roles and responsibilities for collaborative practice	Use the knowledge of each profession's role to assess and address the populations served	Demonstrate collaboration of team members in a scenario to clearly communicate with each other and provide the best holistic care to meet the needs of the individual or population	• Disaster drill simulation • Prehospital injury requiring ambulance transport to the emergency department
Interprofessional communication	Communicate in a team approach with individuals, families, and communities in a responsive and responsible manner to support well-being and quality of life	1. Communicate with confidence, clarity, and respect to promote understanding of information and management of issues 2. Actively listen and encourage sharing or input from others 3. Recognize one's uniqueness and role within the team and contribute to effective communication, conflict resolution, and positive interprofessional working relationships	Scenarios that require multiple professions in diagnosis and planning the care of a patient: • Code situation • Respiratory decline of patient with unknown etiology
Interprofessional teamwork and team-based service	Apply relationship-building values and the principles of team dynamics to perform effectively in different team roles to plan and deliver services that are safe, timely, efficient, effective, and equitable	1. Work with others to develop consensus on the ethical principles to guide all aspects of interaction with individuals and teamwork 2. Use process improvement strategies 3. Reflect on individual and team performance for individual as well as team performance improvement	• Home health scenario that requires collaboration via phone • Focus the debriefing process on improvement of any interprofessional simulation
Values and ethics for interprofessional practice	Work with individuals of other professions to maintain a climate of mutual respect and shared values	1. Provide care for the community 2. Demonstrate high standards of ethical conduct 3. Act with honesty and integrity in relationships with all team members and clients 4. Maintain competence in one's profession	Complex scenarios that include moral or ethical decision making and counseling with the patient or family: • Organ transplant decisions • Hospice care • Cultural themes

IPE, Interprofessional education.

students, IPE simulations are an excellent way to learn how to function and adapt practices to achieve the best outcomes.

Simulation is a strategy to assist team members with effective communication and promote collaboration with other professionals. According to an INACSL survey in 2010, only about half of the respondents provided any IPE. Of the programs providing IPE experiences, only a few institutions stated that the practice was used more than occasionally in the simulation community.[44] Challenges to this type of education exist. In particular, the logistics of scheduling multiple professions for simulation is one of the major obstacles for IPE experience.[67-70] The Institute of Medicine (IOM) also called for the federal government and professional organizations to study the approaches and foci to determine their contribution to improving the workforce.[21,22] The professional organizations have a responsibility to determine the best resources and methods for improving the education of the healthcare workforce, both in initial education and in continuing professional development.

Example

The following scenario was used in a doctorate of nursing practice program to evaluate nurse practitioner students' ability to assess and develop a differential diagnosis with a patient presenting with angina. Students participated in this experience at the end of their clinical diagnostics course and this was used for summative evaluation purposes. Prior to any simulation experience, a curricular simulation integration form was used to document objectives, evaluation measures, and the specific details related to the scenario (Fig. 29-2). This plan mapped out the specific details related to the simulation experience and contributed to a successful simulation experience for both the faculty and the students. To prepare, the students received the evaluation rubric to review prior to entering the simulation lab for testing (Fig. 29-3).

<u>**Course Title: Diagnosis and Management of Adults II**</u>

<u>**Scenario Topic:**</u> Caring for a patient experiencing chest pain progressing to unstable angina

<u>**Time Allotment:**</u> 15 minutes for scenario

<u>**Instructor:**</u> Dr. Ross and Dr. Howard

<u>**Facilitation Method:**</u> No Facilitator Prompting

<u>**Student Level (# of participants, role descriptions)**</u>
One DNP–NP student per scenario demonstrating the role of the NP

<u>**Scenario Objectives and Evaluation Criteria**</u>
Upon completion of this scenario, the student will be able to:
   Obtain pertinent subjective and objective data from history related to chest pain
   Perform a focused physical exam related to complaints of cardiac-related chest pain
   Identify clinical manifestations associated with multiple etiologies of chest pain
   Consider differential diagnosis related to chest pain
   Recognize stable angina progressing to unstable angina
   Maintain a safe environment during patient consult
   Initiate an appropriate diagnostic work-up
   Prescribe appropriate pharmacologic therapy
   Provide patient education regarding treatment regimen
   Document appropriate SOAP note regarding clinical consult

<u>**Set-up/Equipment**</u>
- High fidelity patient simulator
- BP cuff
- Stethoscope
- Thermometer

<u>**Prescenario Learning Activities**</u>
Attend class lectures and participate in clinical sharing on coronary artery disease (CAD) and chest pain
Review PowerPoint materials and participate in Discussion Board conversation related to cardiac conditions
Review competency evaluation form

<u>**Instructions for Starting Scenario**</u>
Introduction to Scenario:
Mr. Pat Tassium 50 y/o obese male with history of stable angina reports to the office with the following complaints. He recently noticed increased SOB when ambulating up to his second floor bedroom. He noticed that he has to stop one time before reaching the top of the stairs. Mr. Tassium experienced tightness in his chest X 2 last week as he climbed the stairs to bed. What brings him into the office is when he was mowing his lawn he had to stop twice and take SL NTG. This is different than his past action of just resting and the chest pain would subside.

<u>**Social History**</u>
Married with three children
Works as the dean in the school of business for the local university
Smokes a pack of cigarettes in three days; this is a considerable decrease from a pack a day a year ago
Admits to social drinking only; one to two drinks on weekends
Currently on the following medications:
   ASA a day
   Lopressor 50 mg 1 tablet daily for HTN
   NTG 0.4 mg SL prn for chest pain

FIG 29-2 Simulation integration and planning form. *ASA,* Acetylsalicylic acid; *BP,* blood pressure; *DNP,* doctor of nursing practice; *HTN,* hypertension; *NP,* nurse practitioner; *prn,* as needed; *SL NTG,* sublingual nitroglycerin; *SOAP,* subjective, objective, assessment, and plan; *SOB,* shortness of breath. (Developed by C. Ross, PhD, RN, and V. Howard, EdD, RN. Courtesy of RMU Regional RISE Center.)

Simulator Actions (Vital Signs/Simulator Controls)	Expected Student Interventions/Events
Initial State **Pulse:** 62 **BP:** 140/92 **RR:** 16 **Pulse oximeter:** 96% **Heart rhythm:** regular with occasional unifocal PVC	Obtains pertinent subjective and objective data from history related to chest pain Performs focused physical exam related to complaints of cardiac related chest pain Identifies clinical manifestations associated with multiple etiologies of chest pain Considers differential diagnosis related to chest pain Recognizes stable angina progressing to unstable angina Maintains safe environment during patient consult Initiates appropriate diagnostic work-up Prescribes appropriate pharmacologic therapy Provides patient education regarding treatment regimen Documents appropriate SOAP note regarding clinical consult

Relevant Debriefing Points (Event Management)
- Problem Recognition
- Prioritization

- Problem Intervention
- Rationales

Positive Feedback and Areas for Improvement

Application to Clinical Practice

Simulation Evaluation Survey

Procedure
1. Students given copy of competency evaluation form with general categories one week prior to exam
2. Schedule students for 15-minute time frame
3. Arrive at simulation room and conduct scenario 9 times
4. All students return for 30 minutes upon completion for debriefing:
   - Perception of simulation experience
   - Scenario specifics
   - Simulation evaluation form
5. Other NP faculty view scenarios and complete student performance evaluation forms

FIG 29-3 Student evaluation rubric. *BP*, Blood pressure; *NP*, nurse practitioner; *PVC*, premature ventricular contraction; *RR*, respiratory rate; *SOAP*, subjective, objective, assessment, and plan.

The detailed evaluation rubric (Fig. 29-4) was used by the faculty member to evaluate the students and provide summative feedback. After the scenario the students completed a Scenario Evaluation Form to evaluate the quality of the learning experience (Fig. 29-5).[7] These evaluation data were reviewed by the simulation facilitators after the scenario activity to ensure that the scenario met the needs of the students and reflected the highest quality and evidence.

SIMULATION RESOURCES

Organizations

INACSL was founded after discussions by several attendees of the annual Learning Resource Center Conference in 2001. The nonprofit organization has grown to more than 1500 members worldwide. The organization's mission statement is to promote research and disseminate evidence-based standards for clinical simulation methodologies and learning environments. Its vision is to be nursing's portal to the world of clinical simulation pedagogy and learning environments. The majority of members are nurses, although anyone is

welcome to become a member. Institutional membership is also available. The organization is affiliated with SSH and a founding member of the Global Network for Simulation in Healthcare (GNSH), an organization composed of the leadership of simulation organizations worldwide.

SSH was founded in 2004 and has a membership of approximately 3000 healthcare providers in all specialty areas. SSH began offering a program to accredit simulation laboratories in 2010. The most recent benefit offered by SSH is the ability to receive certification as a simulation educator. Box 29-5 lists additional organizations that support simulation in health education.

Leaders

There are many experts in the field of simulation; however, some deserve special recognition for the work they have done to further the use of this teaching modality. Asmund S. Laerdal may be the most recognized name in simulation, as he was the founder of the Laerdal Company, now known as Laerdal Medical. Initially making partial and full mannequins to further the education of cardiopulmonary resuscitation,

Evaluation Rating			Performance Criteria	Comments
Exceeds Expectations	Meets Expectations	Does Not Meet Expectations		
			Initial Encounter	2 pts
			Assessment/ History Taking/ Differential Diagnosis	8 pts
			Physical Examination	5 pts
			Interventions	6 pts
			Evaluation of Patient Responses	2 pts
			Documentation	2 pts

FIG 29-4 Detailed faculty evaluation rubric.

Evaluation Rating			Performance Criteria	Comments
Exceeds Expectations	**Meets Expectations**	**Does Not Meet Expectations**		
			Initial Encounter	**2 pts**
			Introduces self to patient	
			Checks and verifies patient's identification	
			Validates demographic data	
			Obtains or validates vital signs	
			Assessment/ History Taking/ Differential Diagnosis	**8 pts**
			Asks important questions to elicit cardiovascular risk factors	
			Asks important questions to characterize chest pain; may use PQRST	
			Able to differentiate between stable and unstable angina	
			Considers differentials related to chest pain	
			Identifies clinical manifestations associated with multiple etiologies of chest pain	
			Informs patient of possible differential diagnosis	
			Physical Examination	**5 pts**
			General appearance and validation of vital signs	
			Examination of skin, eyes, carotid pulse, & JVD	
			Chest wall examination: heart & lungs	
			Abdomen	
			Lower extremities	
			Neurologic exam for focal deficits	
			Correlates abnormal assessment findings with differential diagnoses	
			Interventions	**6 pts**
			Ensures patient safety and safe environment by staying with patient or having co-worker stay with patient	
			Orders appropriate immediate interventions	
			Initiates orders for appropriate diagnostic studies: Imaging Laboratory	
			Prescribes appropriate pharmacological therapy	
			Provides patient education and health promotion	
			Evaluation of Patient Responses	**2 pts**
			Evaluates patient's response to all interventions Follow up & referral	
			Documentation	**2 pts**
			Writes an appropriate SOAP note from patient encounter	

FIG 29-4, cont'd *JVD*, jugular venous distention; *PQRST*, provokes, quality, radiates, severity, time; *SOAP*, subjective, objective, assessment, and plan.

Please circle the best response to each of the following questions.

Please circle the response that best describes how you feel about the simulation experience:

	Strongly Disagree	Disagree	Agree	Strongly Agree
1. The simulation experience helped me to better understand advanced nursing concepts.	1	2	3	4
2. The simulation was a valuable learning experience.	1	2	3	4
3. The simulation helped to stimulate critical thinking abilities.	1	2	3	4
4. The simulation was realistic.	1	2	3	4
5. The knowledge gained through the simulation experiences can be transferred to the advanced practice clinical setting.	1	2	3	4
6. I was nervous during the simulation experience.	1	2	3	4
7. Because of the simulation experience, I will be less nervous in the primary care setting when providing care for similar patients.	1	2	3	4
8. Simulation experiences can be a substitute for clinical experiences in the primary care clinical areas.	1	2	3	4
9. Simulation experiences should be included in our DNP education.	1	2	3	4

10. Now, please add any additional comments regarding the simulation experience:

FIG 29-5 Simulation evaluation. *DNP*, Doctor of nursing practice. (Developed by V. Howard. 2010. Courtesy of RMU Regional RISE Center.)

BOX 29-5 U.S. ORGANIZATIONS THAT SUPPORT SIMULATION IN HEALTH EDUCATION

International Nursing Association for Clinical Simulation and Learning (INACSL): www.inacsl.org
Society for Simulation in Healthcare (SSH): www.ssih.org
National League for Nursing (NLN): www.nln.org
American Association of Colleges of Nursing (AACN): www.aacn.nche.edu
The Joint Commission (TJC): www.jointcommission.org
Institute of Medicine (IOM): www.iom.edu
National Council of State Boards of Nursing (NCSBN): www.ncsbn.org
Agency for Healthcare Research and Quality (AHRQ): www.ahrq.gov

---

the company branched out into mannequins and supplies for all areas of patient simulation. Dr. J.S. Gravenstein from the University of Florida led the team that created the Human Patient Simulator (HPS), the first and only full-body simulator that responded to gas inhalation, making it an appropriate tool for anesthesia education. Dr. David M. Gaba, Associate Dean for Immersive and Simulation-based Learning at Stanford University School of Medicine, has experience and opinions regarding patient simulation that are sought after by clinicians worldwide. Pamela Jeffries, PhD, RN, contributed the first framework for the development of simulation experiences through her work with the NLN and Laerdal. All of these leaders have made significant contributions to the education of clinicians, including graduate nurses. There are many others whose expertise and contributions could also be mentioned here.

CONCLUSION AND FUTURE DIRECTIONS

The use of simulation is rapidly emerging as a preferred way to train healthcare professionals in a safe, controlled manner with no risk to patients. One of the reasons for its emergence is that simulation can ameliorate current barriers with traditional clinical experiences. There is a shortage of clinical sites, patients can have complex conditions that a novice learner is unprepared to manage, and clinical sites may have limited student experiences for EHRs, administering medications to pediatric patients, and other situations. These factors, combined with a nursing and nurse educator shortage and the aging population, will further increase the need to teach healthcare providers in a simulation environment.

Newer approaches that reflect the advances in technology are virtual reality computer-based simulations and gaming. Gaming is a type of simulation technique that meets the needs of millennial learners. However, this new approach has not yet been as fully developed as the approaches discussed in this chapter. The emergence of technology for educational purposes creates a need for faculty and health science educators to understand how to not only operate the technology but also implement it within the academic and service settings while still using sound academic principles. Standards of Best Practice: Simulation will continue to serve as a foundation for all types of simulation-based teaching methodologies.

A potential future step is the integration of EHRs into simulation experiences. Simulation experiences that include EHRs are less common and only a few simulation centers have embedded EHRs and other clinical information systems. In the future the entire suite of technical experiences will be available in a simulation center experience.

REFERENCES

1. International Nursing Association for Clinical Simulation and Learning Board of Directors. Standards of best practice: simulation. *Clinical Simulation in Nursing.* 2011;7(4S):S1-S2.
2. Benner P. *From Novice to Expert: Excellence and Power in Clinical Nursing Practice.* Menlo Park, CA: Addison-Wesley; 1984.
3. Kolb DA. *Experiential Learning.* Englewood Cliffs, NJ: Prentice Hall; 1984.
4. Robinson-Smith G, Bradley P, Meakim C. Evaluating the use of standardized patients in undergraduate psychiatric nursing experiences. *Clinical Simulation in Nursing.* 2009;5(6):e203-e211. doi:10.1016/j.ecns.2009.07.001.
5. Maran NJ, Glavin RJ. Low- to high-fidelity simulation: a continuum of medical education. *Med Educ.* 2003;37(Suppl 1):22-28.
6. Alinier G. A typology of educationally focused medical simulation tools. *Med Teach.* 2007;29(8):1-8. doi:10.1080/01421590701551185.
7. Howard V, Ross C, Mitchell A, Nelson G. Human patient simulators and interactive case studies: a comparative analysis of learning outcomes and student perceptions. *Comput Inform Nurs.* 2010;28(1):42-48.
8. Lapkin S, Levett-Jones T, Bellchambers H, Fernandez R. Effectiveness of patient simulation manikins in teaching clinical reasoning skills to undergraduate nursing students: a systematic review. *Clinical Simulation in Nursing.* 2010;6(6):e207-e222. doi:10.1016/j.ecns.2010.05.005.
9. McGaghie W, Issenberg SB, Petrusa E, Scalese R. A critical review of simulation-based medical education research: 2003–2009. *Med Educ.* 2009;44:50-63.
10. Kameg K, Howard V, Clochesy J, Mitchell AM, Suresky J. Impact of high fidelity human simulation on self-efficacy of communication skills. *Issues Ment Health Nurs.* 2010;31(5):315-323.
11. Cooper S, Cant R, Porter J, et al. Simulation based learning in midwifery education: a systematic review. *Women Birth.* 2011; 25(2):64-78. doi:10.1016/j.wombi.2011.03.004.
12. Kirkpatrick DL, Kirkpatrick JD. *Evaluating training programs.* 3rd ed. San Francisco, CA: Berrett-Koehler Publishers; 2006.
13. Barsuk JH, McGaghie WC, Cohen ER, Balachandran JS, Wayne DB. Use of simulation-based mastery learning to improve the quality of central venous catheter placement in a medical inten-

sive care unit. *J Hosp Med.* 2009;4(7):397-403. doi:10.1002/jhm.468.
14. Draycott T, Crofts J, Ash J, et al. Improving neonatal outcome through practical shoulder dystocia training. *Obstet Gynecol.* 2008;112(1):14-20.
15. McCarthy J. Malpractice insurance carrier provides premium incentive for simulation-based training and believes it has made a difference. *Anesthesia Patient Safety Foundation Newsletter.* http://www.apsf.org/newsletters/html/2007/spring/17_malpractice.htm. 2007.
16. Kotter JP. *Leading Change.* Boston, MA: Harvard Business Review Press; 1996.
17. Gantt L. Strategic planning for skills and simulation labs in colleges of nursing. *Nurs Econ.* 2010;28(5):308-313.
18. Kneebone R. Evaluating clinical simulations for learning procedural skills: a theory-based approach. *Acad Med.* 2005;80(6):549-553.
19. Cronenwett L, Sherwood G, Barnsteiner J, et al. Quality and safety education for nurses. *Nurs Outlook.* 2007;55(3):122-131.
20. Institute of Medicine (IOM). *Crossing the Quality Chasm: A New Health System for the 21st Century.* Washington, DC: National Academies Press; 2001.
21. Institute of Medicine (IOM). *Health Professions Education: A Bridge to Quality.* Washington, DC: National Academies Press; 2003.
22. Wachter RM. The end of the beginning: patient safety five years after "to err is human." *Health Affair.* 2004;W4-534-545. http://content.healthaffairs.org/content/early/2004/11/30/hlthaff.w4.534.short.
23. Clapper TC. Beyond Knowles: what those conducting simulation need to know about adult learning theory. *Clinical Simulation in Nursing.* 2010;6(1):e7-e14. doi:10.1016/j.ecns.2009.07.003.
24. Onda EL. Situated cognition: its relationship to simulation in nursing education. *Clinical Simulation in Nursing.* In press. doi:10.1016/j.ecns.2010.11.004.
25. Paige JB, Daley BJ. Situated cognition: a learning framework to support and guide high-fidelity simulation. *Clinical Simulation in Nursing.* 2009;5(3):e97-e103. doi:10.1016/j.ecns.2009.03.120.
26. Knowles MS. Andragogy, not pedagogy. *Adult Leadership.* 1968;16(10):350-352, 386.
27. Knowles MS. *The Adult Learner: A Neglected Species.* 3rd ed. Houston, TX: Gulf; 1984.
28. Kolb DA. *Organizational Behavior: An Experiential Approach to Human Behavior in Organizations.* Englewood Cliffs, NJ: Prentice Hall; 1995.
29. Waldner MH, Olson JK. Taking the patient to the classroom: applying theoretical frameworks to simulation in nursing education. *Int J Nurs Educ Scholarsh.* 2007;4(1):1-14.
30. Lasater K. High-fidelity simulation and the development of clinical judgment: students' experience. *J Nurs Educ.* 2007;46(6):269-276.
31. Lasater K. Clinical judgment development: using simulation to create an assessment rubric. *J Nurs Educ.* 2007;46(11):498-503.
32. Jeffries PR. Preface. In: Jeffries PR, ed. *Simulation in Nursing Education: From Conceptualization to Evaluation.* New York, NY: National League for Nursing; 2007:xi-xii.
33. Gaba DM. The future vision of simulation in health care. *Qual Saf Health Care.* 2004;13:i2-i10. doi:10.1136/qshc.2004.009878.
34. Clark CC. *Classroom Skills for Nurse Educators.* Sudbury, MA: Jones and Bartlett; 2008:161-227.
35. Decker S, Gore T, Feken C. Simulation. In: Bristol T, Zerwehk J, eds. *Essentials of e-Learning for Nurse Educators.* Philadelphia, PA: FA Davis; 2011:277-294.

36. Howard VM, Englert N, Kameg K, Perozzi K. Integration of simulation across the undergraduate curriculum: student and faculty perspectives. *Clinical Simulation in Nursing.* 2011;7(1):e1-e10. doi:10.1016/j.ecns.2009.10.004.

37. International Nursing Association for Clinical Simulation and Learning Board of Directors. Standard I: terminology. *Clinical Simulation in Nursing.* 2011;7(4S):S3-S7. doi:10.1016/j.ecns.2011.05.005.

38. International Nursing Association for Clinical Simulation and Learning Board of Directors. Standard II: professional integrity of participants. *Clinical Simulation in Nursing.* 2011;7(4S):S8-S9. doi:10.1016/j.ecns.2011.05.006.

39. International Nursing Association for Clinical Simulation and Learning Board of Directors. Standard III: participant objectives. *Clinical Simulation in Nursing.* 2011;7(4S):S10-S11. doi:10.1016/jecns.2011.05.007.

40. International Nursing Association for Clinical Simulation and Learning Board of Directors. Standard IV: facilitation methods. *Clinical Simulation in Nursing.* 2011;7(4S):S12-S13. doi:10.1016/j.ecns.2011.05.008.

41. International Nursing Association for Clinical Simulation and Learning Board of Directors. Standard V: simulation facilitator. *Clinical Simulation in Nursing.* 2011;7(4S):S14-S15. doi:10.1016/j.ecns.2011.05.009.

42. International Nursing Association for Clinical Simulation and Learning Board of Directors. Standard VI: the debriefing process. *Clinical Simulation in Nursing.* 2011;7(4S):S16-S17. doi:10.1016/j.ecns.2011.05.010.

43. Childs J, Sepples S. Clinical teaching by simulation: lessons learned from a complex patient care case scenario. *Nursing Education Perspectives.* 2006;27(3):154-158.

44. Gore T, Van Gele P, Ravert P, Mabire C. A 2010 survey of the INACSL membership about simulation use. *Clinical Simulation in Nursing.* 2012;8(4):e125-e133. doi:10.1016/j.ecns.2012.01.002.

45. Waxman KT. The development of evidence-based clinical simulation scenarios: guidelines for nurse educators. *J Nurs Educ.* 2010;49(1):29-35.

46. International Nursing Association for Clinical Simulation and Learning Board of Directors. Standard VII: evaluation of expected outcomes. *Clinical Simulation in Nursing.* 2011;7(4S):S18-S19. doi:10.1016/j.ecns.2011.05.011.

47. Jeffries PR, McNelis AM. Evaluation. In: Nehring WM, Lashley FR, eds. *High-Fidelity Patient Simulation in Nursing Education.* Boston, MA: Jones and Bartlett; 2010:405-424.

48. Hayden J. Use of simulation in nursing education: national survey results. *Journal of Nursing Regulation.* 2010;1(3):52-57.

49. Kardong-Edgren S, Willhaus J, Bennett D, Hayden J. Results of the National Council of State Boards of Nursing National Simulation Survey: Part II. *Clinical Simulation in Nursing.* 2012;8(4):e117-e123. doi:10.1016/j.ecns.2012.01.003.

50. National Council of State Boards of Nursing (NCSBN). NCSBN National Simulation Study. NCSBN. https://www.ncsbn.org/2094.htm. 2011.

51. Kardong-Edgren S, Adamson KA, Fitzgerald C. A review of currently published evaluation instruments for human patient simulation. *Clinical Simulation in Nursing.* 2010;6(1):e25-e35. doi:10.1016/j.ecns.2009.08.004.

52. Leighton KL. Clinical learning environment comparison survey. In: Learning Needs in the Traditional Clinical Environment and the Simulated Clinical Environment: A Survey of Undergraduate Nursing Students [doctoral dissertation]. Paper AAI3271929. Lincoln, NE: University of Nebraska–Lincoln; 2007.

53. Todd M, Manz JA, Hawkins KS, Parsons ME, Hercinger M. The development of a quantitative evaluation tool for simulations in nursing education. *Int J Nurs Educ Scholarsh.* 2008;5(1):Article 41. http://www.bepress.com/ijnes/vol5/iss1/art41/.

54. Jeffries P, Rizzolo M. *NLN/Laerdal Project Summary Report, Designing and Implementing Models for the Innovative Use of Simulation to Teach Nursing Care of Ill Adults and Children: A National Multi-Site Study.* New York, NY: National League for Nursing; 2006.

55. De Giovanni D, Roberts T, Norman G. Relative effectiveness of high- versus low-fidelity simulation in learning heart sounds. *Med Educ.* 2009;43(7):661-668.

56. Friedman Z, Siddiqui N, Katznelson R, Devito I, Bould MD, Naik V. Clinical impact of epidural anesthesia simulation on short- and long-term learning curve: high- versus low-fidelity model training. *Reg Anesth Pain Med.* 2009;34(3):229-232.

57. Kardong-Edgren S, Lungstrom N, Bendel R. VitalSim versus SimMan: a comparison of BSN student test scores, knowledge retention, and satisfaction. *Clinical Simulation in Nursing.* 2009;5(3):e105-e111. doi:10.1016/j.ecns.2009.01.007.

58. Kinney S, Henderson D. Comparison of low fidelity simulation learning strategy with traditional lecture. *Clinical Simulation in Nursing.* 2008;4(2):e15-e18. doi:10.1016/j.ecns.2008.06.005.

59. Lee KHK, Grantham H, Boyd R. Comparison of high- and low-fidelity mannequins for clinical performance assessment. *Emerg Med Australas.* 2008;20(6):508-514.

60. Faran JM, Paro JAM, Rodriguez RM, et al. Hand-off education and evaluation: piloting the observed simulated hand-off experience (OSHE). *J Gen Intern Med.* 2010;25(2):129-134.

61. Ham K, O'Rourke E. Clinical preparation for beginning nursing students. *Nurse Educ.* 2004;29(4):139-141.

62. Hoadley T. Learning advanced cardiac life support: a comparison study on the effects of low- and high-fidelity simulation. *Nurs Educ Perspect.* 2009;30(2):91-95.

63. Radhakrishnan K, Roche JP, Cunningham H. Measuring clinical practice parameters with human patient simulation: a pilot study. *Int J Nurs Educ Scholarsh.* 2007;4(1):1-11.

64. Tiffen J, Corbridge S, Shen BC, Robinson P. Patient simulator for teaching heart and lung assessment skills to advanced practice nursing students. *Clinical Simulation in Nursing.* 2010; 7(3):e91-e97. doi:10.1016/j.ecns.2009.10.003.

65. Kardong-Edgren S, Anderson M, Michaels J. Does simulation fidelity improve student test scores? *Clinical Simulation in Nursing.* 2007;3(1):e21-e24. doi:10.1016/j.ecns.2009.05.035.

66. Interprofessional Education Collaborative Expert Panel. *Core Competencies for Interprofessional Collaborative Practice: Report of an Expert Panel.* Washington, DC: Interprofessional Education Collaborative; 2011.

67. Alinier G. Enhancing trainees' learning experience through the opening of an advanced multiprofessional simulation training facility at the University of Hertfordshire. *British Journal of Anaesthetic and Recovery Nursing.* 2007;8(2):22-27.

68. Angelini DJ. Interdisciplinary and interprofessional education: what are the key issues and considerations for the future? *J Perinat Neonatal Nurs.* 2011;25(2):175-179.

69. Leonard B, Shuhaibar EL, Chen R. Nursing student perceptions of intraprofessional team education using high-fidelity simulation. *J Nurs Educ.* 2010;4(11):628-631. doi:10.3928/0148483420100730-06.

70. Reese CE, Jeffries PR, Engum SA. Learning together: using simulations to develop nursing and medical student collaboration. *Nurs Educ Perspect.* 2010;31(1):33-37.

DISCUSSION QUESTIONS

1. You are a graduate teaching assistant at the local university. A faculty member approaches you to "do" a simulation for class. What information do you need prior to developing the simulation? Provide a rationale for the information needed.
2. As a faculty member facilitating a debriefing, list five questions that you would ask to promote self-reflection.
3. Provide an example of an interprofessional simulation that would facilitate your graduate-level education. List the specific learning objectives, the team members, the participants' experience level and learning, and the type of facilitation and debriefing to guide this simulation scenario.
4. You are a faculty member struggling with generating support for your simulation program. You are experiencing resistance from faculty members and administration with the implementation of this new technology. What can you do to enhance buy-in?

CASE STUDY

You have been hired to teach in a graduate health program. Your newly developed course has an objective that states: *Upon completion of this course, the learner will be able to demonstrate interprofessional team building concepts.* As a new educator, you would like to include simulation as a teaching methodology.

After you are hired, you find a rarely used, high-fidelity Human Patient Simulator in the corner of your skills lab. You inquire about using it for your course but are met with resistance from other faculty members, who tell you that "there is no reason to use simulation. We've always taught our content using written case scenarios and we're doing just fine."

Discussion Questions

1. Use Kotter's eight steps leading to successful change to develop a plan to implement simulation for teaching team concepts.
2. What information should you incorporate when developing the scenario?
3. Unfortunately, students who experienced the scenario at 8 a.m. are sharing information with students scheduled later in the day. Which INACSL standard addresses this issue and how can you deter this behavior?
4. Which published document can assist you in clarifying interprofessional competencies?

UNIT 8

International Informatics Efforts

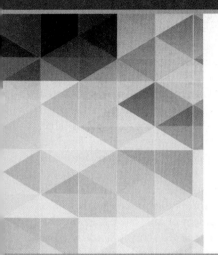

International Efforts, Issues, and Innovations

Hyeoun-Ae Park

To promote international development in health and nursing informatics it is necessary to provide tools for the development of national and regional ehealth initiatives and strategies.

OBJECTIVES

At the completion of this chapter the reader will be prepared to:

1. Outline key international health informatics initiatives

2. Describe key organizations leading international health informatics initiatives

3. Discuss the role of health practitioners such as nurses in international health informatics initiatives

KEY TERMS

Derived classifications, 482

eHealth initiatives, 474

Reference classifications, 482

Related classifications, 482

ABSTRACT

This chapter highlights international health informatics initiatives, international organizations involved in these initiatives, and how health practitioners such as nurses are involved in the activities of these organizations. There are numerous international health informatics–related activities that have been initiated across the different regions of the world. In addition academic societies within these regions are pursuing health informatics theory and practice developments. These international health informatics initiatives, along with associated academic organizations, are introduced here with brief histories and the key activities of each region. There are also several international organizations involved in the development of health informatics, such as the World Health Organization, the International Medical Informatics Association, the International Organization for Standardization, the International Council of Nurses, the International Health Terminology Standards Development Organisation, and Health Level Seven. These organizations are introduced with a short description of health practitioners' contributions to their activities. Finally, global issues in health informatics initiatives are also described.

INTRODUCTION

In many parts of the world healthcare is one of the largest sectors of the economy. As a result, health spending plays a major role in economic policy throughout the world with growing pressure on the healthcare industry to streamline costs, gain efficiency, and become more innovative in improving and maintaining the health of the population. Today the health industry around the world is looking for better ways of providing healthcare and improved health for all. The application of health information technology (health IT), called information and communication technology or ICT in international settings, to healthcare is seen as key to realizing this aim. The World Health Organization (WHO) uses ehealth as an umbrella term to cover all aspects of the use of ICT in healthcare. While the terminology differs—from health IT to ICT to ehealth—the goal of using technology to effectively and efficiently improve the health of individuals, families, and communities remains the same. An important difference exists between the meaning of these terms and the term *health informatics*. Health informatics is a broader term that refers to the discipline as a whole. The terms *ehealth*, *ICT*, and *health IT* refer to the use of technology in meeting healthcare needs and reflect international differences in how the terminology evolved in different areas. In this chapter all three terms are used in an attempt to reflect the terminology of the different regions of the world.

However, whichever term is used—ehealth, health IT, or ICT—the use of technology to improve health faces many challenges, many of which are international. A concerted effort is necessary if these challenges are to be overcome. This chapter highlights international ehealth initiatives and describes the work of health practitioners such as nurses and others in meeting these challenges.

KEY INITIATIVES IN WORLD REGIONS

The following section of the chapters explores key initiatives in health IT and informatics throughout the world by dividing the world into recognized regions. Within each region government supported ehealth initiatives are described. This is followed by a description of the health informatics activities within the region using the IMIA framework.

eHealth Initiatives in Europe

Given the increasing importance of the health and computer industries, the European Union (EU) introduced ehealth as one component of the Digital Agenda for Europe.[1] The history of ehealth in Europe dates back to the beginnings of health informatics in the late 1950s and early 1960s. Since its formation under the Maastricht Treaty in the 1990s the EU has provided more than €500 million in research funding to develop ehealth tools and systems. These EU-supported projects have helped to establish Europe as a world leader in the use of national and regional health networks and electronic health records (EHRs), especially in primary care, and in the deployment of digital health cards.[1]

In 2004 the EU adopted the first ehealth action plan (for 2004 to 2010) to facilitate a more harmonious and complementary European approach to ehealth. The action plan covered everything from electronic prescriptions and digital health cards to new information systems that reduce wait times and errors. The plan identified necessary actions for a widespread European adoption of ehealth technologies and encouraged individual members to customize strategies to their own needs. Thus each member state has developed its own national or regional road map for ehealth. These strategies are directed at addressing the challenges of providing citizen-centered healthcare services to meet the rising expectations of Europeans while concomitantly dealing with the issues that are raised by increasing mobility, aging populations, and budgetary constraints.

National and regional strategies are now focused on deploying ehealth systems, ensuring interoperability, using EHRs, reimbursing ehealth services, and other related issues. To meet these goals the EU has set up a database of European ehealth priorities and strategies to enhance knowledge and facilitate cooperation between states and regions. It includes documents about national ehealth priorities, strategies, road maps, and research programs.

The progress of the first ehealth action plan was evaluated in 2011.[2] Soon after, the European Commission launched the second eHealth Action Plan (eHAP) for 2012 to 2020. This plan combines—and improves when possible—previous actions implemented while looking toward the future of ehealth in Europe.

In addition, the EU supports ehealth research activities under its Research Framework Programme. Furthermore, the EU supports the deployment of innovative ehealth solutions into concrete services that are actually used by those who need them. The ehealth subgroup began in 2005 as an ehealth working group to provide expert ehealth-related advice. Members of the subgroup are key decision makers and leaders in the definition and implementation of national ehealth initiatives. They work in concert with the eHealth Stakeholder Group, whose members are expert representatives of European umbrella organizations active in the ehealth sector, such as telecommunications ministries, health authorities, healthcare professional associations, and industry, as well as patient and citizen groups. The ehealth subgroup is also expected to contribute to the development of ehealth-related legislation and policy. Additional information about these groups can be found at https://ec.europa.eu/digital-agenda/node/1103. Since 2003 member states' health ministers and state secretaries have met yearly to discuss and move ehealth initiatives forward. These annual conferences provide an opportunity to develop and improve European ehealth services.

Another key European initiative to promote ehealth within the region is the European Patients Smart Open Services (epSOS) initiative (www.epsos.eu). The goals related to this effort include building and evaluating a service infrastructure for cross-border interoperability between EHR systems in Europe. This initiative promotes a European health information network and has already influenced member states and provided opportunities in business.

To provide input on legal, ethical, and regulatory issues crucial to ehealth implementation across the EU, the member states proposed SEHGovIA (Supporting the European eHealth Governance Initiative and Action; http://ihe-europe.net/eu-projects/57/sehgovia-thematic-network). SEHGovIA addresses semantic interoperability, terminology, identification, and authentication standardization issues that are vital to successful information exchange of health data across the EU.

With the goal of cross-border interoperability in mind the Healthcare Interoperability Testing and Conformance Harmonisation (HITCH) project was established in the EU for testing and certification of ehealth systems (www.hitch-project.eu). The project encourages the development and approval of common guidelines for testing quality and the organization of a testing tool development infrastructure to fill critical gaps for tools and test plans. A European

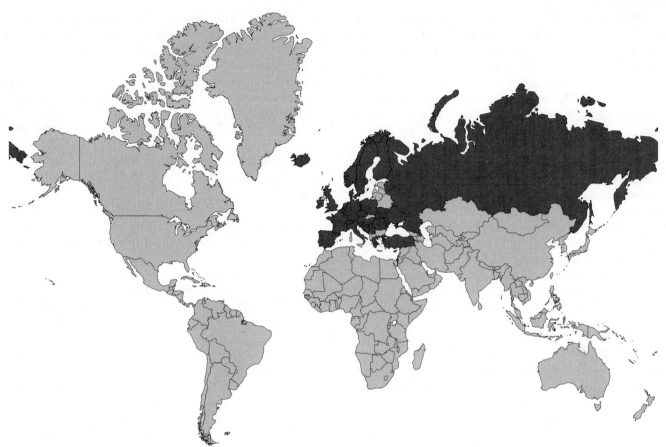

FIG 30-1 European Federation for Medical Informatics (EFMI) member countries: Austria, Belgium, Boznia-Herzegovina, Croatia, Cyprus, Czech Republic, Denmark, Finland, France, Germany, Greece, Hungary, Iceland, Ireland, Israel, Italy, Republic of Moldova, Netherlands, Norway, Poland, Portugal, Romania, Russian Federation, Serbia, Slovenia, Spain, Sweden, Switzerland, Turkey, Ukraine, and United Kingdom.

interoperability framework with an objective set of profiles based on interoperability standards is required before proceeding with testing, projected for piloting in 2014.

HITCH proposes that this common foundation be used by national or regional ehealth projects across Europe to organize their own testing and certification. The common testing tools and test plans found in the foundation would permit products to be tested at the European level and additionally tested only for regional and national extensions to the European interoperability framework. Ideally this would increase consistency, reduce costs, and significantly accelerate deployment across multiple national and regional ehealth projects, improving on the current inconsistent and fragmented approach.

The European Federation for Medical Informatics

The European Federation for Medical Informatics (EFMI) was created in 1976 with the assistance of the WHO Regional Office for Europe. Its main purpose was to enhance European health sciences by encouraging the implementation of information science in the field. Each European country is entitled to be represented in EFMI by a suitable health informatics society. As of this writing, 30 countries in Europe have joined EFMI. The footprint for these countries can be seen in Figure 30-1.

The objectives of EFMI are as follows:
- To advance the international cooperation and dissemination of information in medical informatics within Europe
- To promote high standards in the application of medical informatics
- To promote research and development in medical informatics
- To encourage high standards in education in medical informatics
- To function as a regional member of the International Medical Informatics Association (IMIA)

While the term *medical informatics* is used in stating these goals, it is meant to include the whole spectrum of health informatics and all disciplines concerned with health and informatics. EFMI is a regional member of the International Medical Informatics Association (IMIA) and has formal liaison relations with WHO as well as the Council of Europe. Activities of EFMI include academic conferences and publications, including organizing the Medical Informatics Europe

(MIE) congresses. These take place in 2 of every 3 years in order not to clash with IMIA's triennial MedInfo conferences. The first such congress, MIE 78, was held in Cambridge, England. The proceedings of these congresses are usually published as a series: *Lecture Notes in Medical Informatics* and *Studies in Health Technologies and Informatics*. A selection of the best papers from the MIE conferences is published in special volumes of the *International Journal of Medical Informatics* and *Methods of Information in Medicine*. Open access to the latest MIE conference proceedings is provided on the EFMI website located at http://www.helmholtz-muenchen. de/ibmi/efmi/. Less well known but equally important are the Special Topic Conferences. A Special Topic Conference is organized by a member society in combination with its annual meeting. The topic of the conference is defined by the needs of the member society. Relevant EFMI working groups are engaged for content selection. The EFMI's working groups also organize their own working conferences or business meetings. Currently there are 16 working groups within the EFMI (Box 30-1).

eHealth Initiatives in the APEC Region

Health IT is one of three projects overseen by the Health Working Group (www.apechwg.org) of the Asia-Pacific Economic Cooperation (APEC) oversees. The APEC ehealth collaboration started as a health IT project when leaders accepted the ecommerce agenda at an APEC summit meeting in 1999. At the 2000 APEC summit meeting this group recognized the digital divide among member countries and began to support services for underprivileged populations within the region. In 2001 leaders of member countries addressed basic health

issues within the region and recommended the use of health IT to extend healthcare services to a wider community. In 2003 APEC leaders called for health security and established a health surveillance network to monitor disease outbreaks and bioterrorism. At a meeting in 2005, health ministers underscored the importance of the use of health IT to better face threats to health in the region and welcomed ehealth initiatives. In 2006 to 2009, as part of the APEC e-Health Initiative, annual APEC e-Health Seminars occurred and in 2006 to 2008 an APEC e-Health Action Project was held.

Participants of the e-Health Seminars indicated that it was difficult to do the following:

- Share information through only an annual conference
- Reflect outcomes in relevant industrial areas immediately
- Include public sector involvement in legislation and policy planning, standardization, and human resource development for ehealth services

Based on this feedback the APEC e-Health Community was introduced in 2009. The Community made it possible for APEC member countries to share information and exchange ehealth human and material resources through a connection between developed and underdeveloped economies. It is now possible for industries to reflect the outcomes of seminars immediately by inducing participation from hospitals, clinics, and global companies that deal in relevant health IT and health areas. The APEC e-Health Community also made it possible to promote government participation in the development of policy, legislation, and standards and encourage member country participation by arranging for each country to take turns hosting seminars.

The APEC e-Health Community holds an annual meeting called the APEC e-Health Community Forum. Key objectives of the APEC e-Health Community Forum include the following:

- Bridging the gap between APEC member countries through seminars, capacity building in information sharing, and acknowledging high-value cases related to ehealth
- Stimulating ehealth-focused industries within the region

The main activities of the e-Health Community Forum are technical presentations, exhibitions of ehealth products, and poster presentations. Experts from industry, academe, and research institutes actively participate in these activities. Activities of the e-Health Community Forum include the following:

- Sharing knowledge, skills, and models of the ehealth service system to help collaboration between the public and private health sectors in the APEC region
- Enabling APEC regional governments to maximize ICT applications for healthcare, respond more effectively to epidemic diseases, and vitalize ehealth fields
- Establishing guidelines for the level of ehealth in the region and collaborating with other forums to stimulate ehealth within the region
- Publishing *The Current Status and Future Prospects of eHealth in APEC Regions*

The APEC e-Health Community Forum supports its member countries with a detailed plan that depends on the

---

BOX 30-1 EUROPEAN FEDERATION FOR MEDICAL INFORMATICS (EFMI) WORKING GROUPS

Education in Health Informatics (EDU)
Electronic Health Records (EHR)
Assessment of Health Information Systems (EVAL)
Health Informatics for Interregional Cooperation (HIIC)
Health Information Management (PG HIME)
Human and Organizational Factors of Medical Informatics (HOFMI)
Informatics for the Disabled and Rehabilitation (IDR)
Libre/Free and Open Source Software in Health Informatics (LIFOSS)
Minimum Basic Data Set, Case Mix, Resources Management and Outcomes of Care (MCRO)
Medical Image Processing (MIP)
Natural Language Understanding; Nursing Informatics in Europe (NLU)
Nursing Informatics (NURSIE)
Primary Care Informatics (PCI)
Personal Portal Devices (PPD)
Security, Safety and Ethics (SSE)
Traceability of Supply Chains (TRACE)

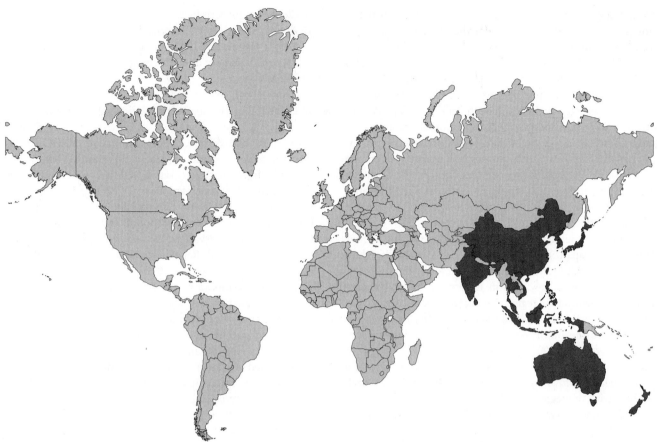

FIG 30-2 Asia Pacific Association for Medical Informatics (APAMI) member countries: Australia, China, Hong Kong Special Administrative Region, India, Japan, Korea, Malaysia, New Zealand, Pakistan, Philippines, Singapore, Sri Lanka, Taiwan, Thailand, and Vietnam. Observer Members: Bangladesh, Indonesia, and Kazakhstan.

current status of ehealth within a particular country. The Forum implements this plan on the following three levels:

- *Initiative level.* Health IT technology and sharing information on and awareness of the current status of ehealth
- *Middle level.* Development of technology through attainment of relevant advanced health IT information
- *Advanced level.* Introduction of current status of technology and newest ehealth technology[3]

Asia Pacific Association for Medical Informatics (APAMI)

To promote the theory and practice of health informatics within the APEC region, the Asia Pacific Association for Medical Informatics (APAMI) began in 1993 as a regional group within IMIA (www.apami.org). Currently it has 15 society members as seen in Fig. 30-2 and listed in Box 30-2.

APAMI activities include triennial conferences and working groups. The inaugural APAMI triennial conference was held in Singapore in 1994. Over the last several years these conferences have been held in seven different Asian countries, including China in 2012. The four working groups within APAMI include Standardization, Health Informatics for Developing Countries, Decision Support, and Nursing

---

BOX 30-2   ASIA PACIFIC ASSOCIATION FOR MEDICAL INFORMATICS (APAMI) MEMBER COUNTRIES

Australia	Singapore
China	Sri Lanka
Hong Kong Special	Taiwan
Administrative Region	Thailand
India	Vietnam
Japan	
Korea	**Observer Members**
Malaysia	Bangladesh
New Zealand	Indonesia
Pakistan	Kazakhstan
Philippines	

Informatics. Each hosts a workshop during the APAMI triennial conference.

APAMI actively promotes telemedicine, bioinformatics, and public health informatics. Because of the large size of its countries, the low specialist-to-population ratio, the affordable cost of technology and telecommunication, and the high penetration rate of health IT for equitable distribution of healthcare services, telemedicine is an important aspect of ehealth within the Asia-Pacific region. One example is the National Telemedicine Initiative of the Thai Ministry of Public Health started in 1998. Thai telemedicine supports remote, underserved populations in Thailand. This system links the Ministry of Public Health and 19 hospitals with about 60 district hospitals. Another example is oncology telemedicine in Japan, which connects 14 cancer centers throughout Japan. High-resolution images are transferred among centers as part teleconference services. Asia-Pacific countries with active telemedicine projects include China, Korea, Australia, India, Bhutan, Singapore, Indonesia, Hong Kong SAR, and New Zealand.

Many countries in the Asia-Pacific region including China, Hong Kong, Japan, Korea, Singapore, India, Malaysia, Thailand, and the Philippines are actively promoting bioinformatics. APAMI plays a key role in facilitating and advancing cooperation within the region. China, Hong Kong, Singapore, and Taiwan have been especially active in public health informatics since the outbreak of severe acute respiratory syndrome (SARS) in 2003. The SARS outbreak provided an opportunity for APAMI to demonstrate the importance of a public health informatics approach to the health of each country with the region. APAMI continues to address public health informatics research and development through contact tracing, epidemiologic reporting, and monitoring for acute disease outbreaks, as was seen with SARS.

eHealth Initiatives in the Pan American Health Organization (PAHO) Region

The Pan American Health Organization (PAHO) initiated the PAHO eHealth Program to improve public health in the Americas through the use of innovative health IT tools and methodologies.[4] The PAHO eHealth Program is the strategic response to the Health Agenda for the Americas presented by the Ministers of Health of the Americas in 2007.[5] This program introduced a conceptual model based on the following three components:

1. Access to information such as PAHO and WHO content and public health content
2. Access to educational material such as training, lectures, web conferences, and open educational resources
3. Interaction management in the Web 2.0 context, which includes the physician–patient relationship and all aspects of telemedicine and telehealth[5]

These follow a strategic pathway consisting of six steps:

- Identification of needs
- Development of innovative solutions
- Adoption of the solution(s)
- Training for implementation
- Implementation and use
- Recording of lessons learned

As of 2013 the PAHO eHealth Program consists of nine projects:

1. Personal health card
2. Digital clinical history
3. Electronic prescriptions
4. Appointment via the Internet
5. Health portals and the social web
6. Risk management and patient security
7. Telemedicine
8. Regional call center
9. Digitalization of clinical and administrative documentation[5]

PAHO is expected to move its ehealth program forward with PAHO and WHO Corporate Initiatives. PAHO Corporate Initiatives include the Regional Health Observatory, desktops, intranet and extranet, Web 2.0, web conferences, social media, *Pan American Journal of Public Health*, Virtual Campus, Virtual Health Library, and the PAHO Institutional Repository. WHO Corporate Initiatives such as the Global Health Observatory, Web 2.0, Global Health Library, Global Institutional Repository, and multilingualism will be used.

Expected results from the PAHO eHealth Program have been established as follows:

- "Support for the formulation and adoption of people-centered ehealth public policies at the national and regional level of the member states.
- Improved organizational and technology infrastructure promoting epidemiologic surveillance services and sustainable, interoperable development of ehealth-centered programs and initiatives
- Intersectoral cooperation, both within each country and among countries with electronic mechanisms for sharing best practices, regional resources, and lessons learned
- Established training in information and communication technologies in universities and among health professionals"[6]

Sample indicators to evaluate whether expected results are achieved include metrics on the use of tools by patients and on the use of web-based collaboration tools by citizens, public health workers, and public health institutions from dispersed or disadvantaged populations.

IMIA-LAC

The Regional Federation of Health Informatics for Latin America and the Caribbean, called IMIA-LAC (www.imia-lac.net), was founded in 1996 to promote theory development and the practice of health informatics within Latin America and the Caribbean (LAC). The IMIA-LAC board proposed the following goals to develop health informatics within the region and strengthen regional ties:

1. Strengthen the network of health informatics societies in Latin America and the Caribbean
2. Define the main health informatics topics to promote and the best groups to engage in such initiatives[7]

Member societies of IMIA-LAC include Argentina, Brazil, Chile, Cuba, Mexico, Uruguay, and Venezuela as shown in Fig. 30-3.

Activities include regional congresses, national conferences, and working groups. An inaugural regional congress of IMIA-LAC was held in Buenos Aires, Argentina, in 2008, organized by Asociación Argentina de Informática Médica

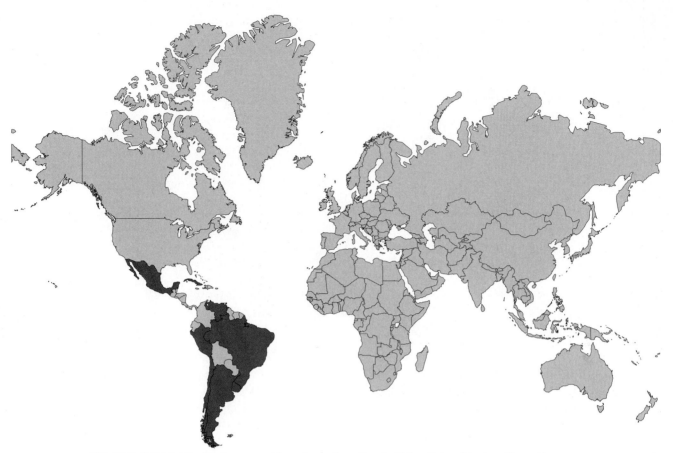

FIG 30-3 IMIA-LAC member countries: Argentina, Brazil, Chile, Cuba, Mexico, Peru, Uruguay, and Venezuela.

(AAIM) with the help of several other organizations working in health informatics in Argentina. As part of the conference IMIA held its board meeting demonstrating its support for the IMIA-LAC regional congress. In addition, the IMIA Health and Medical Informatics Education workgroup held its business meeting there, coordinated by the group from the Hospital Italiano de Buenos Aires. Both the Spanish (SEIS) and the American (AMIA) health informatics societies have supported and participated in the regional congress and coordinated other activities with IMIA-LAC.

The two main working groups within IMIA-LAC are the Health and Medical Informatics Education workgroup and the Health Information Systems workgroup, coordinated by Argentinean, Brazilian, and Cuban experts, with participation from several countries in the region. The Health and Medical Informatics Education workgroup has devised a work plan, including an assessment of the situation in each country and a coordination of health informatics education. Three additional working groups have been established by experts working in these areas. These include:

- Bioinformatics workgroup
- Nursing Informatics workgroup
- Informatics and Quality in Healthcare workgroup

eHealth Initiatives in Africa

Africa has been identified as one of the least economically developed areas in the world. The wealth of a nation depends on the health of its population making healthcare an area of high developmental priority in Africa. In many African countries continued health challenges reveal slow progress toward achieving WHO's Millennium Development Goals related to health.[8] For example, a majority of the population in sub-Saharan Africa still has limited access to modern health facilities. It is hoped that implementing new ehealth and mhealth (mobile health) solutions will allow African countries to use ehealth to deliver higher quality healthcare services.

According to the WHO regional office in Africa, health IT can play a significant role in strengthening national health systems to accelerate progress toward the Millennium Development Goals and improving health outcomes in the region.[9] Needed are strengthened health information systems, public health surveillance systems, mobile devices at the point of care, EHRs, and other applications that provide patient billing, patient scheduling, and the electronic transmission of prescriptions. Telehealth would also contribute to improving equity for underserved populations in rural areas.

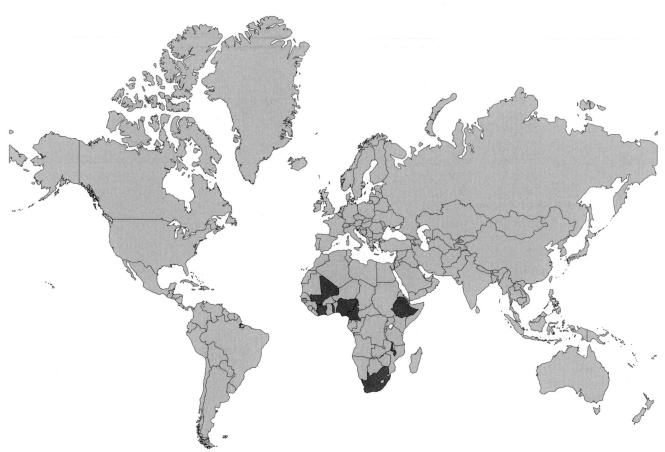

FIG 30-4 HELINA member countries: Cameroon, Ethiopia, Ivory Coast, Malawi, Mali, Nigeria, South Africa, and Togo.

Key challenges impeding the wide-scale implementation of ehealth solutions in Africa include:
- the "digital divide," as demonstrated by the need for increased awareness of ehealth among health professionals and patients
- a cohesive policy environment, providing leadership and coordination with improved financial and human resources
- a technical infrastructure and services within the health sector with monitoring and evaluation systems

Health IT knowledge and expertise is needed to deploy and adopt ehealth technologies. One strategy recommended by ehealth solutions in the African region is to introduce health informatics into the curriculum of institutions thereby systematically developing widespread familiarity and comfort with ehealth.

Health Informatics in Africa (HELINA)

HELINA, IMIA's African regional arm, was created in 1993 with three main goals:
1. to create and implement education and research programs specific to the African perspective
2. to bridge the gap between the public sector and the private sector

3. to plan for the continued development of informatics and ehealth in Africa (www.helina-online.org)

Currently eight countries are members of HELINA: Cameroon, Ethiopia, Ivory Coast, Malawi, Mali, Nigeria, South Africa, and Togo, as shown in Fig. 30-4. Countries such as Algeria, Democratic Republic of the Congo, Egypt, Kenya, Madagascar, Tanzania, Uganda, Zambia, and Zimbabwe are corresponding members. HELINA organizes conferences within the African region. The first was held in Nigeria in 1993 and five more conferences have been organized since that inaugural meeting. These conferences revealed a broader view of local initiatives within Africa. However, the use of health IT in Africa remains very low due to the lack of health information systems suitable for the African requirements and the lack of qualified healthcare personnel to develop, implement, and maintain such systems

Recognizing the need for education, an educational opportunity called Health Informatics Building Blocks (HIBBs) was introduced in 2008 with the goal of offering practical educational tools for applied informaticists, public health workers, policy makers, and healthcare practitioners in low-resource settings.[10] HIBBs modules are open educational resources designed to be portable, reusable, and adaptable to local needs. The program focuses on foundational health

TABLE 30-1	MODULES OF HEALTH INFORMATICS BUILDING BLOCKS (HIBBs)
TOPIC AREA	**MODULES**
Fundamental skills	Introduction to Computers
	Introduction to Word 2010
	Introduction to PowerPoint 2010
	Information Retrieval: Access to Knowledge-Based Resources
Introduction to informatics	Introduction to Medical Informatics
	Health Informatics Terminologies
Health information systems	Introduction to Electronic Medical Records
	Routine Health Information Systems
	EMR Implementation Considerations
Ethics and legal issues	Ethics and Integrity in Data Use and Management
	Privacy, Confidentiality, and Security
Data quality	Data Quality: Out-of-Range Values
	Data Quality: Missing Data
	Data Quality: Data Cleaning
	Data Quality: Introduction to Form Design
Research	Preparing Research Datasets
	Introduction to Bioinformatics
Leadership and management	Managing Change in Healthcare IT Implementations
Training tools	Game-based Assessment Quiz Template

From the South African Institute for Distance Education (Saide) (nd) HIBBs Modules. Retrieved from http://www.oerafrica.org/hibbs/Modules/tabid/1884/Default.aspx.

informatics concepts and related skills that are needed to develop and manage systems in these environments. HIBBs currently offers 19 modules covering 8 different topic areas as outlined in Table 30-1. The leadership for the development of the HIBBs modules is provided by the Global Health Informatics Partnership (GHIP), in partnership with AMIA. Individuals and organizations around the world continue to contribute ideas and expertise to the HIBBs project.

INTERNATIONAL ORGANIZATIONS WITH INFORMATICS IMPLICATIONS

From its beginnings international health-related organizations have played a major role in the development of health informatics. This section of the chapter provides an overview of key organizations that are providing that leadership along with a brief description of their programs and efforts.

eHealth and Health Informatics at WHO

WHO plays a key global role in the development of global health informatics (www.who.org). The vision of WHO knowledge management, one of its programs, is a world with better and more equitable health outcomes through the use of information and communication technologies to improve health services and systems. WHO uses ehealth as an umbrella term that covers all aspects of the use of information and communication technology in healthcare and has promoted its use for many years. In more recent years WHO

has taken steps to make ehealth a priority in strengthening health systems worldwide.

The eHealth Resolution

The 58th World Health Assembly took a historical step toward supporting ehealth by adopting a resolution for a global movement that recognizes the role of ICT to strengthen health systems and improve the safety, quality, and efficiency of services.[11] The resolution urges member states to do the following:

- Create a lasting plan for ehealth development
- Create health IT infrastructure
- Encourage private and non-profit collaboration
- Broaden the reach of ehealth services
- Encourage universal collaboration to determine ehealth standards supported by evidence-based practice
- Create centers and networks for sharing best practices, policies, technical innovations, service improvement, communications, capacity building, and surveillance
- Think about developing national public health information systems
- Enhance surveillance and response to public health emergencies through increased flow of information[12]

Major Activities and Projects in WHO

Global Observatory for eHealth. In direct response to the World Health Assembly ehealth resolution, the Global Observatory for eHealth (www.who.int/kms/initiatives/ehealth/) was established in 2005 to monitor and analyze ehealth and to support national planning through the provision of strategic information in member countries. Two global surveys were conducted, the first in 2005 to establish a baseline and the second in 2009.[13] Key findings of the first survey include the following:

- A digital divide exists in ehealth
- Member states are looking to WHO and its partners for assistance and guidance in the ehealth domain
- Many countries expect to implement ehealth policies in the near future and will need support
- Development of national ehealth governance mechanisms within countries is necessary
- Public-private partnerships for ehealth projects are on the increase and effective management practices should be promoted
- Citizen protection policies should be put into place to ensure patient data confidentiality; interoperability issues should be made a priority by member states
- Health information in electronic formats should be provided in relevant community languages

The second survey, conducted in late 2009, was designed to build on the knowledge base generated by the first survey and identify and analyze trends in ehealth, including the following:

- The uptake of ehealth foundation policies and strategies
- Deployment of mhealth initiatives
- Application of telehealth solutions and adoption of elearning for health professionals and students
- Collection, processing, storage, and transfer of patient information
- Legal and ethical frameworks for electronic patient information
- Legislation and initiatives concerning online child safety, Internet pharmacies, and health information on the Internet
- Governance and organization of ehealth within countries[14]

The second survey proved to be a rich source of data, which have been used to create a series of publications titled the Global Observatory for eHealth series.[14] A list of the publications is included in Table 30-2. Additional information about these surveys as they relate to international privacy and security of personal health data is included in Chapter 19.

WHO Family of International Classifications. WHO is responsible for developing, disseminating, and maintaining international classifications on health called the WHO Family of International Classifications (WHO-FIC) to promote a consensual, meaningful, and useful framework that governments, healthcare providers, and consumers can use as a common language in health information systems (www.who.int/classifications/). Internationally endorsed classifications facilitate the storage, retrieval, analysis, and interpretation of data as well as allow data within and between populations to be compared.

The classifications within the WHO-FIC fall into two main categories: reference classifications and derived and related classifications. Reference classifications are classifications of the basic parameters of health. Derived classifications

TABLE 30-2	GLOBAL OBSERVATORY FOR EHEALTH SERIES
TITLE	**VOLUME NUMBER AND DATE OF PUBLICATION**
Atlas—eHealth country profiles	Volume 1 (2010)
Telemedicine—Opportunities and developments in Member States	Volume 2 (2011)
mHealth: New horizons for health through mobile technologies	Volume 3 (2011)
Safety and security on the Internet: Challenges and advances in Member States	Volume 4 (2011)
Legal frameworks for eHealth	Volume 5 (2012)
Management of patient information: Trends and challenges in Member States	Volume 6 (2012)

From WHO(ND) Global Observatory for eHealth: Publications. Retrieved from http://www.who.int/goe/publications/en/.

are developed by modifying or rearranging reference classifications. Related classifications are associated with the reference classification at specific levels of structure only. Box 30-3 provides a list of the WHO classifications and their related type.

Collaborating with Terminology Standards Development Organizations. In 2010 WHO collaborated with IHTSDO to develop and sustain classification and terminology systems to more efficiently and effectively use public resources with less duplication of efforts.[15] Thus mappings and linkages between International Classification of Diseases (ICD) and Systematized Nomenclature of Medicine Clinical Terms (SNOMED CT) are being developed for automated processing of data to improve coding and information exchange. Additional information on these classification systems is provided in Chapter 22.

International Medical Informatics Association (IMIA)

IMIA is the world body for health and biomedical informatics (www.imia-medinfo.org), originating in 1967 as Technical Committee 4 of the International Federation for Information Processing (IFIP; www.ifip.org). It evolved from a Special Interest Group of IFIP to its current status in 1979. IMIA is connected with WHO as a nongovernmental organization (NGO) and with the International Federation of Health Information Management Associations (IFHIMA). Membership in IMIA is limited to organizations, societies, and corporations. For example, each country can be represented by

BOX 30-3   WORLD HEALTH ORGANIZATION FAMILY OF INTERNATIONAL CLASSIFICATIONS (WHO-FIC)

Reference Classifications

Main classifications based on basic parameters of health. These classifications have been prepared by the World Health Organization (WHO) and approved by WHO's governing bodies for international use.

- International Classification of Diseases (ICD)
- International Classification of Functioning, Disability and Health (ICF)
- International Classification of Health Interventions (ICHI)

Derived Classifications

Those based on reference classifications (i.e., ICD and ICF). Derived classifications may be prepared either by adopting the reference classification structure and categories and providing additional detail beyond that provided by the reference classifications or by rearranging or aggregating items from one or more reference classifications.

- International Classification of Diseases for Oncology, 3rd edition (ICD-O-3)
- ICD-10 for Mental and Behavioral Disorders Clinical Descriptions and Diagnostic Guidelines
- ICD-10 for Mental and Behavioral Disorders Diagnostic Criteria for Research
- Application of the International Classification of Diseases to Neurology (ICD-10-NA)
- Application of the International Classification of Diseases to Dentistry and Stomatology, 3rd edition (ICD-DA)

Related Classifications

Those that partially refer to reference classifications or are associated with reference classifications at specific levels of structure only.

- International Classification of Primary Care (ICPC-2)
- International Classification of External Causes of Injury (ICECI)
- Technical Aids for Persons with Disabilities: Classification and Terminology (ISO9999)
- Anatomical Therapeutic Chemicals Classification with Defined Daily Doses (ATC/DDD)
- International Classification for Nursing Practice (ICNP)

Adapted from World Health Organization (WHO). Derived and related classifications in the WHO-FIC. WHO. http://www.who.int/classifications/related/en/index.html. 2012.

only one member society. As of May 2012 there were 57 member societies. The regional members, with the exception of the North America member countries shown in Figure 30-5 and the Middle East Association for Health Informatics (MEAHI) member countries included in Figure 30-6 were discussed earlier in the sections dealing with informatics regions of the world. In a country where no representative society exists, IMIA accommodates involvement through corresponding members, especially within developing countries. As of May 2012 there were 32 corresponding members.

IMIA is an important player in ensuring that information science and technology are integrated into all fields of healthcare. Its main goals are as follows:

- To promote informatics in healthcare and research in health, bio, and medical informatics
- To advance and nurture international cooperation
- To stimulate research, development, and routine application
- To move informatics from theory into practice in a full range of health delivery settings, from the clinician's office to acute and long-term care
- To further the dissemination and exchange of knowledge, information, and technology
- To promote education and responsible behavior
- To represent the medical and health informatics field with WHO and other international professional and governmental organizations

In its function as a bridge organization, IMIA's goals are as follows:

- To move theory into practice by linking academic and research informaticists with caregivers, consultants, vendors, and vendor-based researchers
- To lead the international medical and health informatics communities throughout the twenty-first century
- To promote the cross-fertilization of health informatics information and knowledge across professional and geographical boundaries
- To serve as the catalyst for ubiquitous worldwide health information infrastructures for patient care and health research.[16]

IMIA provides networking opportunities as well as an international platform for health IT providers, consultants, and publishers. IMIA organizes the World Congress on Medical and Health Informatics, commonly known as MedInfo. The event provides an opportunity to share and exchange ideas and research as well as hold formal meetings and facilitate informal networking of members. From 2015 onward MedInfo will be held every 2 years. IMIA also publishes the annual *IMIA Yearbook of Medical Informatics* and three additional official journals. Since its inception in 1992 the *IMIA Yearbook of Medical Informatics* has been one of the most valuable products that IMIA provides to its members and the health informatics community. IMIA's three official journals are *Applied Clinical Informatics* (www.aci-journal.org), *International Journal of Medical Informatics* (www.ijmijournal.com/home), and *Methods of Information in Medicine* (www.methods-online.com).

IMIA pursues its scientific activity in specific fields of the wider domain of health and biomedical informatics through Working Groups (WGs) and Special Interest Groups (SIGs). A WG or SIG consists of a group of experts with a specific interest. Currently there are 24 WGs and SIGs (Box 30-4). Activities of WGs and SIGs include organizing business meetings at IMIA triennial conferences or IMIA regional meetings, publishing papers related to WG activity written by members of WGs and SIGs, and collaborating with other organizations within IMIA or IMIA regional or member

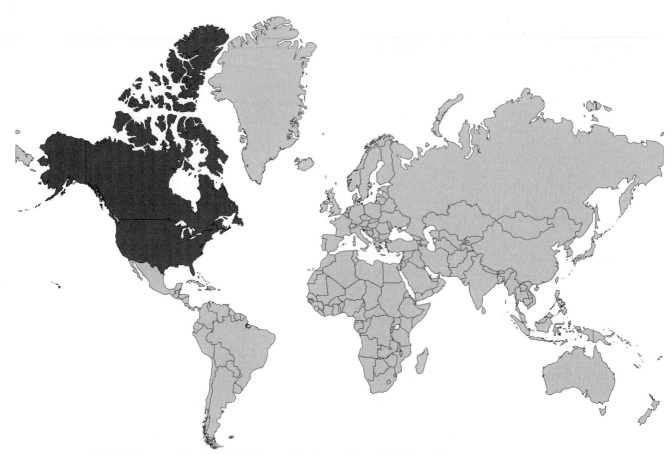

FIG 30-5 International Medical Informatics Association (IMIA) North America member countries: United States and Canada.

societies. The Nursing Informatics SIG (IMIA-NI) is one of the initial and most consistently active SIGs.

IMIA-NI

The Nursing Informatics component of IMIA, IMIA-NI (http://www.imia-medinfo.org/new2/node/151), was originally called Working Group 8 in 1983. The main goals of IMIA-NI are listed in Box 30-5.

IMIA-NI currently has 33 members from 33 member societies of IMIA. IMIA-NI pursues its scientific activity in specific fields of the wider domain of nursing informatics through WGs. Currently there are four IMIA-NI WGs: Consumer/Client Health Informatics, Education, Evidence-Based Practice, and Health Informatics Standards.

IMIA-NI organizes an International Congress on Nursing Informatics. The event occurs every 3 years and provides a scientific exchange of current research and thinking in nursing informatics, formal meetings on nursing informatics topics, and informal networking. The first meeting of IMIA-NI was held in 1982 in London, England, as an international open forum titled "The Impact of Computers on Nursing." Starting in 2012 the conferences are being held every other year. A list

of the IMIA-NI conferences with locations and themes is included in the Evolve resources for this chapter.

INTERNATIONAL STANDARDS EFFORTS

Over the past 2 decades significant efforts have been made in terminology development and standards. This section summarizes international work in this area and students are referred to Chapter 22 for more details where noted.

International Organization for Standardization (ISO)

The International Organization for Standardization (ISO) is the world's largest developer and publisher of international standards (www.iso.org). It is managed by a Central Secretariat in Geneva, Switzerland, and includes national standards institutes of 164 countries. This organization is not affiliated with governments and provides a link between the public and private sectors. Though many member institutes belong to the governmental structure of their countries (or are mandated by their government), others have private sector

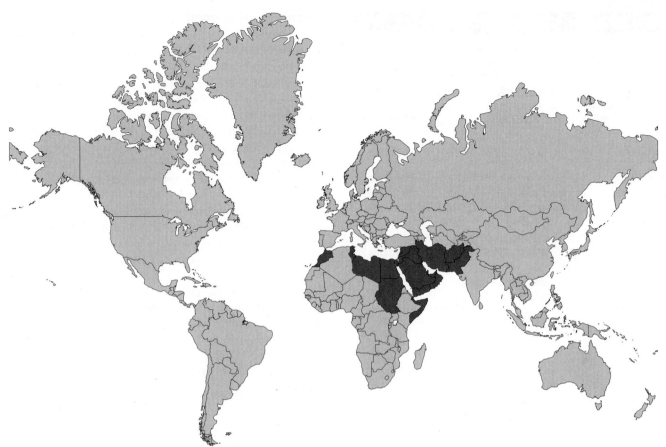

FIG 30-6 Middle East Association for Health Informatics (MEAHI) member countries: Afghanistan, Bahrain, Djibouti, Egypt, Iran, Iraq, Jordan, Kuwait, Lebanon, Libya, Morocco, Oman, Pakistan, Palestine, Qatar, Saudi Arabia, Somalia, South Sudan, Sudan, Syrian Arab Republic, Tunisia, United Arab Emirates, and Yemen.

BOX 30-4	INTERNATIONAL MEDICAL INFORMATICS ASSOCIATION (IMIA) WORKING GROUPS AND SPECIAL INTEREST GROUPS

Biomedical Pattern Recognition
Consumer Health Informatics
Critical Care Informatics
Dental Informatics
Francophone Special Interest Group (SIG)
Health and Medical Informatics Education
Health Informatics for Development
Health Informatics for Patient Safety
Health Information Systems
Human Factors Engineering for Healthcare Informatics
Health Geographical Information Systems (GIS)
Informatics in Genomic Medicine (IGM)
Intelligent Data Analysis and Data Mining
Medical Concept Representation

Mental Health Informatics (inactive)
Open Source Health Informatics
Organizational and Social Issues
Primary Health Care Informatics
Security in Health Information Systems
SIG NI Nursing Informatics
Smart Homes and Ambient Assisted Living
Social Media
Standards in Health Care Informatics
Technology Assessment & Quality Development in Health Informatics
Telehealth
Wearable Sensors in Healthcare

Data from IMIA: Working Groups. http://www.imia-medinfo.org/new2/WG.

origins (i.e., they were established through national partnerships of industry associations). Therefore the ISO is uniquely able to establish a consensus on standards-related solutions for business and the broader needs of society. Currently there are more than 200 technical committees (TCs) developing standards in different domains.

ISO TC 215 is the ISO's TC on health informatics. The scope of ISO TC 215 is to achieve compatibility and interoperability between independent systems, achieve compatibility and consistency of data for comparative statistical purposes (classifications), and reduce duplication of effort and redundancies through standardization. Currently there are 32 active participating (P-member) countries and 24 observing (O-member) countries. As of May 2012 the number of published ISO standards under the direct responsibility of TC 215 (including updates) was 94. ISO TC 215's current work program comprises more than 140 items, comprehensively covering the contemporary health information standards spectrum. Table 30-3 presents ISO TC 215's working groups and their activities. Figure 30-7 illustrates the current structure of ISO TC 215 and its eight working groups.

Many health professionals are involved in ISO. For example, nurses have played an active and important role in different WGs of ISO TC 215 in the development and testing of ISO 18104: Integration of a Reference Terminology Model for Nursing. This defines nursing diagnoses and nursing actions.[17] Nurses can participate in ISO activities by providing comments on an ISO deliverable by becoming a member of their own country's delegation, participating as an expert, providing feedback to appropriate organizations about ISO standards, and participating in related organizations.

International Council of Nurses

The International Council of Nurses (ICN) is a compilation of more than 130 national nurses associations (NNAs) representing the more than 13 million nurses globally (www.icn.ch). ICN began in 1899 with the goal of encouraging quality healthcare, solid health policies, advanced health knowledge, and a respected global nursing presence.

ICN has three key program areas, or Pillars, that are pivotal in implementing quality nursing care: Professional Practice, Regulation, and Socio-Economic Welfare. eHealth is one of three significant ICN projects under the Professional Practice pillar.

The ICN ehealth program encompasses a range of ICN activities, including the International Classification for Nursing Practice (ICNP), which provides a standard for comparing nursing practice locally, regionally, nationally, and internationally, and the Telenursing Network, which encourages and assists nurses in the development and use of telehealth. ICN also participated in other international terminology standards development activities, such as the ISO reference terminology standard and the International Nursing Minimum Data Set (i-NMDS). The i-NMDS builds on the Nursing Minimum Data Set work of Werley and Lang explained in Chapter 22.

International Classification for Nursing Practice (ICNP)

The ICNP is a vocabulary system developed by the ICN after the ICN Congress passed a resolution to begin work on developing ICNP terminology in 1989.

The ICNP provides a systematic way of describing nursing practice across the world, to improve communication within nursing and with other disciplines. Using the ICNP, reliable information about nursing practice can be generated in order to influence decision making, education, and policy; better meet the needs of individuals and groups; deliver more effective interventions; improve health outcomes; and better use resources. The actual implementation of ICNP terminology is underway around the world. For example, there are ICNP-based electronic nursing record systems in Portugal and Korea.[18,19]

ICNP C-Space. The aim of the ICN eHealth Programme is to transform nursing through the visionary application of information and communication technologies. Collaboration is a key to success but is also a big challenge at ICN, since it is a global organization working to connect nurses around the world. C-Space is a web-based collaborative workspace supporting the ICNP, where a group can meet to engage in meaningful dialog, work together on information resources, and publish those resources, without physically coming together (http://icnp.clinicaltemplates.org).

Groups within C-Space currently focus on a variety of topics, including the implementation, research and development, and translation of the ICNP. C-Space also provides a way to easily distribute the ICNP and its derived and associated products in a timely fashion to a range of people across

TABLE 30-3	SCOPE AND STANDARD WORKS OF ISO TC 215 ON HEALTH INFORMATICS	
WORKING GROUP (WG)	**SCOPE**	**STANDARD WORK**
WG 1 Data structure	To develop standards that establish the structure of health information in order to facilitate the sharing of information and data among enterprises, organizations, and information systems	Health summary record dataset, quality requirements and methodology for detailed clinical models, health indicators for conceptual framework, a clinical data warehouse, EHR communication standards series, healthcare provider identification, identification of subjects of care, and service architecture
WG 2 Data interchange	To accomplish messaging and communication in health informatics such that the electronic exchange of information between individual systems and organizations is facilitated	Telehealth and teleradiology, clinical genomics pedigree, clinical document registry, web access to DICOM, web access reference manifest, data type harmonization for information interchange, clinical document architecture, and IHE global standards adoption
WG 3 Semantic content	To develop standards for semantic representation of content in the healthcare domain, for the development and use of ontology and terminology systems, and for the representation and management of knowledge	Categorization and nomenclature of medical devices, semantic harmonization across information models and terminologies, clinical knowledge resources, metadata, mapping of terminologies to classification, common terminology services, maintenance of terminology systems, concepts to support continuity of care, and traditional oriental medicine
WG 4 Security	To define health informatics security and privacy protection standards to protect and enhance the confidentiality, availability, and integrity of health information; to prevent health information systems from adversely affecting patient safety; to protect privacy in relation to personal information; and to ensure the accountability of users of health information systems	Data protection for personal health information, VPN for health information infrastructure, EHR security and audit trails, privilege management and access control, clinical risk management of patient safety, public key infrastructure, pseudonymization, and functional and structural roles
WG 5 Pharmacy and medicines business	To establish standards in the domain of pharmacy and medication (e.g., research, development, regulation, supply, use, and monitoring) to improve the efficiency and interoperability of information systems affecting patient safety	International coding system for medicinal products, individual case safety reports, test names and units for reporting laboratory results, data elements and structure for the exchange of product information, pharmaceutical product identifiers, structures and controlled vocabularies for ingredients and units of measurement, and a prescriber support system
WG 6 Devices	To standardize the application of ICT to health device informatics and device interoperability in support of medicine, healthcare, and wellness	ISO/IEEE 11073 series supporting real-time plug-and-play interoperability, point-of-care medical device communication, personal health device communication, a medical waveform format, device terminology and information modeling, transport and application service profiles, and risk management associated with device ICT
WG 7 Business requirements for electronic health records	To standardize the identification of business requirements for all of the health informatics aspects applied to health records for persons	Business requirements for public health standards, personal health records definition, scope and context, knowledge management of health information standards, requirements for EHR architecture, an EHR system functional model, and architecture for developing countries
WG 8 SDO harmonization	To harmonize work with other standard development organizations, including the Joint Initiative Council	

DICOM, Digital Imaging and Communications in Medicine; *EHR*, electronic health record; *ICT*, information and communication technology; *IEEE*, Institute of Electrical and Electronics Engineers; *IHE*, International Health Exchange; *ISO*, International Organization for Standardization; *SDO*, standard development organization; *VPN*, virtual private network.

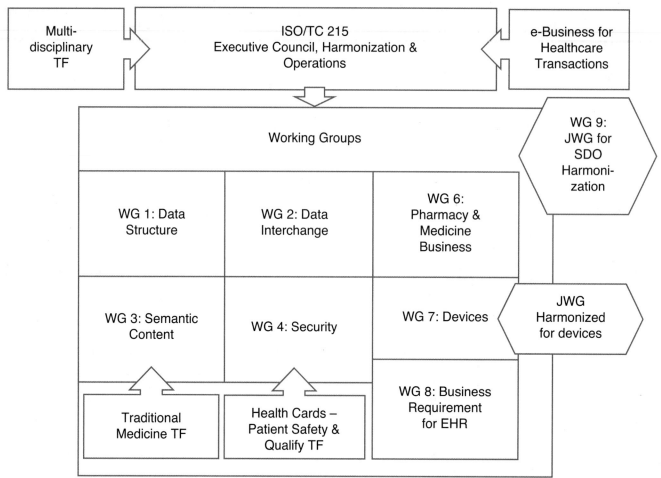

FIG 30-7 The current structure of ISO TC 215 and its eight working groups. *EHR,* Electronic health record; *ISO,* International Organization for Standardization; *JWG,* Joint Working Group; *SDO,* standard development organization; *TC,* technical committee; *TF,* task force; *WG,* working group.

the world. This allows the ICNP to stay responsive and dynamic in representing nursing practice.

The Telenursing Network

The Telenursing Network is one of 11 networks that ICN introduced as a mechanism to provide opportunities for nurses to communicate and pursue common professional interests (www.icn.ch/networks/telenursing-network/). ICN acknowledges that telenurses using health IT extend nursing's reach and improve access to care. Telenursing represents an advance in healthcare delivery and is ideal for addressing health system challenges (e.g., aging population and chronic illness community- and home-based care; geographic, social, and financial circumstances; increasing costs and reduced funding; nursing shortages). Telehealth is defined and described in Chapter 8.

The history of the Telenursing Network dates back to early 2000. ICN published a monograph on telenursing in 2000 titled *Telehealth and Telenursing: Nursing and Technology*

Advance Together and in 2001 published *International Professional Standards for Telenursing Programmes.*[20] Through publications like *International Competencies for Telenursing* in 2007, telenursing was recognized as an important contributor to the ICN's mission of advancing nursing and health worldwide.

The Telenursing Network was launched in 2009 with the aim of seeking, educating, supporting, and collaborating with nurses and other telenursing supporters worldwide. The overarching goal of the Telenursing Network is to improve healthcare services for individuals and institutions worldwide. As an evolving and dynamic resource, the Telenursing Network does the following:

- Provides a global forum for addressing issues related to telenursing and telehealth
- Promotes awareness of telenursing so that the roles and expertise of telenurses are understood, respected, and optimized
- Promotes telenursing as an accepted means for nurses to extend their reach to patients

- Assists with the development and sharing of knowledge, tools, and guidelines, which nurses can use to embed telenursing skills and competencies in their practice
- Establishes links between ICN's Telenursing Network and international organizations that promote and support the use of telehealth and advanced technologies for telenurses
- Provides opportunities for the exchange of knowledge and experience to develop the science and practice of telenursing
- Organizes meetings and conferences[21]

Health Level Seven (HL7)

HL7 (www.hl7.org) is an international community composed of healthcare subject matter experts and information scientists. Its goal is to create and sustain standards for the exchange, management, and integration of data that facilitate patient care and management, delivery, and evaluation of healthcare services. As explained in Chapter 22, HL7 encourages the use of such standards within and among healthcare organizations to optimize healthcare delivery for all.

International Health Terminology Standards Development Organisation (IHTSDO)

IHTSDO (www.ihtsdo.org) is an international nonprofit organization based in Denmark. It owns and administers the rights to SNOMED CT and related terminology standards. The goal of IHTSDO is to establish and maintain optimum interoperability and harmonization between SNOMED CT and standards produced by other international standards development organizations (e.g., American Academy of Ophthalmology; GS1; HL7; ICN; Institute of Electrical and Electronics Engineers; Logical Observation Identifiers Names and Codes; Nomenclature, Properties and Units; openEHR; WHO; and World Organization of National Colleges, Academies). Additional details on SNOMED CT are included in Chapter 22.

GLOBAL CHALLENGES TO EHEALTH

There are multiple challenges facing the use of health IT, at both the local level and the national and international levels. This section explores some of the more important challenges.

Global Interoperability

A key problem in achieving global interoperability in health IT is the lack of semantic (the meaning of terms) interoperability. Key barriers include issues related to the terminology used in describing and documenting healthcare such as cost and accessibility, gaps in exhaustiveness, and lack of granularity.[22] There are many international efforts to solve this problem, such as the development of an international standard clinical terminology, development of clinical data models such as HL7 Clinical Document Architecture (CDA) documents, openEHR Archetypes, and integration of standard data models with terminologies such as SNOMED CT.[23] Harmonization activities among international standards development organizations, such as ISO TC 215, HL7, and European Committee for Standardization (CEN) TC 251, are occurring and are necessary.

Human Resources for eHealth

According to the first global survey on ehealth carried out in 2005 by WHO, and described above, all respondents expressed a need for education and training in ehealth.[13] The lack of human resources with the necessary skills and competencies is a problem for the introduction and use of ehealth in many parts of the world. Different types of professionals with an appropriate mix of skills are needed for the best use of ICT in healthcare (e.g., health informatics professionals, health information management professionals, and others with specialized informatics skills). Current shortages of skilled workers in the healthcare profession demand a human resource strategy and long-term plan for the education and training of ehealth personnel to ensure the quality of collected health data and its security and confidentiality and to manage and maintain the systems and data in the future.[24]

Based on the 2005 WHO survey data, elearning programs and professional development for professional education were recommended in the health sciences. In addition, collaborations need to be developed that can establish databases of existing elearning courses and WHO should advocate for the inclusion of ehealth courses within university curricula.[25]

Information and Communications Technology Infrastructure

eHealth depends on health IT infrastructure and services. Obviously, if infrastructure or services are missing or deficient, ehealth becomes less effective. The digital divide is the result of a gap in information exchange between different demographics and remains a major problem in terms of Internet and especially broadband uptake.[26] This divide continues to expand as healthcare systems and providers increasingly depend on information from the Internet to guide day-to-day care. This is most evident in comparing fixed broadband penetration in Europe and the Americas (10% to 15%) to that in Africa (less than 0.5%).[27] There is also a significant gap in the percentage of Internet users; compared to countries such as Norway and Sweden (which have Internet use of 97.2% and 92.9%, respectively). Many others lag significantly behind these high numbers of Internet use. In Africa only 13.5% of the population is online and although the number of users in China jumped from 22.5 million to 513.1 million between 2000 and 2011, this represents a mere 38.4% of the total population of China.[28]

As with the solutions to problems caused by a lack of knowledgeable personnel, awareness of the disparity and its impact on healthcare is the first step in narrowing the information gap. Education programs will prove beneficial in the attempt to close the digital divide. On the other hand, developments in the mobile sector have been phenomenal. Nearly 1 in 2 people worldwide had a mobile phone by the end of

2007. In Europe penetration has reached nearly 100%, in Asia it has surpassed 33%, and in Africa it has surpassed 25%. This particular digital divide was reduced due to a high level of competition and a decrease in prices.[27] However, having a tool does not necessarily indicate that functionality is available and the lack of data communication services prevents mobile phones from being an effective tool for health management. Improved infrastructure to store data and transfer data securely and in a cost-effective manner and full compatibility, interoperability, and possibly integration with other services would be the best solutions to this challenge.

Legal and Regulatory Framework for eHealth

Patient privacy is a core element of good healthcare practice and legislation and regulation are key tools in protecting privacy. According to the second global survey on ehealth by WHO, a reasonably high level of legal protection of the general privacy of health-related information exists. However, the number of countries adopting more specific ehealth-related privacy protection legislation is still low.[29]

Legal and regulatory ehealth challenges vary from ambiguous legal frameworks to poor data management (e.g., access to personal data and lack of data security rules). A lack of regulations in the transfer of data leads to any number of challenges at the international level, including the following:

- Misinformation
- Unethical use
- Concealed bias
- Covert self-dealing
- Fraudulent practices
- Evasion of legitimate regulation

Security is another area within ehealth that presents many challenges. eHealth applications using mobile terminals and Internet services require authentication methods that are both convenient and highly secure. The increasing use of technology such as biometric authentication for identification is generating new challenges in security, safety, and privacy protection for healthcare providers and consumers alike. Additional information concerning international privacy and security issues is included in Chapter 19.

CONCLUSION AND FUTURE DIRECTIONS

To promote international development in health informatics, it is necessary to provide tools for the development of national and regional ehealth initiatives and strategies. The health IT and health services sectors as well as the various health professions must work together to develop national and international ehealth initiatives and strategies. Successful ehealth services require more than just technology. They require collaboration between countries and professional groups with a focus on improving the health of all.

Many international organizations are ready to assist their members in strengthening their ehealth capacity to increase the impact and effectiveness of their investment in this field. It is also important to promote cooperation among member countries and facilitate information exchange.

Many global efforts are underway to improve the uptake and adoption of health IT. Clearly health IT has become a pan-national phenomenon, as demonstrated by the international efforts and organizations described in this chapter. Global interoperability and standards efforts will continue. It is likely that mhealth efforts will expand, connectivity will increase, and all countries including those with lower levels of resources will begin to maximize the benefits offered by health IT and informatics.

REFERENCES

1. Europe's Information Society. *eHealth: ICT for better healthcare in Europe.* Europe's Information Society. http://ec.europa.eu/ehealth. 2012. Accessed May 20, 2012.
2. Kotsiopoulos I, Whitehouse D. *Assessing the progress of the eHealth Action Plan for the period 2004–2010.* European Commission. http://ec.europa.eu/information_society/activities/health/docs/policy/ehap_assess082011.pdf. August 2011. Accessed May 20, 2012.
3. Korea e-Health Association (KeHA). *Driving growth through health IT: a case study report—promotion for APEC e-Health Community Forum.* Asia-Pacific Economic Cooperation. http://aimp.apec.org/Documents/2010/LSIF/LSIF3/10_lsif3_011.pdf. September 24, 2010. Accessed November 6, 2012.
4. D'Agostino M, Novillo-Ortiz D. PAHO/WHO: eHealth conceptual model and work programme for Latin America and the Caribbean. In: Novillo-Ortiz D, Jadad AR, eds. *The Global People-Centred eHealth Innovation Forum.* London, England: Affinity; 2011 [serial online]. http://group.bmj.com/group/affinity-and-society-publishing/Satellite_18_Global_People_Centred_eHealth.pdf.
5. Pan American Health Organization. Health agenda for the Americas. Paper presented at: 37th General Assembly of the Organization of American States; June 2007; Panama City, Panama.
6. Pan American Health Organization (PAHO). *Expected results.* PAHO. http://new.paho.org/ict4health/index.php?option=com_content&view=article&id=12&Itemid=9&lang=en. 2010. Accessed November 6, 2012.
7. International Medical Informatics Association (IMIA). *IMIA LAC: Regional Federation of Health Informatics for Latin America and the Caribbean.* IMIA. http://www.imia-medinfo.org/new2/node/159. 2010. Accessed November 27, 2012.
8. World Health Organization (WHO). *Millennium Development Goals.* 2000. http://www.who.int/topics/millennium_development_goals/en/. Accessed May 23, 2012.
9. World Health Organization Regional Office for Africa. *Health Solutions in the African Region: Current Context and Perspectives.* 2010. Retrieved from http://www.afro.who.int/en/downloads/doc_download/5728-afrrc60r3-ehealth-solutions-in-the-african-region-current-context-and-perspectives.html.
10. OER Africa. HIBBs: Health Informatics Building Blocks. OER Africa. http://www.oerafrica.org/hibbs/. Accessed May 24, 2012.
11. World Health Organization (WHO). *eHealth resolutions and decisions.* 2005. http://www.who.int/healthacademy/media/WHA58-28-en.pdf. Accessed June 2, 2012.

12. Al-Shorbaji N. *eHealth and health informatics @WHO/HQ*. Pan American Health Organization. http://new.paho.org/ict4health/index.php?option=com_content&view=article&id=32%3Aehealth-and-health-informatics-whohq-by-najeeb-al-shorbaji-director-of-the-department-of-knowledge-management-and-sharing-world-health-organization-who-&catid=17%3Aentrevistas&Itemid=16&lang=en. 2010. Accessed November 16, 2012.

13. World Health Organization (WHO). *Global Observatory for eHealth: Alphabetical list of the ehealth country profiles*. WHO. http://www.who.int/goe/data/country_report/en/index.html. 2005. Accessed June 20, 2012.

14. World Health Organization (WHO). Global Observatory for eHealth: Publications. WHO. http://www.who.int/goe/publications/en/. Accessed June 20, 2012.

15. World Health Organization (WHO). *A collaborative arrangement between the International Health Terminology Standards Development Organization and the World Health Organization*. http://www.who.int/classifications/AnnouncementLetter.pdf. 2010. Accessed May 20, 2012.

16. International Medical Informatics Association (IMIA). General. 2013. http://www.imia-medinfo.org/new2/node/1. Accessed January 31, 2012.

17. International Organization for Standardization (ISO). *ISO 18105: Integration of a Reference Terminology Model for Nursing*. Geneva, Switzerland: ISO; 2003.

18. Cho I, Park HA. Evaluation of the expressiveness of an ICNP-based nursing data dictionary in a computerized nursing record system. *J Am Med Inform Assoc*. 2006;13(4):456-464.

19. Lee YS, Park KO, Bong MR, Park HA. Development and evaluation of ICNP-based electronic nursing record system. *Stud Health Technol Inform*. 2009;146:498-502.

20. Hunter KM. *International Professional Standards for Telenursing Programmes*. Geneva, Switzerland: International Council of Nurses; 2001.

21. International Council of Nurses (ICN). *Goals and benefits*. ICN. http://www.icn.ch/networks/goals-and-benefits/. 2011. Accessed November 16, 2012.

22. Hammond W. Semantic interoperability issue of standardizing medical vocabularies. In: Mohammed S, Fiaidhi J, eds. *Ubiquitous Health and Medical Informatics: The Ubiquity 2.0 Trend and Beyond*. Hershey, PA: IGI Global; 2010:19-42.

23. Qamar R. *Semantic Mapping of Clinical Model Data to Biomedical Terminologies to Facilitate Interoperability*. [doctoral thesis]. Manchester, England: University of Manchester; 2008. http://www.openehr.org/publications/archetypes/RQamar-PhD-Thesis-Mar2008.pdf. Accessed May 20, 2012.

24. Gibson CJ, Covvey HD. *Demystifying e-health human resources*. Information Resources Management Association. http://www.irma-international.org/viewtitle/53656/, DOI:10.4018/978-1-60960-561-2.ch501. 2010. Accessed May 20, 2012.

25. World Health Organization (WHO) Global Observatory for eHealth. *eHealth Tools and Services: Needs of the Member States*. Geneva, Switzerland: WHO; 2006. http://www.who.int/kms/initiatives/tools_and_services_final.pdf.

26. Coverdell M, Utley R. The health care information gap: a global and national perspective. *Online Journal of Nursing Informatics*. 2005;9(1). http://ojni.org/9_1/coverdell.htm. Accessed May 20, 2012.

27. International Telecommunication Union (ITU). ICT Data and Statistics (IDS): Global ICT developments. 2008. http://www.itu.int/ITU-D/ict/statistics/ict/index.html. Accessed May 20, 2012.

28. Internet World Stats. *Usage and populations statistics: 2011*. Internet World Stats. http://www.internetworldstats.com/. 2011. Accessed May 28, 2012.

29. World Health Organization (WHO). Legal frameworks for ehealth. WHO. http://whqlibdoc.who.int/publications/2012/9789241503143_eng.pdf. 2012. Accessed May 20, 2012.

DISCUSSION QUESTIONS

1. What ehealth initiatives exist in different regions of the world? Compare and contrast their aims and activities.
2. Discuss two international organizations involved in ehealth initiatives. Describe their roles and provide a sample of their activities.
3. What kinds of international academic organizations are available in different regions of the world? Based on your specialty, choose which conferences are most appropriate for you to attend and explain why.
4. What kinds of roles can a health practitioner in your specialty play in the ehealth initiatives?
5. How can the different disciplines in health informatics use the current international efforts to work together with an interprofessional approach to improving the health of individuals, families, and communities?

CASE STUDY

You have been awarded a scholarship to visit South Korea for the next 6 months as an international student in healthcare informatics. The following description was included in the materials you received with the announcement of your award.

Health IT (with more recent focus on ehealth) infrastructure in the Republic of Korea has come a long way within a short period since the establishment of the Korea e-Health Association (KeHA) in 2003 by the Korean Ministry of Commerce, Industry, and Energy. Since then, four related government departments in the Ministry of Health and Welfare; Ministry of Knowledge and Economy; Ministry of Education, Science, and Technology; and the Ministry of Public Administration and Security have started planning and promoting their own strategies for ehealth applications. The departments have defined standardization, law and policy planning, human resources development, research and development (R&D) for ehealth products, and international collaboration as the five core pillars for the development of successful ehealth. In 2008, through the reorganization of the Korean government, ehealth has become an even more important growth engine for the Korean economy. Consequently, relevant government ministries produced more concrete and robust action plans for the realization of ehealth on the ground. Korean ehealth reached an important turning point with the establishment of KeHA in 2003. KeHA became the focal point of a national effort to develop ehealth in the Republic of Korea, with a focus on policy research, regulation, standardization, ehealth R&D, and ehealth best practices. KeHA and the Ministry of Knowledge and Economy collaborated internationally through Asia-Pacific Economic Cooperation (APEC) because ehealth was no longer considered a merely local concept. Korea hosted the APEC eHealth Seminar from 2004 to 2009, with support and sponsorship from the APEC Health Working Group and the Republic of Korea. Through this international collaboration, Korea began sharing information, knowledge, experience, and solutions regarding ehealth with countries around the world.

Discussion Questions

1. What universities, medical centres, professional organizations, government agencies, and individuals would you include on your "must visit" list?
2. How did you identify the list from question 1 as being important to your study of health informatics?
3. How would you learn about the history, culture, values, and health-related challenges of Korea before your visit?

The Present and Future

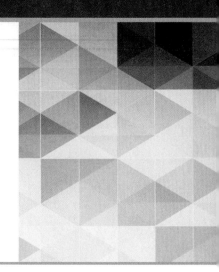

Future Directions and Future Research in Health Informatics

Nancy Staggers, Ramona Nelson, and David E. Jones

Health informatics can be described as an interprofessional discipline that is grounded in the present while planning for the future.

OBJECTIVES

At the completion of this chapter the reader will be prepared to:
1. Explore major trends and their implications for future developments in healthcare, health informatics, and informatics research
2. Analyze techniques and challenges of planning for future directions and trends
3. Apply futurology methodologies in identifying trends and possible, probable, and preferred futures
4. Describe the field of nanotechnology and its subdisciplines, the role of informatics in nanotechnology, and implications for healthcare
5. Analyze the advantages and disadvantages of nanotechnology in health and health informatics

KEY TERMS

ABSTRACT

This chapter expands on the future directions sections included in the individual chapters to provide broad guidance about the future of informatics. First, healthcare trends in society are outlined. Second, futures studies or futurology (methods to analyze probable future directions in any field) is discussed. Third, an overview of potential future directions in informatics are discussed, including the following informatics trends: (1) patient engagement, consumerism, and informatics; (2) electronic health records (EHRs) 2.0; (3) usability and improving the user health information technology (health IT) experience; (4) big data and data visualization; and (5) nanotechnology and nanoinformatics. The last trend is discussed in more detail as an example of the major influence each of these trends will likely have on the future of healthcare and society as a whole. The organization and depth of the nanotechnology-related content also provides a guide for readers to develop similar material in informatics areas of specific interest.

INTRODUCTION

Informatics will play a large role in the future of healthcare. Which informatics trends will prevail and in what depth is unclear. In each of the chapters in this book authors outlined expanding areas of influence, from knowledge discovery to the epatient, from cloud computing to standards integration with public health data sharing, and from initial EHR installations to mobile health. In this chapter unequivocal healthcare trends are listed, followed by methods that readers may use to predict likely trends in the future. These techniques are called futurology or futures research methods. Subsequently, five major trends are discussed: (1) patient engagement, consumerism, and informatics; (2) EHRs 2.0; (3) usability and improving the user experience for health IT; (4) big data and data visualization; and (5) nanotechnology and nanoinformatics. Special attention is given to nanotechnology and nanoinformatics.

The purpose of informatics is to provide support for clinical care, public health, and other practices. Thus to understand the future of health informatics, major health trends need to be acknowledged. Examples of unequivocal trends in society include:

- *Rising healthcare costs.* In the U.S. alone, costs are expected to nearly double to $4.5 trillion by 2019, up from $2.5 trillion in 2009.[1]
- *Aging populations.* By 2050 the global population of those aged 60 years or older will be more than 2 billion.[2]
- *Increase in patients with chronic diseases.* By 2030 chronic diseases will be the leading cause of deaths worldwide.[3] Diabetes rates alone will increase by 2.8% to 4.4%.[4]
- *Predicted shortage of healthcare providers.* By 2025 the U.S. will have a shortage of an estimated 260,000 registered nurses[5] and 124,000 physicians.[6]
- *Health insurance reform.* Several health reform measures are scheduled to take effect in 2014, according to the provisions of the Patient Protection and Affordable Care Act signed into law on March 10, 2010.[7]

These trends clearly have implications for informatics support in the future but how does one determine or perhaps even create future trends? Futures research or futurology, the methods used to determine future trends in any field, may help to answer this question.

FUTURES RESEARCH OR FUTUROLOGY

Health informatics can be described as an interprofessional discipline that is grounded in the present while planning for the future. Health informatics specialists are selecting and implementing today's healthcare information systems, thereby creating the foundation for the systems of tomorrow. By reviewing current trends and predictions, as well as employing tools for predicting and managing the future, health informatics specialists can prepare for their leadership role in planning for the effective and innovative healthcare information systems of the future. This section introduces the reader to levels of change that can be anticipated in future trends. By analyzing methodologies and tools for predicting, planning for, and managing the future, health informatics specialists are introduced to the kind of leadership roles they will play in planning future healthcare information systems. With a better understanding of the potential future, informatics professionals can make better current decisions.

Defining Futures Research or Futurology

Futures research is the rational and systematic study of the future with the goal of identifying possible, probable, and preferable futures. The formal study of the future goes by a number of names, including *foresight and futures studies, strategic foresight, prospective studies, prognostic studies,* and *futurology.* Using a research approach to formally study the future began after World War II. Since that time a number of institutes, foundations, and professional associations were established supporting the field of futures studies. Examples of these are included in Box 31-1. However, from the beginning, this field of study aroused skepticism. Today researchers and corporate strategists may use numerous concepts, theories, principles, and methods that are based on the field of futures research but they may not associate these methods with the field of futurology.[8] A number of educational programs related to futures studies now use the various futurology terms to describe their programs. Box 31-2 includes examples of educational programs related to this field. Despite the initial skepticism about the topic, today the futures studies techniques are accepted, educational programs are available, and these methods can be very useful for informaticists.

The focus of futures studies has evolved over time. Initially, futures studies tended to focus on a longer time horizon of at least 10 years. Today researchers are typically studying the world anywhere from 5 to 50 years from now.[9] This creates an overlap of futures studies with traditional forecasting and planning disciplines that examine political, economic, and market trends on a 1- to 5-year horizon.

Health informatics can use traditional forecasting and planning methods in combination with futures studies methods as well as futures studies. Strategic planning in health informatics typically focuses on projects 1 to 3 years in the future. Institutional long-range planning tends to focus on 5 to 10 years in the future. For example, vendor contracts for major healthcare informatics systems often cover a 5- to 10-year period spanning both strategic and long-range planning. However, there are some differences between forecasting and futures studies.

First, forecasters focus on incremental changes from existing trends while futurists focus on systemic, transformational

> ### BOX 31-1 FUTURES STUDIES: SELECTED ASSOCIATIONS, INSTITUTES, AND FOUNDATIONS
>
> - Acceleration Studies Foundation, http://accelerating.org/index.html
> - Copenhagen Institute for Future Studies, www.cifs.dk/en/
> - Foresight Canada, www.foresightcanada.ca/
> - Fullerton and Cypress Colleges, and School of Continuing Education: Center for the Future, http://fcfutures.fullcoll.edu
> - The Arlington Institute, www.arlingtoninstitute.org
> - Association of Professional Futurists, www.profuturists.org
> - The Club of Rome, www.clubofrome.org
> - *The Futurist,* www.wfs.org/futurist/about-futurist
> - Institute for the Future, www.iftf.org/home
> - The Millennium Project, www.millennium-project.org
> - World Future Society, www.wfs.org/node/920
> - World Futures Studies Federation (WFSF), www.wfsf.org

change. Second, futurists do not offer a single prediction. Rather, they describe alternative, possible, and preferable futures, keeping in mind that the future will be created, in most part, by decisions made today. The technical, political, and sociocultural infrastructure being built today will have a major impact on the choices of tomorrow. Both types of change are key to planning health informatics products.[10] Understanding the impact of future trends and using this information for planning begins by understanding the degree and scope of change that occurs over time.

Future Directions and Level of Change

The 1890 United States census count was finished months ahead of schedule and far under budget by using a punch card counting machine. This technology continued to be used by the U.S. Census Bureau well into the 1950s because the problem to be solved remained basically unchanged. Each decade, the Census Bureau was challenged to count the number of people in the population and certain characteristics about the population. Over the decades the population characteristics to be counted changed but the need to count these data remained the same.

In the 1950s the Census Bureau introduced new technology in the form of computers and magnetic computer tape. The basic problem remained the same but new technology offered more efficient and effective methods for solving that problem. The Census Bureau's introduction of new technology is an example of a first-level change. With a first-level change a new technology solves a problem in a more efficient or effective manner.

For example, replacing a typewriter with a word processer is an example of a first-level change. One is still producing a document but the technology makes the process more effective and efficient. Another example is the use of Bar Code Medication Administration (BCMA) methods. Scanning a bar code before administering medication can make the process of administering medication safer. However, scanning bar codes does not change the basic role or responsibility of healthcare providers. Within the levels of change, first level change is the least disruptive and the most comfortable level of change. In many ways requests that new technology be designed to fit the work-flow of healthcare providers is, in reality, a request, or perhaps a demand, for first-level change only. In fact, if the equipment and related procedures do not support the current roles and responsibilities of the healthcare providers, they quickly develop workarounds to meet their requirements that the degree of change be limited to a first-level change.

A second-level change involves changing how a specific outcome is achieved. For example, historically the peer review process used by professional journals involved sending a submitted manuscript to a limited number of selected experts for an anonymous opinion. The goal was to ensure that only the highest quality articles were published. The process of review and revision could take several weeks or months. In addition, with a limited number of experts screening what is published, some degree of professional censorship existed. Articles representing a paradigm shift in thinking risked being rejected as not on target by a limited set of reviewers. Today, professional online journals, where all readers can comment on material, are changing who is involved and how the peer review process is completed, with comments from readers assuming a more important role than in the past. Similarly, patient groups within social media applications are changing how patients learn about their health problems. Groups of patients help each other to read and interpret the latest research to create a whole new level of health literacy within these groups. Social media interactions not only change the process for achieving an outcome, but also change the relationships between the participants. For example, as patients become organized and knowledgeable, they take a more active role in their own care and move from the role of patients needing education about their diseases into more of a colleague role, sharing new and innovative findings with healthcare providers.

The scope of change at this level creates both excitement and anxiety within professional groups and among individual healthcare providers. The scope of practice, policies, procedures, and established professional customs, such as professional boundaries, are challenged and resistance to this challenge can be expected. For example, in healthcare the goals of improved health for individuals, families, groups, and communities have not changed but technology is changing the roles and responsibilities related to how these goals might be achieved.

A third-level change alters the process and can also refocus the goal. For example, a hyperlinked multimedia journal, with a process for adding reader comments and linking to related publications, may change not only the definition of an expert, but also the historical gold standard for review of new information and knowledge. Another example can be seen in the use of knowledge discovery and data mining with big data to discover clusters and relationships, as opposed to using a theory and hypothesis to develop a traditional clinical trial, thereby redefining (or at least expanding) the concept of research. Third-level change involves changes at the societal and institutional level, typically occurring over long periods of time. For instance, the evolving role of the nurse from a handmaiden for the physician to a leader in healthcare delivery can be seen as a third-level change.

Today, innovations in healthcare and computer technology are interactively creating first-, second-, and third-level changes, creating the future of healthcare within a society that is also undergoing change at all levels. Informatics experts are among the key leaders managing and guiding these change processes within healthcare. However, they face a number of challenges in achieving these goals.

The Challenge of Anticipating Future Directions

In 1970 Alvin Toffler published the book *Future Shock*.[11] One of the themes in the book was "what happens to people when they are overwhelmed by change. It is about how we adapt or fail to adapt to the future."[11(p1)] Interestingly, *Future Shock* was written long before the widespread use of personal computers or the Internet. Today innovations in practice and technology are changing healthcare delivery at an ever-increasing speed. As Toffler identified many decades ago in a slower-paced world, for many the degree and speed of change is overwhelming. This includes people in healthcare in the midst of a knowledge explosion who must do more than just adjust to overwhelming change.

While there are no research methods for predicting the future with absolute certainty, techniques can be used to rationally predict future directions and trends. A historical example of this is the publication of the book *Megatrends* by John Naisbitt in 1982, well before the general population was even aware of the Internet or the potential of owning a computer. Megatrends are trends that affect all aspects of society. The 10 trends identified by Naisbitt are listed in Box 31-3. These trends, identified many years ago, continue to have a major influence on health informatics today.

While health informatics specialists clearly recognize the importance of planning and the long-term implications of building today's healthcare information systems, there are immediate challenges in thinking about the future. First, present issues are often more pressing and take a higher

priority over tasks that can wait for another day. This type of thinking is sometimes referred to as "putting out fires." For example, a health informatics specialist may spend an afternoon answering users' questions but as the number of communications increases, the notes documenting these calls can become increasingly sparse. Trends and patterns that could be used as a basis for a new education and training program, or for upgrading functions in the current healthcare informatics system, can be lost in the pressing demands of the moment.

Second, small rates of growth often seem insignificant. However, major trends start from small, persistent rates of growth. This is especially true when dealing with exponential growth. A few years ago very few patients asked for copies of their health reports and a very small percentage of those patients would have considered accessing their healthcare data via the Internet. In August 2012 the Veterans Health Administration (VHA) reported that the one millionth patient had used the Blue Button application to download data from his or her personal health record (PHR).[12]

Third, there are intellectual, imaginative, and emotional limits to the amount of change that individuals and organizations can anticipate. The imagined future is built on assumptions developed in the past and therefore includes gaps and misinterpretations. Future predications can seem vague and the farther one looks into the future, the more disconnect there is between the present and the significance of the future. For example, nurses educated in small diploma schools 50 years ago usually called a physician to restart an intravenous (IV). Nurses from that time period would have struggled to anticipate the high levels of responsibility common in today's staff nursing role.

Approaches for Predicting

Qualitative and quantitative methods are used in traditional forecasting and planning as well as by futurists to foresee, manage, and create the future. The use of established research methods separates these researchers from soothsayers. Multiple methods used in concert are needed to identify and address future challenges. Selected examples of these methods are presented here. In addition, Box 31-4 includes resources for exploring a number of other methodologies used in this field of study.

Trend Analysis and Extrapolation

Trend analysis involves looking at historical data and identifying trends over time in those data. For example, a log of help desk calls may demonstrate that over the past 2 months there has been an increasing number of calls from clinical managers and department heads concerning the institution's newly introduced budget software. The new software offers a number of options and levels of analysis that were not used in the past and it is more robust and complex. Initially there were several calls from three managers who work in the same division. However, these managers are now making very few calls. Instead, the majority of the calls are coming from a different division. Extrapolation consists of extending these historical data into the future. For example, if the trend line is sloping upward, one

---

BOX 31-3	**NAISBITT'S MEGATRENDS FOR THE 1980s**

Industrial society → Information society
Forced technology → High tech/High touch
National economy → World economy
Short term → Long term
Centralized → Decentralized
Institutional help → Self-help
Representative democracy → Participatory democracy
Hierarchies → Networking
North → South
Either/Or → Multiple options

would continue this line at the same degree of slope into future time periods. Needless to say, this historical upward trend line will not continue forever. Eventually the growth will start to slow and an S curve will develop. With an S curve the growth is slow initially but then becomes very rapid. Once the event begins to reach its natural limit the rate of growth slows again.

A potential example of this pattern is the future use of PHRs by the general public. Initially only a small number of people were using this resource. Google, an early entrant in PHR development, withdrew from this market because of lack of interest by the general public. However, the current Blue Button data from the VHA suggests that the use of PHRs may be at the beginning of an S curve, with the possibility of very rapid growth in the next few years. The expected patterns of growth can be used to plan educational programming as well as support services. The need for these services can be expected to grow and then level off.

While trend analysis and extrapolation demonstrate using quantitative methods to foresee the future, qualitative methods

are also important. One example of qualitative methods is content analysis.

Content Analysis

Content analysis was the major research approach used to identify the trends in the book *Megatrends*.[13] Content analysis within the futures research realm involves reviewing a number of information resources and noting what topics are discussed, what is being said about these topics, and what topics are not discussed. A current example of this type of analysis can be seen in the application MappyHealth (www.mappyhealth.com). MappyHealth uses an automated process to search Twitter posts, looking for trends related to a specific list of diseases. A screenshot showing the types of data being tracked is provided in Figure 31-1. The assumptions made in identifying resources, topics, and trends to monitor can have a major impact on determining the forecasts produced. For example, the initial version of MappyHealth was limited to a list of specific diseases. This is one of the reasons why it is important that informatics specialists review several different resources from several different perspectives to analyze trends.

Scenarios

Scenarios involve asking individuals to envision possible futures within a certain context. For example, people may be asked to describe the EHR one might expect to see 10 to 15 years in the future. This can be done as a group process or individually. Participants should be encouraged to envision scenarios that are multifaceted and holistic, internally consistent, and free of personal bias. Elements in the scenario should not be contradictory or improbable. A well-constructed scenario may suggest events and conditions not presently being considered.

The following three major approaches can be used to construct a scenario:

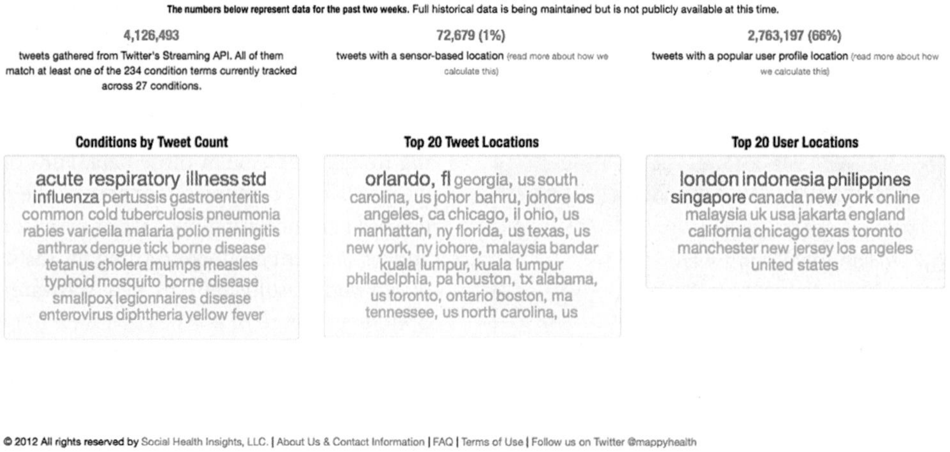

BOX 31-4   FUTURES STUDIES METHODOLOGIES RESOURCES

- Methods and Approaches of Futures Studies, http://crab.rutgers.edu/~goertzel/futuristmethods.htm
- World Future Society:
  - Methods, www.wfs.org/methods
  - Methodologies Forum, www.wfs.org/method.htm
- Futures Research Methodology Version 3.0, www.millennium-project.org/millennium/FRM-V3.html
- Five Views of the Future: A Strategic Analysis Framework, www.tfi.com/pubs/w/pdf/5views_wp.pdf
- Methodologies for Studying Change and the Future, www.csudh.edu/global_options/IntroFS.HTML#FSMethodols

---

FIG 31-1 MappyHealth home page. (Copyright Mappyhealth.org.)

1. The Delphi method can be used to elicit expert forecasts for a specific time frame. A combination or synthesis of opinions is used to develop the scenario.
2. Experts develop scenarios that reflect the viewpoint of their disciplines. These are modified and combined to produce an overall scenario.
3. A cross-impact technique is used to test the effect of one aspect of the scenario on all of its contributing parts.

The creation of scenarios can be used in concert with backcasting.

Backcasting

With backcasting one envisions a desired future end point and then works backward to determine what activities and policies would be required to achieve that future. Backcasting involves the following six steps:
1. Determine goals or the desired future state
2. Specify objectives and constraints
3. Describe the present system
4. Specify exogenous variables
5. Undertake scenario analysis
6. Undertake impact analysis

The end result of backcasting is to develop alternative images of the future, thoroughly analyzed as to their feasibility and consequences.[14]

With the rapid changes in informatics, the use of futures research methods is likely to increase. For the first generation of EHRs and data warehouses, informatics specialists have concentrated more on initial implementations than on forecasting future needs. For the next generations of health IT products, futurology can more readily be incorporated in the health informaticist's suite of skills.

Application of Futures Research

The health informatics specialist uses methodologies and strategies from futures studies in two primary ways. First is foreseeing or predicting future trends and directions. For example, in the 1970s and 1980s much of healthcare was financed via fee-for-service funding approaches. Health information systems were designed to capture charges but not to measure the cost of care. A number of items, including nursing and other services, are included in the patient's charge for a hospital room. In a fee-for-service approach, the contribution of each of these items to the total cost was irrelevant. Cost and charges did not need to correlate. The charge could be whatever the market would bear.

The introduction of the prospective payment system in the 1980s and managed care in the 1990s required that healthcare institutions capture costs rather than just charges. Existing information systems were totally ineffective in capturing costs. The ability to predict these kinds of major changes in healthcare delivery could be a significant advantage to vendors and healthcare institutions alike. By predicting the potential costs and benefits, one is better prepared to manage these events. Cost–benefit analysis is an example of using futures studies for management.

Creating the future is the second way in which health informatics specialists use futures studies methods. By thinking of possible futures scenarios, the informatics specialist can work toward creating the environment in which these futures might be possible. By using the work of futurists, as well as applying futures studies tools, it is feasible to imagine possible future trends and directions and thereby work to create preferable future directions.

THE FUTURE OF INFORMATICS

Health informatics is and will remain a dynamic and complex field. Thus accurately predicting precise directions for the future of health informatics is inherently uncertain. An informal survey of health informatics experts at Medical Informatics Europe 2012 and NI2012 resulted in the following interesting list of projected topics with little overlap (listed in no particular order):
- Robotics
- Cloud computing and "drops from clouds"
- Big data, analytics, and meta-analytics
- Data visualization and information synthesis
- Usability, participatory design, and usability labs
- Augmented reality
- Interprofessional collaboration and cooperation within facilities, across diverse fields inside and outside of informatics, including their implications
- Process modeling with biomedical engineering
- Risk analysis
- eHealth indicators for countries and across nations
- Modularized health informatics systems (available functions or applications versus whole systems)
- Mobile devices for health applications (mhealth)
- Evaluation studies on the impacts of health informatics products
- Personal health, patient-centered health system and applications (moving away from a provider-centered health system), and their implications for informatics
- Ontologies and interoperability, version 2.0
- Health reform and how informatics supports it
- Data reuse for policy-making and decision making
- Theoretical and model-based informatics
- Research-based healthcare using informatics tools
- Increased emphasis on guidelines and protocols to improve care
- EHRs 2.0, redesigned and rethought
- Research and scholarly outlets limited by vendor-support EHRs
- Policy and education role for informaticists[15]

Formal literature does not provide consensus about emerging or future directions for informatics. Most recently, authors wrote about the future of academic biomedical informatics in 2012[15]; a nursing informatics research agenda for 2008 to 2018[16]; medical informatics past, present, and future in 2010[17]; harnessing information and communication technologies for nurses worldwide in 2008[18]; informatics

TABLE 31-1	TRENDS IN HEALTHCARE IMPORTANT TO HEALTH IT
TREND	**DESCRIPTION**
Wellness first	Focus on wellness versus illness
ePower to the patient	Patients take on a larger, more active role in managing their wellness and health
Earlier detection	Earlier detection maximizes options for successful treatment, leading to a speedier return to good health
High-tech healing	New technologies can significantly boost outcomes and quality of life
Resources: more but different	Solving the healthcare resource puzzle requires new players and new care models
Global healthcare ecosystem emerges	More information, more connected, leads to better care and better research.

Adapted from Forum LE. *The Future of Healthcare: It's Health, Then Care.* Falls Church, VA: Computer Sciences Corporation (CSC); 2010.

directions from an IT consulting firm (Table 31-1); and an agenda for nursing informatics in 2006.[19] Within informatics and nursing, major past efforts internationally have centered on terminology development.[20] Beyond that, a consensus of themes is not apparent across articles and little collaboration to develop future directions across disciplines is evident.

Outside the field of healthcare, contemporary issues of *The Futurist* (www.wfs.org/futurist) list its annual outlook on trends for society. Trends pertinent to healthcare include the following:

- *New leader skills.* These will be shaped by those with social networking, content management, data mining, and data meaning skills. New job titles include Chief Content Officer and Chief Data Scientist.[21]
- *Nanotechnology products.* Buckypaper is composed of industrial-grade carbon nanotubes and is 100 times stronger than steel per unit of weight. It conducts electricity like copper and disperses heat like steel or brass.[22]
- *Nanorobots or nanobots.* These carry molecule-sized elements, can detect cancer, and are being developed by researchers at Harvard University.[23]
- *Full-body firewalls.* These are necessary to prevent hackers from tampering with wireless medical devices and internal drug delivery systems. Researchers at Purdue and Princeton universities are developing a medical monitor (MedMon) designed to identify potentially malicious activity.[24]
- *Ubiquitous computing environments.* Workplaces will become ubiquitous computing environments that include computing capabilities and connectivity.[25]
- *Image-driven communication.* Graphics and images will be more heavily relied on for communication, allowing faster comprehension and possibly new ways of thinking but at the cost of eloquence and precision.[26]
- *Living data.* Connectivity will expand to millions of things and sensors will gather more data that will be processed by more computers. Data may become too big, so channeling the power of data will become important.[27]
- *The intelligent "cloud."* This will become not just a place to store data but will evolve into an active resource providing analysis and contextual advice.[28]

Due to the lack of consensus on trends, this chapter weaves threads from available publications, chapter authors' thoughts,

and other current informatics perspectives into the following five major themes:

- Consumerism and informatics
- EHRs 2.0
- Usability and improving the user experience for health IT
- Big data and data visualization
- Nanotechnology and nanoinformatics

A substantial part of the chapter is devoted to nanotechnology and nanoinformatics because the topic is likely new to most readers. Also, given its potential impact on society and funding largess in the billions of dollars worldwide, nanotechnology is currently underemphasized in health education and health informatics.

Consumerism and Informatics

A shift is occurring away from provider-centric care toward patient-centered or consumer-centered care.[19,21,29] Through current informatics tools, consumers are being supported as they assume more responsibility for their own care, especially those consumers with chronic diseases. The importance of this shift is underscored in several chapters of this book: Chapter 8 (telehealth), Chapter 9 (home health), Chapter 13 (the evolving epatient), Chapter 14 (social media and social networking), and Chapter 15 (PHRs). This future direction is clear and will only grow over time. For example, the design of tailored, mhealth (mobile health) PHRs could include the following:

- Theory-based studies on the impact of consumer health IT products
- The integration of consumer and provider health IT products to increase care collaboration

EHRs 2.0

Clearly, the billions of dollars in Health Information Technology for Economic and Clinical Health (HITECH) Act funding directed at healthcare provider incentives will drive development of future EHRs and correlated topics of interoperability and impact. The HITECH Act funding will continue to increase the number of implemented EHRs, especially among eligible professionals and ambulatory practices, the main target for the HITECH Act funds. What is less clear is how these systems will affect the quality of care and the practice of healthcare. There has been a rush to implement EHRs and attend to Meaningful Use to receive financial incentives. Healthcare providers and sites could easily experience detrimental impacts to workflow and patient care, especially initially, instead of the projected benefits of EHRs. The HITECH Act did not include funding for research to assess EHR impacts,[15] so this kind of evaluative research constitutes a future direction for informatics practice as well as needed informatics research. In fact, Shortliffe[15] claims that future academics in informatics will find this kind of research one of the only research avenues available to them for EHR-related activities.

Clinicians are disgruntled with the current offerings from EHR vendors. In an editorial for *The New England Journal of Medicine*, Mandl and Kohane argue that EHR vendors propagate a myth of complexity that precludes innovation and a myth that EHRs are different than more flexible and robust consumer technology.[30] With most sites using vendor-supported EHRs, this kind of impatience from users will likely drive important changes for EHR offerings. One change might be that vendors no longer are full-service providers of EHRs. Instead, they may become smaller service and application providers, allowing sites to pick and choose best options among vendors, including nontraditional vendors such as Google or Microsoft.

Newer infrastructure, such as cloud computing, middleware, and mobile applications, could allow more robust integration efforts at the healthcare provider and consumer end of computing. Consumer demand may force EHR vendors to incorporate newer tools in their offerings, such as more robust clinical documentation tools with integrated graphics and drawing capabilities and even a basic spell-checker, which is currently lacking in today's EHRs. Mandl and Kohane indicate that disruptive technologies for EHRs are needed to displace the current model of EHRs. This suggests another future direction for EHRs.

Interoperability efforts will continue, especially in the U.S., where the diversity of products and EHR components has caused the nation to lag behind others in creating integrated, national, longitudinal patient EHRs. Regional integration efforts have helped in the effort to share data. Interoperability beyond regions will be a continued, costly future direction for the U.S. No doubt informatics research and operational efforts on ontologies will continue to facilitate this work, although efforts have been ongoing for decades. What is needed is consensus about ontologies, especially for nursing.

As EHR implementations increase, it is possible that the traditional view of EHRs may fade. EHRs may be less organization- and site-specific, becoming dispersed with data owners related to roles (patient, healthcare provider, insurer, lab, pharmacy, etc.) and data pulled and integrated from geographic or other defined areas. A particular need for the future is more interdisciplinary views and collaborations for EHRs. Given the importance of teams in healthcare, the next generation of EHRs, no matter how they are instantiated, should offer collaborative workflow tools and methods for synthesizing data and information for "at-a-glance" views

across disciplines, sites, types of agencies, and traditional EHR modules.

Potential areas for future research include the following:
- Evaluative research on the impacts of EHRs from various viewpoints of patients, healthcare providers, teams, care outcomes, and quality of care
- Impacts of integrative views of patient-centered data across traditional EHR modules and disciplines
- Cost-effectiveness research and comparative effectiveness for EHR designs

Usability and Improving the User Experience for Health IT

In the U.S., recent efforts will likely ensure that improving the user experience is a future trend in health IT. As noted in Chapter 21, two federal agencies are currently involved in EHR usability initiatives: the National Institute of Standards and Technology and the Office of the National Coordinator for Health Information Technology, whose Meaningful Use Stage 2 language includes a section on EHR usability. In June 2012 the Food and Drug Administration released draft language called "Applying Human Factors and Usability Engineering to Optimize Medical Device Design," available at www.fda.gov/ MedicalDevices/DeviceRegulationandGuidance/Guidance Documents/ucm259748.htm. These kinds of regulations are likely to proliferate in the future and become more stringent because of patient safety issues.

Given healthcare provider and consumer voices, health IT usability is a much needed future trend. Federal requirements will continue to expand and vendors will have to respond to the need for improved products. Organizations will need to increase their knowledge about and skills for improving the user experience. An excellent resource for meeting this challenge is the Healthcare Information and Management Systems Society (HIMSS) Usability Maturity Model.[31] Additional information on this model can be found at HIMSS.org by searching the terms *usability* and *maturity*.

Research directions for improving the user experience are many. Examples include the following:
- Comparative effectiveness research on EHR and device designs, especially for complex patient views, such as clinical summaries, care transitions, and Electronic Medication Administration Records (eMARs).
- Developing and implementing best design practices agnostic of vendors. Perhaps decoupling user views from underlying code could occur so that optimal designs could be downloaded by healthcare providers and layered onto their local data.
- Determining outcomes for varying application designs. For instance, improved displays can positively affect clinicians' situation awareness and performance in intensive care units (ICUs).[32-34] Similar studies for other applications could be completed.

Big Data and Data Visualization

The term big data was initially defined in 2000 by Francis Diebold, an economist at the University of Pennsylvania (see his paper at http://utpl.academia.edu/nopiedra/Papers/131 6242/Big_DataDynamic_Factor_Models_for_Macro economic_Measurement_and_Forecasting). Big data resulted from vast quantities of available data due to advances in storage technology. Initially downplayed as ambiguous, the term became popular after an October 2010 information management conference featuring IBM and Oracle.[35] For health practitioners the important concept is that huge amounts of data are being generated and relatively inexpensive storage technology will make them even more available in the future.

No matter what term is used, the world is generating mass amounts of data. IBM estimates that 2.5 quintillion bytes of information are generated each day. That is three times the equivalent of the Library of Congress each second.[36] In the life sciences, genomic data have created large datasets for analyses. Biomedical informatics efforts are underway to integrate data across disparate fields. For example, the National Center for Integrative Biomedical Informatics from the National Institutes of Health is developing interactive, integrated, analytic, and modeling technologies from molecular biology, experimental data, and published literature.[37]

Within healthcare, local data warehouses combine longitudinal EHR, administration, and financial data into a searchable database. Sensor data and input from mobile and remote technologies could be integrated with EHR data in the near future. Personalized medicine efforts and nanotechnology promise the expansion of these kinds of databases. Regional efforts and interoperability will also add to the amount of available data. Healthcare providers and informaticists will become familiar with the term *big data* and using big data will become a reality.

With large datasets an unparalleled opportunity exists to examine data and issues across thousands of data points and patients for data integrated across fields (population data, genomics, etc). However, current efforts are hampered by issues in data quality, missing clinical concepts, lack of standard terminology, and the need for specialized tools.

Analytics

One of the pressing issues with big data is making sense of vast amounts of stored data. Chapter 4 discussed one method for achieving this goal—knowledge discovery and data mining—but others are available, including analytics. The goal of data analytics is to understand big data, develop predictive models, and discover new insights. Analytics help in sense making by revealing patterns in the dataset. Figure 31-2 provides an example from biology and computer science. At the intersection of science, design, and data, data visualization involves understanding principles of human perception, design, and computing capabilities.[38]

In the life sciences, interdisciplinary teams of biologists and computer scientists developed interactive visualization tools like MulteeSum to compare genes in fruit flies.[39] In healthcare, analytic tools for searching data warehouses are emerging and are called business intelligence tools. Because analyzing data and making conclusions from stored data can

affect organizational and patient care decisions, the data visualization effort will be an important future trend.

Many analytic tools are available in the marketplace to assist healthcare practitioners. See, for example, a white paper by Gartner Consulting that compares currently available tools at http://www.qlikview.com/us/explore/resources/analyst-reports/gartner-magic-quadrant-business-intelligence-bi-platform.

Research directions for big data and analytic tools include the following:
- Developing interactive visualization tools for health practitioners, especially for nursing, pharmacy, and those less often emphasized
- Developing big data sets combining published literature, population data, and regional data warehouses
- Detecting patterns for interventions and outcomes in regional data warehouses

Nanotechnology

The statement "Big things come in small packages" is appropriate to the field of nanotechnology. Nanotechnology is the study of controlling and altering matter at the atomic or molecular level.[40] The focus of the field is the creation of materials, devices, and other structures at the nanoscale (1 to 1000 nm). The produced items are referred to as nanomaterials, which are composed of smaller subunits called nanoparticles. Nanotechnology is a diverse field that requires a collaborative environment across multiple domains (e.g., surface engineering, physics, organic chemistry, molecular biology, and materials science).

History of Nanotechnology

Even though the majority of research in the field of nanotechnology has been conducted in the past few decades, the field began in 1959 when Richard P. Feynman presented a lecture titled "There's Plenty of Room at the Bottom."[41] In this talk he discussed being able to manipulate individual atoms, which would allow for more flexibility and use in synthetic chemistry.

The field expanded in the 1980s with the invention of the scanning tunneling microscope and the discovery of fullerenes. With the scanning tunneling microscope, scientists could visualize particles at the nanoscale. In 1985 Harry Kroto and his collaborators discovered a molecule composed solely of carbon, which they named Buckminsterfullerene.[42] Buckminsterfullerene is a spherical molecule composed of 60 carbon atoms. This gives the molecule a high structural integrity and makes it very stable. This discovery laid the foundation for the development of one of the most well-recognized nanoparticles, the carbon nanotube. A carbon nanotube is a nanoparticle composed of carbon atoms bound to one another to form a tubelike structure (Fig. 31-3). Carbon nanotubes are a member of the fullerene family of molecules. They have a unique combination of thermal conductivity, mechanical properties, and electrical properties

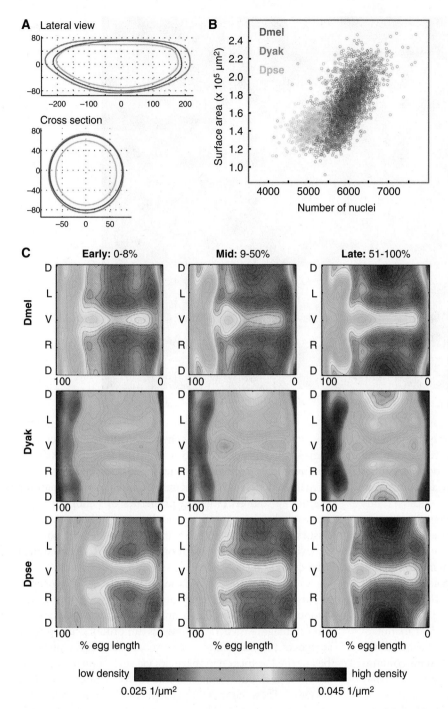

FIG 31-2 Example of visualization tools used to compare fruit fly attributes. (From Fowlkes CC, Eckenrode KB, Bragdon MD, et al. A conserved developmental patterning network produces quantitatively different output in multiple species of Drosophila. *PLoS Genet.* 2011;7[10]:e1002346.)

that makes them useful in the development of structural materials.

Nanofabrication and Nanomedicine

Nanomaterials and nanoparticles are used in electronics, biomaterials, and healthcare. Some claim that this area of science and technology has the opportunity to revolutionize our world. Manipulation of particles at the nanoscale allows the creation of unique materials with special properties (e.g., unique chemical, physical, or biologic properties, such as increased electrical conductivity or strength). The special properties are due to the particles' incredibly small size, which allows absorption or unique movement, and also due to increased surface areas that interact with their environments, creating increased interactions of materials.

Nanofabrication. Nanofabrication is the development of materials used in structures, electronics, and commercial products. Fabricated nanoparticles are typically added to larger physical structures to enhance them, resulting in increased strength, elasticity, conductivity, or antimicrobial properties. Much work has been done with carbon nanotubes because the tubelike structure provides increased material

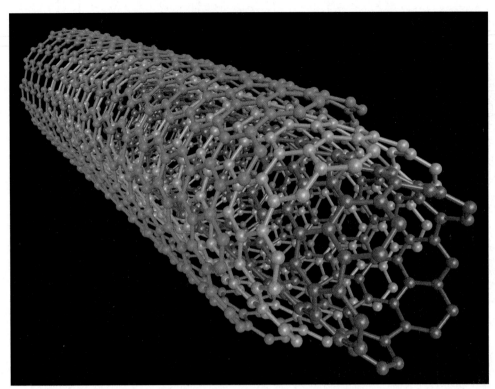

FIG 31-3 A carbon nanotube. (Copyright Owen Thomas/123RF Stock Photo.)

strength. Carbon nanotubes are now commonly used in electronics as wiring for electrical components. For example, a research group at Rice University bound carbon nanotubes to Kevlar fibers to make durable, conductive wires that can be used in wearable electronics and battery-heated body armor.[43] Quantum dots, whose elements move in all three dimensions, are another nanoparticle often used in electronics as semiconductors.

The number of commercially available items containing nanoparticles has increased at an aggressive pace over the past two decades. When the Project on Emerging Nanotechnologies (PEN) began its inventory in 2006, 212 products were listed. Now PEN estimates that more than 1300 manufactured, nanotechnology-enabled products have entered the commercial marketplace around the world.[44] Items containing nanoparticles are very diverse, ranging from everyday items such as nonstick cookware and lotions to unique items such as self-cleaning window treatments. Probably the most commonly used and commercially available product is silver nanoparticles, due to its antimicrobial properties.

Nanomedicine. Nanomedicine centers on the application of nanoparticles and nanoscience techniques to healthcare and clinical research.[45] Its primary goal is the use of nanotechnology for the diagnosis, treatment, and prevention of diseases. Applications include nanoparticles as delivery devices for pharmaceutics, diagnostic devices, and tissue replacement.[46] Due to their size and design, nanoparticles behave differently than traditional particles since they avoid the body's immune defense mechanisms, avoid filtration by the body, and interact more with tissues. Antibodies and a variety of other surface-engineered materials can be conjugated to

the surface of nanoparticles, increasing their specificity for individual cell types (e.g., tumors). Importantly, the use of nanomaterials reduces medication dosages and effects on nontargeted tissues. Current research focuses on exploiting the highly soluble, targeting properties of nanoparticles to improve the delivery of cancer drugs to tumor-containing tissues[47] and on using nanoparticles to deliver nonviral genes and small interfering ribonucleic acid (RNA) to combat viruses and cancer.[48]

Another very intriguing area of nanomedicine research is advanced imaging and thermotherapy. Quantum dot nanoparticles are used in conjunction with magnetic resonance imaging (MRI) techniques to produce exceptional images of tumorous tissues. Chemical or physical groups can be attached to these nanoparticles via surface engineering, so that they seek out tumor cells and increase the resolution of images.[49] These same nanoparticles can then be used in the treatment of tumor cells using techniques such as thermotherapy. The process aggregates nanoparticles in tumorous tissues and then excites the nanoparticles using targeted radio waves, lasers, or focused magnetic waves. The excitation causes the metals in these nanoparticles to heat up, raising the temperature of nearby tissues (localized hyperthermia) and causing targeted cell death.[50]

Work is being done to develop in vitro early detection methods using nanoparticles. Thus nanoparticles are being used as diagnostic tools. One example is the use of a dime-sized microfluidic device containing a network of carbon nanotubes coated with tumor-specific antibodies.[51] A patient's blood sample passes through the device and any tumor cells are bound to the nanotubes. Another sensor includes chips containing thousands of nanowires able to detect proteins and other biomarkers produced by cancerous cells. These types of advances could, in the future, enable the widespread detection and diagnosis of cancer in very early stages.

Cautions about Nanotechnology

Even though nanoparticles are incredibly effective and useful, caution is warranted. Unintended consequences of nanomaterials are due to secondary effects, such as cytotoxicity. For the same reasons that nanoparticles are effective (i.e., their size and increased surface interactions), they also can cause toxicity to the environment and humans. This is a key area of concern and current research in the nanoscience and nanomedicine community.[52,53] Many authors discuss inherent toxicity due to nanomaterials' cationic surface charge.[52-55] This surface charge is necessary for cellular uptake. If the charge is too high, it can create holes within the cell membranes, resulting in membrane degradation, erosion, and ultimately cell lysis. Clearance of nanoparticles from the human body is another key area of concern because nanoparticles may be rapidly eliminated by the kidneys or, alternatively, remain in circulation for long periods of time, increasing exposure and potential toxicity.

Synthetic methods such as the use of surface engineering and biodegradable components to construct nanoparticles are being employed to counteract the inherent toxicity of nanoparticles. These processes are used to alter the cationic surface charge of most nanoparticles by reducing the cationic charge, making it neutral or completely changing it to an anionic charge. However, if the surface charge of nanoparticles is reduced too much, the bioavailability of the nanoparticles is also decreased. Because of potential toxicity, nanoparticles must be evaluated carefully before they are approved for routine use in the clinical arena.[55-56]

Nanoinformatics

Nanoinformatics was created in an effort to help manage the large volumes of data being produced by the field of nanotechnology. The foundations for nanoinformatics began in 2007 by the U.S. National Science Foundation.[57] The focus of nanoinformatics is the use of biomedical informatics techniques and tools for nanoparticle data and information. In October 2011 the U.S. National Nanotechnology Initiative (NNI) document was developed, which outlined the following three major goals for nanoinformatics:

1. Enhance the quality and availability of data about nanoparticles
2. Expand nanotechnology theory, modeling, and simulation
3. Develop an informatics infrastructure[58]

The first goal has received the most attention to date. A number of groups are standardizing nanotechnology terms and developing ontologies to represent the relationships between the terms. The two most recognized standards organizations in nanotechnology are the Nanotechnology Standards Panel of the American National Standards Institute and the Nanotechnology Technical Committee of the International Organization for Standardization. The National Cancer Institute leads one of the most well-recognized ontology programs in nanotechnology, the NanoParticle Ontology.

Some progress has been made on the second and third NNI goals. The U.S. National Science Foundation hosts a site named nanoHUB that offers a wide variety of nanotechnology simulation tools for use by the general public and researchers. Overall, good progress has been made in the young field of nanoinformatics. However, the future will include much more work in this area.

In the future, one of the most pressing goals is to create an available public database of easily computable, nanoparticle data. To accomplish this, the extensive available literature on nanoparticles needs to be mined for relevant properties matched to existing standards systems or ontologies. This kind of database could then be used for future data mining and model development. Beyond that, a next goal could be to develop predictive modeling software for developing quantitative structure activity relationships for nanoparticles. This would allow researchers to develop computer-generated structural images of nanoparticles and test them in a simulated environment, allowing toxicity predictions and estimates of bioavailability.

Issues in Regulation and Ethics

Authors are debating the regulatory and ethical implications of nanomaterials because of the unique properties and potential toxicity inherent in these materials. While some indicate that current frameworks are adequate to allow regulatory and ethical assessments,[59,60] pressing considerations are evident. For example, current cosmetic products such as sunscreens are seldom labeled as containing nanomaterials,[61,62] leaving consumers uninformed. No regulations require such labeling as yet.

Scientists can manufacture completely new materials with nanoscience yet reliable information about the safety of nanomaterials lags behind their fabrication.[62] Exact risks for patients, employees, and scientists are not yet known. The potential applications for nanomaterials are enormous; likewise, their risks and regulatory and ethical implications are equally grand. Future applications could enhance oxygen storage in blood. This would, of course, be a boon to patients with emphysema but it has implications for ethics and regulation of sports competitions, as well as general use in humans.[63] More alarming findings are emerging. For instance, researchers found that nanoparticle uptake by salmon negatively altered feeding behavior and lipid metabolism.[64] This finding is of particular concern because this kind of nanoparticle ingestion mimics typical feeding activity in the food chain. Whether regulatory controls will keep pace with discoveries such as these is an issue.

Once nanomaterials are more commonplace in healthcare, ethical issues arise for the workplace related to hazards, risks, and projected controls.[65] Ethically, workers will need to be informed about potential exposure to nanomaterials and risks related to inhalation, skin absorption, or unintended ingestion. This implies a responsibility for accurate assessment by employers, communication about risks, and perhaps even a form of informed consent by workers. For patients, expanded informed consent may be needed for nano-based medications because all interactions are unlikely to be identified during testing.[46,66] Clearly, safety, regulatory, and ethical concerns are paramount for nanomaterials.

The field of nanotechnology is exciting but caution is warranted. By virtue of the rapid advancements, nanotechnology is a major future direction for informatics, informatics research, commercial product development, health products, and impact assessment.

CONCLUSION AND FUTURE DIRECTIONS

Health informatics specialists and leaders cannot afford to leave the future to chance. They must proactively and systematically identify future trends and directions in society, healthcare, technology, and informatics. This information and knowledge can provide the foundation for designing and building the health information systems of the future. The methods and trends discussed in this chapter provide tools and thoughts for health informaticists to use to identify important trends locally and regionally.

Acknowledgement: David E. Jones's contribution was supported by Grant Number T15LM007124 from the National Library of Medicine.

REFERENCES

1. Centers for Medicare & Medicaid Services. *National Health Expenditure Projections 2009–2019.* Baltimore, MD: Centers for Medicare & Medicaid Services; 2009.
2. World Health Organization (WHO). *What are the public health implications of global ageing?* WHO. http://www.who.int/features/qa/42/en/index.html. 2011. Accessed October 15, 2012.
3. Pellerin C. *Global causes of death move from infectious to chronic diseases.* America.gov. http://www.america.gov/st/health-english/2008/June/20080612141457lcnirellep0.7136347.html. June 12, 2008. Accessed January 7, 2013.
4. Wild S, Roglic G, Green A, Sicree R, King H. Global prevalence of diabetes: estimates for the year 2000 and projections for 2030. *Diabetes Care.* 2004;27(5):1047-1053.
5. American Association of Colleges of Nursing (AACN). *Nursing shortage.* AACN. http://www.aacn.nche.edu/media/FactSheets/NursingShortage.htm. August 6, 2012. Accessed October 15, 2012.
6. Association of American Medical Colleges. *The complexities of physician supply and demand: projections through 2025.* Texas Healthcare Trustees. http://www.tht.org/education/resources/AAMC.pdf. 2008. Accessed October 15, 2012.
7. HealthReform.gov. *Fact sheet: The Affordable Care Act.* Health Reform.gov. http://healthreform.gov/newsroom/new_patients_bill_of_rights.html. 2010. Accessed October 15, 2012.
8. Institute for Futures Studies and Knowledge Management. EBS Business School. http://www.ebs.edu/11866.html?&L=1.
9. Nordlund G. Time-scales in futures research and forecasting. *Futures.* 2012;44(4):408-414.
10. Nelson R. Future directions in health care informatics. In: Nelson SER, ed. *Health Informatics: An Interdisciplinary Approach.* St. Louis: Mosby; 2002:505-518.
11. Toffler T. *Future Shock.* New York, NY: Bantam Books; 1970.
12. U.S. Department of Veterans Affairs (VA). *Blue Button: download my data.* VA. http://www.va.gov/bluebutton/. 2012.
13. Naisbitt, J. *Megatrends.* New York: Warner Communication Company; 1982.
14. Goertzel T. *Methods and approaches of future studies.* Camden Computing Services, Rutgers Camden. http://crab.rutgers.edu/~goertzel/futuristmethods.htm. n.d.
15. Shortliffe EH. The future of biomedical informatics: a perspective from academia. *Stud Health Technol Inform.* 2012;180:19-24.
16. Bakken S, Stone PW, Larson EL. A nursing informatics research agenda for 2008–18: contextual influences and key components. *Nurs Outlook.* 2012;60(5):280-288, e283.
17. Haux R. Medical informatics: past, present, future. *Int J Med Inform.* 2010;79(9):599-610.
18. Abbott PA, Coenen A. Globalization and advances in information and communication technologies: the impact on nursing and health. *Nurs Outlook.* 2008;56(5):238-246, e232.
19. McCormick KA, Delaney CJ, Brennan PF, et al. Guideposts to the future—an agenda for nursing informatics. *J Am Med Inform Assn.* 2007;14(1):19-24.
20. Hovenga EJ. Milestones of the IMIA-NI history and future directions. *St Heal T.* 2009;146:3-10.
21. Colon J. Shakeups in the "C suite": hail to the new chiefs. *The Futurist.* 2012;46(4):6-7.
22. Bisk T. Unlimiting energy's growth. *The Futurist.* 2012;46(3):31.
23. World Future Society. World trends & forecasts. *The Futurist.* 2012;46(3):15-16.
24. World Future Society. Blocking bodyhackers. *The Futurist.* 2012;46(4):2.
25. World Future Society. The best predictions of 2011. *The Futurist.* 2012;46(1):30.
26. Baines L. A future of fewer words?: five trends shaping the future of language. *The Futurist.* 2012;46(2):46.
27. Johnson BD. The secret life of data in the year 2020. *The Futurist.* 2012;46(4):21-23.
28. Carbone C, Nauth K. From smart house to networked home. *The Futurist.* 2012;46(4):30.
29. Forum LE. *The Future of Healthcare: It's Health, Then Care.* Falls Church, VA: Computer Sciences Corporation; 2010.
30. Mandl KD, Kohane IS. Escaping the EHR trap—the future of health IT. *New Engl J Med.* 2012;366(24):2240-2242.
31. Healthcare Information and Management Systems Society (HIMSS). *Promoting Usability in Health Organizations: Initial Steps and Progress toward a Healthcare Usability Maturity Model.* Chicago, IL: HIMSS; 2011.
32. Koch SH, Weir C, Haar M, et al. Intensive care unit nurses' information needs and recommendations for integrated displays to improve nurses' situation awareness. *J Am Med Inform Assn.* 2012;19(4):583-590.
33. Gorges M, Staggers N. Evaluations of physiological monitoring displays: a systematic review. *J Clin Monit Comput.* 2008;22(1):45-66.
34. Drews FA, Westenskow DR. The right picture is worth a thousand numbers: data displays in anesthesia. *Hum Factors.* 2006;48(1):59-71.
35. McBurney V. *The origin and growth of big data buzz.* Toolbox for IT/Topics/Business Intelligence/Blogs. Available from: http://it.toolbox.com/blogs/infosphere/the-origin-and-growth-of-big-data-buzz-51509. 2012. Accessed January 16, 2013.
36. Silver N. The weatherman is not a moron. *The New York Times.* September 9, 2012.

37. Athey BD, Cavalcoli JD, Jagadish HV, et al. The NIH National Center for Integrative Biomedical Informatics (NCIBI). *J Am Med Inform Assn.* 2012;19(2):166-170.

38. Meyer M. *Visualizing data: why an (interactive) picture is worth 1000 numbers. Gould lecture series: technology and the quality of life.* University of Utah, September 5, 2012.

39. Meyer M, Munzner T, DePace A, Pfister H. MulteeSum: a tool for comparative spatial and temporal gene expression data. *IEEE Trans Vis Comput Graph.* 2010;16(6):908-917.

40. National Nanotechnology Initiative. *What is nanotechnology?* Nano.gov. http://www.nano.gov/nanotech-101/what/definition. 2012.

41. Feynman RP. There's plenty of room at the bottom. *Caltech Engineering and Science.* 1960;23(5):22-36.

42. Kroto HW, Heath JR, O'Brien SC, Curl RF, Smalley RE. C60: buckminsterfullerene. *Nature.* 1985;318(6042):162-163.

43. Xiang C, Lu W, Zhu Y, et al. Carbon nanotube and graphene nanoribbon-coated conductive Kevlar fibers. *ACS Appl Mater Interfaces.* 2012;4(1):131-136.

44. The Project on Emerging Nanotechnologies (PEN). *Nanotech-enabled consumer products continue to rise.* PEN. http://www.nanotechproject.org/news/archive/9231/. 2012.

45. de la Iglesia D, Maojo V, Chiesa S, et al. International efforts in nanoinformatics research applied to nanomedicine. *Methods Inf Med.* 2011;50(1):84-95.

46. Staggers N, McCasky T, Brazelton N, Kennedy R. Nanotechnology: the coming revolution and its implications for consumers, clinicians, and informatics. *Nurs Outlook.* 2008;56(5):268-274.

47. Zhao P, Wang H, Yu M, et al. Paclitaxel loaded folic acid targeted nanoparticles of mixed lipid-shell and polymer-core: in vitro and in vivo evaluation. *Eur J Pharm Biopharm.* 2012;81(2):248-256.

48. Zhou J, Liu J, Cheng CJ, et al. Biodegradable poly(amine-co-terpolymers for targeted gene delivery. *Nat Mate.* 2012;11(1):82-90.

49. Pericleous P, Gazouli M, Lyberopoulou A, Rizos S, Nikiteas N, Efstathopoulos EP. Quantum dots hold promise for early cancer imaging and detection. *Int J Cancer.* 2012;131(3):519-528.

50. Ma M, Chen H, Chen Y, et al. Au capped magnetic core/mesoporous silica shell nanoparticles for combined photothermo-/chemo-therapy and multimodal imaging. *Biomaterials.* 2012;33(3):989-998.

51. Veetil JV, Ye K. Development of immunosensors using carbon nanotubes. *Biotechnol Prog.* 2007;23(3):517-531.

52. Elsaesser A, Howard CV. Toxicology of nanoparticles. *Adv Drug Deliv Rev.* 2012;64(2):129-137.

53. Fadeel B, Garcia-Bennett AE. Better safe than sorry: understanding the toxicological properties of inorganic nanoparticles manufactured for biomedical applications. *Adv Drug Deliv Rev.* 2010;62(3):362-374.

54. Mukherjee SP, Davoren M, Byrne HJ. In vitro mammalian cytotoxicological study of PAMAM dendrimers—Towards quantitative structure activity relationships. *Toxicol In Vitro.* 2010;24(1):169-177.

55. Adiseshaiah PP, Hall JB, McNeil SE. Nanomaterial standards for efficacy and toxicity assessment. *Wiley Interdiscip Rev Nanomed Nanobiotechnol.* 2010;2(1):99-112.

56. Blobel B. Architectural approach to ehealth for enabling paradigm changes in health. *Methods Inf Med.* 2010;49(2):123-134.

57. U.S. National Science Foundation. Workshop on nanoinformatics strategies. http://128.119.56.118/~nnn01/Workshop.html. 2007. Accessed 2012.

58. National Nanotechnology Initiative (NNI). NNI 2011 Environmental, Health, and Safety Research Strategy. October 20, 2011. Available at: http://www.nano.gov/node/681. Accessed June 6, 2012.

59. Litton P. "Nanoethics"? What's new? *Hastings Cent Rep.* 2007;27(1):22-27.

60. Godman M. But is it unique to nanotechnology?: reframing nanoethics. *Sci Eng Ethics.* 2008;14(3):391-403.

61. White GB. Missing the boat on nanoethics. *Am J Bioeth.* 2009;9(10):18-19.

62. Hristozov DR, Gottardo S, Critto A, Marcomini A. Risk assessment of engineered nanomaterials: a review of available data and approaches from a regulatory perspective. *Nanotoxicology.* 2012;6:880-898.

63. Toth-Fejel T. Nanotechnology will change more than just one thing. *Am J Bioeth.* 2009;9(10):12-13.

64. Cedervall T, Hansson LA, Lard M, Frohm B, Linse S. Food chain transport of nanoparticles affects behaviour and fat metabolism in fish. *PLoS One.* 2012;7(2):e32254.

65. Schulte PA, Salamanca-Buentello F. Ethical and scientific issues of nanotechnology in the workplace. *Environ Health Perspect.* 2007;115(1):5-12.

66. Resnik DB, Tinkle SS. Ethical issues in clinical trials involving nanomedicine. *Contemp Clin Trials.* 2007;28(4):433-441.

DISCUSSION QUESTIONS

1. In your setting, which future trends are likely to have the largest effect on patient care and related information systems?

2. The 10 trends identified by Naisbitt are listed in Box 31-3. Add two columns to this box. In the first new column project where these trends will be in the next 10 years. In the second new column describe how your projected impact might influence future directions in informatics.

3. Select one of the chapter topics in this book. For example, you might select PHRs in Chapter 15. Use the three levels of change to describe how your selected area of informatics might evolve over the next several years.

4. Use Box 31-4 to access and explore a futures research methodology that was not discussed in this chapter. Describe the methodology and how it could be used in health informatics.

5. Compare and contrast the trends of EHR directions and consumer-centered health informatics. Where do they overlap and where do they differ?

6. Describe how nanomaterials might affect your own life in the near future. Consider the consumer products you use and your role in healthcare.

7. Using futures research methods, identify how you think nanotechnology might impact both health IT and health informatics.

CASE STUDY

You have just been hired as the chief informatics officer (CIO) for a new health system. The health system has 23 acute care facilities and 36 outpatient clinics. It serves as a regional referral center for three states in the Midwest. Your installed base includes a vendor-supplied EHR from a national firm. Work on the data warehouse is just beginning. You have more than 300 varying applications across sites, including everything from a stand-alone pharmacy application for drug interactions to a cancer registry. Your goal is to provide IT support for the organizational vision of being the premier health organization in patient safety for the region. One of the first things you want to do is to plan for the future of IT.

Discussion Questions

1. Given the future directions discussed in this chapter, select the two directions you want to emphasize. Provide rationale for your choices.
2. Discuss how you can use methodologies from futures research to plan for your preferred future with the future directions you selected in Question 1.
3. Outline steps to introduce the chief executive officer to nanotechnology and its potential impact on the organization.
4. You want to increase collaborative work with a local university. What future directions for education do you think are most important as CIO?

A

Academy Higher education in general with an emphasis on the institution as a society of scholars, scientists, and artists.

Accounts payable The monies that are owed to companies such as vendors and suppliers for items purchased on credit.

Advanced practice nurse Nurses educated at the graduate level and authorized to practice as a specialist with advanced expertise in a specialty of nursing.

Adverse event An unintended and unfavorable event associated with the provision of medical care, use of a medical product or treatment protocol.

Ancillary systems Software applications used by patient care support departments such as laboratory, radiology, and pharmacy.

Application A software program designed to help the user to perform specific tasks.

Application service provider (ASP) A company, located remotely, that hosts an electronic health record or departmental system solution for a healthcare enterprise and provides access to the application via a secure network.

Architecture The formal description and design of information technology components, the relationships among them, and their implementation guide.

Attributes The characteristics or properties of the components of a system. Attributes are used to describe a system.

Availability A general term used to describe the amount of time that computer system resources are available to users. This is usually calculated for a one-year period.

Avatar A graphic image representing a person or other entity, usually on the Internet or in a video game.

B

Backcasting A technique for predicting the future by envisioning a desired future end point and then working backward to determine what activities and policies would be required to achieve that future.

Bar Code Medication Administration (BCMA) A method for administering medications using medication administration software, bar codes, and scanners with the goal of reducing errors during the medication administration process.

Bayesian knowledge base A knowledge base built using decision trees and a branch of statistical inference that permits the use of prior knowledge in assessing the probability of an event in the presence of new data. For example, if a patient has a fever and increased white blood cells, the Bayesian knowledge base provides the probability that the patient has an infection versus another disorder that also creates an inflammatory process.

Best of breed An approach to selecting applications involving reviewing vendors' products to determine the "best" for a department or setting.

When this approach is used, each department selects the "best" and the organization is tasked with achieving interoperability among them all.

Big bang A go-live approach in which all applications or modules are implemented at once.

Big data Very large datasets.

Biomedical informatics The interdisciplinary scientific field that studies and pursues the effective uses of biomedical data, information, and knowledge for scientific inquiry, problem solving, and decision making, motivated by efforts to improve human health (AMIA); http://www.amia.org/biomedical-informatics-core-competencies.

Bolt-on system A software program or application that is used in association with a larger application to give users their full required functionality. Users often require interfaces between the primary and bolt-on system. An example is an application for U.S. Mail address verification used in conjunction with a billing system.

Boundary The demarcation between a system and the environment of the system.

Business continuity The process created to ensure that essential functions and services continue during an adverse event.

Business intelligence Automated tools for analyzing massive amounts of data with the goal of improved decision making, typically at the organizational or departmental level.

C

Channel A physical element that carries a message between a sender and a receiver. Examples of channels are radio waves, fiber optic lines, and paper.

Charge description master file A list of all prices for services (e.g., diagnosis-related group, Healthcare Common Procedure Coding, and Current Procedural Terminology 4) or goods provided to patients that serves as the basis for billing.

Claims processing and management The submission of an insurance claim or bill to a third party payer, either manually or electronically, and the follow-up on the payment from the payer.

Classification A single hierarchical terminology that aggregates data at a prescribed level of abstraction for a particular domain.

Clicker A device that is part of a classroom or audience response system that allows real-time feedback to an instructor on, for example, comprehension of presented material.

Clinical application A software program used to perform specific tasks supporting the clinical aspects of healthcare, for example, documentation or orders management.

Clinical data repository The storage component for all patient clinical records data.

Clinical decision support (CDS) Tools and applications that assist the healthcare provider with some aspect of clinical decision making.

Clinical documentation Software that provides a medium for recording, managing, and reporting patient care activities by a variety of disciplines.

Clinical informatics The application of informatics and information technology to deliver healthcare services.

Clinical practice guidelines (CPGs) Statements and recommendations created from evidence-based practice or consensus-based processes and used to guide patient care.

Clinical scenario The plan of an expected and potential course of events for a simulated clinical experience. The clinical scenario provides the context for the simulation and can vary in length and complexity, depending on the objectives.

Closed system A system that is enclosed in an impermeable boundary and does not interact with the environment.

Cloud computing A model for enabling convenient, on-demand network access to a shared pool of computing resources that can be rapidly provisioned and released with minimal management effort or service provider interaction.

Cold site A relocation site for a company pending a disaster (e.g., fire, flood, terrorist event). It usually does not include backed-up copies of data from the original location. Hardware may be available but may need to be configured.

Comparative effectiveness research Studies designed to determine which methods to prevent, diagnose, treat, and monitor a health condition work best in terms of both benefit and harm, for which patients, and under what circumstances.

Complexity theory Complexity theory builds on chaos theory using a qualitative approach to the study of dynamic nonlinear social systems that change with time and demonstrate complex relationships.

Comprehensive educational information system The hardware, applications, data, and integrated functionality designed for managing an academic setting such as a university.

Computer science The "systematic study of algorithmic methods for representing and transforming information, including their theory, design, implementation, application, and efficiency. ... The roots of computer science extend deeply into mathematics and engineering. Mathematics imparts analysis to the field; engineering imparts design." (University at Buffalo School of Engineering and Applied Sciences, n.d., para 1.)

Computerized provider order entry (CPOE) Software designed to allow clinicians to enter and manage a variety of patient care orders, such as medications, laboratory, nutrition care, and other diagnostic tests, via the computer.

Concept A term that represents a group of ideas or items. It may represent an abstract idea, such as love, or be concrete, such as fruit.

Confidentiality Ensuring that data or information is disclosed only to authorized personnel.

Configuration management database (CMDB) A data repository containing all related components of an information system or information technology (IT) environment. A CMDB represents the authorized configuration of the significant components of the IT environment. A key goal of a CMDB is to help an organization understand the relationships between these components and track their configuration.

Confusion matrix Classification is a data mining function that assigns items in a collection to target categories or classes. A confusion matrix is an array used to test the specific classification model used for classifying the items by showing relationships between true and predicted classes.

Content management system An educational application that is used to create, edit, store, and deliver learning objects and materials such as PowerPoint slides, videos, diagrams etc. These learning objects and materials can be used in different courses for different purposes.

Course management system (CMS) A software program or application that permits a faculty member to design and deliver a course without knowing programming code. Students use the CMS to learn the concepts and skills being taught.

Covered entity A health plan, a healthcare clearinghouse, or a healthcare provider that transmits health information in electronic form.

Critical (key) application Defined by the stakeholders as an application that must be recovered first in the case of a disaster or downtime, as it is critical to some aspect of the organization and its operations (business).

Crowdsourcing The process of tapping into the collective intelligence of a group to complete business-related tasks that a company would normally either perform itself or outsource to a third party provider.

Cytotoxicity The property of an agent being toxic to cells.

Dashboard An application designed to provide a visual display of specific data points, for example, for organizational performance data.

Data Uninterpreted elements such as a person's name, weight, or age. Because they are uninterpreted, they do not have meaning.

Data center A housing facility for computer systems, applications, and related components (e.g., servers and storage systems).

Data dictionary Stores standard terms for healthcare. Defines the terms and structure in a database and is used to control and maintain integration in large databases. It records (1) what data is stored, (2) the description and characteristics of the data, (3) relationships among data elements, and (4) access rights and frequency of terms.

Data exchange The sharing of data among systems using an agreed-upon standard electronic communication, convention, or "rule."

Data integrity The accuracy and consistency of stored and transmitted data. Data integrity can be compromised when information is entered incorrectly or deliberately altered or when the system protections are not working correctly or suddenly fail.

Data mining A step in the knowledge discovery process of finding correlations or patterns among dozens of fields in large relational databases.

Data standards Data processes that have been approved by a recognized body and provide for common and repeated use, rules, guidelines, or characteristics for activities or their results, aimed at achieving the optimum degree of order in a given context.

Data visualization Using software tools to detect visual patterns in large datasets.

Debriefing A review and self-reflection activity led by a facilitator following a simulation or other IT-related experience.

Decision making The process of considering available data and information which is then matched with available knowledge to reach a conclusion or to make a judgment.

Denial management The tracking and follow-up of denials for payment from insurance companies.

Dental informatics The application of computer and information sciences to improve dental practice, research, education, and management.

Derived classifications World Health Organization classifications based on reference classifications but adapted by either providing additional detail or becoming a compilation of multiple reference classifications.

Digital divide The gap between groups of users in the adoption and use of personal electronic devices and the Internet.

Digital literacy The ability to operate and understand digital devices of all types including the technical skills to operate these devices, the conceptual knowledge to understand their functionality, and the ability to creatively and critically use these devices to access, manipulate, evaluate, and apply data, information, knowledge, and wisdom in activities of daily living.

Disaster recovery Plans and procedures that organizations use when essential services or systems will not be available for an extended period of time or when it is expected that the disaster or event will have a significant impact on operations. Includes plans for response during the event or disaster as well as plans for recovery.

Discount usability evaluations Cost-effective methods to determine usability issues for applications. These methods require minimal human resources and time yet still find about 80% of critical design issues.

Disruptive technology An innovation that replaces long-held traditional ideas and ways of doing things. A technology that abruptly causes a change in thinking or direction.

Distance education Instruction and learning that takes place when the teacher and the learner are in two different settings and possibly teaching and learning at two different times.

Distance learning The process of learning using distance education technology, which separates the learner in time and space from his or her peers and instructor.

Distributed learning Learning that occurs through the use of technologies (such as video and Web 2.0 tools) and interactive activities and that may include augmented classrooms, hybrid courses, or distance education courses.

Distributive education A change in pedagogy where the course developer uses technology to customize the learning environment to the learning styles of the learners; the learners may be taking distance, hybrid (combination of online and face to face), or on-site courses. Includes interactive activities using available technologies.

Downtime A time during which a computer or software is not available or not functioning due to hardware, operating system, or application program failure.

Dynamic homeostasis The constantly changing processes used by a system to maintain a steady state or balance. The normal fluctuations seen in body chemistry levels demonstrate dynamic homeostasis.

Dynamic system A system that is in a constant state of change in response to a reiterative feedback loop.

eBooks Books in a digital format that may or may not require a proprietary device to read (e.g., Kindle, Nook).

Education games Games that engage students in active learning. They generally include some sort of competition related to teams and winning a contest.

eHealth Electronic communication and information technology related to health information and processes accessible through online means.

eHealth initiatives Efforts and programming implemented to standardize and transform the use of technology in healthcare with the goal of improving patient care.

eLearning A change in the learner's knowledge and/or skills that is attributable to an experience with an electronic device.

Electronic data interchange (EDI) The standards or act of transferring data via computer technology between organizations (trading partners).

Electronic health record (EHR) A longitudinal electronic record of patient health information produced by encounters in one or more care settings.

Electronic health record (EHR) adoption The depth and breadth of use or penetration of EHRs in healthcare provider organizations and practices.

Electronic medical record (EMR) A digital version of a patient's chart used in a clinician's office or other healthcare setting.

Electronic Medication Administration Record (eMAR) Software used to view and document patient medications.

Enterprise resource planning (ERP) Facilitates the flow of data or information for business functions inside an organization and manages the connections to outside vendors or stakeholders. Most often associated with the supply chain functions.

Entropy A measure of the disorder or unavailability of energy within a system.

ePatient A person who uses technology to actively engage in his or her healthcare and manages the responsibility for his or her own health and wellness.

ePatient movement A movement in which patients play an increasing role in their own healthcare and contribute to the care of others.

ePortfolio A portfolio that is maintained in a digital format.

Equifinality The tendency of open systems to reach a characteristic final state from different initial conditions and in different ways.

Ergonomics In the U.S. this focuses on the physical design and implementation of equipment, tools, and products as they relate to human safety, comfort, and convenience. The term is used interchangeably with *human factors* in Europe and elsewhere.

Evidence-based practice (EBP) The use of research, data, and scientific evaluation as a basis for clinical decision making and the provision of patient care.

Expert system A computer system that uses knowledge and a set of rules or procedures to interpret data and information and make decisions. Such a system differs from a decision support system in that the final decision is made by the computer as opposed to the provider. This term has also been used to refer to a type of clinical decision support system that provides diagnostic or therapeutic advice in a manner consistent with a clinical domain expert.

Extrapolation Extending historical data to create future predictions and trend lines.

F

Fat client A personal computer with full functionality and disk storage that exists in a client–server environment. It contrasts with a thin client that is, in essence, solely a terminal with no embedded software (e.g., a dummy terminal).

Fidelity Believability or the degree to which a simulated experience approaches reality; as fidelity increases, realism increases.

Financial information system (FIS) A system that records, stores, and manages financial operations within an organization for the purposes of reporting and decision making.

Fixed asset management The management of objects that cannot be easily converted to cash or sold or used for the care of a patient.

Focused ethnographies Research methods borrowed from anthropology and sociology in which the focus is on the person's point of view and his or her experiences and interactions in social settings.

Formative evaluation Feedback provided with the goal of improving a program or a person's performance, typically given in the early or middle portion of the program.

Fractal type patterns Irregular geometric shapes that are repeatedly subdivided into parts that are a smaller copy of the whole (e.g., a snowflake).

Framework A basic conceptual structure for organizing ideas.

Futures research A rational and systematic approach to identifying possible, probable, and preferable futures. The formal study of the future is also called foresight and futures studies, strategic foresight, prospective studies, prognostic studies, and futurology.

G

General ledger A listing of all financial transactions made by the healthcare organization.

Generalist nurse A professional nurse educated at the undergraduate level for the broad practice of nursing in primary, secondary, and tertiary healthcare.

Guided discovery A process by which clinicians engage epatients in developing a shared hypothesis and plan of care based on data and reported experiences.

H

Harmonization The process of adjusting for differences and inconsistencies among different measurements, terms, methods, procedures, schedules, specifications, or systems to make them uniform or mutually compatible.

Health 1.0 Use of the Internet to search for health-related information. The user can read but cannot interact in any way with the website or the information.

Health 2.0 Internet-based healthcare resources that allow interactive communication with other patients and healthcare resources across the country and around the world.

Health 3.0 Anticipated Internet-based healthcare resources that learn from a user's behaviors and search activities.

Health advocacy Supports and promotes patient's healthcare rights as well as enhances community health and policy initiatives that focus on the availability, safety, and quality of care.

Health communication A process whereby practitioners create social change by changing people's attitudes and external structures, modify or eliminate certain behaviors using multiple behavioral and social learning theories and models to advance program planning, and identify steps to influence audience attitudes and behavior.

Health informatics An interdisciplinary specialty and scientific discipline focused on integrating the health sciences, computer science, and information science to discover, manage and communicate data, information, knowledge, and wisdom supporting the provision of healthcare for individuals, families and communities.

Health information exchange (HIE) The process of reliable and interoperable electronic health-related information sharing conducted in a manner that protects the confidentiality, privacy, and security of the information.

Health information organization (HIO) An organization that oversees and governs the exchange of health-related information among organizations according to nationally recognized standards.

Health information technology (health IT) The use of electronic methods for managing health-related date and information.

Health Information Technology for Economic and Clinical Health (HITECH) Act A law that established programs designed to improve healthcare quality, safety, and efficiency using health information technology.

Health IT governance The process of establishing an overarching structure for health IT in organizations, including establishing goals and objectives; creating policies, standards, and services; and developing mechanisms and processes for the oversight, enforcement, and coordination of the policies, standards, and services.

Health IT support personnel Individuals who assist in the design, development, implementation, ongoing support, and maintenance of the health IT hardware and software.

Health policy Includes the decisions, plans, and actions that guide the achievement of healthcare goals within a society.

Heuristic evaluations Assessments of a device or product against accepted guidelines or published usability principles.

High availability Processes that allow full functioning of systems during downtimes. Includes a redundant system in place, configured and waiting in standby mode if the primary production node fails. Requires manual intervention for end-users to access it.

Home health Healthcare and social services provided by free-standing and facility-based community agencies at patients' residences, work sites, or other locations.

Hot site An alternative site that is an exact duplication of the original site with real-time synchronization to allow an organization to relocate with minimal losses.

Human factors The scientific discipline concerned with the understanding of interactions among humans and other elements of a system. The term also refers to the profession that applies theory, principles, data, and methods to product design to optimize human well-being and overall system performance.

Human resources information system (HRIS) A computerized information system and applications used to record, store, and manage human resource data and information.

Human–computer interaction (HCI) The study of how people design, implement, and evaluate interactive computer systems in the context of users' tasks and work. Used interchangeably with the term *ergonomics* in Europe and elsewhere.

Human-made disaster A disaster created by humans that results in significant injuries, deaths, or damage to property.

I

Immunization information system (IIS) A confidential, population-based, computerized database that records all immunization-related data and information, such as doses administered by participating healthcare providers to persons residing within a given geopolitical area. Can be used at the healthcare provider, patient, and population level.

Incentive management Use of monetary and point-based rewards for staff who volunteer to meet institutional needs, such as staffing needs.

Incident response team (IRT) A group of people from the organization who prepare for and respond to incidents, downtimes, or other emergencies.

Informatics The study and use of information processes and technology in the arts, sciences, and the professions.

Informatics nurse specialist A nurse formally educated at the graduate level in nursing informatics, health informatics, or biomedical informatics.

Informatics researcher and innovator A nurse educated in a doctoral-level education program who uses health data, information, knowledge, and wisdom to generate new knowledge and best practices or to develop new technologies to continuously improve health outcomes.

Information A collection of data that has been processed to produce meaning.

Information ecology A science that studies the laws governing the influence of information summary on the formation and functioning of biosystems, including those of individuals, human communities, and humanity in general, and on the health and psychological, physical, and social well-being of the human being, and that undertakes to develop methodologies to improve the information environment.

Information science The discipline that investigates the properties and the means of processing information for optimum accessibility and usability. It is concerned with the origination, collection, organization, storage, retrieval, interpretation, transmission, transformation, and use of information.

Information supply chain A full set of elements (technology based, process specific, and organizational in nature) that is necessary to support logistics and supplies in organizations. It includes (1) collecting information from discrete processes, (2) transforming this information from data to knowledge, and (3) distributing this information efficiently and in a timely manner to the appropriate data consumers.

Information system A combination of information technology, data, and human activities or processes that support operations and decision making.

Informed consent Permission given by an individual who has been provided with an understanding of the risks, benefits, limitations, and potential implications of the consent.

Infrastructure The hardware and software used to connect computers and users, including cables; equipment such as routers, repeaters, and other devices that control transmission paths; software used to send, receive, and manage the signals that are transmitted; and often the computers themselves, although this component is not consistently considered infrastructure.

Integrated system A fully integrated health information system or a fully interoperable system. It may be monolithic (from one vendor) or best of breed.

Interactive whiteboard An interactive display controlled by a computer, typically with a touch screen, video conferencing, and note-taking functionality.

Interface engine Software that transforms or maps data from one application to a receiving application's (or system's) requirements while a message is in transit to allow it to be accepted. The software is built with one-to-many concepts in mind. These import-export modules then are connected to an interface engine so that the mapping, routing, and monitoring are managed by this system.

Interface terminology A set of designations or representations structured to support representation of concepts for data entry and display on the graphical user interface.

Interoperability The ability for systems to reliably exchange data and operate in a coordinated, seamless manner.

Interprofessional education (IPE) An environment in which students from two or more disciplines learn from, with, and about each other to enable effective collaboration and improve health outcomes.

Intervention scheme A comprehensive, hierarchical taxonomy designed to organize patient assessment.

Intrusion detection Involves software, policies, and procedures used to detect attempted entry or inappropriate access to a computer or network.

J

Joint cognitive systems Systems in which information is shared or distributed among humans and technology.

K

Knowledge Created when data and information are identified and the relationships between the data and information are formalized.

Knowledge base A component, typically within an electronic health record, that stores and organizes a healthcare enterprise's information and

knowledge used by the enterprise for clinical operations.

Knowledge discovery and data mining (KDDM) An approach to identifying patterns in large datasets that entails methods such as statistical analysis, machine learning methods, and data visualization. In some literature the terms *knowledge discovery* and *data mining* are used interchangeably. Also the terms *knowledge discovery* and *knowledge discovery in data* are sometimes used to refer to the broad process of finding knowledge in data.

Knowledge transformation Converting knowledge from research results, to evidence summary, to practice guidelines, to integration and then evaluation of the impact.

L

Lead part The unit of a system that plays the dominant role in the operation of the system.

Learning An increase in knowledge, a change in attitude or values, or the development of new skills.

Learning health system (LHS) A health system in which science, informatics, incentives, and culture are aligned for continuous improvement and innovation, with best practices seamlessly embedded in the delivery process and new knowledge captured as a by-product of the delivery experience.

Learning management system (LMS) An educational application used to address educational functions ranging from class administration and document and grade tracking to report generation and delivery of online courses. While these applications are mainly used as course management systems delivering hybrid or online courses they can also be used for other group activities such as setting up access to online advising and other university services for enrolled students.

Learning theory A theory that describes the process by which people learn and the factors that influence the learning process. Currently there are several different learning theories.

Logic model A graphical depiction of the logical relationships between the resources, activities, outputs, and outcomes of a program.

M

Machine learning Adjustment of a computer model or algorithm based on exposure to training examples.

Master person index (MPI) The information used to uniquely identify each person, patient, and customer of a healthcare enterprise. Synonyms for this term include *master patient index*, *master member index*, and *patient master index*.

Material management The storage, inventory control, quality control, and operational management of supplies, pharmaceuticals, equipment, and other items used in the delivery of patient care or the management of the patient care system. Material management is a subset of the larger function of supply chain management; the supply chain also includes the acquisition of materials of care and the logistics or movement of those materials to caregiving facilities and organizations.

Meaningful Use Sets of specific objectives that must be achieved to qualify for federal incentive payments. Meaningful Use means that healthcare providers must show that they are using certified electronic health record technology in ways that can be measured using specific criteria.

Medical informatics The branch of informatics that focuses on disease diagnosis and management.

Microblogging A form of blogging (online journaling of an author's thoughts) in which entries are kept brief using character limitations (e.g., Twitter).

N

Nanofabrication The development of nanomaterials used in structures, electronics, and commercial products.

Nanoinformatics The use of informatics techniques and tools for nanomaterial or nanoparticle data management and storage; information to improve research in the field of nanotechnology.

Nanomedicine A subspecialty of nanotechnology centering on the application of nanoparticles and nanoscience techniques to healthcare and clinical research.

Nanotechnology The study of controlling and altering matter at the atomic or molecular level.

Nationwide Health Information Network (NwHIN) A set of standards, services, and policies that enable secure health information exchange over the Internet and across diverse settings.

Natural disaster A disaster created by nature.

Natural language processing Computer processing of text written or spoken by humans.

Negentropy A measure of energy that can be used by a system for maintenance as well as growth.

Networked personal health record A personal health record that is electronically linked to multiple data sources (e.g., electronic health records, pharmacies, labs). Entities that are linked to the networked record may provide services to the user (e.g., secure messaging). These systems also allow for the storage of personally entered data.

Niche applications Specialty software applications created to address the requirements of specific departments and groups of users.

Noise Anything that is not part of a message but occupies space on the channel and is transmitted with the message.

Nurse-managed health center A site that primarily offers outpatient clinic and primary healthcare and social services provided by nurses.

Nursing informatics A specialty that integrates nursing science, computer science, and information science to manage and communicate data, information, knowledge, and wisdom in nursing practice, education, research and administration.

O

Omaha System A research-based taxonomy designed to support documenting client care from admission to discharge in various settings. It exists in the public domain and can be used without licensing fees. Its primary application has been in the home health arena.

Online education A version of distance education that requires the use of the Internet to deliver the educational materials.

Ontology A model of a domain that defines the concepts existing in that domain as well as taxonomic and other relationships existing between the concepts. Within health informatics an ontology would be a formal, computer-understandable description of a domain.

Open shift management A web-based self-scheduling solution in which the manager uses a variety of instant communication tools to announce openings in the schedule and staff members respond by tendering schedule and shift requests for consideration and approval.

Open system A system that is enclosed in a semipermeable boundary and interacts with the environment.

Outcome and Assessment Information Set (OASIS) A standardized assessment tool and core dataset mandated by the Centers for Medicare & Medicaid Services for use by Medicare-certified home health agencies.

Outcomes-based quality improvement (OBQI) A risk-adjusted outcome reporting tool that is based on Outcome and Assessment Information Set and mandated by the Centers for Medicare & Medicaid Services for use by Medicare-certified home health agencies.

P

P4 Medicine Medicine that is predictive, preventive, personalized, and participatory.

Palliative care and hospice Healthcare and social services provided to those with life-threatening or terminal illnesses.

Participatory health and medicine A healthcare model that includes patients, caregivers, and healthcare professionals working together in all aspects of a patient's health.

Patient accounting A process for collecting and tracking debits and credits for patient care provided by clinicians that is billed to insurance companies and/or the patient.

Patient safety Freedom from accidental injury due to healthcare, medical care, or medical errors, where error is defined as the failure of a planned action to be completed safely or as intended or the use of a wrong plan to achieve an aim.

Patient-centered care An essential partnership between interprofessional care providers and the individuals, families, and communities that are the recipients of care.

Pay for performance A strategy to pay healthcare providers for high-quality care as measured by selected evidence-based standards and procedures.

Payroll system An application that creates and disburses compensation payments to employees. This is also referred to as a disbursement system.

Phased go-live A gradual go-live approach within an institution by service line, selected areas, or departments.

Phenomenon An observable fact or event.

Picture archiving and communication system (PACS) A combination of hardware and software configured to provide for the storage, retrieval, management, distribution, and presentation of radiological images.

Point of care Patient care and procedures that are performed at or near the patient care site.

Practice management system (PMS) An application designed to assist in the management of a practice by collecting patient demographic information, insurance information, appointment scheduling, reason for the visit, patient care procedures done for the patient, charging information for the billing process, and collection and follow-up.

Practice-based evidence A specific research design using observations and cohorts of patients. Used to answer questions of treatment effectiveness that involves meticulous prospective data collection in a naturalistic clinical setting of multiple interventions and outcomes, with rigorous statistical control of relevant patient differences.

Predictive scheduling Resource scheduling based on a predictive model used to forecast bed demand changes in patient acuity, workload distribution, and variability caused by shift, day of the week, month, and seasonality.

Preprocessing (of data) Preparation of data for data mining—data cleaning, transformation, replacement of missing values, etc.

Privacy The capacity to control when, how, and to what degree information about oneself is communicated to others.

Problem classification scheme A comprehensive, hierarchical taxonomy designed to identify diverse patients' health-related concerns.

Problem rating scale for outcomes A comprehensive, recurring evaluation framework designed to measure patient progress.

Program evaluation The systematic collection of information about the activities, characteristics, and results of programs to make judgments about the program, improve or further develop program effectiveness, inform decisions about future programming, and increase understanding.

Protected health information (PHI) Personally identifiable health information, such as name, birth date, and Social Security number, created or received by a covered entity.

Public health The science and art of protecting and improving the health of communities through education, promotion of healthy lifestyles, and research for disease and injury prevention.

Public health informatics The application of informatics in areas of public health, including disease or condition surveillance, reporting, and health promotion. Public health informatics and its corollary, population informatics, are concerned with groups rather than individuals.

Public health surveillance Collecting, analyzing, and interpreting health-related data for the planning, implementation, and evaluation of public health.

Q

Quality of care The degree to which health services for individuals and populations increase the likelihood of desired health outcomes and are consistent with current professional knowledge.

Quantified self A person invested in using tools and data to quantify and monitor his or her daily experiences using personal metrics.

R

Radio frequency identification (RFID) Technology that uses electronic tags to track and monitor equipment and activities. Typically used in patient bands, lab specimens, or surgical sponges.

Randomized controlled trial A specific research design involving random assignment of subjects to experimental and control groups and other design features to assure as much variable control as possible. With this research design approach, the differences between the groups are most likely related to the treatment each group received.

Receiver A device or individual that receives a message that has been sent over a channel.

Reference classifications Main terminology classifications based on basic parameters of health.

Reference terminology A set of atomic level designations, representing a domain knowledge of interest, structured to support representations of both simple and compositional concepts independent of human language (within machine) that facilitates data collection, processing, and aggregation.

Regional Health Information Organization (RHIO) Characterized as a quasipublic, nonprofit organization whose goal is to share secure health-related data within a region.

Reiterative feedback loops Feedback loops where the effect of the system's actions or output are continuously returned to the system as input, thereby effecting the system's future output.

Related classifications World Health Organization classifications that partially refer to reference classifications, or are associated with the reference classification at specific levels of structure only.

Remote hosting An application hosted off-site, typically by a vendor, at a site with vendor-owned hardware.

Request for information (RFI) A document that is developed and sent to vendors requesting basic or overview information to determine which vendors are most likely to meet the institution's requirements for a new information system. Not as formal as a request for proposal (RFP). Both RFP and RFI are used as part of the purchasing process.

Request for proposal (RFP) A detailed document developed and sent to vendors outlining the institution's requirements to request a proposal describing the vendors' capabilities to meet the listed requirements and the related costs. RFPs and requests for information (RFIs) are used as part of the purchasing process.

Revenue cycle All business components (administrative and clinical) dealing with patient service revenue.

Reverberation The process of change throughout a system that occurs in response to change in one part of a system.

Risk analysis A systematic process for examining an information system to identify the security vulnerabilities and potential risks to an information system or organization. Also referred to as risk assessment.

S

Scope creep Occurs when requirements are added on after the initial project was defined and approved. Added requirements are substantial enough to affect the project costs and/or timeline.

Security The administrative, technical, and physical safeguards in an organization or information system to prevent privacy breaches.

Sender The originator of a message to be sent over a channel.

Service level agreement (SLA) An agreement made between information technology and a key stakeholder where the level of service is formally defined and agreed upon. This can include uptime guarantees, response time to issues, and even disaster recovery timelines.

Service-oriented architecture (SOA) An architecture design configuration where services are business oriented, loosely coupled with other services and system components, vendor and platform independent, message based, and encapsulated with internal architecture and program flow that are hidden from the service user.

Simulation A pedagogy, or instructional method, using one or more teaching strategies to promote, improve, and validate a participant's progression from novice to expert.

Simulation experience A term often used synonymously with *simulated clinical experience* or *scenario*.

Simulation learning environment An atmosphere that is created by the facilitator to allow for sharing and discussion of participant experiences without fear of humiliation or punitive action. The goals of the simulation learning environment are to promote trust and foster learning.

Social media An application used to create an online environment that is established for the purpose of mass collaboration.

Social networking The use of social media and online platforms that enable groups and individuals to connect with others sharing similar interests.

Sociotechnical Refers to complex systems recognizing the interaction between people and technology in work settings, particularly settings such as healthcare.

Stakeholders People affiliated with an organization (internal and external) who share a vested interest in the outcomes produced by that organization.

Stand-alone personal health record A personal health record that is not electronically linked to other data sources and can serve as a portable electronic store of personally entered data.

Standardized terminology Terms and definitions adopted by a national or international standardizing and standards organization and made available to the public.

Standards of Best Practice: Simulation Seven sets of definitions and principles developed by the International Nursing Association for Clinical Simulation and Learning that should be considered and incorporated when developing all simulation-based learning experiences for learners (terminology, professional integrity, participants' objectives, facilitation methods, facilitator, debriefing process, and evaluation of outcomes).

Strategic alignment The process of matching two or more organizational strategies to ensure that they synergistically support the organization's goals and vision.

Strategic vision The desired future state of an organization or institution.

Subsystem Any system within the target system.

Summative evaluation An evaluation that determines the effects or outcomes of a person's, program's, or organization's performance; a program's impact; or a technology's effectiveness. The goal is to determine the merit of the evaluation target.

Supersystem The overall system in which the target system exists.

Supply chain management (SCM) The acquisition, movement of, storage, inventory control, quality control, and operational management of supplies, pharmaceuticals, equipment, and other items used in the delivery of patient care or the management of the patient care system.

Supply item master file A list (hard copy or electronic) of all items used in the delivery of care for a health organization that can be requested by healthcare providers and managers. This file typically contains between 30,000 and 100,000 items.

Systems life cycle A conceptual model or framework used to describe each stage in the life of a living or nonliving system, such as an information system.

T

Tall Man lettering The use of mixed case lettering, allowing easy differentiation of similar terms such as look-alike medication names.

Target system The system of interest.

Task analysis A suite of well-known usability methods to decompose and understand users' actions and behaviors. Composed of more than 100 different methods, it is used to determine goals, tasks, issues with interactions, the flow of work, and other activities in sociotechnical systems.

Telehealth The use of telecommunication methods to provide patient care and education as well as public health and health administration.

Telehealth competency Having and using knowledge, understanding, and judgment when providing telehealth.

Telemedicine The use of medical information exchanged from one site to another via electronic communications for the health and education of the patient or healthcare provider and for the purpose of improving patient care, treatment, and services.

Telenursing The use of telehealth technology to deliver nursing care and conduct nursing practice.

Terminology cross-mapping Assigning an element or concept in one set to an element or concept in another set through semantic correspondence.

Terminology harmonization A process of ensuring consistency of terms and the definitions of those terms within and across different terminologies.

Tethered personal health record A personal health record that is electronically linked to the clinical information systems of a given healthcare provider or organization. It may include functions such as secure messaging and online scheduling as well as storage of personally entered data.

Theory A scientifically acceptable explanation of a phenomenon.

Thin client A centrally managed computer workstation without a hard drive that has its operating system and application delivered from a central server via the network and all data stored on network storage. This is in contrast to a fat client, which has software embedded in the client.

Think-aloud protocol A usability method in which users talk aloud about what they are doing as they interact with a product. These interactions are observed or recorded and then analyzed.

Threat An act of man or nature that has the potential to cause harm to an informational asset.

Transaction history file A running log of all material transactions of the healthcare organization.

Transparency Indicates that the policies, procedures, and technologies affecting health information use for individuals' health information are easily accessed and understood.

Trend analysis The process of analyzing historical data and identifying trends over time.

U

uHealth Ubiquitous health technologies that integrate core components of computers, wireless networks, sensors, and other modalities, such as mhealth (mobile) devices, to create an environment that can monitor, respond to, and assist in meeting healthcare needs of individuals.

Unintended consequences Unplanned and unexpected consequences from a device, process, or event such as the adoption of health IT.

Usability The extent to which a product can be used by specific users in a specific context to achieve specific goals with effectiveness, efficiency, and satisfaction.

User experience A person's perceptions and responses that result from the use or anticipated use of a product, system, or service.

User interface A boundary between users and products, typically a display or computer screen or interaction device. It allows humans and products to cooperatively perform tasks.

V

Vendor A person or business that sells products, goods, or services to a company or institution.

Vendor master file A list of all manufacturers and distributors (vendors) who provide materials needed for the healthcare organization that also contains the associated contract terms and prices for specific items. This file typically contains between 200 and 500 different vendors and suppliers.

Virtual community An online community that shares many characteristics with traditional social groups.

Vulnerability A weakness in an information system, system security procedures, internal controls, or implementation that could be exploited.

W

Web 2.0 Sophisticated web functionality with social engagement, interaction, and networking capabilities.

Web 3.0 Emerging functionality in which browsers learn from user search behavior and adapt accordingly.

Wisdom The appropriate use of knowledge in managing or solving human problems. It involves knowing when and how to use knowledge in managing a client need or problem.

Workaround A temporary and potentially unsafe fix for a problem which fails to provide a genuine solution to the problem.

Page numbers followed by *f* indicate figures; *t*, tables; *b*, boxes.